The Pathology of Vessels

Springer-Verlag France S.A.R.L

Phat N. Vuong
Sir Colin Berry

The Pathology of Vessels

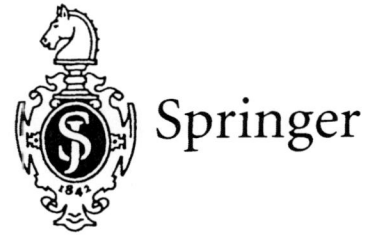

Springer

Phat N. Vuong,
MD, PhD, DHDR
Unité d'Anatomie et de Cytologie Pathologiques
Hôpital Saint-Michel
33, rue Olivier-de-Serres, 75015 Paris, FRANCE

Sir Colin Berry
DSc, MD, PhD, FRCPath, FRCP, FFPM
St. Bartholomew's and the Royal London School of Medecine and Dentistry
Department of Morbid Anatomy and Histopathology
Whitechapel, London, E1 1BB, UNITED KINGDOM

ISBN 978-2-8178-0788-1   ISBN 978-2-8178-0786-7 (eBook)
DOI 10.1007/978-2-8178-0786-7

© Springer-Verlag France 2002
Originally published by Springer-Verlag France,Berlin, Heidelberg in 2002

SPIN : 10701454

PREFACE

Vascular pathology is essentially based on a transverse, multi-organ approach to pathology. It has been the subject of only a few reference works as it tends to be ignored by organ specialists. However, the vascular system is widely distributed in all tissues ; it is modelled very early during organogenesis by haemodynamic factors, it possesses a remarkable reactivity and plasticity, and it is involved in a large number of pathological processes. General pathologists are often poorly equipped to interpret morphological features encountered during histological examination and to integrate these findings into a rational approach.

This book by Doctor Phat N. VUONG and Professor Colin BERRY presents an exhaustive, precise, and concise interpretation of a whole range of different lesions, which are sometimes difficult to interpret. After describing normal structure, age-related changes, and the main basic lesions, this book provides precise descriptions in all of the main areas : atherosclerotic, inflammatory, dysplastic, and traumatic diseases, etc. Throughout this book, the lesions are precisely described with identification of the various recognized syndromes and discussion of the main established pathophysiological interpretations, together with a complete bibliography.

We hope this book, based on the authors' medical and scientific knowledge, has the success it deserves. We would like to thank them for giving us a very well documented book, which will be useful to both students and experienced pathologists.

Pr Jean-Pierre CAMILLERI
Director of the Medical Division
of Institut Curie

INTRODUCTION

The adverse outcomes produced by vascular diseases are a major part of the workload of almost all clinicians and pathologists, but the pathological investigation and description of vascular lesions is often less carefully considered than are changes in other systems.

The reasons for this are complex. Many outcomes depend on the complications of one major disease – atherosclerosis, which has been well studied and well characterised at particular sites. However, there are very few studies in other vascular fields which match the thoroughness and complexity of those of Stary on the coronary circulation. Many of the specimens obtained following intervention for serious illness are inadequately examined in terms of proper evaluation of their vascular lesions, for example, amputation specimens and resected ischaemic bowel. The vasculitis syndromes are clinically complex and overlapping; the vascular pathology often fails to be distinctive in a way which allows definitive diagnosis to be made from small biopsies. These considerations have led to an uncritical view of the information to be obtained from these specimens; there is seldom the kind of close contact between vascular surgeons and pathologists that there is between renal physicians and their pathologists.

It is now possible to intervene in a number of ways in the vascular tree, at all levels from the microcirculation to the aortic root and grafts, stents, mechanical dilatation, biochemical interventions and genetic manipulation are all used. In the acutely ill patient, considerable damage may be caused to the vascular tree by the necessary supportive interventions. The pathological problems resulting from all these events need to be better described.

This book attempts to provide information for the general pathologist who will see a number of these specimens on a daily basis, and the practising cardiologist or vascular surgeon who takes an interest in the pathological process in the diseases which call for their intervention. Related texts deal with particular areas in detail, for example, vascular lesions in transplantation (Current Topics in Pathology, vol 92) and lesions produced by cardiac pacer leads (Current Topics in Pathology, vol 86). This volume is for the non-specialist pathologist who will, perforce, have to deal with a number of the lesions described within it. We hope it will be a useful bench-side book.

PNV-CLB

"A really new and really original book would be one that makes people love the old truths"

(Un livre bien neuf et bien original serait celui qui ferait aimer les vieilles vérités)

Vauvenargues.

To the patients for their forbearance and their living lessons ;
to our teachers for their generosity and devotion ;
to our colleagues, surgeons, clinicians and pathologists for
their encouragement and cooperation ;
to our families for their patience.
PNV-CLB

ACKNOWLEDGEMENTS

We would especially like to thank many colleagues who have allowed us to use material from their collections. Their names are directly cited under the documents.

Pr Jean-Pierre Camilleri wrote the preface. Pr Paul P. de Saint-Maur provided us with useful comments and advice. Mrs Gloria Girton reviewed the text with patience. Mrs Touria Benassavy, Elisabeth Charpentier, Béatrice Larcher prepared all the histological slides. Mrs Lien Horn drew the illustrations. Mr Michel Paing took the photographs. We are grateful for their contributions.

The use of new techniques, in particular E-mail, has made communication between the authors a pleasure rather than a chore, but both of us have depended heavily on Miss Lorraine Singer and Ms Sylvaine Dezègue, whose invaluable help we would like to acknowledge.

PNV-CLB

TABLE OF CONTENTS

I	Histology of vessels	1
II	Vascular ageing	25
III	Fundamental lesions in vascular pathology	35
IV	Atherosclerosis	69
V	Non-atherosclerotic and non-vasculitic diseases	89
VI	Vascular trauma	119
VII	Effects of physical and chemical agents on vessels	139
VIII	Vessels and infectious diseases	163
IX	Thrombosis and embolism	199
X	Aneurysms and other changes in vascular dimensions	215
XI	Vasculitis	237
XII	Operative pathology	289
XIII	The pathology of veins, lymphatics, arteriovenous anastomoses and the erectile vascular tissue	327
XIV	Developmental anomalies and hereditary diseases of vessels	351
XV	Vascular changes in metabolic and endocrine disorders	393
XVI	Hypertension and vessels	417
XVII	Vascular tumours and tumour-like conditions	431
XVIII	Tumours of vessel wall components and vascular related structures	479
Annex I	Laboratory handling of vascular specimens	503
Annex II	Pathological interpretation of vascular specimens and immunohistochemistry of vessels	519
Index		527

I
Histology of vessels

1 – The structure of vessels

Blood vessels

The cardiovascular system consists of four main types of vessel: arteries, veins, capillaries and the less well defined sinusoids. No vessel (small or large) should be seen as a simple conduit; all have distinct functional characteristics, which, in turn, will affect organ function profoundly, and their structure is modified by the functional demands they must satisfy. As an arbitrary definition we can say that any vessel whose diameter is larger than 250 to 300 μm and visible to the naked eye belongs to the macrocirculation and that the microcirculation is made up of vessels measuring less than 250 μm in diameter [1].

Arteries

The basic structural plan of large arteries is presumably a biologically sound one; it is highly conserved from lower vertebrates and has persisted for more than 350 million years. The walls of arteries are well-organised connective tissue structures composed of cell and matrix arranged in the three transmural zones or tunicae, the intima, media and adventitia.

The intima

In normal arteries, the intima encompasses an endothelium, a subendothelial layer and a basement membrane. The intima consists of a narrow region bounded on the luminal side by a single continuous layer of endothelial cells and peripherally by a fenestrated sheet of elastic fibres, the internal elastic lamina. In the subendothelium, smooth muscle cells and various components of the extracellular connective tissue matrix are present.

Endothelial cells (ECs) form a monolayer that lines the entire vascular system. They are elongated or polygonal cells (length: 25-50 μ, width: 10-15 μ, thickness: 0,1-1 μ) and form junctional complexes with their neighbouring endothelial cells and with cells in the media. Their morphology varies depending on their location [2]. They are flat, elongated in the direction of blood flow and with a nucleus causing a focal luminal protrusion. Numerous pinocytic vesicles are seen close to the plasma membrane and present a flask-shaped invagination of the luminal and abluminal cell membrane. The cytoplasm of endothelial cells contains Weibel-Palade (WP) bodies in

addition to usual intracellular organelles [3]. WP bodies (Fig. 1) are around 0.1 μm wide, 3 μm long, membrane-bound structures that represent the storage organelle for von Willebrand's factor (vWF). Intermediate filaments of vimentin type are present in the endothelial cells, sometimes abundant and present as fascicles, or as whorls filling the cell cytoplasm. An excess of this type of filament has been regarded as a regressive change associated with aging and disease [4]. Actin filaments may also be found in endothelial cells close to the cell membrane with a few in the cytoplasm. Adjacent endothelial cells are interconnected by junctional complexes made up of tight junctions, intermediate junctions and gap (nexus) junctions [5, 6]. Tight junctions (Fig. 2) and intermediate junctions (Fig. 3) serve to prevent the free passage of molecules across an endothelium. In the re-

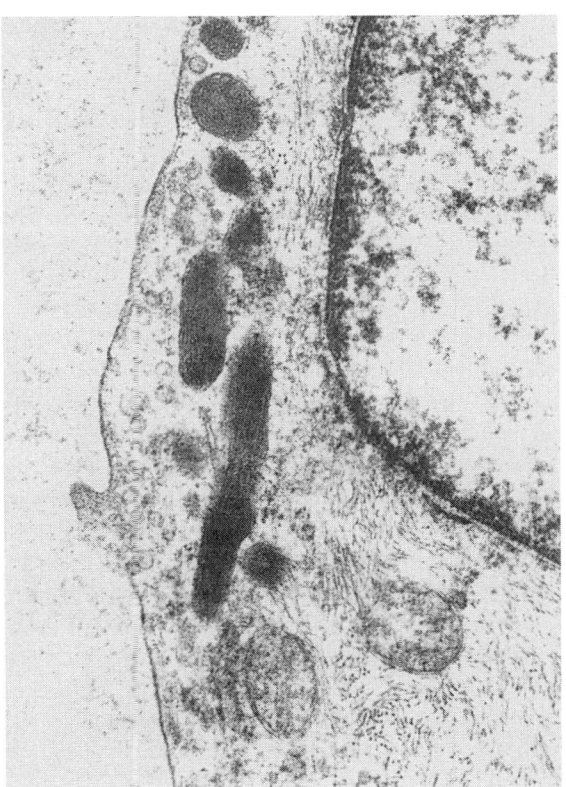

Fig. 1. Ultrastructural appearance of a Weibel-Palade body. X 24 140

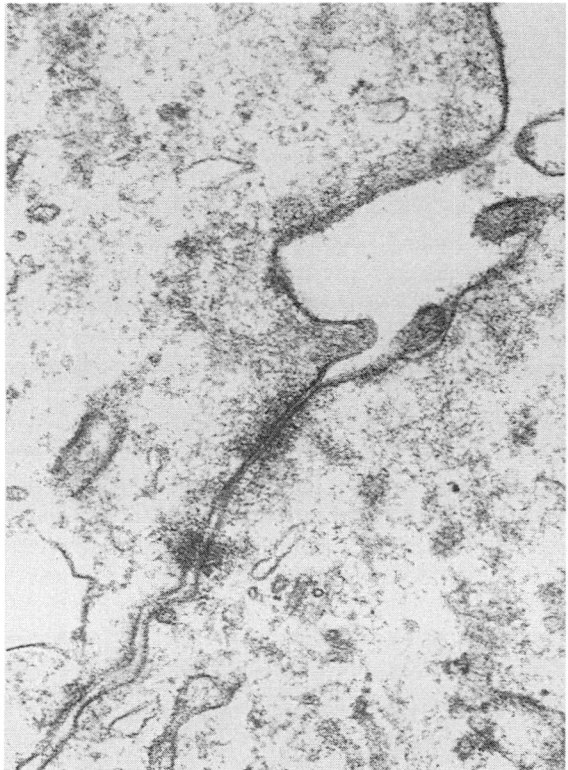

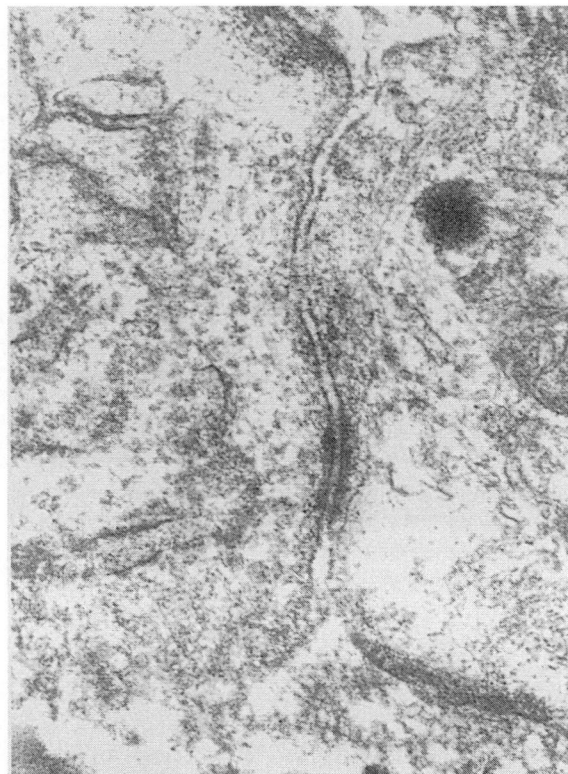

Fig. 2. Two tight junctions between endothelial cells. X 34 800

Fig. 3. An intermediate junction between two endothelial cells. X 37 310

gion of a tight junction, the plasma membranes of two adjacent endothelial cells are fused. For complete sealing, the junction has to extend as a continuous band or belt around the entire circumference of a cell. How effectively a tight junction acts as a seal depends on the number of strands in the junction. The greater their number, the less permeable the junction and on this basis, they may be categorised from very leaky to very tight. In some arteries, endothelial cells have up to 5 continuous strands. However, in most capillaries (except capillaries of the blood-brain barrier) the strands are staggered and often discontinuous. Tight junctions and intermediate junctions are relatively labile structures, which may widen under the influences of haemodynamic factors, such as high blood pressure [7, 8] and, possibly, of vasoactive agents [9]. Gap junctions are membrane specialisations that provide a cell-to-cell low resistance conduction pathway for co-ordination of tissue function. They are composed of nonselective channels that allow passage of ions, nucleotides and other small molecules with molecular masses up to 1200 Da [10]. The presence of nexus junctions between arterial endothelial cells is essential for metabolic co-operation in this cell layer and plays a role in transmitting some signals to the underlying smooth muscle cells (Fig. 4-5). Coupled endothelial cells in arteries may act as a unit and this interaction, along with that of myoendothelial contacts, may help explain the ability of an intravascular compound to affect vascular tone without gaining direct access to all cells of the vascular wall.

The subendothelial layer, 0.3 to 0.5 mm thick, is composed mainly of type III collagen fibers and a population of connective tissue cells (myofibroblasts, histiocytes and mast-cells) which are all capable of proliferation.

The media

This is the main load-bearing component of the arterial wall. The main constituents of this layer include smooth muscle cells, myofibroblasts, connective tissue containing elastic fibers, and collagen fibers, arranged in an orderly way in an amorphous ground substance. The mechanical properties of elastic arteries depend

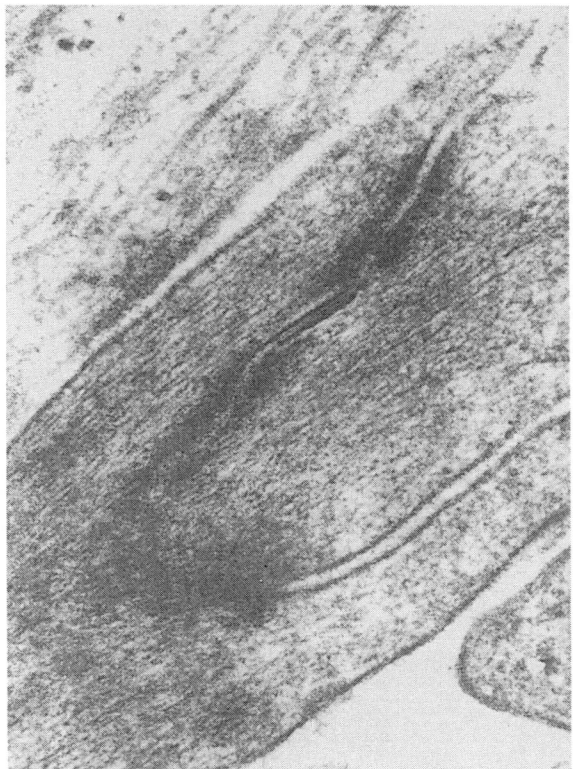

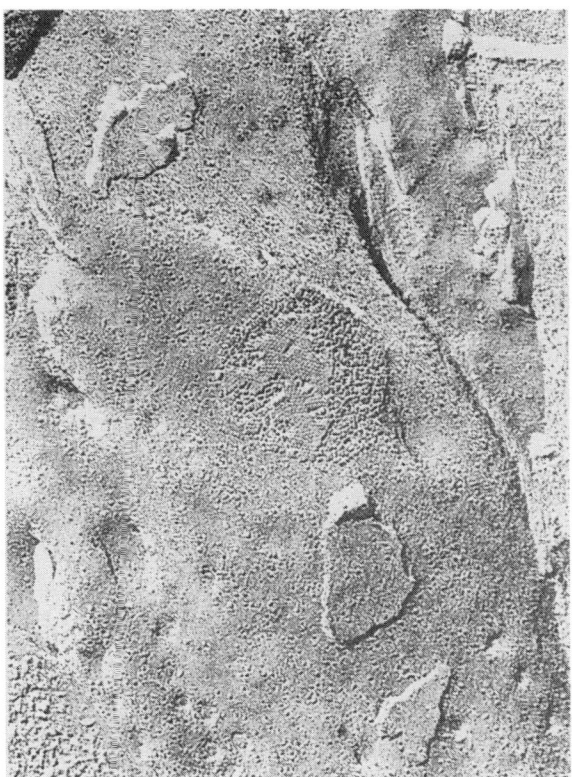

Fig. 4. Nexus junction between an endothelial cell and a smooth muscle cell. X 52 230

Fig. 5. Ultrastructural aspect of a nexus junction after freeze fracture. X 52 230

largely on this coat which is composed of numerous layers of strong, concentrically arranged, elastic lamellae, which alternate with interlamellar zones. The zones are formed by sheets of smooth muscle cells containing fine elastic fibers and ground substance rich in mucopolysaccharides. One lamella and an adjacent interlamellar zone form a lamellar unit [11]. In the human aorta, there are about 40 lamellar units at birth [12] and up to 52 in young adults [13] (Fig. 6-7). The increase in number is accompanied by an increase in thickness of the lamellar units from 8.2 µm at four years of age to 10.6 µm in young adults. Wolinsky and Glagov [14] showed that the number of lamellar units in the media of the adult mammalian aorta is almost proportional to the radius regardless of the species or variations in the wall thickness. Hence, the average tension per lamellar unit of the media is remarkably constant regardless of the radius or the species. A similar pattern is seen in other elastic arteries: pulmonary (Fig. 8), subclavian, axillary, common iliac and common carotid. The smooth muscle cells (SMCs) of the aortic media are smaller than

those elsewhere (20 µ in length, 5 µ in diameter). They contract actively and are able to synthesise collagen fibers, elastic fibers and components of the extracellular matrix. Vascular smooth muscle cells are capable of considerable proliferative activity after injury and in certain pathological states. Vascular muscle cells contain thick (myosin), thin (actin) and intermediate (10 nm) filaments, and the filamentous organisation of actin and myosin are compatible with a sliding filament mechanism of contraction, as in skeletal and cardiac muscle [15].

The major intermediate filament protein present in vascular smooth muscle cells is vimentin [16] but SMCs of the arterial wall are heterogeneous as far as their content of vimentin and desmin are concerned [17, 18]. More desmin positive cells are present in the aorta towards the iliac arteries than at the arch [19, 20]. These filaments are associated with the typical structures of the vascular smooth muscle cells, dense bodies and dense bands.

The cells are surrounded by an extracellular matrix and are interconnected by gap junctions whose

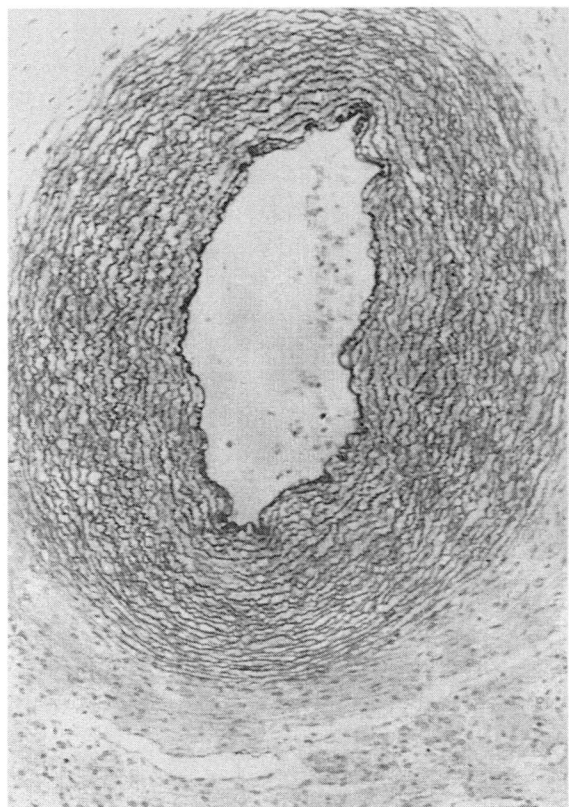

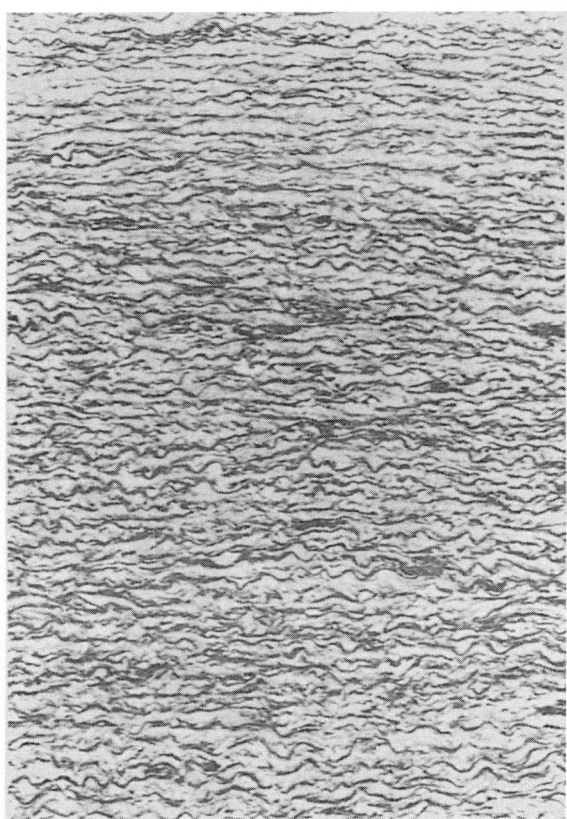

Fig. 6. Elastic frame of the aortic media of a baby suffering from sudden death. Orcein elastic stain (Orcein)

Fig. 7. Elastic frame of the aortic media in a young adult. Orcein

number depends on the type of blood vessel. In addition, intermediate junctions – sites of direct adherence between smooth muscle cells – allow transmission of stress directly from one cell to another [21, 22]. In response to this load, smooth muscle cells produce scleroproteins, which are arranged in a way that distributes the load in the wall. These intermediate junctions are symmetrical structures formed by two electron dense areas that match each other in adjacent smooth muscle cells. Vascular SMCs are capable of many functions, including vasodilatation or constriction in response to normal or pharmacological stimuli; synthesis of various types of collagen, elastin, and proteoglycans; elaboration of growth factors and cytokines; migration and proliferation.

In muscular arteries SMCs are the predominant component of the media, arranged in concentric layers whose number varies from 3-4 in small to 10-40 in large arteries. The elastic fibers are condensed into membranes in the inner and the outer parts. The external elastic lamella, whose fibers are gathered in

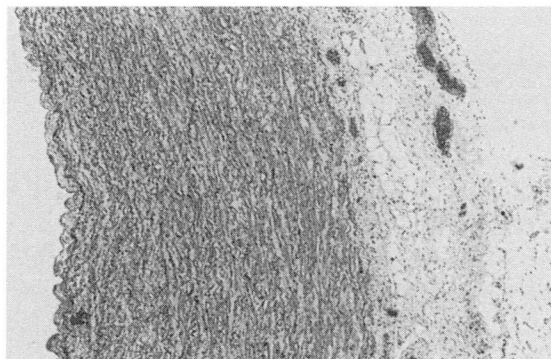

Fig. 8. Pulmonary artery. Orcein

loose bundles, is less well defined than the internal. In muscular arteries (Fig. 9), the wall thickness is about one-fourth of the lumen size. As the resistance of a blood vessel to blood flow is proportional to the fourth power of the diameter, small changes in the lu-

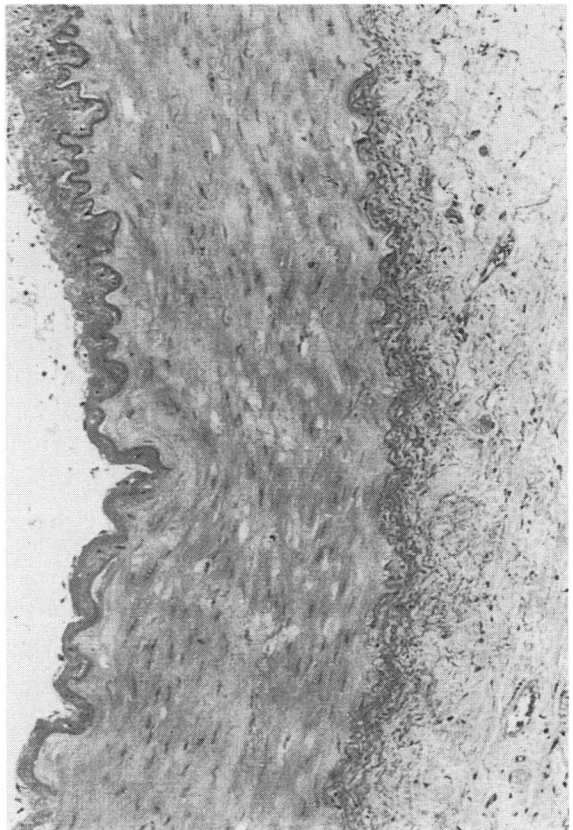

Fig. 9. Muscular artery. Orcein

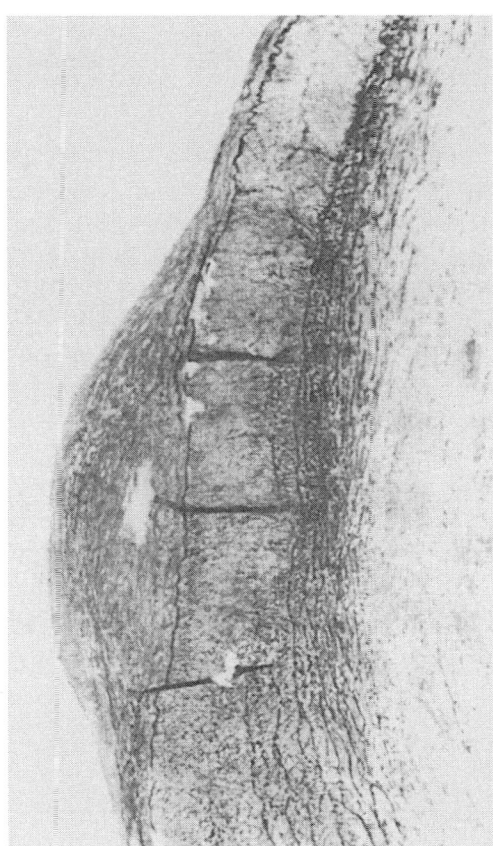

Fig. 10. Transitional zone between the aorta and the renal artery. Orcein

men size produced by muscular activity may lead to a marked flow-limiting effect.

It is important to note that there are transitional forms between muscular and elastic arteries. In these vessels the media show smooth muscle layers progressively replacing the elastic lamellae. In the common iliac and axillary arteries, this segment is circumscribed and measures between 1 to 3 cm in length. The junction between major aortic visceral arteries (renal, superior mesenteric celiac trunk) is generally short – measuring less than 1 cm [23] and is even shorter in the coronary vessels. Distortion of elastic fibers in the transitional segment should not be considered to be pathological (Fig. 10-11).

The adventitia

Beyond the media is the adventitia, a poorly defined layer of investing connective tissue in which nerve fibers, some smooth muscle cells, fibroblasts and the vasa vasorum are found (Fig. 12-13).

Peri-adventitia

This is an ill-defined sheath of loose connective and adipose tissue that surrounds the vessel and at some sites separates it from the tissues and viscera. The peri-adventitia is prominent in vessels that expand or extend markedly, such as the pulmonary arteries.

Architectural variations in arteries

The internal mammary artery, commonly used for an aorto-coronary bypass graft, is of the elastic type (Fig. 14). The external elastic lamina is either lacking or poorly developed in intracranial and intraosseous arteries (Fig. 15-16), as well as in systemic bronchial arteries. In the lungs, elastic arteries contain a more continuous elastic frame; muscular arteries have a thinner media than their extrapulmonary counterparts. Smooth muscle cells may extend into distal small arteries.

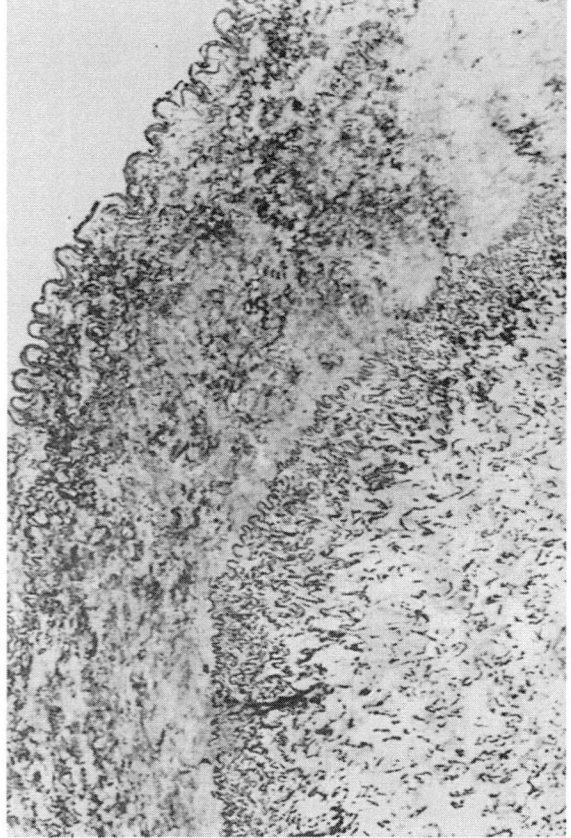

Fig. 11. Transitional zone between the aorta and the renal artery. Note normal distortion of the elastic fibers. Orcein

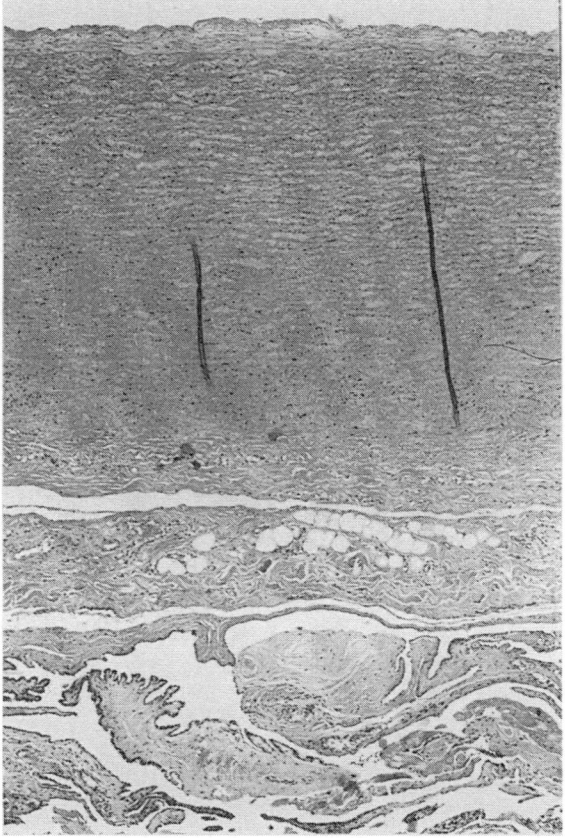

Fig. 12. Aortic adventitia partially covered by mesothelium. Haematoxylin, eosin and saffron stain (HES)

Vascularity and innervation of vessels

Large vessels are supplied with their own vasa vasora. These nutrient blood vessels branch into an arteriolar-capillary-venous network, and send vascular buds that penetrate as far as the outer half of the media. They perfuse the outer two-thirds of the media. In large and medium-sized arteries, nutrition of the smooth muscle cell layers of the inner third of the media depends on direct diffusion from the lumen. Interstitial fluid flows outward in adventitial capillaries and venules that do not penetrate into the media. In large vessels, lymphatic vessels have an arrangement similar to that of the vasa vasora. Non-myelinated motor nerve fibers arise from sympathetic ganglia. These fibers leave plexuses located in the peri-adventitia, cross the adventitia and penetrate the media or the intima. Afferent myelinated fibers give rise to sensory nerve endings in the adventitia. Sympathetic ganglia are present in the adventitia of some large ves-

sels. Arterioles are richly supplied by nerves providing autonomic control of blood flow.

Veins

Structure

The structure of veins reflects both low intraluminal pressure and their function as a major reservoir. In normal conditions, the volume of blood contained in veins is four to five times greater than that in corresponding arteries. In the walls of veins the major layers are less well demarcated than in arteries.

1. The intima is composed of an endothelial lining on a scanty connective tissue layer, bounded by a poorly defined internal elastic membrane. Venous endothelial cells have a mitotic potential greater than their arterial counterparts; it is thought that endothelial cells from small vein segments in adults have a growth capacity to cover areas com-

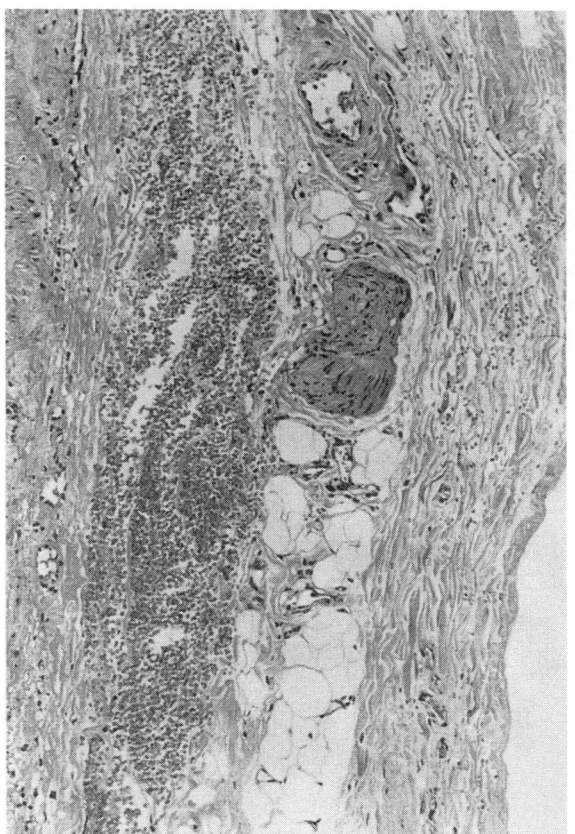

Fig. 13. Aortic adventitia criss-crossed by vasa vasora and nerve bundles. HES

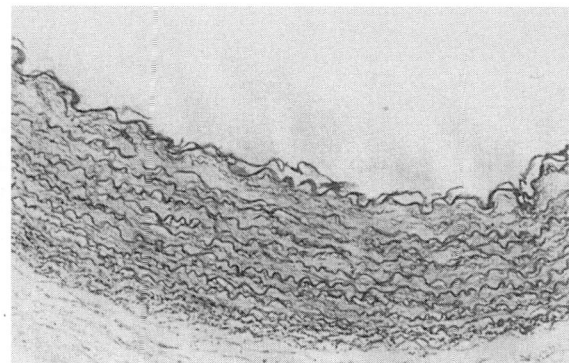

Fig. 14. Internal mammary artery. Orcein

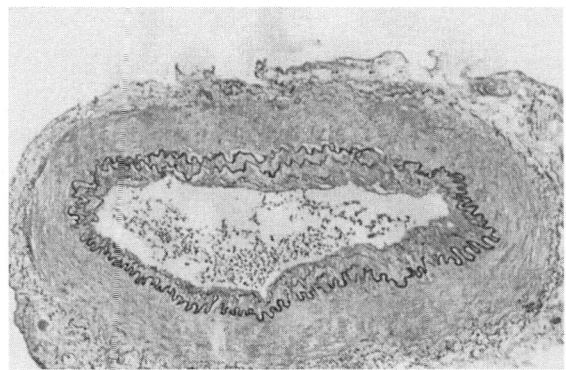

Fig. 15. Intracranial artery. Orcein

parable in size to the luminal areas of vascular prostheses commonly used in arterial surgery [2, 24].

2. The media is not well defined, as it is in arteries. It is capable of supporting the hydrostatic pressure of the blood in the leg vein, for example, but is relatively non-compliant. Smooth muscle cells are fewer, arranged into 3 layers intertwined with loose connective tissue, elastic fibers and some lymphocytes.

3. The adventitia is markedly thicker than in arteries and is made up of connective tissue criss-crossed by vasa vasora. In superficial veins, these nutrient vessels originate from perforating arteries coming from several levels and receive many anastomoses [25]. Collagen fibers (type III IV and I) are much more abundant than elastin. The nerve supply is provided by unmyelinated fibers that penetrate as far as the intima but the innervation is less dense than that of arteries.

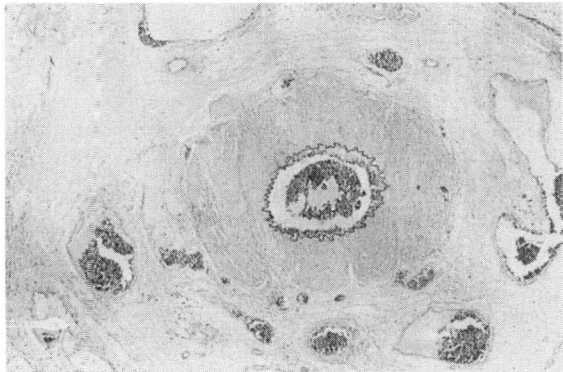

Fig.16. Intraosseous artery. Orcein

Infracardiac and supracardiac veins.

1. In infracardiac veins flow is resisted by gravity. They are thus characterised by the presence of semilunar valves (Fig. 17) which serve to minimise

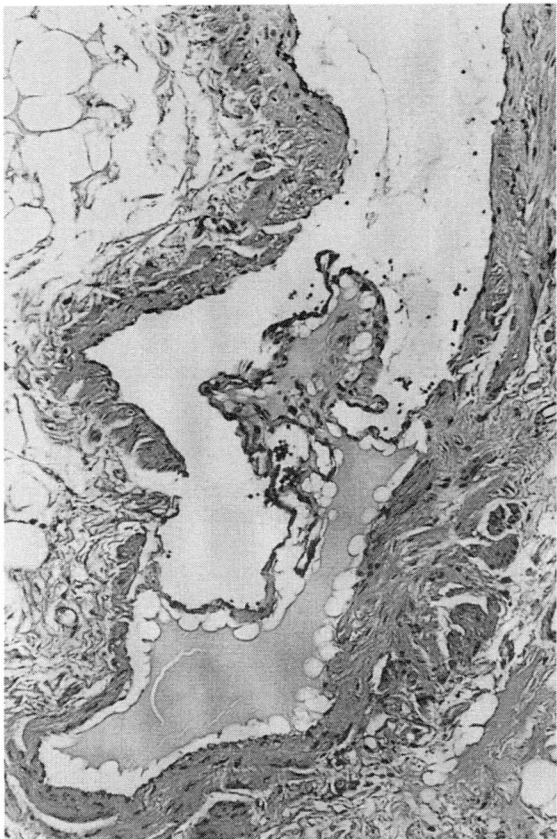

Fig. 17. Infracardiac vein. Note the semilunar valves. HES

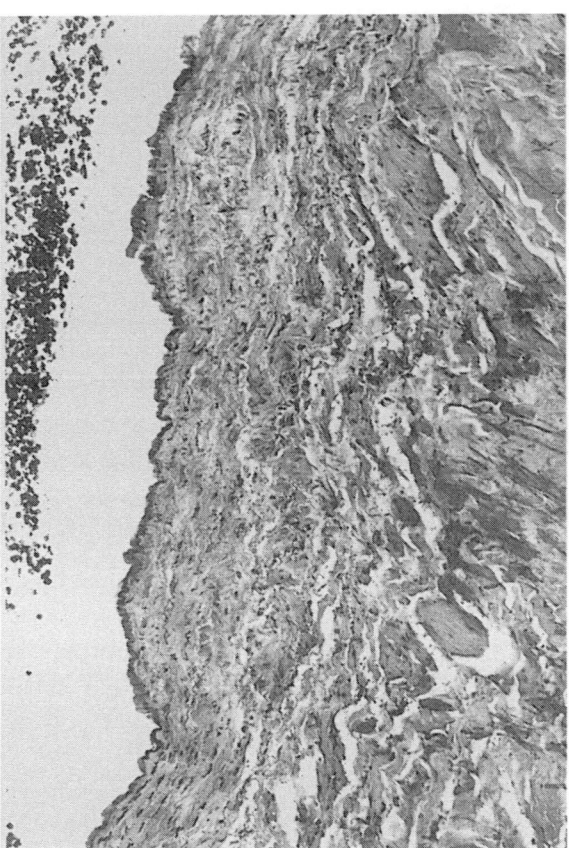

Fig. 18. Infracardiac fibromuscular vein. HES

back flow. These valves, generally arranged in pairs, are a focal enfolding of the intima and an adjacent portion of the vein wall. Both sides of the valve cusp are covered by endothelial cells (ECs) and the core is supported by an axis containing some elastic fibers and a few smooth muscle cells. There is an increase in fibrous tissue in the valve implantation site [26]. Above each valve, the vein calibre is slightly increased to form a pocket or sinus. In the media, smooth muscle cells present an oblique or plexiform orientation. Propulsive veins may contain either a great amount of collagen fibers (the deep fibromuscular veins of the arm, Fig. 18) or a greater number of smooth muscle cells arranged in longitudinal and circular layers (musculo-elastic veins, Fig. 19). A delicate network of collagen and elastic fibers encloses these cells (Fig. 20).

2. Supracardiac veins are either fibrous (intracranial dural venous sinuses) or fibroelastic; they contain elastic fibers in the wall. Their walls are thinner than those of propulsive veins. Semilunar valves are less well developed or absent. In jugular veins, the valve root is devoid of smooth muscle cells and is made up entirely of fibrous tissue (Fig. 21).

Architectural variation in veins

Veins that are rich in smooth muscle cells may form true sphincters (for example, the supra-hepatic veins). In the juxta-cardiac segment of the vena cava and pulmonary veins, myocardial cells extend into the adventitia (Fig. 22, 23), and the proximal vein may contract during systole. Pulmonary veins have an attenuated external elastic membrane (Fig. 24) [27]. Venous plexuses consist of small convoluted veins displaying discrete, sack-like, funnel-shaped or serpiginous ectasias. They exist in the submucosa of the anal canal and surround some pelvic viscera, such as the uterus or urinary bladder. Connections with arteries give rise to arteriovenous anastomoses that allow rapid passage

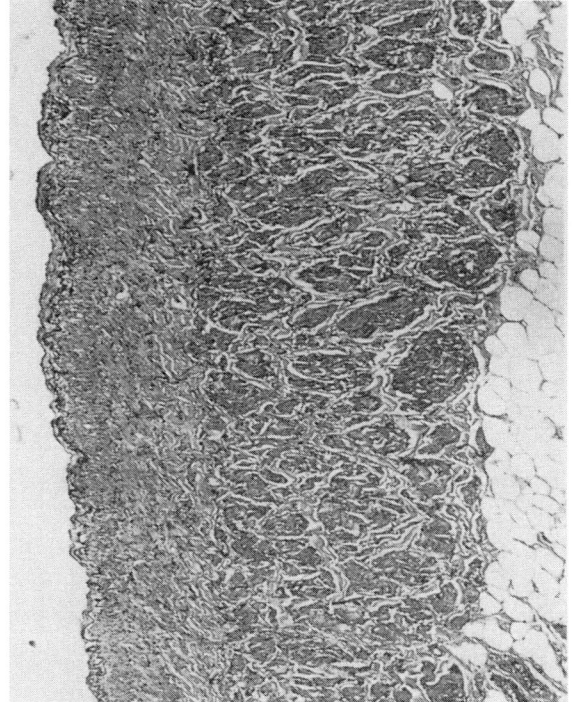

Fig. 19. Infracardiac musculo-elastic vein. HES

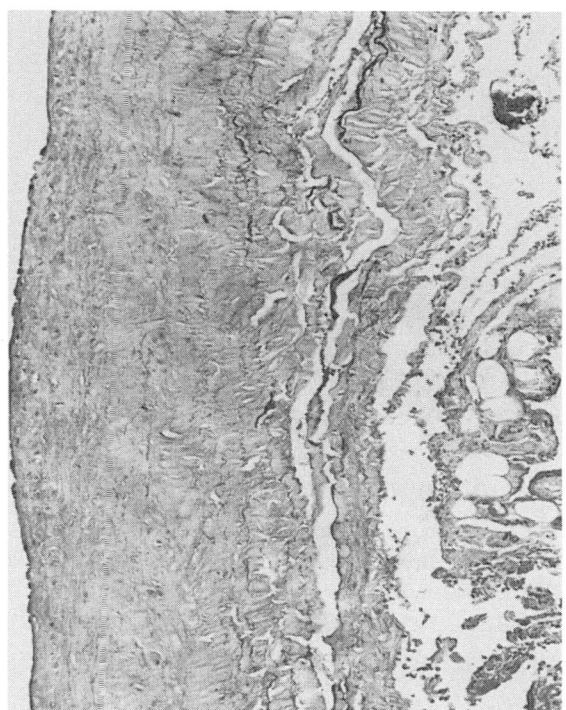

Fig. 20. Infracardiac musculo-elastic vein. Note the delicate elastic fibers of the media. Orcein

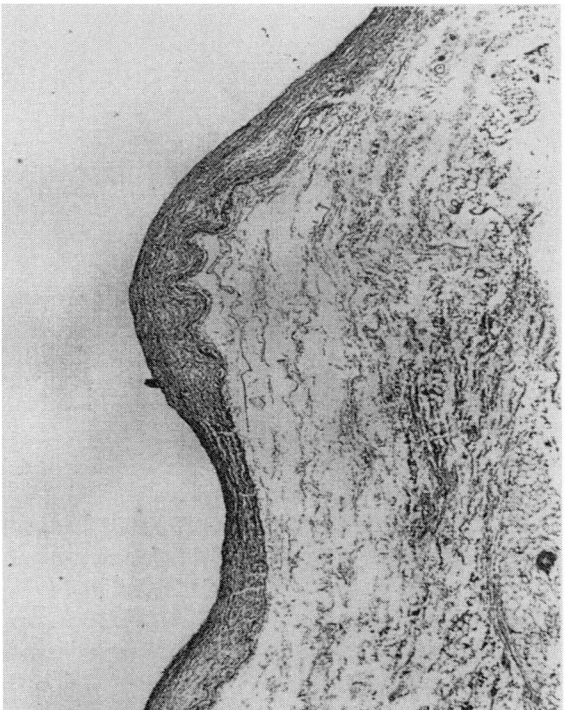

Fig. 21. Supracardiac jugular vein devoid of semilunar valves. HES

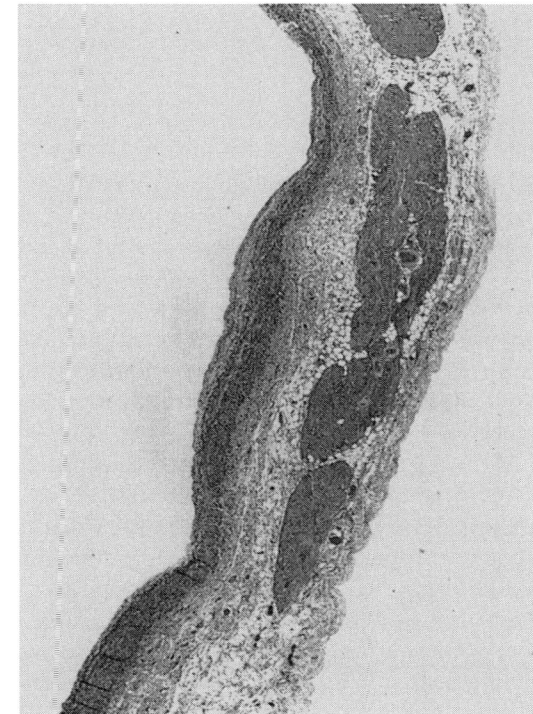

Fig. 22. Juxtacardiac segment of the vena cava. Note extension of myocardial cells into the adventitia. HES

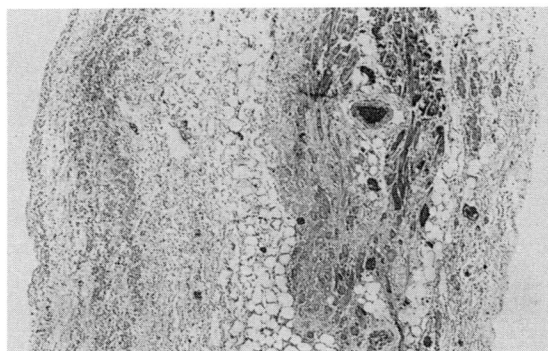

Fig. 23. Juxtacardiac segment of the pulmonary vein harbouring myocardial cells in the adventitia. HES

of arterial blood into the venous system and contribute to thermoregulation. This process is particularly evident in the skin and nasal mucosa [28, 29].

Microcirculation

The microcirculation contains around 10% of the total blood volume (around 4% of this is in the lungs). It is divisible into three compartments: arterioles, capillaries and post-capillary venules, but the transition between the systemic and the microcirculation is gradual.

Arterioles

Vessels with the structure of arterioles may measure from 250 μm to less than 50 μm [28] in diameter (Fig. 25). In the intima, a well-defined internal elastic membrane is often lacking and the basement membrane of the endothelial cells separates the endothelium from the media, which is composed of a single layer of SMCs (Fig. 26). This layer becomes discontinuous at the end of the arteriole, the meta-arteriole or precapillary sphincter. This portion is 10 to 100 μm in length and presents a gradual transition to junctional capillaries.

Various structures form protuberances that dramatically reduce the lumen of the arterioles. These are variously described as cushions, columns or bolsters, sleeves and sphincters and develop from the intima and the media. An endothelial lining, supported by smooth muscle cells and elastic fibers arising from the inner portion of the media covers them. Often clustered in groups of 3 to 4, they are generally located at the origin of a collateral arteriole. They are frequently found in the lungs. Numerous unmyelinated vasomotor nerve fibers are observed in the adventitia of arte-

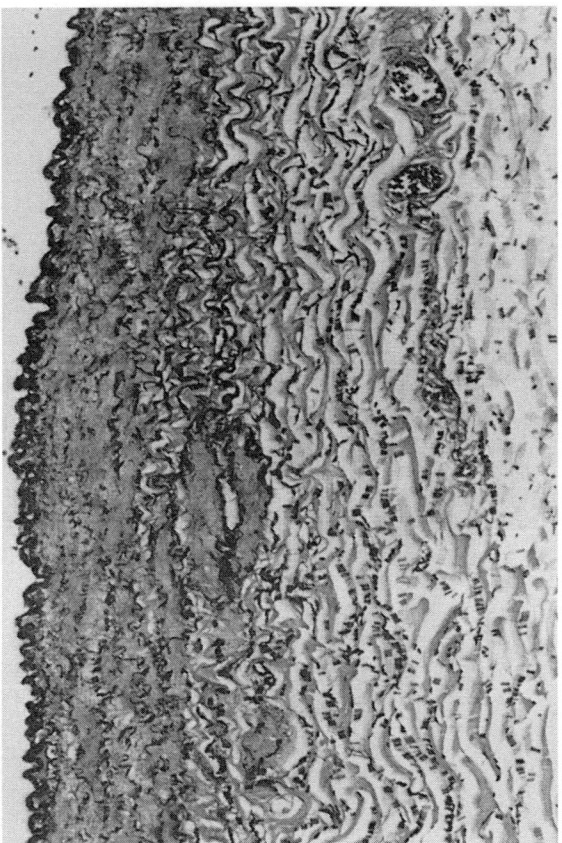

Fig. 24. Pulmonary vein showing an attenuated external elastic membrane. Orcein

rioles. Arterioles are the principal areas of normal resistance to blood flow, inducing both a changes from pulsatile to steady flow and a sharp reduction in pressure as blood passes from arterioles to capillaries. The small arteries and the arterioles bear the brunt of blood pressure changes; these changes may alter their structure.

Capillaries

These vessels form a regular network of anastomosing narrow channels. Their diameter ranges from 5 to 10 μm, approximately the size of a red blood cell (7 to 8 μm). Some authors [30] include postcapillary "venules" up to 50 μm or more in the capillary bed. In the renal glomerulus, the capillaries are essentially part of the arterial system and in the hepatic lobule represent part of the venous system. Their densities vary in different tissues or organs; there are none in normal cartilage but other tissues are criss-crossed by very dense networks (myocardium 2000/mm^2,

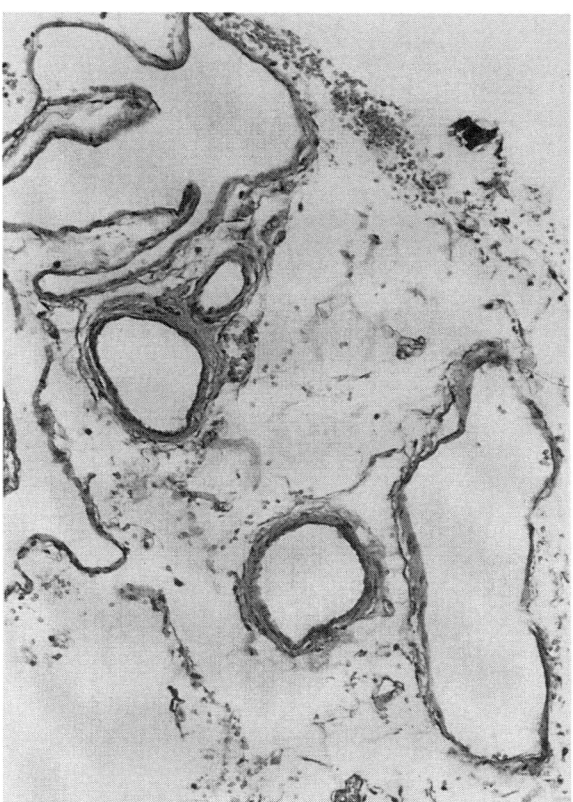

Fig. 25. Two arterioles surrounded by capillaries. HES

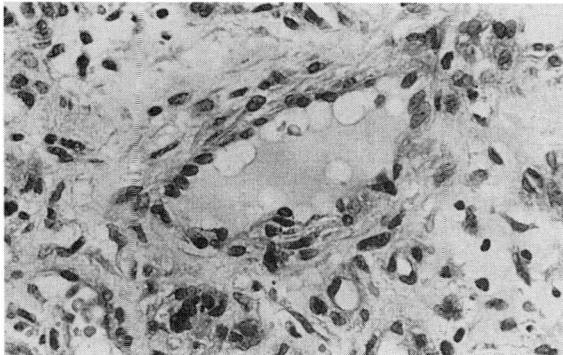

Fig. 26. Arteriole. HES

pulmonary parenchyma, endocrine glands, skeletal muscle 600 to 1200/mm^2, cerebral cortex 1000/mm^2).

Structure

Capillaries are supported on the outside by a thin basement membrane providing some mechanical strength, made up mostly of type IV collagen and a thin sheath of cells, the peri-endothelium, at the periphery. Like other vessels they are lined by endothelial cells. There is no media. The peri-endothelium or peri-capillary layer is composed of a discontinuous layer of undifferentiated mesenchymal cells or pericytes. In some capillaries (and venules), pericytes lie outside the endothelial cells but are enveloped in their own basal lamina, which may fuse with the endothelial basement membrane. Capillaries at different sites have different structures distinguished by the degree of continuity of endothelium and of basement membrane as observed by electron microscopy: continuous, fenestrated and sinusoid.

1. In continuous capillaries, the endothelium and the basement membrane are continuous (Fig. 27). They are found in the muscle, heart, lungs, skin, and the nervous system. The permeability of these capillaries is highly regulated through control of transport across and between endothelial cells. Some authors have described 4 subtypes [31, 32]: capillaries with or without pericytes, having turgescent or flat endothelium but it is not clear that these have any functional significance.

2. Fenestrated capillaries have a sieve-like endothelium that is covered with orifices or pores (Fig. 28). Most endocrine glands, renal glomeruli, and some vessels of the gastrointestinal tract have fenestrated endothelia, which allow more rapid transport. These gaps, whose diameters range from 20 to 30 µm (endocrine glands) and from 50 to 100 µm (renal glomeruli), may be blocked by a single or double layer of basal membrane.

3. Some capillary vascular channels (sinusoids or sinusoid capillaries) have a discontinuous endothelium with partial (red pulp of the spleen) or absent basement membrane (bone marrow or liver) and the endothelial cells lie directly on the collagen fibers (Fig. 29). Such structures facilitate the passage of cells across the walls.

The capillary bed has two patterns of flow, through true capillaries and direct capillaries. True capillaries control intermittent circulation by the contraction of precapillary sphincters. Direct capillaries, which are numerous in glandular organs and in muscles, provide continuous circulation between arterioles and venules and empty directly into venules.

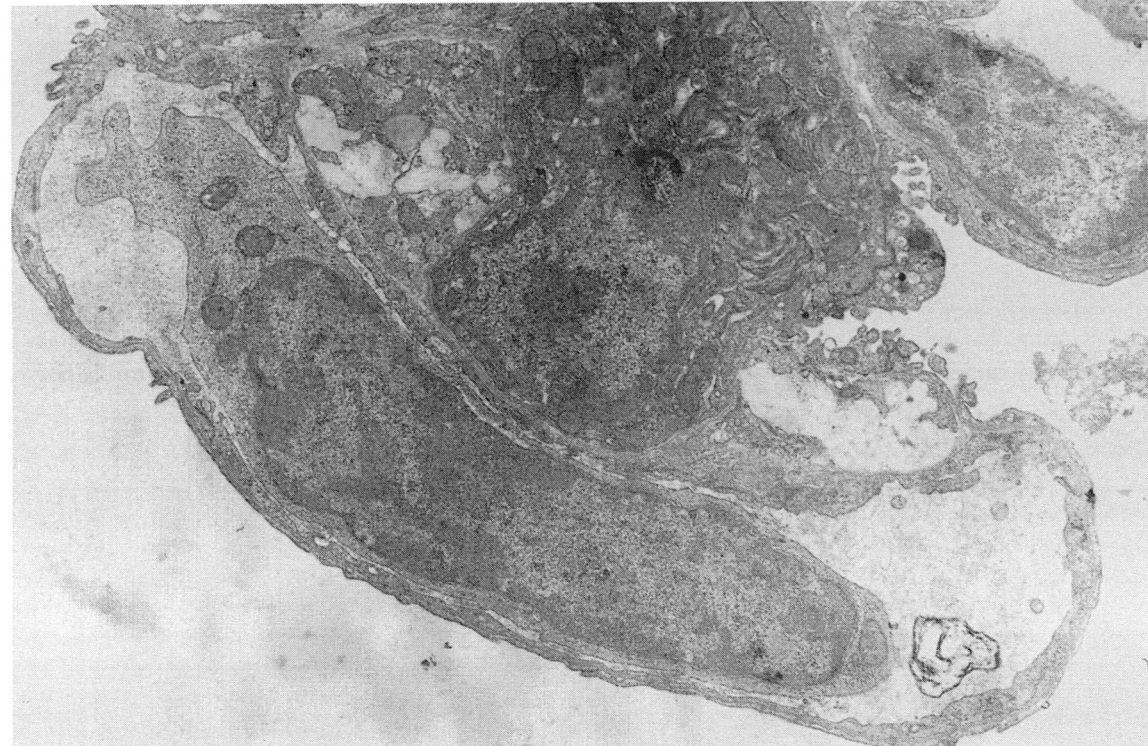

Fig. 27. Continuous capillary. X 9 000 (Courtesy Dr Y.Boulard)

Venules

Structure

In general venules have a structure very similar to that of capillaries, but their diameter is greater for a given anatomical location.

1. Pericytic venules are characterised by the presence of pericytes similar to those of capillaries, although they appear to become activated more readily on stimulation. Their diameter ranges from 10 to 50 μm and their length from 50 to 700 μm. The endothelium is generally continuous. The basal lamina is thin and penetrated by pericytes, which form a continuous layer. A true media is absent. The adventitia is relatively thin with few connective fibers. Pericytic venules play an important role in the exchange between blood and interstitial fluid. In the brain, gap junctions have been visualised between endothelial cells and pericytes [33].

2. Muscular venules have a calibre ranging from 50 to 200 μm in diameter. At greater diameters, the muscular layer becomes continuous and the ve-nule becomes a small vein. Just as in arterioles, venules may contain intimal structures such as columns and sphincters but these are less numerous than in arterioles, however, they provide local control of blood flow. In the lungs, it may be difficult to distinguish venules from arterioles [27].

3. Postcapillary venules are an important point of interchange between the lumen of the vessels and the surrounding tissues. They are lined by tall, almost cuboidal endothelial cells in some sites. Fluid and leukocytic exudation occur preferentially in these venules in many types of inflammation.

Specialized vascular structures

Arteriovenous anastomoses

These are direct connections between small-calibre arteries and veins. Some are vestigial remnants of the embryonic circulation; others are present in the normal physiological state and are precisely localised. Two types may be distinguished.

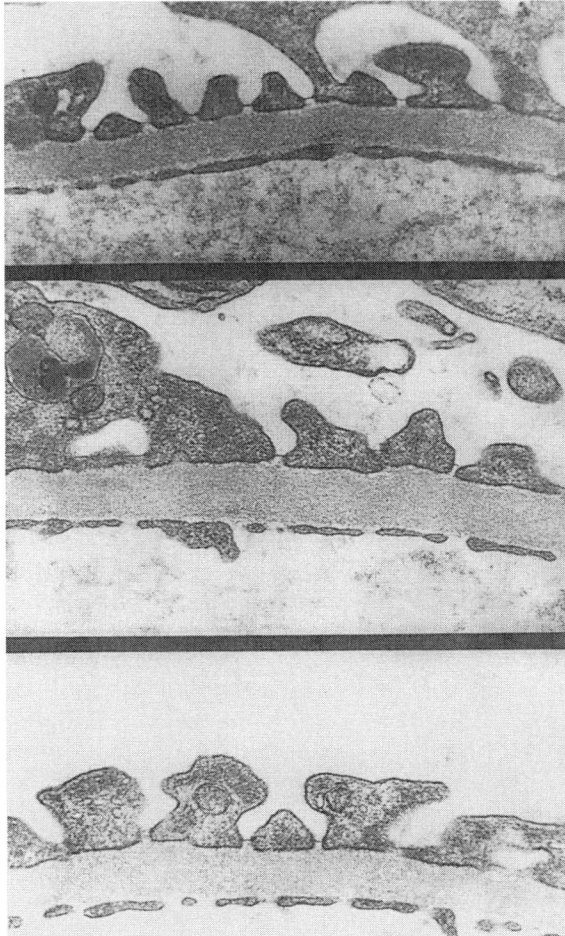

Fig. 28. Fenestrated capillary. X 26 950 (Courtesy Pr P. Bruneval)

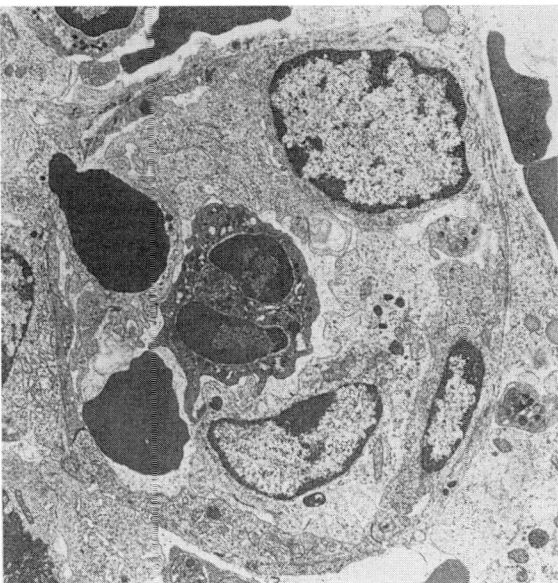

Fig. 29. Discontinuous capillary. X 9 000 (Courtesy Dr Y. Boulard)

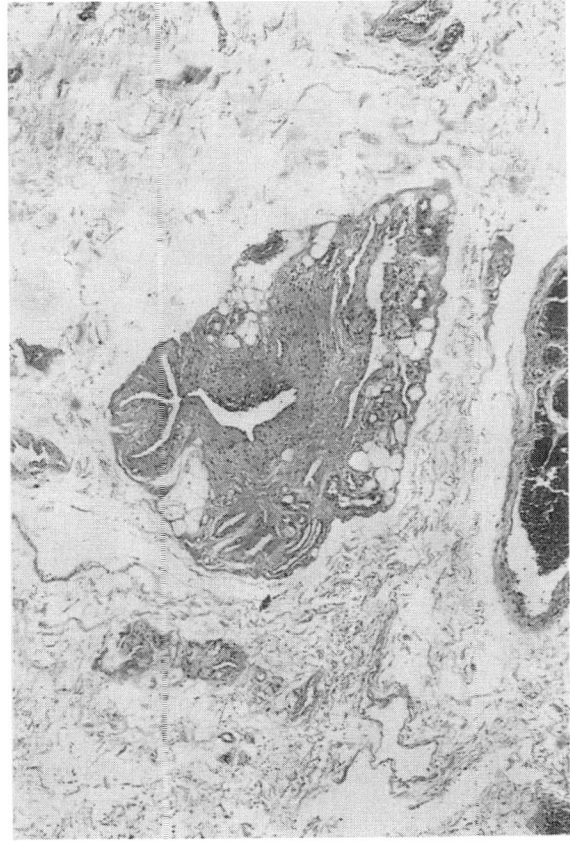

Fig. 30. Recto-anal cross-over arteriovenous anastomosis. HES

Cross-over arteriovenous anastomosis

This is a direct connection between an arteriole and a venule. The arterial side of the anastomosis presents a sphincter developed from the media and this may be capable of complete closure, in haemodynamic terms. This type of anastomosis exists in the anal canal (Fig. 30) where the small terminal branches of the rectal arteries connect with the submucosal venous plexus and form numerous arteriovenous anastomoses or "anal glomeruli." These structures are anchored to the internal anal sphincter by collagen fibers and smooth muscle cells from the musculus mucosa (Fig. 31, 32). The whole system has been referred to as the "corpus cavernosum recti" [34]. Symptomatic haemorrhoids appear when the supporting and anchoring structures

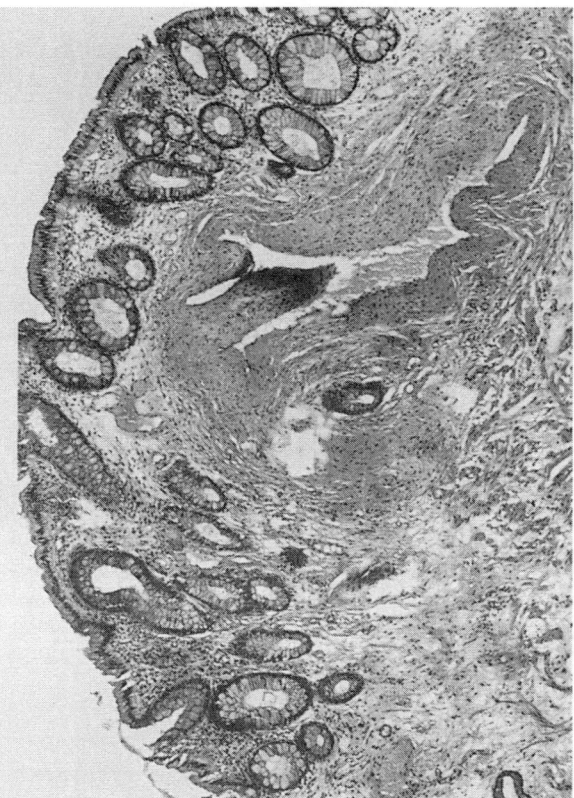

Fig. 31. Cross-over arteriovenous anastomosis in the upper portion of the anal canal. HES

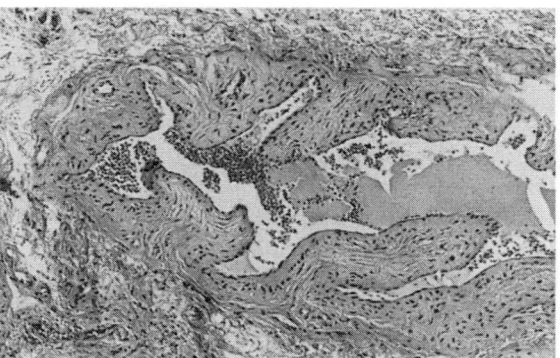

Fig. 32. Recto-anal cross-over arteriovenous anastomosis or "anal glomeruli" or "corpus cavernosum recti". HES

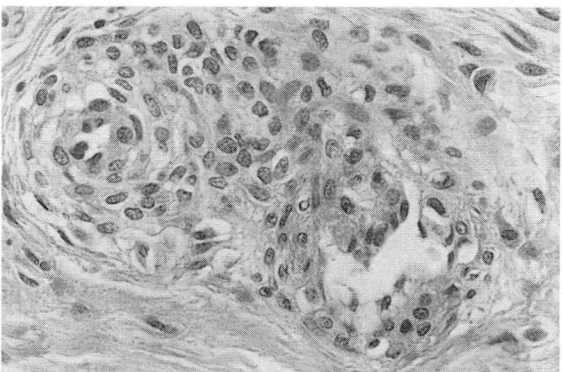

Fig. 33. H-shaped arteriovenous anastomosis. Glomic cells are present around the intermediate segment. HES

of these anastomoses deteriorate. Collagen fibers undergo degenerative changes, together with replacement of muscle cells by collagen. The result is venous stasis and dilation, anal cushion formation and haemorrhoid prolapse [35].

H-shaped arteriovenous anastomosis

In this type, the arteriole is connected to a venule through an intermediate segment. In its longest part, the segment is like an arteriole – its media contains smooth muscle cells with some epithelioid glomic cells in the periphery (Fig. 33). The remaining juxtavenous part resembles a venule. This type of anastomosis is frequently observed in areas where there are intense variations in blood flow (pinna of the ear, nasal mucosa) where there are intense variations in blood flow [36, 37]. It is a major part of a neurovascular glomi.

Erectile vascular tissue

Erectile tissue is found in the nasal mucosa (Fig. 34), the corpora cavernosa and corpus spongiosum in the male penis (Fig. 35, 36), and the clitoris (Fig. 37). It is composed of specialised anastomotic vascular spaces having variable calibre and irregular contour. These vessels appear more venous than arterial. They are lined with endothelial cells and surrounded by a thin layer of smooth muscle cells, which coalesce into extraluminal cushions or bolsters. They are widely interconnected, a change which should not be mistaken for congenital angiodysplasia [38, 39]. These vascular spaces are small slits in the flaccid state. In penile erection, their diameter increases several times because of engorgement of venous cavities produced by contraction of smooth muscle of the trabecular structures against the penile tunica albuginea. The interstitial loose connective tissue contains the usual type of nu-

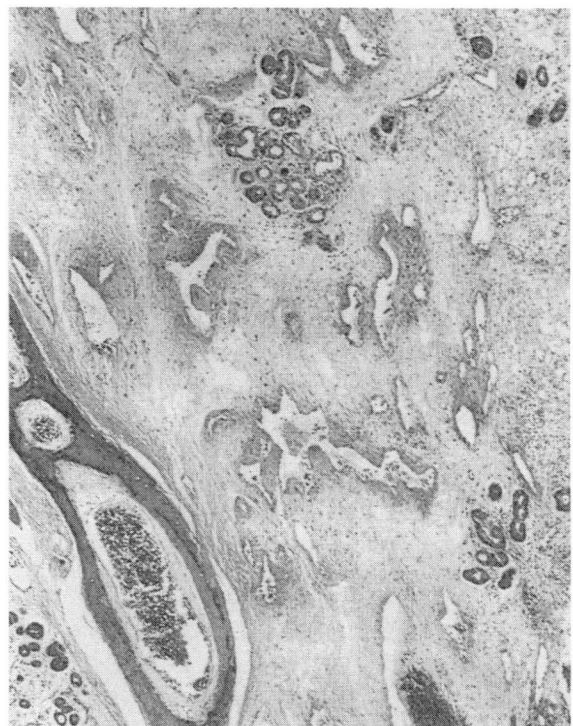

Fig. 34. Erectile vessels of the nasal mucosa. HES

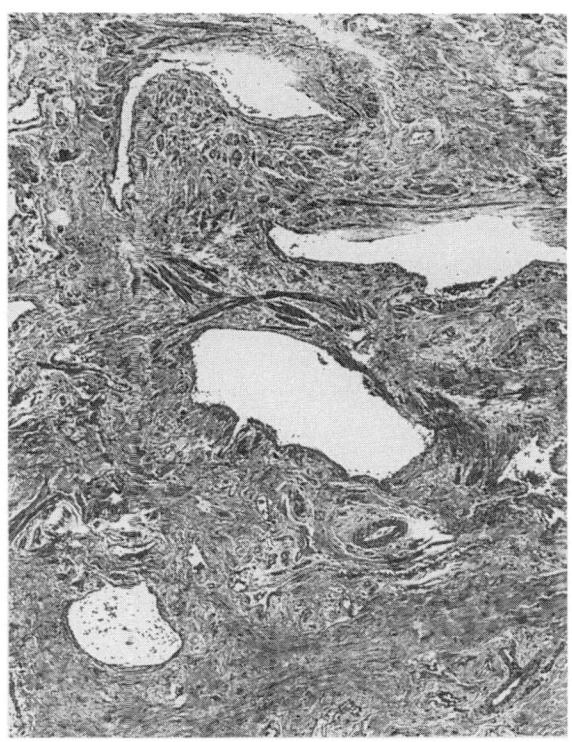

Fig. 35. Erectile vessels of the penile corpora cavernosa. HES

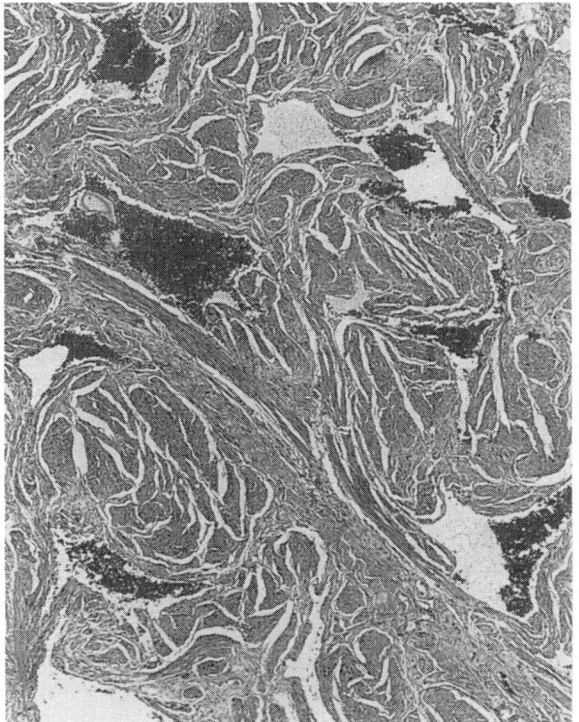

Fig. 36. Erectile vessels of the penile corpus spongiosum. HES

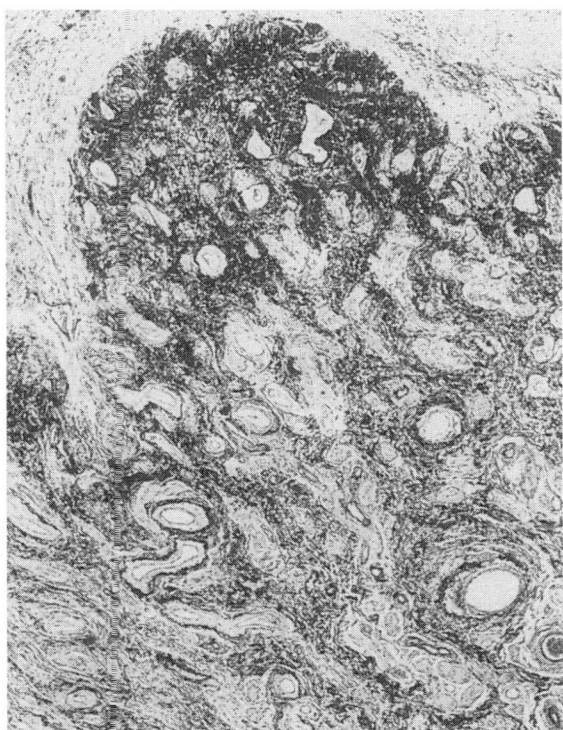

Fig. 37. Clitoral erectile vessels enclosed by an abundant elastic network. Orcein

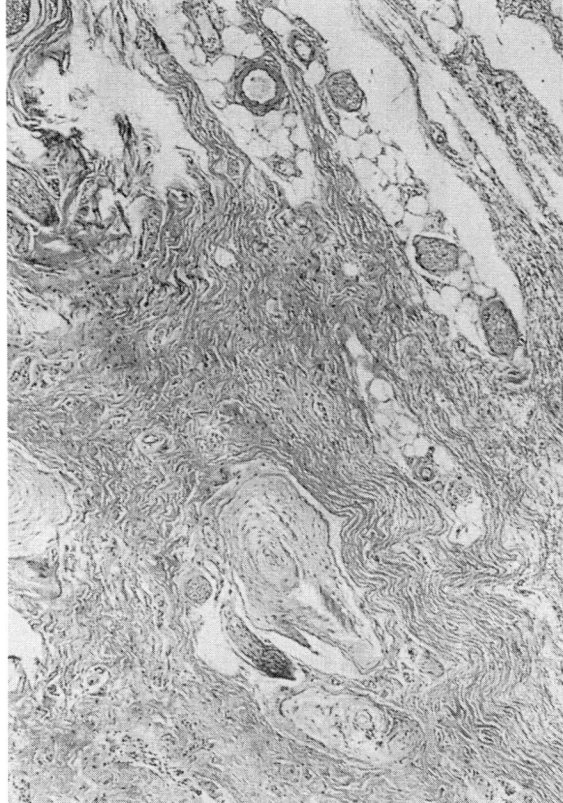

Fig. 38. Nerve endings and sensory corpuscles in the clitoral interstitial connective tissue. HES

tritive blood vessels, lymph vessels and numerous nerve endings and some sensory corpuscles (Fig. 38). Autonomic nerve transmitters and substances released by the endothelium-including acetylcholine, bradykinin, vasoactive intestinal polypeptide (VIP), and endothelium - derived relaxing factor (EDRF), control trabecular smooth muscle tone. Endothelium-derived nitric oxide leads to smooth muscle relaxation [40, 41].

Vaso active tissues

Paraganglia

These are distributed throughout the body, notably in the adrenal medulla, the organs of Zuckerkandl, along para-vertebral sympathetic nerve ganglia, and in some cranial nerves (including the paraglosso-pharyngeal and vagus nerves). They are also found in the retroperitoneal space and in some viscera (heart, kidney, testis, and ovary). Their organoid arrangement consists of wide vascular sinusoid circumscribed by neuro-ectodermal cells, mixed with nerve endings in contact with cells. There are two types of paraganglia:

1. Chromaffin-positive paraganglia secreting catecholamines, innervated by efferent cranial nerve innervation but devoid of chemoreceptor function.
2. Chromaffin-negative paraganglia, which do not secrete catecholamines, but which have efferent cranial nerve innervation and a chemoreceptor function. They are scattered from the base of the skull to the aortic arch and found in the jugular glomus, in the tympanic membrane, carotid body, and paraganglia of the vagus nerve and along the aorta (Fig. 39, 40).

The carotid sinus

The sinus is a swelling formed by the terminal part of the common carotid artery and the origin of the internal carotid. Baroreceptor or chemoreceptor nerve endings thicken the adventitia and represent the main components of the "reflexogenic" area. Nerve endings are not encapsulated; their structural arrangement resembles that of Messner's touch corpuscles (Fig. 41).

Neurovascular glomus

A typical neurovascular glomus is an ovoid structure, visible with a magnifying glass, measuring 200 to 300 μm in diameter and sheathed in a capsule of connective tissue. It corresponds to a specialised form of arteriovenous anastomosis that serves to regulate local blood flow. Glomi are particularly frequent in the nail bed and in skin areas exposed to variations in temperature [42]. Intravisceral glomi (lungs, heart, kidneys, spleen, stomach, intestine, and lymph nodes) should not be miss-interpreted as metastases of cellular blue nevi. Histologically, a glomus is comprised of two parts: the glomus body and the arteriovenous anastomosis proper (Fig. 42). The first structure is made up of an afferent convoluted arteriole that branches into preglomic arterioles. The second is composed of irregular thick-walled segments known as the Sucquet-Hoyer canals. These canals, corresponding to the arteriovenous anastomoses, have a narrow lumen delineated by a thick layer of SMCs intermingled with several sets of glomic globular or epithelioid cells (Fig. 43). Collecting veins are located at the periphery. Immunoelectron microscopy reveals two types of glomic cells: type I cells contain loose arrays of alpha smooth muscle actin positive microfilaments, sometimes arranged in small bundles, type II cells have tightly packed actin filaments. Immunoreactivity for cathepsin D is much greater in type I cells than in type II cells [43]. Routine immunohistochemical

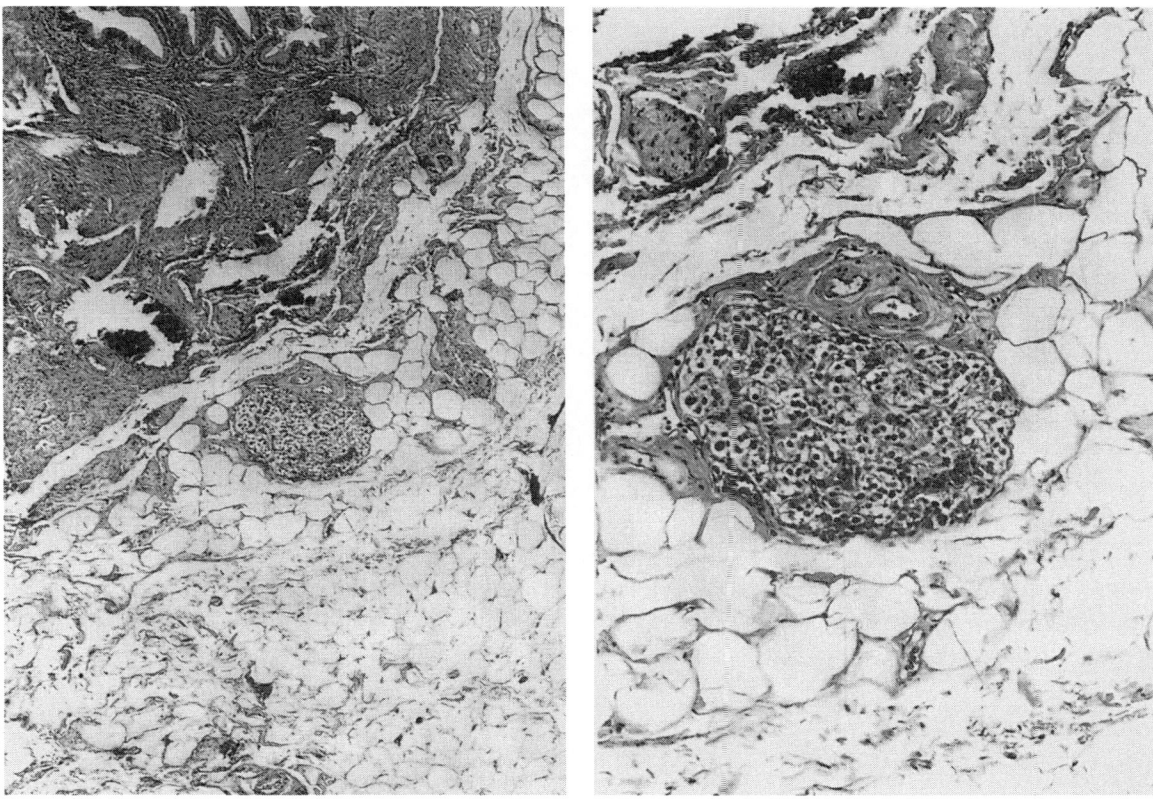

Fig.39-40. Chromaffin-negative paraganglion located in the serosa of a gallbladder. HES

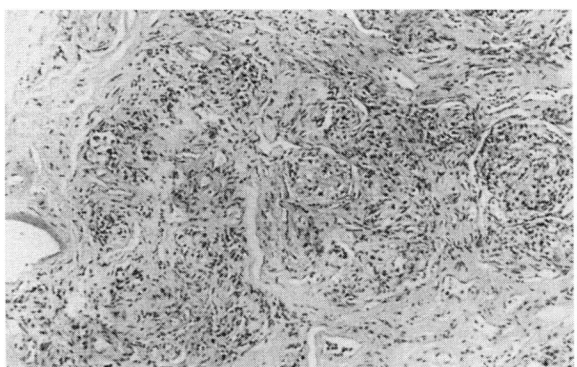

Fig. 41. Carotid sinus. HES

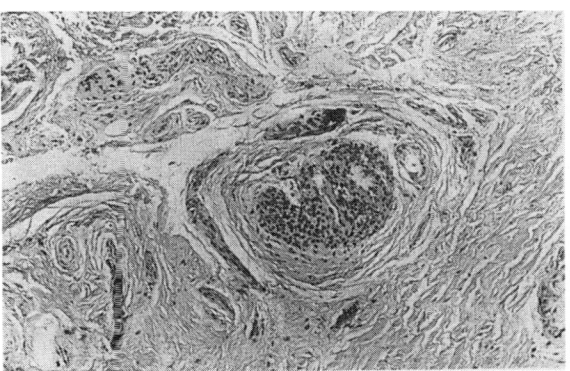

Fig. 42. Neurovascular glomus. HES

study confirms the immunopositivity of both smooth muscle cell types for alpha-smooth muscle actin, vimentin, and smooth muscle myosin. There is no internal elastic membrane in these arterioles, which drain into a short, thin-walled venous segment. The initial part of this segment contains various intimal structures in the form of cushions or columns. The arterioles act as a sphincter. The entire entity is surrounded by lamellae of collagenous tissue containing numerous myelinated and unmyelinated nerve fibers and vessels. There is a reticulin meshwork, radiating from the vascular basement membrane

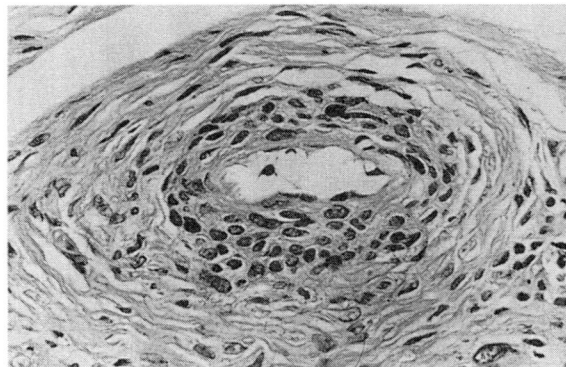

Fig. 43. Neuromuscular glomus. Note glomic cells intermingled with smooth muscle cells in a thick-walled arteriovenous anastomosis. HES

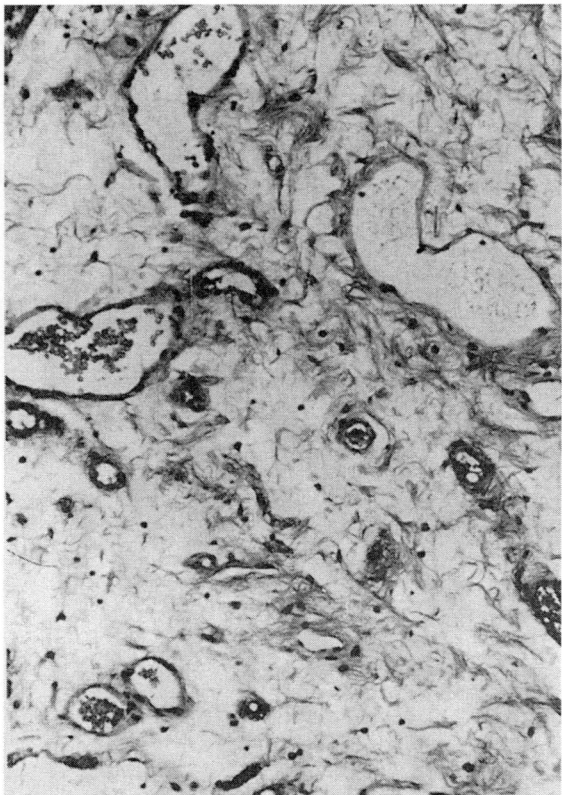

Fig. 44. Lymphatic capillaries. HES

and surrounding each glomic cell. Sensory structures such as Messner's, Pacinian's or Ruffini's corpuscles are frequently found at the periphery of the glomus.

Lymphatic vessels

The collection of tissue fluid by the lymphatic tree is leisurely compared with the flow of blood. An average trip from the distal lower extremity through the lymphatics and back to the general circulation via the thoracic duct takes about 20 minutes [44]. The system begins in the tissues as blind-ended capillaries that drain into larger collecting lymphatics and thence into two main lymphatic trunks. Lymphatic vessels are absent from the bone marrow, the central nervous system, much of the eyes, the internal ear, the fetal placenta, cartilage, and the endocrine glands with the exception of the thyroid. Lymphatic/venous anastomoses have been observed to form rapidly when there is proximal obstruction, which suggests to some that lymphovenous anastomoses normally exist. This has been thought to explain occasional deaths following injection of dye for lymphangiography [44].

Lymphatic capillaries

These start from the lymph canaliculi, which are thin-walled, blind-ended spaces. These channels branch and anastomose freely to form a dense capillary network within connective tissue. They are difficult to identify except when the connective tissue is oedematous and may be mistaken for artefactual spaces. In tissue sections, lymphatic capillaries are identified as collapsed thin-walled, endothelium-lined channels devoid of blood cells (Fig. 44). They are wider and

have a more irregular contour than blood capillaries. Reticulin staining technique helps to demonstrate a discontinuous basement membrane. No pericytes are found externally. The whole vessel is surrounded by a small amount of connective tissue. While differences exist between the structure and function of the blood and lymphatic capillaries, lymphatic endothelium, like that of blood vessels, synthesises Factor VIII-related antigen and fibronectin. Ultrastructurally, lymphatic endothelial cells show Weibel-Palade bodies, overlapping intercellular junctions and anchoring. However, differentiation of lymphatics and blood vessels has been possible with histochemical proof of alkaline phosphatase and 5'-nucleotidase in the endothelium [45, 46].

Small lymphatics

These have an ill defined, thin media containing SMCs arranged in bundles. The lumen is lined with endothelial cells which, in some areas, are in direct contact with the adventitia (Fig. 45).

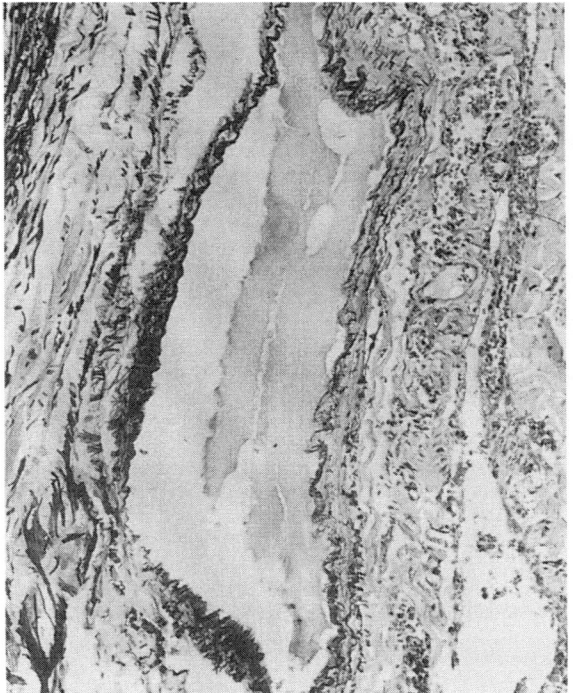

Fig. 45. Small lymphatic. HES

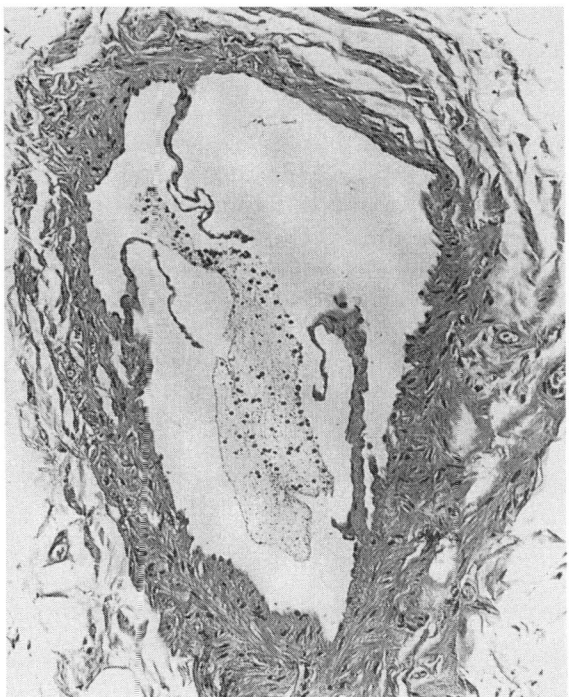

Fig. 46. Collecting lymph vessel. HES

Collecting lymph vessels

Larger lymphatics are visible to the naked eye. They have delicate unidirectional valves (Fig. 46) and it is noteworthy that peripheral lymphatics have been observed to pulsate weakly – these pulsations contribute to flow partly because of the presence of valvules on the collectors (Fig. 47). However, the arterial pulse, voluntary muscle contraction, the pressure of adjoining tissues and the drop in intrathoracic pressure on inhalation alll contribute to flow [47, 48]. Like arteries large lymphatics have three coats – intima, media and adventitia – but these are not clearly delineated. In the intima, a thin network of longitudinally arranged elastic fibers supports the endothelium. SMCs with a predominantly circular arrangement compose the media (a few fine elastic fibers are found among the smooth muscle cells). The adventitia forms the thickest coat and consists of bundles of collagen fibers, elastic fibers and some SMCs, all of which are longitudinally oriented. Valves are numerous in lymphatic vessels and are located at closer intervals than in veins. They consist of an endothelial fold with some muscle at their base [49].

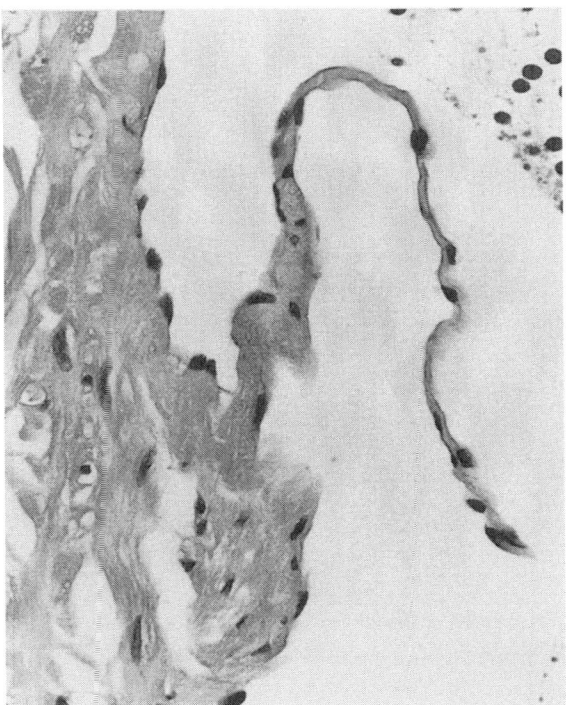

Fig. 47. Collecting lymph vessel. A semilunar valve supported by a delicate connective core. HES

Lymphatic trunks

These ultimately gather into two main trunks, the thoracic duct and the right lymphatic duct. The thoracic duct opens into the venous system at the junction of the left jugular and subclavian veins. The right lymphatic duct receives lymph only from the upper right portion of the body and empties it into the right brachiocephalic vein. The histological structure of these trunks resembles that of a large vein (Fig. 48). However, some differences exist. The media is the thickest component of the wall and differs from that of large veins in containing a great deal of muscle. The SMCs have a predominately circular arrangement and are separated by abundant connective tissue and some elastic fibrils. The wall of the thoracic duct contains nutrient blood vessels similar to the vasa vasora of large blood vessels.

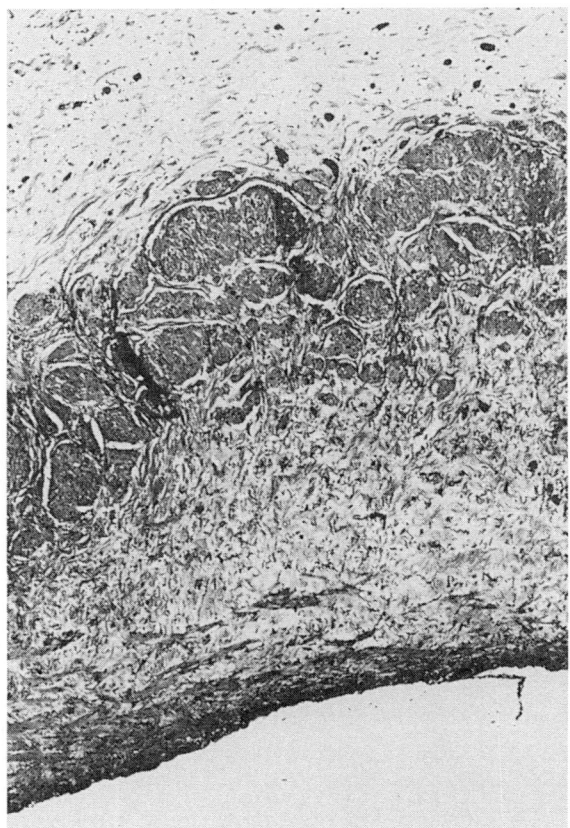

Fig. 48. Lymphatic trunk. HES

Bibliography

1. Krause WJ, Cutts JH (1981) Concise text of histology. Williams & Wilkins, Baltimore, London p. 429
2. Romanov YA, Balyasnikova IV, Bystrevskaya VB, Byzova TV, Ilyinskaya OP, Krushinky AV, Latsis RV, Soboleva EL, Tararak EM, Smirnov VN (1995) Endothelial heterogeneity and intimal blood-borne cells. Relation to human atherosclerosis *In* Numano F, Wissler RW (eds.) Atherosclerosis III. Recent advances in atherosclerosis research. The 3rd Saratoga international conference on atherosclerosis in Nekoma. Ann NewYork Acad (vol 748) p. 12
3. Takamizawa K, Hayashi K (1988) Uniform strain hypothesis and thin-walled theory in arterial mechanics. Biorheology 25: 555-65
4. Hayashi KK, Ide K, Matsumoto T (1994) Aortic walls in atherosclerotic rabbits – mechanical study. J Biomech Eng 116: 284-93
5. Dobrin PB (1983) Handbook of Physiology – The Cardiovascular System III (Am Physiol Soc, Bethesda, 1983), Chap 3, pp. 65-102
6. Han HC, Fung YC (1995) Longitudinal strain of canine and porcine aortas. J Biomech 28: 637-41
7. Sato M, Hayashi K, Niimi H, Moritake K, Okumura A, Handa H (1979) Axial mechanical properties of arterial walls and their anisotropy. Med Biol Eng Comput 17: 170-6
8. Fronek K, Fung YC (1980) Mechanical properties of arteries as a function of topography and age. Biorheology 17: 227-34
9. Vito RP (1980) Mechanical properties of soft tissues – I: a mechanical system for biaxial testing. J Biomech 13: 947-50
10. Humphrey JD, Kang T, Sakarda P, Anjanappa M (1993) Computer aided vascular experimentation: a new electromechanical test system. Ann Biomed Eng 21: 33-43
11. Halpern W, Osol G, Coy GS (1984) Mechanical behaviour of pressurised in vitro prearteriolar vessels determined with a video system. Ann Biomed Eng. 12: 463-79
12. Weizsaecker HW, Pinto JG (1988) Isotropy and anisotropy of the arterial wall J Biomech 21: 477-87
13. Carmines DV, McElhaney JH, Stack R (1991) A piecewise non-linear elastic stress expression of human and pig coronary arteries tested in vitro. J Biomech 24: 899-906
14. Wolinsky H, Glagov S (1967) A lamellar unit of aortic medial structure and function in mammals Circ Res 20: 99-111
15. Hayashi KK, Sato M, Handa H, Moritake K (1974) Exp Mech 14: 440-4
16. Papageorgiou GL, Jones NB (1985). Photoelectric transducer for measuring the length and diameter of elastic vessels. J Biomed Eng 7: 295-300
17. Brant AM, Shah SS, Rodgers VGJ, Hoffmeister J, Herman I, Kormos RL, Borovetz HS (1988) Biomechanics of the arterial wall under simulated flow conditions J Biomech 21: 107-13
18. Newman DL, Gosling RG, Bowden NLR (1971) Changes in aortic distensibility and area ratio with the development of atherosclerosis. Atherosclerosis 14: 231-40
19. Pagani M, Mirsky I, Baig H, Manders WT, Kerkhof P, Vatner SF (1979) Effects of age on aortic pressure-diameter and elastic stiffness-stress relationships in unanesthetized sheep. Circ Res 44: 420-9
20. Gross DR, Hwang NHC (1981) The Rheology of Blood, Blood Vessels and Associated Tissues. Sijthoff and

Noordoff, Alphen aan den Rijn, The Netherlands, pp. 319-36

21. Gentile BJ, Chuong CJC, Ordway GA (1988) Regional volume distensibility of canine aorta during treadmill exercise. Circ Res 63: 1012-19

22. Langewouters GL, Wesseling KH, Goedhard WJA (1981) Advances in Physiological Sciences, Vol. 8 Cardiovascular Physiology, Heart, Peripheral Circulation and Methodology (Akademiai Kiado, Budapest, and Pergamon, Oxford), pp. 271-81

23. Janzen J, Lanzer P, Rothenberger-Janzen K, Vuong PN (2000) The transitional zone in the tunica media of renal arteries has a maximal length of 10 millimetres. Vasa 29: 168-72

24. Watkins MT, Sharefkin JB, Zajtchuk R, Maciag TM, D'Amore PA, Ryan US, Van Wart H, Rich NM (1984) Adult human saphenous vein endothelial cells: assessment of their reproductive capacity for use in endothelial seeding of vascular prostheses. J Surg Res 36: 588-96

25. Lefebvre D, Lescalie F (1996) Vascularization of the wall of the superficial veins. Anatomic study of the vasa vasorum. J Mal Vasc 21: S245-S48

26. Butterworth DM, Rose SS, Clark P, Rowland P, Knight S, Haboubi NY (1992) Light microscopy, immunohistochemistry and electron microscopy of the valves of the lower limb veins and jugular veins. Phlebology 7: 27-30

27. Colby TV, Yousem SA (1991) Lungs In Sternberg SS (ed) Histology for pathologists. Raven Press, New York 479-97

28. Fawcett DW (1986) Bloom and Fawcett, A textbook of histology. WB Saunders Company, Philadelphia, London, Toronto, Mexico City, Rio de Janeiro, Sydney, Tokyo, HongKong, 1017 p.

29. Widdicombe J (1997) Microvascular anatomy of the nose. Allergy 52: S7-S11

30. Lie JT (1980) The structure of the normal vascular system and its reactive changes. In Juergens JL, Spittell JA, Fairbairn II JF (ed) Peripheral vascular diseases. Saunders, Philadelphia, London, Toronto 51-81

31. Czyba JC, Girod C (1970) Cours d'histologie et embryologie (tome 1). Siemp, Lyon p. 230

32. Simionescu N, Simionescu M (1977) The cardiovascular system In Weiss L, Greep RO (eds.) Histology. Mac Graw-Hill, New York pp 373-431

33. Cuevas P, Gutierrez-Diaz JA, Reimers D, Dujovny M, Diaz FG, Ausman JI (1984) Pericyte endothelial gap junctions in human cerebral capillaries. Anat Embryol (Berl) 170: 155-9

34. Stelzner F, Staubesand J, Machleidt H (1962) Das corpus cavernosum recti – die Grundlage der inneren hämorrhoiden. Langenbecks Arch Klin Chir 299: 302-12

35. Datsun IG, Mel'man EP (1992) Role of glomus shunts of the anorectal cavernous bodies in the mechanism of hemorrhoid development. Arkh Patol 54: 28-31

36. Passali D, Buccella MG, Vetuschi A, Bellussi L (1990) Arteriovenous anastomosis in nasal cavities using microcorrosion technique. Acta Otorhinolaryngol Ital 10: 453-63

37. Skladzien J, Litwin JA, Nowogrodzka-Zagorska N, Miodonski AJ (1995) Corrosion casting study on the vasculature of nasal mucosa in the human fetus. Anat Rec 242: 411-6

38. Krantz KE (1977) The anatomy and physiology of the vulva and vagina In Philipp EE, Barnes J, Newton M eds. Scientific foundation of obstetrics and gynaecology, 2nd ed. Heinemann, London p 65-78

39. Benson SG, McConnell JA, Schmists WA (1981) Penile polsters: Functional structures or atherosclerotic changes? J Urol 125: 800-3

40. Furchgott RF (1996) The 1996 Albert Lasker Medical Research Awards. The discovery of endothelium-derived relaxing factor and its importance in the identification of nitric oxide. JAMA 276: 1186-8

41. Choi YD, Mah SY, Xin ZC, Choi HK (1997) The distribution of nitric oxide synthase in human corpus cavernosum on various impotent patients. Yonsei Med J 38: 125-32

42. Sick H, Wolfram-Gabel R (1993) Vascular networks of the periphery of the finger nail. Arch Anat Histol Embryol 75: 47-60

43. Kasper M, Golfert F, Funk RH (1997) Immunoelectron microscopical characterization of the epithelioid type of smooth muscle cells in human glomus organs. Ultrastruct Pathol 21: 425-30

44. Stark RE, Kaplan JM, Kittredge RD (1984) Lymphedema In Haimovici H: Vascular surgery, Principles and techniques. Appleton-Century-Crofts, Norwalk, Connecticut pp. 1071-84

45. Witte MH, Witte CL (1987) Lymphatics and blood vessels, lymphangiogenesis and hemangiogenesis: from cell biology to clinical medicine. Lymphology 20: 257-66

46. Petersen W, Tillmann B (1995) Age-related blood and lymph supply of the knee menisci. A cadaver study. Acta Orthop Scand 66: 308-12

47. Gruffaz J (1984) Anatomy and physiology of the lymphatic system. Phlebologie 37: 189-93

48. Puckett CL, Silver D (1984) Complications of lymphadenectomy and lymphedema In Greenfield LJ (ed): Complications in surgery and trauma. JB Lippincott Company Philadelphia pp 91-101

49. Borisov AV, Anichkov NM (1992) Lymphangion in health and in lymphedema. Arkh Patol 54: 27-32

II
Vascular ageing

Introduction

Changes in the morphology and composition of the vascular system start before birth, continue through childhood, and are maintained into old age. The critical developmental period of the blood vessels falls between the 5th and 16th weeks of intrauterine life. In this period, the basic wall structure characteristic of the particular vessel type (i. e. the elastic and muscular arteries, large veins, limb veins, and lymphatics) is formed [1]. The ageing process is associated with predictable anatomic and physiologic alterations in the cardiovascular system [2-4]. It is important to separate the alterations in structure and function that occur during growth from those that occur in adult life, some of which may be associated with disease. Arteries continue to increase in diameter, length and wall thickness in adulthood [5], when the dimensions of the body as a whole change little. Despite assertions to the contrary, occlusive vascular disease is not ubiquitous and should, therefore, be distinguished from the universal alterations in structure, composition and mechanical properties that occur in all of us In early life elastic arteries, large muscular arteries and conduit veins increase in length, diameter and wall thickness allometrically. The dimensions of arterioles and venules as well as capillaries are determined by the rheological properties of blood and the chemistry of haemoglobin [6] and do not change with age.

Arteries

Two processes should be distinguished: changes in early life and ageing.

Changes in early life

The intima thickens because of the migration and proliferation of vascular smooth muscle cells (VSMCs) followed by synthesis of scleroprotein and extracellular matrix [7]. It should be emphasised that intimal thickening is often eccentric and has been observed in fetal circulation [8] and in children. It is thought to be adaptive in nature, often occurring near junctions where shear stresses are changing during growth [9-13]. In later life, VSMCs continue to migrate towards the intima where they proliferate and synthesise scleroprotein to produce a more widely distributed intimal thickening [14]. It has been argued that this process may also be adaptive in nature,

compensating for changes in lumen diameter due to medial remodelling [15] and driven by the requirement to maintain shear stress at an optimum value [16]. Under these conditions the intimal structure resembles that of the media, containing regular layers of smooth muscle cells and elastic laminae [7, 17] and may well contribute to the ability of the vessel to withstand circumferential stress [15]. Increased shear stress disrupts the glycocalyx on the luminal side of vessels, and releases plasminogen activator and metalloproteinases, causing disruption of the basement membrane, migration and proliferation of endothelial cells [18]. If the shear stress is not normalised, because of, for instance, the presence of an occlusion downstream, the proliferation continues, resulting in a progressive reduction in lumen diameter. The intimal proliferation occurring under these circumstances has a much less ordered structure [15]. During growth and development, the elastic laminae of the media become thicker, although their number appears to be fixed at birth [9, 19]. Collagen content increases, as does the number of myofilaments and extracellular fibres, which, over time, will gradually replace specialist cellular junctions with a mesh of extracellular fibres [20].

Changes in ageing

In later life, a series of structural, architectural and compositional modifications take place in the vasculature. Elastic laminae become thinner and more fragmented [21] (Fig. 1) while collagen, ground substance and areas of calcification become more prominent [22]. The number of projections seen on VSMC membranes, which are thought to be points of attachment to elastin fibres, is increased and the VSMCs become less rounded in cross section and more irregularly shaped [23, 24]. In the subendothelial space, blood-derived leukocytes and extracellular matrix rich in glycosaminoglycans accumulate. The decrease of the transarterial wall oxygen gradient, together with accumulation of lipid peroxides caused by senile functional decay of cells and membrane damage, underlines the possible role of ischemia and free radicals. However, in the normal architecture of the vessel wall, these changes, which can be referred to as "the vasculopathy of ageing", are likely to be the consequence of adaptive mechanisms to maintain normal conditions of flow, mechanical stress and/or wall ten-

Fig. 1. Thinning and fragmentation of the elastic laminae of the aortic media in an elderly person. Haematoxylin, eosin and saffron stain (HES)

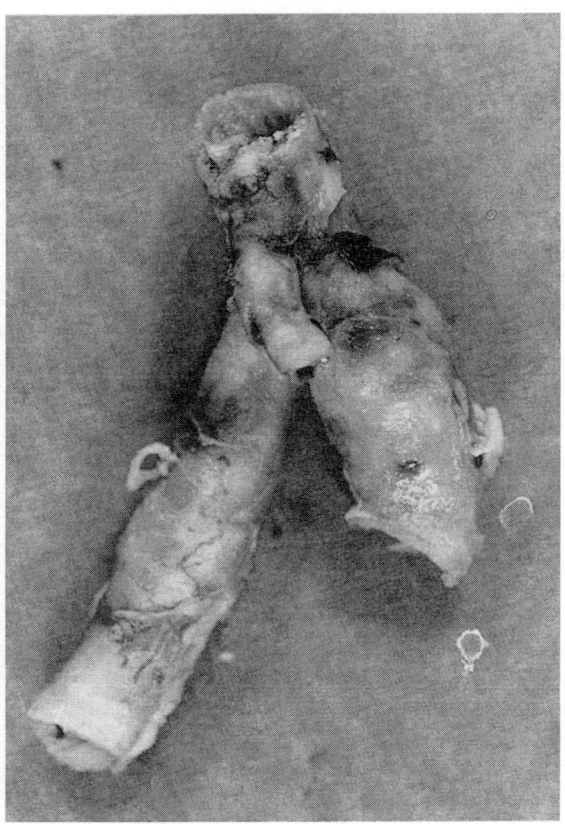

Fig. 2. Polyaneurysmal dystrophy of the femoral tripod

sion [25]. In the large elastic arteries, hypertension and ageing are associated with increased collagen content and concomitant increases in relative wall thickness [26], both of which tend to cause a reduction in distensibility [27, 28]. In the aorta, intimal thickness increases with advancing age and is maximal in the abdominal segment [29]. Until recently, it had been assumed that increased relative wall thickness in more distal vessels, such as the radial, brachial and femoral, would lead to similar decreases in distensibility and elastic modulus. However, there is now an increasing body of evidence to show that, when compared at a given pressure or total strain, the compliance of these vessels in patients with untreated essential hypertension is, in fact, lower than that in normotensives [30-34], and that this reduction may be due to changes in the properties of the wall material itself [35]. Thus, the regional differences in the response of the arterial system to hypertension echo those seen with ageing and lend support to the idea that, in the context of vascular structure and function,

hypertension may be thought of as accelerated ageing [36]. Nichols and O'Rourke [26] have also suggested that the arterial wall, being subjected to continual cyclic stress, undergoes material fatigue. This will affect all components but it is only the elastin that cannot be re-synthesised. The end result of this process is a gradual replacement of elastin with collagen [37], leading to a progressive increase in the elastic modulus of the wall material with age. It is worth noting that since large conduit arteries contain more elastin in early life than do smaller muscular vessels, this may account for the greater reduction in stiffness with age seen in the large elastic arteries. Once the conduit arteries start to become stiffer, their characteristic impedance, and hence the pulse pressure for a given mean pressure, will increase. This, in turn, leads to increased circumferential stress, which, assuming no change in distensibility, will result in increased circumferential strain and a tendency to synthesise more collagen, leading to further increases in elastic modulus.

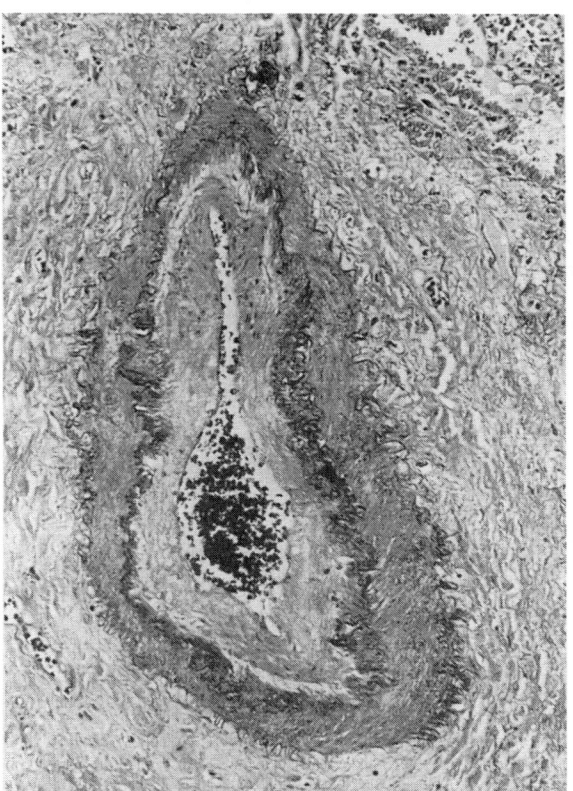

Fig. 3. Calcific depositions along the internal elastic membrane. HES

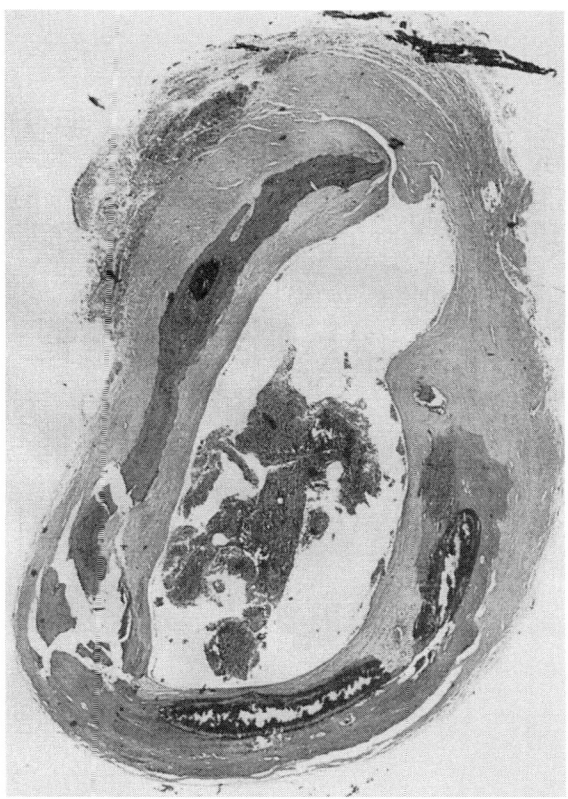

Fig. 4. Monckeberg's medial calcific sclerosis with osseous metaplasia. HES

Other consequences

Atrophy of the smooth muscle cells of the media

This process produces thinning and weakening of this layer. This process may be important in the sub-renal aorta and large peripheral arteries (iliac, femoral, and popliteal arteries). The vessels thus become tortuous and enlarged (dolichomega-arteries) (Fig. 2), leading to polyaneurysmal dystrophy [38, 39].

Degradative alterations of elastin provoke mineralization in the vascular wall

The amount of P and Ca increases, approaching in some places 9% and 20%, and mineral deposits appear in the media [40], resulting in Monckeberg's medial calcific sclerosis (pipestem arteries). Calcification of the media attracts considerable attention clinically, although its pathological significance is limited. This lesion often involves the peripheral arteries but may affect larger arteries. In small arteries such as superficial temporal arteries, calcification often develops along the medial aspect of the internal elastic membrane (Fig. 3), extend to the underlying media and may undergo osseous metaplasia (Fig. 4).

Hyalinosis

Accumulation of hyaline material within the wall of small muscular arteries and arterioles gives rise to hyalinosis. This glassy, homogenous and slightly eosinophilic material (Fig. 5) stains positively by Periodic Acid Schiff (PAS) technique. It is made up of a variety of plasma proteins (fibrinogen, immunoglobulins), lipoproteins, intercellular connective material, and cellular debris. The hyaline material accumulates first, then spills over into the media, suffocating the myocytes. This process thickens the vascular wall, and reduces its lumen. In capillaries, this material thickens the basement membrane, enclosing pericytes, which undergo degenerative changes. Frequent with age, hyalinosis is also observed in children [41], and in some pathological conditions such as atherosclerosis, benign nephroangiosclerosis (juxta-glomerular arte-

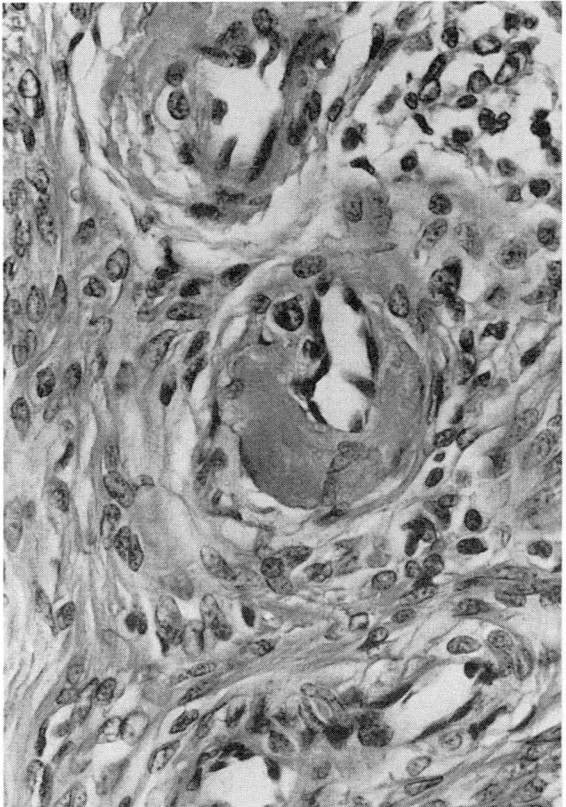

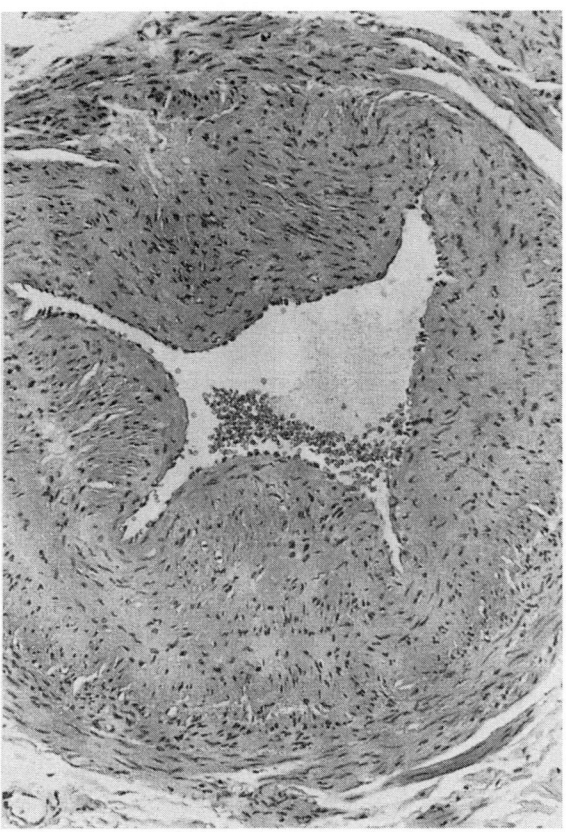

Fig. 5. Arteriolar hyalinosis. HES

Fig. 6. Phlebosclerosis involving a medium-sized vein. HES

rioles), diabetes mellitus (retinal and dermis capillaries) [42, 43], cerebral hypertension [44] and porphyria. Hyalinosis should be distinguished from deposits of glassy, eosinophilic PAS-negative material, accumulated around capillaries, arterioles and venules. These deposits result from organisation of non-resorbed oedema caused by chronic stasis. Elastin staining technique allows us to locate these deposits, which surround the adventitia.

Veins

With age, the amount of basic fibroblast growth factor (bFGF) and platelet-derived growth factor (PDGF) decreases. These factors are known to modulate the synthesis of extracellular matrix components and to stimulate the proliferation of the vein smooth muscle cells [45]. In veins, aging changes are more evident in the fifth to the sixth decades [46] when they become sinuous, fibrous, hardened or atrophic. Their general architecture remains recognisable while they develop a larger lumen with an irregular contour

and poor parietal flexibility. "Phlebosclerosis" (venofibrosis, fibrous endophlebitis, hyperplastic phlebitis, hypertrophy of veins, endophlebosclerosis) involves all three venous coats, resulting in atrophy of the wall (Fig. 6-7). This age-related phenomenon mostly affects veins subject to stasis or to increased luminal pressure. Elastic fibers in the wall become thin and fragmented with areas of irregular thickening. In the media, the middle muscular layer undergoes atrophy while the outermost layer hypertrophies. The wall of an aged vein contains less collagen I and III than does a normal vein, while the total quantity of collagen IV, V VI remains unchanged [46]. Loss of elasticity and contractility facilitates gradual dilation of the vein, but age is not a factor in the development of varicose veins [47].

Microvasculature

This process has been mostly assessed in the cutaneous and cerebral microvasculatures. A marked loss in dermal nutritional vessel density and surface area

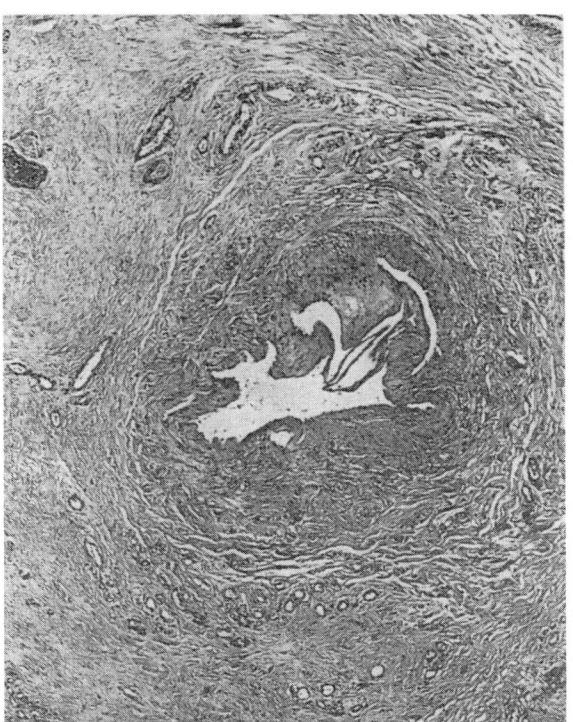

Fig. 7. Atrophy of a small calibre vein. HES

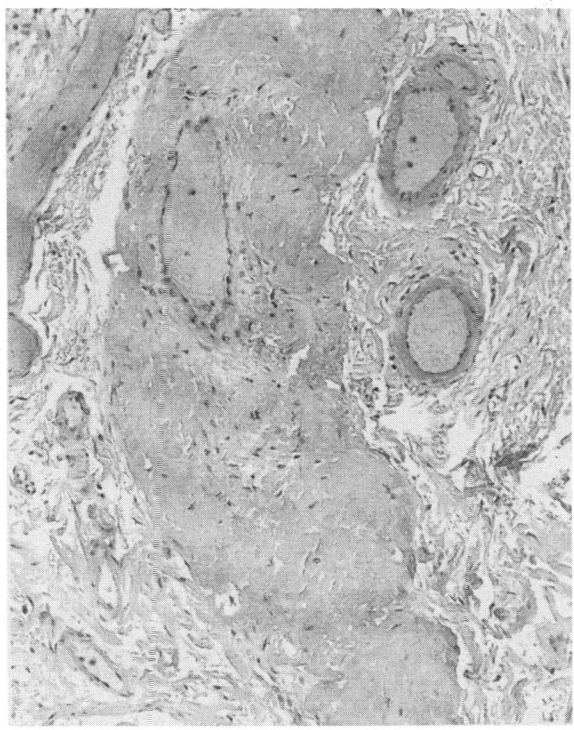

Fig. 8. Amorphous deposits around the basement membrane of a capillary. HES

for exchange is characteristic of ageing. Dermal papillary loops are significantly reduced in old skin compared to young skin (forehead by 40%; forearm by 37%). Rarefaction of pericytes leads to dilation of capillaries, which become fragile, and to senile purpura [48-50]. Leakage of plasma material leads to amorphous deposits around the basement membrane (Fig. 8). This material should be differentiated from amyloid. Venules become sinuous and beaded because of the development of microaneurysms (Fig. 9), which resemble those described in the course of diabetic microangiopathy. In the brain, several reports have demonstrated that cerebral blood flow decreases with age and may contribute to neurodegenerative changes found in ageing animals and man. Decreases in cerebral microvasculature are associated with the decline in growth hormone and insulin-like growth factor 1 [51].

Erectile tissue

Vascular sclerosis (Fig. 10) is a systemic phenomenon correlated to age, and the cavernosal tissue (penis, cli-

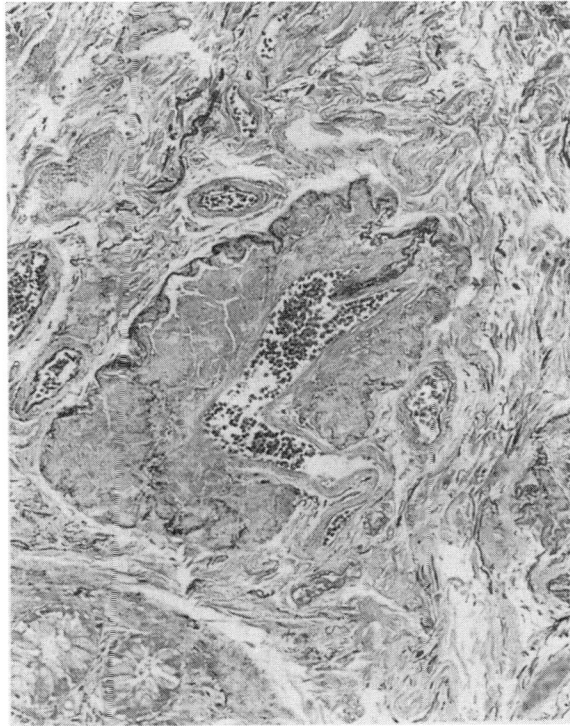

Fig. 9. Venule deformity with aneurysmal dilation. Orcein elastic stain (Orcein)

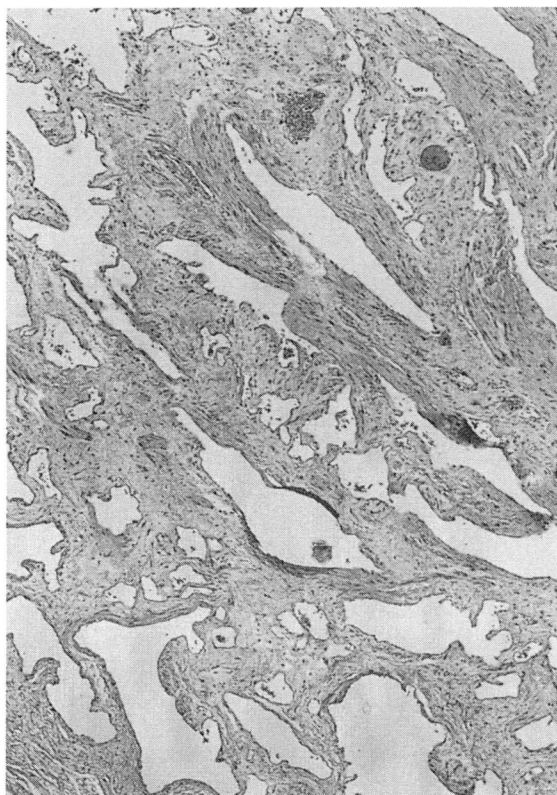

Fig. 10. Erectile tissue sclerosis. HES

toris) is not exempt. This phenomenon, if it appears at an early age, can induce vasculogenic impotence [52-55].

Lymph vessels

Progressive involution of lymph vessels occurs with age. It is characterised by a reduction in the number of branches of lymph vessels, and an abnormal pattern with meanders and changes in the wall structure, which becomes thinner with formation of sac-like dilations realising lymphangiectases [56, 57]. The presence of atherosclerotic changes in the intima of lymph vessels reported by Evsevyev and Shadanov is debatable [58]. Morphometric study demonstrates a reduction in media musculature and an increase in collagen connective tissue, resulting in a lymphangiosclerosis [59], similar to the phlebosclerosis seen in veins. This change also involves the valves of the collecting lymph vessels. Differentiation between age-related lymphangiosclerosis and post-lymphangitic changes can be difficult. In lymph vessels with marked varicosity, the thinned vascular wall may be almost free of muscle cells.

Bibliography

1. Kocova J, Tesar Z (1979) The development of the vascular system in man. Cor Vasa 21: 124-7
2. Berry CL (1973) Growth, development and healing of large arteries. Ann Roy Coll Surg Engl 53: 246-57
3. Vuong PN, Desoutter P, Houissa-Vuong S, Body J, Benigni J-P, Sevestre J-P (2000) : Aspect morphologiques de la sénescence vasculaire. Angéiologie 52 : 13-9
4. Duncan AK, Vittone J, Fleming KC, Smith HC (1996) Cardiovascular disease in elderly patients. Mayo Clin Proc 71: 184-96
5. Berry CL (1989) Organogenèse de la paroi artérielle. *In* Camilleri JP, Berry CL, Fiessinger J-N, Bariéty J (eds) Les maladies de la paroi artérielle. Flammarion, Paris, p 44-59
6. Vogel S (1992) Vital Circuits. On Pumps, Pipes and the Workings of the Circulatory System, Oxford University Press, New York
7. Glagov S, Zarins CK, Masawa N, Xu CP, Bassiouny H, Giddens DP (1993) Mechanical functional role of non-atherosclerotic intimal thickening. Front Med Biol Eng 5: 37-43
8. Matonoha P, Zechmeister A (1992) Structure of the coronary arteries in the prenatal period in man. Funct Devel Morph 2: 209-12
9. Clark JM, Glagov S (1985) Transmural organisation of the arterial media. The lamellar unit revisited. Haemodynamics and atherosclerosis. Insights and perspectives gained from human arteries. Arteriosclerosis 5: 19-34
10. Resnick N, Gimbrone MA Jr (1995) Hemodynamic forces are complex regulators of endothelial gene expression. FASEB J 9: 874-82
11. Resnick N, Yahav H, Khachigian LM, Collins T, Anderson KR, Dewey FC, Gimbrone MA Jr (1997) Endothelial gene regulation by laminar shear stress. Adv Exp Med Biol 430: 155-64
12. Papadaki M, Eskin SG (1997) Effects of fluid shear stress on gene regulation of vascular cells. Biotechnol Prog 13: 209-21
13. Chien S, Li S, Shyy YJ (1998) Effects of mechanical forces on signal transduction and gene expression in endothelial cells. Hypertension 31: 162-9
14. Michel JB, De RN, Plissonnier D, Anidjar S, Salzmann JL, Levy BJ (1990) Pathophysiological role of the vascular smooth muscle cell. Cardiovasc Pharmacol 16: S4-S11
15. Masawa N, Glagov S, Zarins C K (1994) Quantitaive morphologic study of intimal thickening at the human carotid bifurcation; 1 Axial and circumferential distribution of maximal intimal thickening in asymptomatic, uncomplicated plaques. Atherosclerosis 107: 137-46
16. Glagov S, Vito R, Giddens DP, Zarins CK (1992) Microarchitecture and composition of artery walls: relationship to location, diameter and the distribution of mechanical stress. J Hypertens Suppl 10: S101-4
17. Glagov S (1994) Intimal hyperplasia, vascular modeling, and the restenosis problem. Circulation 89: 2888-91
18. Hudlicka O, Brown MD (1996) Postnatal growth of the heart and its blood vessels. J Vasc Res 33: 266-87
19. Berry CL, Sosa-Melgarejo JA, Greenwald SE (1993) The relationship between wall tension, lamellar thickness, and intercellular junctions in the fetal and adult aorta: its relevance to the pathology of dissecting aneurysm. J Path 169: 15-20
20. Clark JM, Glagov S (1979) Structural integration of the arterial wall. 1 Relationships and attachments of medial

smooth muscle cells in normally distended and hyperdistended aortas. Lab Invest. 4: 587-602

21. Lakatta EG, Mitchel JH, Pomerance A, Rowe GG (1987) Human ageing; changes in structure and function. J Am Coll Cardiol 10: 42A-47A

22. Everhart JE, Pettitt DJ, Knowler WC, Rose FA, Bennett PH (1988) Medial arterial calcification and its association with mortality and complications of diabetes. Diabetologia 31: 16-23

23. Gerrity RG, Cliff WJ (1975) The aortic tunica media of the developing rat. I. Quantitative stereologic and biochemical analysis. Lab Invest 32: 585-600

24. Toda T, Tsuda N, Nishimori I, Leszczynski DE, Kummerow FA (1980) Morphometric analysis of the ageing process in human arteries and the aorta. Acta Anat (Basel) 106: 35-44

25. Bilato C, Crow MT (1996) Atherosclerosis and the vascular biology of aging. Aging (Milano) 8: 221-34

26. Nichols WW, O'Rourke MF (1990) In McDonald's Blood Flow in Arteries, Edward Arnold, London, pp 398-420

27. Belz GG (1995) Elastic properties and Windkessel function of the human aorta. Cardiovasc Drugs Ther 9: 73-83

28. Robert L, Jacob MP, Fulop T (1995) Elastin in blood vessels. Ciba Found Symp 192: 286-99

29. Virmani R, Avolio AP, Mergner WJ, Robinowitz M, Herderick EE, Cornhill JF, Guo SY, Liu TH, Ou DY, O'Rourke M (1991) Effect of aging on aortic morphology in populations with high and low prevalence of hypertension and atherosclerosis. Comparison between occidental and Chinese communities. Am J Pathol 139: 1119-29

30. Boutouyrie P, Laurent S, Benetos A, Girerd XJ, Hoeks AP, Safar ME (1992) Opposing effects of ageing on distal and proximal large arteries in hypertensives. J Hypertens Suppl 10: S87-91

31. Benetos A, Laurent S, Hoeks AP, Boutouyrie PH, Safar ME (1993) Arterial alterations with ageing and high blood pressure. A non-invasive study of carotid and femoral arteries. Arteriosclerosis & Thrombosis 13: 90-97

32. Benetos A, Asmar R, Gautier S, Salvi P, Safar M (1994) Heterogeneity of the arterial tree in essential hypertension; a non-invasive study of the terminal aorta and the common carotid artery. J Hum Hypertension 8: 501-7

33. Laurent S, Girerd X, Mourad JJ, Lacolley P, Beck L, Boutouyrie P, Mignot JP, Safar M (1994) Elastic modulus of the radial artery wall material is not increased in patients with essential hypertension. Arteriosclerosis & Thrombosis 14: 1223-31

34. Safar M, Girerd X (1996) Arterial hypertension, aging and cardiac decompensation. Ann Cardiol Angeiol (Paris) 45: 439-44

35. Laurent S (1994) Reduction of arterial wall mechanical stress as a goal for antihypertensive therapy. J Cardiovasc Pharmacol 23: S35-S41

36. Wolinsky H (1972) Long term effects of hypertension on the rat aortic wall and their relation to concurrent ageing changes. Morphological and chemical studies. Circ Res 30: 301-9

37. Ooyama T, Sakamoto H (1995) Arterial ageing of aorta and atherosclerosis—with special reference to elastin. Nippon Ronen Igakkai Zasshi 32(5): 326-31

38. Tilson MD (1992) Aortic aneurysms and atherosclerosis. Circulation 85: 205-11

39. Powell J, Greenhalgh RM (1989) Cellular, enzymatic and genetic factors in the pathogenesis of abdominal aortic aneurysms. J Vasc Surg 9: 297-304

40. Cichocki T, Heck D, Jarczyk L, Rokita E, Strzalkowski A, Sych M (1989) Artery wall calcification: correlation of atherosclerosis with mineralization. Pathologica 81: 139-49

41. Rambaud JC, Galian A, Touchard G, Morel-Maroger L, Mikol J, Van Effenterre G, Leclerc JP, Le Charpentier Y, Haut J, Matuchansky C, et al (1986) Digestive tract and renal small vessel hyalinosis, idiopathic nonarteriosclerotic intracerebral calcifications, retinal ischemic syndrome, and phenotypic abnormalities. A new familial syndrome. Gastroenterology 90: 930-8

42. Lysenko LV (1990) Diabetic macro- and microangiopathy of the lungs. Arch Pathol 52: 31-6

43. Saltykov BB, Kaufman OIa, Velikov VK, Shubina OI (1991) Morphogenesis of diabetic microangiopathy. Arkh Patol 53: 60-5

44. Amano S (1977) Vascular changes in the brain of spontaneously hypertensive rats: hyaline and fibrinoid degeneration. J Pathol 121: 119-28

45. Drubaix I, Giakoumakis A, Robert L, Robert AM (1998) Preliminary data on the age-dependent decrease in basic fibroblast growth factor and platelet-derived growth factor in the human vein wall and in their influence on cell proliferation. Gerontology 44: 9-14

46. Bouissou H, Pieraggi MT, Julian M, Maurel E, Thiers J-C (1994) Anatomo-pathologie de la veine variqueuse. In Barthelemy P, Lefebvre D (eds) Insuffisance veineuse des membres inférieurs. Masson, Paris 17-25

47. Merlen JF, Coget JM (1986) Vieillissement de la veine et de la venule. Phlébologie 39: 795-804

48. Shadanov DA (1966) On senile changes in lymphatic capillaries and vessels. J Cardiovasc Surg 7: 108-16

49. Yan Y (1990) Age-related microvascular changes in human skin. Chung Kuo I Hsueh Ko Hsueh Yuan Hsueh Pao 12: 9-12

50. Kelly RI, Pearse R, Bull RH, Leveque JL, de Rigal J, Mortimer PS (1995) The effects of aging on the cutaneous microvasculature. J Am Acad Dermatol 33: 749-56

51. Sonntag WE, Lynch CD, Cooney PT, Hutchins PM (1997) Decreases in cerebral microvasculature with age are associated with the decline in growth hormone and insulin-like growth factor 1. Endocrinology 138: 3515-20

52. Conti G, Virag R (1989) Human penile erection and organic impotence: normal histology and histopathology. Urol Int 44 303-8

53. Fontana D, Rolle L, Lacivita A, Porpiglia F, Del Noce G, Tamagnone A (1993) Anatomo-functional changes in the cavernous body in the elderly. Arch Ital Urol Androl 65: 483-6

54. Feldman HA, Goldstein I, Hatzichristou DG, Krane RJ, McKinlay JB (1994) Impotence and its medical and psychosocial correlates: results of the Massachusetts Male Aging Study. J Urol 151: 54-61

55. Tarcan T, Park K, Goldstein I, Maio G, Fassina A, Krane RJ, Azadzoi KM (1999) Histomorphometric analysis of age-related structural changes in human clitoral cavernosal tissue. J Urol 161: 940-4

56. Andriushin IuN, Trofimova TM (1976) Senile changes in the intraorganic lymphatic bed of human facial skin. Arkh Anat Gistol Embriol 71: 114-7

57. Pena JM, Ford MJ (1996) Cutaneous lymphangiectases associated with severe photoaging and topical corticosteroid application. J Cutan Pathol 23: 175-81

58. Rabinowitz AJ, Saphir O (1965) The thoracic duct. Significance of age-related changes and of lipid in the wall. Circulation 31: 899-905

59. Cluzan R.-V (1995) Physiopathologie In Janbon C, Cluzan R.-V. Lymphologie. Masson, Paris 17-25 28-39

III
Fundamental lesions in vascular pathology

1 – Stenosis and occlusion

Thrombosis

Thrombosis is defined as the formation of a solid mass in the circulatory system from the elements of the blood during life.

Pathology

Thrombosis may occur in arteries, veins, and the microcirculatory bed. Three types are generally described:

1. White (conglutination) thrombus. Grossly, this appears greyish-red and friable. Histologically, it consists of conglomerates of platelets forming distinct bands or lamellae surrounded by fibrin and leukocytes. Red blood cells are scattered among these structures (Fig. 1). The whole mass resembles the lines on sand seen on a tidal beach. The bands form perpendicular to the axis of blood flow (Fig. 2).
2. Red (coagulation) thrombus. Made up of fibrin lamellae formed parallel to the vascular axis and filling the entire vascular lumen. These lamellae are intermingled with numerous red blood cells and some leukocytes (Fig. 3).
3. Mixed. Grossly, these thrombi are firm, red or greyish-red (Fig. 4). The head is essentially a white thrombus firmly adherent to the vascular wall. The tail is a friable, non-adherent, homogenous red thrombus, floating in the vascular lumen; it is easily detached under the pressure of blood flow. The body consists of alternating white and red zones called Zahn bands (Fig. 5). Zahn bands are made up of masses of platelets, and the red bands of fibrin lamellae and red blood cells. These bands lie perpendicular to the blood flow in an occluding thrombus, and parallel to the blood flow in a parietal one.

Ante-mortem thrombi should be distinguished from agonal and post-mortem clots. An agonal clot is red, or whitish-red and devoid of characteristic Zahn bands. A post-mortem clot may either resemble an agonal clot or present a mixed pattern with a red band at the bottom and a whitish-yellow band on the surface, a pattern particularly apparent in cardiac cavities and great vessels and resulting from the effects of gravity on the constituents of the blood. Whatever the type, an agonising or post-mortem clot remains elastic to the touch, and non-adhe-

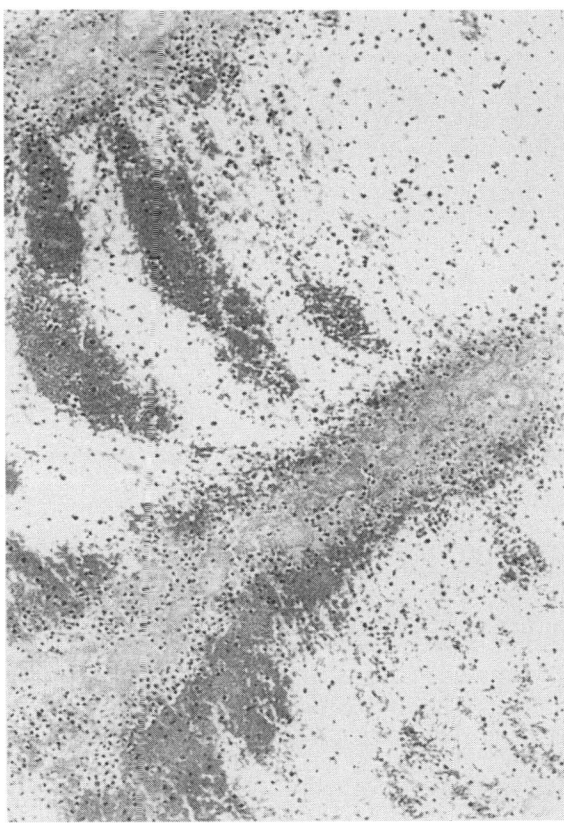

Fig. 1. Lamellar aspect of a white thrombus. Haematoxylin, eosin and saffron stain (HES)

rent to the vascular wall; its diameter is less than that of the vessel. In contrast, a thrombus is friable, adherent to the vascular wall, and frequently occludes the entire vascular lumen.

Evolution of a thrombus

Four events may occur:

Thrombolysis

Plasminogen, absorbed by the thrombus from the circulatory flow, is transformed into plasmin, destroys fibrin fibers and induces liquefaction of the thrombus before it undergoes organisation. Thrombolysis can occur in a fresh, 4-to-5 day old thrombus.

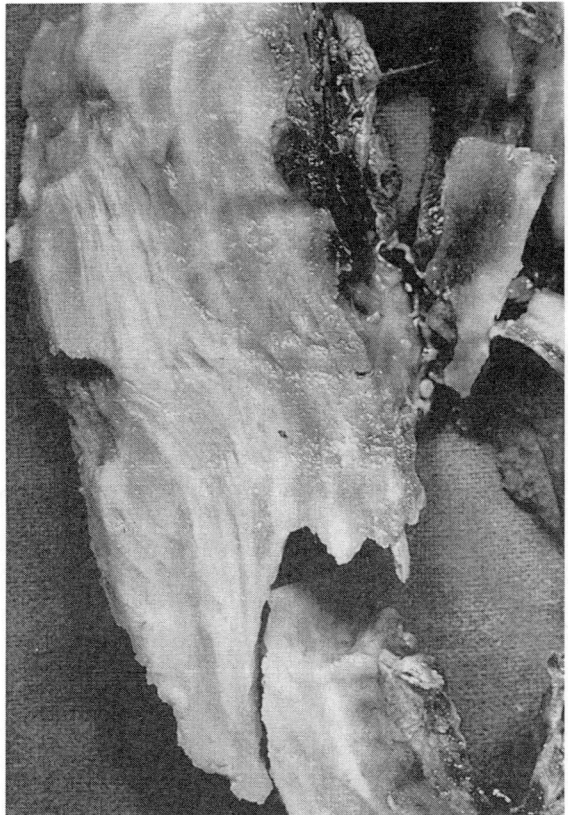

Fig. 2. Cut section of a white thrombus. Note band-like pattern

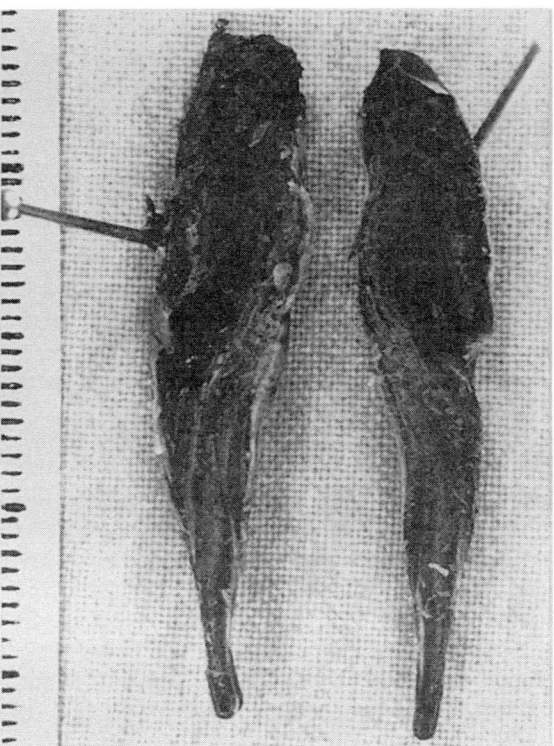

Fig. 3. Longitudinal section of a red thrombus

Homogenisation

Proteolytic enzymes released by leukocytes destroy platelets, red blood cells and fibrin, transforming the thrombus into an homogenised mass. Its central part undergoes liquefaction and gives rise to a pus-like liquid (Fig. 6). This process may start at the centre of the clot and extends peripherally two days after the formation of the thrombus. Superimposed infection will lead to suppuration with sepsis [1].

Embolism

A fragment of thrombus can detach, move through the bloodstream and become an embolus. This risk diminishes from around the 10th day after thrombus formation, as fibroblasts penetrate its base and begin synthesising collagen fibers. However, embolism can occur at any time while the thrombotic material persists. Recurrent micro-emboli can lead to occlusion of small pulmonary arteries resulting in pulmonary hypertension and right heart insufficiency.

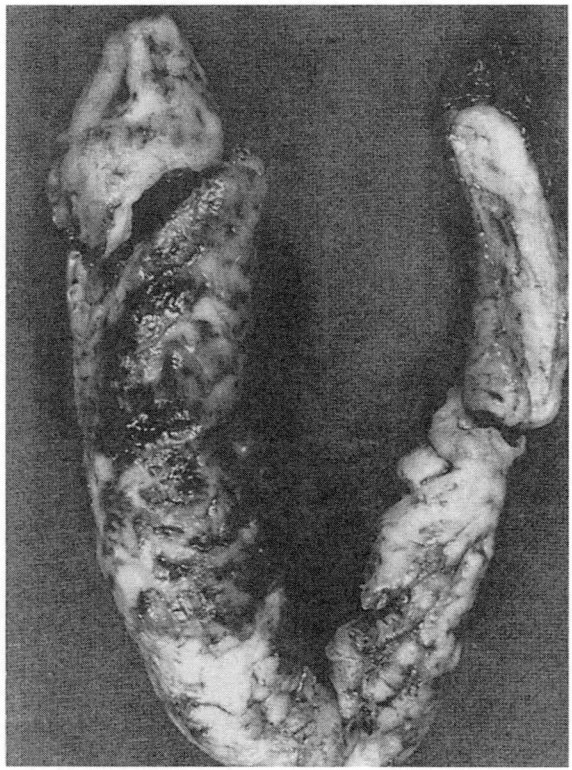

Fig. 4. Mixed thrombus

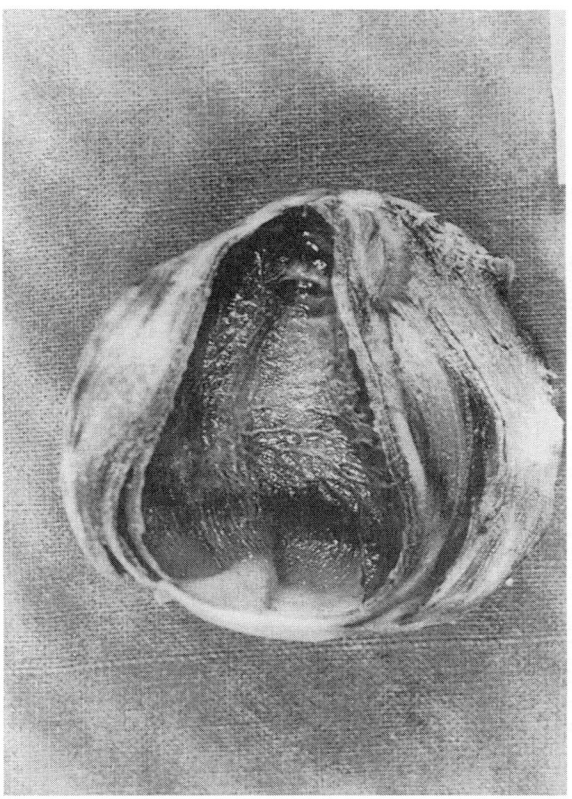

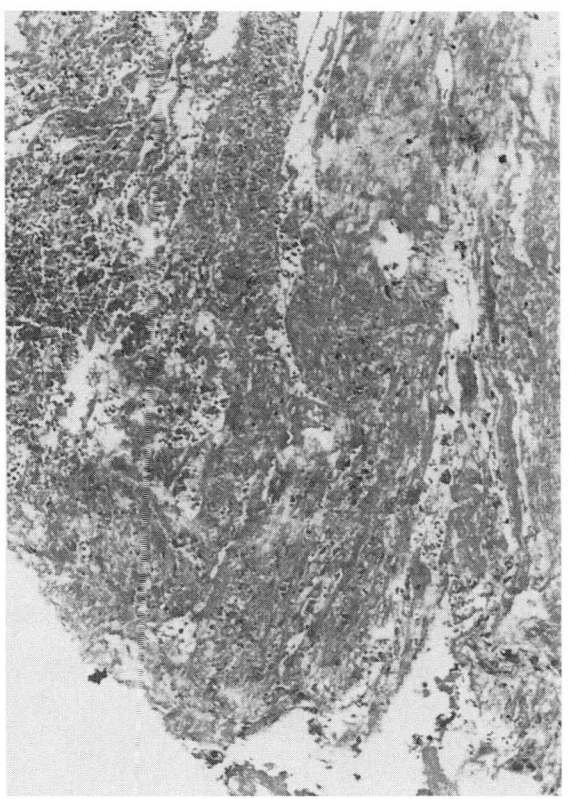

Fig. 5. Cut section of a mixed thrombus showing Zahn bands

Fig. 6. Homogenised thrombus. HES

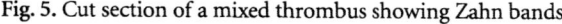

Organisation

From the first day, neighbouring endothelial cells proliferate, covering the thrombus and penetrating its base (Fig. 7). Endothelial buds form capillaries from the 10th day (Fig. 8). Fibroblasts penetrate the base of the thrombus from the 5th day, synthesise collagen fibers from the 10th day and some elastic fibers from the 28th day attaching the thrombus to the venous wall (Fig. 9). From that time, it is difficult to remove by thrombectomy. Granulation tissue breaks down all of the different components of a thrombus whatever its state and replaces it by connective tissue and finally produces fibrosis from the 4th to 6th week (Fig. 10). Table 1 summarises the different steps of early organisation of a thrombus. These steps allow us to determine the age of a thrombus with relative precision during its first 28 days.

An occlusive thrombus is thus gradually transformed into a block of fibrous tissue (Fig. 11) adhering to the intima and containing haemosiderin-laden macrophages, capillaries and myofibroblasts. Next, fibroblasts surrounding the enclosed vascular slits differentiate into smooth muscle cells (Fig. 12). Some vascular slits then become newly-formed vessels allowing the thrombosed vessel to be recanalised. These vessels occasionally have a well defined intima and media and a well defined internal elastic lamina (Fig. 13). A partially occlusive thrombus may be incorporated into the intima. Newly-formed elastic lamellae may develop on its luminal aspect (Fig. 14). For a small thrombus, however, the only residual evidence of a previous lesion is a localised and moderate thickening of the intima at the thrombotic site (Fig. 15). An exuberant but localised form of an organising vascular thrombus may lead to the so-called "intravascular papillary endothelial hyperplasia" or Masson's tumour (See Chapter XVII).

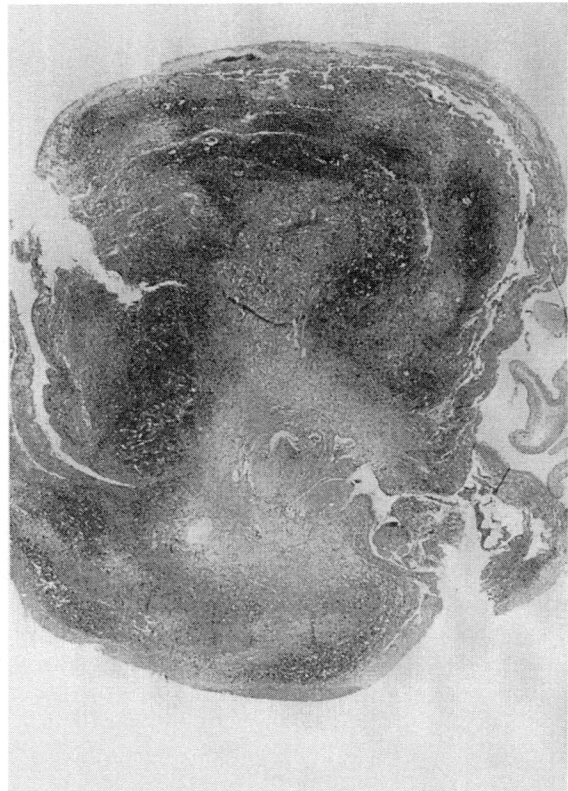

Fig. 7. Occluding venous thrombus with partial organisation. HES

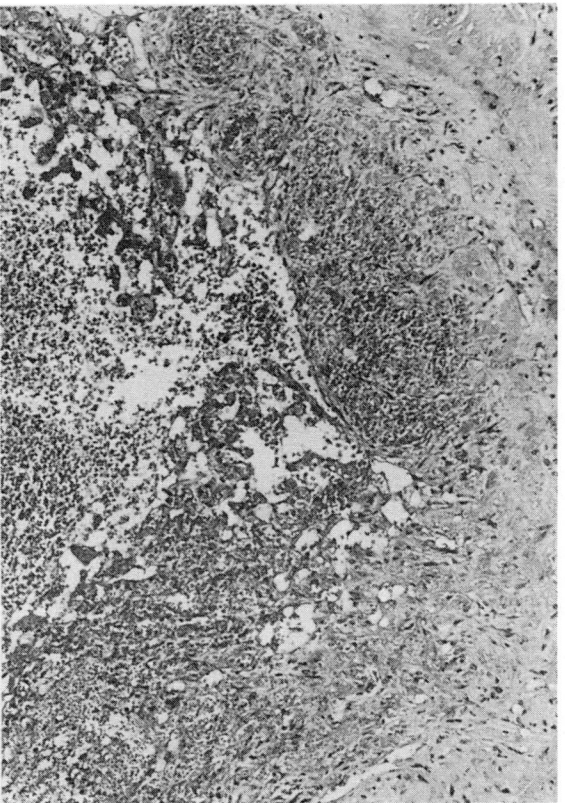

Fig. 8. Endothelial buds are apparent in the thrombus at day 10. HES

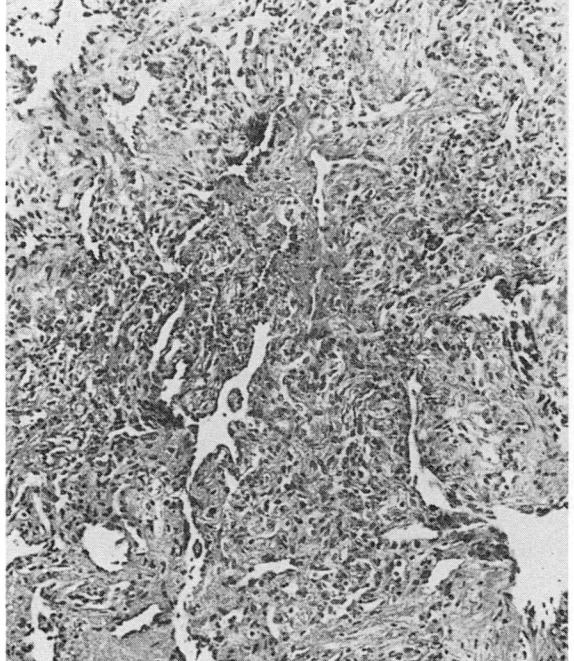

Fig. 9. Endothelial buds and proliferation of fibroblasts in a thrombus at day 28. HES

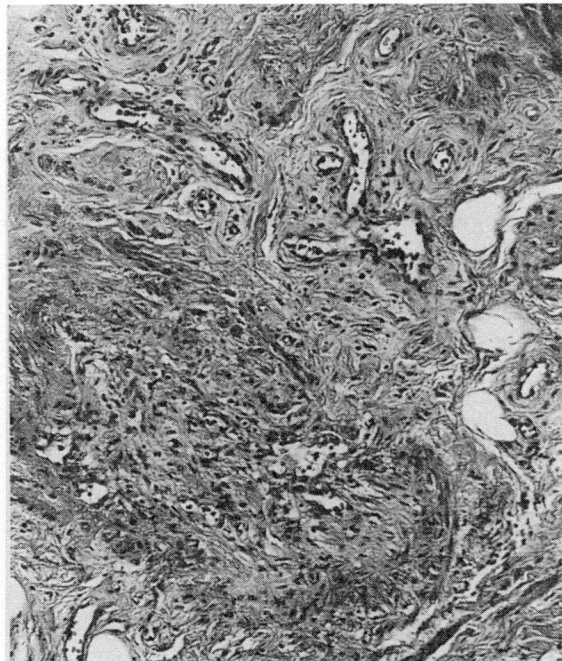

Fig. 10. Occlusive organised thrombus. HES

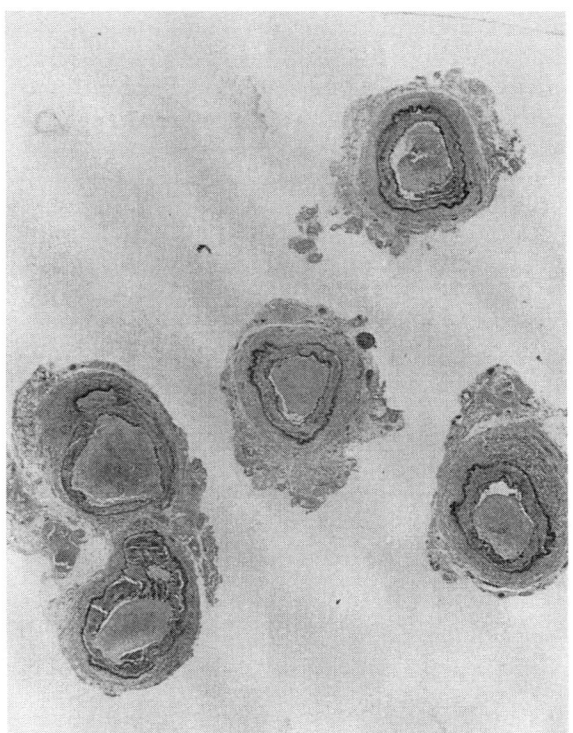

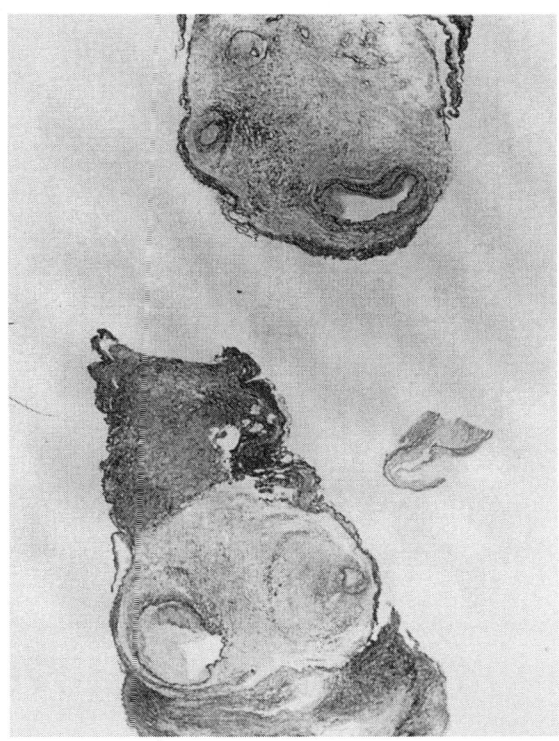

Fig. 11. Cut sections of an artery showing an extensive occlusive thrombus. Orcein elastic stain (Orcein)

Fig. 12. A recanalised thrombus with newly-formed vessels. Orcein

Table 1. Different steps in the organisation of a thrombus (d :day)

ORGANISATION OF A THROMBUS	d2	d5	d10	d28	d42	d>42
Endothelial cells cover the thrombus	+	+	+	+	+	
Endothelial cells penetrate the thrombus	+	+	+			
Endothelial cells form capillary buds			+	+	+	
Fibroblasts penetrate the thrombus		+	+	+	+	
Fibroblasts produce collagen fibers			+	+	+	
Fibroblasts produce elastic fibers				+	+	
Fibrosis						+

Embolism

An embolus is a solid or semi-solid mass, often derived from the constituents of the blood, actively transported in the circulation. It may lodge in any vessel. Anatomo-clinical syndromes are classified accor-

ding to the vessels involved (peripheral arteries, pulmonary vessels) and the nature of the embolus. Direct consequences include acute ischemia with infarction [2]; indirect consequences depend on the nature of the embolus (blood clot, cholesterol crystals, air and gas bubbles, foreign bodies, parasitic

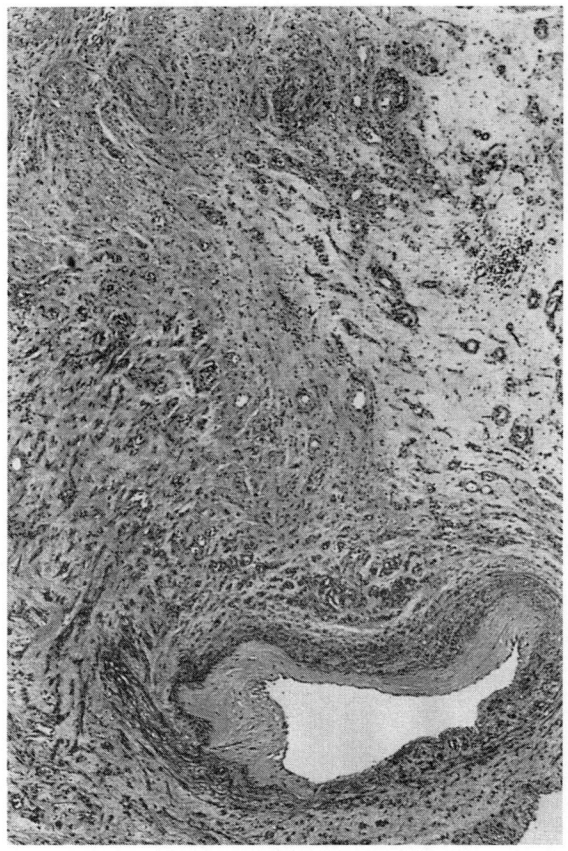

Fig. 13. Newly-formed vessels inside an organised thrombus. HES

parts, fat globules, clumps of bacteria, tumour cells, bone marrow, amniotic material and so-on [3, 4]. Alteration of the endothelium caused by contact with the embolus may initiate formation of a thrombus thereby accelerating occlusion of the vessel.

Lesions of different components of the vascular wall

Rupture

Veins and lymphatics are clearly more susceptible to rupture than arteries. Rupture may involve one, two or all of the vascular layers [5]. Vascular ruptures are of four types:

Rupture of the intima

The intima is the most fragile layer of a vessel. Grossly, the wound is often linear and parallel with or perpendicular to the blood flow, much more rarely circumferential, resulting in a ring defect. Histologically, the break is characterised by laceration of the endothelial lining together with disruption of the internal elastic membrane, exposing the underlying tissue (Fig. 16). Leukocytes and monocytes infiltrate the edges of the break while the crater is filled by a thrombus (Fig. 17).

Rupture of the intima and media

Ruptures usually disrupt the intima, including the internal elastic lamina and the media in whole or part (Fig. 18). Leukocytes infiltrate the edges, which are distorted by haemorrhage. Medial smooth muscle cells bordering the medial break undergo necrosis. A thrombus fills the parietal defect.

Complete rupture of the three layers

The artery is clearly disrupted and there is haemorrhage when a large artery is involved (Fig. 19). Elastin staining helps identify complete break of the internal and external elastic membranes (Fig. 20). In a small artery, the stumps may retract and occluding thrombi may stop the haemorrhage, at least temporarily.

Rupture of the adventitia alone or of the external elastic lamina

This lesion, caused by an abrupt stretching of the vessel, often goes unnoticed and becomes manifest only when complications develop. The parietal weakness may result in herniation of the intima into the adventitia. Histologically, the external elastic lamina is disrupted or absent and is replaced by fibrotic tissue.

Endothelial cell changes

Swelling

Endothelial cells of the microcirculatory bed become turgescent, and epithelial-like, with prominent nuclei protruding into the vascular lumen (Fig. 21) in acute inflammation, infectious vasculitis, vascular neoplasms (epithelioid hemangioma) and anoxia.

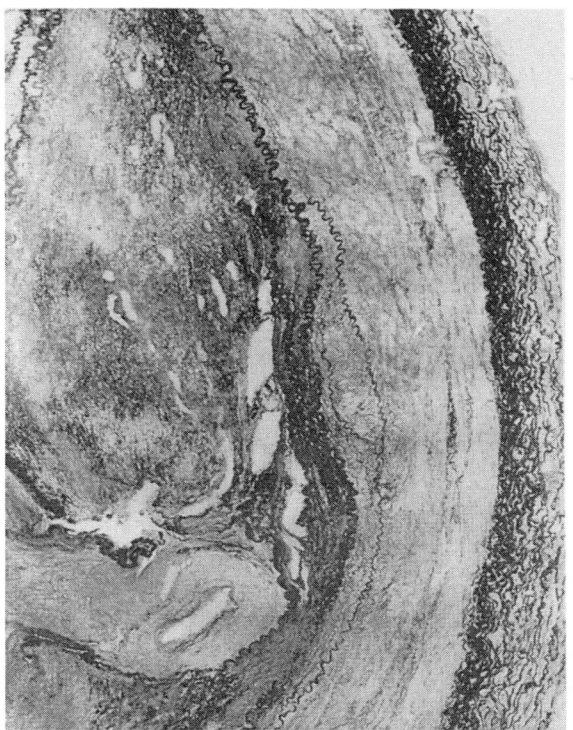

Fig. 14. Newly-formed vessels inside an organised thrombus. Orcein

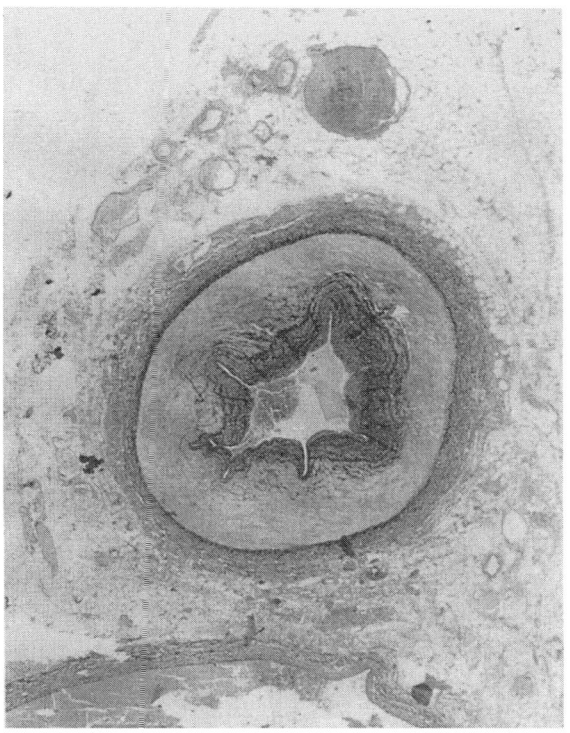

Fig. 15. Incorporated thrombus with intimal thickening in a small calibre artery. Orcein

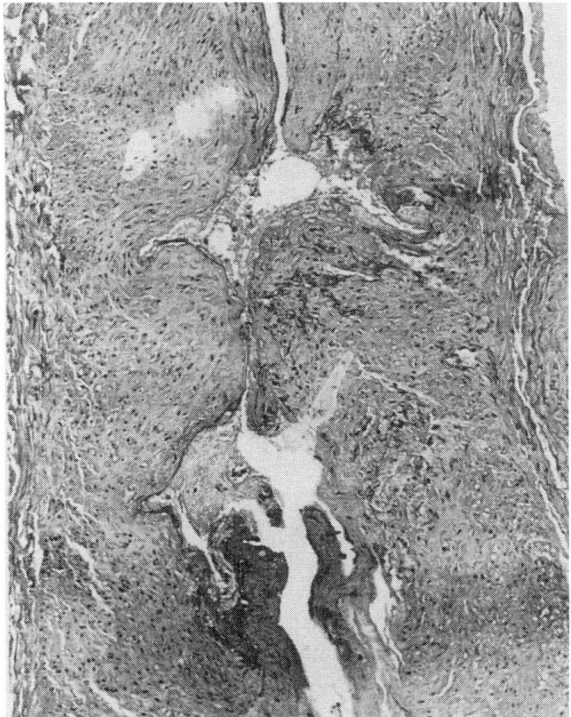

Fig .16. Rupture of the intima. Orcein

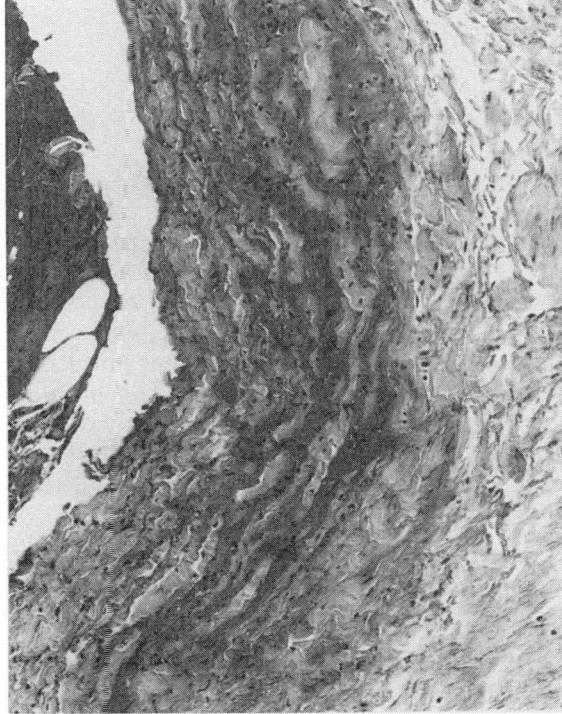

Fig. 17. Rupture of the intima. Intimal break infiltrated by haemorrhage and neutrophils. HES

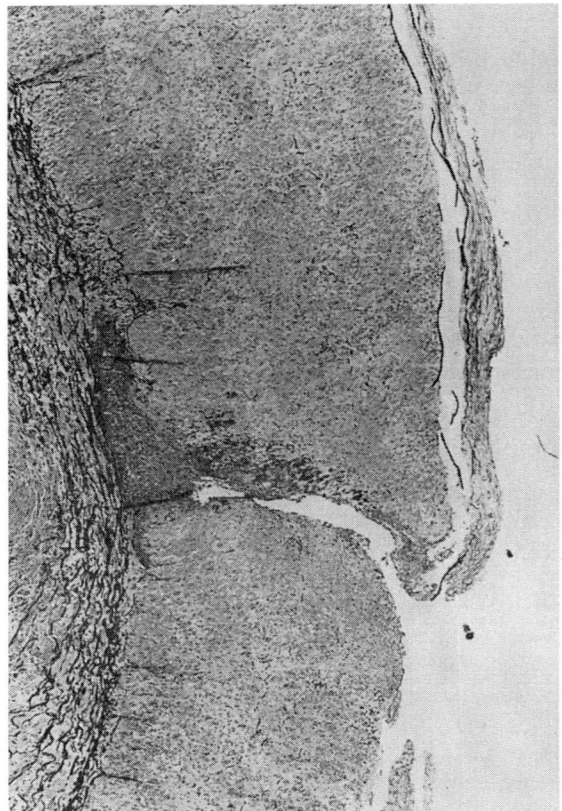

Fig. 18. Rupture of the intima and media. Orcein

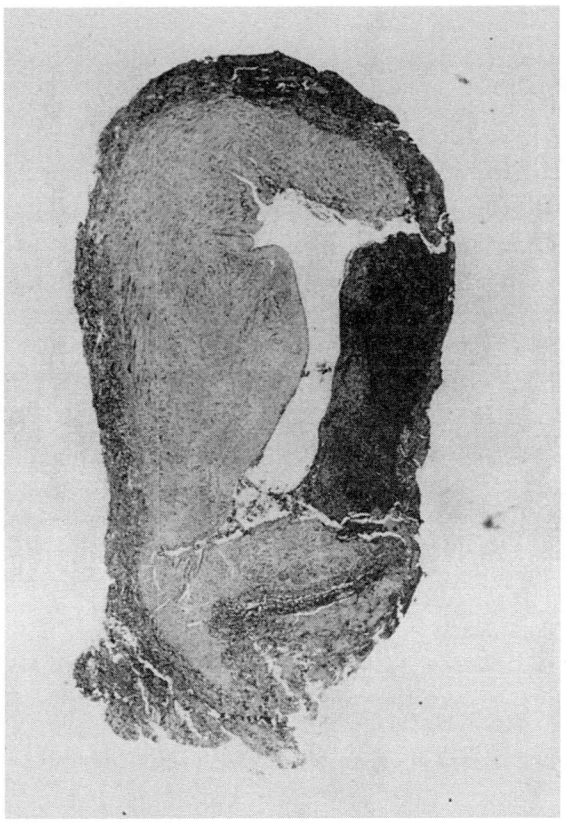

Fig. 19. Complete rupture of the three vascular layers sealed by an haematoma. Orcein

Endothelial cell loss

Cell loss may occur as focal (Fig. 22) or widespread (Fig. 23) denudation, exposing the subendothelial space. Causes include local trauma (vein puncture), balloon angioplasty or X-irradiation. Focal endothelial loss is repaired by migration and proliferation of neighbouring endothelial cells [6]. Thrombin inhibits endothelial cell monolayer repair and proliferation [7, 8].

Intimal thickening (intimal hyperplasia, obstructive endarteritis)

Here the acellular subendothelial layer of the intima is thickened (Fig. 24) by fibrosis with proliferation of myofibroblasts or dedifferentiated smooth muscle cells migrating from the media (Fig. 25) and with the synthesis and lamellar deposition of extracellular matrix (Fig. 26). Elastic fibers may be present (Fig. 27) and, at times, a true newly-formed internal elastic

membrane underlies the endothelium (Fig. 28). This condition may reduce the vascular lumen dramatically [9, 10] and is potentiated by injury to the smooth muscle cells of the media. The differential diagnosis includes an incorporated thrombus.

Intimal hyperplasia may occur in thrombosis, after vascular trauma (rupture, compression, angioplasty and other surgical procedures such as anastomosis), immunological injury (transplant vasculopathy), and in conditions as varied as ageing, atherosclerosis, fibromuscular dysplasia, and neurofibromatosis [11, 12]. During healing, endothelial cell coverage preceeds intimal hyperplasia [13]. Smooth muscle cells undergo dedifferentiation, lose the capacity to contract and gain the capacity to divide and synthesize extracellular matrix. Thus the "contractile" phenotype shifts to the "proliferative-synthetic" phenotype. Ultrastructurally, thick myosin-containing filaments disappear while organelles involved with protein synthesis (rough endoplasmic reticulum and

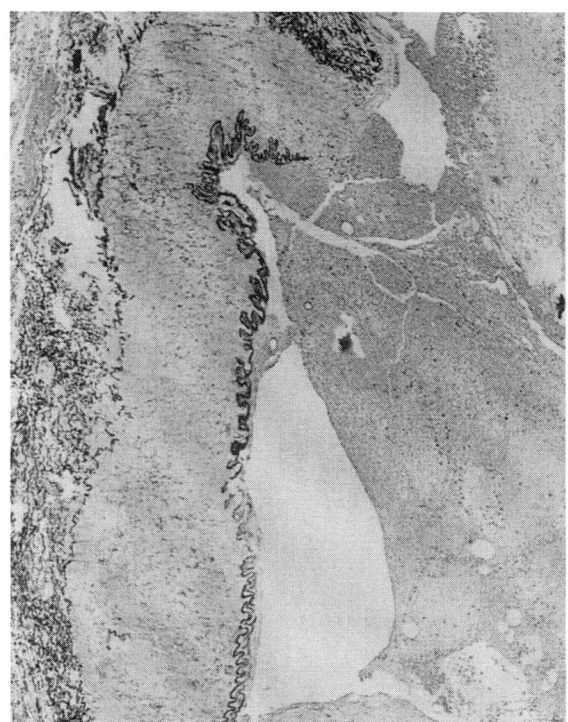

Fig. 20. Complete rupture of the three vascular layers. Note clear cut edges of the internal and external elastic membranes. Orcein

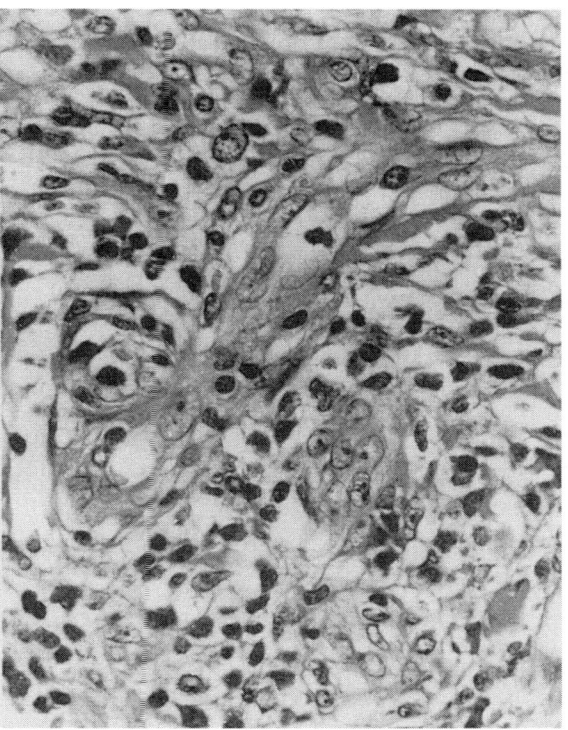

Fig. 21. Swollen endothelial cells lining newly-formed capillaries inside an inflammatory granuloma. HES

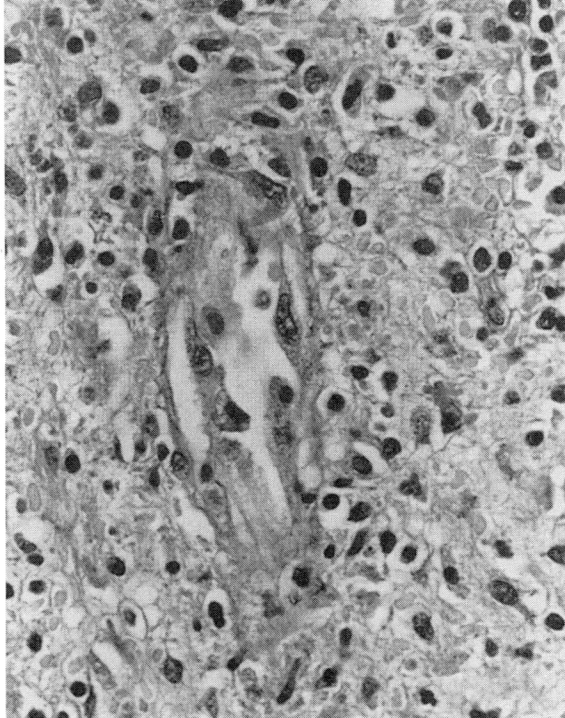

Fig. 22. Endothelial detachment. HES

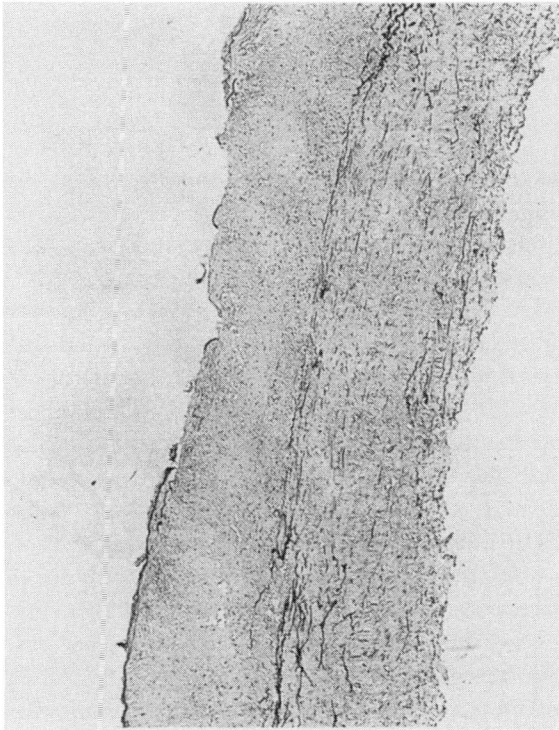

Fig. 23. Widespread denudation of the endothelium with abrasion of the internal elastic membrane after balloon angioplasty. Orcein

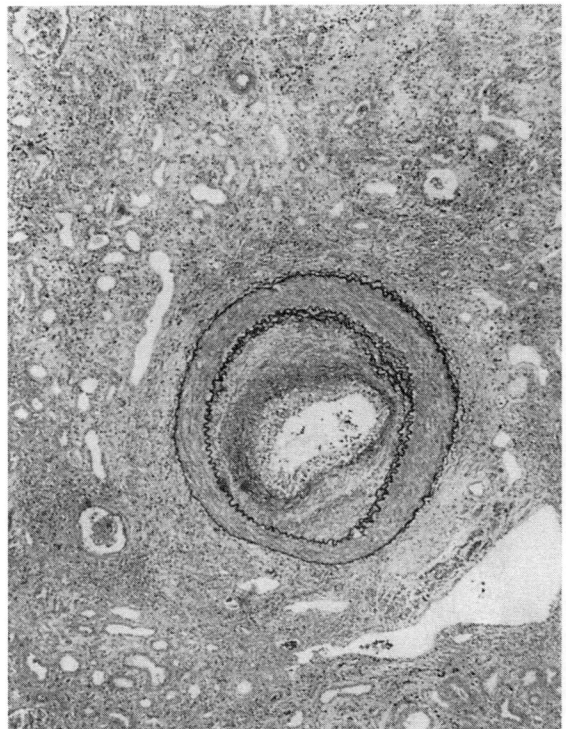

Fig. 24. Renal transplant. Intimal thickening of an intraparenchymal artery. Orcein

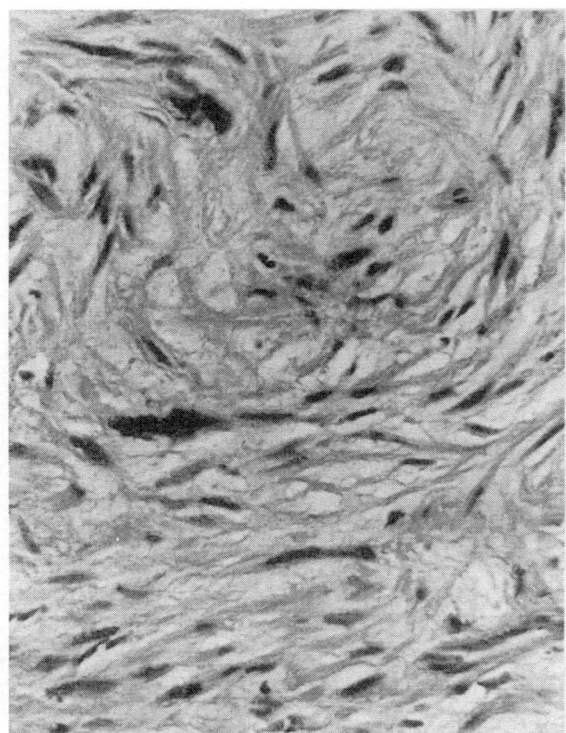

Fig. 25. Intimal thickening. Alpha smooth muscle actin-labelled myofibroblasts. Peroxidase antiperoxidase immunohistochemical technique (PAP)

Golgi apparatus) increase in number. Normally, smooth muscle cells rarely divide. In experimental arterial injury, approximately 15 to 40% of cells have undergone mitosis within 48 hours after trauma [9]. Intimal smooth muscle cells may return to a nonproliferative state when either the overlying endothelial layer is totally covered or the chronic endothelial stimulation ceases. Migration and proliferation of smooth muscle cells are both regulated by growth promoters and inhibitors [14-17]. Inhibitors include heparan sulfates, interferon-gamma, nitric oxide (NO)/endothelial-derived relaxing factor (EDRF) and transforming growth factor-beta (TGF-β). Promoters include platelet-derived growth factor (PDGF) derived from platelets, macrophages and endothelial cells, basic fibroblast growth factor (bFGF), and IL-1. Some inhibitors and promoters are endogenous to the vascular wall (PDGF, heparan sulfates, and TGF-β); others, such as IL-1, are not.

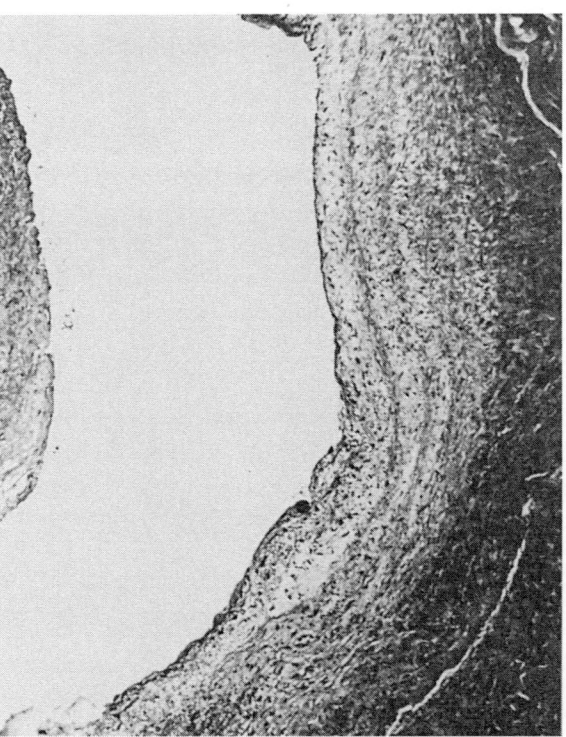

Fig. 26. Intimal thickening. Lamellar deposition of extracellular matrix. Masson's trichrome stain

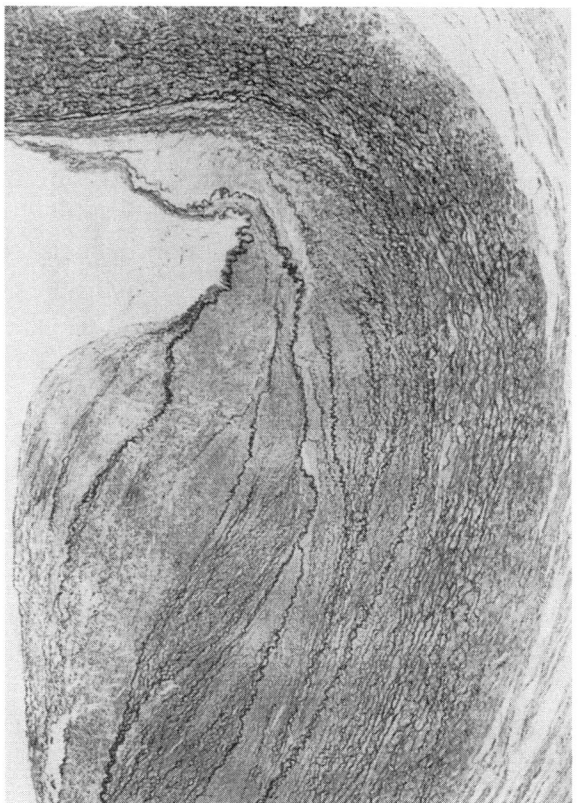

Fig. 27. Intimal thickening. Stratified newly-formed elastic fibers interspersed with the extracellular matrix. Orcein

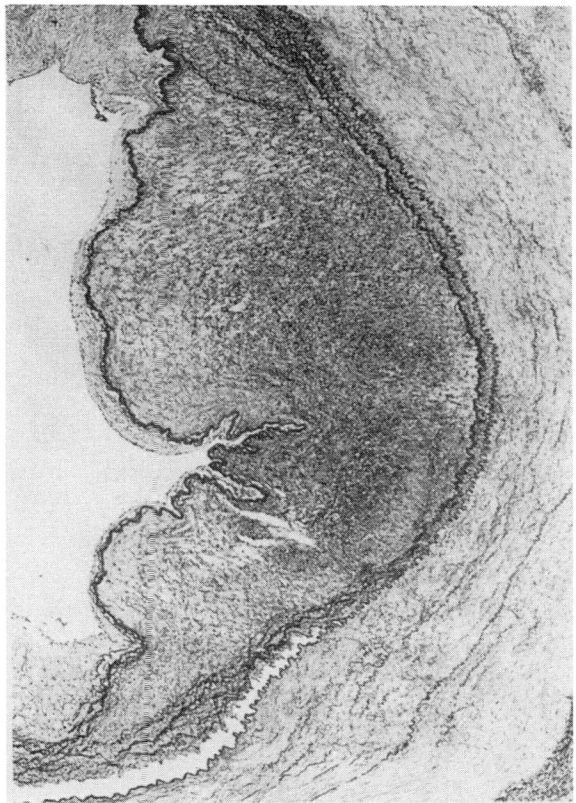

Fig. 28. Newly-formed internal elastic lamella covering an intimal thickening plaque. Note duplication of the former internal elastic membrane. Orcein

Medial changes

Thickening

This change affects both muscular arteries and veins. In arteries, the thickened media is made up of enlarged smooth muscle cells, with elongated nuclei (Fig. 29). These cells are concentrically arranged around a pinpoint lumen, in an "onion bulb" pattern. Myofibroblasts proliferate, resulting in exuberant fibrosis enclosing smooth muscle cells. In veins, smooth muscle cells undergo hypertrophy and present a leiomyomatous-like pattern. This change is seen most often in the adventitial vasa vasora running alongside dissecting haematoma or aneurysm. Causes include arteriosclerosis, medial fibromuscular dysplasia, hypertension, altered flow and pressure.

Thinning

Thinning of the media is rarely primary. Causes include medial fibromuscular dysplasia (Fig. 30) and "fatigue" changes in venous vascular grafts [18-20].

Adventitial thickening

Fibrotic thickening of the adventitia (Fig. 31) occurs in ageing, hypertension, the fibrotic stages of some vasculitides (Takayasu's disease) injury induced by radiation and angioplasty [21], and adventitial fibromuscular dysplasia [22, 23]. Hypertrophy of adventitial smooth muscle bundles may occur in pedicular vessels of atrophic viscera or accompany lesions of fibromuscular dysplasia of the media.

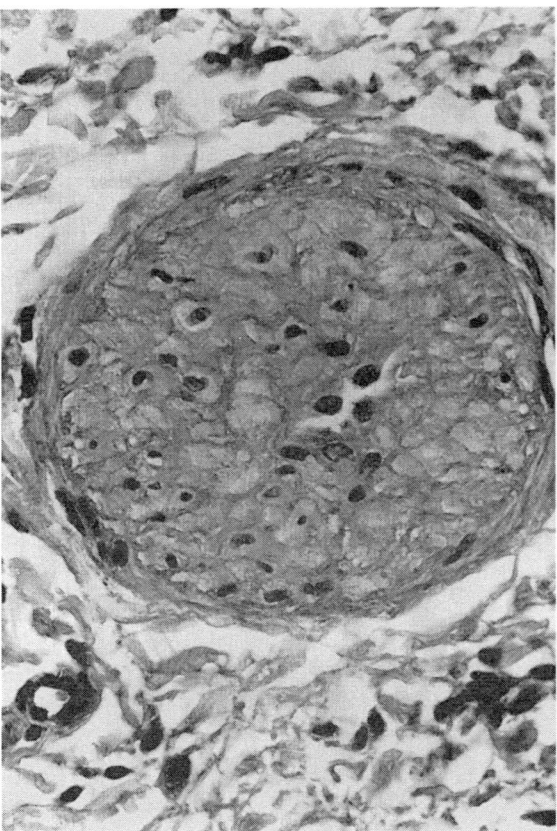

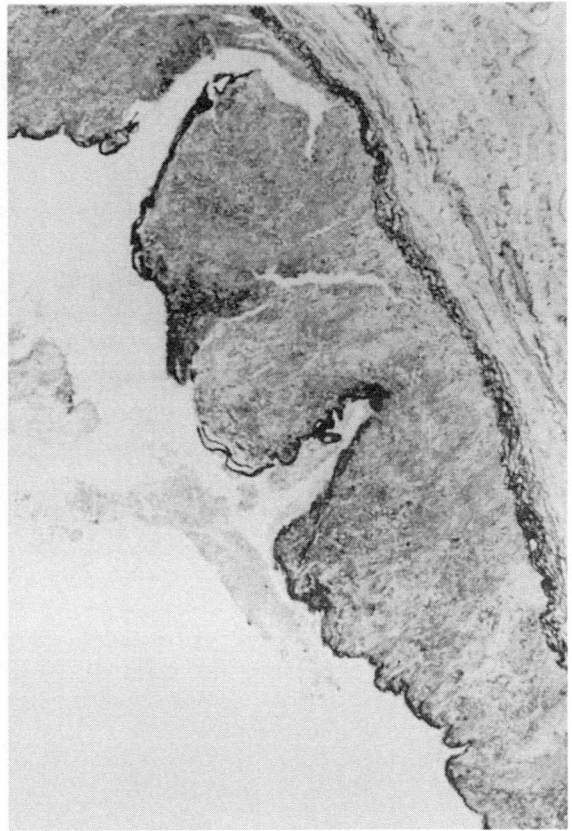

Fig. 29. Concentric hypertrophy of the media of an arteriole. HES

Fig. 30. Focal thinning of the media with inflexion of the internal elastic lamella caused by fibromuscular dysplasia. Orcein

Abnormal deposits

Fibrinoid deposits

Fibrinoid is a granular substance having a staining reaction like that of fibrin (Fig. 32). It consists of disintegrated fibrin, lipids and extravasated plasma proteins including complement fraction C3, and immunoglobulins. These are intermingled with more-or-less fragmented red blood cells and the debris of myocytes [24]. Arterioles are frequently involved. Fibrinoid material is more eosinophilic and less homogenous than the hyaline change seen with ageing [25]. In malignant hypertension, fibrinoid material thickens the media of arterioles and when an inflammatory reaction develops around the affected vessel a necrotizing vasculitis is seen, with superimposed haemorrhages and oedema. The presence of fibrinoid material in the vascular wall results from endothelial damage or a parietal rupture. The lesion may

develop as a result of leukocytoclastic vasculitis or periarteritis nodosa and in the arteritides of other collagen diseases (lupus erythematosus, rheumatoid arthritis, dermatomyositis, scleroderma). It may be associated with giant cell arteritis or amyloid angiopathy [26, 27]. The now happily rare malignant hypertension used to be an important cause with involvement of the microcirculatory bed a major feature [28]. Radiation vasculitis is frequently accompanied by fibrinod necrosis [23].

Calcification

Diffuse calcification is common with increasing age and was, in the past, described as an entity (Monkeberg's medial calcific sclerosis or pipestem arteries) [29, 30]. This lesion has no clinical significance and is not indicative of occlusive arterial disease. It may involve the aorta and large arteries of the extremities and medium-sized visceral arteries (Fig. 33). Mediacalcosis of veins is rare and association with ar-

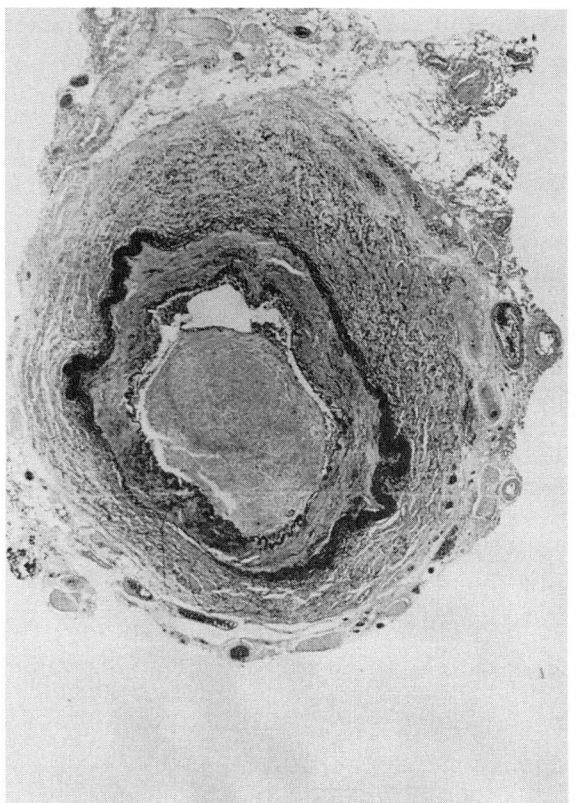

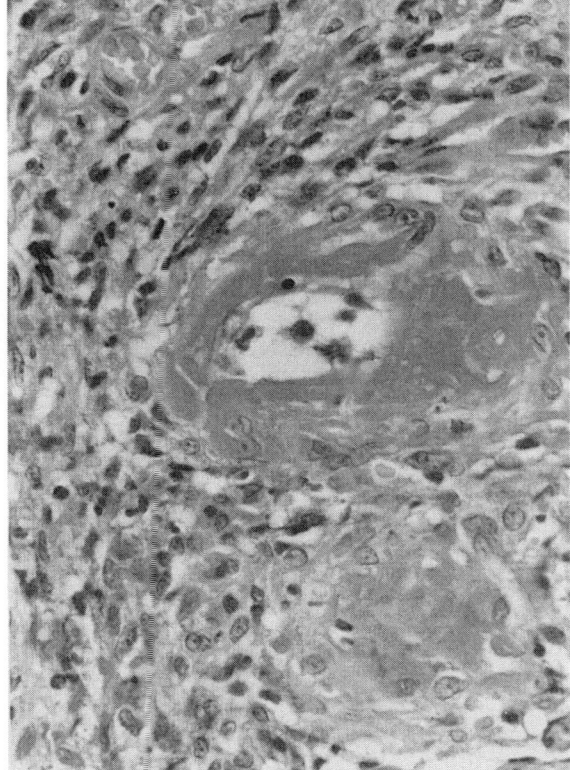

Fig. 31. Marked fibrotic thickening of the adventitia with occlusive thrombosis caused by adventitial fibromuscular dysplasia. Orcein

Fig. 32. Fibrinoid deposit thickening an arteriole wall. HES

terial calcification is not the rule. There is thickening and irregularity of the media resulting in tortuosity and lengthening. In elastic arteries, the elastic frame of the media degenerates and fragments; smooth muscle cells disappear and are replaced by fibrous tissue. Calcium deposits and focal haemorrhage occur secondarily. In muscular arteries, calcium deposits often distort the media at the junction of its innermost and outermost part. This process is frequently limited to a sector of the arterial wall but can extend to its entire circumference. Foci of osseous metaplasia can be seen (Fig. 34). In veins, calcifications may be diffuse and are frequently associated with phlebosclerosis. Mediacalcosis should be distinguished from intimal calcified atherosclerotic plaques and idiopathic arterial calcifications of infancy [31]. Sometimes, calcifications may line up along the internal elastic membrane with subsequent foreign body granulomata simulating giant cell arteritis or Horton's disease. However, these two lesions may coexist.

Elderly subjects are mostly affected (senile medial calcinosis) but young and middle-aged individuals may occasionally be involved (juvenile and presenile medial calcinosis). Mönckeberg's sclerosis may follow arterial hyalinosis in the course of the ageing process. But it may result from various pathological conditions: primary or secondary hyperparathyroidism, possible toxic injury with calcification as an attempt at repair, or long-term treatment with corticosteroids in arthritic patients [32]. Pseudoxanthoma elasticum, an uncommon hereditary disorder, may also be accompanied by degeneration and fragmentation of arterial elastic fibers and by roentgenographic evidence of premature calcification of the peripheral arteries [33].

Other deposits

Deposits such as oxalate crystals, and amyloid are discussed in the chapter XV.

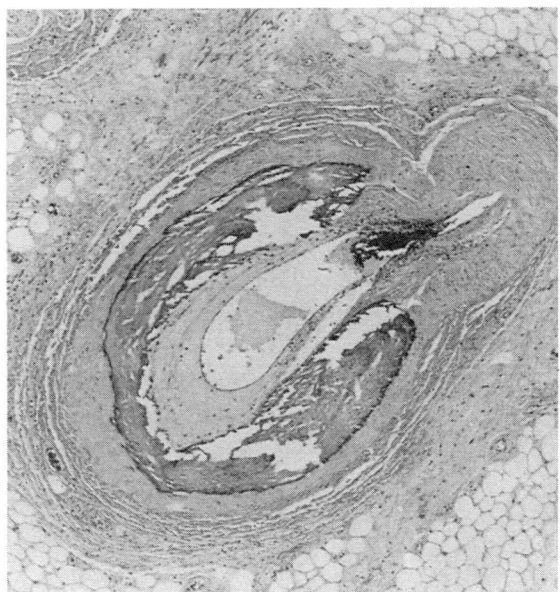

Fig. 33. Monkeberg's medial sclerosis with calcification in the media. HES

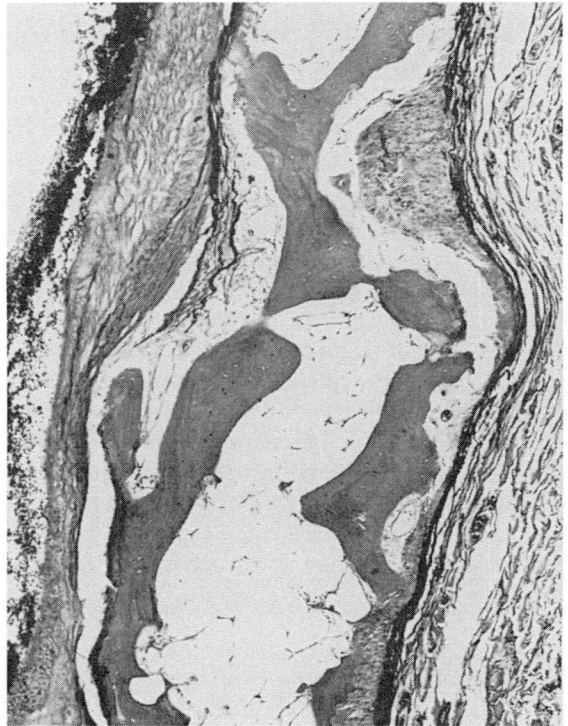

Fig. 34. Osseous metaplasia inside a medial calcification. Orcein

Alterations in caliber

Ectasia

Telangiectasia

This term describes dilatation or prominence of normal blood vessels: capillaries, arterioles, arteries, small venules (Fig. 35). There is no clinical problem apart from cosmetic concern. The change is particularly noticeable in the skin because of the rich blood supply of the dermis and subcutaneous tissue. Telangiectasia may be congenital or acquired. Acquired exaggeration of the normal capillary and venous pattern (simple telangiectasia) occurs in many conditions, including acne rosacea, idiopathic cutaneous atrophy, xeroderma pigmentosum, morphoea, syphilis and lupus erythematosus. Simple telangiectasia of palmar surfaces of the hands and fingers may be indicative of scleroderma months, and even years, before the cutaneous changes of the disease appear.

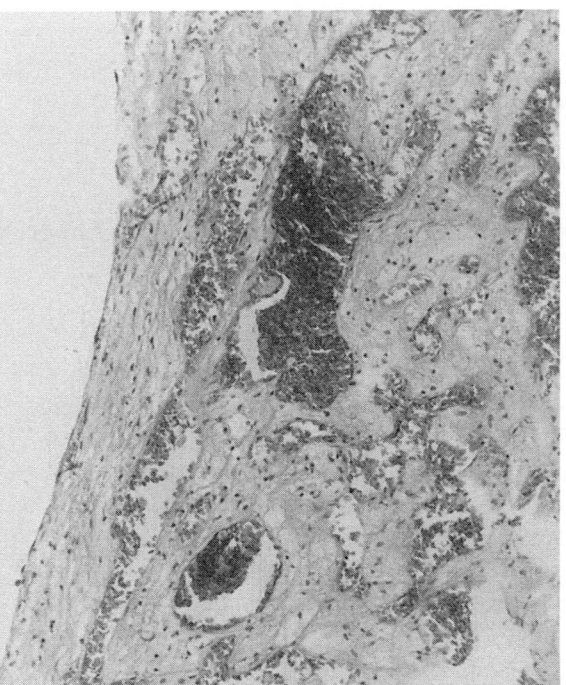

Fig. 35. Blood capillary telangiectasia. HES

Lymphangiectasia

Dilatation of lymph vessels may occur in various pathological conditions and lymphostasis. The condition may be acquired (Fig. 36) or congenital (Fig. 37) (See chapter 13 "The pathology of veins, lymphatics, arteriovenous anastomoses and the erectile vascular tissue").

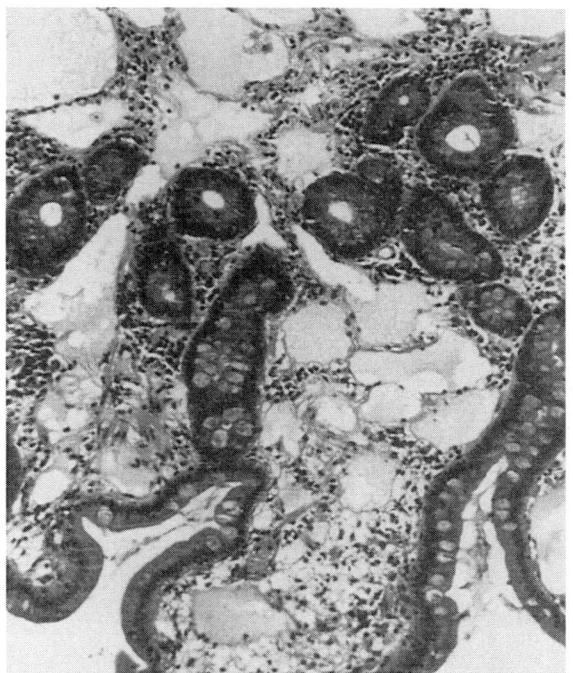

Fig. 36. Acquired intestinal lymphangiectasia in a patient suffering from malabsorption syndrome. HES

Aneurysm

An aneurysm is a localised dilatation of all of the component layers of a vessel resulting from loss of the normal physical characteristics of the wall and is thus differentiated from the dilatation and tortuosity of arteries that occurs with age. Aneurysms may be saccular (Fig. 38) or fusiform (Fig. 39) Histologically, the wall of an established aneurysm is made up of fibrous tissue in which the remnants of elastic laminae and areas of inflammation may be seen. The luminal aspect will commonly show confluent atherosclerotic plaques in larger vessels and thrombosis is common (Fig. 40). Operative specimens containing a non-aneurysmal area are the only way to identify the primary lesion which may vary according to the type of vessel involved.

Any condition that interferes with the mechanical integrity of the vessel wall may allow aneurysms to develop. The factors involved include atherosclerosis, fibromuscular dysplasia, hereditary dystrophy of the connective and elastic tissue of the arterial wall (as, for example, in Marfan's syndrome), congenital defects (berry aneurysms and microaneurysms of Charcot-Bouchard), trauma, septic embolism or local sepsis [34], vasculitis (syphilis, lupus erythematosus) and collagen diseases, for example, relapsing polychondritis. Less well defined genetic abnormalities than Marfan's syndrome may also play a role [35-37].

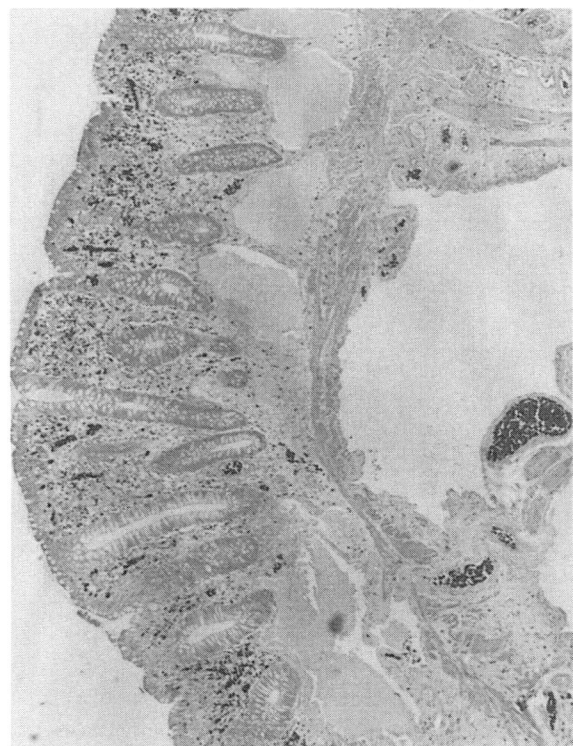

Fig. 37. Congenital colonic lymphangiectasia with underlying submucosal angiodysplasia. HES

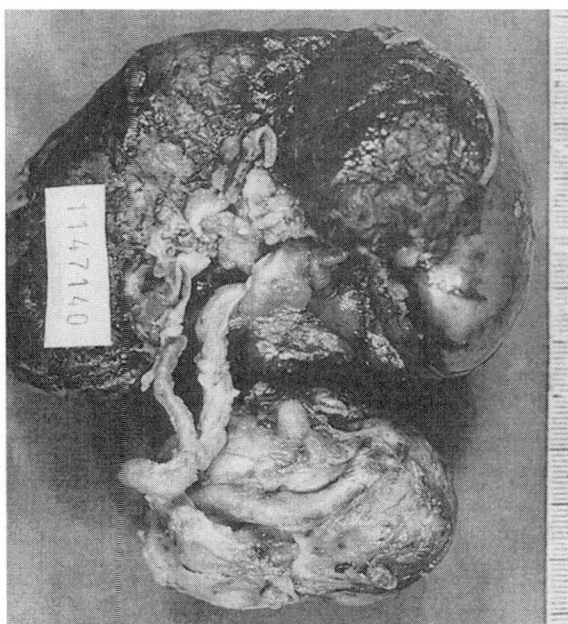

Fig. 38. Sacciform aneurysm of the splenic artery

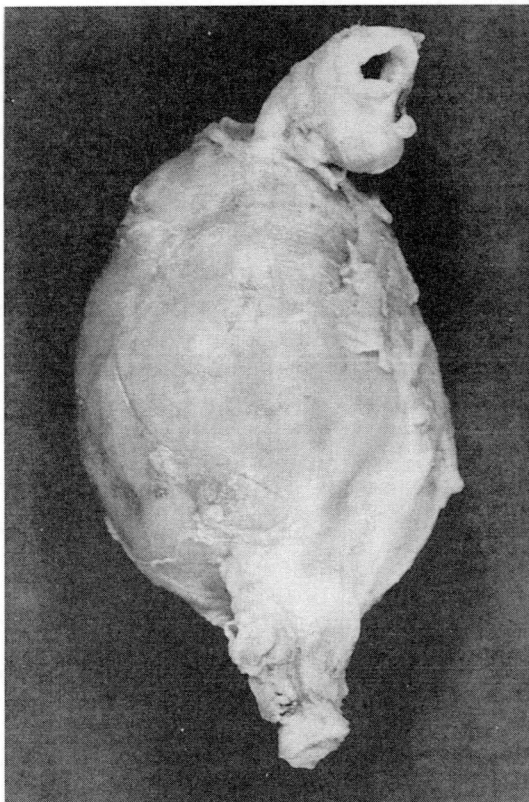 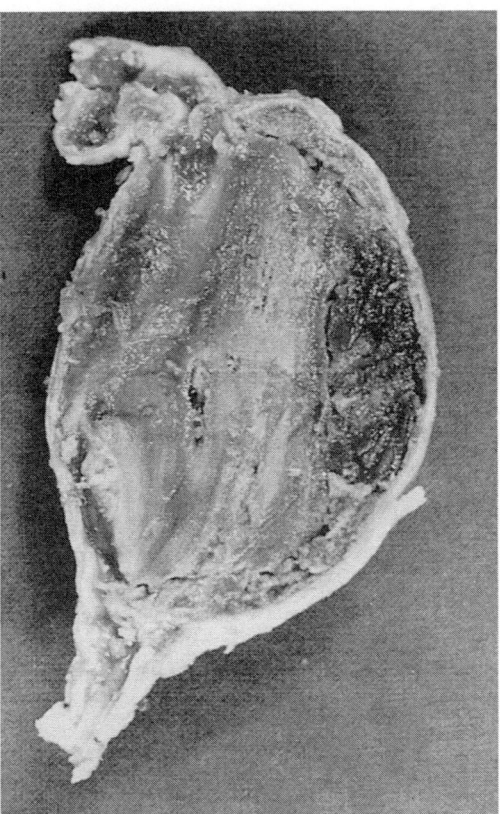

Fig. 39-40. Fusiform aneurysm of the popliteal artery showing occlusive thrombus on cut section (Fig.39). Note luminal atheromatous calcified plaques (Fig.40)

Post stenotic dilatation

Grossly, this mimics a sack-like aneurysm (Fig. 41-42) and is characterised on the endothelial aspect of the vessel by a "jet-lesion", a corrugated patch developed on the surface of the intima (Fig. 43), lying distal to the stenosis. Histologically, it consists of localized fibrous intimal thickening. The medial architecture is usually distorted, with loss of elastic tissue leading to dilatation (Fig. 44). Superimposed atherosclerotic plaques and intraluminal thrombosis may develop. Thrombosis is frequent. All acquired or congenital stenotic lesions may produce post-stenotic dilatation. The clinical manifestations depend on the vessels involved, but the thoracic outlet syndrome is an example.

Post traumatic or false aneurysm

This lesion involves arteries and/or veins. Clinically, they present as a pulsatile mass of variable size resulting from an organised haematoma within the wall of the vessel following rupture of the intima and media.

Grossly, the lesion mimics a true aneurysm with the vascular lumen frequently occluded. Histological examination may reveal remnants of the vascular coats within the organised haematoma (Fig. 45). Elastin staining helps identify the damaged internal elastica lamina, while the external elastic lamella is often unaffected (Fig. 46). A false aneurysm may develop after a vascular rupture from any cause [38].

Dissecting aneurysm

Penetration of the blood into the media of an artery, almost always as a result of an intimo-medial rupture, produces a dissecting hematoma which forms an aneurysm [39]. The term "dissecting aneurysm" is a misnomer, since there is no arterial dilatation; a more accurate term is «dissecting haematoma». The haematoma developed in the vascular wall can occlude the lumen or extend to the adventitia resulting in fatal haemorrhage. Arterial dissection may be spontaneous, traumatic or iatrogenic [5, 40]. The majority of patients have a history of hypertension. Dissection rarely affects veins.

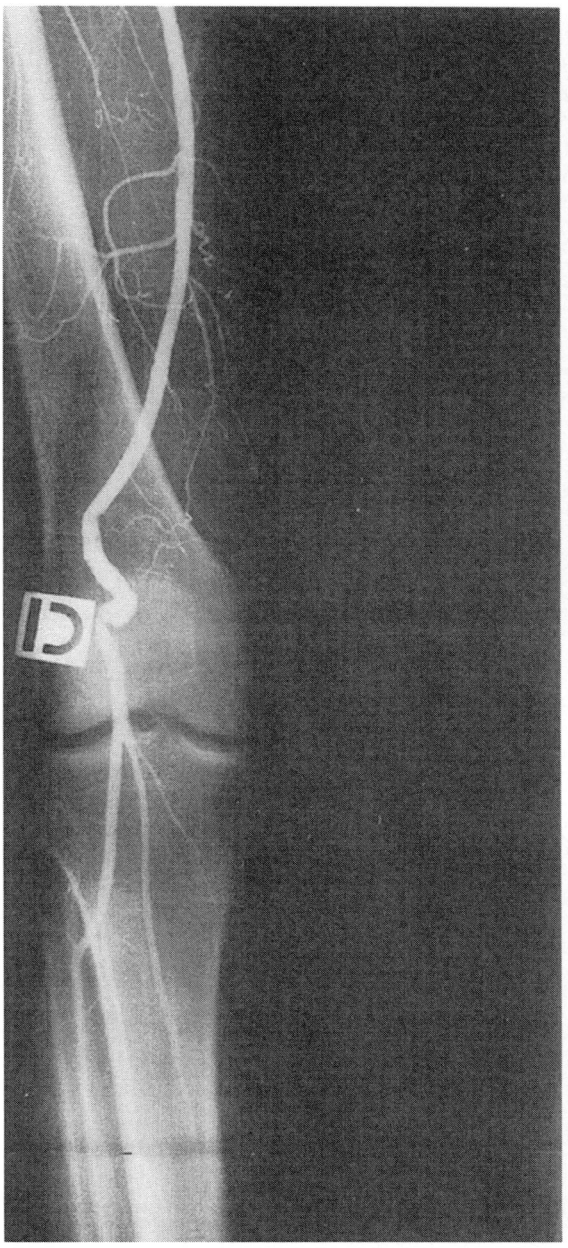

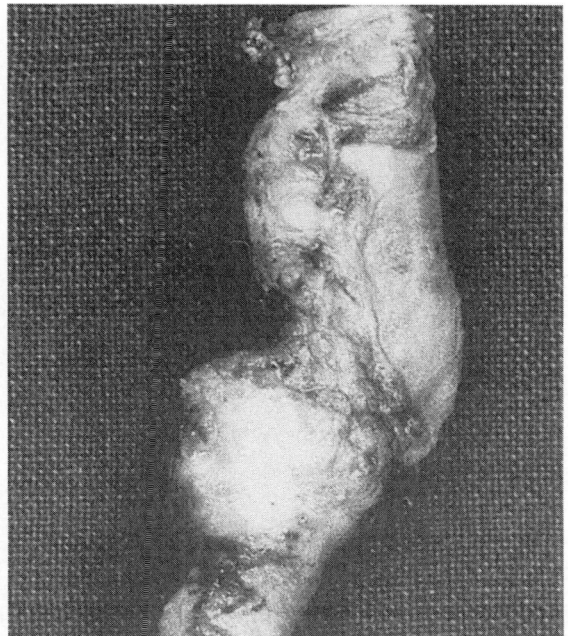

Fig. 42. Sack-like post-stenotic dilatation

Fig. 41. Angiographic aspect of a post-stenotic dilatation of an entrapped popliteal artery (Courtesy Dr F.Cheilan)

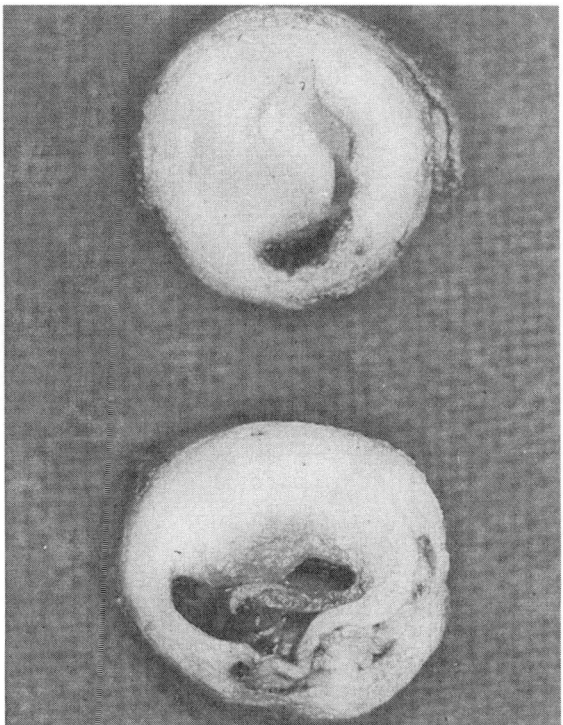

Fig. 43. Intimal "jet-lesion" developed in a post-stenotic dilatation

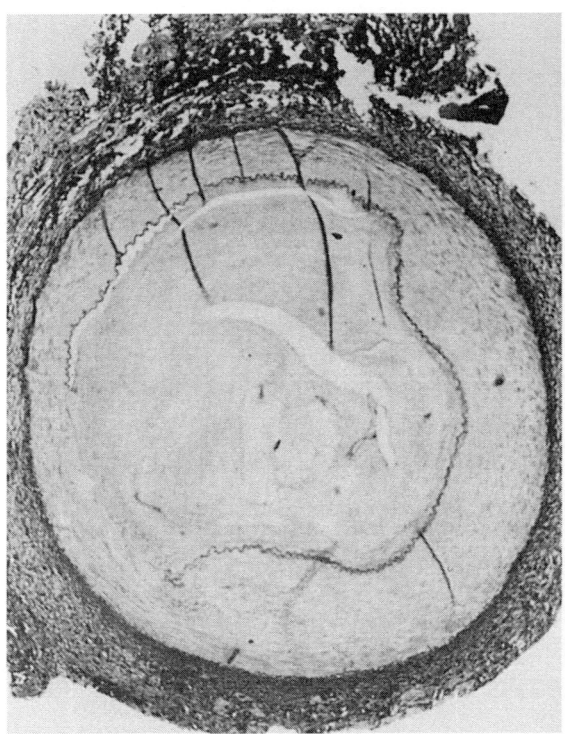

Fig. 44. Marked intimal fibrotic thickening with partial disappearance of the underlying internal elastic lamella of a "jet-lesion". Orcein

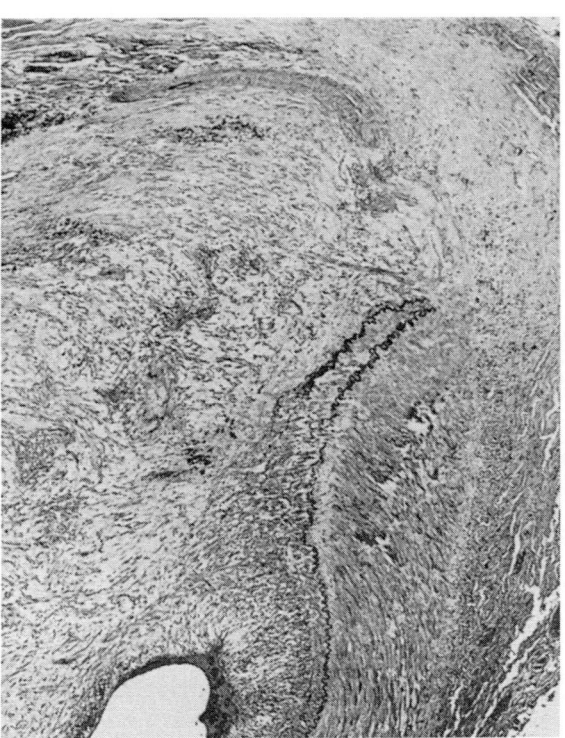

Fig. 46. Remnant of the internal elastic membrane in the post-traumatic aneurysm wall. Orcein

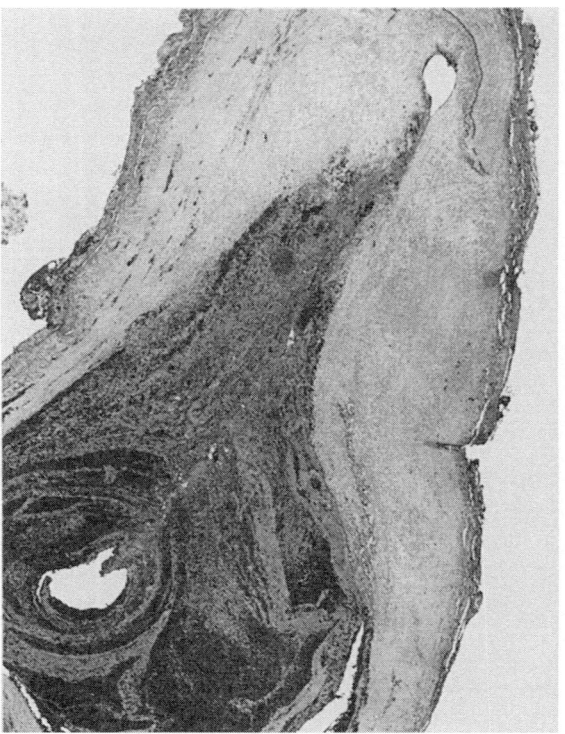

Fig. 45. Thrombosed post-traumatic aneurysm of a temporal artery. Orcein

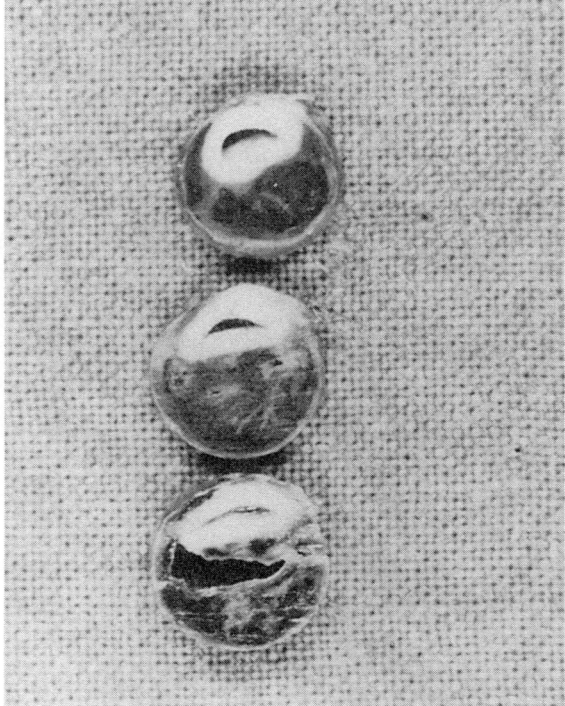

Fig. 47. Dissecting aneurysm. Fresh dissecting haematoma collapsing the arterial lumen

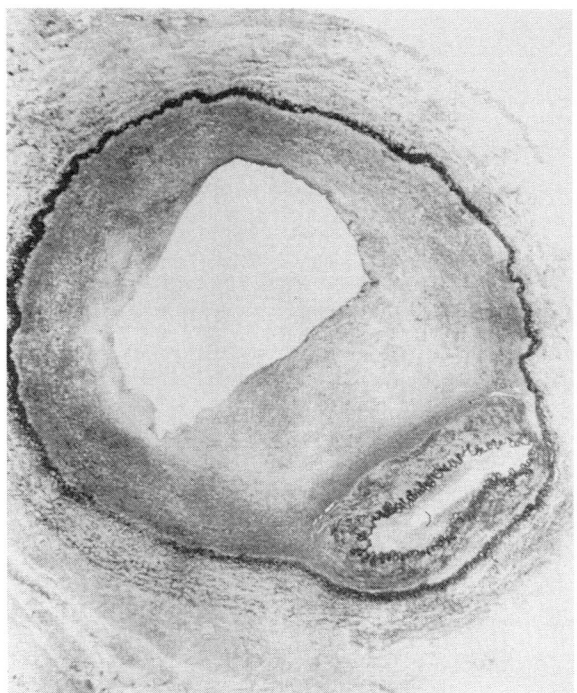

Fig. 48. Dissecting aneurysm. Organisation of the cleavage plane with double-barrelled aspect. Orcein

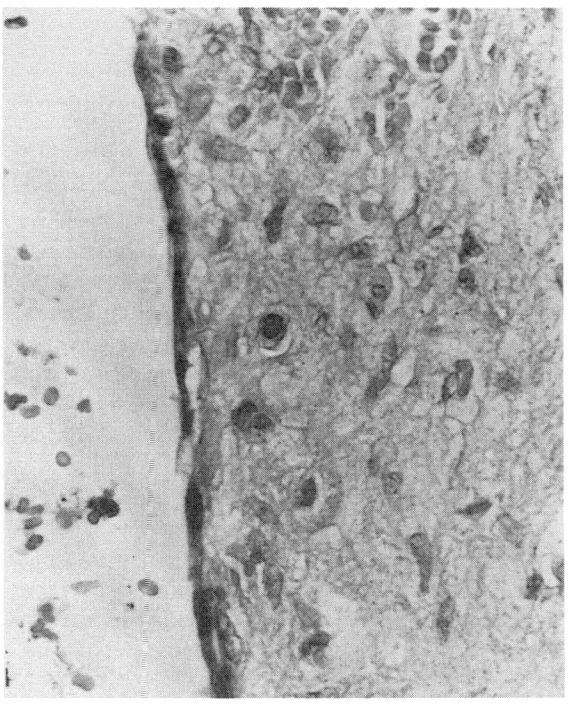

Fig. 49. Dissecting aneurysm. Organised cleavage plane invested by CD34-labeled endothelial cells. PAP

Grossly, the dissected area may resemble a fusiform aneurysm. On cut section, the vascular lumen encompasses two lumina with the dissection beginning in the media roughly at the junction of the inner third and outer two-thirds of the media (Fig. 47). This site is determined by the nature of cell/cell and cell/stroma attachments, which drop rapidly in density at this level [41]. The dissection usually extends for one third to two thirds of the circumference of the artery but when the whole circumference is involved, these two concentric cylinders are seen with the true lumen partially collapsed [42]. The hematoma may penetrate the adventitia and give rise to bleeding. Organisation of the cleavage plane results in a vascular section reveals a double-barrelled aspect (Fig. 48). Histologically, the collapsed true lumen is bordered by the intima supported by a ruptured internal elastic lamina. In the acute stage, the cleavage plane is infiltrated by neutrophils and haemorrhage. In the subacute stage, this plane is lined with granulation tissue containing haemosiderin-laden macrophages, fibroblasts, loose fibrous tissue and newly-formed capillaries. The organised cleavage plane may be colonized by endothelial cells, whose morphology can be confirmed by immunohistochemical markers (Fig. 49). In the chronic stage, the cleavage plane is frequently sealed by scarring fibrotic tissue. When a re-entry orifice is present, it allows the dissecting channel to communicate with the arterial lumen (Fig. 50).

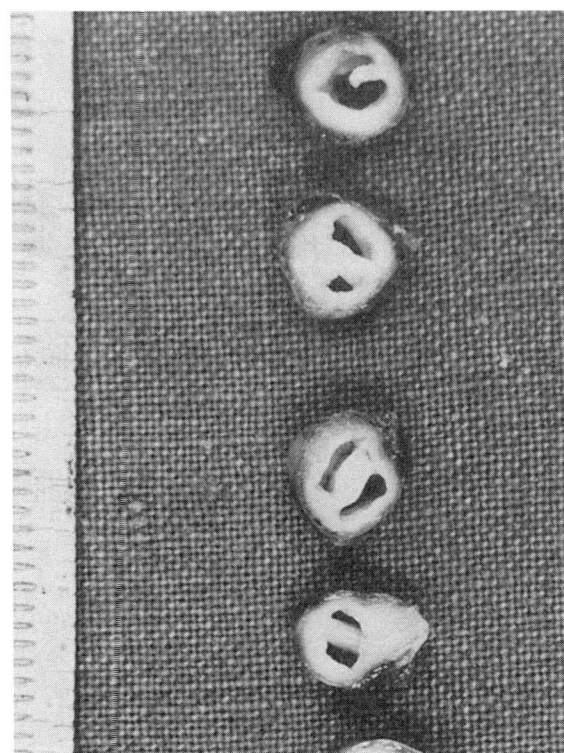

Fig. 50. Dissecting aneurysm. Chronic dissection with re-entry orifice

Arteriovenous fistulae

An arteriovenous fistula is an abnormal communication between an artery and a vein. Lymphatic vessels are rarely involved.

Congenital arteriovenous fistulae

Congenital arteriovenous fistulae result from failure of the common capillary network to differentiate into a normal definitive vascular tree. Anastomotic channels thus form between otherwise normally developed arterial and venous trunks. Congenital arteriovenous fistulas may be isolated, or belong to complex haemangiomatous syndromes (for example, the Osler-Weber-Rendu, Sturge-Weber and Klippel-Trenaunay syndromes).

Histologically, these lesions are represented by collections of anomalous patulous vessels having a structure that is atypical for either artery or vein but which represents something intermediate between them (Fig. 51-52). Small precapillary arteriovenous communications are present. In some cases, haemangiomatous changes may be associated (Fig. 53).

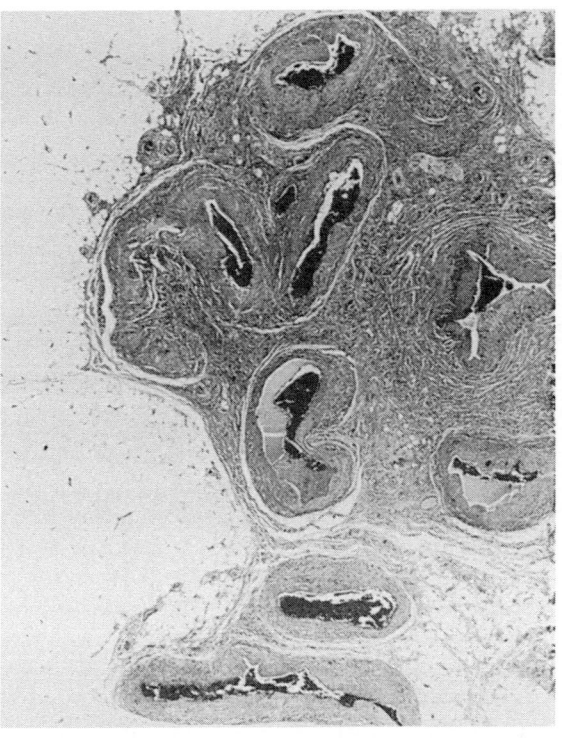

Fig. 52. Congenital arteriovenous fistula. Note patoulous vessels mimicking either arteries or veins. HES

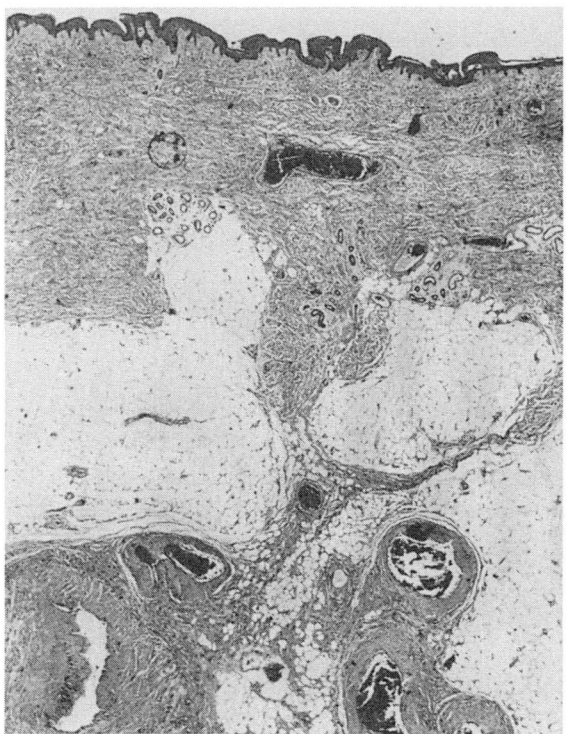

Fig. 51. Congenital arteriovenous fistula. HES

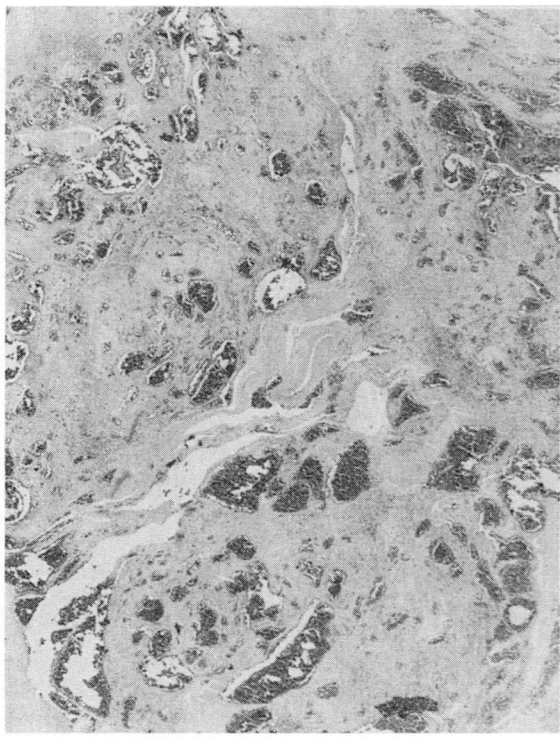

Fig. 53. Congenital arteriovenous fistula with associated hemangiomatous changes. HES

Surrounding tissue often presents local haemorrhages, haemosiderin deposits and fibrosis. In the lungs, fistulae often develops away from the bronchial tree. A-V fistulae should be distinguished from a normal arteriovenous shunts, which occur more frequently after embolism, and in patients with pulmonary stenosis and sickle cell anaemia. They appear in the pleura in cirrhotic patients and are analogous to spider angiomas of the skin.

Acquired arteriovenous fistulae

Most acquired fistulae are caused by trauma, rarely by rupture of an arterial aneurysm into its satellite vein. Grossly, the vein shows fusiform dilatation on either side of the fistula. The lumen of the artery is dilated above the orifice and there is narrowing below it. The histological features of an arteriovenous fistula are similar, whatever the cause (Fig. 54). The orifice is surrounded by fibrotic tissue containing newly-formed blood vessels and haemosiderin-laden macrophages. On the arterial side, elastic stains reveal the remnants of internal and external elastic membranes (Fig. 55). On the venous side, the intima exhibits cushion-like thickening, and harbours numerous newly formed elastic fibers arranged in a circular layer (Fig. 56). Thickening of the media is evident with fibrosis, hy-

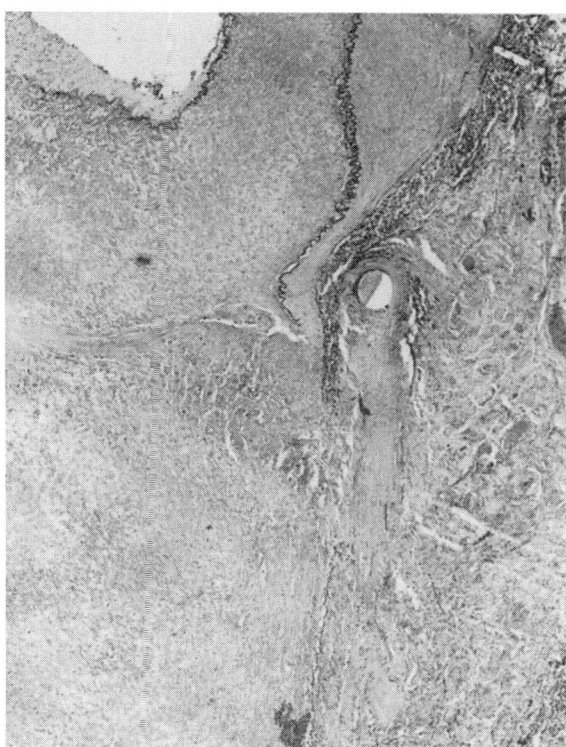

Fig. 55. Acquired cubital arteriovenous fistula. Fistular orifice evidenced by a suture thread. Note well-preserved internal elastic lamella on the arterial side. Orcein

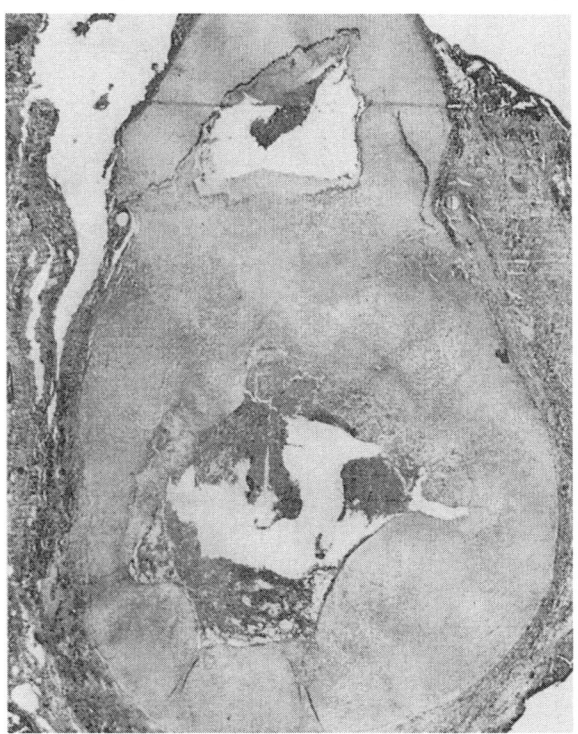

Fig. 54. Acquired cubital arteriovenous fistula as a permanent vascular access for haemodialysis. Note well-preserved internal elastic lamella of the cubital artery. Orcein

pertrophy of smooth muscle cells, and production of elastic fibers A transition into an artery ("arterialisation") cannot readily be recognized. In the chronic stage, the venous wall is distorted by fibrotic strands surrounding islets of hypertrophied myocytes, intermingled with elastic fibers. A true internal elastic membrane may develop in the intima (Fig. 57). The arterial wall below the orifice thins and smooth muscle cells and scleroproteins are lost from the media.

Coarctation

This term defines a constriction of a vessel. The condition most frequently involves the aorta and may be congenital or acquired; both forms may produce symptoms of arterial insufficiency: intermittent claudication, coldness of the extremities, and reduction or disappearance of the pulsations in the distal arteries [43]. Congenital coarctation is responsible for a shelf-like obstruction in the aortic lumen (Fig. 58) the coarctation ridge consisting of intimal thickening with some infolding of the media (Fig. 59).

Coarctation may be associated with other malformations including bicuspid aortic valve, hypoplasia of the proximal part of the aortic arch and more rarely

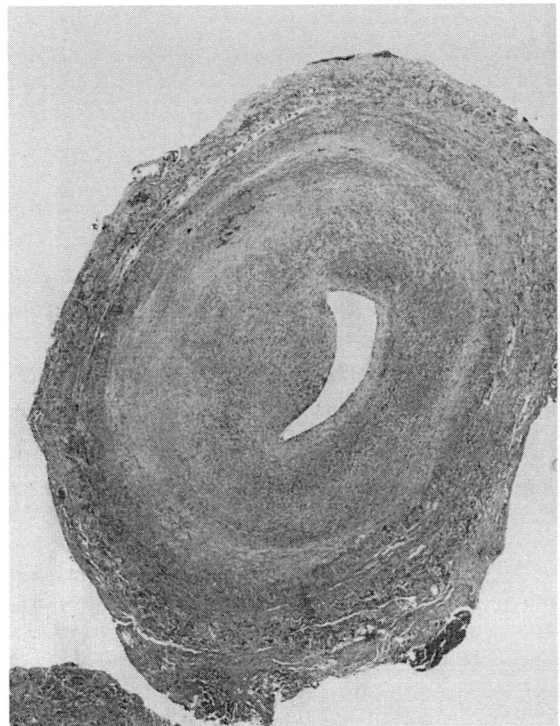

Fig.56. Acquired cubital arteriovenous fistula. Marked intimal fibrotic thickening on the venous side. HES

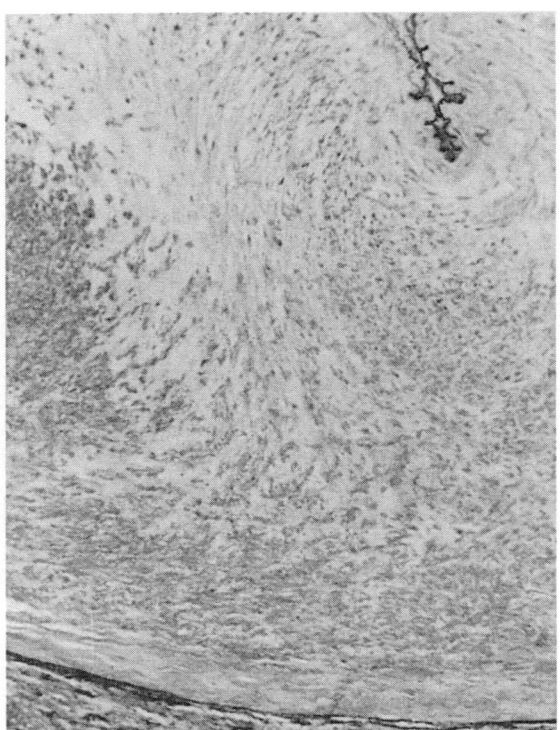

Fig. 57. Acquired cubital arteriovenous fistula. "Arterialised" venous side with intimal fibrosis and a newly-formed internal elastic lamella. Orcein

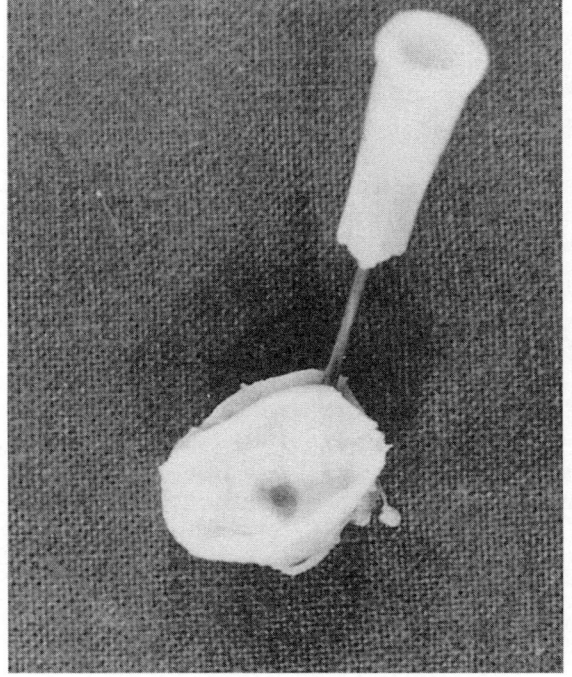

Fig. 58. Sieve-like congenital coarctation of the aortic isthmus

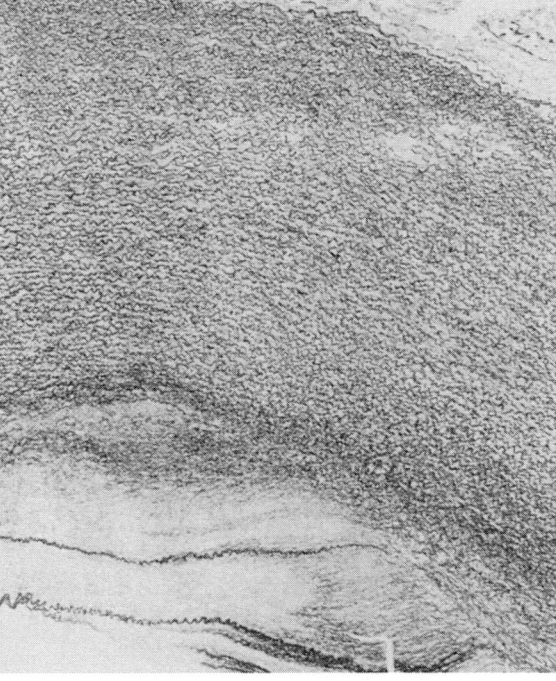

Fig. 59. Congenital coarctation of the aortic isthmus. Coarctation ridge consisting of intimal thickening with some infoldings of the media. Orcein

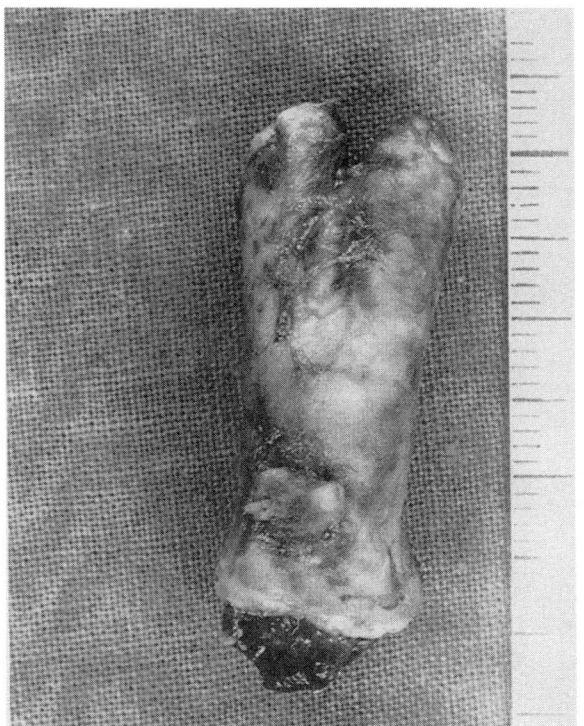
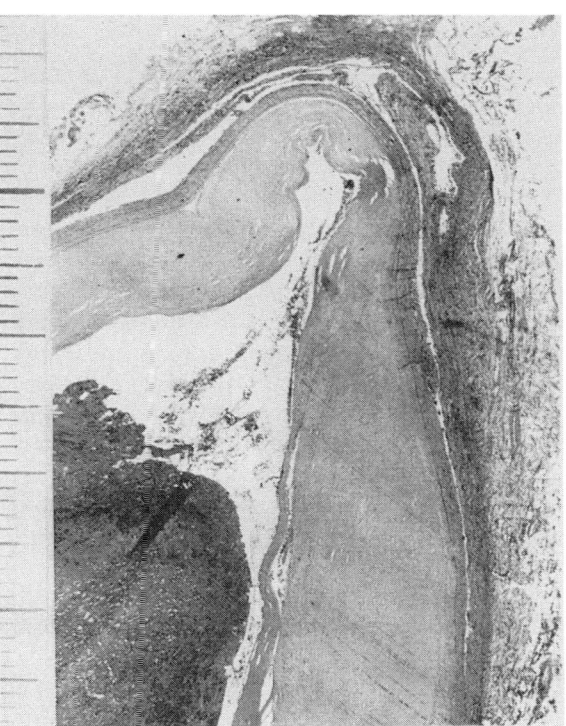

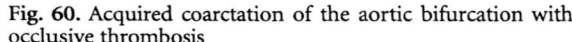

Fig. 60. Acquired coarctation of the aortic bifurcation with occlusive thrombosis

Fig. 61. Acquired coarctation of the aortic bifurcation caused by atherosclerosis. HES

the iliac-femoral system. It has been found in association with cerebellar hypoplasia and neurofibromatosis [44-48]. It is a feature of some forms of fibromuscular dysplasia [49, 50].

Acquired coarctation may result from extensive atherosclerosis with or without thrombosis [51, 52]. An old embolic occlusion or an incomplete aortic rupture may temporarily reduce the lumen of the aorta and, if healing occurs, may cause persistent coarctation (Fig. 60-61) Other causes include Takayasu's arteritis and external compression by benign or malignant tumours [53]. These acquired conditions are less frequently associated with hypertension in the upper extremities than in congenital coarctation.

Dilatation and tortuosity of vessels

Arteries

Elongation with dilatation and tortuosity of arteries is often referred to as a specific entity, for example the "dolichomega-arteries" of Leriche [54] or "arteriomegaly" [55-56].

Grossly, the vessel extends and meanders. The histological patterns of ectatic arteries are variable; they may be normal, or show atherosclerotic changes, or thinning of the media.

Aetiological factors include age-related degenerative changes leading to polyaneurysmal dystrophy, or congenital developmental defects such as the Beckwith-Wiedemann syndrome [57-59].

Veins

Dilatation of veins is rarely diffuse and is caused by the incompetence of venous valves. Varicoceles and pelvic congestion syndrome are two characteristic examples. The venous plexus is tortuous, and dilated. Histologically, the venous wall has a pattern similar to that of a varicose vein. Slim elastic fibres of widely varying orientation are present in the media and adventitia [60].

Lymphatics

Lymph cysts and lymphoceles may lead to chylous effusion, ascites, dilatation of the lymph vessels in the retroperitoneal space and, rarely, to symptoms such as chylous metrorragia or vaginal discharge [61-63].

Grossly, the size of a lymph cyst or a lymphocele varies between a few millimetres and up to 20 cm in diameter. Histologically, lymph cysts and lymphoceles are surrounded by smooth muscle cells. Differentiation between these structures and lymphangiectasia may be difficult and is often only possible from the clinical and peroperative findings. Differential diagnoses include enterogenic, pancreatogenic, nephrogenic cysts, true angiomata, parasitic cysts, false cyst following necrosis, and old hematomata.

Abnormal cellular infiltrations

Primary vascular tumors are considered elsewhere.

Leukocytoclastic vasculitis

This vasculitis, often confined to a single viscus, is characterised by a heavy infiltrate of neutrophils in the vascular wall. Nuclear debris is seen in and around blood vessels associated with haemorrhage and fibrinoid necrosis in larger vessels (Fig. 62). Immunoglobulins and complement components can be detected by direct immunofluorescence in the vascular walls. The lesion results from an immune complex-mediated process with infections (hepatitis C virus), drugs, and foreign proteins (staphylococcal protein A) as triggers. It occurs as a part of a number of auto-immune diseases including Henoch-Scholein purpura, erythema elevatum diutinum (Bury's disease), erythema nodosum, granuloma faciale, hypocomplementemic vasculitis, Wegener's disease, Behcet's disease, polyarteritis nodosa and neoplasia [64-69].

Eosinophilic vasculitis

This condition is characterised by the presence of eosinophils in the walls of blood vessels and may involve arteries, capillaries and veins (Fig. 63). Fibrinoid necrosis is rare. The wall of the vessel may be thickened and the lumen occluded. Cutaneous eosinophilic necrotizing vasculitis can

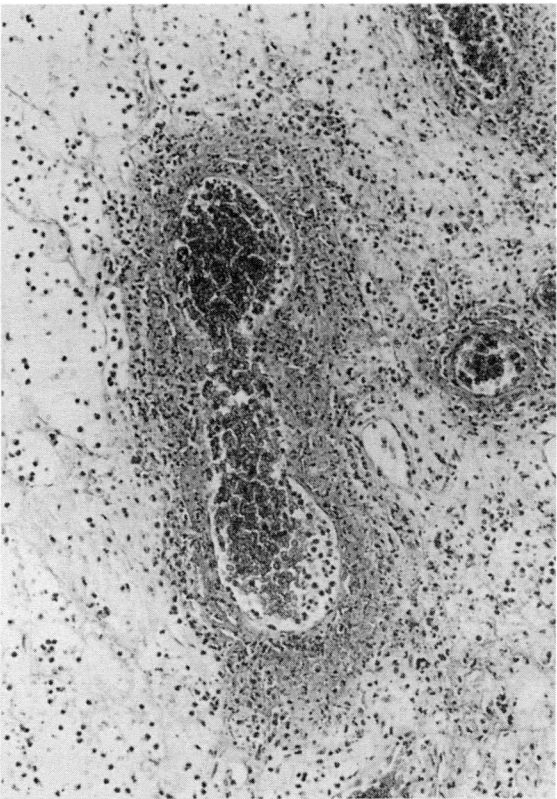

Fig. 62. Leukocytoclastic vasculitis. HES

be associated with common widespread pruritic, erythematous papules and angioedema of face and hands associated with peripheral blood eosinophilia [70-72]. Immunofluore-scence studies may evidence marked deposition of the cytotoxic eosinophil granule major basic protein, eosinophil adhesion molecule-1 on the endothelium of the affected vessels. Eosinophilic vasculitis occurs in eosinophilic granuloma, allergy (interstitial eosinophilic pneumoconiosis associated with asthma), connective tissue diseases and parasitic diseases. Churg-Strauss granulomatosis may show eosinophilic vasculitis.

Lymphocytic vasculitis

Lymphocytic vasculitis is characterised by the presence of lymphocytes within the vessel walls (Fig. 64). This lesion should be differentiated from ubiquitous perivascular infiltration of lymphocytes frequently

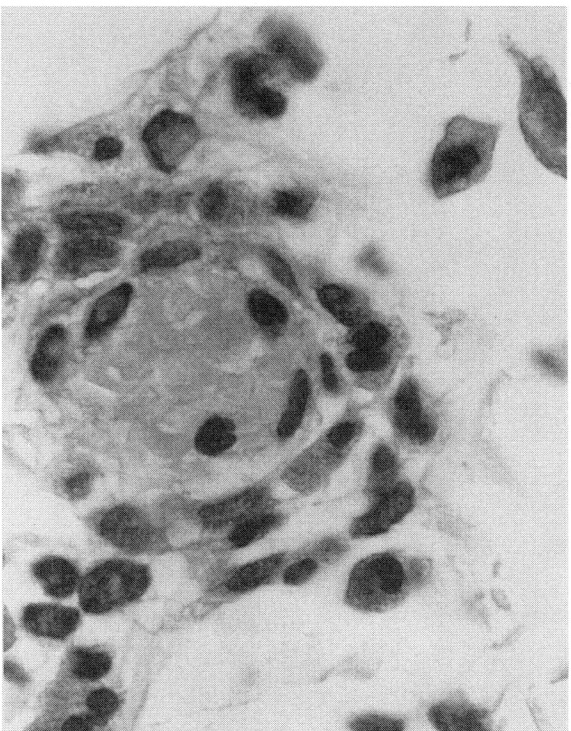

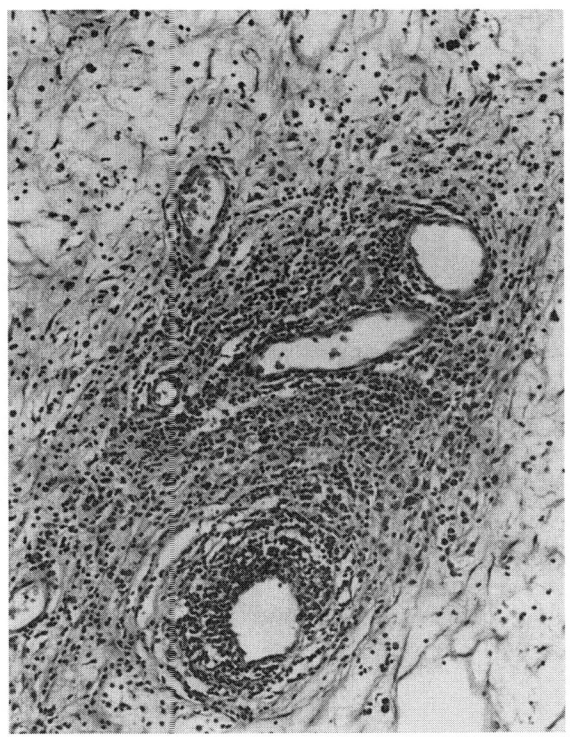

Fig. 63. Eosinophilic vasculitis. HES

Fig. 64. Lymphocytic vasculitis. HES

noted in an inflammatory process [73]. Lymphocytic vasculitis is commonly seen in lymphoproliferative disorders, whether they are benign, premalignant or malignant. Lymphocytic vasculitis occurs in allergies, Wegener's disease, erythema nodosum, lupus erythematosus, Behcet's disease, chronic ulcerative colitis, pityriasis lichenoides, mycobacterial, rickettsial and fungal infections and bacterial toxins [74-79].

Rejection-type vasculitis

In some forms of organ rejection the walls of vessels in the transplant are infiltrated with lymphocytes, plasma cells, immunoblasts and eosinophils. Small lymphocytes penetrate the subendothelial space and detach the endothelial cells, which undergo hyperplasia and degeneration, a change referred to as endothelialitis [80]. Immunohistochemistry has revealed that the lymphocytes are mostly T cells (UCHL1+). In reality, the lesions are complex in form and aetiology and have been recently reviewed in a number of organ systems [81]. The mechanism responsible for this vascular change is thought to be immunological; however, direct confirmation of this mechanism is lacking [82].

Endothelialitis is not specific to rejection phenomenon. This lesion can be noted in tertiary syphilis, Mediterranean boutonneuse fever, or in Sneddon syndrome, a condition characterised by the combination of skin lesions (livedo racemosa) and cerebral infarctions [83-87]. Endothelialitis also mimics uteroplacental vasculopathy in patients experiencing recurrent spontaneous abortions [88].

Granulomatous vasculitis

The term "granulomatous vasculitis" is confusing. It is used to designate various types of vasculitis: visceral giant cell arteritis [89], allergic eosinophilic vasculitis [90], necrotising polyarteritis nodosa in Wegener's granulomatosis [91], fibrinoid change or haemorrhage (or both) and granulomatous inflammation in and around vessel walls [92]. Granulomatous vasculitis may involve arteries, veins, lymphatics or capillaries.

Giant cell vasculitis is a variant of granulomatous vasculitis characterised by a predominance of giant multinucleated cells, often seen around fragmented elastic tissue (Fig. 65). Immunohistochemical tech-

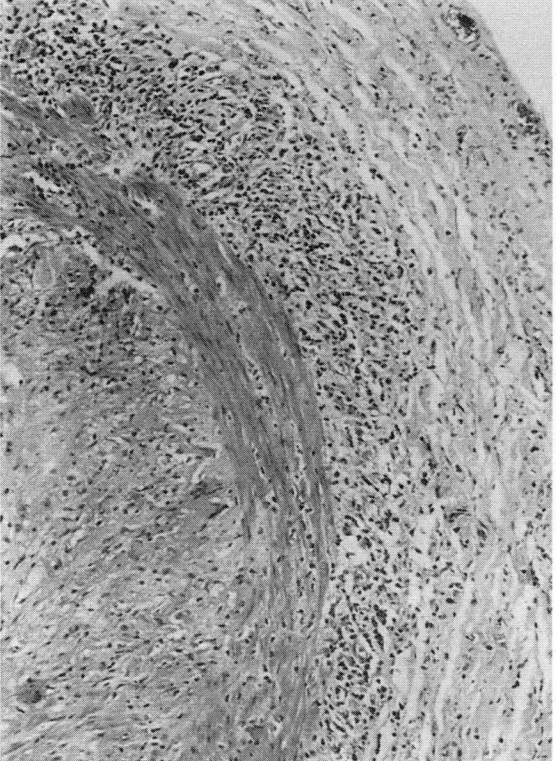

Fig. 65. Giant cell vasculitis. HES

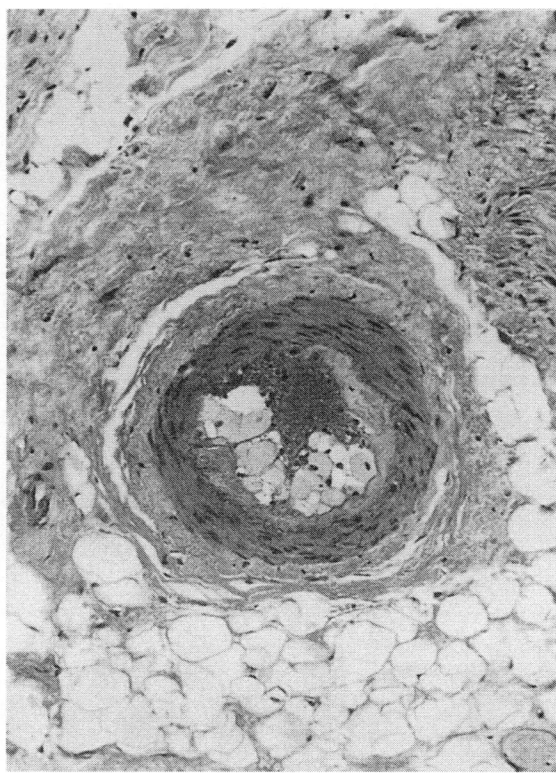

Fig. 66. Foam-cell vasculitis. HES

niques show tumour necrosis factor (TNF) in up to 60% of the cells (giant cells and macrophages) in all areas of inflamed arteries, suggesting that their predominant source is from the monocyte lineage [93]. However, the inflammatory infiltrate of GCA is tightly regulated, and cell accumulation in the granulomata is an active, not a passive, mechanism. The inflammatory pathway in GCA is focused on T cells and macrophages and excludes B cells [94]. This lesion should be differentiated from foreign body granulomata developed around intravascular foreign material from surgical procedures. This type of vasculitis can be part of polyarteritis nodosa, Wegener's granulomatosis, Churg-Strauss angiitis, or Takayasu's arteritis.

Foam-cell vasculitis

This lesion may involve arteries, veins, or capillaries. Grossly, the accumulation of foam cells results in yellowish, flat or mildly prominent areas where, histologically, macrophage foam cells infiltrate the intima and/or the media (Fig. 66). In chronic graft rejection and XR-induced or post-radiation vasculopathy, elas-

tic and muscular arteries have areas of intimal thickening with foam cell infiltration, oedema, myofibroblastic proliferation and fibrosis [23, 95].

Incorporation of foreign material within the vascular wall

Whatever the type of material used, fundamental lesions are similar. Generally, the inserted material is refringent to polarised light.

Suture threads

The severity of the granulomatous inflammatory process seen depends on the type of suture thread employed. Foreign body granulomata persist for a long time with non-resorbing threads (linen, silk, nylon, tergal, covered thread, stiff cotton thread). Absorbable sutures seldom disappear completely, but, whatever the type of suture material employed, fibrosis finally develops, making the sutured area stiff and sometimes stenotic (Fig. 67).

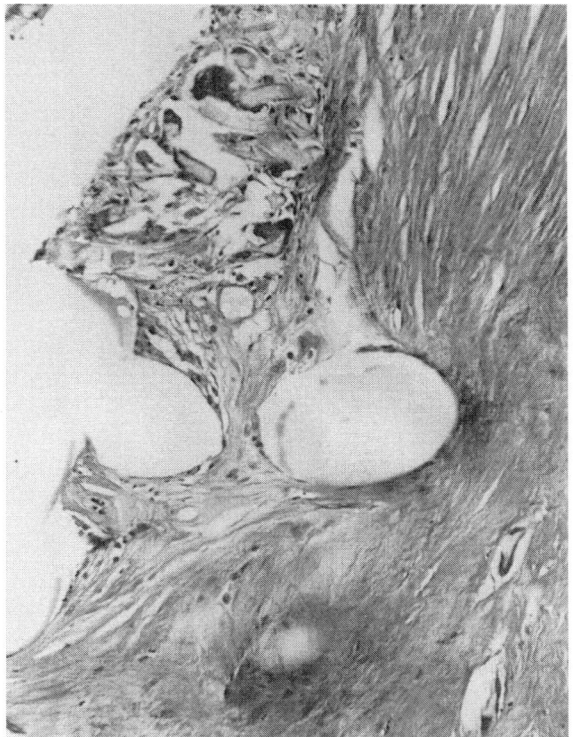

Fig. 67. Foreign body granulomata developed around a suture thread and a Dacron patch-graft. HES

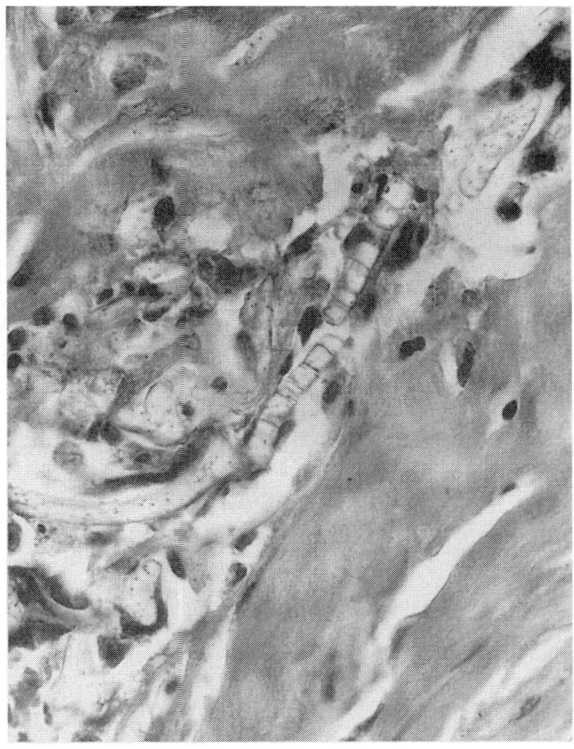

Fig. 68. Foreign body granuloma disintegrating a synthetic prosthetic fibre. HES

Patch-grafts

A patch-graft is used to close a vascular defect (arterial autografts, venous autografts, and synthetic materials may be used). Identification of the stitches enables the pathologist to locate the margins of the patch. Foreign body granulomata develop around synthetic materials which may undergo fragmentation (Fig. 68).

Vascular grafts and prostheses

Changes at anastomotic lines

On the luminal aspect, the recipient artery develops an intimal thickening which is often in a flap-like form extending over the edge of the graft or prosthesis (Fig. 69). Foreign body granulomata develop around suture threads in the recipient artery.

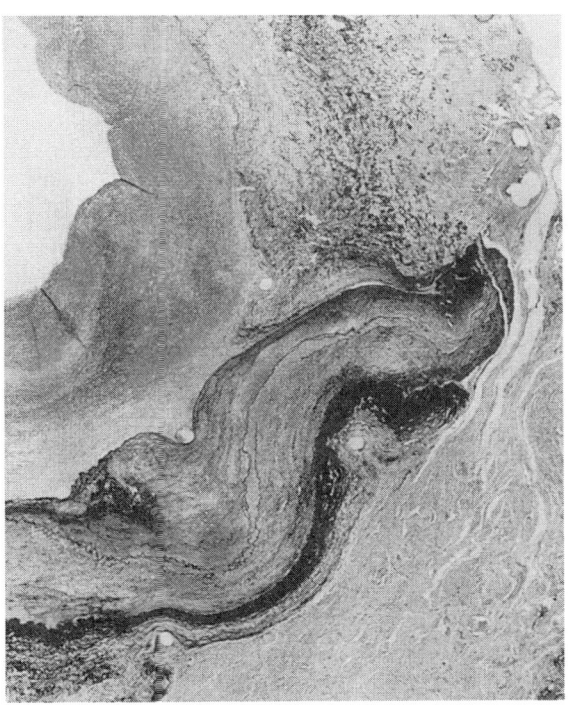

Fig. 69. Venous graft. Anastomotic intimal flap developed in the arterial side and sliding over the venous side. Note well-organised internal and external elastic lamellae of the recipient artery. Orcein

Adaptation of synthetic bypass grafts to the neighbouring tissue and the recipient artery

The bed or external capsule of the bypass is made up of connective tissue that connects the bypass to the surrounding tissue. There is an inflammatory reaction with fibrosis and foreign body granulomata may develop.

At the interface with the blood, changes occur differently in the middle part of the bypass and at its anastomoses. Immediately after implantation, the luminal aspect of the middle portion of the graft is covered with a thin layer of fibrin containing some platelets, monocytes, and leukocytes. Organisation of this layer in the 1st to 3rd weeks gives rise to a pseudo-intima. At the line of anastomosis, endothelial cells coming from the endothelium of the recipient artery slide over the anastomosis and effect a partial re-endothelialisation for a few millimetres. Endothelial cell markers (factor VIII, major blood group antigens) document this phenomenon. Development of a definitive endothelium far from the line of anastomosis is not always seen; the endothelium does not appear as a continuous sheet. Later, intimal hyperplasia of the recipient vessel leads to a "flap" overlapping the anastomotic line, which may cause stenosis with thrombosis [96-99].

Glues

Some adhesive agents have been used to treat acute dissection of the aorta, to control bleeding from prostheses or to anastomose microvessels [100-103]. Biological gelatin-resorcinol-formaldehyde (GRF) and fibrin (Tissucol, Tisseel) glue have been tested experimentally. GRF glue permits perfect anatomical repair and glue sealing seems to prevent recurrent dissection [104, 105]. The early histological changes in "sealed" areas are unknown except from experimental studies. On operative specimens from recurrent aortic dissection, the glue-sealed areas appear as hyaline fibrotic patches without inflammation. Elastin staining permits identification of this area, which is devoid of elastic fibers (Fig. 70).

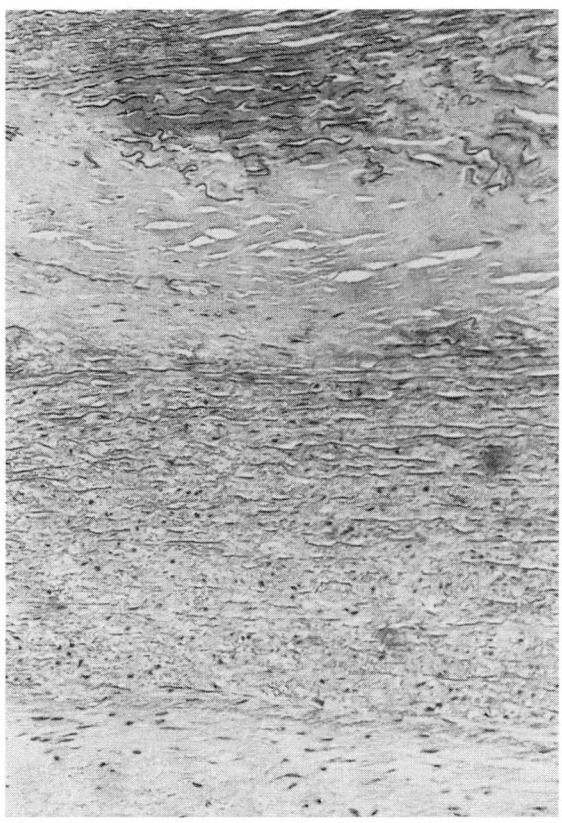

Fig. 70. Aortic dissection. Glue-sealed cleavage plane filled with fibrotic tissue devoid of elastic fibres. Orcein.

Bibliography

1. Lefebvre P, Motte S, Wautrecht JC, Cornez N, Delplace J, Dereume JP (1996) Livedo vasculitis: report of a case. J Mal Vasc 21: 50-3

2. Duong van Huyen JP, Fornes P, Iliou MC, Pagny JY, Guermonprez JL, Bruneval P (1996) Fatal coronary embolization following high-speed rotational atherectomy. Histopathology 29(1): 73-6

3. Matsuba T, Sujiura T, Irei M, Kyan Y, Kunishima N, Uchima H, Miyagi S, Iwata Y, Matsuba K (1994) Acute pneumonitis presumed to be silicone embolism. Intern Med 33: 481-3

4. Vuong PN, Cogan M, Nguyen PC, Colin JP, Piriou L (1995) Myxoma of the left atrium disclosed by femoral embolism. Value of anatomo-pathological study of the vascular desobstruction product (Letter) Presse Med 24: 1222

5. Vuong PN, P Lagneau P (1987) Pathologie artérielle traumatique In Camilleri JP, Berry CL, Fiessinger JN, Bariéty J: Les maladies de la paroi artérielle, Flammarion, Paris, p. 579

6. Lajvardi A, Trerotola SO, Strandberg JD, Samphilipo MA, Magee C (1995) Evaluation of venous injury caused by a percutaneous mechanical thrombolytic device. Cardiovasc Intervent Radiol 18: 172-8

7. DiMuzio PJ, Pratt KJ, Park PK, Carabasi RA (1994) Role of thrombin in endothelial cell monolayer repair in vitro. J Vasc Surg 20: 621-8

8. Silber S (1997) Rapid hemostasis of arterial puncture sites with collagen in patients undergoing diagnostic and interventional cardiac catheterization. Clin Cardiol 20: 981-92

9. Clowes AW, Clowes MM, Reidy MA (1986) Kinetics of cellular proliferation after arterial injury. III. Endothelial

and smooth muscle growth in chronically denuded vessels. Lab Invest 54: 295-303

10. Bjornsson TD, Dryjski M, Tluczek J, Mennie R, Ronan J, Mellin TN, Thomas KA (1991) Acidic fibroblast growth factor promotes vascular repair. Proc Natl Acad Sci U S A 88: 8651-5

11. Ettenson DS, Gotlieb AI (1994) Endothelial wounds with disruption in cell migration repair primarily by cell proliferation. Microvasc Res 48: 328-37

12. Schwartz SM, Majesky MW, Murry CE (1995) The intima: development and monoclonal responses to injury. Atherosclerosis 118: S125-S140

13. Doornekamp FN, Borst C, Post MJ (1996) Endothelial cell recoverage and intimal hyperplasia after endothelium removal with or without smooth muscle cell necrosis in the rabbit carotid artery. J Vasc Res 33: 146-55

14. Muller DW (1997) The role of proto-oncogenes in coronary restenosis. Prog Cardiovasc Dis 40: 117-28

15. Papadaki M, Eskin SG (1997) Effects of fluid shear stress on gene regulation of vascular cells. Biotechnol Prog 13: 209-21

16. Resnick N, Yahav H, Khachigian LM, Collins T, Anderson KR, Dewey FC, Gimbrone MA Jr (1997) Endothelial gene regulation by laminar shear stress. Adv Exp Med Biol 430: 155-64

17. Chien S, Li S, Shyy YJ (1998) Effects of mechanical forces on signal transduction and gene expression in endothelial cells. Hypertension 31: 162-9

18. Powell J, Greenhalgh RM (1989) Cellular, enzymatic and genetic factors in the pathogenesis of abdominal aortic aneurysms. J Vasc Surg 9: 297-304

19. Tilson MD (1992) Aortic aneurysms and atherosclerosis. Circulation 85: 205-11

20. Desoutter P, Vuong PN, Nguyen P-C, Bensenane J, Chemla E (1996) Anévrysme développé au niveau d'un pontage fémoro – poplité par greffon veineux ex-situ de dix ans (Lettre) Presse Med 25: 1039

21. Wilcox JN, Scott NA (1997) Potential role of the adventitia in arteritis and atherosclerosis. Int J Cardiol 54: S21-S35

22. Lagneau P, Michel JB, Vuong PN (1987) Surgical treatment of Takayasu's disease. Ann Surg 205: 157-66

23. Zidar N, Ferluga D, Hvala A, Popovic M, Soba E (1997) Contribution to the pathogenesis of radiation-induced injury to large arteries. J Laryngol Otol 111: 988-90

24. Takahashi H, Shibata Y, Fujita S, Okabe H (1996) Immunohistochemical findings of arterial fibrinoid necrosis in major and lingual minor salivary glands of primary Sjogren's syndrome. Anal Cell Pathol 12: 145-57

25. Itoh Y, Yamada M (1997) Cerebral amyloid angiopathy in the elderly: the clinicopathological features, pathogenesis, and risk factors. J Med Dent Sci 44: 11-9

26. Baldursson O, Steinsson K, Bjornsson J, Lie JT (1994) Giant cell arteritis in Iceland. An epidemiologic and histopathologic analysis. Arthritis Rheum 37: 1007-12

27. Bertrand E, Kuczynska-Zardzewialy A, Palasik W, Chorzelski T (1995) Rare vascular changes in the brain in a case of subacute cutaneous lupus erythematosus. Folia Neuropathol 33: 235-40

28. Gustafsson F (1997) Hypertensive arteriolar necrosis revisited. Blood Press 6: 71-7

29. Mönckeberg JG (1903) Über die reine Mediaverkalkung der Extremitätenarterien und ihr Verhalten zur Arteriosklerose. Virchows Arch (Pathol Anat) 171: 141-67

30. Cichocki T, Heck D, Jarczyk L, Rokita E, Strzalkowski A, Sych M (1989) Artery wall calcification: correlation of atherosclerosis with mineralization. Pathologica 81: 139-49

31. Stuart G, Wren C, Bain H (1990) Idiopathic infantile arterial calcification in two siblings: failure of treatment with diphosphonate. Brit. Heart J 64: 156-9

32. Kalbak K (1972) Incidence of arteriosclerosis in patients with rheumatoid arthritis receiving long-term corticosteroid therapy. Ann Rheum Dis 31: 196-200

33. Lie JT, Juergens JL (1980) Degenerative arterial diseases other than atherosclerosis In Juergens JL, Spittell JA, Fairbairn II JF (ed) Peripheral vascular diseases. Saunders, Philadelphia, London, Toronto 237-51

34. Semba CP, Sakai T, Slonim SM, Razavi MK, Kee ST, Jorgensen MJ, Hagberg RC, Lee GK, Mitchell RS, Miller DC, Dake MD (1998) Mycotic aneurysms of the thoracic aorta: repair with use of endovascular stent-grafts. J Vasc Interv Radiol 9: 33-40

35. Anderson LA (1994) An update on the cause of abdominal aortic aneurysms. J Vasc Nurs 12: 95-100

36. Halloran BG, Baxter BT (1995) Pathogenesis of aneurysms. Semin Vasc Surg 8: 85-92

37. Ghorpade A, Baxter BT (1996) Biochemistry and molecular regulation of matrix macromolecules in abdominal aortic aneurysms. Ann N Y Acad Sci 800: 138-50

38. Vuong PN, Escourrou J, Desoutter P, Houissa H (1986) Posttraumatic false aneurysm of the superficial temporal artery. Apropos of a case report and review of the medical literature. J Mal Vasc 11: 375-8

39. Meszaros I (1997) Aortic dissection. Orv Hetil 138: 843-9

40. Basso C, Morgagni GL, Thiene G (1996) Spontaneous coronary artery dissection: a neglected cause of acute myocardial ischaemia and sudden death. Heart 75: 451-4

41. Berry CL, Sosa-Melgarejo JA, Greenwald SE (1993) The relationship between wall tension, lamellar thickness, and intercellular junctions in the fetal and adult aorta: its relevance to the pathology of dissecting aneurysm. J Pathol 169: 15-20

42. Kodera K, Sakai A, Masakazu A, Lin ZB, Oosawa M (1997) A case report of chronic dissecting aortic aneurysm (Stanford type A) with circumferential detachment of the intima. Nippon Kyobu Geka Gakkai Zasshi 45: 2011-5

43. Nobrega J, Rosa M R, Santos RM, da Gama D, Ravara L (1997) Subisthmic aortic coarctation. Apropos a rare case of arterial hypertension. Rev Port Cardiol 16: 777-84

44. Goh WH, Lo R (1993) A new 3C syndrome: cerebellar hypoplasia, cavernous haemangioma and coarctation of the aorta. Dev Med Child Neurol 35: 637-41

45. Kurien A, John PR, Milford DV (1997) Hypertension secondary to progressive vascular neurofibromatosis. Arch Dis Child 76: 454-5

46. Mickley V, Lang G, Fleiter T, Sunder-Plassmann L (1997) Atypical aortic coarctations in type I neurofibromatosis. Zentralbl Chir 122: 735-42

47. Rossi MA (1997) Infrarenal aortic coarctation and diffuse hypoplasia of the aortoiliac-femoral system. Acta Cardiol 52: 273-9

48. Sarigul A, Yurdakul Y, Isbir S, Mercan S, Celiker A (1997) Bicuspid aortic valve and coarctation of aorta. Turk J Pediatr 39: 429-32

49. Vuong PN, Janzen J, Bical O, Susa-Uva M (1995) Fibromuscular dysplasia causing atypical coarctation of the thoracic aorta: Histologic presentation of a case. Vasa 24: 194-198

50. Suarez WA, Kurczynski TW, Bove EL (1999) An unusual type of combined aortic coarctation due to fibromuscular dysplasia Cardiol Young 9: 323-6

51. Bonhoeffer P, Bonnet D, Sidi D, Kachaner J (1997) Thrombus in coarctation of the aorta masquerading as an interrupted aortic arch. Heart 77: 183-4

52. Froelich JJ, Drude L, Klose KJ (1997) Severe calcifying atherosclerosis of the thoracic aorta with symptoms of aortic isthmus stenosis. Case report. Radiologe 37: 173-6

53. Janzen J, Vuong PN, Rothenberger-Janzen K (1999) Takayasu's arteritis and fibromuscular dysplasia as causes of acquired atypical coarctation of the aorta: retrospective analysis of seven cases. Heat Vessels 14: 277-82.

54. Leriche R (1943) Dolicho-méga artères et dolicho-méga veines: Allongement et dilatation, sans obstacles, de l'artère et de la veine iliaques primitives simulant un anévrysme. Presse Méd 38: 554-5

55. D'Andrea V, Malinovsky L, Bartolo M, Todini A, Biancari F, Catania A, Di Matteo FM, Manfredi RM, Bartolucci R, De Antoni E (1996) Arteriomegaly in the aorto-iliac-femoral area with or without associated aneurysm. Ann Ital Chir 67: 411-5

56. D'Andrea V, Malinovsky L, Cavallotti C, Benedetti Valentini F, Malinovska V, Bartolo M, Todini AR, Biancari F, Di Matteo FM, De Antoni E (1997) Angiomegaly. J Cardiovasc Surg (Torino) 38: 447-55

57. Hamazaki M, Saito A (1979) Beckwith-Wiedemann's syndrome – a report of an autopsied case –. Acta Pathol Jpn 29: 99-107

58. Kapur S, Kuehl KS, Midgely FM, Chandra RS (1985) Focal giant cell cardiomyopathy with Beckwith-Wiedemann syndrome. Pediatr Pathol 3: 261-9

59. Elliott M, Bayly R, Cole T, Temple IK, Maher ER (1994) Clinical features and natural history of Beckwith-Wiedemann syndrome: presentation of 74 new cases. Clin Genet 46: 168-74

60. D'Andrea V, Malinovsky L, Cavallotti C, Bartolo M, Todini A, Malinovska V, Di Matteo G (1992) Venous wall ultrastructure in generalized venomegaly. Cor Vasa 34: 265-72

61. Jimenez Cossio JA, San Martin P (1985) Chylous metrorrhea. Lymphology 18: 107-10

62. Junod JM (1985) Chylous metrorrhagia. J Cardiovasc Surg (Torino) 26: 107-9

63. Shahlaee AH, Burton EM, Sabio H, Plouffe L Jr, Teeslink R (1997) Primary chylous vaginal discharge in a 9-year-old girl: CT-lymphangiogram and MR appearance. Pediatr Radiol 27: 755-7

64. Abu-Shakra M, Koh ET, Treger T, Lee P (1995) Pericardial effusion and vasculitis in a patient with systemic sclerosis. J Rheumatol 22: 1386-8

65. Arbiser JL, Dzieczkowski JS, Harmon JV, Duncan LM (1995) Leukocytoclastic vasculitis following staphylococcal protein A column immunoadsorption therapy. Two cases and a review of the literature. Arch Dermatol 131: 707-9

66. Buezo GF, Garcia-Buey M, Rios-Buceta L, Borque MJ, Aragues M, Dauden E (1996) Cryoglobulinemia and cutaneous leukocytoclastic vasculitis with hepatitis C virus infection. Int J Dermatol 35: 112-5

67. Bohn S, Buchner S, Itin P (1997) Erythema nodosum: 112 cases. Epidemiology, clinical aspects and histopathology. Schweiz Med Wochenschr 127: 1168-76

68. Calabrese LH, Duna GF (1996) Drug-induced vasculitis. Curr Opin Rheumatol 8: 34-40

69. Gyselbrecht L, De Keyser F, Ongenae K, Naeyaert JM, Praet M, Veys EM (1996) Etiological factors and underlying conditions in patients with leucocytoclastic vasculitis. Clin Exp Rheumatol 14: 665-8

70. Chen KR, Su WP, Pittelkow MR, Leiferman KM (1995) Eosinophilic vasculitis syndrome: recurrent cutaneous eosinophilic necrotizing vasculitis. Semin Dermatol 14: 106-10

71. Chen KR, Su WP, Pittelkow MR, Conn DL, George T, Leiferman KM (1996) Eosinophilic vasculitis in connective tissue disease. J Am Acad Dermatol 35: 173-82

72. Ohwada S, Yanagisawa A, Joshita T, Yanagisawa T, Iino Y, Izumi M, Inoue T, Komiya J, Morishita Y (1997) Necrotizing granulomatous vasculitis of transverse colon and gallbladder. Hepatogastroenterology 44: 1090-4

73. Carlson JA, Mihm MC Jr, LeBoit PE (1996) Cutaneous lymphocytic vasculitis: a definition, a review, and a proposed classification. Semin Diagn Pathol 13: 72-90

74. Farrell AM, Gooptu C, Woodrow D, Costello C, Bunker CB, Cream JJ (1996) Cutaneous lymphocytic vasculitis in acute myeloid leukaemia. Br J Dermatol 135: 471-4

75. Chen KR, Kawahara Y, Miyakawa S, Nishikawa T (1997) Cutaneous vasculitis in Behcet's disease: a clinical and histopathologic study of 20 patients. J Am Acad Dermatol 36: 689-96

76. Chergui MH, Vandeperre J, Van Eeckhout P (1997) Enterocolic lymphocytic phlebitis: a case report. Acta Chir Belg 97: 293-6

77. Kao GF, Evancho CD, Ioffe O, Lowitt MH, Dumler JS (1997) Cutaneous histopathology of Rocky Mountain spotted fever. J Cutan Pathol 24: 604-10

78. Williamson RM, Walker NI, Searle JW, Stitz RW (1997) Large intestinal lymphocytic phlebitis and venulitis in chronic ulcerative colitis. Pathology 29: 12-6

79. Abe Y, Nakano S, Aita K, Sagishima M (1998) Streptococcal and staphylococcal superantigen-induced lymphocytic arteritis in a local type experimental model: comparison with acute vasculitis in the Arthus reaction. J Lab Clin Med 131: 93-102

80. Koskinen P, Lemstrom K, Bruggeman C, Lautenschlager I, Hayry P (1994) Acute cytomegalovirus infection induces a subendothelial inflammation (endothelialitis) in the allograft vascular wall. A possible linkage with enhanced allograft arteriosclerosis. Am J Pathol 144: 41-50

81. Ahsan N, Holman MJ, Katz DA, Abendroth CS, Yang HC (1997) Successful reversal of acute vascular rejection in a renal allograft with combined mycophenolate mofetil and tacrolimus as primary immunotherapy. Clin Transplant 11: 94-7

82. Hosenpud JD, Shipley GD, Wagner CR (1992) Cardiac allograft vasculopathy: current concepts, recent developments, and future directions. J Heart Lung Transplant 11: 9-23

83. Scaffidi L, Scaffidi A (1981) Characteristics of the rash in Mediterranean boutonneuse fever. Minerva Med 72: 2085-96

84. Zelger B, Sepp N, Stockhammer G, Dosch E, Hilty E, Ofner D, Aichner F, Fritsch PO (1993) Sneddon's syndrome. A long-term follow-up of 21 patients. Arch Dermatol 129: 437-47

85. Canta LR, Koedijk FH, Tijssen CC (1994) Sneddon's syndrome: an unusual cause of cerebral infarct at a relatively young age. Ned Tijdschr Geneeskd 138: 963-7

86. Drobacheff C, Moulin T, Van Landuyt H, Merle C, Vigan M, Laurent R (1994) Cutaneous tertiary syphilis with neurological symptoms. Ann Dermatol Venereol 121: 34-6

87. Sepp N, Zelger B, Schuler G, Romani N, Fritsch P (1995) Sneddon's syndrome—an inflammatory disorder of small arteries followed by smooth muscle proliferation. Immunohistochemical and ultrastructural evidence. Am J Surg Pathol 19: 448-53

88. Kohut KG, Anthony MN, Salafia CM (1997) Decidual and placental histologic findings in patients experiencing spontaneous abortions in relation to pregnancy order. Am J Reprod Immunol 37: 257-61

89. Alguacil-Garcia GF, Moreno-Requena J, Martinez-Albadalejo M, Hallal-Hachem H, Gonzalez-Pina B, de Paco-Moya M (1995) Idiopathic granulomatous vasculitis: response to immunosuppressive therapy. J Clin Pathol 48: 579-82

90. Alwie ML, Wakaki K, Kurashige Y, Koizumi F (1995) Experimental granulomatous vasculitis induced by sensitization with Ascaris suum antigen in mice. Pathol Int 45: 914-24

91. Aoki N, Soma K, Owada T, Ishii H (1995) Wegener's granulomatosis complicated by arterial aneurysm. Intern Med 34: 790-3

92. Gibson LE, el-Azhary RA, Smith TF, Reda AM (1994) The spectrum of cutaneous granulomatous vasculitis: histopathologic report of eight cases with clinical correlation. J Cutan Pathol 21: 437-45

93. Field M, Cook A, Gallagher G (1997) Immuno-localisation of tumour necrosis factor and its receptors in temporal arteritis. Rheumatol Int 17: 113-8

94. Martinez-Taboada V, Brack A, Hunder GG, Goronzy JJ, Weyand CM (1996) The inflammatory infiltrate in giant cell arteritis selects against B lymphocytes. J Rheumatol 23: 1011-4

95. Deligeorgi-Politi H, Wight DG, Calne RY (1994) Chronic rejection of liver transplants revisited. Transpl Int 7: 442-7

96. Camilleri JP, Phat VN, Bruneval P, Tricottet V, Balaton A, Fiessinger JN, Cormier JM (1985) Surface healing and histologic maturation of patent polytetrafluoroethylene grafts implanted in patients for up to 60 months. Arch Pathol Lab Med 109: 833-7

97. Shi Q, Wu MH, Onuki Y, Ghali R, Hunter GC, Johansen KH, Sauvage LR (1997) Endothelium on the flow surface of human aortic Dacron vascular grafts. J Vasc Surg 25: 736-42

98. Vuong PN, Cormier JM (1987) Pathologie de l' artère opérée In Camilleri JP, Berry CL, Fiessinger J-N, Bariéty J: Les maladies de la paroi artérielle, Flammarion, Paris, 591

99. Vuong PN, Cheilan F, Houissa-Vuong S (1999) Pathologie des prothèses vasculaires. Ann Pathol 19: 195-202

100. Olivier A, Leandri J, Loisance D (1982) Experimental test of two tissue adhesives (GRF and IBC 2) in vascular microsurgery in the rat. J Chir (Paris) 119: 261-6

101. Citrin P, Doscher W, Wise L, Margolis IB (1985) Control of needle hole bleeding with ethyl-cyanoacrylate glue (Krazy Glue). J Vasc Surg 2: 488-90

102. Wadstrom J, Wik O (1993) Fibrin glue (Tisseel) added with sodium hyaluronate in microvascular anastomosing. Scand J Plast Reconstr Surg Hand Surg 27: 257-61

103. Werker PM, Kon M (1997) Review of facilitated approaches to vascular anastomosis surgery. Ann Thorac Surg 63: S122-S127

104. Guilmet D (1990) Chirurgie des dissections aiguës de l'aorte. Encycl Med Chir (Elsevier, Paris). Instantanés Médicaux 9: 1-12

105. Latremouille C, Fabiani JN (1996) Dissection aortique. Encycl Med Chir (Elsevier, Paris). Cardiologie – Angéiologie, 11-650-A-10, 10p

IV
Atherosclerosis

1 – Definition

Atherosclerosis (AS) is a progressive disease resulting from "an association of variable alterations of the intima of arteries, which consists of a focal accumulation of lipids, complex glucids, blood and its products, fibrotic tissue and calcium deposition" [1]. These alterations lead to fibrosis, calcification, narrowing, occlusion and structural weakening of the arterial wall.

2 – Epidemiology

No disease is responsible for more deaths in developed countries than atherosclerosis. In the United States of America in 1987, 976,706 of the 2,127,000 deaths (46%) were attributed to diseases of the heart and blood vessels, most of these to atherosclerosis and its complications [2]. The widespread variation in incidence in different nations indicates the role of a number of personal and environmental factors that have been widely studied over many years, resulting in the identification of a number of risk factors for the manifestations of the disease.

This work began in 1948 with the Framingham studies established by Dawber in the USA and Ancel Key's Seven Countries Study, carried out mainly in Europe [3, 4]. Multifactorial causation was accepted by the 1960's and the risk factors of age, gender, hypercholesterolaemia, hypertension and cigarette smoking were established. In addition, these longitudinal studies established the importance of myocardial infarction as a cause of sudden death, the dangers of arrhythmia and the role of ischaemia in heart failure, none of which had previously been fully appreciated.

3 – Risk factors

Firmly established risk factors for atherosclerotic disease now include age, gender, hypercholesterolaemia, hypertriglyceridaemia, decreased high-density lipoprotein, diabetes mellitus, arterial hypertension, elevated plasma homocysteine, some hypercoagulable states, tobacco use and a sedentary life-style. A corollary of certain of these hypotheses is that atherosclerosis may be attenuated by adequate modification of diet and physical exercise, and the constant surveillance of the patient [5].

Risk factors not readily modified

Age

It is often asserted – wrongly – that early lesions of atherosclerosis appear in childhood [6]. Misinterpretation of growth and remodelling events in development has resulted in confusion about what constitutes the early stages of the disease. The careful studies of Stary and his American Heart Association groups [7-9] have documented the evolution of intimal lesions in infancy and childhood through to a classification of complicated lesions (see Table 1). Although a number of studies have shown that risk factors probably operate from early in life [10] it is clear that clinically significant manifestations of the disease, including myocardial infarction (MI), increase with age; this complication rises with each decade except in the very young. Five percent of MI occur in people under age 40, and 45% occur under age 65 [11]. Autopsy reveals atherosclerosis to some degree in nearly all people over 50 years of age, suggesting to some that it should be regarded as part of the normal ageing process as well as a disease [12]. Any investigation of the aetiology of atherosclerosis requires a distinction between atherosclerosis related to ageing and pathological atherosclerosis causing disease and/or death.

Sex

Males are more severely affected than females. Protection is clearly oestrogen related and post-menopausal females appear to show progression of the disease in a trajectory closely comparable to that seen in males. The cardiovascular protective action of estrogen is reported to be mediated indirectly by an effect on lipoprotein metabolism and by a direct effect on the vessel wall itself. Estrogen is active both in vascular smooth muscle and endothelium. Functionally competent estrogen receptors have been identified in vascular smooth muscle cells, and specific binding sites have been demonstrated in endothelium.

Estrogen administration promotes vasodilatation in part by stimulating prostacyclin and nitric oxide synthesis. Both the prostaglandin synthase and the constitutive nitric oxide synthase are induced by estrogen treatment. In vitro, estrogen exerts a direct inhibitory effect on the smooth muscle by inhibiting calcium influx. In addition, estrogen inhibits vascular smooth muscle cell proliferation [13-17]. Experimentally, oral contraceptive treatment may inhibit atherogenesis by decreasing arterial LDL degradation [18]. Myocardial infarction is uncommon in premenopausal women unless a number of the well-defined risk factors are present. This finding is equally valuable for blacks and whites [11].

Familial predisposition

The work of Barker and others [19-21] has shown that the role of genetics and development is expressed as complex interactions in determining familial predisposition to atherosclerosis. Some classical risk factors, including hereditary disorders of lipoprotein metabolism and the familial dyslipoproteinaemias [22, 23], and elevation in plasma homocysteine [12, 24], are of major significance in small groups of the population. In general, however, familial histories of IHD often occur against a background of polygenic or multifactorial causation. In familial hypercholesterolaemia more than 350 mutations at the locus for the receptor for LDL have been found. Most are specific to particular families, but some are concentrated in particular population groups, such as French Canadians [25]. Certain mutations appear more common in some geographical areas – Glasgow, Scotland, is one such site [26].

Hypertension

Although well defined causes of hypertension exist, it is clear that in most instances blood pressure is determined polygenically and that levels of pressure may be set, in terms of a place in centiles, very early in life [27, 28]. Thus a relatively high arterial pressure will enhance the accumulation of cholesterol in the vessel wall at higher-pressure centiles in individuals. Endothelial cells are subjected to both fluid shear stress and cyclic hoop stretch forces that influence cell function [29, 30]. These loads induce cell elongation and the formation of stress fibers, increase the production of tissue plasminogen activator, and enhance von Willebrand factor release with subsequent platelet aggregation, increased permeability, pinocytosis and lipoprotein transfer [31, 32].

Acquired risk factors

Hyperlipidaemia

Hyperlipidaemia clearly plays a significant role in the genesis of atherosclerosis; the many strands of evidence include the following briefly summarised factors. The major lipid components in atheromatous plaques are cholesterol and cholesterol esters derived from the plasma [33]. In Man, particularly within defined population groups, there is a significant correlation between the total plasma cholesterol or low-density lipoprotein (LDL) level and the mortality rate from IHD. There is no clear threshold separating persons at risk from those free of risk but, in general, symptoms are uncommon when the total serum cholesterol levels are below 150mg/dl. The major component of the lipid composition of the atheromatous lesions derives from the circulating cholesterol and other lipids, particularly in the form of low-density lipoproteins (LDL) [34]. Increased blood pressure and vessel radius predispose to the local insudation of lipid and there is a close relationship between sites where turbulent blood flow occurs and the prevalence of raised plaques. As we have seen, hereditary disorders, and some acquired causes of hypercholesterolaemia (diabetes mellitus) lead to premature and more extensive atherosclerosis. Many groups have shown that high-cholesterol diets can produce atherosclerotic lesions in a wide variety of experimental animals. Atherosclerotic plaques regress or fail to progress when levels of serum cholesterol are lowered by diet or drugs in a number of experimental models. Genetic manipulation of mice producing various abnormalities of lipid metabolism, including apolipoprotein E deficiency, leads to abnormal lipid metabolism and atherosclerotic plaques. These lesions also represent an attractive target for the development of somatic gene transfer (gene therapy) intended to modulate systemic factors with the goal of inhibiting disease progression [35, 36].

Smoking

The death rate from IHD doubles when the patient consumes one or more packs of cigarettes per day for several years. Smoking greatly augments atherosclerosis of the abdominal aorta, and has a major role in formation of abdominal aortic aneurysms [37]. The effects of heavy smoking are independent of blood pressure, serum cholesterol and body weight and depend on adverse effects on the intima and on platelet activity [38, 39].

Diabetes mellitus

This condition induces hypercholesterolaemia and leads to atherosclerosis of greater severity at an earlier age than in non-diabetic patients [40]. The question of whether diabetes mellitus acts independently or in conjunction with hyperlipoproteinemia in the development of atherosclerosis has not been resolved [39, 41].

Local metabolic factors

Endothelial permeability is not a passive phenomenon and the endothelium is a metabolically active organ, exhibiting respiration, glycolysis, and oxidative phosphorylation. In this active tissue complex glycosylation adducts form with time and advanced glycosylation end (AGE) products accumulate on long-lived molecules, such as collagen and nucleic acids. There they may trap soluble plasma proteins covalently and act as signals for macrophage recognition and uptake. Recognition and uptake of AGE-proteins by macrophages further contribute to the process of atherogenesis by stimulating release of macrophage secretory products, including macrophage-derived growth factor [42-45].

Other factors

Although well documented in a number of studies, the role of a number of other factors, including lack of physical exercise, a "stressful" life style, psychic state, obesity, oral contraceptive use, hyperuricaemia and infections on the genesis of atherosclerotic lesions suggests that none of them is a major component. They may be of more significance in the production complications of established disease (for example, thrombosis).

4 – Pathogenesis

Historically, there have been two main hypotheses

The "thrombogenic" theory of von Rokitansky (1852), based on observations in Man, postulated that fibrinous substances deposited from the lumen upon the arterial surface undergo metamorphosis into a mass composed of large numbers of cholesterol crys-

tals and of fatty globules. Intimal thickening results from a deposit of fibrin associated with the subsequent organisation of fibroblasts and vascularization leading to a secondary accumulation of lipids.

The "imbibition" theory arose from the results of experimental studies conducted by Ignatovski in 1908, and Anitschkov and Chalatov in 1913 [46,-48]. Following Anitschkow's production of atheromatous lesions in rabbits by cholesterol feeding, a large body of accumulated clinical and experimental evidence suggests those atherosclerosis results from changes in lipid metabolism. Anitschkow attributed this disorder to either excessive consumption of lipids or impaired control of lipid metabolism by an endocrine organ [49]. It is clear that the lipid theory, which evolved through various stages from a simplistic view to a series of sophisticated biochemical arguments, retains a central importance in the pathogenesis of atherosclerosis. Nevertheless there is little doubt that the thrombogenic mechanism plays a prominent part in the progression of plaque stage atherosclerosis. Ulceration of the plaque breaks the endothelial cover and blood interacts with the deeper components of the lesion leading to adhesion, activation and aggregation of platelets with thrombosis. The thrombotic material may become overgrown by endothelium and incorporated into the intima [48, 50].

An "Inflammatory" mechanism

More recently it has been suggested that the processes of adhesion of monocytes and lymphocytes to the endothelial cell surface, migration of monocytes into the sub-endothelial space and differentiation into macrophages, all of which are part of the pathogenesis of atherosclerosis, occur as a result of infection. The subsequent ingestion of low density lipoproteins and modified or oxidised low density lipoproteins by macrophages leads to accumulation of cholesterol esters, the formation of foam cells and calcification [51,52]. Vascular dendritic cells (VDCs) are also found to be distributed throughout atherosclerotic lesions and to be in contact with other intimal cells, including macrophages, smooth muscle cells, foam cells and lymphocyte-like cells [53-55]. A large number of growth factors, cytokines and vasoregulatory molecules regulate these processes and approaches to modifying specific cellular interactions, growth-regulatory molecules or controlling the expression of genes encoding these molecules may provide opportunities for lesion prevention or regression [56-58].

The current interest in a possible link between infectious diseases and atherosclerosis had its roots in several studies published in the late 1980s. Patients with myocardial infarction were reported to carry antibodies related to *Chlamidia pneumoniae* [59-61]. This pathogen has been identified in coronary atherosclerotic plaques [62] and, in vitro, human umbilical vein endothelial cells (HUVEC) can serve as hosts to *C. pneumoniae* [63]. Recently, two strains of *Helicobacter pylori* have been found in association with an increased incidence of heart disease [64-66] but the significance of these findings is problematic. The presence of herpes simplex viral mRNA has been demonstrated in human artery wall tissue in individuals with evidence of atherosclerosis [67, 68] but to the authors this seems to be co-incidental. The same is probably true of cytomegalovirus infection(CMV), which shows tropism for the vascular tree [69-71].

The "Response-to-injury" hypothesis

Focal endothelial damage leads to increased endothelial permeability or other evidence of endothelial dysfunction [72]. Increased permeability of the endothelium and insudation of platelet factors, plasma lipoproteins and other plasma constituents at these sites of injury lead to many focal cellular interactions. These may involve endothelial cells, smooth muscle cells of intimal and medial origin, monocytes, macrophages, T lymphocytes and their surrounding connective matrix. Activated endothelium also promotes the adhesion of monocytes and their transmigration into the intima. The co-ordinated expression of adhesion molecules of the selectin, integrin or immunoglobulin superfamily on the surface of endothelial cells and of monocytes modulates these events. Having migrated into the intima, monocytes undergo morphological and functional modifications leading to the generation of the polypeptide mediator network instrumental in the migration, differentiation and proliferation of smooth muscle cells.

5 – Pathology and differential diagnosis

Macroscopy

Grossly, lesions are classified into five types (Table 1): the lipid deposits, the lipid or fatty streaks, the gelatinous plaques, the fibrolipidic plaques or fibroathero-

mas, and the complicated lesions. All these lesions may develop in the same area of an artery.

Lipid deposits

Lipid deposits are seen as yellowish, flat or mildly prominent, well-circumscribed oval points measuring about 0.5mm in diameter (Fig. 1). Lipid deposits in the aorta are noticed in 43% of infants under 1. Beyond this age, they are always present [73, 74].

Lipid or fatty streaks

These are discrete prominent linear lesions, 1 to several mm long, parallel to the blood flow axis (Fig. 1). The lesions can interconnect in a reticulate network. Lipid streaks can resorb, remain stable or develop further. Their outcome depends on the site, the patient's age and the ethnic group [75, 76].

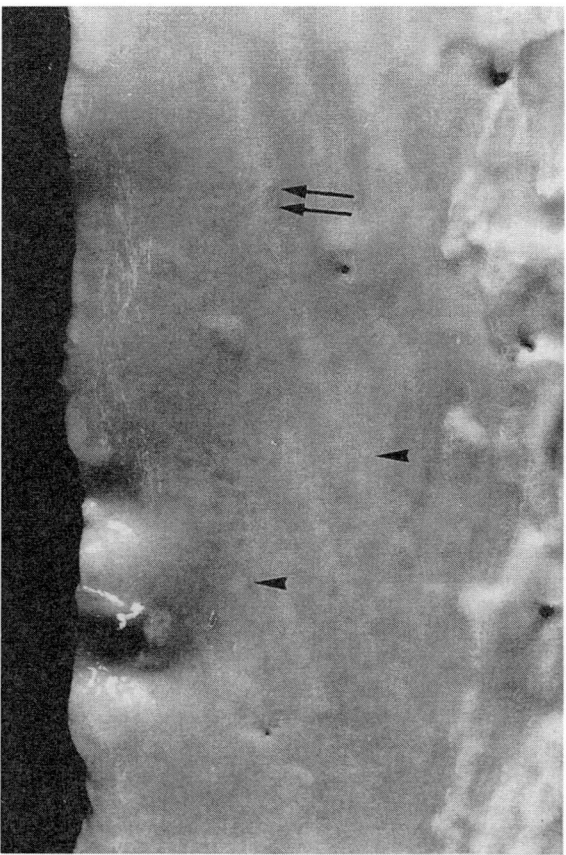

Fig. 1. Atheromatous aorta. Note lipid deposits (arrow heads) and lipid or fatty streaks (arrows) disseminated in the intima

Table 1. Classification of human atherosclerotic lesions by macroscopical and histological patterns, sequences of progression, growth mechanism and onset, with clinical correlation according to the Committee on Vascular Lesions of the Council on Arteriosclerosis, American Heart Association (9). NB : types Vb and Vc of this classification correspond respectively to type VII* and VIII* lesions of classifications published elsewhere (7, 8).

Types	Histology	Sequence in progression	Main growth mechanism	Age of onset and clinical correlation
Type I (initial) lesion	Isolated macrophage foam cell	I-> II	Lipid accumulation	Infants and children (1st decade)
Type II (fatty streak) lesion	Intracellular lipid accumulation	II->III	Lipid accumulation	Infants and children (1st-2nd decades)
Type III (intermediate) lesion	Type II lesion + Extracellular lipid pools	III->IV	Lipid accumulation	Adolescents and young adults (3rd decade)
Type IV (atheroma) lesion	Type II lesion + core of extracellular lipid	IV->V IV-VI	All lesions that disrupt intimal structure : Lipid accumulation and thrombus incorporation	Adults (3rd decade). Potentially symptom-producing lesion
Type V (fibro-atheroma)	Va : multiple lipid cores and fibrotic layers Vb : mainly calcific (type VII*) Vc : mainly fibrotic (typeVIII*)	V->VI	Accelerated proliferation of smooth muscle and deposit of collagen. Accumulation of lymphocytes, macrophages and macrophage foam cells	Older persons (after 3rd decade). Potentially symptom-producing lesion
Type VI (complicated) lesion	VIa :disruption of the surface VIb : haematoma, haemorrhage VIc : Thrombosis VIabc :VI(a+b+c)		Thrombosis, Haematoma	Older persons (after 3rd decade). Potentially symptom-producing lesion

Gelatinous plaques

These plaques are translucid, greyish, surelevated areas of the intima (Fig. 2). They are frequently isolated and measure from 0.8 mm to 1-cm. gelatinous plaques can resorb. Their presence at the periphery of advanced lesions indicates progression of the disease [77].

Fibrolipidic plaques or fibroatheromas

These structures are whitish-grey and surelevated lesions whose size varies from 1 to 3 cm (Fig. 3). Cross section reveals a yellow core sandwiched between the intima and the intima-media transitional zone. Fibrolipidic plaques are permanent and irreversible, and can be stabilised or may develop further [78].

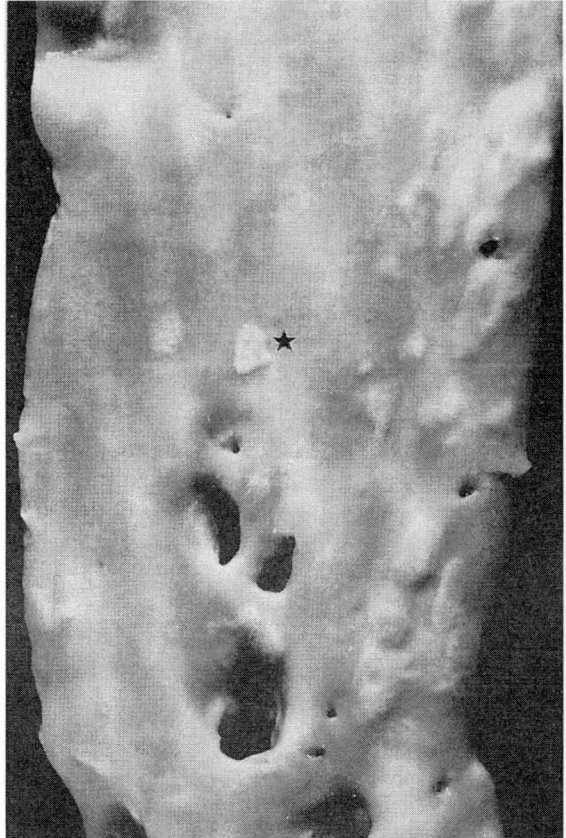

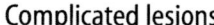

Fig. 2. Atheromatous aorta. Gelatinous plaque (star)

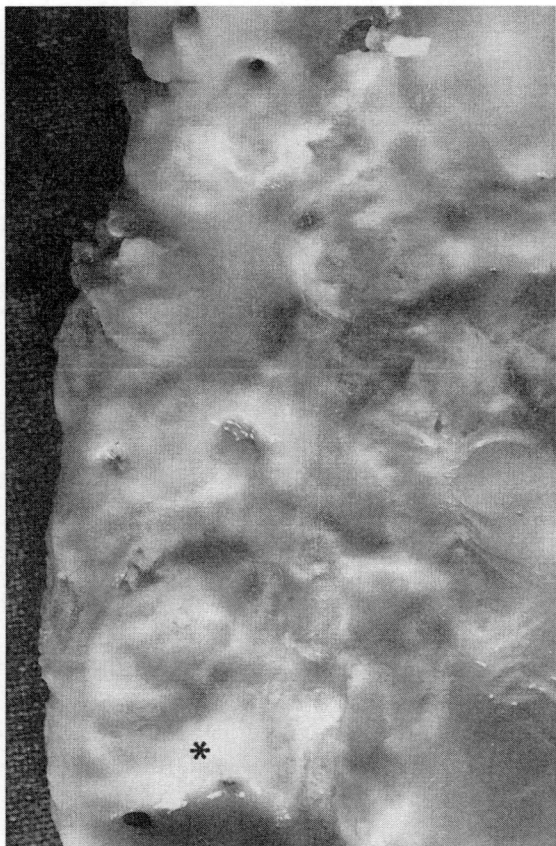

Fig. 3. Atheromatous aorta. Fibrolipidic plaque or fibroatheroma (asterisk)

Complicated lesions

These include calcification (Fig. 4), intra-plaque hae-morrhage, ulceration, thrombosis (Fig. 5) and embolism.

Histology

Atherosclerotic lesions initially involve the intima alone. According to the Committee on Vascular Lesions of the Council on Arteriosclerosis of the American Heart Association [9], histological atherosclerotic lesions can be resolved into six (I-VI) types, each characterised by its cells, matrix, composition and architecture, or other specific features, which may account for the variable risk for further complications [8, 9, 79 ,80]. This classification attempts to correlate the appearance of lesions noted in clinical imaging studies with histological lesion types and corresponding clinical syndromes. In the histological classification, lesions are designated by Roman numerals, which indicate the usual sequence of lesion progres-sion. The numerals I-VI represent the usual sequence in which lesions develop and progress from the initial accumulations of lipoproteins and macrophages to atheroma and fibroatheroma stages, which are susceptible to thrombotic deposits and ischaemic clinical episodes.

Type I lesion

This initial lesion is made up of small infiltrates of macrophage foam cells containing esterified cholesterol. This lesion is more marked at sites of adaptive intimal thickening. These lesions are generally not a precursor of atherosclerosis.

Type II lesion

This consists of layers of macrophage foam cells and lipid-laden smooth muscle cells; the definition includes lesions grossly designated as fatty streaks (Fig.6).

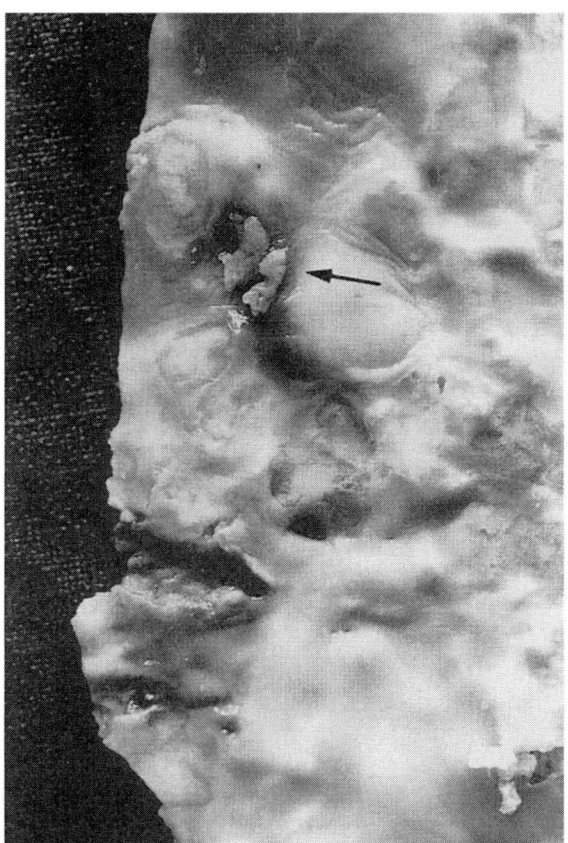

Fig. 4. Atheromatous aorta. Calcified plaque (arrow)

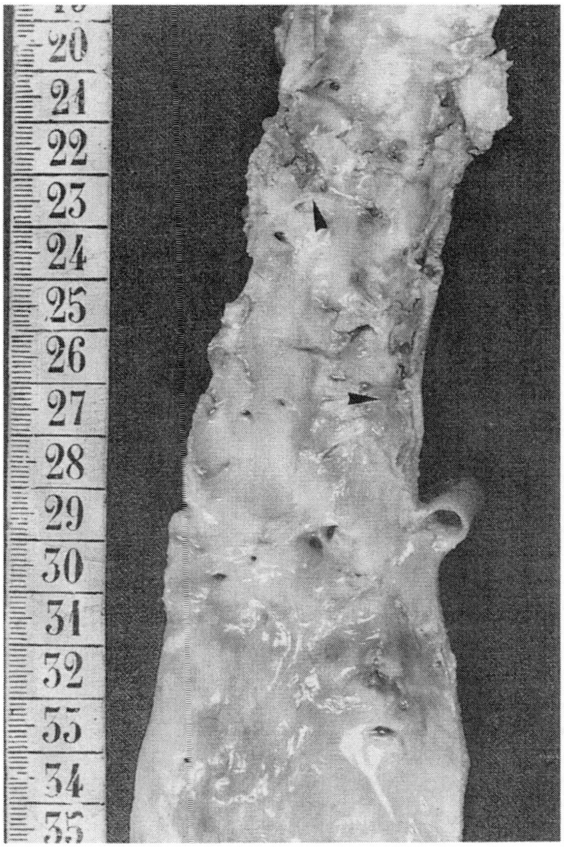

Fig. 5. Atheromatous aorta. Ulcerated plaque with overlying thrombosis (arrow heads)

Type III lesion

Type III lesions occur mainly in adolescents and young adults and are morphologically intermediate between the small lesions of children (I and II) and the potentially symptom-producing type IV lesion. In addition to the lipid-laden cells of type II, type III lesions contain scattered collections of extracellular lipid droplets and particles that disrupt the coherence of some intimal smooth muscle cells (Fig. 7). Type III lesions include gelatinous plaques. Fibrosis occurs when the plaque enlarges [78].

Types IV, V and VI lesions

The type IV lesion (fibrolipid plaque or fibroatheroma) is characterised by a larger, confluent, and more disruptive core of extracellular lipid made up of cholesterol and its esters, neutral lipids in great amounts and cellular debris, interspersed with lipid-loaded myocytes. This structure is covered by a fibrous cap containing glycosaminoglycans (GAG) and

elastic fibers. The entirety lifts up the endothelium and compresses the underlying media. First appearing around the fourth decade of life, type IV lesions may also contain thick layers of loose and dense fibrotic tissue (type V lesion) and/or complications such as disruption of the lesion surface or fissures, haematoma or haemorrhage, and thrombosis (type VI lesion). Type V lesions are subdivided into three subgroups according to the lesion patterns: Va type having multiple lipid cores and fibrotic layers, Vb type being mainly calcific and Vc type mainly fibrotic. Types Vb and Vc of this classification correspond respectively to types VII* and VIII* lesions of other previous classifications published elsewhere [7, 8, 81]. Calcification may undergo osseous metaplasia with haematopoiesis present (Fig. 8). A polypoid lesion projecting into the lumen may occur, but this is rare, although the tendency for the complication to occur at sites of dilatation permits development of post-dilatation stenosis [82].

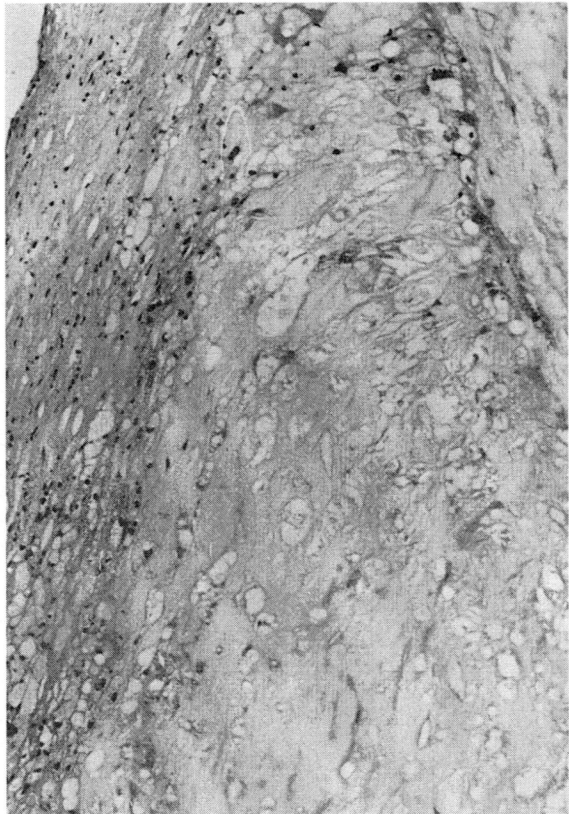

Fig. 6. Type II lesion made up of infiltrates of foam cells and lipid-laden smooth muscle cells. Haematoxylin, eosin and saffron stain (HES)

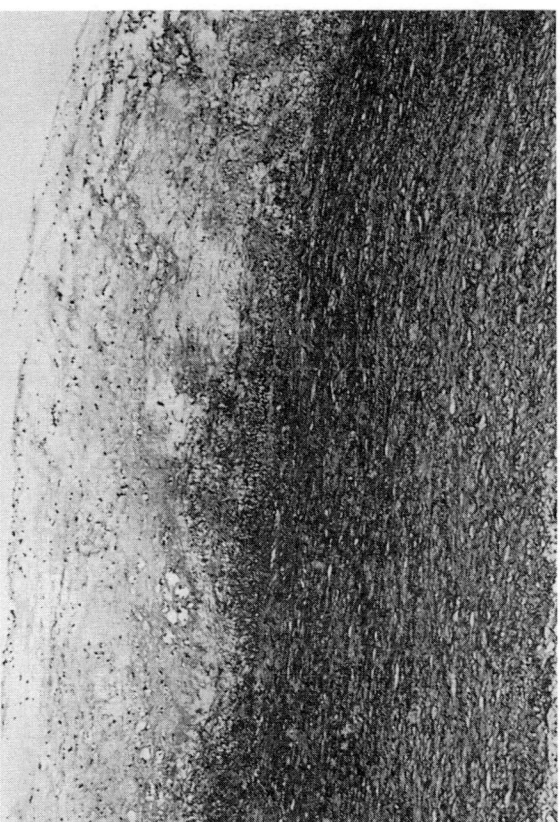

Fig. 7. Type III lesion. Note disruption of the intima. Orcein elastic stain (Orcein)

Type VI (complicated) lesion

Complications include ulceration, haemorrhage, haematoma formation and thrombosis. Type VI encompasses 4 subgroups: VIa type presenting ulceration or disruption of the lesion surface, VIb type distorted by haematoma or haemorrhage, VIc type capped by thrombosis and VIabc type when all the complications are concomitant.

Plaque disruption or ulceration

Necrosis of the cap of a plaque with rupture and subsequent thrombosis (Fig. 9) is the basis of most of the severe clinical consequences of atherosclerosis. Bleeding from the vasa vasora or the granulation tissue around it may contribute to this process [83]. However, the propensity of atherosclerotic plaques to disrupt is influenced by their lipid content and the distribution of these lipids within the plaque [33]. Plaques with increased lipid content appear more prone to rupture, particularly when the lipid pool is localised eccentrically within the intima. Macrophages, perhaps by participating in the uptake and metabolism of lipoproteins, secretion of growth factors, and production of enzymes and toxic metabolites, may facilitate plaque rupture. The particular composition or configuration of a plaque and the haemodynamic forces to which it is exposed may determine its susceptibility to disruption. Cellular processes, possibly including apoptosis, may destabilise the plaque and promote rupture [84-86]. Exposure of collagen, lipids, and smooth muscle cells after plaque rupture leads to the activation of platelets and the coagulation cascade system. Acute changes in coronary plaque morphology (plaque disruption, thrombus or both) are found in 57% of cases of sudden coronary death [87, 88].

Haemorrhage

An intra-plaque haemorrhage with haematoma formation accelerates stenosis by displacing the plaque into the lumen, thus causing obstruction, a downstream embolism, or a parietal dissection (Fig. 10).

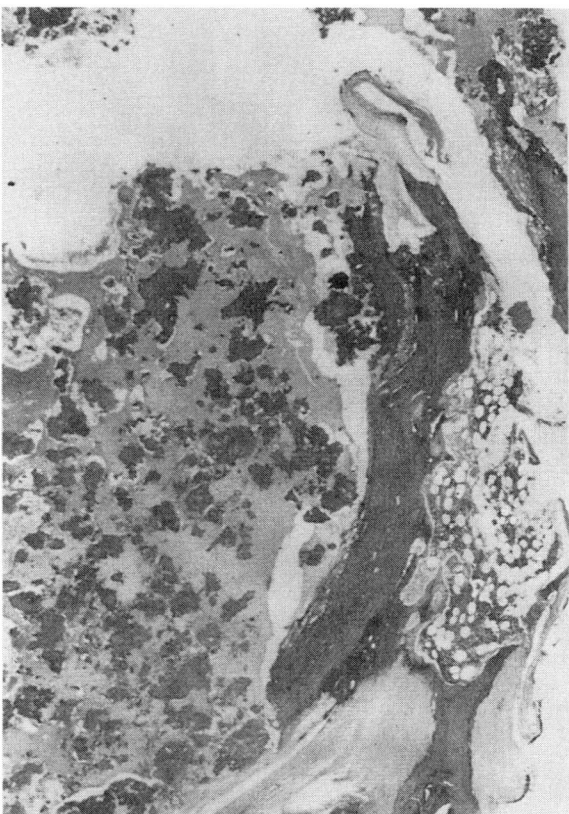

Fig. 8. Calcified plaque with underlying osseous metaplasia. HES

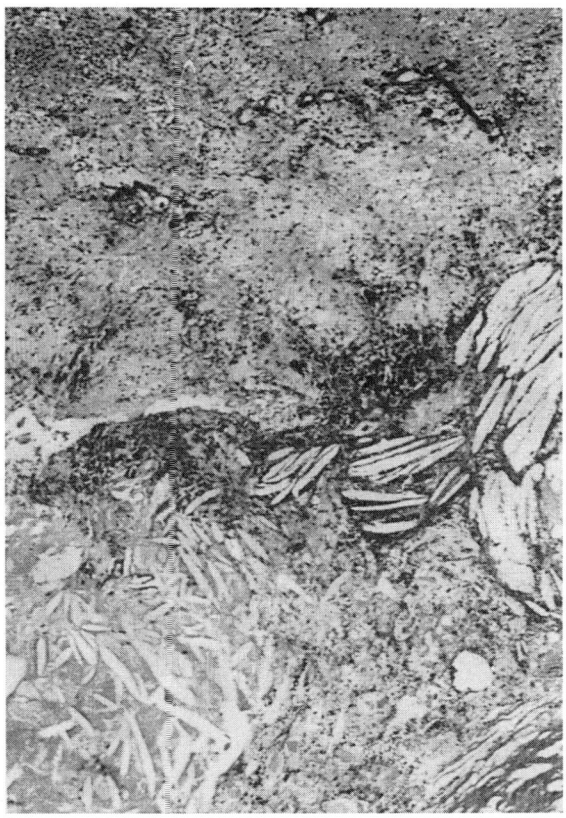

Fig. 9. Plaque disruption with bleeding. HES

Thrombosis

Ulceration of the plaque disrupts the endothelial cover and blood is in direct contact with the highly thrombogenic atheromatous material, leading to adhesion, activation and aggregation of platelets at the breach [89]. Parietal thrombi, formed in flowing blood, are rarely occlusive and are frequently incorporated into the plaque, thus increasing its thickness. However, these thrombi may be dislodged in whole or in part to cause an arterial embolism. Although the mechanisms of ulceration remain unclear, the resulting mural thrombosis contributes to the progression and complications of atherosclerosis.

6 – Outcome

Regression of atherosclerosis

Experimental studies show that atherosclerotic lesions induced by cholesterol feeding may regress if the atherogenic diet is discontinued, and regression after administration of anticholesterol drugs has been demonstrated in a number of laboratory models. These experimental data suggest the potential reversibility of human atherosclerosis, and evidence for this has been found [90]. A quantitative, statistical analysis of angiograms in patients aggressively treated with lipid-lowering agents, such as HMGCoA reductase inhibitors, has shown atherosclerosis to regress [57, 80, 91]. Early lesions are clearly more, readily reversible (fatty streaks, fibrous plaques), but prevention of progression of these lesions may represent the best therapeutic target [3, 92, 93].

Stenosis

The local risk is mainly correlated with the degree of stenosis and increases with the extent of atherosclerosis, the presence of ulceration and thrombosis (Fig. 11). As an example, atherosclerotic carotid stenosis leads to ipsilateral stroke only in circumstances

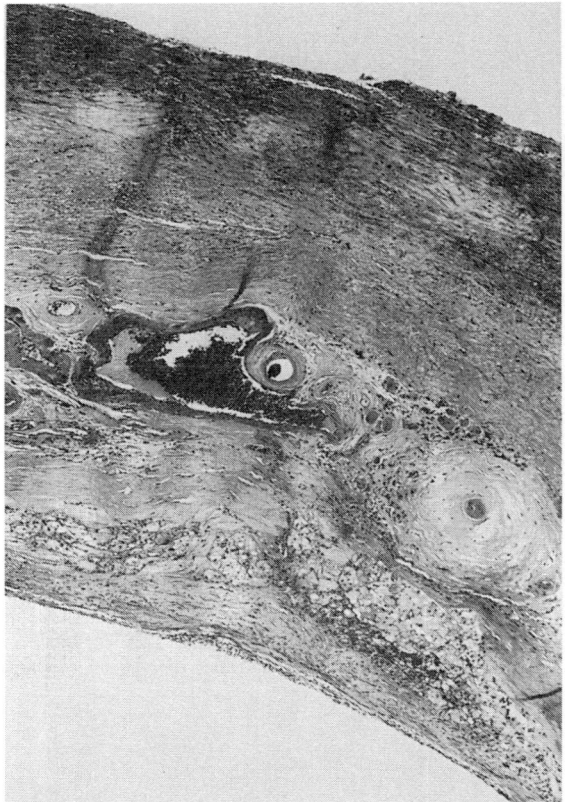

Fig. 10. Intra-plaque haemorrhage displaying the start of organisation. HES

Peripheral embolization

Atheromatous material is the most frequent source of peripheral embolization. Obstruction of multiple small arteries by cholesterol crystals may be spontaneous or induced by trauma, surgery or imaging procedures [99-101]. Recent reports have discussed the possible influence of anticoagulant therapy in promoting peripheral cholesterol embolization [102-105]. Symptomatic distal embolization of dislodged large plaques is rare.

Frequently, the discovery of atheromatous emboli in tissues is an incidental finding in surgical pathology or at autopsy. Microemboli may produce variable clinical manifestations, skin necrosis and ischaemia of the digestive tract, but sudden ischaemia in limb extremities (acrocyanosis) or permanent organ damage (acute renal failure, hypertension, acute pulmonary oedema, digestive

where stenosis is greater than 30% and then reaches 17% per year in symptomatic stenoses of 70 to 90% [94-96].

Dilatation

Human arteries dilate as a result of the changes produced by the lesions of atherosclerosis with an increase in arterial size that is proportional to the cross-sectional area of plaque that has accumulated in the vessel [97]. Intravascular ultrasound demonstrates that this is a focal compensatory enlargement at discrete sites of atherosclerotic narrowing immediately adjacent to more normal areas in which arterial size is smaller [98]. Finally, underlying compression of the media and atrophy of the arterial wall leads to the formation of an aneurysm (Fig. 12).

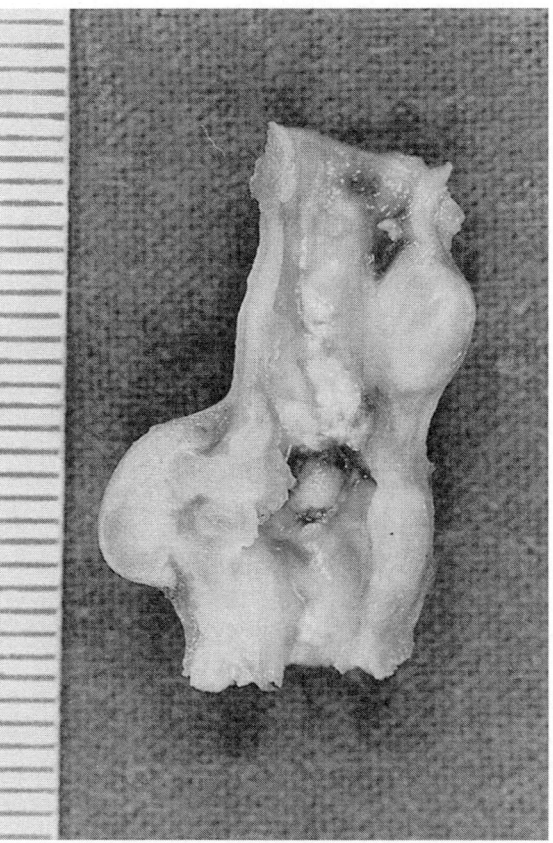

Fig. 11. Iliac artery displaying stenotic atherosclerotic lesions with a neighbouring thrombosed sack-like aneurysm

perforation) when the embolism is massive is rare [106]. Lesions in the skin, chiefly that of the digits or digestive manifestations (haemorrhage) [107] are not rare. A combination of cerebrovascular accidents and generalised broken ("racemose") livedo reticularis in the skin is sometimes referred to as "Sneddon's syndrome" [108]. Livedo reticularis may be position dependent, becoming prominent with the patient standing, but completely vanishing after several minutes of lying supine [109]. In some cases the clinical picture may resemble a vasculitis with a clinical and biological inflammatory syndrome simulating periarteritis nodosa or polymyositis [110-112].

The gross aspect of cholesterol embolization varies. For example, in the digits infarctions may be total or partial, affecting a part of the extremity

(Fig. 13). In the digestive tract, the mucosa may present punch-out ulcerations scattered along the anti-mesenteric border. These lesions may undergo necrosis and perforation [106] (Fig. 14). In solid viscera, such as the kidneys and spleen, the appearance of small infarcts scattered in the cortex is highly suggestive. Histologically, small arteries and the microcirculatory bed are usually involved. Their occluded lumina shows pear-shaped slits corresponding to cholesterol crystals interspersed with lipophages and blood clot debris. Cholesterol emboli are surrounded by a foreign-body granuloma made up of neutrophils, histiocytes and multinucleated giant cells (Fig. 15). The entirety leads to a block of fibrous tissue enclosing some slits during resolution.

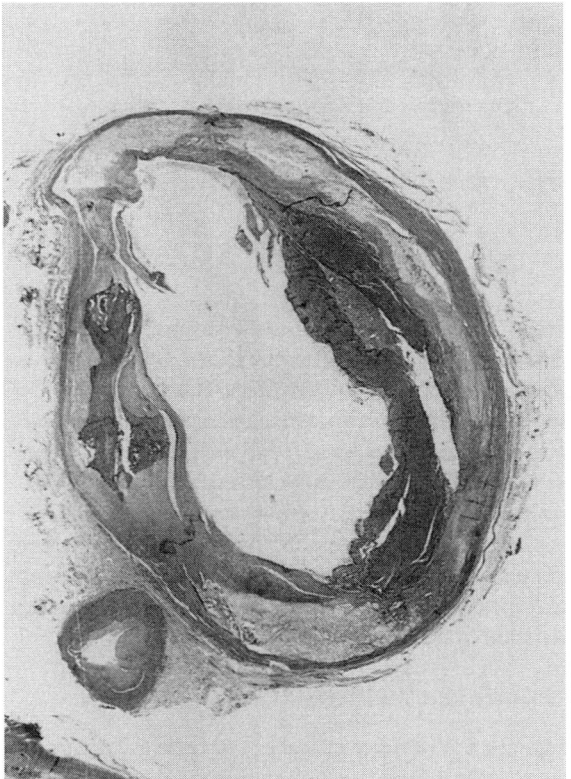

Fig. 12. Atherosclerotic fusiform aneurysm. Masson's trichrome stain

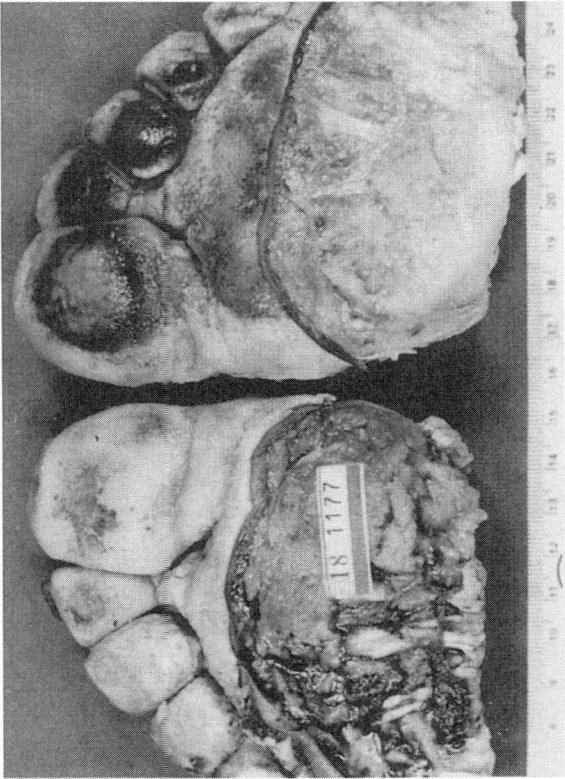

Fig. 13. Peripheral cholesterol embolism with gangrene of both forefeet imposing bilateral guillotine amputation (Courtesy Pr J-M Cormier)

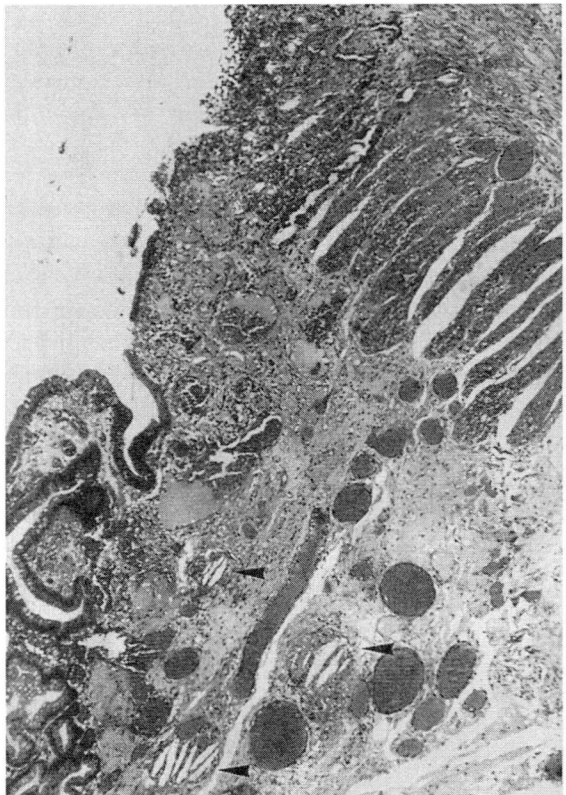

Fig. 14. Ischaemic enteritis with perforation caused by multiple cholesterol emboli (arrow heads).HES

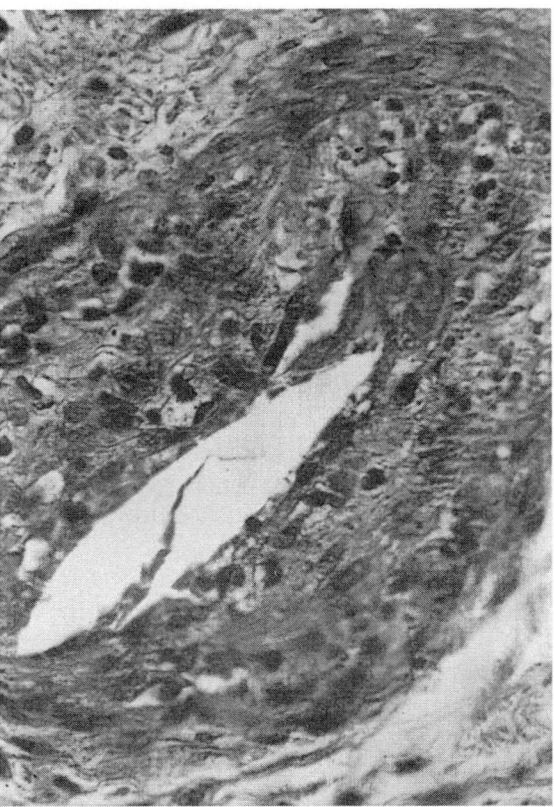

Fig. 15. Foreign body granuloma engulfing a cholesterol embolus. HES

7 – Location of advanced lesions and clinical presentations

Location

Atheroslerotic lesions do not develop at the same rate in all parts of the arterial system; some parts are more vulnerable or more susceptible to atherosclerosis than others. In the aorta, the abdominal segment is generally found to be more extensively involved by complicated atherosclerotic lesions than is the thoracic. Medium-sized arteries (coronary vessels, Circle of Willis, peripheral arteries of the limbs) are the most severely involved, while the internal mammary artery and the inferior epigastric arteries are generally well protected from atherosclerosis [113].

Aorta

Aortic lesions are predominantly found in the ascending segment and the arch, but those developed in the abdominal segment, in particular from the renal arteries to the iliac bifurcations, are more advanced and complicated in any given case. Atherosclerosis of the thoracic aorta is highly associated with risk for distal embolic events (transoesophageal studies) [114]. Lesions in the aorta frequently compromise the ostia of branches, including the coronary arteries, cervical trunks, intercostal arteries, coeliac trunk, and mesenteric and renal vessels.

Coronary atherosclerosis

There are a number of excellent reviews of the pattern of atherosclerosis in coronary vessels and its consequences. Most observers accept two well-characterised findings. These are that coronary artery stenosis is more severe in men than in women (the coronary arteries are larger in males and the heart weight is greater) [115] and that more than 90% of patients with ischaemic heart disease (IHD) have advanced stenosing coronary atherosclerosis. Most have one or more lesions causing at least 75% reduction of the cross-sectional area of at least one of the major epicardial arteries. However, the onset and prognosis of IHD do not depend entirely on the extent and severity of fixed, chronic anatomic lesions. Dynamic changes (haemorrhage, fissuring, or ulceration) in coronary plaque morphology play a critical role in the natural history. Such vascular injury precipitates the development of the acute coronary syndromes– unstable angina, acute myocardial infarction, or sudden ischaemic death in most patients [88] (Table 2).

Clinically significant stenosing plaques may be located anywhere within the three major vessels but tend to predominate within the first 2 cm of the left anterior descending (LAD) (40-50%), the left circumflex (LCX) (15-20%) and the proximal and distal thirds of the right coronary (RC) (30-40%) artery [11]. At least one coronary artery exhibiting 25-100% narrowing is found in 74% of adult autopsies [115] and although only a single major coronary epicardial trunk may be affected, more often two or all three– LAD, LCX, and RC arteries are involved [11]. The left coronary arterial branches are

more severely involved than those of the right in about are two thirds of patients [116, 117]. Sometimes the major secondary (but still epicardial) branches are also involved (diagonal branches of the LAD, obtuse marginal branches of the LCX, or posterior descending branch of the RC). Diagram 1 summarises the coronary artery changes in autopsy patients with myocardial infarction.

Carotid and vertebral arteries

Stenosis and occlusion of the extracranial arteries have long been recognised as major causes of strokes. Angiographic and pathological studies show that there are certain anatomic sites of predilection for severe lesions that lead to clinical disease. The topographic distribution of carotid and vertebral disease seems to be independent of age, sex and country [118]. In the carotid arteries, the lesions may be bilateral (66%) but not symmetrical [119, 120]. The maximum prevalence is at the bifurcation, the bulb or sinus portion and siphon region, and the first 1-cm of the internal branch. The minimum prevalence occurs at the second segment of the internal carotid. Clinical risk seems to correlate more closely with plaque morphology and surface characterisation than with the degree of stenosis [121, 122].Variations in plaque composition can

Table 2. Correlation between coronary artery atherosclerosis and ischaemic heart syndromesæ

CORONARY ARTERY PATHOLOGY	ISCHAEMIC HEART SYNDROMES
>75% stenoses	Stable angina
Plaque rupture with mural thrombus, often thromboemboli	Unstable angina
Plaque rupture, complete thrombosis	Myocardial infarction -LAD : anterior wall of left ventricle near apex ; anterior two-thirds of interventricular septum -RC : inferior/posterior wall of left ventricle ; posterior one-third of interventricular septum ; posterior right ventricular free wall in some cases -LCX : lateral wall of left ventricle
Severe multi-vessel disease, often plaque rupture with thrombus or thromboemboli	Sudden death

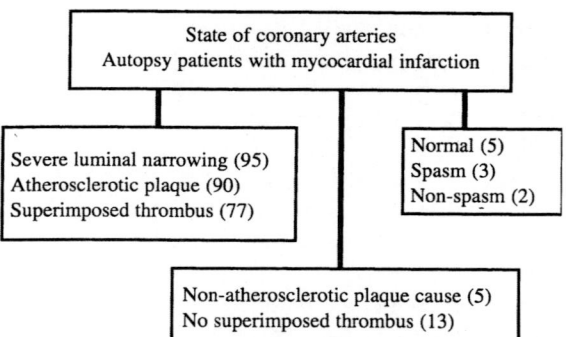

Diagram 1. Pathological status of the coronary arteries of patients dying of myocardial infarction

make carotid artery plaques prone to ulceration, subintimal haemorrhage, plaque progression, or embolization, and thus increase the risk of ipsilateral ischaemic neurologic events [123]. The origin of the vertebral artery is particularly susceptible to severe atherosclerosis; so is the intracranial segment. In the neck, lesions tend to develop in the slightly ectatic segments between the foramina of the transverse processes of the cervical vertebrae [124].

Intracranial arteries

Involvement of all parts of the arterial tree may occur and the circle of Willis is always involved, at least in part. Stenotic lesions usually involve the three main points of the vertebro-basilar axis: the ostia, the endocranial segment of the vertebral artery, and the basilar trunk [125].

Visceral arteries

In the pulmonary arteries, atherosclerosis is a common autopsy finding only in pulmonary hypertension of some duration. Lesions remain discrete and localised at branching sites. In the coeliac trunk and mesenteric arteries, atherosclerotic plaques develop at the ostia and in the first few centimetres [126]. In the renal arteries, lesions are most severe at the proximal part, often leading to stenosis. Progression of atherosclerotic renal artery stenosis occurs at an average rate of 7% per year [127] but atherosclerotic plaques in the renal artery are often found both clinically and at autopsy in normotensive subjects. Foster et al [128] observed that in only 39 % of hypertensive patients with renal artery atherosclerosis was hypertension of renal origin.

Peripheral arteries

In the lower limbs, patients with clinical symptoms have lesions that are mostly stenotic. They develop in areas of rapid haemodynamic change at the iliac branching site, in Hunters canal and in the tibial arch.

8 – Atherosclerosis in veins

Low pressure vessels do not normally develop atherosclerosis; where high pressure in the venous system persists over a period of time, for example, vein grafts, fistulae, portal hypertension or in the normally low pressure pulmonary arteries in pulmonary hypertension, lesions will develop with time but rarely reach advanced stages of development. Normal venous ageing, parietal thrombus incorporation, effects of hypercholesterolaemia combined with mechanical stress and special local structural factors (thrombotic breakdown) [129, 130] may produce lesions. Atherosclerotic changes are seen in venous grafts in arterial situations. Experimental studies have been carried out by Friedman [131, 132]. Some authors have suggested that these lesions may result from an immune-mediated process [133], but the reasons for this increased susceptibility and the role of hyperlipidaemia are not known.

Pathology and differential diagnosis.

Atherosclerotic plaques mostly develop in areas submitted to an increase in venous pressure: pulmonary veins, the portal trunk, and the iliac veins (Fig. 16). Grossly, the plaques are yellowish-white, slightly raised lesions, whose principal axis is longitudinal, measuring a few millimetres to a few centimeters in length. Softening with ulceration rarely occurs. Histologically, the lesions resemble those in arteries but the main difference is the occurrence of a large number of lesions and the high number of T lymphocytes (UCHL-1+, MT-1+) and macrophages (HAM-56+) found in these sites [134]. The plaques are usually superimposed on intimal hyperplasia (Fig. 16) with massive proliferation of smooth muscle cells (HHF-35+). The proliferation of smooth muscle cells and the nature of the surrounding extracellular matrix determine the liability of plaques to rupture and the precipitation of vein graft occlusion [135]. This exceptional lesion should be distinguished from lipid deposits seen in an organised thrombus.

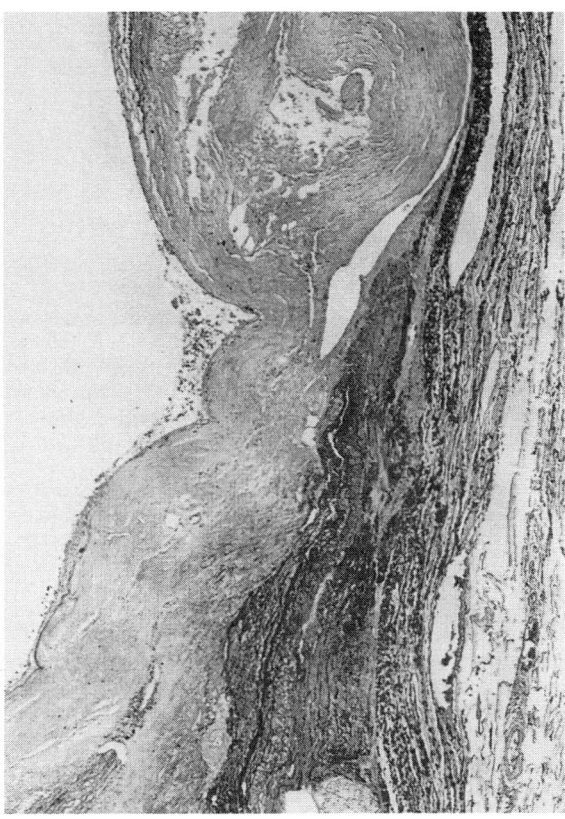

Fig. 16. Florid atherosclerotic plaque developed in the iliac vein. Orcein

Bibliography

1. WHO Study Group (1958) Classification of atherosclerotic lesions. WHO Technical Report Series, Lipids in atherosclerosis
2. Consigny PM (1995) Pathogenesis of atherosclerosis. Am J Roentgenol 164: 553-8
3. Kannel WB (1995) Clinical misconceptions dispelled by epidemiological research. Circulation 92: 3350-60
4. Kornitzer M (1996) 20 years of cardiovascular epidemiology. The epidemiologist's viewpoint. Rev Epidemiol Santé Publique 44: 563-76
5. Glasser SP, Selwyn AP, Ganz P (1996) Atherosclerosis: risk factors and the vascular endothelium. Am Heart J 131: 379-84
6. Haust MD (1978) Atherosclerosis in childhood. Perspect Pediatr Pathol 4: 155-216
7. Stary HC (1992) Composition and classification of human atherosclerotic lesions. Virchows Arch A Pathol Anat Histopathol 421: 277-90
8. Stary HC (1994) Changes in components and structure of atherosclerotic lesions developing from childhood to middle age in coronary arteries. Basic Res Cardiol 89: S17-S32
9. Stary HC, Chandler AB, Dinsmore RE, Fuster V, Glagov S, Insull W Jr, Rosenfeld ME, Schwartz CJ, Wagner WD, Wissler RW (1995) A definition of advanced types of atherosclerotic lesions and a histological classification of atherosclerosis. A report from the Committee on Vascular Lesions of the Council on Arteriosclerosis, American Heart Association. Circulation 92: 1355-74 and Arterioscler Thromb Vasc Biol 15: 1512-31
10. Berenson GS, Srinivasan SR, Bao W (1997) Precursors of cardiovascular risk in young adults from a biracial (black-white) population: the Bogalusa Heart Study. Ann NY Acad Sci 817: 189-98
11. Schoen FJ (1994) The heart *In* Cotran RS, Humar V, Robbins SL, Schoen FJ: Robbins Pathologic basis of disease. WB Saunders Company, Philadelphia, 5th ed, pp 517-82
12. Nehler MR, Taylor LM Jr, Porter JM (1997) Homocysteinemia as a risk factor for atherosclerosis: a review. Cardiovasc Surg 5: 559-67
13. Farhat MY, Lavigne MC, Ramwell PW (1996) The vascular protective effects of estrogen. FASEB J 10: 615-24
14. Maffei S, De Caterina R (1996) Hormone replacement therapy and cardiovascular risk. G Ital Cardiol 26: 899-940
15. Chae CU, Ridker PM, Manson JE (1997) Postmenopausal hormone replacement therapy and cardiovascular disease. Thromb Haemost 78: 770-80
16. Nathan L, Chaudhuri G (1997) Estrogens and atherosclerosis. Annu Rev Pharmacol Toxicol 37: 477-515
17. Roque M, Heras M, Roig E, Masotti M, Rigol M, Betriu A, Balash J, Sanz G (1998) Short-term effects of transdermal estrogen replacement therapy on coronary vascular reactivity in postmenopausal women with angina pectoris and normal results on coronary angiograms. J Am Coll Cardiol 31: 139-43
18. Wagner JD, Adams MR, Schwenke DC, Clarkson TB (1993) Oral contraceptive treatment decreases arterial low density lipoprotein degradation in female cynomolgus monkeys. Circ Res 72: 1300-7
19. Dennison E, Fall C, Cooper C, Barker D (1997) Prenatal factors influencing long-term outcome. Horm Res 48: S25-S29
20. Godfrey KM (1998) Maternal regulation of fetal development and health in adult life. Eur J Obstet Gynecol Reprod Biol 78: 141-50
21. Godfrey K, Robinson S (1998) Maternal nutrition, placental growth and fetal programming. Proc Nutr Soc 57: 105-11
22. Angelin B, Rudling M (1992) Molecular aspects of human lipid metabolism. Eur J Clin Nutr 46: 153-60
23. Hegele RA (1997) The genetic basis of atherosclerosis. Int J Clin Lab Res 27: 2-13
24. Tang L, Mamotte CD, Van Bockxmeer FM (1998) The effect of homocysteine on DNA synthesis in cultured human vascular smooth muscle. Atherosclerosis 136: 169-73
25. Vohl MC, Moorjani S, Roy M, Gaudet D, Torres AL, Minnich A, Gagne C, Tremblay G, Lambert M, Bergeron J, Couture P, Perron P, Blaichman S, Brun LD, Davignon J, Lupien PJ, Despres JP (1997) Geographic distribution of French-Canadian low-density lipoprotein receptor gene mutations in the Province of Quebec. Clin Genet 52: 1-6
26. Lee WK, Haddad L, Macleod MJ, Dorrance AM, Wilson DJ, Gaffney D, Dominiczak MH, Packard CJ, Day IN, Humphries SE, Dominiczak AF (1998) Identification of a common low density lipoprotein receptor mutation (C163Y) in the west of Scotland. J Med Genet 35: 573-8
27. Berry CL (1978) Hypertension and arterial development. Long-term considerations. Br Heart J 40: 709-17

28. Corea L, Bentivoglio M, Savino K, Zollino L (1991) Recent findings on the physiopathology of hypertension. Cardiologia 36: S51-S58

29. Moore JE Jr, Burki E, Suciu A, Zhao S, Burnier M, Brunner HR, Meister JJ (1994) A device for subjecting vascular endothelial cells to both fluid shear stress and circumferential cyclic stretch. Ann Biomed Eng 22: 416-22

30. Cucina A, Sterpetti AV, Pupelis G, Fragale A, Lepidi S, Cavallaro A, Giustiniani Q, Santoro D'Angelo L (1995) Shear stress induces changes in the morphology and cytoskeleton organisation of arterial endothelial cells. Eur J Vasc Endovasc Surg 9: 86-92

31. Reinhart WH (1994) Shear-dependence of endothelial functions. Experientia 50: 87-93

32. Zhao S, Suciu A, Ziegler T, Moore JE Jr, Burki E, Meister JJ, Brunner HR (1995) Synergistic effects of fluid shear stress and cyclic circumferential stretch on vascular endothelial cell morphology and cytoskeleton. Arterioscler Thromb Vasc Biol 15: 1781-6

33. Felton CV, Crook D, Davies MJ, Oliver MF (1997) Relation of plaque lipid composition and morphology to the stability of human aortic plaques. Arterioscler Thromb Vasc Biol 17: 1337-45

34. Grundy SM (1995) Role of low-density lipoproteins in atherogenesis and development of coronary heart disease. Clin Chem 41: 139-46

35. Dzau VJ, Gibbons GH, Kobilka BK, Lawn RM, Pratt RE (1995) Genetic models of human vascular disease. Circulation 91: 521-31

36. Rader DJ (1997) Gene therapy for atherosclerosis. Int J Clin Lab Res 27: 35-43

37. McGill HC Jr (1990) Smoking and the pathogenesis of atherosclerosis. Adv Exp Med Biol 273: 9-16

38. Wald N, Idle M, Bailey A (1978) Carboxyhaemoglobin levels and inhaling habits in cigarette smokers. Thorax 33: 201-6

39. Chesebro JH, Fuster V, Frye RL (1978) Smoking, family history and shortened platelet survival in coronary disease patients age 50 and under (abstract). Circulation 58: S221

40. Valek J (1997) Prevention of atherosclerosis in diabetics. Cas Lek Cesk 136: 523-6

41. Colwell JA, Winocour PD, Lopes-Virella M, Halushka PV (1983) New concepts about the pathogenesis of atherosclerosis in diabetes mellitus. Am J Med 75: 67-80

42. Cerami A, Vlassara H, Brownlee M (1986) Role of nonenzymatic glycosylation in atherogenesis. J Cell Biochem 30: 111-20

43. Greco AV, Mingrone G, Metro D (1987) Lipid lipoperoxidation and atherosclerosis. Minerva Med 78: 1139-45

44. Harrison DG, Ohara Y (1995) Physiologic consequences of increased vascular oxidant stresses in hypercholesterolaemia and atherosclerosis: implications for impaired vasomotion. Am J Cardiol 75: 75B-81B

45. Munzel T, Harrison DG (1997) Evidence for a role of oxygen-derived free radicals and protein kinase C in nitrate tolerance. J Mol Med 75: 891-900

46. Yatsu FM, Fisher M (1989) Atherosclerosis: current concepts on pathogenesis and interventional therapies. Ann Neurol 26: 3-12

47. Kritchevsky D (1995) Dietary protein, cholesterol and atherosclerosis: a review of the early history. J Nutr 125: S589-S593

48. Capron L (1996) Evolution des théories sur l'athérosclérose. Rev Prat (Paris) 46: 533-7

49. Anitschkow N, Chalatow S (1913) On experimental cholesterin steatosis and its significance in the origin of some pathological processes (translated by Mary Z. Pelias) In Classics in arteriosclerosis research. Arteriosclerosis (1983) 3: 178-82

50. Duguid JB (1948) Thrombosis as a factor in the pathogenesis of aortic atherosclerosis J Pathol Bacteriol 60: 57-61

51. Watanabe T, Haraoka S, Shimokama T (1997) Inflammatory and immunological nature of atherosclerosis. Int J Cardiol 54: S51-S60

52. Schmitz G, Herr AS, Rothe G (1998) T-lymphocytes and monocytes in atherogenesis. Herz 23: 168-77

53. Bobryshev YV, Lord RS (1995) Ultrastructural recognition of cells with dendritic cell morphology in human aortic intima. Contacting interactions of Vascular Dendritic Cells in athero-resistant and athero-prone areas of the normal aorta. Arch Histol Cytol 58: 307-22

54. Nagornev VA, Maltseva SV (1996) The phenotype of macrophages which are not transformed into foam cells in atherogenesis. Atherosclerosis 121: 245-51

55. Nagornev VA, Rabinovich VS (1997) The role of immune inflammation in atherogenesis. Vopr Med Khim 43: 339-48

56. Van der Wal AC, Becker AE, Das PK (1993) Medial thinning and atherosclerosis—evidence for involvement of a local inflammatory effect. Atherosclerosis 103: 55-64

57. Ross R (1993) Atherosclerosis: current understanding of mechanisms and future strategies in therapy. Transplant Proc 25: 2041-3

58. Ross R (1997) Cellular and molecular studies of atherogenesis. Atherosclerosis 131: S3-S4

59. Saikku P, Leinonen M, Tenkanen L, Linnanmaki E, Ekman MR, Manninen V, Manttari M, Frick MH, Huttunen JK (1992) Chronic Chlamydia pneumoniae infection as a risk factor for coronary heart disease in the Helsinki Heart Study. Ann Intern Med 116: 273-8

60. Saikku P (1997) Chlamydia pneumoniae and atherosclerosis—an update. Scand J Infect Dis 104: S53-S56

61. Laurila A, Bloigu A, Nayha S, Hassi J, Leinonen M, Saikku P (1997) Chronic Chlamydia pneumoniae infection is associated with a serum lipid profile known to be a risk factor for atherosclerosis. Arterioscler Thromb Vasc Biol 17: 2910-3

62. Grayston JT (1993) Chlamydia in atherosclerosis. Circulation 87: 1408-9

63. Kaukoranta-Tolvanen SS, Laitinen K, Saikku P, Leinonen M (1994) Chlamydia pneumoniae multiplies in human endothelial cells in vitro. Microb Pathol 16: 313-9

64. Mendall MA, Goggin PM, Molineaux N, Levy J, Toosy T, Strachan D, Camm AJ, Northfield TC (1994) Relation of Helicobacter pylori infection and coronary heart disease. Br Heart J 71: 437-9

65. de Luis DA, Lahera M, Canton R, Boixeda D, Roman AL, Aller R, de La Calle H (1998) Association of Helicobacter pylori infection with cardiovascular and cerebrovascular disease in diabetic patients. Diabetes Care 21: 1129-32

66. Pasceri V, Cammarota G, Patti G, Cuoco L, Gasbarrini A, Grillo RL, Fedeli G, Gasbarrini G, Maseri A (1998) Association of virulent Helicobacter pylori strains with ischaemic heart disease. Circulation 97: 1675-9

67. Fabricant CG, Fabricant J, Litrenta MM, Minick CR (1978) Virus-induced atherosclerosis. J Exp Med 148: 335-40

68. Benditt EP, Barrett T, McDougall JK (1983) Viruses in the etiology of atherosclerosis. Proc Natl Acad Sci U S A 80: 6386-9

69. Hendrix MGR, Daemen M, Bruggeman CA (1991) Cytomegalovirus nucleic acid distribution within the human vascular tree. Am J Pathol 138: 563-7

70. Bayad J, Galteau MM, Siest G (1993) Viral theory of atherosclerosis. Role of cytomegalovirus. Ann Biol Clin (Paris) 51: 101-7

71. Kol A, Sperti G, Maseri A (1997) Association between prior cytomegalovirus infection and the risk of restenosis after coronary atherectomy. N Engl J Med 336: 587-8

72. Ross R (1993) The pathogenesis of atherosclerosis: a perspective for the 1990s. Nature 362: 801-9

73. Schwartz CJ, Ardlie Ng, Carter RF, Paterson JC (1967) Cross aortic sudanophilia and hemosiderin deposition. A study in infants, children and young adults. Arch Pathol 83: 325-36

74. Stary HC (1985) Macrophage foam cells in the coronary artery intima of human infants. Ann NY Acad Sci 454: 5-8

75. McGill HC Jr (1968) The geographic pathology of atherosclerosis. Williams and Wilkins. Baltimore, pp 1-93

76. Restrepo C, Tracy RE (1975) Variations in human aortic fatty streaks among geographic locations. Atherosclerosis 21: 179-93

77. Berry CL (1987) Définition des lésions d'athérosclérose. In Camilleri JP, Berry CL, Fiessinger J-N, Bariety J (eds): Les maladies de la paroi artérielle. Flammarion, Paris, p 143

78. Bouissou H, Pieraggi MT, Julian (1987) Progression, aspects topographiques et régression des lésions athéroscléreuses In Camilleri JP, Berry CL, Fiessinger J-N, Bariety J (eds): Les maladies de la paroi artérielle. Flammarion, Paris, p 214

79. Brasen JH, Niendorf A (1997) Atherosclerosis. Formal pathogenesis, classification and functional significance. Pathologe 18: 218-27

80. Fuster V (1997) Human lesion studies. Ann N Y Acad Sci 811: 207-24

81. Spencer T, Ramo MP, Salter DM, Anderson T, Kearney PP, Sutherland GR, Fox KA, McDicken WN (1997) Characterisation of atherosclerotic plaque by spectral analysis of intravascular ultrasound: an in vitro methodology. Ultrasound Med Biol 23: 191-203

82. Qvarfordt PG, Reilly LM, Sedwitz MM, Ehrenfeld WK, Stoney RJ (1984) "Coral reef" atherosclerosis of the suprarenal aorta: a unique clinical entity. J Vasc Surg 1: 903-9

83. Williams JK, Heistad DD (1996) The vasa vasorum of the arteries. J Mal Vasc 21: S266-S269

84. Bjorkerud S, Bjorkerud B (1996) Apoptosis is abundant in human atherosclerotic lesions, especially in inflammatory cells (macrophages and T cells), and may contribute to the accumulation of gruel and plaque instability. Am J Pathol 149: 367-80

85. Bauriedel G, Schmucking I, Hutter R, Luchesi C, Welsch U, Kandolf R, Luderitz B (1997) Increased apoptosis and necrosis of coronary plaques in unstable angina. Z Kardiol 86: 902-10

86. Konstadoulakis MM, Kymionis GD, Karagiani M, Katergianakis V, Doundoulakis N, Pararas V, Koutselinis A, Sehas M, Peveretos P (1998) Evidence of apoptosis in human carotid atheroma. J Vasc Surg 27: 733-9

87. Fuster V, Stein B, Ambrose JA, Badimon L, Badimon JJ, Chesebro JH (1990) Atherosclerotic plaque rupture and thrombosis. Evolving concepts. Circulation 82: SII47-SII59

88. Farb A, Tang AL, Burke AP, Sessums L, Liang Y, Virmani R (1995) Sudden coronary death. Frequency of active coronary lesions, inactive coronary lesions, and myocardial infarction. Circulation 92: 1701-9

89. Ambrose JA (1992) Plaque disruption and the acute coronary syndromes of unstable angina and myocardial infarction: if the substrate is similar, why is the clinical presentation different? J Am Coll Cardiol 19: 1653-8

90. Hodis HN (1995) Reversibility of atherosclerosis-evolving perspectives from two arterial imaging clinical trials: the cholesterol lowering atherosclerosis regression study and the monitored atherosclerosis regression study. J Cardiovasc Pharmacol.25: S25-S31

91. Schaefer S, Hussein H, Gershony GR, Rutledge JC, Kappagoda CT (1997) Regression of severe atherosclerotic plaque in patients with mild elevation of LDL cholesterol. J Investig Med 45: 536-41

92. Weber G, Fabbrini P, Resi L, Tanganelli P, Sforza V, Vesselinovitch D, Wissler RW (1986) Ultrastructural aspects of cynomolgus atherosclerotic carotid artery lesions on cholestyramine 'regression' treatment. Appl Pathol 4: 225-32

93. Foubert L, Deiager S, Bruckert E, Turpin G (1997) Lipid risk factors of atherosclerosis: who, when, how to treat? Ann Endocrinol (Paris) 58: 275-82

94. Bousser MG (1993) What are high-risk atherosclerotic carotid stenoses? Rev Prat 43(19): 2487-92

95. Agapitos E, Kavantzas N, Bakouris M, Pavlopoulos PM, Kassis K, Liapis C, Sechas M, Davaris P (1996) Estimation of the percentage of carotid atheromatous plaque components and investigation of a probable correlation with the neurologic status of the patients. Gen Diagn Pathol 142: 105-8

96. Kardoulas DG, Katsamouris AN, Gallis PT, Philippides TP, Anagnostakos NK, Gorgoyannis DS, Gourtsoyannis NC (1996) Ultrasonographic and histologic characteristics of symptom-free and symptomatic carotid plaque. Cardiovasc Surg 4: 580-90

97. Glagov S, Weisenberg E, Zarins CK, Stankunavicius R, Kolettis GJ (1987) Compensatory enlargement of human atherosclerotic coronary arteries. N Engl J Med 316: 1371-5

98. Nomura M, Wang J, Ando T, Kimura M, Kurokawa H, Ishii J, Kinoshita M, Iwase M, Watanabe Y, Hishida H (1996) Lumen and wall morphology of mild coronary dilatation assessed by in vivo intravascular ultrasound. J Cardiol 27: 41-7

99. Moses S, Motro M, Shoenfeld Y (1997) Blunt trauma causing emboli from friable atherosclerotic plaques. Harefuah 133: 355-6

100. Mitusch R, Stierle U, Sheikhzadeh A (1998) Atherosclerosis of the aorta as a source of arterial embolisms. Z Kardiol 87: 789-96

101. Prat C, Loko M, Devoize JL (1998) Post-arteriography cholesterol embolism. J Neurol Neurosurg Psychiatry 65: 564

102. Arko F, Buckley C, Baisden C, Manning L (1997) Mobile atheroma of the aortic arch is an underestimated source of embolization. Am J Surg 174: 737-9

103. Belenfant X, d'Auzac C, Bariety J, Jacquot C (1997) Cholesterol crystal embolism during treatment with low-molecular-weight heparin. Presse Med 26: 1236-7

104. Dressler FA, Craig WR, Castello R, Labovitz AJ (1998) Mobile aortic atheroma and systemic emboli: efficacy of anticoagulation and influence of plaque morphology on recurrent stroke. J Am Coll Cardiol 31: 134-8

105. Rauh G, Spengel FA (1998) Blue toe syndrome after initiation of low-dose oral anticoagulation. Eur J Med Res 3: 278-80

106. Iung B, Baudouy Ph, Vuong PN, Faucher B, Borie H, Longueville G, Valleteau de Moulliac M (1992) Perforation jéjunale par embolie de cholestérol: à propos d'un cas traité chirurgicalement. Rev Med Interne 13: 371-4

107. Balian A, Gaudric M, Guimbaud R, Sogni P, Couturier D, Chaussade S (1998) Cholesterol crystal embolization in the digestive tract. Gastroenterol Clin Biol 22: 290-7

108. Schellong SM, Weissenborn K, Niedermeyer J, Wollenhaupt J, Sosada M, Ehrenheim C, Lubach D (1997) Classification of Sneddon's syndrome. Vasa 26: 215-21

109. Sheehan MG, Condemi JJ, Rosenfeld SI (1993) Position dependent livedo reticularis in cholesterol emboli syndrome. J Rheumatol 20: 1973-4

110. Haygood TA, Fessel J, Strange DA (1968) Atheromatous microembolism simulating polymyositis. JAMA 203: 423-5

111. McCalmont CS, McCalmont TH, Jorizzo JL, White WL, Leshin B, Rothberger H (1992) Livedo vasculitis: vasculitis or thrombotic vasculopathy? Clin Exp Dermatol 17: 4-8

112. Cruz Vicente JM (1997) Atheroembolic disease. An Med Interna 14: 257-62

113. Sons HJ, Godehardt E, Kunert J, Losse B, Bircks W (1993) Internal thoracic artery: prevalence of atherosclerotic changes. J Thorac Cardiovasc Surg 106: 1192-5

114. Montgomery DH, Ververis JJ, McGorisk G, Frohwein S, Martin RP, Taylor WR (1996) Natural history of severe atheromatous disease of the thoracic aorta: a transesophageal echocardiographic study. J Am Coll Cardiol 27: 95-101

115. Stehbens WE (1995) Atherosclerosis and degenerative diseases of blood vessels In Stehbens WE and Lie JT: Vascular pathology, Chapman&Hall Medical,London p.175-269

116. Kimura BJ, Russo RJ, Bhargava V, McDaniel MB, Peterson KL, DeMaria AN (1996) Atheroma morphology and distribution in proximal left anterior descending coronary artery: in vivo observations. J Am Coll Cardiol 27: 825-31

117. Harrer J, Lonsky V, Dominik J, Zacek P, Sistek J, Harrerova L, Knap J (1997) Coronary revascularization in diffuse atherosclerosis of the anterior descending coronary artery. Rozhl Chir 76: 342-8

118. Haimovici H (1984) Atherosclerosis: biological and surgical considerations. In Haimovici: Vascular surgery. Principles and techniques. Appleton-Century-Crofts, Norwalk, Connecticut p.135-62

119. Dixon S, Pais SO, Raviola C, Gomes A, Machleder HI, Baker JD, Busuttil RW, Barker WF, Moore WS (1982) Natural history of nonstenotic, asymptomatic ulcerative lesions of the carotid artery. A further analysis. Arch Surg 117: 1493-8

120. Ricota JJ, Schenk EA, Ekhom SE, Deweese JA (1986) Angiographic and pathologic correlates in carotid artery disease. Surgery 99: 284-92

121. Wasserman BA, Haacke EM, Li D (1994) Carotid plaque formation and its evaluation with angiography, ultrasound, and MR angiography. J Magn Reson Imaging 4: 515-27

122. Park AE, McCarthy WJ, Pearce WH, Matsumura JS, Yao JS (1998) Carotid plaque morphology correlates with presenting symptomatology. J Vasc Surg 27: 872-8

123. Seeger JM, Barratt E, Lawson GA, Klingman N (1995) The relationship between carotid plaque composition, plaque morphology, and neurologic symptoms. J Surg Res 58: 330-6

124. Meyer WW (1964) Über die rhythmishe Lokalisation der atherosklerotischen Herde im cervicalen Abschmitt der Vertebralarterie. Beitr Path Anat 130: 24-39

125. Liudkovskaia IG (1994) Pathologic aspects of disorders of cerebral circulation in arterial hypertension and atherosclerosis. Arkh Patol 56: 8-11

126. Jarvinen O, Laurikka J, Sisto T, Salenius JP, Tarkka MR (1995) Atherosclerosis of the visceral arteries. Vasa 24: 9-14

127. Zierler RE, Bergelin RO, Davidson RC, Cantwell-Gab K, Polissar NL, Strandness DE Jr (1996) A prospective study of disease progression in patients with atherosclerotic renal artery stenosis. Am J Hypertens 9: 1055-61

128. Foster JH, Dean RH, Pinkerton JA, Rhamy RK (1973) Ten years experience with the surgical management of renovascular hypertension. Ann Surg 177: 755-66

129. Zwolak RM, Kirkman TR, Clowes AW (1989) Atherosclerosis in rabbit vein grafts. Arteriosclerosis 9: 374-9

130. Boerboom LE, Olinger GN, Rodriguez ER, Ferrans VJ, Kissebah AH (1991) Atherogenic effect of barotrauma on in situ saphenous veins in monkeys. J Thorac Cardiovasc Surg 102: 448-53

131. Stehbens WE, Karmody AM (1975) Venous atherosclerosis associated with arteriovenous fistulas for hemodialysis. Arch Surg 110: 176-80

132. Orcel L (1978) Vaisseaux. Pathologie non tumorale des vaisseaux sanguins. Chapitre V In Delarue J, Laumonier R (eds) Anatomie pathologique.Pathologie spéciale. Flammarion, Paris, p.154

133. Ratliff NB, Myles JL (1989) Rapidly progressive atherosclerosis in aortocoronary saphenous vein grafts. Possible immune-mediated disease. Arch Pathol Lab Med 113: 772-6

134. van der Wal AC, Becker AE, Elbers JR, Das PK (1992) An immunocytochemical analysis of rapidly progressive atherosclerosis in human vein grafts. Eur J Cardiothorac Surg 6469-73

135. Newby AC, George SJ (1996) Proliferation, migration, matrix turnover, and death of smooth muscle cells in native coronary and vein graft atherosclerosis. Curr Opin Cardiol 11: 574-82

V
Non-atherosclerotic and non-vasculitic diseases

1 – Fibromuscular dysplasia

First reported by Leadbetter and Burkland in 1938 [1], fibromuscular dysplasia (FMD) is a segmental, non-atheromatous and non-inflammatory disease affecting mostly intermediate size arteries. It is manifest by consistent alterations in the smooth muscle cells of arteries, associated with modifications of the extracellular ground substance. Recent progress in diagnostic imaging allows more precise diagnosis of the location and type of lesions and, in general, pathologists have few opportunities to study fibromuscular dysplasia. X-ray-controlled angioplasty or embolization [2-4] now deals with most of the lesions and operative surgery is carried out only when angioplasty fails. The morphological pattern of fibromuscular dysplasia now seen by the pathologist is a mixture of the primary lesions plus the changes produced by the complications of angioplasty. Many so-called natural complications (dissecting haematoma, aneurysm, A-V fistula) result directly from the invasive techniques.

The incidence of FMD is difficult to determine since only symptomatic patients are investigated [5]. It may be an incidental finding at autopsy [6] or be revealed by trauma; it is clear that many FMD lesions may stay clinically asymptomatic. While FMD involves patients of all ages the renal artery lesions mostly affect young and middle-aged women [7]. Clinically, fibromuscular dysplasia is one of the most frequent causes of renovascular hypertension [8], second in frequency only to atherosclerosis. In the renal arteries, lesions involve the trunk and the main branches; the right renal artery is most often involved. Extrarenal lesions may cause cerebral, visceral and peripheral ischaemia with various clinical syndromes; locked-in syndrome, thoracic outlet syndrome, stroke and sudden death [9-13].

The cause of FMD is unknown. Abnormalities of the vasa vasora and haemodynamic disorders have been proposed as causative factors [14, 15]. Leung et al [16] suggested a mechanical factor since involvement of the right renal artery which is under greater tension, is more frequent than that of the left. The disease is most common in young women; however, a possible role for estrogens acting on fibroblasts or smooth muscle cells is disputed [17] and, more recently, estrogen has been reported to inhibit vascular smooth muscle cell proliferation [18]. Systemic prolonged vasoconstriction has been invoked in pathogenesis as some patients treated with ergotamine tartrate for migraine [19-21] or harbouring adrenal phaeochromocytoma or adenoma, develop FMD [22, 23].

The disease may involve multiple arterial fields (renal, gastro-duodenal, iliac, coronary, aortic) and may be associated with congenital disorders (neurofibromatosis, Bourneville's tuberous sclerosis, Williams syndrome, bone fragility, brachysyndactyly, Hirschsprung's disease, and congenital cardio-vascular malformations). It may co-exist with metabolic disorders (alpha 1-antitrypsin deficiency and persistent hypokalaemia, antiphospholipid autoantibodies). Cases involving neonates and occurrence in twins or several siblings of the same family favour a possible hereditary factor [24-44] and a defect in the synthesis of connective tissue proteins [45, 46] or of fibromyoblast metabolism have been suggested [47-50, 51]. However, the occurrence of FMD in a variety of connective tissue disorders (such as Marfan's disease) suggests that FMD may be a non-specific disorder of multifactorial origin [52, 53]. FMD has been detected recently in veterinary medicine [54]; however, attempts to produce the lesions experimentally have failed [55].

Pathology and differential diagnosis

The list of affected arteries is long; aorta [56-58, 59, 60, 61], intracranial vessels [62, 63], carotid [64-66], coronary [52, 67, 68], axillary, subclavian, brachial, iliac, femoro-popliteal, superior mesenteric, coeliac, splenic, hepatic, colonic and peripheral and subcutaneous arteries have all been documented [69-87]. Simultaneous involvement of multiple arteries has been noted [88-96]. However, it is rare for fibromuscular dysplasia to present as a generalized arterial disease [97-99]. An affected artery may display multifocal lesions [100]. Non-invasive imaging fails to detect associated venous and lymphatic lesions [101].

Grossly, the affected artery presents an uneven calibre (Fig. 1) with variable thickness and outpouchings. In some areas, partial detachment of the intima gives rise to either intraluminal pedunculated polyps or fence-like formations (Fig. 2-3). The succession of stenotic areas explains the angiographic images of a string of beads or a pile of dishes (Fig. 4) produced by extensive medial FMD [102].

Histologically, there are 3 types of lesions [103-105]. In the intimal form, the intima is thickened by a

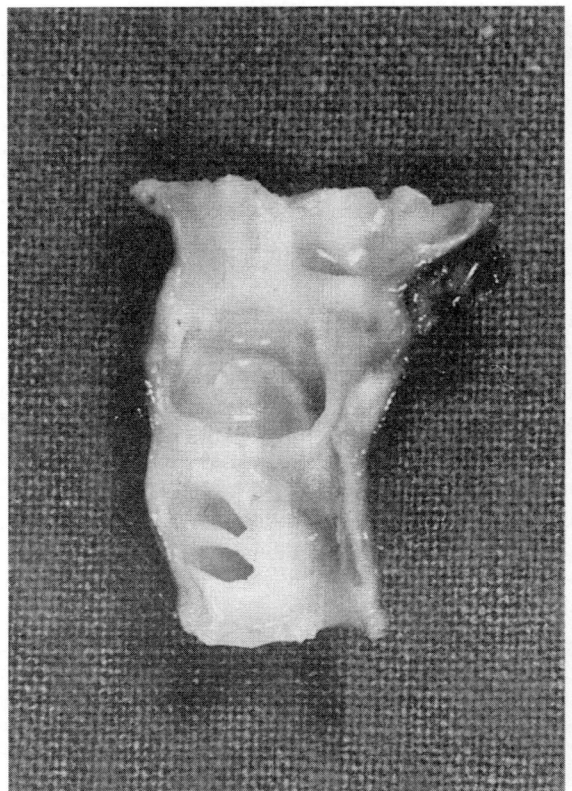

Fig. 1. Renal artery fibromuscular dysplasia. Gross aspect

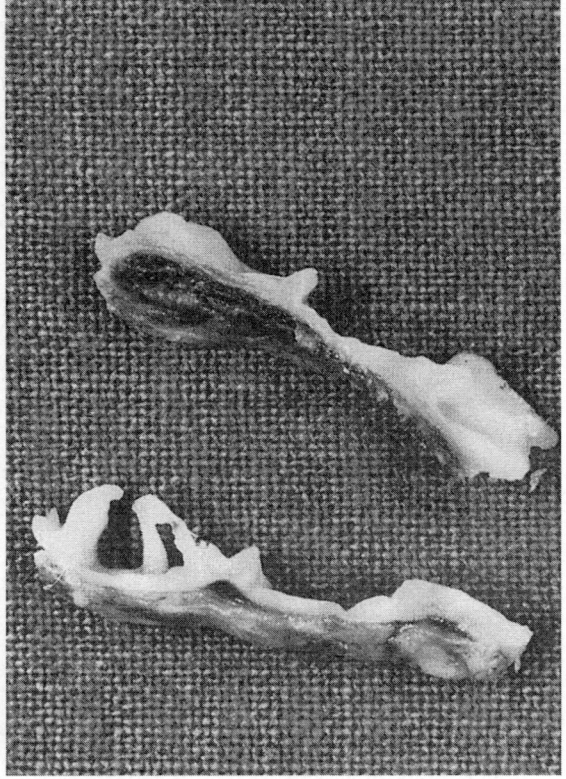

Fig. 2. Renal artery fibromuscular dysplasia. Gross aspect. Note uneven wall thickness with protruding pseudo-polyp

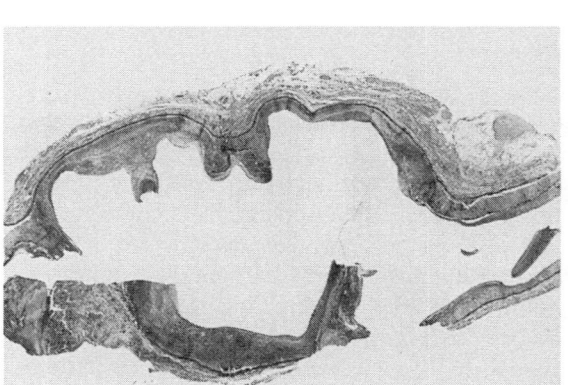

Fig. 3. Renal artery fibromuscular dysplasia with cushion-like thickening of the intima. Orcein elastic stain (Orcein)

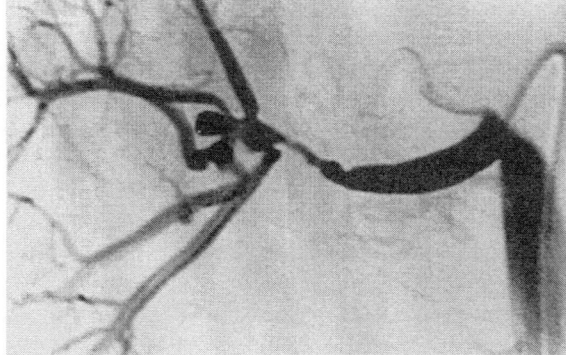

Fig. 4. Angiographic "pile of dishes" pattern of a renal artery involved by medial fibromuscular dysplasia (Courtesy Dr P.Lagneau)

fibroblastic proliferation (Fig. 5). This lesion may be diffuse and affect many viscera, leading to multi-organ failure [106, 107]. Prinzmetal's angina may be produced by coronary artery involvement [108]. As the intimal form may simulate endarteritis obliterans, localised intimal hyperplasia adjacent to an atherosclerotic plaque, or an intimal flap at an anastomotic line, the reported frequency varies greatly in different series. The medial form encompasses three subtypes; fibromuscular hyperplasia [109], extensive with aneurysm formation, and perimedial involvement leading to subadventitial fibrosis. In extensive medial FMD, fibrosis distorts and crushes the medial smooth muscle cells (Fig. 6), which show cytoplasmic vacuolization and nuclear pyknosis (Fig. 7). In places, the smooth muscle cells are few or absent (Fig.8), and the media is replaced by a fibrotic lamina [103, 104, 110]. In areas of parietal thinning, the intima lies directly on the external elastic lamella and this zone may become aneurysmal (Fig. 9). In perimedial FMD, changes in the external part of the media predominate [111, 112]. Nodular fibrosis develops, distorting the external elastic lamellae and lifting the adventitia. Staining with orcein reveals the angular contours of the external elastic lamella and enables identification of the unchanged adventitia (Fig. 10). With time, the fibrosis tends to surround the outer part of the media, giving rise to a fibrotic ring (Fig. 11). In some areas, fibrosis extends medially, compressing the smooth muscle cells giving rise to combined extensive and perimedial changes (Fig. 12-13). In adventitial FMD, fibrosis may engulf nutrient vessels, nerves and lymph nodes and compresses the remaining arterial layers (Fig. 14). This fibrosis must be distinguished from post-traumatic change, post-angioplastic scarring, peri-aortic involvement of Takayasu's disease [113, 114] and perivascular extension of retroperitoneal fibrosis. Table 1 lists the histological types and subtypes of fibromuscular dysplasia (FMD) with their frequencies in renal arteries.

Other histological variants exist. Perimedial and intimal types may coexist in the same arterial segment giving rise to multifocal stenoses [115]. In the renal artery, the perimedial subtype may be the initial change with subsequent progression to extensive disease, as the mean age of the patients for the two entities is 27.8 and 33.9 yr respectively [51, 59, 116, 117]. In our experience, arteries with medial FMD often present with hyperplasia of the smooth muscle fibres criss-crossing the adventitia (Fig. 15). This process thus thickens the vascular wall. We believe this to be a compensatory process to improve the function of the arterial wall as the media is replaced by fibrosis, especially when it is under tension (renal, splenic, hepatic arteries in particular).

The natural history of the disease is not understood, although it is clearly progressive. Repeated angiography will detect new lesions [118-120]. In the kidneys, unsuspected fibromuscular dysplasia may continue to progress in the intraparenchymal arteries (Fig. 16) of an implanted graft causing hypertension in the recipient [121]. Cases involving the aorta have been reported [59, 60] and atypical coarctation may be produced (Fig. 17-18).

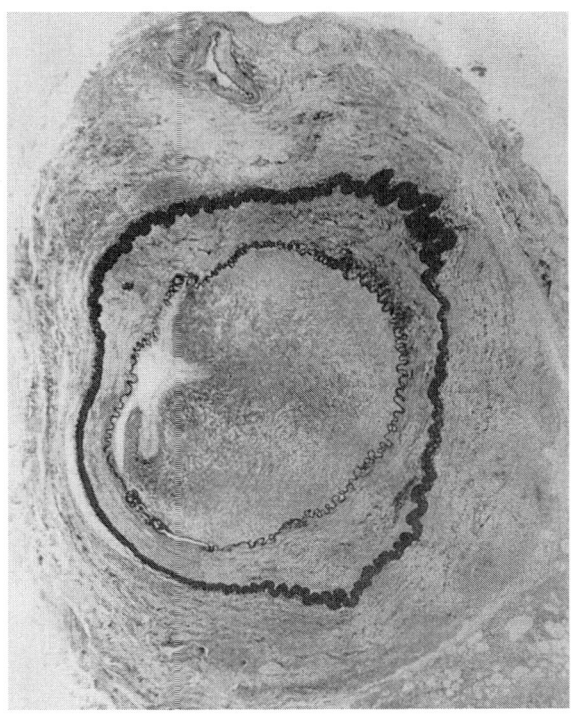

Fig. 5. Intimal form of fibromuscular dysplasia. Orcein

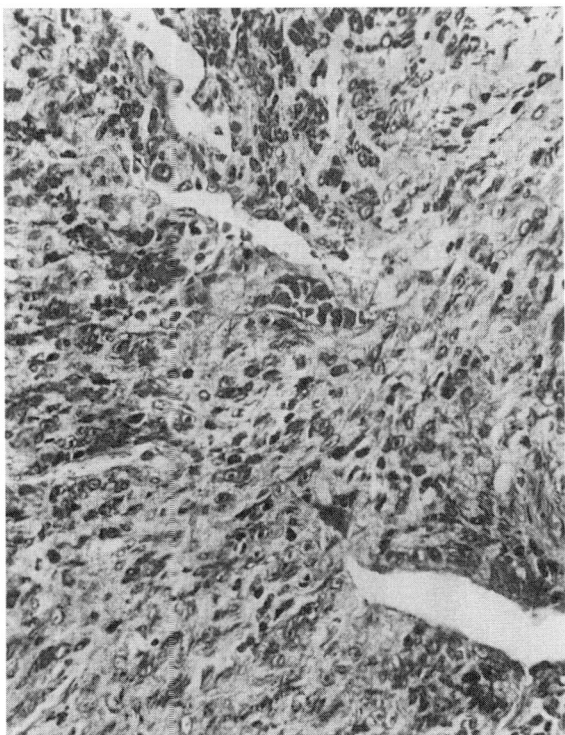

Fig. 6. Extensive medial fibromuscular dysplasia. Note fibrosis suffocating smooth muscle cells. Masson's trichrome stain (Masson's trichrome)

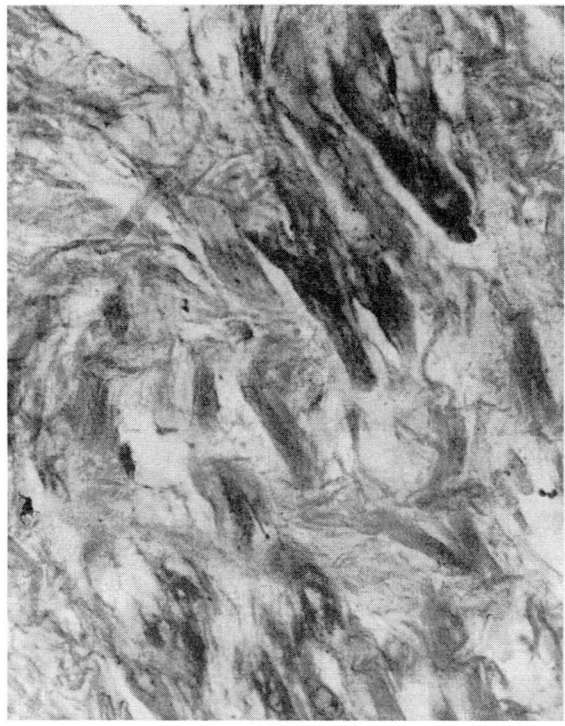

Fig. 7. Extensive medial fibromuscular dysplasia. Dystrophic changes (cytoplasmic vacuolization and nuclear pyknosis) of smooth muscle cells. Masson's trichrome

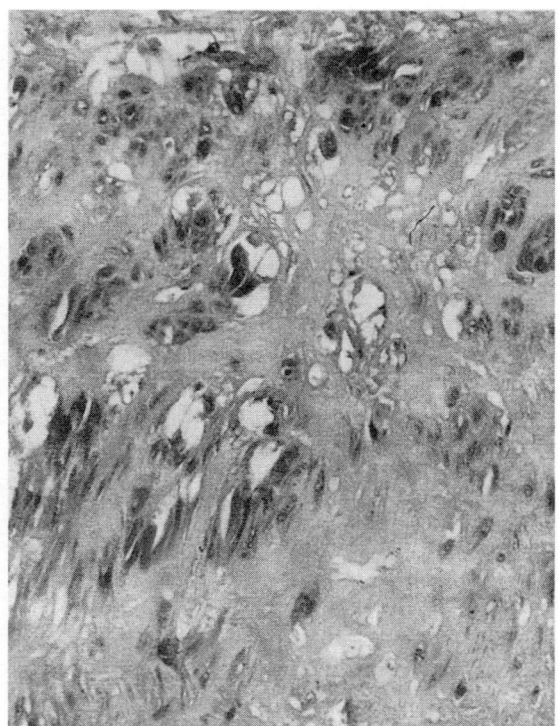

Fig. 8. Extensive medial fibromuscular dysplasia. Predominant fibrosis replacing the smooth muscle cells. Masson's trichrome

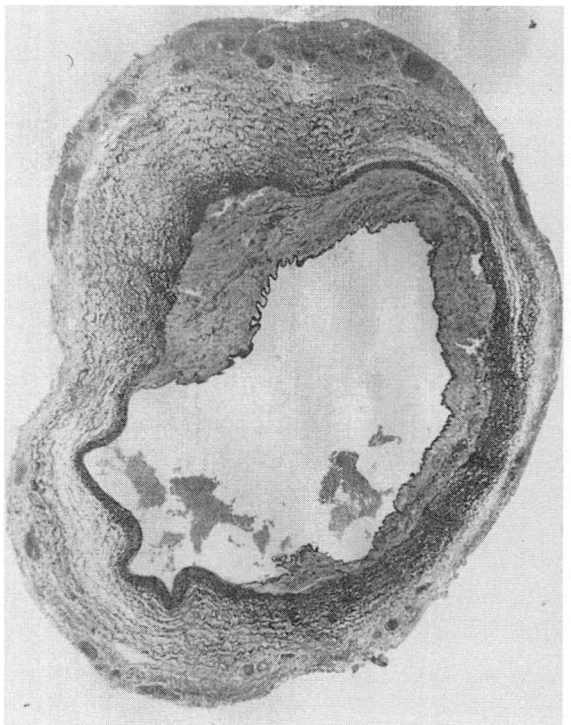

Fig. 9. Extensive medial fibromuscular dysplasia. Thinning wall areas are the starting points for the development of an aneurysm. Orcein

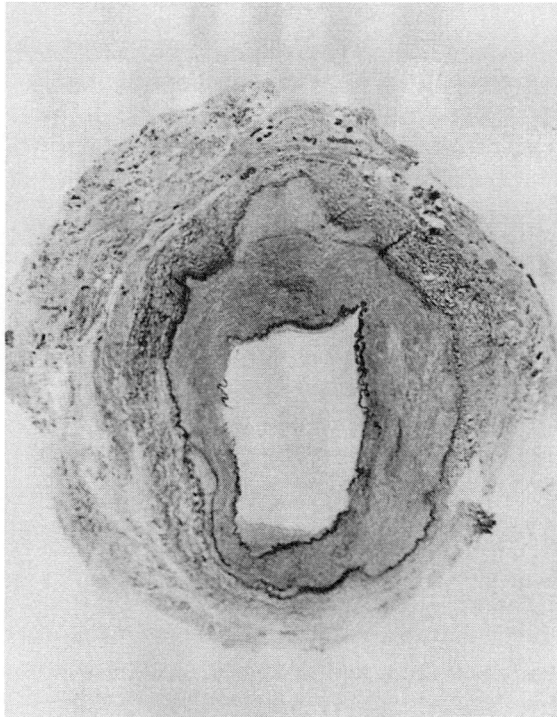

Fig. 10. Perimedial fibromuscular dysplasia. Initial changes with nodular fibrosis distorting the external elastic membrane. Orcein

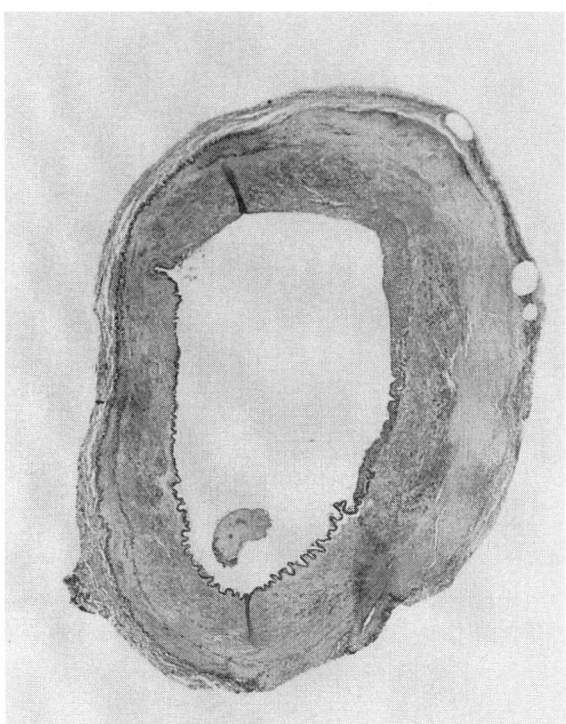

Fig. 11. Perimedial fibromuscular dysplasia. Advanced changes with fibrotic ring strangling the outer part of the media. Orcein

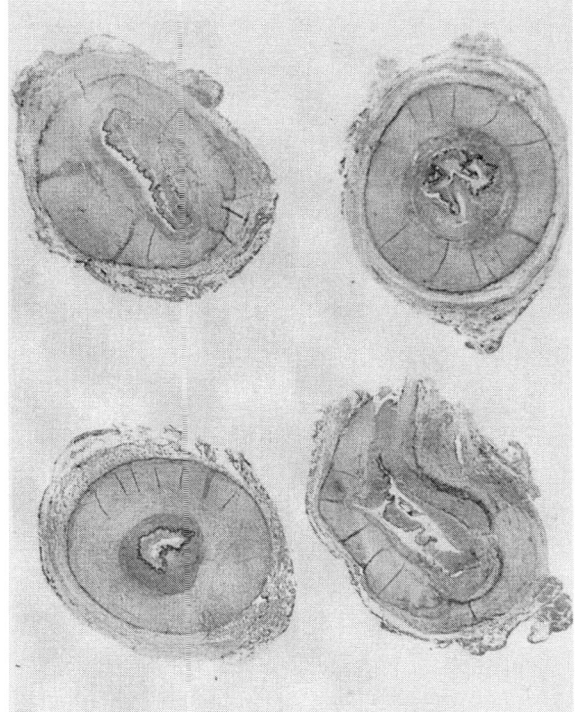

Fig. 12. Medial fibromuscular dysplasia. Combined perimedial and extensive changes in the same artery. Orcein

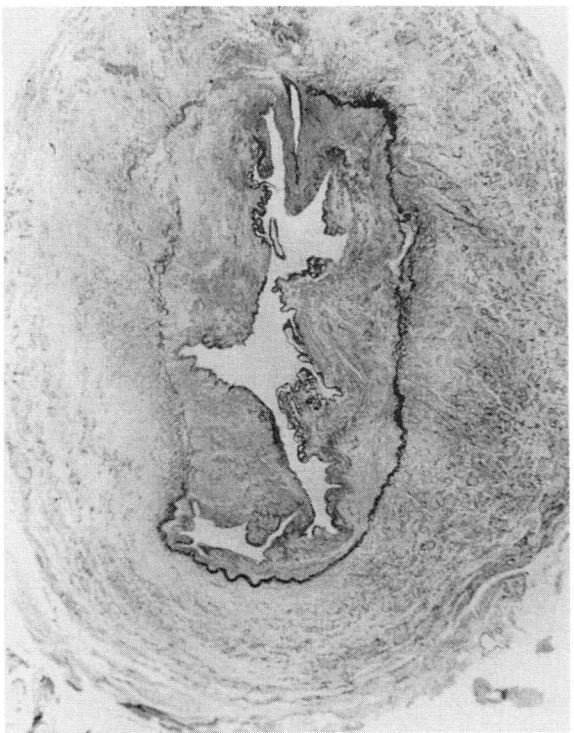

Fig. 13. Medial fibromuscular dysplasia. Combined perimedial and extensive changes. Note the fibrous ring in the outer part of the media. Orcein

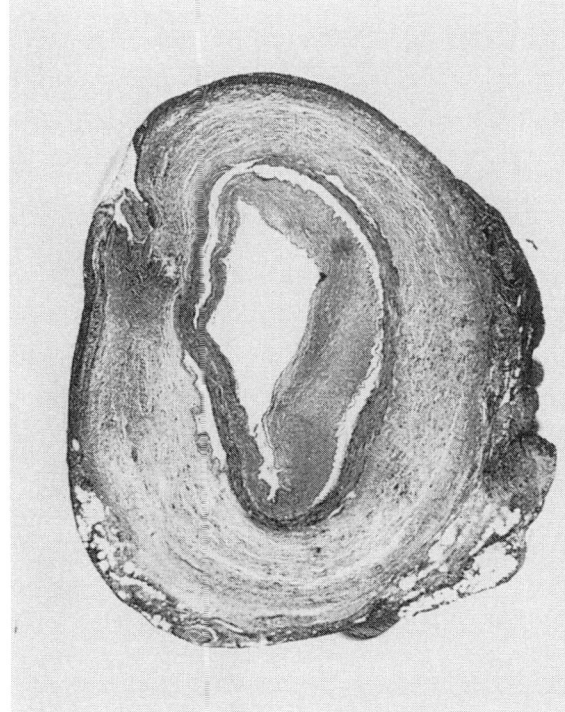

Fig. 14. Adventitial fibromuscular dysplasia. Orcein

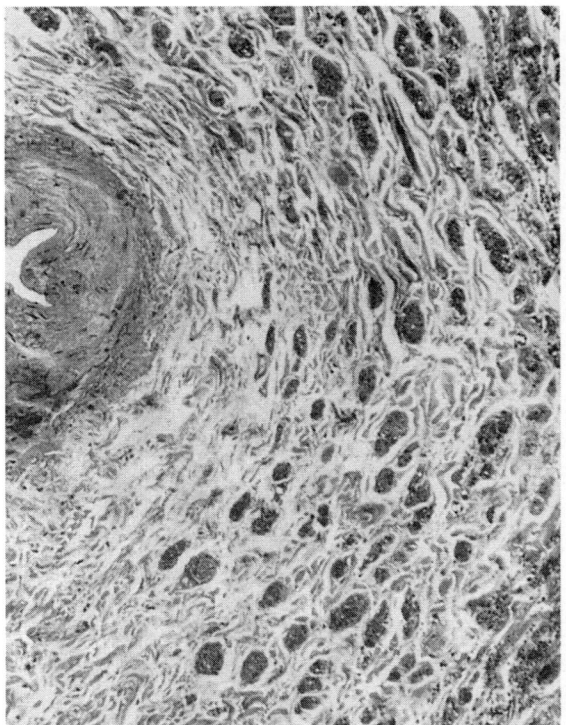

Fig. 15. Medial fibromuscular dysplasia. Reactional hyper-plasia of the smooth muscle fibres in the adventitia. Masson's trichrome

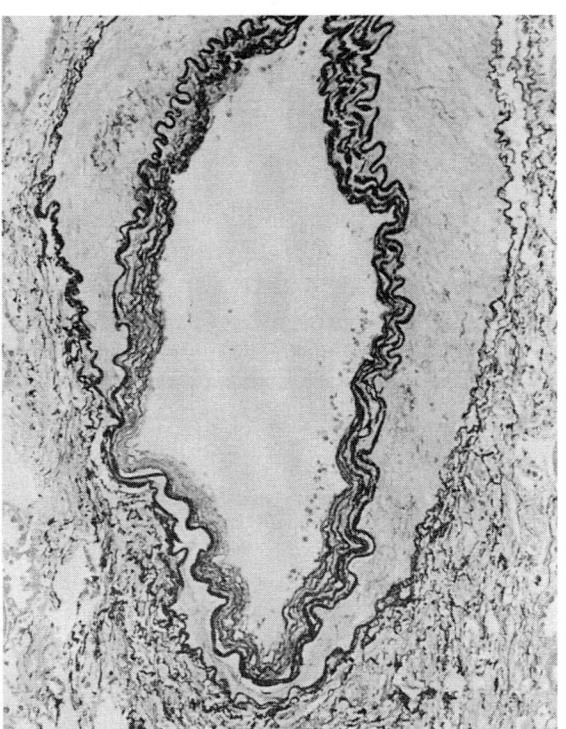

Fig. 16. Extensive fibromuscular dysplasia of the renal artery involving an intra-parenchymal collateral. Orcein

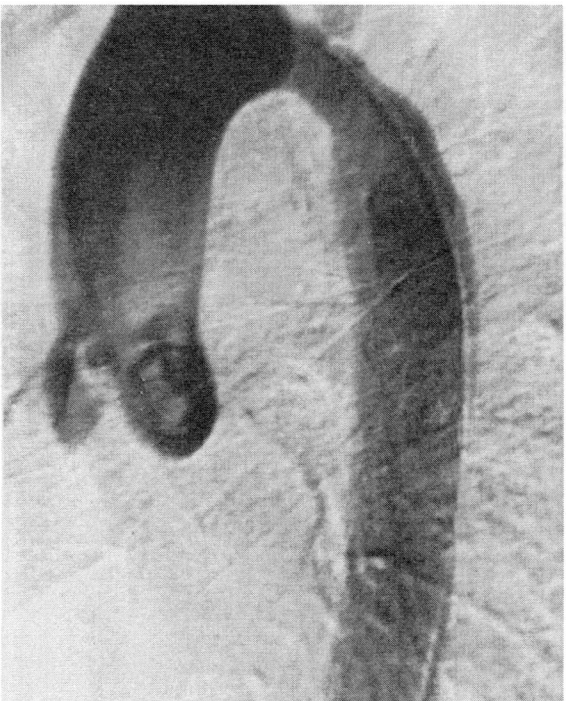

Fig. 17. Atypical coaractation of the aortic isthmus with "string of beads" or "pile of dishes" pattern evidenced by the angiogram (Courtesy Dr O.Bical)

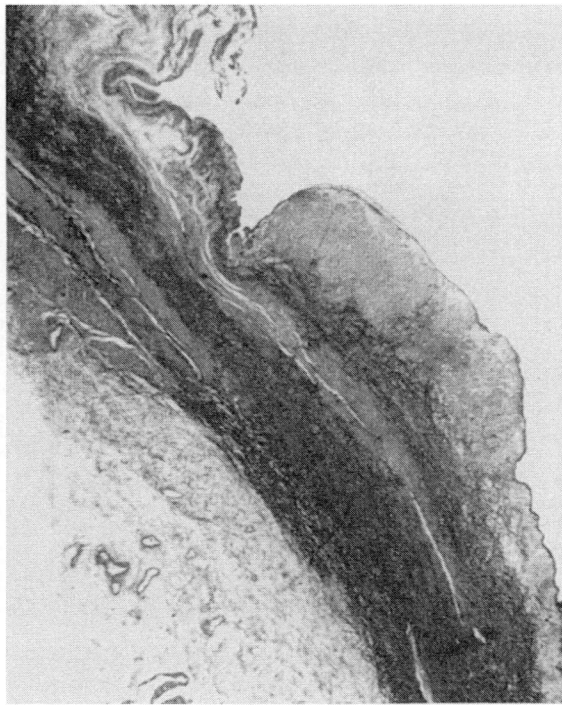

Fig. 18. Atypical coaractation of the aortic isthmus caused by medial fibromuscular dysplasia. Orcein

Table 1. Histological types and subtypes of renal artery fibromuscular dysplasia

ARTERIAL LAYER	FIBROMUSCULAR DYSPLASIA TYPES	SUBTYPES	%
Intima	Intimal	None	1-2
Media	Medial	Localised	1
	Medial	Extensive	60
	Medial	Perimedial/ Subadventitial	39
Adventitia	Adventitial/Periarterial	None	<1

Aneurysms are more frequently seen in the extensive medial subtype [104, 122-124] (Fig. 19-20). They are morphologically unremarkable, their walls being composed of fibrous tissue. The luminal aspect may show atherosclerotic plaques. Operative specimens containing a non-aneurysmal area are necessary to identify the primary FMD. An exceptional complication of aneurysm is rupture into the corresponding vein, giving rise to a fistula [125]. Thrombosis is common and worsens stenosis; it may lead to complete obstruction of the affected artery. Parietal dissection or dissecting haematoma may occur spontaneously after a trauma or angioplasty [126]. The cleavage can involve the intima or, more frequently, the media in its outermost or subadventitial part. Secondary intimal fibrotic thickening often develops in and around stenotic areas and favours thrombosis; it must be distinguished from primary intimal fibrodysplasia.

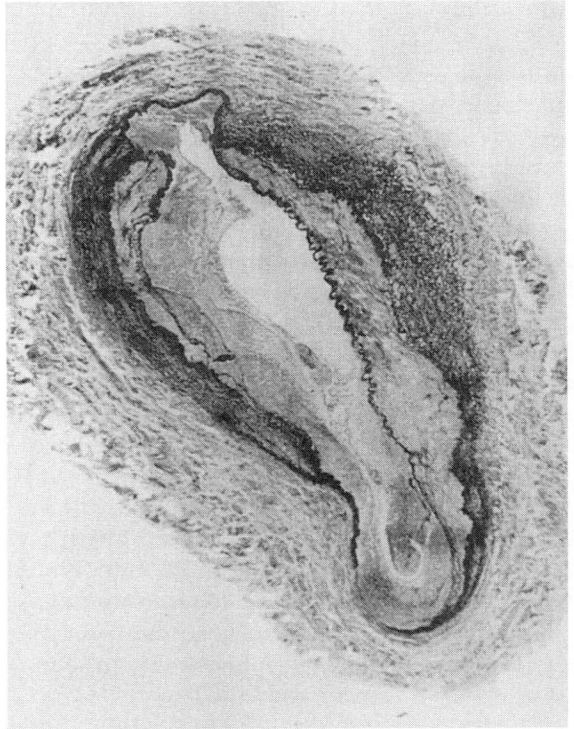

Fig. 19. Extensive fibromuscular dysplasia of a renal artery. Note parietal thinning areas or outpouchings. Orcein

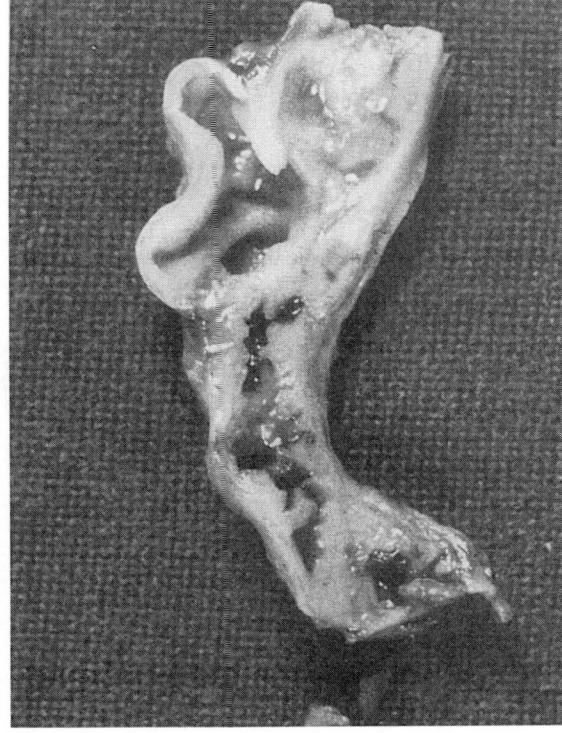

Fig. 20. Extensive fibromuscular dysplasia of a renal artery. Sack-like aneurysm

2 – Moyamoya disease

This condition – of unknown aetiology – was first described by Kawakita in 1963. Its name is derived from the cerebral angiographic patterns of exuberant collateral vessels in the basal ganglia (Fig. 21) and the "puff of smoke" appearance (Fig. 22) which accompanies stenosed and distorted internal carotid arteries with occlusion of their main cerebral branches [127, 128]. Patients complain of being in a "fog", apparently caused by ischaemia. The thin collateral vessels responsible for the typical angiographic appearances arise from the circle of Willis in a wispy, smoke-like pattern (Fig. 22). Intracranial veins (superficial, superior striate, inferior striate), as well as perforating arteries, show various degrees of dilatation. Delayed venous filling may predict an ischaemic attack [129].

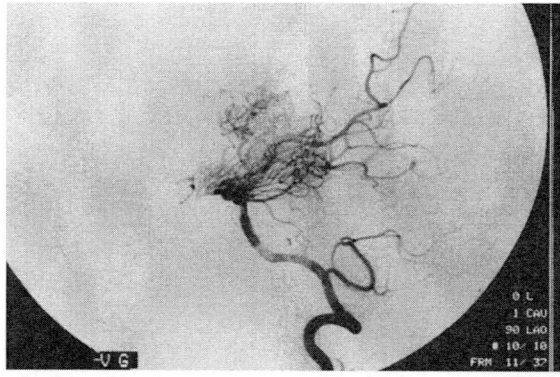

Fig. 21. Moyamoya disease with exuberant collateral vessels in the basal ganglia (Courtesy Pr Ch. Raybaud)

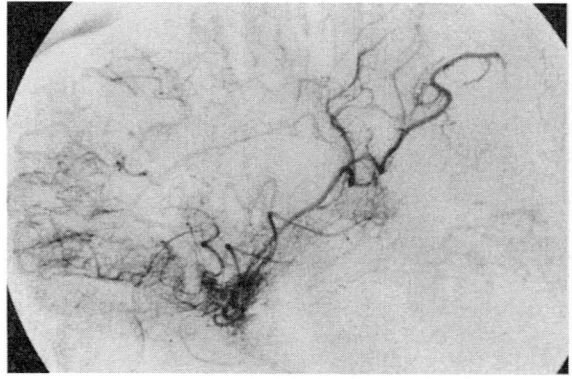

Fig. 22. Angiographic "puff of smoke" appearance in Moyamoya disease (Courtesy Pr Ch. Raybaud)

The disease, frequent in Asia (Japan, China, the Philippines, Korea, Malayasia, India), has been also reported in North America and Europe [130, 131]. The condition affects mostly female children and adolescents [132] but adults may also be affected [133, 134]. Ages range from 5 to 47 years. There is a tendency for familial multifactorial inheritance. Moyamoya disease has been reported in fraternal twins [135]. Mother-to-child inheritance has been observed in most cases [136].

Diffuse stenosis of the internal carotid artery with occlusion of its main branches, and subarachnoid haemorrhage result in infarction and an alteration of the mental state. The mean age at the onset of cerebral ischaemia is 9.7years. Most cases present as recurrent strokes in otherwise healthy children, often following a febrile period, with abrupt onset of hemiparesis, transient aphasia, convulsions and, often, spontaneous resolution. There is no diagnostic laboratory test. Cerebrospinal fluid (CSF) from Moyamoya patients contains significantly higher concentrations of basic fibroblast growth factor (b-FGF) ($P<0.05$) than is found normally. The b-FGF level is apparently elevated in patients with well developed neovascularization after indirect revascularization surgery ($P<0.01$) [137]. Cerebral revascularization surgery may halt clinical progression [138-140].

Association of Moyamoya disease with congenital heart disease (coarctation of the aorta, ventricular septal defect, aortic and mitral valve stenoses, and tetralogy of Fallot) and arterial anomalies (aneurysms, ectasia, fenestration, arteriovenous malformation and fibromuscular dysplasia) have been reported [140-142] but the pathogenesis of remains unclear. An autoimmune mechanism has been evoked, as some patients suffering from SLE, Sjogren's syndrome and twins having this disease present the same HLA type with a high incidence of autoimmune antibody [135, 143-146]. The occurrence of Moyamoya disease in Down syndrome suggests to some that a protein encoded on chromosome 21 may be related to its pathogenesis [147, 148]. Patients with Moyamoya disease present a higher incidence of Epstein-Barr virus (EBV) DNA than normal controls [149] and infection of rats with *Propionibacterium acnes* induces Moyamoya-like changes of the intracranial internal carotid arteries [150]. Other potential mechanisms of producing similar changes include radiation [151, 152] and thrombotic disorders such as hereditary spherocytosis, glycogen storage disease type Ia, sickle cell anemia, and protein S deficiency [153-156].

Pathology and differential diagnosis.

Involvement of the cerebral arteries, including those of the circle of Willis, may be unilateral or bilateral [145, 157]. There may be stenosis of extracranial arteries (renal, coronary, superficial temporal) leading to renal hypertension [158-164].

The cerebral arteries display intimal thickening and defects in the elastic membrane (Fig. 23). Old and recent thrombi with partial recanalization are frequently seen. Intimal hyperplasia may be responsible for infarction, alteration of the mental state and small vessel proliferation in basal ganglia in patients. These changes are not specific, however. The "puff of smoke" pattern on angiography may also be seen in arteriosclerotic occlusive disease, post-radiation arteritis, intravascular tumour proliferation and tuberculous meningitis.

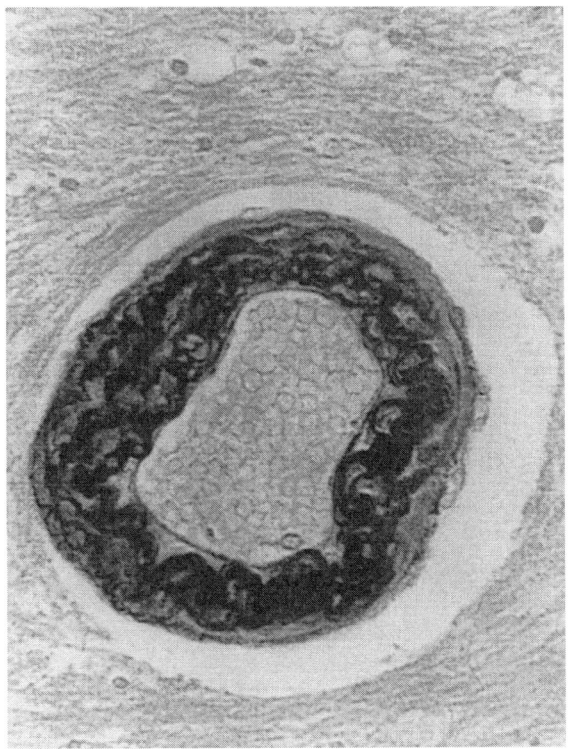

Fig. 23. A medium-sized arteriole in the white matter of a 28 yo woman who died of catastrophic intracerebral haemorrhage in labour. She had presented as a child with an ischaemic stroke, and, after investigation, including angiography, was diagnosed as having moya-moya disease. Elastic van Giesen stain

3 – Adventitial cystic degeneration of vessels

Ejrup and Hiertonn first reported this condition in the popliteal artery in 1954 [165]. It is variously known as cystic degeneration, adventitial mucoid cyst, cystic adventitial disease or degeneration of the popliteal artery. The last two terms are favoured by most authors [166, 167] but are not entirely satisfactory as the mucoid degeneration of the vessels wall takes place in the outermost part of the media, or in the adventitia. This lesion occurs preferentially in arteries; however, some cases of adventitial cystic degeneration have been reported in veins [168-170]. In 1979, Flanigan et al [171] reviewed 115 cases but more than 323 reports dealing with arteries and veins are now available in the literature [172]. The change affects mainly males and the age of the patients has ranged from 11 to 60 years with a mean of 36 [171, 173, 174]. The popliteal artery is by far the most frequent site, 264 cases being reported from 1954 to 1995 [175-177]. Extrapopliteal locations concern the stem vessels in the extremities or a vessel neighbouring a joint (ankle, elbow, wrist), such as the iliofemoral axis, the radial and ulnar arteries, and the saphenous vein [178-186]. Involvement of the aorta has also been reported [187]. The cysts are rarely multiple [188, 189].

Arteriography shows almost complete obstruction of the arterial lumen, which has a smooth, fluted stenosis. This stenosis may be one-sided or have an hourglass appearance with no stenotic dilatation (Fig. 24) [190]. Only exceptionally does the cyst regress spontaneously [98, 191]. The treatment is essentially surgical. Recurrence of cystic adventitial disease in an interposed vein graft has been reported [192].

The pathogenesis remains obscure and three main theories have been proposed. These are:

1. Trauma. Most cases of cystic adventitial disease affect para-articular vessels such as the popliteal artery and its satellite vein, the radial artery, or the saphenous vein. Repeated micro-trauma may be the cause of parietal degenerative changes with cyst formation. Many facts support this hypothesis; the singular sex predilection and age distribution, the anatomical location and the frequent association of adventitial mucoid cyst with local dysmorphic anomalies, such as the "nail-patella syndrome" [193-197].

2. Joint-related theory. The close anatomical contact between vessels and joints supports this hypothesis. Cases of spontaneous rupture of the cyst into the joint have been reported. Moreover, the cystic

contents are rich in hyaluronic acid and protein and stain with alcian blue. Cystic adventitial disease may result either from inclusion of mucus-secreting synovial cells in the vascular wall [191, 192, 198-202], or from a synovial capsular remnant (ganglion) growing along muscles, tendon sheaths and vascular branches with secondary herniation into the adventitia of the adjacent vessel [203-206]. Inclusion of mucus-secreting synovial cells may be congenital or acquired through trauma to the adventitia. The lesion resembles a synovial cyst; however, synovial cells have never been identified in the lumen.

3. Developmental disorder. A recent review by Levien and Benn [172] of 323 cases unveiled that all reported cases of adventitial cystic disease have occurred in the non-axial arteries. Non-axial arteries develop at a later stage than the axial vessels during limb differentiation and development. In the upper limb, the main subclavian-axillary-brachial trunk represents the axial artery. Non axial arteries, located below the elbow, consist of the median, ulnar and radial arteries. In the lower limb, the axial artery persists in the lower leg as the peroneal artery. The anterior and posterior tibial arteries are non-axial. During limb bud development, cell rests derived from condensations of mesenchymal tissue destined to form the knee, hip, wrist, or ankle joints may be incorporated into the nearby and adjacent nonaxial vessels at the 15-22-week stage [207, 208] These cell rests are then responsible for the formation of adventitial cystic disease later in life, when the mucoid material secreted results in a mass within the arterial or venous wall.

Pathology and differential diagnosis

Initially the lesion develops at the junction of the media and the adventitia (Fig. 25). This area is distorted by a pool of mucoid gel staining positively with acid alcian blue and periodic acid Schiff (PAS) and containing some fragmented elastic and collagen fibres. Focal infiltration of macrophages may occur with haemorrhage. Only later does a cyst, devoid of lining, become evident and raise the adventitia (Fig. 26-27). These structures compress the lumen [209, 194, 169] (Fig. 28). The major differential diagnosis is a dissecting haematoma. When thrombosis occurs, differential diagnosis from an entrapped popliteal artery is impossible; surgical exploration ultimately establishes the diagnosis. In veins, lesions always occur near branches and bifurcations.

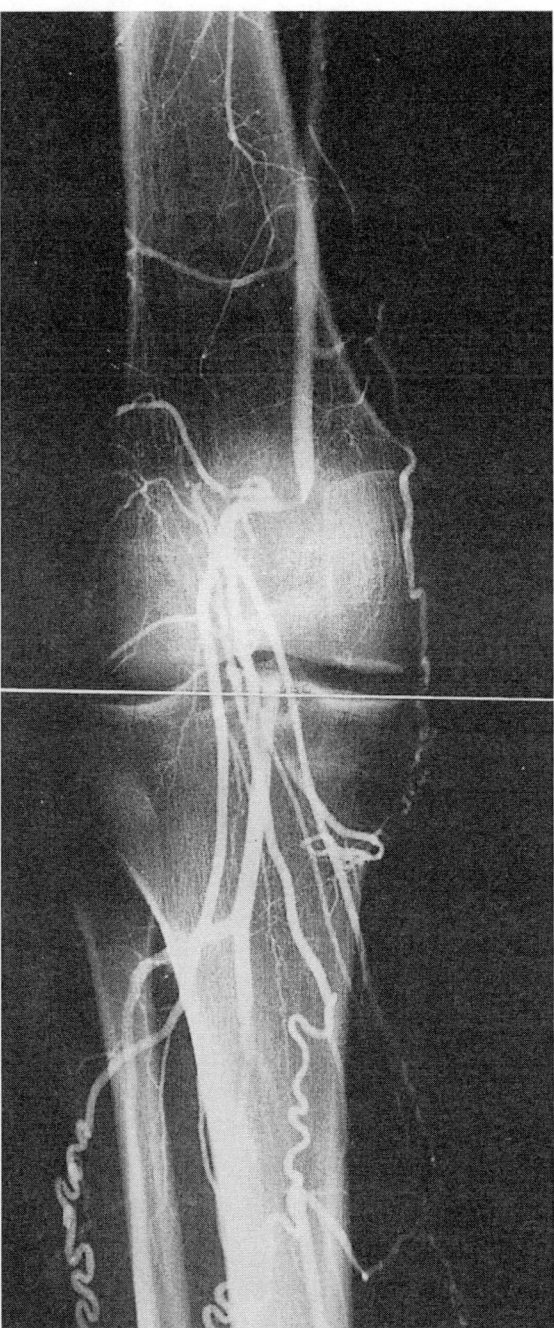

Fig. 24. Degenerative adventitial cyst of the left popliteal artery. Fluted-stenosis angiographic pattern (Courtesy Dr F.Cheilan)

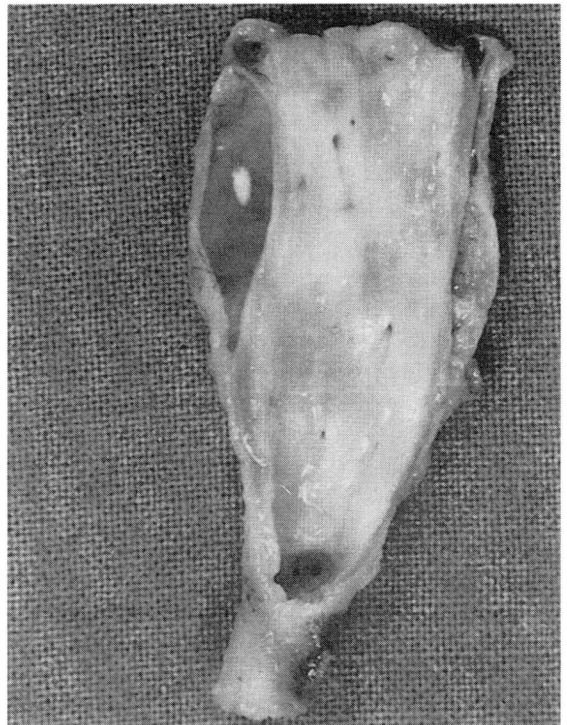

Fig. 25. Degenerative adventitial cyst of the popliteal artery. Note mucoid material in the cystic lumen

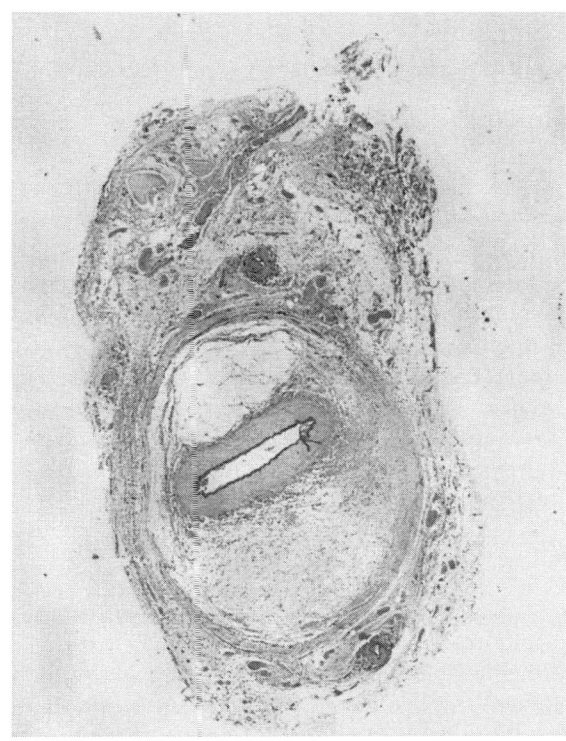

Fig. 26. Accumulation of mucoid material starts at the junction of the media and the adventitia. Orcein

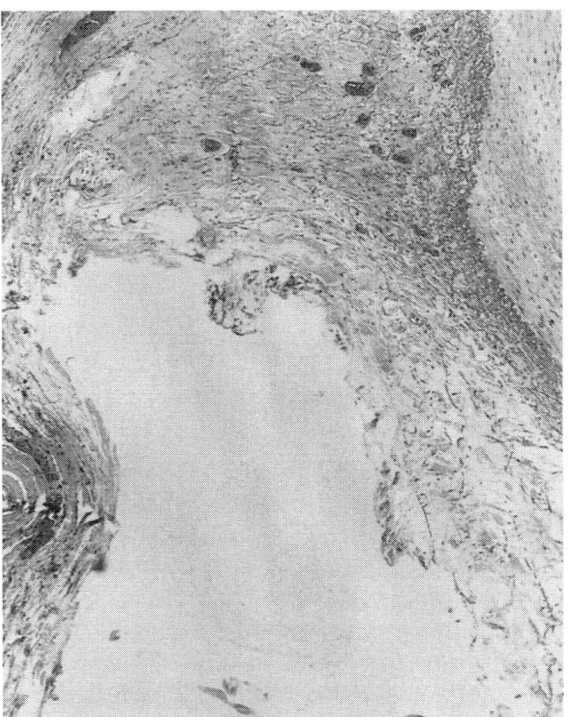

Fig. 27. Degenerative adventitial cyst of the popliteal artery. Histological aspect of the cystic wall devoid of lining. Orcein

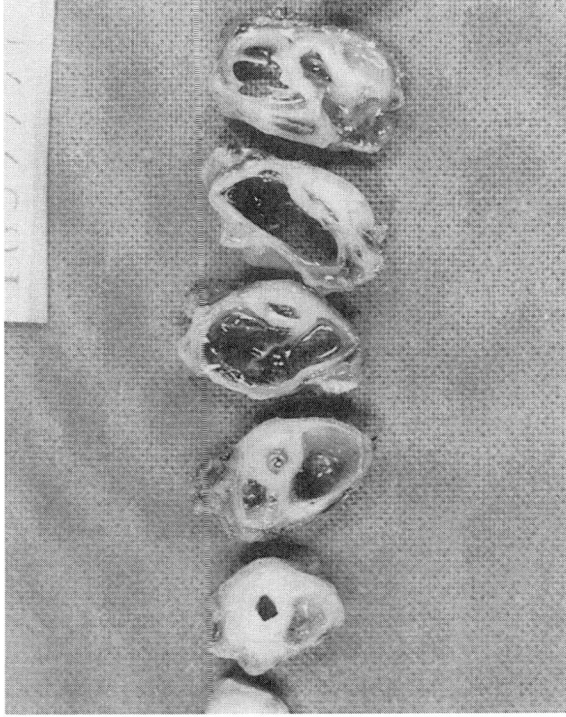

Fig. 28. Large degenerative adventitial cyst of the popliteal artery compressing the arterial lumen

4 – Cystic medial necrosis, mucoid degeneration of the media, medial degeneration

This condition, called "medionecrosis aortae idiopathica cystica" by Erdheim [210], is not a pathological entity but an ageing change [211], characterised by focal pooling of mucoid material, mostly in the middle and outer thirds of the media with degenerative changes of the elastic fibers and/or the myocytes. Schlatmann and Becker [212] have described the change in detail and have argued convincingly for its abolition as a term used to describe a disease.

Pathology and differential diagnosis

With increasing age, metachromatic, PAS positive mucoid material accumulates in elastic arteries, forming cysts of various sizes (Fig. 29), which may fragment and disrupt the elastic frame. Orcein staining shows areas of elastic loss giving rise to a "ti-

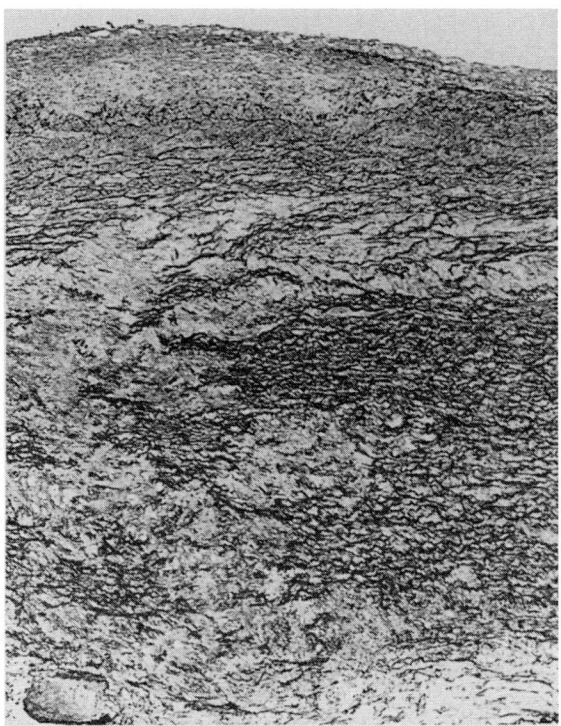

Fig. 30. Cystic medial necrosis of the aorta. "Tiger skin pattern" of the elastic frame. Orcein.

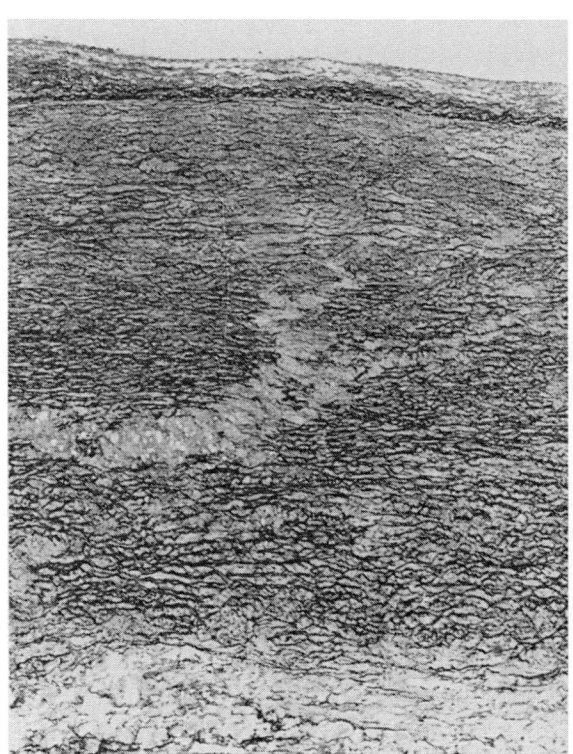

Fig. 29. Cystic medial necrosis of the aorta. Disseminated pooling of mucoid material in the aortic wall. Orcein

ger skin pattern" (Fig. 30). Myocytes decrease in number and are replaced by fibrosis [211, 213]. There is gradual dilatation of the artery. When veins are involved, the media contains numerous cysts filled with mucoid material, distorting the connective tissue and the muscle bundles.

5 – Segmental arterial mediolysis or segmental mediolytic arteriopathy

Formerly known as segmental mediolytic arteritis [214], segmental arterial mediolysis (SAM) or segmental mediolytic arteriopathy begins with necrosis of the outer media, which may extend to the mid– and inner media (Fig. 31-32). The lesion is accompanied by deposits of fibrinous material (Fig. 33) along the medial adventitial junction and replacement of the lysed muscle fibers by fibrin, erythrocytes, and granulation tissue mimicking necrotizing vasculitis [21, 215]. In muscular arteries, organisation of uncomplicated SAM lesions produces an appearance resembling the medial type of FMD and some have

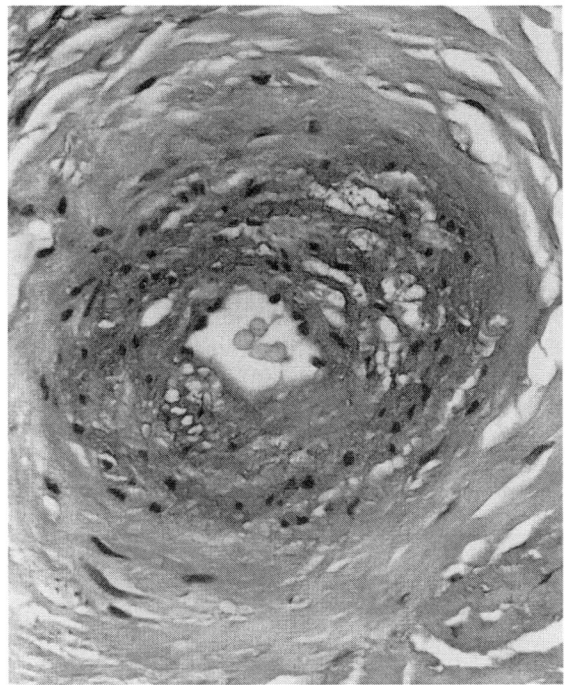

Fig. 31. Segmental arterial mediolysis of a muscular small calibre artery. Haematoxylin, eosin and saffron stain (HES)

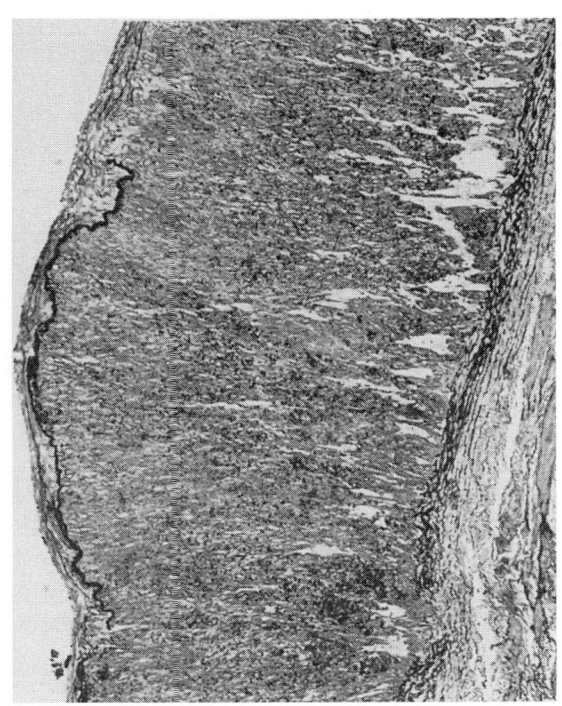

Fig. 32. Segmental arterial mediolysis of a muscular medium calibre artery. Orcein

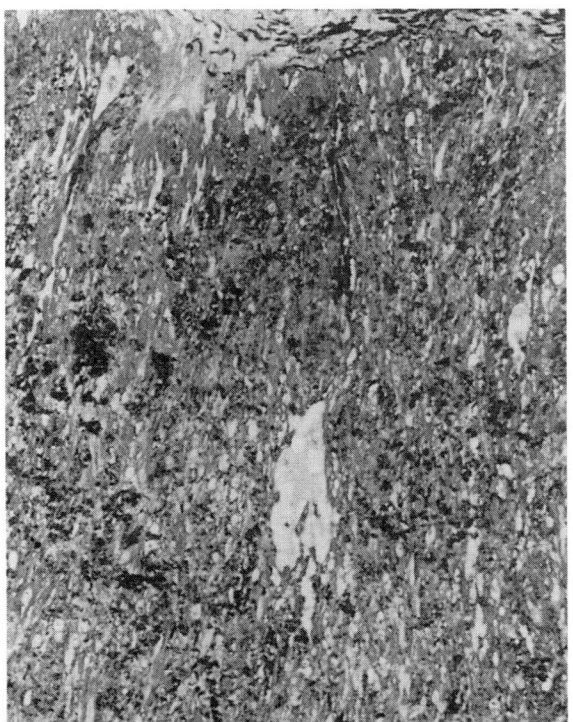

Fig. 33. Segmental arterial mediolysis of a muscular medium calibre artery. Note cyst formation in the outer part of the media. Orcein

considered SAM to be an early variant of fibromuscular dysplasia [21, 86]. The differential diagnosis becomes problematic for elastic arteries; distinction from FMD is impossible, especially when FMD is associated with other aortic changes, for example those of Marfan's disease [38]. Transmural mediolysis leads to thrombosis, dissecting haematoma and aneurysm. Certain morphological features of SAM suggest that this arterial lesion is caused by vasospasm, ascribed to focal endothelial paracrine dysfunction by Slavin [21].

6 – Acquired angiodysplasia (angiodystrophy)

The term angiodysplasia embraces a large variety of vascular changes involving arteries, veins and lymphatics but is mostly used for congenital vascular abnormalities [216]. This term has also been used to describe acquired degenerative changes in vessels [217] and some authors have proposed the term "angiodystrophy" instead of "angiodysplasia" to avoid confusion [218]. The condition mostly affects the digestive tract, the uterus, and the bladder and is responsible for recurrent, often occult, haemorrhages. The cause of angiodysplasia is uncertain but has been attributed to various mechanisms; degenerative changes [218, 219] resulting from aging, a deficiency of mucosal vascular collagen type IV [220], hormonal disorders (involving estrogens, progestogens, parathormone) [221, 222] or mechanical factors operating in the wall of these muscular and contracting viscera.

Digestive tract angiodysplasia

In the digestive tract, angiodystrophy develops after the age of 60 yrs and may cause massive gastrointestinal haemorrhage. Digestive angiodystrophy may be associated with ageing-related vascular degenerative changes, colic diverticulosis [223], rectal prolapse and certain coagulation disorders, such as type II thrombasthenia, Bernard-Soulier's syndrome, congenital platelet dysfunction, type I and immune-mediated von Willebrand and Osler-Rendu-Weber diseases [224-226], end-stage renal disease [221, 227], cryptogenic hepatic cirrhosis [228], and aortic stenosis in 20 to 30 % of cases (Heyde syndrome). The association of caecal angiodysplasia and aortic stenosis remains an enigma. The bleeding ceases after valve replacement by either a mechanical or biological prostheses even though the angiodysplasic lesions remain. Impaired aggregability of thrombocytes does not seem to be the explanation [229, 217, 230, 231]. Angiodysplasic lesions can develop anywhere (colon, stomach, rectum, and small intestine) in the gastrointestinal tract.

In the stomach, angiodysplasia frequently develops in the antrum. Gastric antral vascular ectasia (GAVE) leads to blood loss in the disorders of the so-called "watermelon stomach" [232]. In the lower digestive tract, angiodysplasia develops mainly in the right colon, especially the caecum, but the rectum may also be involved [228, 233, 234]. Normal colic distension and contraction may occlude the submucosal veins that penetrate the muscle wall intermittently, leading to focal dilatation and tortuosity of overlying submucosal and mucosal vessels. The tension in the walls of these organs is a product of intraluminal pressure and diameter. Because the caecum has the widest diameter of the colon, it develops the greatest wall tension, perhaps explaining the preferential distribution of these lesions at this site in the large bowel.

A selective angiogram performed during a haemorrhagic episode allows topographic diagnosis by displaying an arteriolar meshwork (Fig. 34) with early and prolonged opacification of dilated and tortuous veins. Opaque medium may extravasate when the blood flow reaches 0.5 to 3 ml/mn [235]. Other techniques, such as endoscopic ultrasound and digital spectroscopy, may improve detection rates [236, 237]. However, some lesions are only visible during endoscopy. Tortuous dilatation of submucosal and mucosal blood vessels is seen as cherry red, slightly raised patches communicating with a draining vein (Fig. 35). Surgical resection is the treatment of choice [234]. The major problem is how to locate the lesions when arteriographic findings are non conclusive. Per-operative endoscopic identification of the lesion may be helpful.

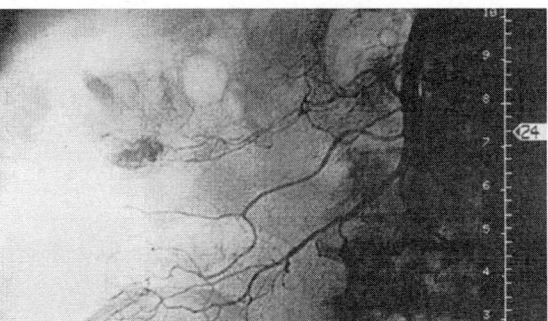

Fig. 34. Cecal angiodysplasia. Angiographic pattern

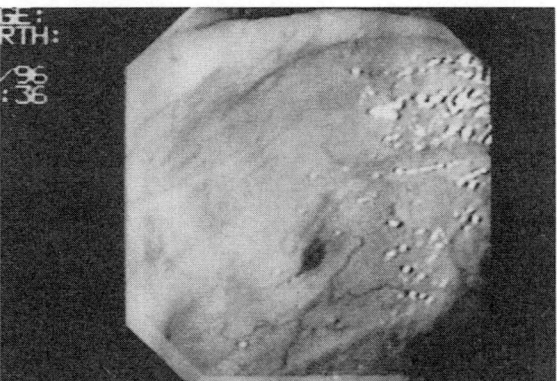

Fig. 35. Cecal angiodysplasia. Endoscopic pattern

Pathology and differential diagnosis

On non-injected operative specimens, angiodystrophic lesions may not be evident to the naked eye and vascular injection techniques carried out on fresh operative specimens are necessary [218]. The combined technique of injecting a dye (india ink) (Fig. 36-37) and a water-soluble contrast medium into the resected specimen reveals areas of dilated vessels, which can be identified histologically [218, 238]. In the di-

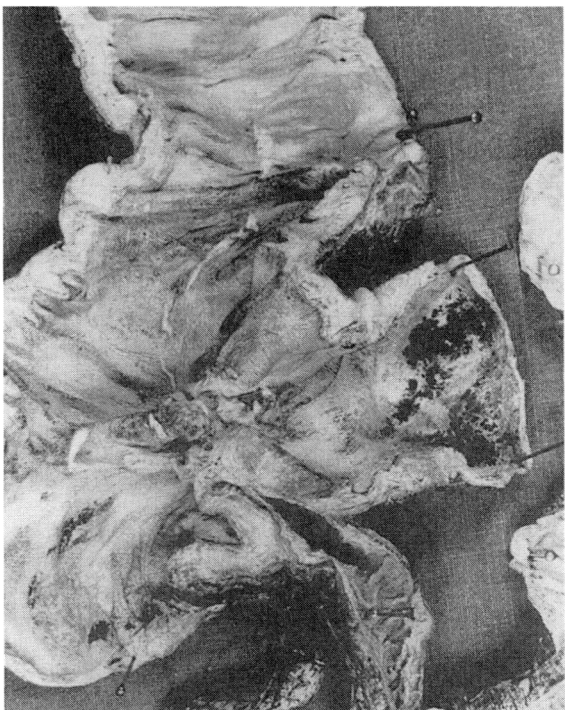

Fig. 36. Cecal angiodysplasia. Ink injection technique helps identify more diffuse lesions

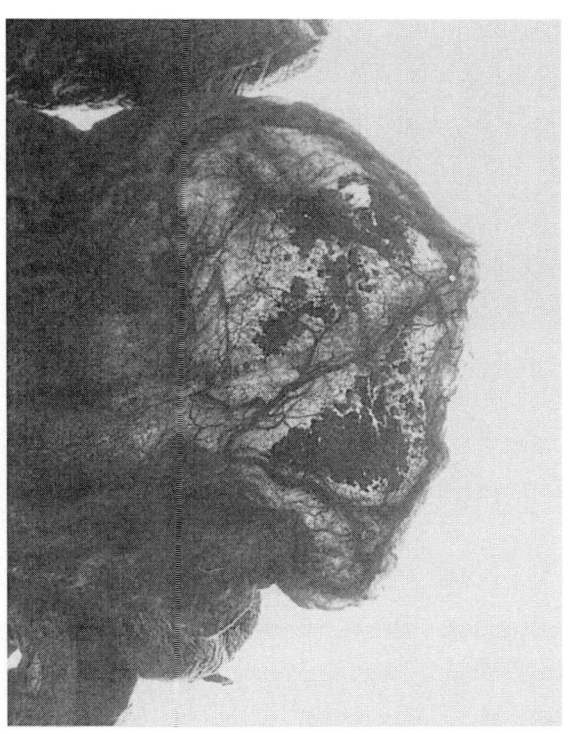

Fig. 37. Cecal angiodysplasia. "Cleared specimen" after ink injection technique

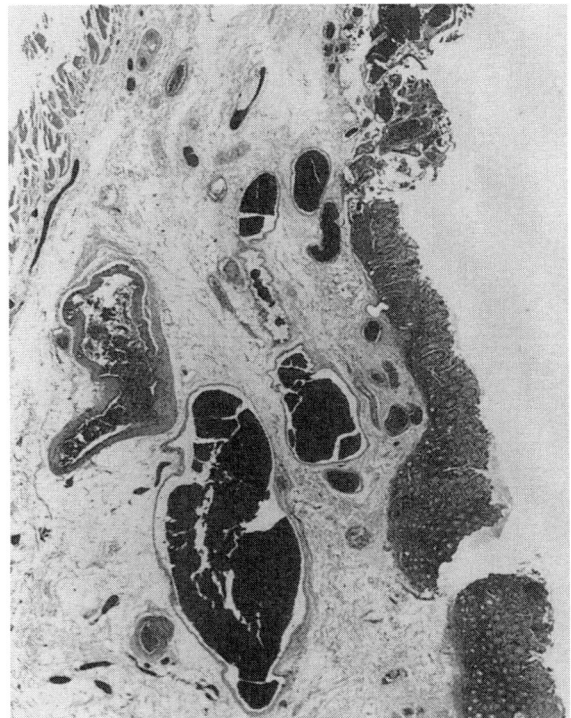

Fig. 38. Cecal angiodysplasia. Abnormal vascular network identified by ink injection technique. HES

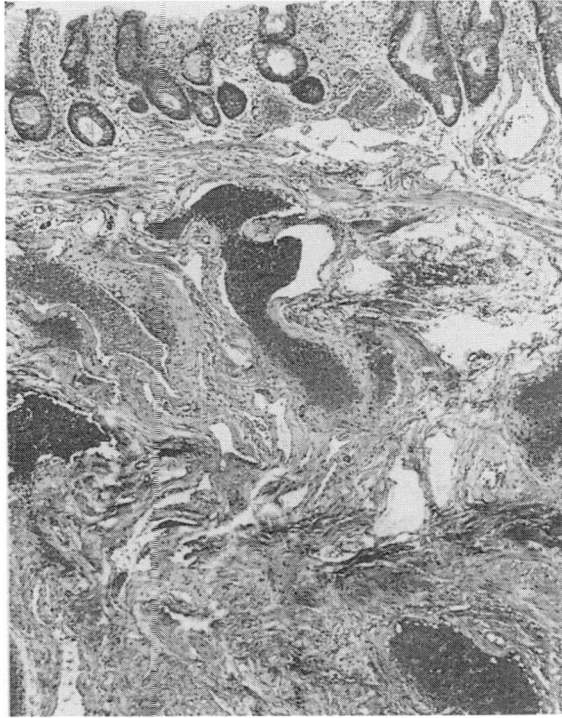

Fig. 39. Cecal angiodysplasia. Ectatic capillaries, venules and veins displaying marked degenerative changes. HES

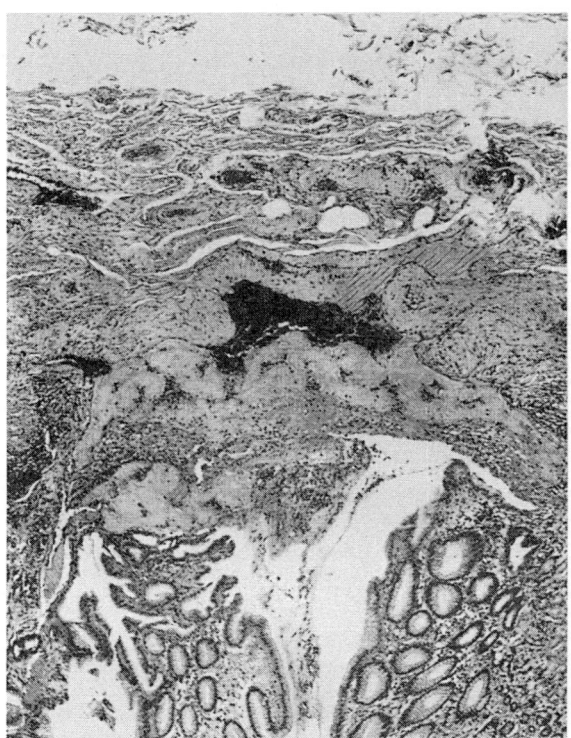

Fig. 40. Gastric antral vascular ectasia or "watermelon stomach" ulceration with underlying angiodysplasia. HES

gestive tract, most angiodysplasias span the mucosa and submucosa, suggesting that they are ectatic nests of pre-existing veins, venules, and capillaries (Fig. 38-39-40). The vascular channels may be separated from the intestinal lumen only by the vascular wall and a layer of attenuated epithelial cells. Immunohistochemical study evidences a decrease in collagen type IV in ectatic vessels in the mucosa as compared to similarly sized vessels in the submucosa and perforating vessels. In many cases these vessels appear to lose staining at the level of the muscularis mucosae [220].

Uterine angiodystrophy (Vuong-Proust Syndrome)

This new anatomical entity is responsible for recurrent unexplained metrorrhagia [218, 219]. The mean age at presentation is 38,5 yrs and bleeding is resistant to medical, haemostatic and/or hormonal treatment. Severe iron deficiency anaemia may result.

Mechanical factors may be the major cause of this condition. Partial compression by leiomyomas or fibrosis developed around mural adenomyomatous foci may cause the dilatation of interstitial myometrial vessels and endometrial venous sinuses and capilla-

ries. Degenerative changes occurring in the vessel walls may result from previous pregnancies or interstitial fibrosis. These changes may sometimes affect the pelvic venous plexuses.

Pathology and differential diagnosis

Grossly, the uterine mucosa shows haemorrhages. Dilated vessels may be prominent in the mucosa and the myometrium (Fig. 41). In haemorrhagic areas of the endometrium, markedly dilated capillaries and dystrophic endometrial venous sinuses are seen. These structures are in continuity with underlying interstitial veins in the myometrium. (Fig. 42). In some areas, endometrial dilated capillaries and venous sinuses thicken the endometrium, and form polypoid masses protruding into the uterine cavity (Fig. 43). The underlying myometrial veins show dystrophic changes with an uneven fibrotic wall with elastin deposition (Fig. 44). Organised thromboses may be present. Vascular injection techniques help to identify these connections in fresh operative specimens (Fig. 45). These lesions are similar to those observed in the angiodysplasia of the digestive tract and are found in 16% of cases of menorrhagia in the experience of one of us [218] and are sometimes associated with leiomyomatosis, adenomyosis, and endometrial hyperplasia.

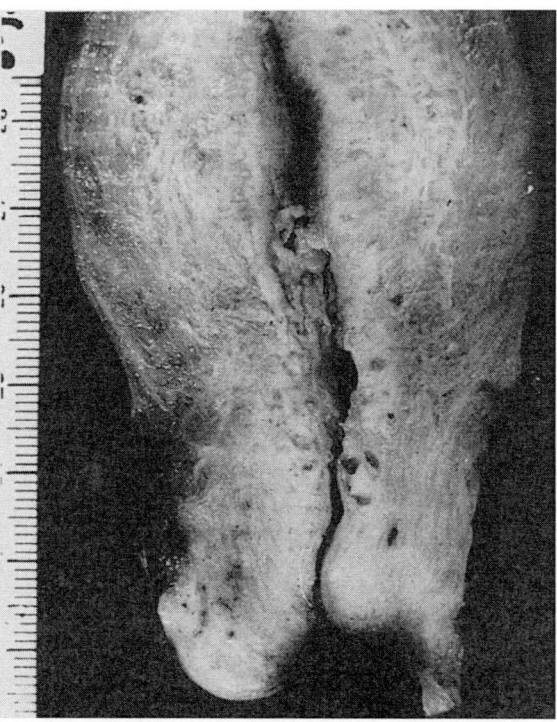

Fig. 41. Angiodystrophy of the uterus. Note ectatic veins in the isthmus and myometrium

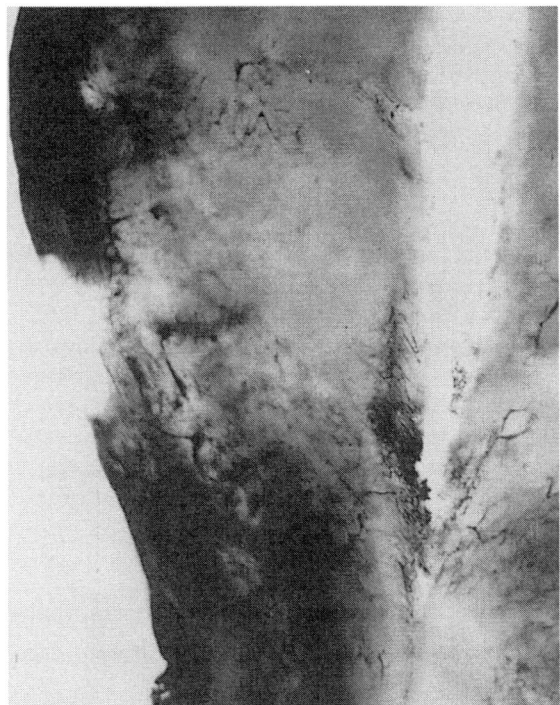

Fig. 42. Angiodystrophy of the uterus. Markedly dilated capillaries and venous plexuses are present in haemorrhagic areas. "Cleared specimen" after ink injection technique

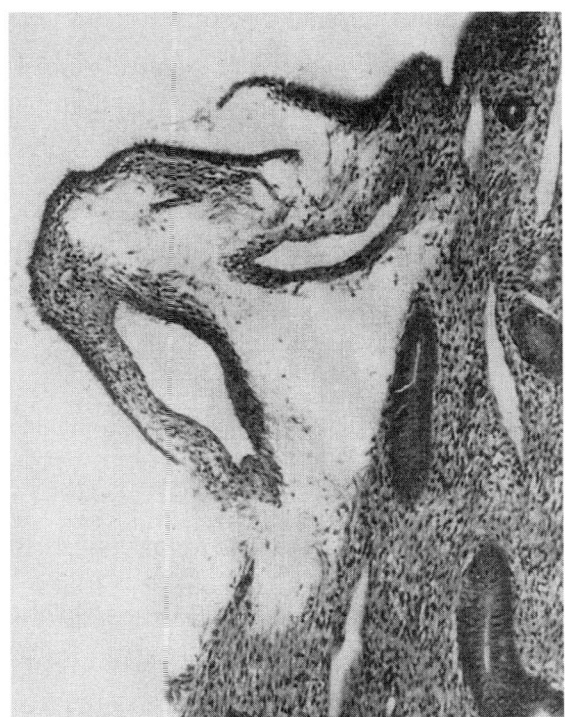

Fig. 43. Angiodystrophy of the uterus. Ectatic capillaries distort the endometrial stroma and protrude into the uterine cavity. HES

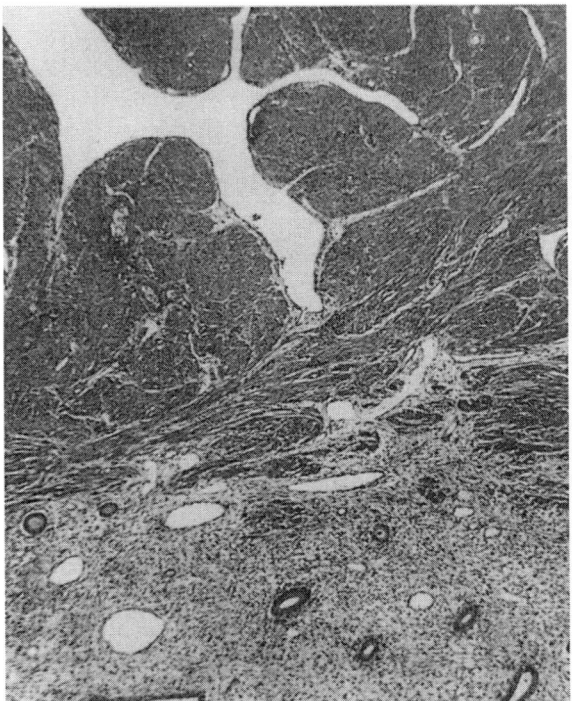

Fig. 44. Angiodystrophy of the uterus. Dystrophic changes in underlying myometrial veins.HES

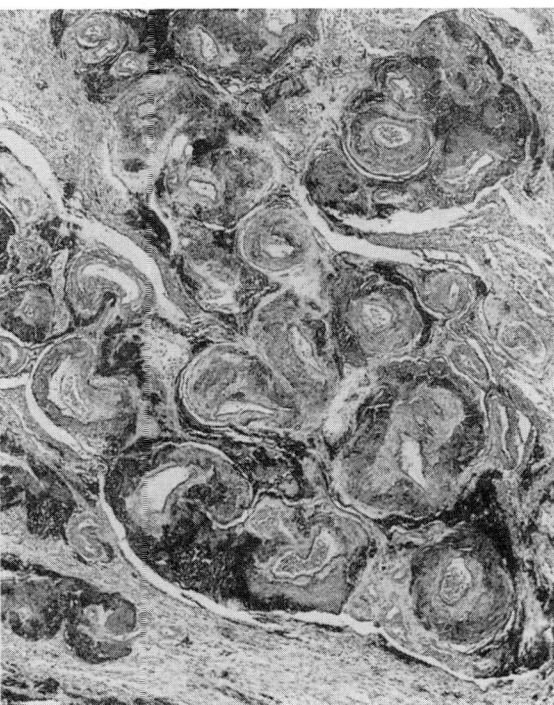

Fig. 45. Angiodystrophy of the uterus. Dystrophic changes in underlying myometrial veins. Note elastin deposits around uterine veins. Orcein

Veno-lymphatic angiodysplasia

This condition may be the cause of recurrent varicose veins [239].

7 – Progressive systemic sclerosis

Progressive systemic sclerosis (PSS) is characterized by inflammatory and degenerative processes leading to excessive deposition of collagen and other connective tissue matrix proteins,resulting in exuberant fibrosis of multiple organ systems [240]. The incidence of PSS ranges from 67 to 265 per 100,000 in different studies [241]. The peak age of onset is in the third and fourth decades. Females are affected three times as often as males, and during childbearing years [242]. There is a weak association with HLA antigens DR3 and DR5 [243, 244]. However, unaffected family members present an increased prevalence of anti-nuclear antibodies (ANA) and anti-Scl-70 and anti-centromere autoantibody positivity [245, 246].

The cause is unknown. Many xenobiotics have been suggested to be causative, including benzene, toluene, vinyl chloride, formaldehyde, bleomycin, pentazocine, cocaine, appetite suppressants, rape seed oil/aniline, silica dust, paraffin, processed-petrolatum jelly and L-tryptophan (which produces a fibrosing condition associated with eosinophic myalgia). The role of breast silicone-gel filled prostheses is now discounted [247-250].

T-lymphocytes and monocytes appear to be the major inducing cells of PSS. Fibroblasts, mast cells, platelets, and endothelial cells act as targets or mediators of the disease. Activated T-cells are believed to release cytokine IL-2 and cause endothelial cell damage. IL-2 then stimulates monocytes to release transforming growth factor (TGF) which activates fibroblasts to secrete cytokine IL-4 and organized elements of the extracellular matrix [251, 252].

The illness involves the skin with localised (morphea, linear or nodular scleroderma) [253, 254] or diffuse changes (generalized morphea or systemic sclerosis). Skin involvement has three distinct phases; initially, the fingers and hands are ooedematous, puffy and stiff, mimicking a carpal tunnel syndrome, then severe induration appears, the skin turning firm and hard and finally, the skin undergoes atrophy, becoming softened. Affected areas then show an increase in mobility.

There are three main subtypes of systemic sclerosis; diffuse systemic sclerosis, the CREST syndrome (Calcinosis cutis, Raynaud's phenomenon, Esophageal dysmotility, Sclerodactyly, and Telangiectasia); and combined diffuse sclerosis and disseminated telangiectasia [255-258]. Overlap syndromes may exist sharing features of polymyositis, systemic lupus erythematosus (SLE), rheumatoid arthritis, mixed connective tissue disease, Sjogren's syndrome, retroperitoneal fibrosis, peripheral neuromuscular manifestations and the eosinophilia-myalgia syndrome [259-264].

Involvement of deep organs is often fatal. Motility disorders of the digestive tract predispose to bacterial overgrowth and malabsorption, ileus, volvulus, pseudodiverticulae, and perforation [265]. Primary biliary cirrhosis occurs in 4% of patients with CREST syndrome [266]. Pulmonary hypertension, cor pulmonae, aspiration pneumonitis, spontaneous pneumothorax and pleural disease, compromising lung involvement, may all occur. "Scleroderma renal crisis" leads to renovascular hypertension and progressive renal failure [267-269]. Vasculogenic impotence by outflow disorder has been reported [46].

Associated neoplasms have been reported in the lungs (alveolar cell and bronchogenic carcinoma) and the digestive tract (colonic adenocarcinoma) [270]. The overall survival rate is 60% at 5 years, and 42% at 10 years.

Criteria for diagnosis of systemic sclerosis may be major (proximal diffuse sclerosis with non-pitting skin induration) or minor (sclerodactyly, digital pitting scars, loss of digital finger pulp pads, and basilar pulmonary fibrosis). The diagnosis should be made when a patient fulfills the major criterion or two minor criteria.

Pathology and differential diagnosis
Virtually all organs may be affected by systemic sclerosis. Lesions are often present in the blood vessels and heart.

In the skin, early changes consist of oedema and perivascular infiltrates containing CD4 + T cells with swelling and degeneration of collagen fibers which become eosinophilic. Capillaries, arterioles and small arteries display thickening of the basement membrane, endothelial cell damage and partial occlusion (Fig. 46-47). With progression, progressive fibrosis appears in the dermis with a marked increase of compact collagen in the dermis, thinning of the epidermis, loss of rete pegs, and atrophy of dermal appendages. Dermal capillaries and arterioles present hyaline thickening of the walls. Telangiectasia and focal subcutaneous calcifications may develop. In advanced stages, loss of

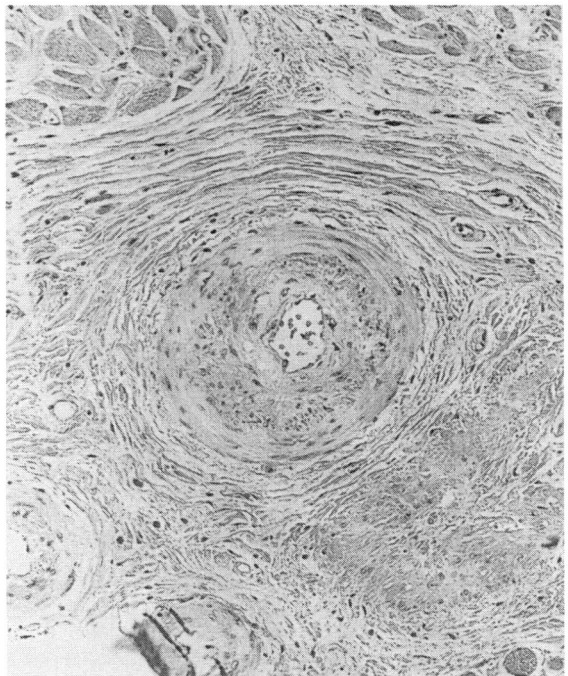

Fig. 46. Progressive systemic sclerosis. Intimal thickening with endothelial damage in a small calibre artery. HES

blood supply leads to peripheral vascular deterioration with distal digital ulceration (Fig. 48-49), and hyper-and hypo-pigmentation [271, 272]. Sometimes the fingertips may undergo autoamputation. In the lungs, fibrous thickening of small pulmonary vessels accompany diffuse interstitial and alveolar fibrosis. In the heart, thickening of intramyocardial arterioles, together with myocardial fibrosis, leads to ischaemic or restrictive cardiomyopathy with severe congestive heart failure. In the kidney, the small arcuate and interlobular arteries display concentric "onion-skin" sub-endothelial/intimal proliferation leading to impaired flow (Fig. 50). Focal segmental glomerulosclerosis resulting from ischaemia of the glomeruli occurs at the end stage (Fig. 46). Constriction of the efferent glomerular arterioles, results in severe systemic hypertension [267]. Vasculitis has also been reported.

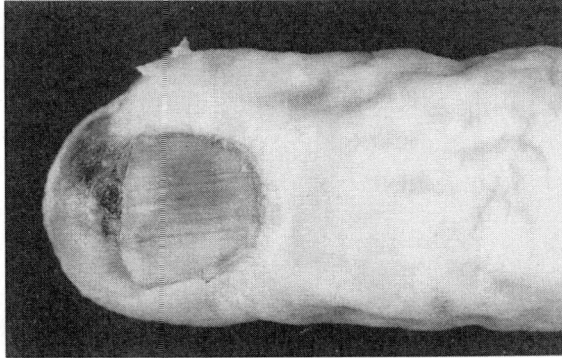

Fig. 48. Progressive systemic sclerosis. Advanced stage with finger gangrene

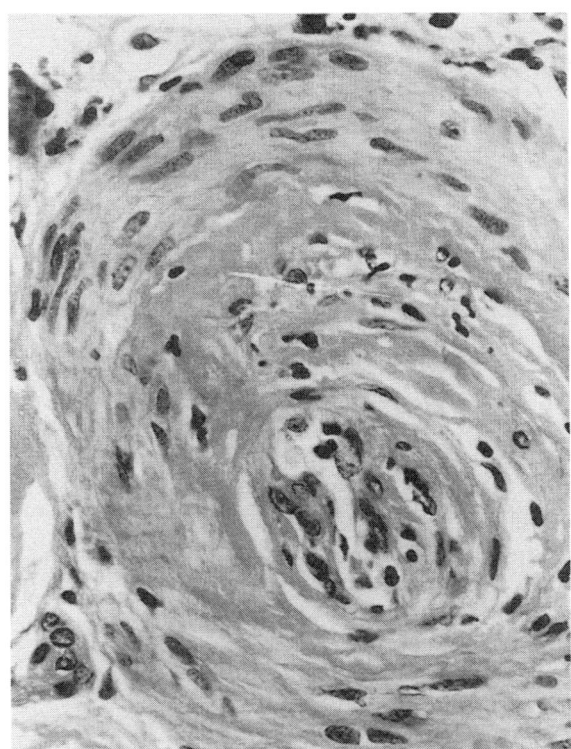

Fig. 47. Progressive systemic sclerosis. Marked endothelial damage with total occlusion of a small calibre artery. HES

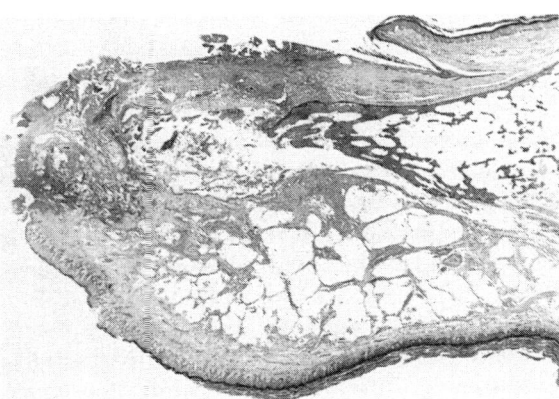

Fig. 49. Progressive systemic sclerosis. Advanced stage with extensive gangrene of the finger extremity. HES

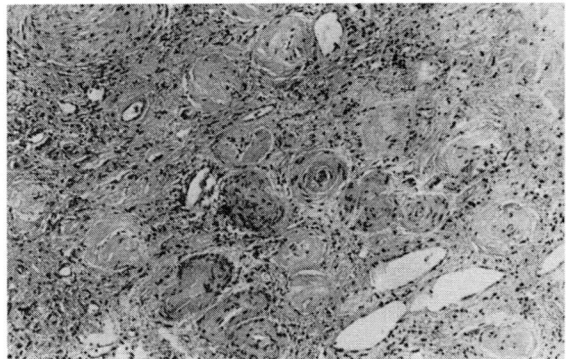

Fig. 50. Progressive systemic sclerosis. "Onion-skin" intimal proliferation of intrarenal arteries. HES

8 – Ainhum

This poorly understood disease is characterised by a spontaneous and slowly progressive fibrous constriction in the digito-plantar fold, usually of the little toe, resulting in gradual spontaneous amputation of the toe.

Messum first reported the condition in 1821 [273], Clark called it "dry gangrene" of the toes in 1860 and da Silva Lima gave the first detailed description in 1867 in Brazil. Wucherer applied the name ainhum in 1872. However, there are many synonyms in the tropical and sub-tropical countries in which it is common. Its incidence is highest in India, Brazil and Panama where the prevalence may reach 2,5 per thousand [274]. Isolated cases of ainhum have been reported in Europe, Canada, and in the United States [275]. Most case reports deal with deeply pigmented male patients, in the fourth and fifth decades.

Clinically, the lesion starts as a deepening of the digito-plantar fold of the fifth toe. An additional lesion may be found on the fourth toe and bilaterality has been reported [276]. Involvement of the fingers is rare. A groove develops and becomes more pronounced, extending medially around the toe over a period of months to years. Ulceration of the floor of the groove follows with progressive resorption of the bone. Fibrosis may lead to a medial rotation of the toe plantar surface and auto-amputation of the toe. Pain is of variable severity, but there are no systemic manifestations. Dent et al [277] reported arteriographic abnormalities of the blood supply to the foot proximal to the groove. Surgical amputation of the diseased toe relieves pain. Z-plasty in the area of the constricting band may be attempted with poor results. Intralesional injection of corticoid (triamcinolone) may help relieve pain with partial resolution of the fibrotic band [278].

Leprosy [279], syphilis, yaws, dermatophytosis, keratoderma hereditarium mutilans (Vohwinkel's syndrome) [280], chiggers, barefootedness, foreign bodies and chronic traumatic arteritis have all been incriminated in the pathogenesis of ainhum [281] and a genetic component is suspected as there is a tendency to geographical clustering of cases and familial occurrence.

Pathology and differential diagnosis

In early and moderately advanced lesions, vessels and nerves remain normal. Advanced lesions display chronic dermatitis with elongation of the epidermal rete pegs and parakeratosis. The leukocytic infiltrate consists mainly of T lymphocytes. The underlying bone undergoes osteoporosis with cortical bone resorption. Foreign body granulomas may be present [282]. Marked fibrosis of the dermis compresses the tendons, vessels, and nerves as the toe approaches auto-amputation. Eventually the constricted band becomes a fibrous cord and the distal portion a fibro-fatty knob. Ainhum must be differentiated from "pseudo-ainhum" which follows burns, frostbite, keratoderma [283], scleroderma [284], psoriasis [285], discoid lupus erythematosus [286], sickle cell disease, and diabetes [287].

Bibliography

1. Leadbetter WF, Burkland CE (1938) Hypertension in unilateral renal disease. J Urol 39 : 611-26
2. Gambini G, Argento R, Esposito S, Fioroni E, Rossi S, Valori C (1990) Transluminal percutaneous angioplasty in renovascular hypertension caused by monolateral fibromuscular dysplasia. Clin Ter 132: 259-65
3. Ishijima H, Ishizaka H, Sakurai M, Ito K, Endo K (1997) Partial renal embolization for pediatric renovascular hypertension secondary to fibromuscular dysplasia. Cardiovasc Intervent Radiol 20: 383-6
4. Imamura H, Isobe M, Takenaka H, Kinoshita O, Sekiguchi M, Ohta M (1998) Successful stenting of bilateral renal artery stenosis due to fibromuscular dysplasia assessed by use of pressure guidewire technique: a case report. Angiology 49: 69-74
5. Fiquet-Kempf B, Grimbert P, Pannier-Moreau I, Vuagnat A, Jeunemaitre X, Plouin PF (1999) Fibromuscular dysplasia of the renal arteries. Néphrologie 20: 13-8
6. Palubinskas AJ, Ripley HR (1964) Fibromuscular hyperplasia in extrarenal arteries. Radiology 82: 451-4
7. Prieto LN, Dyer CB, Thompson PM, Whigham C Jr (1996) The oldest reported patient with fibromuscular dysplasia of the renal artery. South Med J 89: 405-8
8. Wells TG, Belsha CW (1996) Pediatric renovascular hypertension. Curr Opin Pediatr 8: 128-34

9. Shimauchi M, Kaji Y, Goya T, Kinoshita K (1989) A case report of fibromuscular dysplasia presenting symptoms like moyamoya disease: "string of beads" appearance of the pericallosal artery. No Shinkei Geka 17: 981-4

10. Imamura M, Yokoyama S, Kikuchi K (1997) Coronary fibromuscular dysplasia presenting as sudden infant death. Arch Pathol Lab Med 121: 159-61

11. Zurin AA, Houkin K, Asano T, Ishikawa T, Abe H (1997) Childhood ischaemic stroke caused by fibromuscular dysplasia of the intracranial artery—case report. Neurol Med Chir (Tokyo) 37: 542-5

12. Burke AP, Virmani R (1998) Intramural coronary artery dysplasia of the ventricular septum and sudden death. Hum Pathol 29: 1124-7

13. Leventer RJ, Kornberg AJ, Coleman LT, Phelan EM, Kean MJ (1998) Stroke and fibromuscular dysplasia: confirmation by renal magnetic resonance angiography. Pediatr Neurol 18: 172-5

14. Harrisson EGJr, Hunt JC, Bernatz (1967) Morphology of fibromuscular dysplasia of the renal artery in renovascular hypertension. Am J Med 43: 97-112

15. Palubinskas AJ, Newton TH (1965) Fibromuscular hyperplasia of the internal carotid arteries. Radiol Clin (Basel) 34: 365-70

16. Leung DY, Glagov S, Mathews MB (1976) Cyclic stretching stimulates synthesis of matrix components by arterial smooth muscle cells in vitro. Science 191: 475-7

17. Ross R, Klebanoff SJ (1967) Fine structural changes in uterine smooth muscle and fibroblasts in response to estrogen. J Cell Biol 32: 155-67

18. Farhat MY, Lavigne MC, Ramwell PW (1996) The vascular protective effects of estrogen. FASEB J 10: 615-24

19. Fievez M, Koerperich G, Dulieu J (1975) Arterial fibromuscular dysplasia and ergotism. Ann Anat Pathol (Paris) 20: 357-66

20. Paulson GW, Boesel CP, Evans WE (1978) Fibromuscular dysplasia. Arch Neurol 35: 287-90

21. Slavin RE, Saeki K, Bhagavan B, Maas AE (1995) Segmental arterial mediolysis: a precursor to fibromuscular dysplasia? Mod Pathol 8: 287-94

22. de Mendonca WC, Espat PA (1981) Pheochromocytoma associated with arterial fibromuscular dysplasia. Am J Clin Pathol 75: 749-54

23. Mattix H, Dennard DT, Hall WD (1997) Fibromuscular dysplasia of the renal artery and adrenal adenoma in a 36-year-old woman with hypertension. Am J Med Sci 314: 51-3

24. Bloor K, Williams RT (1963) Neurofibromatosis and coarctation of the abdominal aorta with renal artery involvement. Brit J Surg 50: 811-3

25. Halpern HH, Sanford HS, Viamonte M (1965) Renal artery abnormalities in three hypertensive sisters. JAMA 194: 124-5

26. Hansen J, Holter C, Thorbert JV (1965) Hypertension in two sisters caused by so-called fibromuscular hyperplasia of the renal arteries. Acta Med Scand 178: 461-74

27. Rushton AR (1980) The genetics of fibromuscular dysplasia. Arch Intern Med 140: 233-6

28. Gladstien K, Rushton AR, Kidd KK (1980) Penetrance estimates and recurrence risks for fibromuscular dysplasia. Clin Genet 17: 115-6

29. Planche C, Camilleri JP, El Abdel Hafez A, Zannier D, Mercier JN, Artru B (1983) Lesions of the aortic arch in Recklinghausen's disease. Arch Mal Cœur Vaiss 76: 607-13

30. Debure C, Fiessinger JN, Bruneval P, Vuong NP, Cormier JM, Housset E (1984) Multiple arterial lesions in von Recklinghausen's disease. A case. Presse Med 13: 1776-8

31. Taguchi T, Tanaka K, Ikeda K (1985) Fibromuscular dysplasia of arteries in Hirschsprung's disease. Gastroenterology 88: 1099-103

32. Savin H, Jutrin I, Ravid M (1986) Persistant hypokalemia due to bilateral fibromuscular dysplasia of the renal arteries. Clin Nephrol 25: 199-201

33. Dominguez FE, Tate LG, Robinson MJ (1988) Familial fibromuscular dysplasia presenting as sudden death. Am J Cardiovasc Pathol 2: 269-72

34. Finley JL, Dabbs DJ (1988) Renal vascular smooth muscle proliferation in neurofibromatosis. Hum Pathol 19: 107-10

35. Meredith JT, Cerezo L, Alvarez M, Price G, Bourgeois S (1988) Gastrointestinal arterial fibromuscular dysplasia of childhood. Arch Pathol Lab Med 112: 833-7

36. Mandreoli M, Zuccala A, Zucchelli P (1992) Fibromuscular dysplasia of the renal arteries associated with antiphospholipid autoantibodies: two case reports. Am J Kidney Dis 20: 500-3

37. Watanabe S, Tanaka K, Nakayama T, Kaneko M (1993) Fibromuscular dysplasia at the internal carotid origin: a case of carotid web. No Shinkei Geka 21: 449-52

38. Schievink WI, Bjornsson J, Piepgras DG (1994) Coexistence of fibromuscular dysplasia and cystic medial necrosis in a patient with Marfan's syndrome and bilateral carotid artery dissections. Stroke 25: 2492-6

39. Nopajaroonsri C, Lurie AA (1996) Venous aneurysm, arterial dysplasia, and near-fatal hemorrhages in neurofibromatosis type 1. Hum Pathol 27: 982-5

40. Paraf F, Bruneval P (1996) Arterial fibromuscular dysplasia and Bourneville's tuberous sclerosis. Ann Pathol 16: 203-6

41. Szpak GM, Kuczynska-Zardzewialy A, Popow J (1996) Brain vascular changes in the case of primary antiphospholipid syndrome. Folia Neuropathol 34: 92-6

42. Hamed RM, Ghandour K (1997) Abdominal angina and intestinal gangrene—a catastrophic presentation of arterial fibromuscular dysplasia: case report and review of the literature J Pediatr Surg 32: 1379-80

43. Solder B, Streif W, Ellemunter H, Mayr U, Jaschke W (1997) Fibromuscular dysplasia of the internal carotid artery in a child with alpha-1-antitrypsin deficiency. Dev Med Child Neurol 39: 827-9

44. Grange DK, Balfour IC, Chen SC, Wood EG (1998) Familial syndrome of progressive arterial occlusive disease consistent with fibromuscular dysplasia, hypertension, congenital cardiac defects, bone fragility, brachysyndactyly, and learning disabilities. Am J Med Genet 75: 469-80

45. Moreland RB, Traish A, McMillin MA, Smith B, Goldstein I, Saenz de Tejada I (1995) PGE1 suppresses the induction of collagen synthesis by transforming growth factor-beta 1 in human corpus cavernosum smooth muscle. J Urol 153: 826-34

46. Nehra A, Hall SJ, Basile G, Bertero EB, Moreland R, Toselli P, de las Morenas A, Goldstein I (1995) Systemic sclerosis and impotence: a clinicopathological correlation. J Urol 153: 1140-6

47. Ross R (1971) The smooth muscle cell. II. Growth of smooth muscle in culture and formation of elastic fibers. J Cell Biol 50: 172-86

48. Ross R, Klebanoff SJ (1971) The smooth muscle cell. I. In vivo synthesis of connective tissue proteins. J Cell Biol 50: 159-71

49. Sottiurai VS, Fry WJ, Stanley JC (1978) Ultrastructure of medial smooth muscle and myofibroblasts in human arterial dysplasia. Arch Surg 113: 1280-8

50. Bragin MA, Cherkasov AP (1979) Morphogenesis of fibromuscular dysplasia of the renal arteries. Arkh Patol 41: 46-52

51. Camilleri JP (1987) Aspects anatomo-pathologiques et physiopathologiques des dysplasies fibromusculaires *In* Camilleri JP Berry CL, Fiessinger JN, Bariety J (eds): Les maladies de la paroi artérielle. Flammarion, Paris, p 465-474

52. James TN (1990) Morphologic characteristics and functional significance of focal fibromuscular dysplasia of small coronary arteries. Am J Cardiol 65: 12G-22G

53. Schievink WI, Bjornsson J, Parisi JE, Prakash UB (1994) Arterial fibromuscular dysplasia associated with severe alpha 1-antitrypsin deficiency. Mayo Clin Proc 69: 1040-3

54. Braga IS 3rd, Tanaka S, Itakura C, Mizutani M (1996) Fibromuscular dysplasia in intramuscular arteries of Japanese quail (Coturnix coturnix japonica). J Comp Pathol 114: 123-30

55. Rothfield NJH (1969) Experimental fibromuscular arterial dysplasia. Radiology 93: 1291-7

56. Hata J, Hosoda Y (1976) Tubular stenosis of the aorta with aortic fibromuscular dysplasia. Arch Pathol Lab Med 100: 652-5

57. Connolly JE (1978) Fibromuscular hyperplasia of the abdominal aorta. J Cardiovasc Surg (Torino) 19: 563-6

58. Ohteki H, Itoh T, Natsuaki M, Sakurai J, Tazaki H, Watanabe T, Yamada T (1989) Atypical coarctation of the thoracic aorta with fibromuscular dysplasia—report of a successful surgical repair and review of the literature. Nippon Geka Gakkai Zasshi 90: 130-3

59. Vuong PN, Trinh AC, Lagneau P, Camilleri JP (1989) Coarctation of the abdominal aorta and stenosis of the left renal artery with hypertension caused by fibrodysplasia. Arch Pathol Lab Med 113: 809-11

60. Vuong PN, Janzen J, Bical O, Susa-Uva M (1995) Fibromuscular dysplasia causing atypical coarctation of the thoracic aorta: histological presentation of a case. Vasa 24: 194-8

61. Golosovskaia MA, Serov RA, Lebedeva TM (1996) Two cases of fibromuscular dysplasia of the aorta. Arkh Patol 58: 62-6

62. Arunodaya GR, Vani S, Shankar SK, Taly AB, Swamy HS, Sarala D (1997) Fibromuscular dysplasia with dissection of basilar artery presenting as "locked-in-syndrome". Neurology 48: 1605-8

63. Cloft HJ, Kallmes DF, Kallmes MH, Goldstein JH, Jensen ME, Dion JE (1998) Prevalence of cerebral aneurysms in patients with fibromuscular dysplasia: a reassessment. J Neurosurg 88: 436-40

64. Miyauchi M, Shionoya S (1991) Aneurysm of the extracranial internal carotid artery caused by fibromuscular dysplasia. Eur J Vasc Surg 5: 587-91

65. Furie DM, Tien RD (1994) Fibromuscular dysplasia of arteries of the head and neck: imaging findings. AJR Am J Roentgenol 162: 1205-9

66. Manninen HI, Koivisto T, Saari T, Matsi PJ, Vanninen RL, Luukkonen M, Hernesniemi J (1997) Dissecting aneurysms of all four cervicocranial arteries in fibromuscular dysplasia: treatment with self-expanding endovascular stents, coil embolization, and surgical ligation. AJNR Am J Neuroradiol 18: 1216-20

67. Zack F, Terpe H, Hammer U, Wegener R (1996) Fibromuscular dysplasia of coronary arteries as a rare cause of death. Int J Legal Med 108: 215-8

68. Burke AP, Farb A, Tang A, Smialek J, Virmani R (1997) Fibromuscular dysplasia of small coronary arteries and fibrosis in the basilar ventricular septum in mitral valve prolapse. Am Heart J 134: 282-91

69. Wylie EJ, Binkley FM, Palubinskas AJ (1966) Extrarenal fibromuscular hyperplasia. Am J Surg 1122: 149-55

70. Sarles JC, Horta ME, Castelo HB, Delecourt P (1980) Arterial dysplasia of the colonic arteries: a rare cause of hemoperitoneum. Dis Colon Rectum 23: 411-7

71. Iwai T, Konno S, Hiejima K, Satake S, Suzuki S, Hiranuma S, Kamiyama R (1985) Fibromuscular dysplasia in the extremities. J Cardiovasc Surg (Torino) 26: 496-501

72. Herpels V, Van de Voorde W, Wilms G, Verbeken E, Baert A, Lauweryns J, Nevelsteen A (1987) Recurrent aneurysms of the upper arteries of the lower limb: an atypical manifestation of fibromuscular dysplasia—a case report. Angiology 38: 411-6

73. Patra P, De Lajartre AY, Chaillou P, Duveau D, Planchon B, Dupon H (1987) Fibromuscular dysplasia of the arteries of the leg. Apropos of 1 case. J Mal Vasc 12: 185-8

74. van den Dungen JJ, Boontje AH, Oosterhuis JW (1990) Femoropopliteal arterial fibrodysplasia. Br J Surg 77: 396-9

75. Insall RL, Chamberlain J, Loose HW (1992) Fibromuscular dysplasia of visceral arteries. Eur J Vasc Surg 6: 668-72

76. Kanzaki T, Kobayashi T, Shimizu H, Miura Y, Takayasu M, Abe T (1992) Aneurysm in the skin: arterial fibromuscular dysplasia. J Am Acad Dermatol 27: 883-5

77. Lin WW, McGee GS, Patterson BK, Yao JS, Pearce WH (1992) Fibromuscular dysplasia of the brachial artery: a case report and review of the literature. J Vasc Surg 16: 66-70

78. Thevenet A, Latil JL, Albat B (1992) Fibromuscular disease of the external iliac artery. Ann Vasc Surg 6: 199-204

79. Chambers JL, Neale ML, Appleberg M (1994) Fibromuscular hyperplasia in an aberrant subclavian artery and neurogenic thoracic outlet syndrome: an unusual combination. J Vasc Surg 20: 834-8

80. Setoyama M, Shimada T, Kanzaki T, Moriya K, Okahara K, Asakura T (1994) Cutaneous arterial fibromuscular dysplasia: a case report and electron-microscopic study. J Dermatol 21: 205-10

81. Hirooka S, Oshikiri N, Kimura M, Sugawara M, Oguma H, Irisawa T, Kasuya S (1995) A left subclavian arterial aneurysm caused by fibromuscular dysplasia: a case report. Kyobu Geka 48: 221-3

82. Neukirch C, Bahnini A, Delcourt A, Kieffer E (1996) Popliteal aneurysm due to fibromuscular dysplasia. Ann Vasc Surg 10: 578-81

83. Yamaguchi R, Yamaguchi A, Isogai M, Hori A, Kin Y (1996) Fibromuscular dysplasia of the visceral arteries. Am J Gastroenterol 91: 1635-8

84. Kotiloglu E, Ciftci AO, Tanyel FC, Hicsonmez A (1997) Neuronal intestinal and fibromuscular arterial dysplasias associated with intraluminal mucosal web. Eur J Pediatr Surg 7: 52-4

85. Tsatalpas P, Butters M (1997) Aneurysms of the iliac artery in fibromuscular dysplasia as differential diagnostic consideration in acute lower abdominal pain. Zentralbl Chir 122: 413-7

86. Chan RJ, Goodman TA, Aretz TH, Lie JT (1998) Segmental mediolytic arteriopathy of the splenic and hepatic arteries mimicking systemic necrotizing vasculitis. Arthritis Rheum 41: 935-8

87. Vuong PN, Desoutter P, Van T, Houissa-Vuong S (1999) Fibrodysplasie musculaire artérielle revelée par un faux anevrisme traumatique: un cas. J Mal Vasc (Paris) 24: 377-380

88. Lie JT, Kim H-S (1977) Fibromuscular dysplasia of the superior mesenteric artery and coexisting cerebral berry aneurysms. Angiology 28: 256-9

89. Clairbone TS (1979) Fibromuscular hyperplasia: report of a case with involvement of multiple arteries. Am J Med 49: 103-5

90. Ouchi Y, Tagawa H, Yamakado M, Takanashi R, Tanaka S (1989) Clinical significance of cerebral aneurysm in renovascular hypertension due to fibromuscular dysplasia: two cases in siblings. Angiology 40: 581-8

91. Patel KS, Wolfe JH, Mathias C (1990) Left external iliac artery dissection and bilateral renal artery aneurysms secondary to fibromuscular dysplasia: a case report. Neth J Surg 42: 118-20

92. Reilly JM, McGraw DJ, Sicard GA (1993) Bilateral brachial artery fibromuscular dysplasia. Ann Vasc Surg 7: 483-7

93. Ertel B, Schmitt R, Helmberger T, Schnur KP (1994) The multilocular occlusive form of fibromuscular hyperplasia. Radiologe 34: 63-6

94. Tsukamoto S, Ohira M, Okumura H, Narata M, Sezai Y, Ishii K (1995) Bilateral common iliac artery aneurysms secondary to fibromuscular dysplasia accompanied with a coronary aneurysm. A case report. J Cardiovasc Surg (Torino) 36: 587-90

95. Persu A, Dubois C, Pirson Y, de Plaen JF (1997) Renal fibromuscular dysplasia and cerebral aneurysm in a hypertensive patient with a familial history of cerebral vascular complications. Presse Med 26: 1429-31

96. Lee EK, Hecht ST, Lie JT (1998) Multiple intracranial and systemic aneurysms associated with infantile-onset arterial fibromuscular dysplasia. Neurology 50: 828-9

97. Pesonen E, Koskimies O, Rapola J, Jaakelainen J (1980) Fibromuscular dysplasia in a child: a generalized arterial disease. Acta Paediatr Scand 69: 563-6

98. Furunaga A, Zempo N, Akiyama N, Takenaka H, Kuga T, Fujioka K, Esato K (1992) Cystic disease of right popliteal artery with spontaneous resolution. Nippon Geka Gakkai Zasshi 93: 1501-3

99. Fukuhara H, Kitayama H, Yokoyama T, Shirotani H (1996) Thromboembolic pulmonary hypertension due to disseminated fibromuscular dysplasia. Pediatr Cardiol 17: 340-5

100. Pannier-Moreau I, Grimbert P, Fiquet-Kempf B, Vuagnat A, Jeunemaitre X, Corvol P, Plouin PF (1997) Possible familial origin of multifocal renal artery fibromuscular dysplasia. J Hypertens 15: 1797-801

101. Ekelund L, Gerlock AJ, Goncharenko V, Francis R (1977) Renal venographic findings in 29 kidneys with fibromuscular dysplasia of the renal artery. Radiology 125: 631-2

102. Fujimoto S, Kayama T, Ogawa A, Sakurai Y, Yoshimoto T, Suzuki J (1987) Two cases of intracranial fibromuscular dysplasia whose repeated angiography disclosed progression of the lesion. No To Shinkei 39: 937-45

103. Harrison EG Jr, Mc Cormack LJ (1971) Pathologic classification of renal arterial disease in renovascular hypertension. Mayo Clin Proc 46: 161-7

104. Stanley JC, Gewertz BL, Bove EL, Sottiurai V, Fry WJ (1975) Arterial fibrodysplasia. Histopathologic character and current etiologic concepts. Arch Surg 110: 561-6

105. Luscher TF, Lie JT, Stanson AW, Houser OW, Hollier LH, Sheps SG (1987) Arterial fibromuscular dysplasia. Mayo Clin Proc 62: 931-52

106. Wirth FP, Miller WA, Russell AP (1981) Atypical fibromuscular hyperplasia. Report of two cases. J Neurosurg 54: 685-9

107. Stokes JB, Bonsib SM, McBride JW (1996) Diffuse intimal fibromuscular dysplasia with multiorgan failure. Arch Intern Med 156: 2611-4

108. Guermonprez JL, Gueret P, Camilleri JP, Guerinon J, Deloche A, Maurice P (1977) Prinzmetal's angina. Histological study of peroperative coronary specimens. Apropos of 2 cases. Arch Mal Cœur Vaiss 70: 301-8

109. Kanazawa M, Abe K (1997) Renovascular fibromuscular hyperplasia. Ryoikibetsu Shokogun Shirizu 16: 334-7

110. Youngberg SP, Sheps SG, Strong CG (1977) Fibromuscular disease of the renal arteries. Med Clinic North Am 61 623-41

111. McCormack LJ, Noto TJ, Meaney FF (1967) Subadventitial fibroplasia of the renal artery: a disease of young women. Am Heart J 73: 602-6

112. Hata J, Hosoda Y (1979) Perimedial fibroplasia of the renal artery: a light and electron microscopic study. Arch Pathol Lab Med 103: 220-23

113. Vuong PN, Lagneau P (1987) Pathologie artérielle traumatique In Camilleri JP Berry CL, Fiessinger JN, Bariety J (eds): Les maladies de la paroi artérielle. Flammarion, Paris, p579

114. Lagneau P, Michel JB, Vuong PN, Temmar M (1987) Splanchnic arteries and Takayasu's disease In Visceral vascular surgery, Persson AV, Skudder PA Jr (eds). Marcel Dekker, New York, p175

115. James TN, Marshall TK (1976) De subitaneis mortibus. XVII. Multifocal stenoses due to fibromuscular dysplasia of the sinus node artery. Circulation 53: 736-42

116. Fry WJ, Ernst CB, Stanley JC, Arbor EA (1973) Renovascular hypertension in the pediatric patient. Arch Surg 107: 692-8

117. Michel JB, Camilleri JP, Lagneau P, Milliez P (1980) Fibrodysplasies de l'artère rénale. Aspects morphologiques et risques évolutifs. Nouv Presse Med 9: 697-700

118. Goncharenko V, Gerlock AJ Jr, Shaff MI, Hollifield JW (1981) Progression of renal artery fibromuscular dysplasia in 42 patients as seen on angiography. Radiology 139: 45-51

119. Sell JJ, Seigel RS, Orrison WW, Roberts WS (1995) Angiographic pattern change in fibromuscular dysplasia. A case report. Angiology 46: 165-8

120. Langis P, Oliva VL, Harel C (1997) Fibromuscular dysplasia of the renal artery—rapid progression with formation of aneurysm: case report. Can Assoc Radiol J 48: 8-10

121. Nghiem DD, Schulak JA, Bonsib SM, Ercolani L, Corry RJ (1984) Fibromuscular dysplasia: an unusual cause of hypertension in the transplant recipient. Transplant Proc 16: 555-8

122. Castaneda-Zuniga W, Zollikofer C, Valdez-Davila O, Nath PH, Amplatz K (1979) Giant aneurysms of the renal arteries: an unusual manifestation of fibromuscular dysplasia. Radiology 133: 327-30

123. Kalyanaraman UP, Elwood PW (1980) Fibromuscular dysplasia of intracranial arteries causing multiple intracranial aneurysms. Hum Pathol 11: 481-4

124. Radhi JM, McKay R, Tyrrell MJ (1998) Fibromuscular dysplasia of the aorta presenting as multiple recurrent thoracic aneurysms. International journal of Angiology 7: 215-8

125. Poutasse EF (1975) Renal artery aneurysms. J Urol 113: 443-9

126. Eachempati SR, Sebastian MW, Reed RL 2nd (1998) Posttraumatic bilateral carotid artery and right vertebral

artery dissections in a patient with fibromuscular dysplasia: case report and review of the literature. J Trauma 44: 406-9

127. Chauhuri KR, Edwards R, Brooks DJ (1993) Adult moyamoya diseases. An unusual cause of stroke. Br Med J 307: 852-4

128. Houkin K, Yoshimoto T, Kuroda S, Ishikawa T, Takahashi A, Abe H (1996) Angiographic analysis of moyamoya disease—how does moyamoya disease progress? Neurol Med Chir (Tokyo) 36: 783-7

129. Kimura H, Oka K, Ikeda K, Yamamoto M, Tomonaga M (1997) The clinical significance of cerebral veins in moyamoya disease. Clin Neurol Neurosurg 99: S90-S95

130. Peerless SJ (1997) Risk factors of moyamoya disease in Canada and the USA. Clin Neurol Neurosurg 99: S45-S48

131. Yonekawa Y, Ogata N, Kaku Y, Taub E, Imhof HG (1997) Moyamoya disease in Europe, past and present status. Clin Neurol Neurosurg 99: S58-S60

132. Manceau E, Giroud M, Dumas R (1997) Moyamoya disease in children. A review of the clinical and radiological features and current treatment. Childs Nerv Syst 13: 595-600

133. Han DH, Nam DH, Oh CW (1997) Moyamoya disease in adults: characteristics of clinical presentation and outcome after encephalo-duro-arterio-synangiosis. Clin Neurol Neurosurg 99: S151-S155

134. Imaizumi T, Hayashi K, Saito K, Osawa M, Fukuyama Y (1998) Long-term outcomes of pediatric moyamoya disease monitored to adulthood. Pediatr Neurol 18: 321-5

135. Asami N, Miyahara S, Ueda T, Wakisaka S, Kinoshita K (1990) Moyamoya disease in fraternal twins. No To Shinkei 42: 1093-6

136. Yamauchi T, Houkin K, Tada M, Abe H (1997) Familial occurrence of moyamoya disease. Clin Neurol Neurosurg 99: S162-S167

137. Yoshimoto T, Houkin K, Takahashi A, Abe H (1997) Evaluation of cytokines in cerebrospinal fluid from patients with moyamoya disease. Clin Neurol Neurosurg 99: S218-S220

138. Iwama T, Todaka T, Hashimoto N (1997) Direct surgery for major artery aneurysm associated with moyamoya disease. Clin Neurol Neurosurg 99: S191-S193

139. Iwama T, Hashimoto N, Miyake H, Yonekawa Y (1998) Direct revascularization to the anterior cerebral artery territory in patients with moyamoya disease: report of five cases. Neurosurgery 42: 1157-61

140. Lutterman J, Scott M, Nass R, Geva T (1998) Moyamoya syndrome associated with congenital heart disease. Pediatrics 101: 57-60

141. Pilz P, Hartjes HJ (1976) Fibromuscular dysplasia and multiple dissecting aneurysms of intracranial arteries. A further cause of Moyamoya syndrome. Stroke 7: 393-8

142. Voros E, Kiss M, Hanko J, Nagy E (1997) Moyamoya with arterial anomalies: relevance to pathogenesis. Neuroradiology 39: 852-6

143. Wanifuchi H, Kagawa M, Takeshita M, Izawa M, Maruyama S, Kitamura K (1986) Autoimmune antibody in moyamoya disease. No Shinkei Geka 14: 31-5

144. Inoue TK, Ikezaki K, Sasazuki T, Ono T, Kamikawaji N, Matsushima T, Fukui M (1997) DNA typing of HLA in the patients with moyamoya disease. Jpn J Hum Genet 42: 507-15

145. Matsuki Y, Kawakami M, Ishizuka T, Kawaguchi Y, Hidaka T, Suzuki K, Nakamura H (1997) SLE and Sjogren's syndrome associated with unilateral moyamoya vessels in cerebral arteries. Scand J Rheumatol 26: 392-4

146. Leno C, Mateo I, Cid C, Berciano J, Sedano C (1998) Autoimmunity in Down's syndrome: another possible mechanism of Moyamoya disease. Stroke 29: 868-9

147. Mito T, Becker LE (1992) Vascular dysplasia in Down syndrome: a possible relationship to moyamoya disease. Brain Dev 14: 248-51

148. Cramer SC, Robertson RL, Dooling EC, Scott RM (1996) Moyamoya and Down syndrome. Clinical and radiological features. Stroke 27: 2131-5

149. Tanigawara T, Yamada H, Sakai N, Andoh T, Deguchi K, Iwamura M (1997) Studies on cytomegalovirus and Epstein-Barr virus infection in moyamoya disease. Clin Neurol Neurosurg. 99: S225-S228

150. Yamada H, Deguchi K, Tanigawara T, Takenaka K, Nishimura Y, Shinoda J, Hattori T, Andoh T, Sakai N (1997) The relationship between moyamoya disease and bacterial infection. Clin Neurol Neurosurg. 99: S221-S224

151. Rajakulasingam K, Cerullo LJ, Raimondi AJ (1979) Childhood moyamoya syndrome. Postradiation pathogenesis. Childs Brain 5: 467-75

152. Sinsawaiwong S, Phanthumchinda K (1997) Progressive cerebral occlusive disease after hypothalamic astrocytoma radiation therapy. J Med Assoc Thai 80: 338-42

153. Merkel KH, Ginsberg PL, Parker JC Jr, Post MJ (1978) Cerebrovascular disease in sickle cell anemia: a clinical, pathological and radiological correlation. Stroke 9: 45-52

154. Charuvanij A, Laothamatas J, Torcharus K, Sirivimonmas S (1997) Moyamoya disease and protein S deficiency: a case report. Pediatr Neurol 17: 171-3

155. Goutières F, Bourgeois M, Trioche P, Demelier JF, Odièvre M, Labrune P (1997) Moyamoya disease in a child with glycogen storage disease type Ia. Neuropediatrics 28: 133-4

156. Holz A, Woldenberg R, Miller D, Kalina P, Black K, Lane E (1998) Moyamoya disease in a patient with hereditary spherocytosis. Pediatr Radiol 28: 95-7

157. Natori Y, Ikezaki K, Matsushima T, Fukui M (1997) "Angiographic moyamoya": its definition, classification, and therapy. Clin Neurol Neurosurg 99: S168-S172

158. Ashleigh RJ, Weller JM, Leggate JR (1992) Fibromuscular hyperplasia of the internal carotid artery. A further cause of the 'moyamoya' collateral circulation. Br J Neurosurg 6: 269-73

159. Nakano T, Azuma E, Ido M, Itoh M, Sakurai M, Suga S, Kawaguchi H (1993) Moyamoya disease associated with bilateral renal artery stenosis. Acta Paediatr Jpn 35: 354-7

160. Aoyagi M, Fukai N, Yamamoto M, Matsushima Y, Yamamoto K (1997) Development of intimal thickening in superficial temporal arteries in patients with moyamoya disease. Clin Neurol Neurosurg 99: S213-S217

161. Choi Y, Kang BC, Kim KJ, Cheong HI, Hwang YS, Wang KC, Kim IO (1997) Renovascular hypertension in children with moyamoya disease. J Pediatr 131: 258-63

162. Hosoda Y, Ikeda E, Hirose S (1997) Histopathological studies on spontaneous occlusion of the circle of Willis (cerebrovascular moyamoya disease). Clin Neurol Neurosurg 99: S203-S208

163. Yang SH, Li B, Wang CC, Zhao JZ (1997) Angiographic study of moyamoya disease and histological study in the external carotid artery system. Clin Neurol Neurosurg 99: S61-S63

164. Akasaki T, Kagiyama S, Omae T, Ohya Y, Ibayashi S, Abe I, Fujishima M (1998) Asymptomatic moyamoya disease associated with coronary and renal artery stenoses—a case report. Jpn Circ J 62: 136-8

165. Ejrup B, Hiertonn T (1954) Intermittent claudication: three cases treated by free vein graft. Acta Chir Scand 108: 217-30

166. Scobie TK, Curry RH (1975) Cystic adventitial disease of the popliteal artery. Can J Surg 18: 46-50

167. Inoue Y, Iwai T, Ohashi K, Takiguchi N, Sakurazawa K, Muraoka Y, Satoh S, Kasuga T, Endo M (1992) A case of popliteal cystic degeneration with pathological considerations. Ann Vasc Surg 6: 525-9

168. Annetts DL, Graham AR (1980) Cystic degeneration of the femoral vein: a case report. Br J Surg 67: 287-8

169. Lie JT, Jensen PL, Smith RE (1991) Adventitial cystic disease of the lesser saphenous vein. Arch Pathol Lab Med 115: 946-8

170. Yoshii S, Ikeda K, Murakami H (1998) Cystic, myxomatous adventitial degeneration of a saphenous vein. J Vasc Surg 27: 780-2

171. Flanigan DP, Burnham SJ, Goodreau JJ, Bergan JJ (1979) Summary of cases of adventitial cystic disease of the popliteal artery. Ann Surg 189: 165-75

172. Levien LJ, Benn CA (1998) Adventitial cystic disease: a unifying hypothesis. J Vasc Surg 28: 193-205

173. DeLaurentis DA, Wolferth CC Jr, Wolf FM, Naide D, Nedwich A (1973) Mucinous adventitial cysts of the popliteal artery in an 11-year-old girl. Surgery 74: 456-9

174. Ishibashi S, Namiki K, Abe M, Shirahata Y, Ohnishi K, Toyoda T, Ohuchi K (1995) Cystic adventitial disease of the popliteal artery—a case of young boy. Tohoku J Exp Med 176: 173-80

175. Paty PS, Kaufman JL, Koslow AR, Chang BB, Leather RP, Shah DM (1992) Adventitial cystic disease of the femoral vein: a case report and review of the literature. J Vasc Surg 15: 214-7

176. Schraverus P, Dulieu J, Mailleux P, Coulier B (1997) Cystic adventitial disease of the popliteal vein: report of a case. Acta Chir Belg 97: 90-2

177. Tsolakis IA, Walvatne CS, Caldwell MD (1998) Cystic adventitial disease of the popliteal artery: diagnosis and treatment. Eur J Vasc Endovasc Surg 15: 188-94

178. Bollinger A, Pouliadis G (1977) Pathology, clinical correlates, radiology and surgery of cystic adventitial degeneration of the peripheral blood vessels. 2. Clinical correlates and arteriography. Vasa 6: 100-4

179. Absoud EM (1984) Recurrent cystic adventitial disease of the radial artery. Angiology 35: 257-60

180. Ishikawa K (1987) Cystic adventitial disease of the popliteal artery and of other stem vessels in the extremities. Jpn J Surg 17: 221-9

181. Durham JR, McIntyre KE Jr (1989) Adventitial cystic disease of the radial artery. J Cardiovasc Surg (Torino) 30: 517-20

182. Piazza M, Blandamura S, Capitanio G, Previato Schiesari A, Giampalmo A (1991) Cystic adventitial disease: histopathological contribution of a case in the ilio-femoral region. Pathologica 83: 69-73

183. Chakfe N, Beaufigeau M, Geny B, Suret-Canale MA, Vix J, Groos N, Edah-Tally S, Steinmetz E, Kretz JG (1997) Extra-popliteal localizations of adventitial cysts. Review of the literature. J Mal Vasc 22: 79-85

184. Borrelli M, Bracco E, Scarrone A, Belgrano E, Ferro C (1995) Cystic adventitial degeneration of the common femoral artery. A case report. Radiol Med (Torino) 89: 350-2

185. Steffen CM, Ruddle A, Shaw JF (1995) Adventitial cystic disease: multiple cysts causing common femoral artery occlusion. Eur J Vasc Endovasc Surg 9: 118-9

186. Vuong PN, Peze W (1996) Sub-adventitial cystic degeneration of the radial artery. Report of a case (Letter) Presse Med 25: 458

187. Kitzis M, Assens P, Couffinhal JC, Bourgeois P, Weiss AM, Remond P, Andreassian B (1983). Adventitial cyst of the aorta. Sem Hop 59: 2857-60

188. Campbell RT, McCluskey BC, Andrews MI (1970) A case of polycystic adventitial disease of the left external iliac and femoral artery. Br J Surg 57: 865-8

189. Hall RI, Proud G, Chamberlain J, McNeil IF (1985) Cystic adventitial disease of the common femoral and popliteal arteries. Br J Surg 72: 756-8

190. Vuong PN, Laurian Cl (1992) Artère poplitée "piégée". Intérêt de l'imagerie médicale et revue de la littérature. J Radiol 73: 247-52

191. Soury P, Rivière J, Watelet J, Peillon C, Testart J (1995) Spontaneous regression of a sub-adventitial cyst of the popliteal artery. J Mal Vasc 20: 323-5

192. Ohta T, Kato R, Sugimoto I, Kondo M, Tsuchioka H (1994) Recurrence of cystic adventitial disease in an interposed vein graft. Surgery 116: 587-92

193. Holmes JG (1960) Cystic adventitial degeneration of the popliteal artery. JAMA 173: 654-6

194. Hansen JPH (1966) Cystic mucoid degeneration of the popliteal artery. Acta Chir Scand 131: 171-7

195. Mark TM, Rywlin AM, Unger H (1983) Cystic adventitial degeneration of the popliteal artery. Its occurrence in a patient with the nail-patella syndrome. Arch Pathol Lab Med 107: 186-8

196. Schafer K, Sell G, Schafer B, Rumpelt HJ (1995) Cystic degeneration of the adventitia of the popliteal artery as a possible sequela of entrapment syndrome. Chirurg 66: 154-7

197. Sys J, Michielsen J, Bleyn J, Martens M (1997) Adventitial cystic disease of the popliteal artery in a triathlete. A case report. Am J Sports Med 25: 854-7

198. Shute K, Rothnic NG (1973) The aetiology of cystic arterial disease. Br J Surg 60: 397-400

199. Leu HJ, Largiader J, Odermatt B (1984) Pathogenesis of the so-called cystic adventitial degeneration of peripheral blood vessels. Virchows Arch A Pathol Anat Histopathol 404: 289-300

200. Tabata D, Arikawa K, Umebayashi Y, Chosa N, Kinjo T, Nishida S (1991) A case report of cystic adventitial degeneration communicating with the hip joint in the external iliac artery. Nippon Geka Gakkai Zasshi 92: 611-3

201. Mailleux P, Mairy Y, Coulier B, Coppens JP, Joris JP (1992) Adventitial cyst of the common femoral artery: computerized tomography demonstration of the articular origin of this disorder. J Belge Radiol 75: 1-4

202. di Marzo L, Della Rocca C, d'Amati G, Gallo P, Sciacca V, Mingoli A, Cavallaro A (1994) Cystic adventitial degeneration of the popliteal artery: lectin-histochemical study. Eur J Vasc Surg 8: 16-9

203. Devereux D, Forrest H, Mcleod T, Ahweng A (1980) The nonarterial origin of the cystic adventitial disease of the popliteal artery in two patients. Surgery 88: 723-7

204. Jay GD, Ross FL, Mason RA, Giron F (1989) Clinical and chemical characterization of an adventitial popliteal cyst. J Vasc Surg 9: 448-51

205. Bergan JJ (1995) Adventitial cystic disease of the popliteal artery. In Rutherford RB (ed.) Vascular surgery. Philadelphia: WB Saunders; 1995. p. 883-8

206. Urayama H, Ohtake H, Kosugi I, Watanabe Y, Minato H (1998) Distortion of the radial artery by a mucinous cyst. Case reports. Scand J Plast Reconstr Surg Hand Surg 32: 437-40

207. Senior HD (1920) The development of the human femoral artery, a correction. Am J Anat 17: 271-9

208. Larsen WJ (1993) Development of the vasculature *In* Larsen WJ (ed.) Human embryology. New York: Churchill Livingstone p. 181-4

209. Mentha C (1963) La dégénérescence mucoïde des veines. Presse Med 71: 2205-6

210. Erdheim J (1930) Medionecrosis aortae idiopathica cystica. Virchows Arch (Pathol Anat) 276: 187-229

211. Schlatmann IJM, Becker AE (1977) Histologic changes in the normal aging aorta: implication for dissecting aneurysm. Am J Cardiol 39: 13-20

212. Schlatmann IJM, Becker AE (1977) Pathogenesis of dissecting aneurysm of aorta. Comparative histopathologic study of significance of changes. Am J Cardiol 39: 21-6

213. Spina M, Garbin G (1976) Age-related chemical changes in human elastins from non-atherosclerotic areas of thoracic aorta. Atherosclerosis 24: 267-79

214. Slavin RE, Gonzalez-Vitale JC (1976) Segmental mediolytic arteritis: a clinical pathologic study. Lab Invest 35: 23-9

215. Guzman R, Restrepo JF, Lizarazo H, Pena M, Mendez O, Iglesias A (1994) Arterial fibrodysplasia causing occlusive vascular disease simulating primary vasculitis. Rev Invest Clin 46: 67-71

216. Chomette G, Auriol M, Tranbaloc P, de Saint-Maur PP (1983) Anatomopathological aspects of arterial angiodysplasias. Ann Med Interne (Paris) 134: 444-50

217. Marescaux J, Petit B, Pavis d'Escurac X, Aprahamian M, Damge C, Sibilly A (1986) Les malformations vasculaires du côlon. Une cause fréquemment méconnue d'hémorragie digestive basse. Presse Med 15: 2204-7

218. Vuong PN, Proust A, Guillet JL, Benamour JM, Lucas M, Vaury Ph, Baviera E (1994) Angiodystrophie utérine responsable de métrorragies récidivantes, une nouvelle entité anatomo-pathologique. Gynécologie 2: 230-26

219. Janzen J, Rothenberger-Janzen K (2000) Angiodystrophy of the uterus (Vuong-Proust syndrome) responsible for recurrent metrorrhagia: two new cases. Singapore J Obstet Gynaecol 31:161-64

220. Roskell DE, Biddolph SC, Warren BF (1998) Apparent deficiency of mucosal vascular collagen type IV associated with angiodysplasia of the colon. J Clin Pathol 51: 18-20

221. Yorioka N, Hamaguchi N, Taniguchi Y, Asakimori Y, Nishiki T, Oda H, Yamakido M (1996) Gastric antral vascular ectasia in a patient on hemodialysis improved with CAPD. Perit Dial Int 16: 177-8

222. Oliveras A, Aubia J, Cao H, Puig JM, Barbosa F, Lloveras J, Masramon J (1998) Is there a role for parathormone in the pathogenesis of colonic angiodysplasia? (Letter) Nephrol Dial Transplant 13: 1052

223. Bokhari M, Vernava AM, Ure T, Longo WE (1996) Diverticular hemorrhage in the elderly—is it well tolerated? Dis Colon Rectum 39: 191-5

224. Okamura T, Kanaji T, Osaki K, Kuroiwa M, Yamashita S, Niho Y (1996) Gastrointestinal angiodysplasia in congenital platelet dysfunction. Int J Hematol 65: 79-84

225. Bellucci S, Caen JP (1997) Gastrointestinal angiodysplasia in constitutional thrombocytopathies. Int J Hematol 65: 419-20

226. Inbal A, Bank I, Zivelin A, Varon D, Dardik R, Shapiro R, Rosenthal E, Shenkman B, Gitel S, Seligsohn U (1997) Acquired von Willebrand disease in a patient with angiodysplasia resulting from immune-mediated clearance of von Willebrand factor. Br J Haematol 96: 179-82

227. Vujkovac B, Lavre J, Sabovic M (1998) Successful treatment of bleeding from colonic angiodysplasias with tranexamic acid in a hemodialysis patient. Am J Kidney Dis 31: 536-8

228. Sebastian JJ, Lucia F, Botella MT, Yus C, Uribarrena R (1996) Diffuse gastrointestinal angiodysplasia associated with cryptogenic hepatic cirrhosis and coagulopathy simulating von Willebrand disease. Rev Esp Enferm Dig 88: 631-3

229. Boley SJ, Dibiase A, Brandt LJ, Sammartano R (1979) Lower intestinal bleeding in the elderly. Am J Surg 137: 57-64

230. Arcidiacono G, De Domenico C, Battaglia E, Bordignon E, Asmundo GO, Zingali C, Longhitano A, Cuscuna S, Gurgone E, Vigo G, Ossino AM, Di Mauro C (1996) Angiodysplasia of the right colon and aortic stenosis. A case report. Minerva Cardioangiol 44: 173-7

231. Larsen NH (1997) Heyde syndrome. Ugeskr Laeger 159: 4628-30

232. Tobin RW, Hackman RC, Kimmey MB, Durtschi MB, Hayashi A, Malik R, McDonald MF, McDonald GB (1996) Bleeding from gastric antral vascular ectasia in marrow transplant patients. Gastrointest Endosc 44: 223-9

233. Pradel E, de Lalande Ph, Molkhou JM, Fournier P, Vuong P (1989) Les angiodysplasies rectales. Ann Gastroenterol Hépatol 25: 305-6

234. Afifi R, el Alaoui M, Kerkeb O (1997) A rare cause of lower digestive tract bleeding: angiodysplasia of the small bowel. J Chir (Paris) 134: 189-92

235. Raoul J-L (1995) Hémorragies digestives basses abondantes. Approche diagnostique et thérapeutique. Gastroenterol Clin Biol 19: B41-B46

236. Krevsky B (1997) Detection and treatment of angiodysplasia. Gastrointest Endosc Clin N Am 7: 509-24

237. Ottonello M, Fabiano F, Serafini P, Santi F (1997) Intestinal angiodysplasia: diagnosis and therapy. Minerva Chir 52: 971-4

238. Koga H, Iida M, Nagai E, Aoyagi K, Matsumoto T, Takesue M, Yao T, Tsuneyoshi M, Fujishima M (1996) Jejunal angiodysplasia confirmed by intravascular injection technique in vitro. Report of a case and review of the literature. J Clin Gastroenterol 23: 139-44

239. Kohler A, Dirsch O, Brunner U (1997) Veno-lymphatic angiodysplasia as the cause of recurrent inguinal varicose veins. Vasa 26: 52-4

240. van de Water J, Jimenez SA, Gershwin ME (1995) Animal models of scleroderma: contrasts and comparisons. Int Rev Immunol 12: 201-16

241. Maricq HR, Weinrich MC, Keil JE, Smith EA, Harper FE, Nussbaum AI, LeRoy EC, McGregor AR, Diat F, Rosal EJ (1989) Prevalence of scleroderma spectrum disorders in the general population of South Carolina. Arthritis Rheum 32: 998-1006

242. Knupp MZ, O'Leary JA (1971) Pregnancy and scleroderma. Systemic sclerosis. J Fla Med Assoc 58: 28-30

243. DiBartolomeo AG, Rabin BS, Rodnan GP (1981) HLA-D antigens in progressive systemic sclerosis (scleroderma). Immunol Commun 10: 733-40

244. Hietarinta M, Ilonen J, Lassila O, Hietaharju A (1994) Association of HLA antigens with anti-Scl-70-antibodies and clinical manifestations of systemic sclerosis. Br J Rheumatol 33: 323-6

245. Johanet C, Agostini MM, Vayssairat M, Abuaf N(1989) Anti-Scl-70 and anti-centromere autoantibodies. Biological markers of 2 forms of systemic scleroderma. Presse Med 18: 207-11

246. Inaba R, Maeda M, Fujita S, Kashiki N, Komura Y, Nagata C, Yoshida H, Mirbod SM, Iwata H, Shikano Y, et al (1993) Prevalence of Raynaud's phenomenon and specific clinical signs related to progressive systemic sclerosis in the general population of Japan. Int J Dermatol 32: 652-5

247. Varga J, Schumacher HR, Jimenez SA (1989) Systemic sclerosis after augmentation mammoplasty with silicone implants. Ann Intern Med 111: 377-83

248. Hochberg MC, Miller R, Wigley FM (1995) Frequency of augmentation mammoplasty in patients with systemic sclerosis: data from the Johns Hopkins-University of Maryland Scleroderma Center. J Clin Epidemiol 48: 565-9

249. Anderson DR, Schwartz J, Cottrill CM, McClain SA, Ross JS, Magidson JG, Klainer A, Bisaccia E (1996) Silicone granuloma in acral skin in a patient with silicone-gel breast implants and systemic sclerosis. Int J Dermatol 35: 36-8

250. Field T, Bridges AJ (1996) Clinical and laboratory features of patients with scleroderma and silicone implants. Curr Top Microbiol Immunol 210: 283-90

251. Blann AD, Illingworth K, Jayson MI (1993) Mechanisms of endothelial cell damage in systemic sclerosis and Raynaud's phenomenon. J Rheumatol 20: 1325-30

252. Salmon-Ehr V, Serpier H, Nawrocki B, Gillery P, Clavel C, Kalis B, Birembaut P, Maquart FX (1996) Expression of interleukin-4 in scleroderma skin specimens and scleroderma fibroblast cultures. Potential role in fibrosis. Arch Dermatol 132: 802-6

253. Krell JM, Solomon AR, Glavey CM, Lawley TJ (1995) Nodular scleroderma. J Am Acad Dermatol 32: 343-5

254. Mizutani H, Taniguchi H, Sakakura T, Shimizu M (1995) Nodular scleroderma: focally increased tenascin expression differing from that in the surrounding scleroderma skin. J Dermatol 22: 267-71

255. Perez MI, Kohn SR (1993) Systemic Sclerosis. J Am Acad of Dermatol 28: 525-547

256. Isenberg DA, Black C (1995) Raynaud's phenomenon, scleroderma, and overlap syndromes. BMJ 310: 795-8

257. Legerton III CW, Smith EA, Silver RM (1995) Systemic sclerosis: clinical management of its major complications. Rheumatic Disease Clinics of North America 21: 203-16

258. Williamson DJ (1995) Update on scleroderma. Med J Aust 162: 599-601

259. Mansell MA, Watts RW (1980) Retroperitoneal fibrosis and scleroderma. Postgrad Med J 56: 730-3

260. Giordano M, Ara M, Valentini G, Chianese U, Bencivenga T (1981) Presence of eosinophilia in progressive systemic sclerosis and localized scleroderma. Arch Dermatol Res 271: 411-7

261. Shimomura C, Eguchi K, Mine M, Tezuka H, Matsunaga M, Ueki Y, Otsubo T, Nakao H, Migita K, Kawakami A, et al (1989) A case of progressive systemic sclerosis accompanied with rheumatoid arthritis. Ryumachi 29: 284-90

262. LeRoy EC (1992) Raynaud's phenomenon, scleroderma, overlap syndromes, and other fibrosing syndromes. Curr Opin Rheumatol 4: 821-4

263. Hietaharju A, Jaaskelainen S, Kalimo H, Hietarinta M (1993) Peripheral neuromuscular manifestations in systemic sclerosis (scleroderma). Muscle Nerve 16: 1204-12

264. Abu-Shakra M, Koh ET, Treger T, Lee P (1995) Pericardial effusion and vasculitis in a patient with systemic sclerosis. J Rheumatol 22: 1386-1388

265. Monastra Varrica L, Doweck J, Amendola R, Farias R, Schenone L, Bori J, Fiorini A, Musi AO, Corti RE (1994) Esophageal involvement in progressive systemic sclerosis. Acta Gastroenterol Latinoam 24: 245-9

266. Ueno Y, Shibata M, Onozuka Y (1998) Association of extrahepatic autoimmune diseases in primary biliary cirrhosis—clinical statistics and analyses of Japanese and non-Japanese cases. Nippon Rinsho 56: 2687-98

267. Donohoe JF (1992) Scleroderma of the Kidney. Kidney International 41: 462-77

268. Zwettler U, Andrassy K, Waldherr R, Ritz E (1993) Scleroderma renal crisis as a presenting feature in the absence of skin involvement. Am J Kidney Dis 22: 53-6

269. Gonzalez EA, Schmulbach E, Bastani B (1994) Scleroderma renal crisis with minimal skin involvement and no serologic evidence of systemic sclerosis. Am J Kidney Dis 23: 317-9

270. Lefebvre C, Tousignant J, Chartier S, Demers D (1993) Colonic adenocarcinoma and scleroderma. Ann Dermatol Venereol 120: 293-5

271. Fiessinger JN, Camilleri JP, Mignot J, Kazandjian S, Vayssairat M, Housset E (1980) Scleroderma microangiopathy. Physiopathogenic hypothesis. Rev Med Interne 1: 61-4

272. Posner MA, Herness D, Green S (1980) Severe peripheral vascular deterioration in scleroderma. A case report. Acta Orthop Scand 51: 239-41

273. van Zyl ML, van Staden DA (1984) Ainhum. S Afr Med J 66: 107-8

274. Meyers WM (1976) Ainhum In Binford CH, Connor DH (Eds.) Pathology of tropical and extraordinary diseases, AFIP, Washington DC, p 668-71

275. Greene JT, Fincher RM (1992) Case report: ainhum (spontaneous dactylolysis) in a 65-year-old American black man. Am J Med Sci 303: 118-20

276. Genakos JJ, Cocores JA, Terris A (1986) Ainhum (dactylolysis spontanea). Report of a bilateral case and literature review. J Am Podiatr Med Assoc 76: 676-80

277. Dent DM, Fataar S, Rose AG (1981) Ainhum and angiodysplasia. Lancet 2(8243): 396-7

278. Rossiter JW, Anderson PC (1976) Ainhum: treatment with intralesional steroids. Int J Dermatol 15: 379-82

279. Khare AK; Bansal NK; Meena HS (1987) Dapsone syndrome – a case report. Indian J Lepr 59: 106-9

280. Peris K, Salvati EF, Torlone G, Chimenti S (1995) Keratoderma hereditarium mutilans (Vohwinkel's syndrome) associated with congenital deaf-mutism. Br J Dermatol 132: 617-20

281. Kamalam A, Thambiah AS (1981) Ainhum, trichosporiosis and Z-plasty. Dermatologica 162: 372-7

282. Warter A, Audouin J, Sekou H (1988) La dactylolyse spontanée ou ainhum. Etude histopathologique Ann Pathol 8: 305-10

283. Graham RM, James MP (1985) Pseudo-ainhum, angiodysplasia and focal acral hyperkeratosis. J R Soc Med 78: S13-S15

284. Park BS, Hyun Cho K, Youn JI, Chung JH (1996) Pseudoainhum associated with linear scleroderma [letter] Arch Dermatol 132: 1520-1

285. McLaurin CI (1982) Psoriasis presenting with pseudoainhum. J Am Acad Dermatol 7: 130-2

286. Sharma RC, Sharma AK, Sharma NL (1998) Pseudo-ainhum in discoid lupus erythematosus [letter] J Dermatol 25: 275-6

287. Koberich M (1980) Ainhum and a pseudo-ainhum syndrome. Overview with 2 case reports (Ainhum und Pseudo-Ainhum-Syndrom. Eine Ubersicht mit zwei Fallberichten) Z Hautkr 55: 349-54

VI
Vascular trauma

Introduction

The pathological interpretation of vascular trauma should take three factors into account. Firstly, vascular damage depends on the type of injury and each type leaves a distinctive imprint. Secondly, vascular injury may have medico-legal significance, especially when related to surgical manipulations [1-3]. The task of the pathologist may be to determine whether the vascular changes are directly caused by injury or represent a complication of a pre-existing lesion [4, 5]. Finally, traumatic injury to vessels rarely occurs alone and neighbouring tissues are likely to be damaged. The vascular sequelae of injury are often worsened by this injury to surrounding structures [6]. Vascular damage resulting from operative techniques is discussed in chapter XII.

1 – Direct trauma

Four types of injury may occur: rupture of the intima, rupture of the intima and media, rupture of all three layers and rupture of the adventitia alone or of the external elastic membrane. The morphological presentation varies with the mechanism of injury.

Open trauma or wounding

There is usually complete rupture of the three layers of the vessel. The wound may be augmented by small holes if caused by cutting tools or pointed instruments (bullet or missile fragments, knives, bony fragments) [7, 8].

Closed trauma or blunt injury to vessels

Several types of injury occur.

Direct blow

The vessel is either directly crushed or compressed. The severity of the lesion depends on the force of the blow and the location of the vessels. Severe injury is particularly likely when the vessel is compressed against a bony surface (for example the superficial temporal artery and the popliteal artery and subclavian arteries) [9-11].

Compression injury

Concentric crush injury is produced by ligation of the vessel, the accidental hair-thread tourniquet syndrome in infants, and strangulation or hanging [12, 13]. In judicial hanging, the carotid arteries may be occluded and obstruction of vertebral arteries may result from a combination of compression posterior and inferior to the mastoid processes, backward and upward compression on the thyro-hyoid membrane, and vertical traction on the neck. In suicidal hanging, the carotid arteries can be occluded in certain positions of the head and the vertebral arteries may also be compressed in certain positions [14]. However, death in cases of non-judicial hanging result from complex mechanisms combining obstruction (airways and/or vascular), vagal stimulation, and carotid sinus pressure [15]. In closed trauma to the thorax, direct compression may cause injury but the transmission of force to the blood in the aorta may cause additional radial compression injury to the aorta.

Deceleration

Sudden, violent deceleration produces shearing of vessels at the junction between fixed and relatively mobile segments. In the thorax, the aortic arch is held in place by the supra-aortic trunk and the left pulmonary pedicle. The thoracic aorta is secured to the vertebral column by the intercostal arteries and the posterior diaphragmatic arch. During deceleration, the aortic arch is drawn downwards by the heart. The descending aorta, securely held to the vertebral column, is pushed up and forwards. The shearing force occurring at the junction between these two segments may cause a rupture [16] (Fig. 1).

In an automobile crash, passengers who are not wearing seat belts are abruptly thrown forwards and upwards on impact. In addition to the two forces of deceleration, there is a third force of torsion caused by the rotation of the heart to the left. The resultant of these three forces acting together ruptures the aortic arch at the point of insertion of the arterial ligament, in front of the origin of the left subclavian artery. The car driver receives the impact of the steering wheel against his chest, which accentuates this torsion. A second point of rupture of the ascending aorta may occur, just above the aortic valve (Fig. 2). Using a 2-point seat belt system causes abrupt flexion of auto-

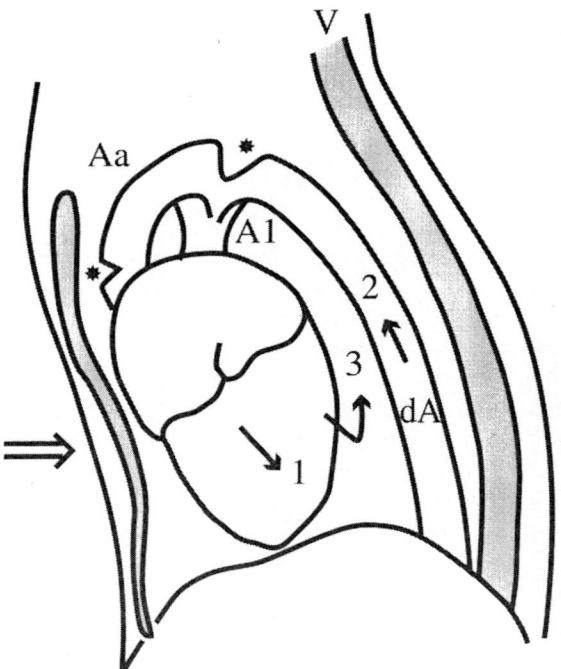

Fig. 1. Mechanism of rupture of the driver's aortic arch caused by an antero-posterior automobile crash. (=>) : impact of steering wheel ; (=> 1,2,3) : deceleration forces ; (*) : rupture sites ; Aa : aortic arch ; Al :arterial ligament ; dA : descending aorta ; V : vertebral column.

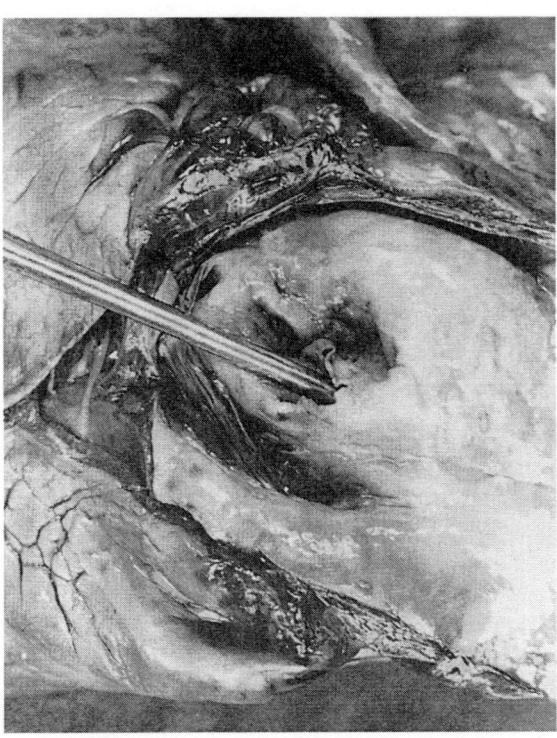

Fig. 2. Dissection with fatal rupture of the aortic arch in an automobile crash victim

mobile accident victims. The area above the area of flexion is carried downwards and forwards, and the inferior segment upwards and forwards. As abrupt flexion is added to compression, the zone of flexion undergoes shearing forces with consequent rupture of the abdominal aorta and the common iliac artery [10, 17].

Stretch and tear injuries

These occur when the initial force abruptly displaces the viscera, while the aorta remains relatively fixed, causing abrupt stretching of the arteries with propagation of a systolic shock wave secondary to increased intra-abdominal pressure [18, 19]. The site of the rupture is frequently at the ostium or in the para-ostial portion of the vessel involved [20]. In victims of automobile crashes with fronto-facial impact, the 3 point seat belt exerts thoracic compression, together with a decrease in anteroposterior diameter [21]. Deceleration tilts the heart and its contents downward

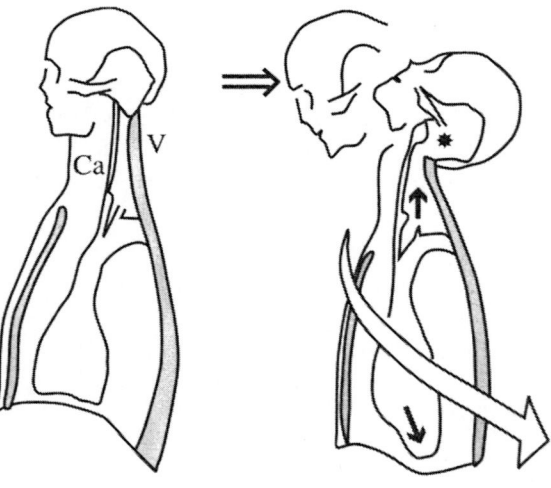

Fig. 3. Mechanism of rupture of internal carotid arteries in a fronto-facial impact of an automobile crash victim wearing a 3-point seat belt. (=>) : fronto-facial impact. (*) : bony structures ; Ca : internal carotid artery, V : vertebral column

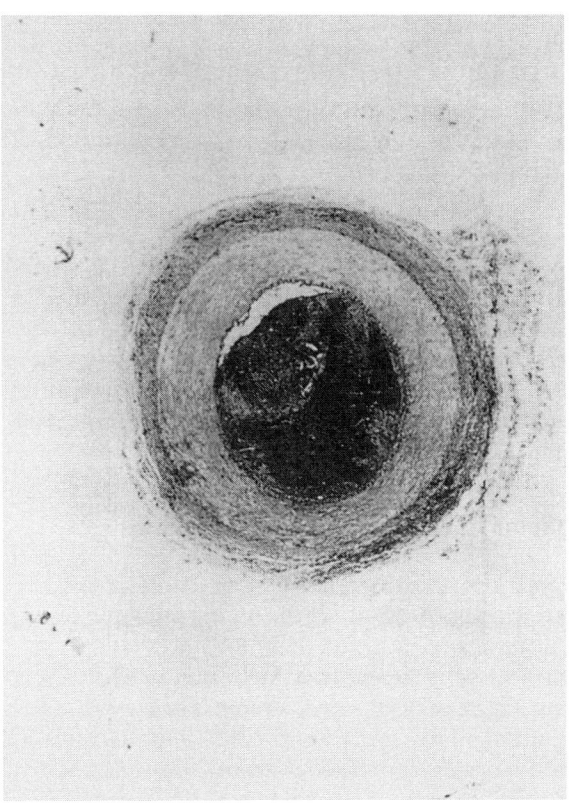

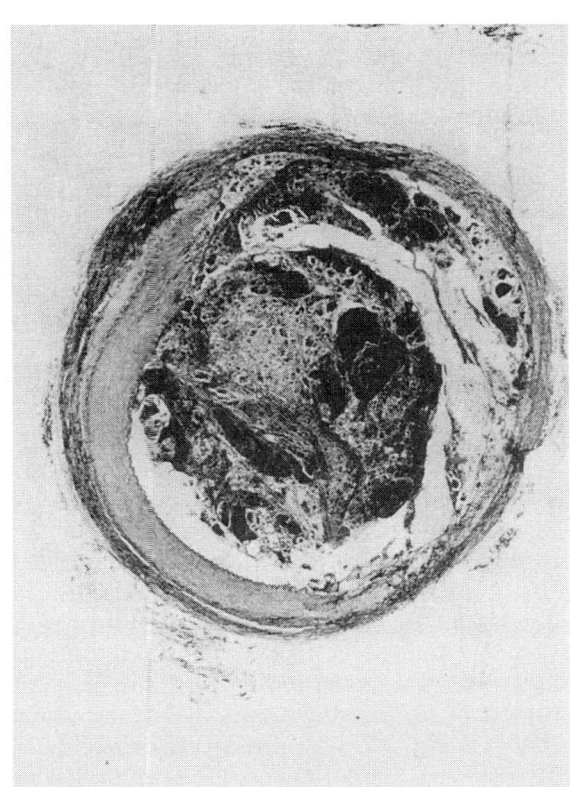

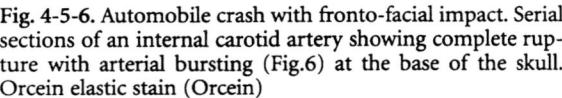

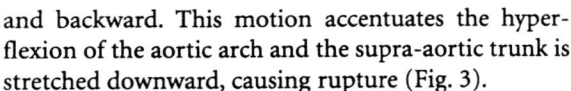

Fig. 4-5-6. Automobile crash with fronto-facial impact. Serial sections of an internal carotid artery showing complete rupture with arterial bursting (Fig.6) at the base of the skull. Orcein elastic stain (Orcein)

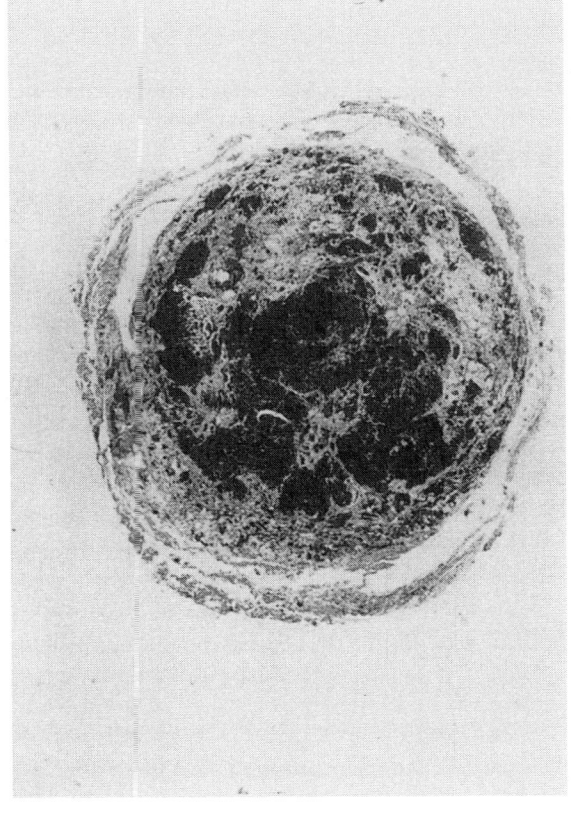

and backward. This motion accentuates the hyperflexion of the aortic arch and the supra-aortic trunk is stretched downward, causing rupture (Fig. 3).

Moreover, deceleration, with thoracic compression, increases the pressure of the circulatory shock wave, which propagates upward. This circulatory wave is transmitted to the carotid vessels, which are already under tension and affects the orifices of the carotid vessels at the base of the skull. At this level the wave of blood strikes non-expandable bony structures, and ampullary dilatation occurs in the internal carotid arteries, with bursting of the intima or intimal and medial layers of the vessel (Fig. 4-5-6). Headrest helps prevent this complication.

Temporary cavitation

Determinants of the wounding effects of a metallic projectile include the velocity (V), mass (M), shape, fragmentation, and deformation of the missile, as well as the characteristics of the tissue it goes through (tissue elasticity, density, thickness of the wounded body part, the type of tissue, its specific gravity, internal cohesiveness and anatomical relationships). In bullet or projectile wounds, vascular lesions are caused by the phenomenon of temporary cavitation, secondary to a sudden release of kinetic energy (KE) when the bullet penetrates the body tissue according to the following formula

$$KE = 1/2 \, MV^2$$

The kinetic energy released is more strongly influenced by velocity (V) than mass (M). The resulting pressure waves cause stretching or even tearing of vessels, which may show one or more ruptures [22-24]. There is a correlation between the number of ruptures produced and the speed of penetration of the bullet; ruptures in the artery are more severe according to their proximity to the centre of the temporary cavity. There are two types of bullets in this context [25, 26]: low (300 m/sec) and high velocity (600 and over m/sec). High velocity projectiles cause large, devastating wounds. Low velocity injuries may push back the artery as the bullet penetrates tissue with rupture of the adventitia alone, and of the external elastic lamella [27]. The microcirculation also suffers. The pathological changes in small vessels include microthrombus formation, endothelial loss, breaks in the internal elastic layer, and necrosis. These lesions directly depend on the quantity of the energy absorbed from the missile. Thus the extent and type of treatment required is determined more by the tissues and organs injured than by the characteristics of the wounding agent [28, 29].

Complications of direct trauma

The immediate consequences of vascular trauma include spasm, haemorrhage, thrombosis and embolism, ischaemia and infection. Delayed complications include false aneurysms, dissection and fistula [30-32].

Despite firmly held beliefs to the contrary spontaneous haemostasis, as a result of vascular spasm, occurs only exceptionally in large arteries [33], although it clearly happens in small vessels. In some anatomical sites, a perivascular haematoma confined by the adjacent structures may ensure haemostasis. Microemboli usually arise from a detached thrombus or an atheromatous plaque shaken loose by the trauma but macroemboli of tissue debris (brain, bone sequestrum, adipose tissue) or foreign bodies (projectile shrapnel, bullet, clothing) are common and often follow an unexpected course [34].

Ischaemia resulting from traumatic thrombosis may be gradual or abrupt in onset [35]. Extensive debridement of damaged soft tissues is necessary to avoid the release of cytokines and cell debris into the circulation, resulting in shock and acute renal tubular necrosis.

Traumatic arterio-venous fistulae are relatively frequent during military conflicts [36]. The time taken for an arterio-venous fistula to develop varies enormously with different patterns of injury; fistulae have been reported from 2 to 16 hr up to 8 days after injury and even periods as long as 3 to 9 years have been recorded [37, 38]. Acquired or traumatic fistulae tend to increase in size rapidly but have a favourable prognosis if corrected promptly.

Trauma of Veins and Lymphatic vessels

Damage to large veins may be a source of massive haemorrhage in blunt or penetrating injury. In limbs, military experience underlines the importance of venous repair in attempts at limb salvage when faced with a high-velocity missile wound. The civilian experience supports the notion that venous ligation in particular circumstances results in little, if any, added morbidity to the patient and may be life-saving in certain instances [39, 40].

Direct trauma to the great lymphatic trunks, especially the thoracic duct, can lead to chylous effusions leading to accumulations of macrophages, lymphocytes, and neovascularization in the surrounding tissue [41, 42]. Rupture may result from contusion, penetrating chest trauma, over-extension of the thorax, severe coughing and major surgery [43-45]. Traumatic chylous effusions occur more often in children and young adults than in the elderly, probably because the flexibility of the juvenile spine permits greater and more intensive extensions and compressions of the duct.

2 – Specific syndromes of chronic injury of vessels

Thoracic outlet syndrome and related conditions

This syndrome embraces all conditions that produce compression of the subclavian artery and/or vein, with or without participation of the brachial plexus.

Galenus and Veaslius first reported compression caused by the cervical rib in the 2nd century A.D. Law described ligaments and other abnormal structures originating in soft tissue associated with this condition in 1920. Adson and Coffey in 1927 emphasized the role of the anterior scalene muscle. In 1956, Peet proposed the term "Thoracic Outlet Syndrome" (TOS) to designate this condition and in 1966, Ross introduced the transaxillary resection of the first rib to relieve TOS [46].

The subclavian vessels and the brachial plexus traverse the thoracic outlet, lying in the retroclavicular fossa, and pass under the clavicle to penetrate the axilla. The subclavian artery leaves the thorax by arching over the first rib, between the insertions of the anterior and middle scalene muscles and becomes the axillary artery. The brachial plexus runs alongside the artery but is posterior to it. The subclavian vein has a similar path, but passes anterior to the anterior scalene muscle.

The neurovascular bundle in the thoracic outlet can be compressed or stretched at three sites: in the costo-clavicular space bound by the clavicle and the first rib, at the interscalene triangle delineated by the anterior scalene and medial scalene muscle and the first rib inferiorly, and in the angle formed by the coracoid process of the scapular and the insertion of the pectoralis minor.

The thoracic outlet syndrome and related conditions may result from an increase in bulk of the scalene and the shoulder girdle muscles (weight-lifters or certain athletes) from an abnormal first rib; from an abnormal clavicle with excessive callus formation after fracture, exostoses, osteomyelitis or a congenital absence of the middle third of this bone. The female clavicle is usually longer than the male, and the shoulder and clavicle tend to descend more in women than in men giving rise to symptoms [47]. Other causes include excessive effort or strain in carrying objects, prolonged use of the arm in an incorrect posture, non-ergonomic techniques, and cervical kyphoscoliosis. Table 1 lists the different types of thoracic outlet syndrome (Fig. 7), their sites and causes, and the structures involved.

The costo-clavicular syndrome is by far the most frequent manifestation. The subclavian artery and brachial plexus are subjected to pressure between the clavicle and first rib. In the scalenus anterior syndrome, the subclavian artery is raised and stretched by the broad ligamentous insertion of the muscle without participation of the first rib. In the cervical rib syndrome, contraction of the scalene muscles raises the first rib, thus crushing the contents of the interscalene triangle (subclavian artery and brachial plexus) against the clavicle. When the arm is hyperabducted (hyperabduction syndrome), the subclavian neurovascular bundle is compressed by the tendinous insertion of the pectoralis minor muscle onto the coracoid process This manœuvre also narrows the costo-clavicular space. In the Paget-von Schrötter syndrome, the cervical rib or anomalous first thoracic rib may compress the subclavian vein where it penetrates the root of the neck [48, 49].

Table 1. Variants of thoracic outlet syndrome

VARIANTS	SITE AND CAUSES OF COMPRESSION	INVOLVED STRUCTURES
Costo-clavicular syndrome	Compression between the clavicle and the first rib in the costo-clavicular space	Subclavian artery, Brachial plexus
Scalenus anticus syndrome	Compression between the anterior and medial scalene muscles	Subclavian artery, Brachial plexus
Cervical rib syndrome	Compression between scalene muscles and the first rib in the interscalene triangle	Subclavian artery, Brachial plexus
Paget – von Schrötter syndrome	Compression between the anterior scalene muscle, the clavicle and the abnormal first rib	Subclavian vein
Hyperabduction syndrome	Compression by tendinous insertions of pectoralis minor onto the scapular coracoid process	Subclavian artery, Brachial plexus

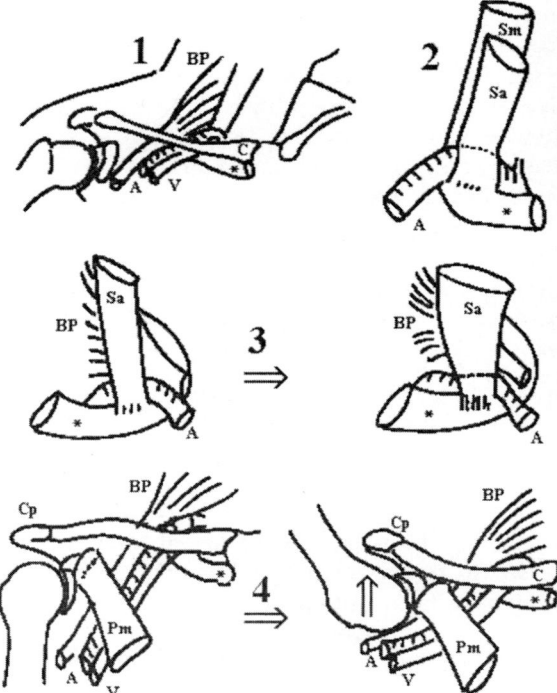

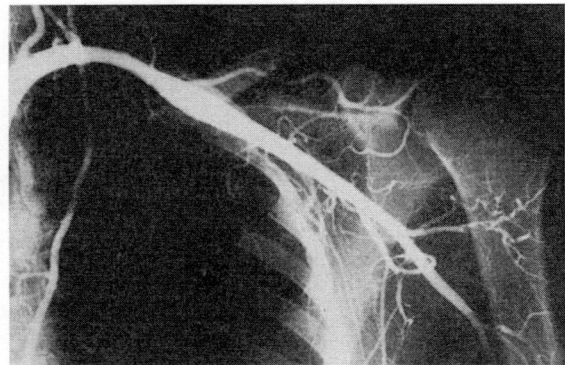

Fig. 8. Angiographic aspect of a post-stenotic dilatation of subclavian right artery in thoracic outlet syndrome

Fig. 7. Thoracic outlet syndromes and related conditions. Major variants: Costo-clavicular (1), Scalenus anticus (2) Cervical rib (3) and Hyperabduction (4) syndromes. A : subclavian artery, BP : brachial plexus, c : clavicle, Cp : coracoid process, Pm : pectoralis minor, Sa : musculus scalenus anticus, Sm : musculus scalenus medius, V : subclavian vein, (*) : first rib

The thoracic outlet syndrome and its related conditions rarely affect children; typically the majority (86%) are young women in early and middle life (average age: 36 years [50-52]. The patient presents with upper extremity pain, varying from minor intermittent aching to severe constant pain, involving the supraclavicular area, the shoulder, and the upper part of the arm. At times, pain can extend to the forearm and hand, causing weakness. Often this symptom is exaggerated when the arm is abducted above the head or when the shoulder is rotated downward and backward. Numbness, tingling, paraesthesia, weakness, and fatigability may be experienced, and swelling and discoloration may be present. Intermittent Raynaud's syndrome affects 15% of patients, but the pallor and coldness of digits are less prominent than in Raynaud's phenomenon caused by other conditions [53]. All these symptoms become permanent when the subclavian artery is occluded.

Oedema of the hand with diffuse pain in the arm and forearm occurs when venous occlusion is present. Radial pulsation changes in amplitude when the arm is hyperabducted (hyperabduction manoeuvre) or when the neck is extended and the chin turned toward the side being examined (scalene manoeuvre). When compression of the subclavian artery is continuous, a soft bruit may be noted in the supraclavicular or infraclavicular space at the middle or distal third of the clavicle. An angiogram may demonstrate a stenosis with post-stenotic dilatation in the subclavian artery (Fig. 8) and an electromyogram (EMG) may display abnormal features in some patients. Magnetic angioresonance displays changes in blood flow on forced arm movement [54]. Spiral computed tomography is expected to be useful for determining the complex pathophysiologic processes that underlie thoracic outlet syndrome [55, 56]. Other vascular impairments may be associated: subclavian artery kinking and vertebral steal syndrome [57]. Post-stenotic dilatation of the subclavian artery is a rare but dangerous complication of TOS. It occurs in patients with cervical ribs (Fig. 9) or abnormal first thoracic ribs [58-61]

Complications include post-stenotic dilatation (Fig. 10), vascular rupture, thrombosis and ischaemia with chronic arm claudication. Thrombosis may occlude the subclavian or axillary artery (Fig. 11). When the syndrome occurs on the right, retrograde extension of the thrombus may cause cerebral embolism. Ulceration and acral necrosis frequently occur in the skin of the fingers [62]. Venous thrombosis results in mild to moderate chronic venous insufficiency in the upper limb. Extension to the axillary vein may result in pulmonary embolism. Most patients who have a

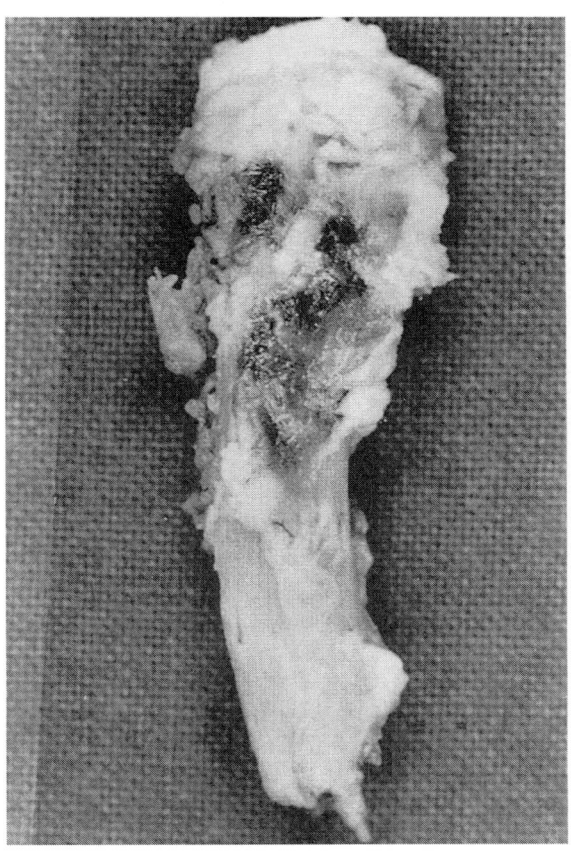

Fig. 9. Hypertrophied first thoracic rib causing thoracic outlet syndrome

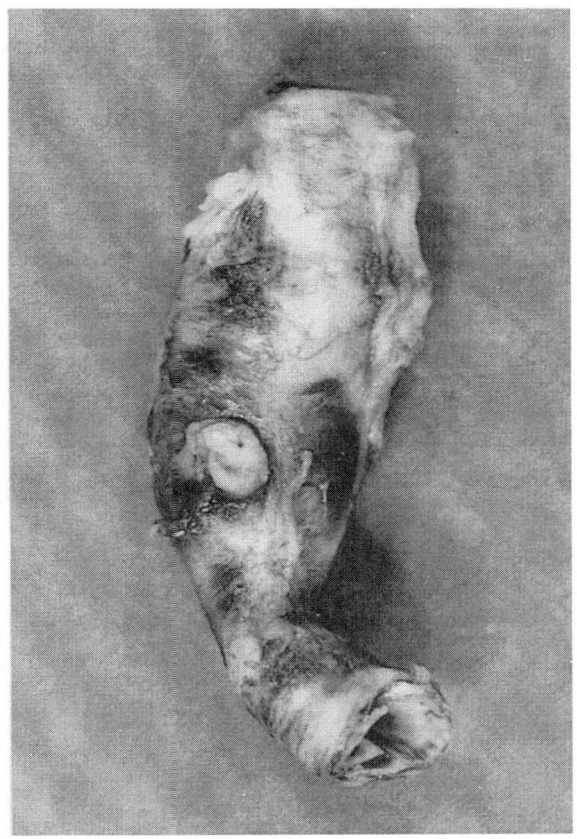

Fig. 10. Subclavian artery showing the compression area with post-stenotic dilatation

cervical rib or an anomalous first thoracic rib do not present symptoms from these abnormalities and no treatment is called for. Surgical treatment is considered when symptoms progress; poststenotic dilatation develops without any increase in symptoms. This treatment may include removal of the cervical rib, section of the anterior scalene muscle, resection of the clavicle, or division of the tendon of the pectoralis minor [63, 64].

Pathology and differential diagnosis

Repeated and intermittent compression of the subclavian artery induces intimal thickening with superimposed luminal thrombus. The media undergoes hypertrophy while the adventitia displays fibrosis. Compression also damages the subclavian venous wall, producing phlebitis with fibrosis leading to stenosis with thrombosis extending into the axillary vein (30-40%). None of these changes is specific.

Popliteal artery entrapment syndrome

The popliteal artery commences at the termination of the femoral artery at the opening in adductor magnus, and crosses the popliteal fossa obliquely downwards and outwards, to the lower border of the popliteus muscle. Superficially, it is covered above by the semimembranosus; in the middle of its course by connective and adipose tissue; and below, is overlapped by the gastrocnemius, plantaris and soleus muscles, the popliteal vein and the internal popliteal nerve. The popliteal vein lies superficial and external to the artery above, then crosses it and runs along its inner side. The internal popliteal nerve crosses the artery below the joint and lies on its inner side. Laterally, the popliteal artery is limited by the muscles which are located on either side of the popliteal space.

Any muscular and/or vascular anomaly can entrap and compress the popliteal vessels, usually the artery [65], rarely the vein [66, 67]. These anomalies are not symmetrical but occasionally the popliteal artery en-

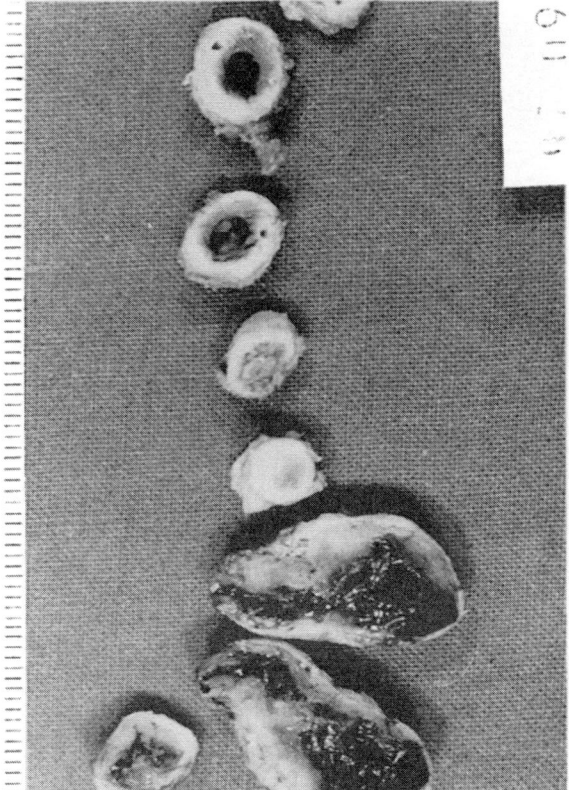

Fig. 11. Subclavian artery compression syndrome with post-stenotic dilatation. Cut sections evidence old and fresh luminal thrombi

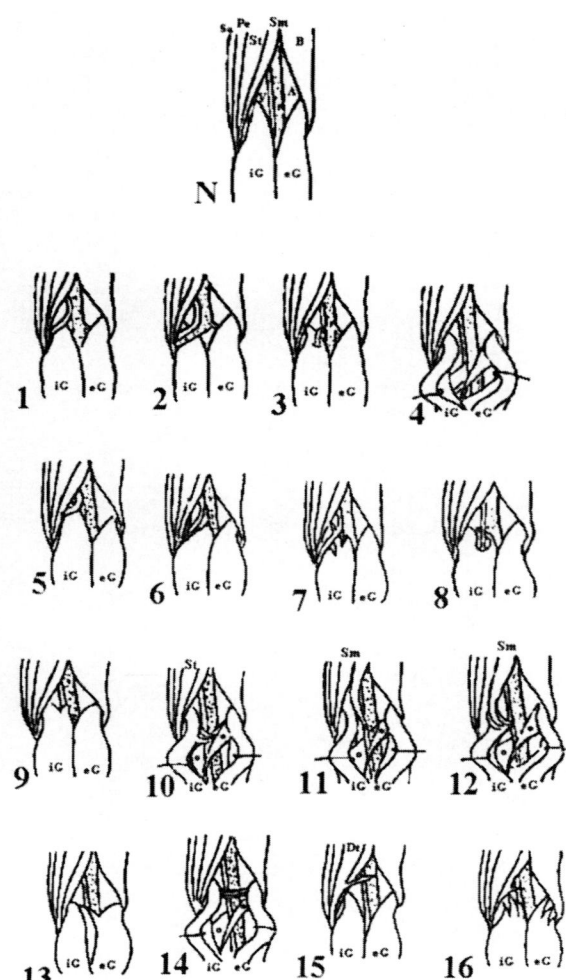

Fig. 12. Various types of the popliteal artery entrapment syndrome. Group I.-Isolated abnormal course of the PA (1-4) Group II.– Abnormal course of the PA associated with one or severe muscular anomalies (5-8) Group III.– Isolated muscular anomalies (9-16) A : popliteal artery, B : biceps femoris, Sm : semimembranosus, St : semitendinosus, eG : outer head of the gastrocnemius muscle, iG : inner head of the gastrocnemius muscle, N : normal state, Pe : pectineus muscle, Sa : sartorius muscle, V : popliteal vein, (*) : plantaris muscle, (o) : popliteus muscle

trapment syndrome may be bilateral [68, 69]. The numerous names attributed to this condition reflect the complexity of the lesions: entrapped popliteal artery syndrome, extrinsic compression of the popliteal artery, occlusion of the popliteal artery caused by muscular entrapment, thrombosis of the popliteal artery secondary to abnormal course, circulatory disorders of the inferior limbs caused by muscular anomaly of the popliteal fossa and popliteal arteriopathy caused by anatomic anomaly. However, these lesions can be classified into three groups: 1°) group I: an isolated abnormal course of the popliteal artery; 2°) group II: an abnormal course of the artery associated with one or several muscular anomalies; and 3°) group III: and isolated muscular anomalies. Table 2 lists the frequency, causes and corresponding types of anomalies described in diverse classifications [70-77]. Fig. 12 illustrates these anomalies.

From the pathogenic standpoint, the popliteal artery is submitted to variations of its curvature and calibre during flexion and extension of the knee. When there is a conflict between the popliteal artery (having a normal or an abnormal course) and a muscle (having an abnormal or normal insertion), the artery is often stretched and/or compressed against osseous structures. Repeated tension applied to the arterial wall is a repeated localised trauma [75] like that of vascular syndromes secondary to compression caused by supporting anatomic structures described above.

Table 2. Causes of entrapment of popliteal artery, frequency and corresponding classifications of each group and type. Classifications (D : Delaney, F : Ferrero, I : Insua, M : Maistre, R : Roussel) ; Mis : Miscellaneous anomaly ; PA : Popliteal artery. PV : Popliteal vein

T	%	CAUSES	I	D	M	R	F
		Group I.-Isolated abnormal course of the PA					
1	35	The PA deviates from its proper course, encircles the internal border of the internal head (iG) of the gastrocnemius muscle	1	1	1	1	1
2	1,5	Idem type 1, the PV runs alongside the PA in its abnormal course			1		
3	0,5	The PA deviates from the medial line, perforates the inner head (iG) of the gastrocnemius muscle				1C	2
4	7	The PA crosses in front of the popliteus muscle (o), separates from the PV which follows its normal course		4	Mis		
		Group II.– Abnormal course of the PA associated with one or several muscular anomalies					
5	28	The PA encircles the internal border of the inner head (iG) of the gastrocnemius muscle, which has an abnormally high insertion into the inner femoral condyle		2	1A		
6	17	The inner head (iG) of the gastrocnemius muscle is inserted abnormally into the outer part of the inner femoral condyle. This structure pushes the artery outside the midline, separating it from the PV			1B	4	
7	0.5	The inner head (iG) of the gastrocnemius muscle encompasses 3 tendons (internal, intermediate and external). The PA encircles the external border of the external tendon			1B		
8	6	The inner head (iG) of the gastrocnemius muscle has an accessory tendon, abnormally inserted into the external border of the muscle femoral condyle, separating the PA from the PV			3		3
		Group III.– Isolated muscular anomalies					
9	0.5	Compression by erratic accessory insertions of the inner head (iG) of the gastrocnemius muscle or both its heads		2	2A		
10	0.5	Compression by fibro-muscular tendons of the inner head of the gastrocnemius muscle. These tendons are inserted into the outer femoral		2	Mis		

		condyle and the plantaris muscle					
11	0.5	Compression by the semimembranosus muscle abnormally inserted into the internal lip of the femoral linae aspera				Mis	3
12	0.5	Compression by the fibrous strands extending from the 3rd adductor ring and linking the gastrocnemius muscle to the semimembranosus muscle					
13	0.5	Compression by the outer head (eG) of the gastrocnemius muscle. This anomaly may be bilateral					9
14	0.5	Compression by fibrous strands stretched between the two heads of the gastrocnemius muscle					6
15	0.5	Compression by an abnormal tendon of the semitendinosus muscle					8
16	0.5	Compression by muscles having abnormal insertions extending vertically from the upper part to the lower part and from the outer to the inner border of the popliteal fossa					10

There is no correlation between the severity of the arteriopathy and the type of anatomical anomaly. Whatever the type of anomaly, this trauma leads to a of the clavicle variably complete arterial obstruction with thrombosis, post-stenotic aneurysm, false aneurysm formation and, distal embolism [78]. A systematic search for this syndrome should be made when any young patient complains of intermittent claudication of the lower limbs.

The first case of popliteal artery entrapment syndrome was reported in 1870 by Stuart [79], when a medical student at the University of Edinburgh. The frequency of the defect is unknown since the anomaly is free of complications and in the presence of a compensated collateral circulation, often remains unnoticed [65, 80]. Any age may be involved; the youngest known patient was 11, the eldest 64 [79, 81, 82]. The disease manifests mostly in highly trained (competitive runners) and normally active young men and women with a male predilection [65]. Computed tomography helps to identify the path of popliteal vessels (Fig. 13). On angiography medial deviation of the proximal popliteal artery, segmental occlusion of the midpopliteal artery, post-stenotic dilatation and notching of the popliteal artery (Fig. 14) upon passive dorsiflexion or active plantar flexion of the foot are seen [80, 83-86]. Complications include post-stenotic aneurysm [72, 73, 75, 87] (Fig. 15), thrombosis, deterioration of the distal vascular bed caused by distal embolism [88] and false aneurysm secondary to rupture of the intima and media, often occurring after physical exercise. In the non-complicated stage, the treatment consists of freeing the vessel from the trap. When complications occur, resection with a venous bypass is indicated. This bypass should always follow the normal course of the popliteal artery in order to prevent a recurrent syndrome [89-91]. New therapeutic approaches, such as combined percutaneous transluminal thrombembolectomy (PTTE), local thrombolysis (LTL) and percutaneous transluminal angioplasty for thrombotic and embolic obstructions

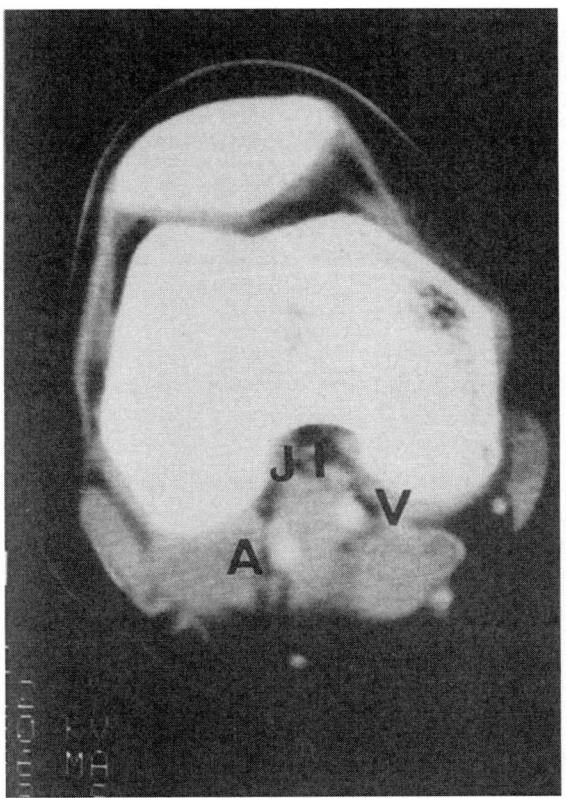

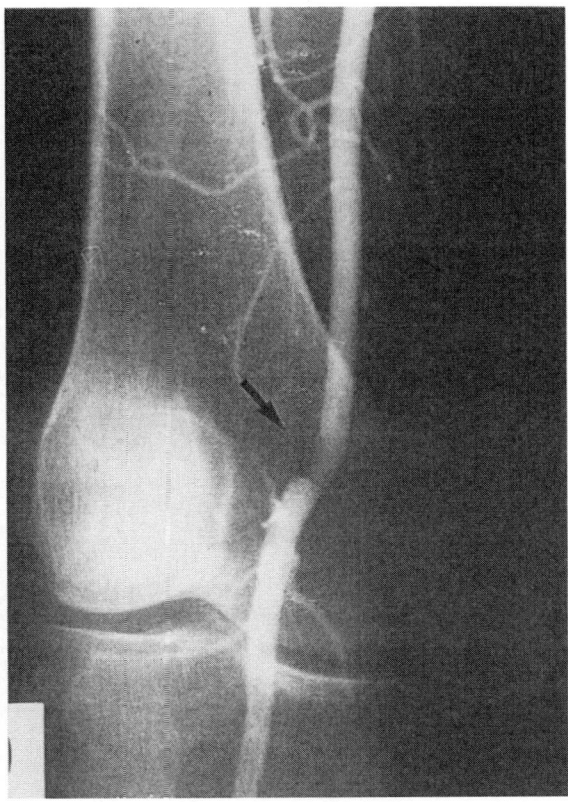

Fig. 13. Type 6 popliteal artery entrapment syndrome: the abnormally inserted inner head of the gastrocnemius (JI) pushes the artery (A) outside the midline, separating it from the vein (V). Computed tomography (Courtesy Dr Cl. Laurian)

Fig. 14. Medial deviation with notching (arrow) of the entrapped proximal popliteal artery identified on an angiogram (Courtesy Dr Cl. Laurian)

(PTA), have been also proposed to avoid direct vascular surgery [92].

Pathology and Differential diagnosis

The morphological appearance of the entrapped popliteal vessel is unremarkable. Most accounts do not desribe the nature of the parietal lesions. Intimo-medial rupture is rare (Fig. 16). In some cases, the artery remains unchanged [93]. In others, the intima is thickened by fibrosis leading to "intimal dysplasia" [73] (Fig. 17). In Rich's case report [94], the satellite vein showed ectasia. The main differential diagnosis is the so-called "adventitial mucoid cyst" of the popliteal artery (See chapter V).

Endofibrosis of the external iliac artery (Competition cyclist arteriopathy)

This newly-identified vascular entity of mechanical origin [95-98] is characterised by intimal thickening with kinking or buckling of the external iliac artery developing during repeated flexion of the thigh on the pelvis. The external iliac artery passes obliquely downwards and outwards along the inner border of psoas major from the bifurcation of the common iliac to Poupart's ligament, where it enters the thigh and becomes the femoral artery. This artery rests against the psoas muscles from which it is separated by the iliac fascia. It is stretched between its upper origin and lower end, near Poupart's ligament; however, it remains mobile between these two fixed points. Besides several small branches to the psoas muscles and the neighbouring lymph nodes, the external iliac artery gives off two branches of considerable size, the deep epigastric artery and deep circumflex iliac artery. Repeated flexion of the thigh on the pelvis induces marked traction and relaxation of the artery. This process results in lengthening and kinking of the mobile segment. The presence of a psoas-bound collateral may limit the lengthening but accentuate the kinking of the artery. Constraints on the greater curva-

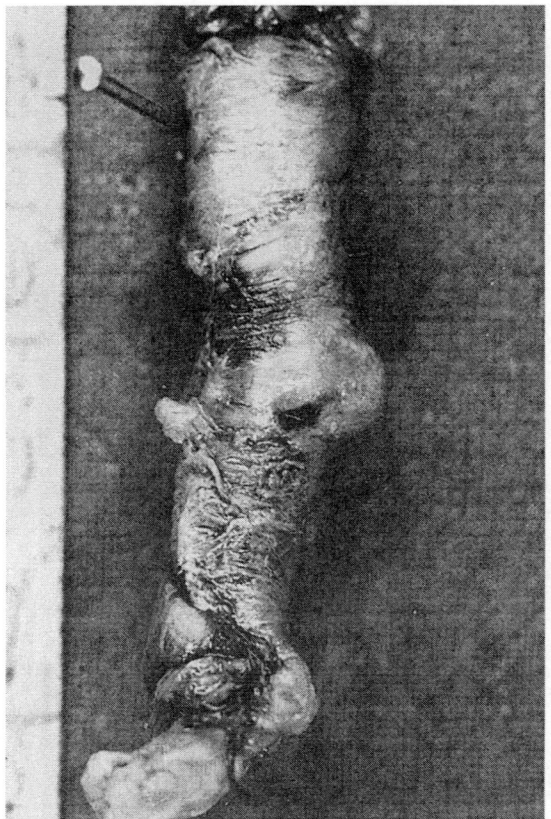

Fig. 15. Entrapped popliteal artery with post-stenotic dilatation

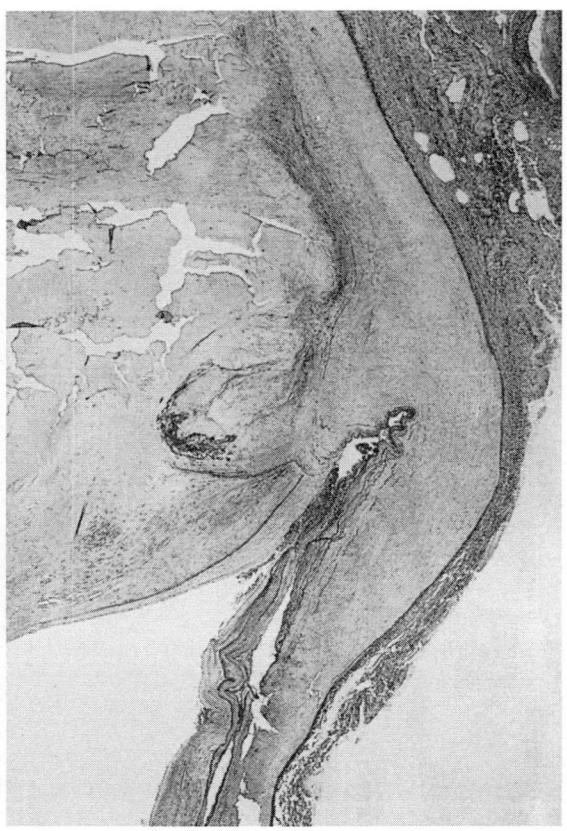

Fig. 16. Intimo-medial rupture with marked intimal proliferation. Orcein

ture of the buckle cause parietal lesions whose severity is enhanced when the arterial pressure increases.

The disease occurs most frequently in young (mean age: 27), high-level, professional cyclists riding at least 15,000 or 20,000 km a year (generally, a minimal total performance of 60,000 km is necessary for the disease to appear). Endurance-trained athletes and body builders are rarely affected [99]. The most frequent symptom is claudication, first limited to the thigh, then extending to the whole limb. More rarely, the patient may present with swelling of the thigh. These symptoms appear during physical exertion and regress at rest. Clinical examination reveals no anomaly except for a mild and inconsistent asymmetry of the thigh. Sometimes an iliac murmur is heard when the thigh is flexed on the pelvis. Ultrasound examinations taken at rest may evidence the lesions in 80% of endofibrotic patients and allow ruling out the diagnosis of popliteal entrapment syndrome during dorsiflexion of the foot. An exer-

cise test on an ergometric bicycle helps to detect stenosis on the aorto-ilio-femoral axis. Invasive investigations (arteriography or angioscopy) with flexion of the thigh on the pelvis frequently show extensive but mild stenoses (less than 40% diameter), sometimes with a buckle or lengthening [100]. Dissecting aneurysm of the external iliac artery is a serious complication [101]. Although long-term results are unknown, most of the surgically treated patients return to competition.

Pathology and differential diagnosis

The artery remains flexible; changes may involve the entire circumference of the artery or only a part of the circumference. Fibrosis thickens the intima but the integrity of the endothelium and other arterial coats are preserved.

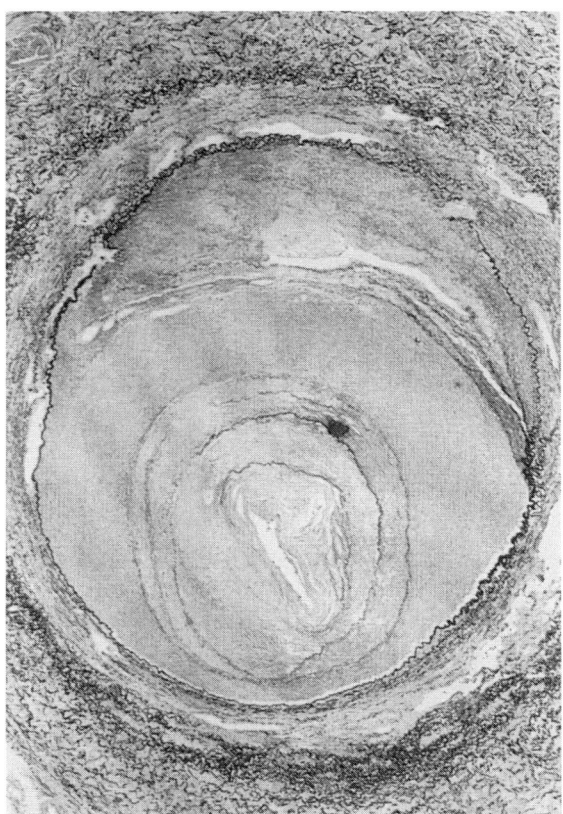

Fig. 17. Occlusive intimal proliferation resembling "intimal dysplasia." Orcein

Coeliac compression syndrome

This syndrome occurs when the median arcuate ligament of the diaphragm and/or periarterial neural tissue causes extrinsic compression of the coeliac axis with upper abdominal angina. The classic triad of coeliac compression syndrome consists of abdominal pain, an epigastric bruit, and angiographic evidence of coeliac compression. Operative therapy consists of thorough exploration, transection of the median arcuate ligament, and either coeliac dilatation or an aortosplenic bypass [102]. Pathological changes are non specific.

Venous compression syndromes

Cockett's syndrome

This is characterised by a partial or complete compression of the left primary iliac vein between the right primary iliac artery and the lumbar vertebrae.

This condition results from an exaggeration of the anatomical development of the right common iliac artery and the left common iliac vein. The latter is displaced forwards against the unyielding artery by the convexity of the lower lumbar vertebrae. There is thus a degree of compression over the termination on the left common iliac vein [103, 104]. Other causes include: abnormal iliocaval junction [104], ectopic kidney [105], retro-iliac ureter [106], and hip algodystrophy [107]. There is a female predominance; the patients' mean age at presentation is around 37 yrs [86]. Generally the condition is asymptomatic; however the most frequent presentation is an inexplicable unilateral swelling and oedema of the distal leg, usually the left, in the presence of an apparently normal venous system. Other complications may also exist: acute or recurrent ilio-femoral thrombosis, obstructive membranes in the inferior vena cava, chronic venous insufficiency with venous claudication, skin pigmentation and venous ulceration [108].

The compression is usually compensated by an increase in the collateral circulation in the lumbar or sacral region. The compression pattern is often less evident in non invasive imaging (ultrasound, particularly colour-duplex) than in phlebography. The compression may be partial, not affecting flow, or there may be total occlusion. Recurrent oedema requires stenting or surgical treatment of the affected segment [109-111]. Constricting fibrous bands or adhesions with severe obstruction need to be freed surgically with end-to-end re-anastomosis in the front of the artery or with reimplantation into the inferior vena cava.

Pathology and differential diagnosis

In some subjects, the compression is severe and may be associated with intimal thickening leading to venous spur formation or a fibrous band with adhesion at the proximal end of the left common iliac vein. These changes favour deep venous thrombosis [111].

Other venous compression syndromes

Compression syndrome of the innominate veins

This is caused by an intermittent compression of the left innominate vein by the supra-aortic trunks, mainly the left subclavian artery, during expiration. The clinical picture is characterised by a superior vena cava syndrome. This anomaly is the thoracic equivalent of Cockett's syndrome [112].

Soleus syndrome

First described by Servelle in 1968 [113], this rare syndrome is characterised by a permanent compression of the tibioperoneal or tibiofibular vein by the tendinous arch of soleus. The syndrome results from abnormal anatomical development of the soleus insertion. Compression of the vein leads to raised pressure in the venous circulation of the calf with sural thrombosis and insufficiency of the perforating veins. The syndrome frequently involves young, active women. Presenting symptoms consist of a heavy feeling in the legs, pain, malleolar oedema, paraesthesia exacerbated in the evening after a long period of standing, or varices. Section of the soleal tendinous arch is necessary to free the vascular bundle.

Pathology and differential diagnosis

The compressed vein displays unremarkable fibrotic thickening of the intima and media. Thrombosis may occur.

Nutcracker syndrome

This syndrome results from compression of the left renal vein between the aorta and the superior mesenteric artery, which leads to painless, intermittent, gross haematuria. Other variants encompass compression of the left renal vein by ureteral varices and extrinsic tumours [114-116]. Physical examination and routine laboratory examinations are often noncontributory. Renal ultrasonographic study, selective left renal angiography, and retrograde left renal venography demonstrate the compression. Pathological changes of the left renal vein are unremarkable, with parietal fibrosis, endovenous thickening and thrombosis.

Bibliography

1. Fruhwirth J, Koch G, Ivanic GM, Seibert FJ, Tesch NP (1997) Vascular lesions in surgery of the hip joint. Unfallchirurg 100: 119-23
2. Kumar SN, Chapman JA, Rawlins I (1998) Vascular injuries in total knee arthroplasty. A review of the problem with special reference to the possible effects of the tourniquet. J Arthroplasty 13: 211-16
3. Goodkin R, Laska LL (1998) Vascular and visceral injuries associated with lumbar disc surgery: medicolegal implications. Surg Neurol 49: 358-70
4. Vuong PN, Lagneau P (1987): Pathologie artérielle traumatique In Camilleri JP, Berry CL, Fiessinger J-N, Bariety J: Les maladies de la paroi artérielle, Flammarion, Paris 579-90
5. Vuong PN, Desoutter P, Van Tan, Houissa-Vuong S (1999) Fibrodysplasie musculaire artérielle révélée par un faux anévrisme traumatique: un cas. J Mal Vasc (Paris) 25: 377-80
6. Waikakul S, Sakkarnkosol S, Vanadurongwan V (1998) Vascular injuries in compound fractures of the leg with initially adequate circulation. J Bone Joint Surg Br 80: 254-8
7. Cameron PA, Dziukas L, Hadj A, Hooper S, Tatoulis J (1998) Aortic transection. Aust N Z J Surg 68: 264-7
8. Modrall JG, Weaver FA, Yellin AE (1998) Diagnosis and management of penetrating vascular trauma and the injured extremity. Emerg Med Clin North Am 16: 129-44
9. Vuong PN, Sebban E, Sobiak S, Houissa-Vuong S, Lagneau P, Camilleri JP (1986) Pseudo-anévrysme traumatique de l'artère temporale superficielle ou complication vasculaire d'une gifle. A propos d'une observation avec revue de la littérature médicale. Sem Hôp Paris 62: 2697-703
10. Roth SM, Wheeler JR, Gregory RT, Gayle RG, Parent FN 3rd, Demasi R, Ribet J, Weireter LJ, Britt LD (1997) Blunt injury of the abdominal aorta: a review. J Trauma 42: 748-55
11. von Segesser LK, Fischer A, Vogt P, Turina M (1997) Diagnosis and management of blunt great vessel trauma. J Card Surg 12: S181-S186
12. Durigon M, Barbet JP, Barres D, Gherardi R, Guillon F, Paraire F, Polivka (1988) Pathologie médico-légale. Masson, Paris, Milan, Barcelone, Mexico 171 p
13. Vazquez Rueda F, Nunez Nunez R, Gomez Meleno P, Blesa Sanchez E (1996) The hair-thread tourniquet syndrome of the toes and penis. An Esp Pediatr 44: 17-20
14. Terazawa K, Wu B, Takatori T (1991) A bibliographic discussion on the obstruction of arteries and the air passage in hanging. Nippon Hoigaku Zasshi 45: 311-7
15. Elfawal MA, Awad OA (1994) Deaths from hanging in the eastern province of Saudi Arabia. Med Sci Law 34: 307-12
16. Kodali S, Jamieson WR, Leia-Stephens M, Miyagishima RT, Janusz MT, Tyers GF (1991) Traumatic rupture of the thoracic aorta. A 20-year review: 1969-1989. Circulation 84: SIII40-6
17. Dell'Erba A, Di Vella G, Giardino N (1998) Seatbelt injury to the common iliac artery: case report. J Forensic Sci 43: 215-7
18. Guerriero WG, Carlton CE Jr, Scott R Jr, Beall AC Jr (1971) Renal pedicle injuries. J Trauma 11: 53-62
19. Clark DE, Georgitis JW, Ray FS (1981) Renal arterial injuries caused by blunt trauma. Surgery 90: 87-96
20. Mitchell GM, McCann JJ, Rogers IW, Hickey MJ, Morrison WA, O'Brien BM (1996) A morphological study of the long-term repair process in experimentally stretched but unruptured arteries and veins. Br J Plast Surg 49: 34-40
21. Richaud J, Lazorthes Y (1980) Pathogénie des lésions traumatiques fermées de la carotide interne du cou. Déductions à propos de 17 cas. J Trauma 3: 161-70
22. Fu XB (1990) Experimental study of multiple organ injuries after high-velocity missiles. Chung Hua Wai Ko Tsa Chih 28: 371-3, 383
23. Mendelson JA (1991) The relationship between mechanisms of wounding and principles of treatment of missile wounds. J Trauma 31: 1181-202
24. Scialpi M, Magli T, Boccuzzi F, Scapati C (1995) Computed tomography in gunshot trauma. I. Ballistics elements and the mechanisms of the lesions. Radiol Med (Torino) 89: 485-94
25. Amato JJ, Rich NM, Billy LJ, Gruber RP, Lawson NS (1971) High-velocity arterial injury: a study of the mechanism of injury. J Trauma 11: 412-6

26. Amato JJ, Rich NM (1972) Temporary cavity effects in blood vessel injury by high velocity missiles. J Cardiovasc Surg (Torino) 13: 147-55

27. Bonath KH, Vannini R, Koch H, Schnettler R (1996) Gunshot wounds—ballistics, physiopathology, surgical treatment. Tierarztl Prax 24: 304-15

28. Briusov PG, Kuznetsov NM, Dolishnii VN (1991) Dynamic microvascular changes in gunshot wounds. Voen Med Zh 7: 4-6

29. Tan YH, Zhou SX, Liu YQ, Liu BL, Li ZY (1991) Small-vessel pathology and anastomosis following maxillofacial firearm wounds: an experimental study. J Oral Maxillofac Surg 49: 348-52

30. Galeon M, Goffette P, Van Beers BE, Pringot J (1997) Post-traumatic intrahepatic pseudoaneurysm: diagnosis with helical CT angiography and management with embolization. J Belge Radiol 80: 287-8

31. Takeshima S, Hatori N, Uryuda Y, Yoshizu H, Tanaka S (1997) A case report of the subclavian pseudoaneurysm due to blunt chest trauma without fracture. Nippon Kyobu Geka Gakkai Zasshi 45: 1884-8

32. Vadlamudi G, Schinella R (1998) Traumatic pseudoaneurysm: a possible early lesion in the spectrum of epithelioid hemangioma/angiolymphoid hyperplasia with eosinophilia. Am J Dermatopathol 20: 113-7

33. Cormier JM, Florent J (1967) Les hématomes rétro-péritonéaux par blessures des vaisseaux iliaques au cours des fractures du bassin. Mem Acad Chir (Paris) 93: 458-62

34. Wascher RA, Gwinn BC 2nd (1995) Air rifle pellet injury to the heart with retrograde caval migration. J Trauma 38: 379-81

35. Hausmann R, Betz P (1997) Delayed death after attempted suicide by hanging. Int J Legal Med 110: 164-6

36. Kalt M, Knipping L, Mangold G (1997) Traumatic arteriovenous fistula between superior thyroid artery and vein. Chirurg 68: 1304-6

37. Stehbens WE (1968) Blood vessel changes in chronic experimental arteriovenous fistulas. Surg Gynecol Obstet 127: 327-38

38. Hewitt RL, Smith AD, Drapanas T (1973) Acute traumatic arteriovenous fistulas. J Trauma 13: 901-6

39. Ierardi RP, Kerstein MD (1995) Venous injuries: military versus civilian experience. Mil Med 160: 396-8

40. Sirbu H, Herse B, Busch T, Dalichau H (1998) Pulmonary vein injury through repetitive clip friction: an unusual cause of hemothorax. Ann Thorac Surg 65: 548-50

41. Coluccio G, Rosato L, Paino O, Fornero G (1997) Chyloperitoneum after traumatic rupture of subdiaphragmatic thoracic duct. A clinical case. Minerva Chir 52: 1367-70

42. Lopez Espadas F, Iribarren Sarrias JL, Martinez Jimenez C, Fernandez Rico R, Lacruz Canas A, Quesada Suescun A (1997) Chylothorax secondary to blunt thoracic trauma. Report of 6 cases. Arch Bronconeumol 33: 168-71

43. Worthington MG, de Groot M, Gunning AJ, von Oppell UO (1995) Isolated thoracic duct injury after penetrating chest trauma. Ann Thorac Surg 60: 272-4

44. Ikonomidis JS, Boulanger BR, Brenneman FD (1997) Chylothorax after blunt chest trauma: a report of 2 cases. Can J Surg 40: 135-8

45. Hart AK, Greinwald JH Jr, Shaffrey CI, Postma GN (1998) Thoracic duct injury during anterior cervical discectomy: a rare complication. Case report. J Neurosurg 88: 151-4

46. Davidovic LB, Lotina SI, Vojnovic BR, Kostic DM, Colic MM, Stanic MI, Djoric PD (1998) Treatment of the thoracic outlet vascular syndrome. Srp Arh Celok Lek 126: 23-30

47. Fairbrain II JF, Campbell JK, Payne WS (1980) Neurovascular compression syndromes of the thoracic outlet In Juergens JL, Spittell JA Jr, Fairbairn II JF: Peripheral vascular diseases 1980, WB Saunders, Philadelphia, London, Toronto 629-53

48. Brancherau A, Winninger AL, Orso A, Devin R (1974) Problèmes nosologiques soulevés par le syndrome de la traversée thoraco-brachiale. A propos de 18 cas. J Chir (Paris) 107: 39-45

49. Adelman MA, Stone DH, Riles TS, Lamparello PJ, Giangola G, Rosen RJ (1997) A multidisciplinary approach to the treatment of Paget-Schroetter syndrome. Ann Vasc Surg 11: 149-54

50. Workum P, Purvis RJ, Thomas GW (1971) A case of thoracic outlet syndrome occurring in infancy. Pediatrics 48: 462-3

51. Jamieson WG, Chinnick B (1996) Thoracic outlet syndrome: fact or fancy? A review of 409 consecutive patients who underwent operation. Can J Surg 39: 321-6

52. Tucciarone L, Anaclerio S, Tomassini A, Papandrea S, Costantino F, Sabbi T (1996) Anterior scalenus syndrome in pediatric age. Report of a case. Minerva Pediatr 48: 461-4

53. Mackinnon SE, Patterson GA, Novak CB (1996) Thoracic outlet syndrome: a current overview. Semin Thorac Cardiovasc Surg 8: 176-82

54. Tobalina I, Alvaro-Gonzalez LC, Garcia-Andrade L (1996) Arterial thoracic outlet syndrome and diagnostic angioresonance. Rev Neurol 24: 1541-2

55. Matsumura JS, Rilling WS, Pearce WH, Nemcek AA Jr, Vogelzang RL, Yao JS (1997) Helical computed tomography of the normal thoracic outlet. J Vasc Surg 26: 776-83

56. Remy-Jardin M, Doyen J, Remy J, Artaud D, Fribourg M, Duhamel A (1997) Functional anatomy of the thoracic outlet: evaluation with spiral CT. Radiology 205: 843-51

57. Bogalho L, Seixas I, Martins JM, Pisco JM (1998) Angiography in thoracic outlet syndrome. Acta Med Port 11: 33-6

58. Desai Y, Robbs JV (1995) Arterial complications of the thoracic outlet syndrome. Eur J Vasc Endovasc Surg 10: 362-5

59. Gruss JD, Geissler C (1997) Aneurysms of the subclavian artery in thoracic outlet syndrome. Zentralbl Chir 122: 730-4

60. Hood DB, Kuehne J, Yellin AE, Weaver FA (1997) Vascular complications of thoracic outlet syndrome. Am Surg 63: 913-7

61. Iida H, Mori H, Mochizuki Y, Okamura Y, Nagai S, Shimada K (1997) A case report of thoracic outlet syndrome with acute arterial obstruction caused by abnormal first rib. Nippon Kyobu Geka Gakkai Zasshi 45: 2026-9

62. Schelo C, Kroger K, Hinrichs A, Rensing N, Rudofsky G (1997) Ischemia of the arm with finger necroses: differential carpal tunnel syndrome and thoracic outlet syndrome diagnosis. Vasa 26: 311-3

63. Thompson RW, Petrinec D, Toursarkissian B (1997) Surgical treatment of thoracic outlet compression syndromes. II. Supraclavicular exploration and vascular reconstruction. Ann Vasc Surg 11: 442-51

64. Wenz W, Husfeldt KJ (1997) Thoracic outlet syndrome—an interdisciplinary topic. Experience with diagnosis and therapy in a 15-year patient cohort (80 transaxillary re-

sections of the 1st rib in 67 patients) and a literature review. Z Orthop Ihre Grenzgeb 135: 84-90

65. Erdoes LS, Devine JJ, Bernhard VM, Baker MR, Berman SS, Hunter GC (1994) Popliteal vascular compression in a normal population. J Vasc Surg 20: 978-86

66. Iwai T, Sato S, Yamada T, Muraoka Y, Sakurazawa K, Kinoshita H, Inoue Y, Endo M, Yoshiba T, Suzuki S (1987) Popliteal vein entrapment caused by the third head of the gastrocnemius muscle. Br J Surg 74: 1006-8

67. Gerkin TM, Beebe HG, Williams DM, Bloom JR, Wakefield TW (1993) Popliteal vein entrapment presenting as deep venous thrombosis and chronic venous insufficiency. J Vasc Surg 18: 760-6

68. Ezzet F, Yettra M (1971) Bilateral popliteal artery entrapment: case report and observation. J Cardiovasc Surg 12: 71-4

69. Gibson MH, Mills JG, Johnson GE, Downs AR (1977) Popliteal entrapment syndrome. Ann Surg 185: 341-8

70. Insua JA, Young JR, Humphries AW (1970) Popliteal artery entrapment syndrome. Arch Surg 101: 771-4

71. Delaney TA, Gonzalez LL (1971) Occlusion of popliteal artery due to muscular entrapment. Surgery 69: 97-101

72. Maistre B, Garnier J, Nosny P (1972) Artériopathie poplitée par compression musculo-tendineuse. Chirurgie 98: 667-73

73. Roussel J, Dietz F, Kieny R (1973) Syndrome ischémique par malposition de l'artère poplitée. J Med Strasbourg 4: 201-9

74. Ferrero R, Barile C, Bretto P, Buzzachino A, Ponzio F (1980) Popliteal artery entrapment syndrome. J Cardiovasc Surg 21: 45-52

75. Vuong PN (1990) "Entrapped" popliteal artery: pathology and pathogenesis. Report of 7 cases with review of the literature Arch Anat Cytol Pathol 38: 72-80

76. Ohta M, Kusaba A, Shrestha DR, Koja K, Kina M, Shiroma H, Ohmine Y (1991) Popliteal artery entrapment syndrome. Report of two cases. J Cardiovasc Surg (Torino) 32: 697-701

77. Banjo AO (1996) Aberrant popliteus muscle: anatomy and clinical consideration. Afr J Med Med Sci 25: 69-73

78. Gyftokostas D, Koutsoumbelis C, Mattheou T, Bouhoutsos J (1991) Post stenotic aneurysm in popliteal artery entrapment syndrome. J Cardiovasc Surg (Torino) 32: 350-2

79. Stuart A (1870) Note on variation in the course of the popliteal artery. J Anat 13: 162

80. Chernoff DM, Walker AT, Khorasani R, Polak JF, Jolesz FA (1995) Asymptomatic functional popliteal artery entrapment: demonstration at MR imaging. Radiology 195: 176-80

81. Hamming JJ, Vink M (1965) Obstruction of the popliteal artery at an early age. J Cardiovasc Surg 6: 516-524

82. Fitze G, Taut H, Rupprecht E, Roesner D (1997) Popliteal artery entrapment syndrome. Case report of an 11-year-old boy. Langenbecks Arch Chir 382: 393-7

83. Cormier JM, Laurian CL, Fichelle JM, Bardi K, Franceschi Cl, Luizy F (1985) Artère poplitée piégée. Apport de l'exploration ultrasonique. Presse Méd 14: 2183-5

84. Engel A, Adler OB, Carmeli R (1991) Computed tomography in the diagnosis of popliteal artery entrapment syndrome. Harefuah 121: 437-8

85. Vuong PN, Laurian C (1992) Entrapped popliteal artery. Value of medical imaging and review of the literature J Radiol 73: 247-52

86. Belcaro G, Nicolaides AN, Veller M (1995) Venous disorders. A manual of diagnosis and treatment. Saunders, London, Philadelphia, Toronto, Sydney, Tokyo, 194 p.

87. Porcellini M, Selvetella L, Bernardo B, Del Viscovo L, Parisi B, Baldassarre M (1997) Popliteal artery entrapment syndrome: diagnosis and management. G Chir 18: 182-6

88. Mazzucchetti S, Marinoni V, Guala A (1992) Popliteal entrapment syndrome with distal embolization. Description of a clinical case. Minerva Med 83: S1-S5

89. Van Damme H, Ballaux JM, Dereume JP (1988) Femoropopliteal venous graft entrapment. J Cardiovasc Surg (Torino) 29: 50-5

90. Zund G, Roggo A, Etter C, Brunner U (1994) Differential surgical therapy of popliteal entrapment syndrome 1967 to 1992. Helv Chir Acta 60: 879-81

91. Neuman M, Rosen MP, Skillman J (1998) Femoral-popliteal bypass graft entrapment: angiographic demonstration. J Vasc Interv Radiol 9: 606-8

92. Steurer J, Hoffmann U, Schneider E, Largiader J, Bollinger A (1995) A new therapeutic approach to popliteal artery entrapment syndrome (PAES). Eur J Vasc Endovasc Surg 10: 243-7

93. Haimovici H, Sprayregen S, Johnson F (1972) Popliteal artery entrapment by fibrous band. Surgery 72: 789-92

94. Rich NM, Hughes CW (1967): Popliteal artery and vein entrapment. Am J Surg 113: 696-8

95. Walder J, Mosimann F, Van Melle G, Mosimann R (1984) A propos de l'endofibrose iliaque chez deux coureurs cyclistes. Chir Acta 51: 793-5

96. Mosimann R, Walder J, Van Melle G (1985) Stenotic intimal thickening of the external iliac artery: illness of competition cyclists? Vasc Surg 19: 258-63

97. Rousselet M-C, Saint-André J-P, L'Hoste P, Enon B, Megret A, Chevalier J-M (1990) Stenotic intimal thickening of the external iliac artery in competition cyclists. Hum Pathology 21: 524-9

98. Abraham P, Saumet JL, Chevalier JM (1997) External iliac artery endofibrosis in athletes. Sports Med 24: 221-6.

99. Khaira HS, Awad RW, Aluwihare N, Shearman CP (1996) External iliac artery stenosis in a young body builder. Eur J Vasc Endovasc Surg 11: 499-501

100. Chevalier JM, Enon B, Walder J, Barral X, Pillet J, Megret A, Lhoste P, Saint-André JP, Davinroy M (1986) Endofibrosis of the external iliac artery in bicycle racers: an unrecognized pathological state (L'endofibrose iliaque externe du cycliste de compétition: une pathologie artérielle méconnue). Ann Chir Vasc 1: 297-303

101. Del Gallo G, Plissonnier D, Planet M, Peillon C, Testart J, Watelet J (1996) Dissecting aneurysm of the external iliac artery. An unusual course of endofibrosis in an athlete. J Mal Vasc 21: 95-7

102. Aburahma AF, Powell MA, Boland JP (1995) A case study of abdominal angina secondary to coeliac compression syndrome. W V Med J 91: 10-2

103. Cockett FB, Thomas ML (1965) The iliac compression syndrome. Br J Surg 52: 816-21

104. Pinsolle J, Videau J (1982) Anomalies du carrefour iliocave: interprétation du syndrome de Cockett d'après 180 dissections. Chirurgie 108:451-8

105. Guegan H, Carles J, Junes F, Plagnol P, Videau J (1992) Cockett's syndrome caused by an ectopic kidney. Apropos of two cases J Chir (Paris) 129: 257-62

106. Morlier D, Jurascheck F, Watteau JP, al Salti R, Belhamou S, Fernandez R, Touraine P, Zeyer B (1990) Cockett's syndrome and retro-iliac ureter. A previously unknown and

original association apropos of a case and review of the literature. J Urol (Paris) 96: 223-6

107. Laroche M, Etchebar F, Carrie JM, Arlet J, Jacquemier JM, Cantarel A, Mazières B (1990) Hip algodystrophy and Cockett's syndrome. Rev Rhum Mal Osteoartic 57: 571-3

108. Verhaeghe R (1995) Iliac vein compression as an anatomical cause of thrombophilia: Cockett's syndrome revisited. Thromb Haemost 74: 1398-401

109. Le Minh T, Bertrand A, De Tœuf J (1992) Pelvic venous compression syndrome: description of a case and literature review. Rev Med Brux 13: 243-7

110. Michel C, Laffy PY, Leblanc G, Bonnet D (1994) Treatment of Cockett syndrome by percutaneous insertion of a vascular endoprosthesis (Gianturco). J Radiol 75: 327-30

111. Buelens C, Vandenbosch G, Stockx L, Raat H, Lacroix R, Verhaeghe R, Wilms G, Baert AL (1996) Cockett syndrome. Initial results with percutaneous treatment in 6 patients. J Belge Radiol 79: 132-5

112. Wurtz A, Quandalle P, Lemaitre L, Robert Y (1990) A superior vena cava syndrome of unusual etiology: compression syndrome of the innominate veins. Ann Chir 44: 642-4

113. Servelle M, Babilliot J (1968) Syndrome du soléaire. Phlébologie 21: 399-405

114. Stassen CM, Weil EH, Janevski BK (1989) Left renal vein compression syndrome ("nutcracker phenomenon"). ROFO Fortschr Geb Rontgenstr Nuklearmed 150: 708-10

115. Lee CC, Lin JT, Deng HH, Lin ST (1993) Haematuria due to nutcracker phenomenon of left renal vein: report of a case. J Formos Med Assoc 92: 291-3

116. Cakir B, Arinsoy T, Sindel S, Bali M, Akcali Z, Uluoglu O (1995) A case of renal vein thrombosis with posterior nut cracker syndrome. Nephron 69: 476-7

VII
Effects of physical and chemical agents on vessels

1 – Physical agents

X-Ray induced or post-radiation vasculopathy

When vessels are exposed to ionising radiation experimentally there is immediate damage to the endothelium, with increased permeability and necrosis followed by healing with intimal proliferation and vascular stenoses. Smooth muscle cells undergo more subtle damage resulting in loss of cellularity of the media and replacement by fibrosis. Radiation also induces a chronic antiangiogenic effect and contributes to growth abnormality, for example, in limb development [1, 2]. In man, long-term complications of radiation injury are still commonly seen despite advances in radiotherapy. Acute effects are largely time dependent and can be controlled by alteration of therapy schedule. For chronic changes, the age at the time of exposure to radiation does not seem to affect the time of the onset of lesions. No direct correlation has been established between the severity of the injury and the dose of radiation and the true incidence of radiation-induced vascular changes is almost certainly underestimated. The duration of time between exposure and development of post-radiation changes varies from months to 24 years, with a mean of 14 years [3-7], and further complications (tissue necrosis, infection, and ulceration) may occur later. The clinical patterns depend on the role of the organ system involved, and ischaemic syndomes, erectile dysfunction [8], aortic arch syndrome or pulseless disease [9], aneurysms, veno-occlusive liver disease [10] and vascular rupture [11] have all been reported. In children, moyamoya syndrome has been reported following radiation therapy for tumours at the base of the brain [12].

Pathology and differential diagnosis

The extent and severity of radiation vasculopathy is generally dependant on the dose and the exposure time although this is not always demonstrable in human tissues. Like other radiation-induced lesions, the morphology in the vessels is not specific, but is often characteristic enough to be recognizable. All blood vessels may be affected [13]; however, radiation most often injures capillaries, sinusoids, and small arteries. The response to radiation is progressive. The initial expression is an increased permeability leading to oedema. Endothelial cell show degenerative changes; some of them may detach in the lumen (Fig. 1). Later,

there is an irregular proliferation of endothelial cells leading to capillaries of irregular diameter and shape and sometimes giving rise to a bizarre granulation-tissue reaction [14]; pleomorphic stromal and endothelial cells should not be misinterpreted as malignant. Small calibre arterioles show fibrinoid infiltration in the wall (Fig. 2). Fibrous proliferation strengthens the blood/tissue barrier and ultimately results in a loss of parenchymal cells. Large arteries suffer least; however, when significant damage does occur, it tends to be clinically significant and even fatal [15, 16]. With conventional therapeutic irradiation, large lymphatic vessels show little alteration [17]. However, lymphoedema may develop in scarred

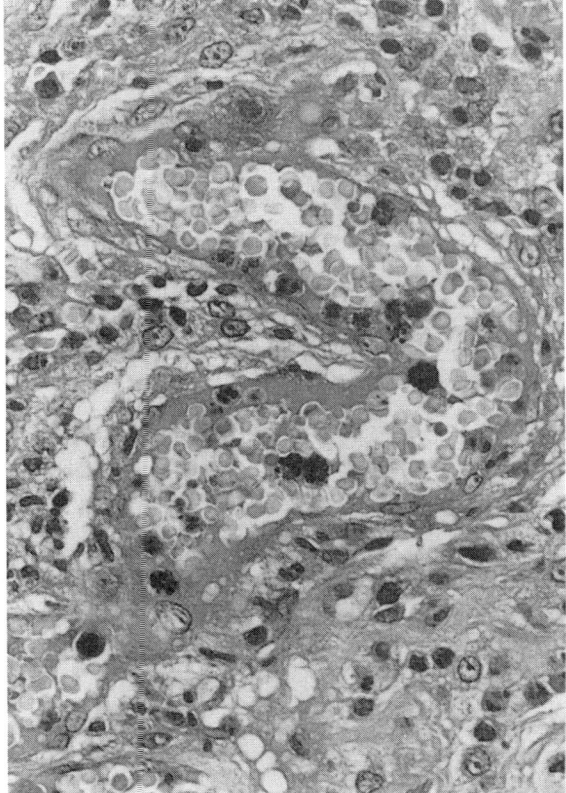

Fig. 1. Vascular effects of X-rays. Initial effects on blood capillaries. Note degenerative changes and detachment of endothelial cells. Haematoxylin, eosin and saffron stain (HES)

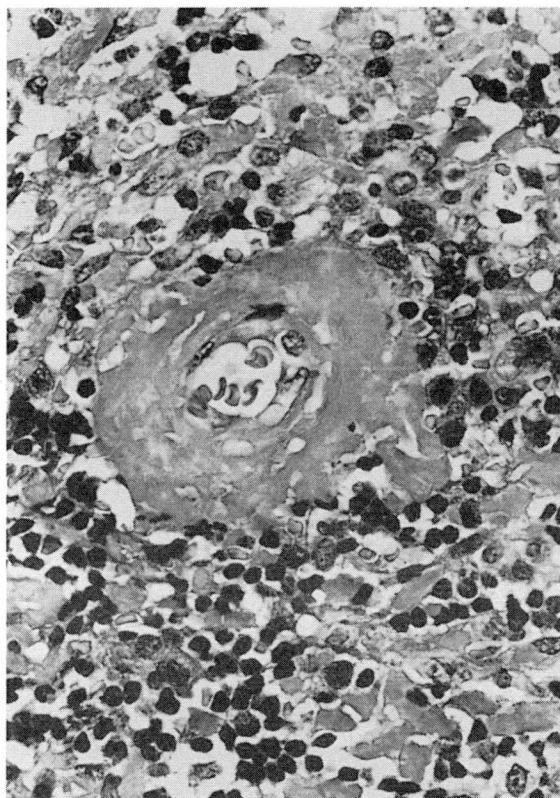

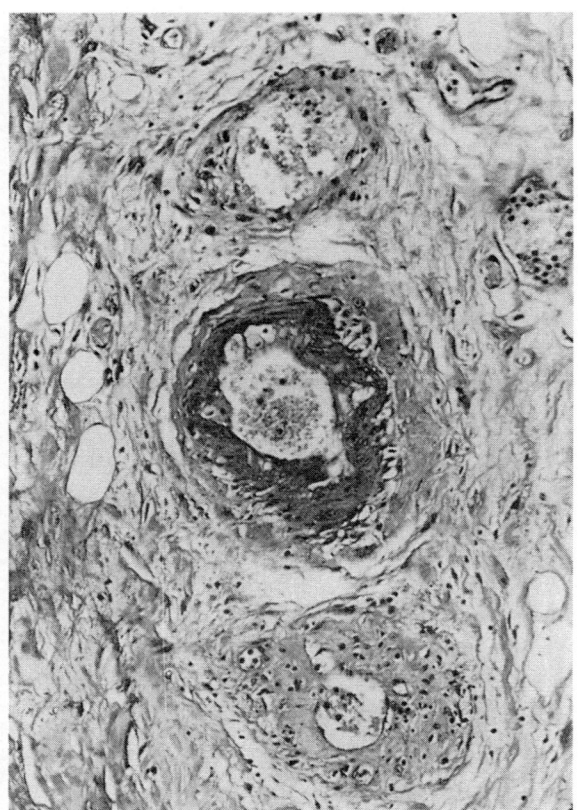

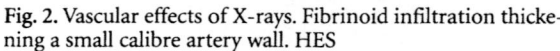

Fig. 2. Vascular effects of X-rays. Fibrinoid infiltration thickening a small calibre artery wall. HES

Fig. 3. Vascular effects of X-rays. Intimal foam cell infiltration. HES

areas, as small lymphatics do not regenerate with the same intensity in fibrotic tissue [18].

Histologically, all three vessel layers are involved [19]. Initially, endothelial cells undergo degenerative changes (cytoplasmic vacuolization, nuclear pyknosis), exfoliate into the lumen, and induce an early inflammatory response. Immunofluorescence staining helps to demonstrate expression of E-selectin on the surface of irradiated endothelial cells [20, 21]. Fibrinoid infiltration distorts the junction between the intima and media and these changes are often associated with oedema and haemorrhages in the perivascular tissue [10, 16]. In large arteries, these changes may also involve the vasa vasora. In the next stage, fibrosis thickens the intima. Foam cells infiltrate this layer (Fig. 3) and, to a lesser degree, the adjacent media (Fig. 4). A fibro-lipid plaque is formed, narrowing the artery (Fig. 5). Later (5 to 10 years) fibrosis is seen mainly in the media (Fig. 6). Atheromatous plaques are found after 10 to 25 years [7, 22-25]. The

arterial lesions in the chronic stage resemble to those of atherosclerosis (Fig. 7). Segmental changes with periarterial fibrosis corresponding to the irradiated area may be found [16, 24]. Damaged vessels may show thrombosis, stenosis, calcification (Fig. 8) or rupture of the arterial wall with aneurysm formation [26-29].

The diagnosis of radiation-induced changes in a vessel, especially in an artery, may be made safely when three conditions are satisfied; the patient is a non-smoker, free of a history of atheroma, hypercholesterolaemia and diabetes mellitus, whose arteries reveal atheromatous plaques and fibrosis involving both vessels and perivascular tissues, and where the vessels adjacent to the irradiated area are within normal limits. Post-radiation changes (cutaneous or visceral) occur in the areas showing the vascular changes [30, 31]. The differential diagnosis includes atherosclerosis and vascular necrosis caused by infiltration of tumour [11, 32-35].

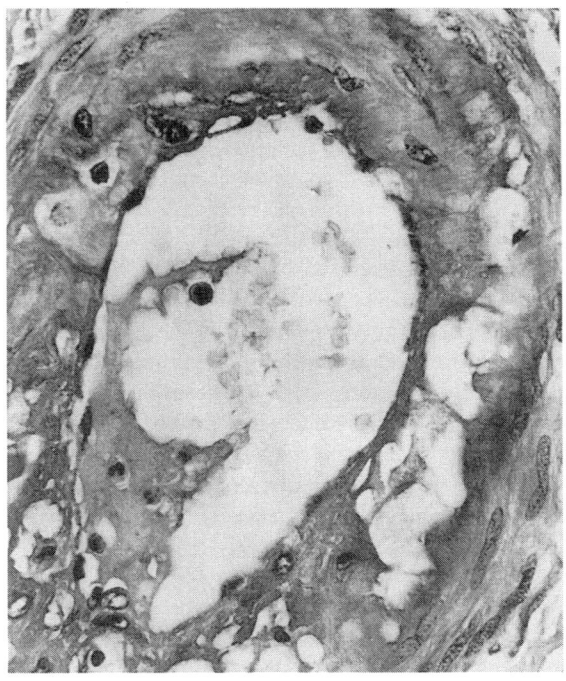

Fig. 4. Vascular effects of X-rays. Intimal and medial infiltration of foam cells. HES

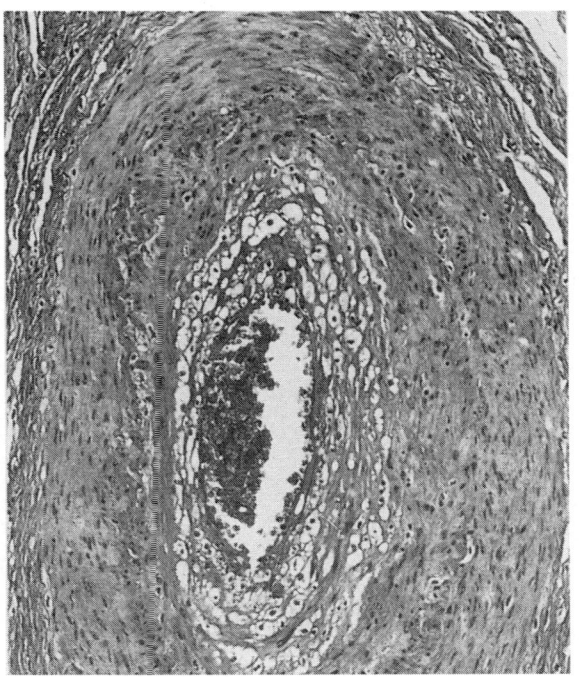

Fig. 5. Vascular effects of X-rays. Radiation-induced fibrolipid plaque (type IV lesion). HES

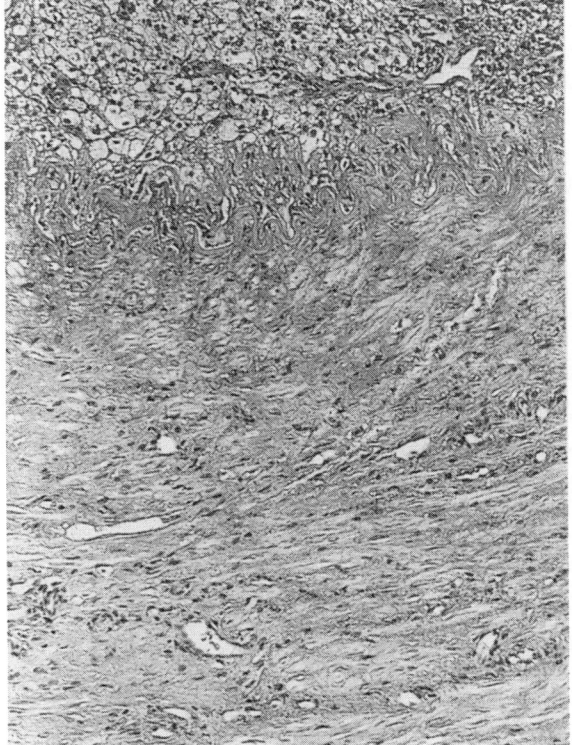

Fig. 6. Vascular effects of X-rays. Radiation-induced fibro-lipid plaque with marked fibrosis of the underlying media (atherosclerotic type V lesion). HES

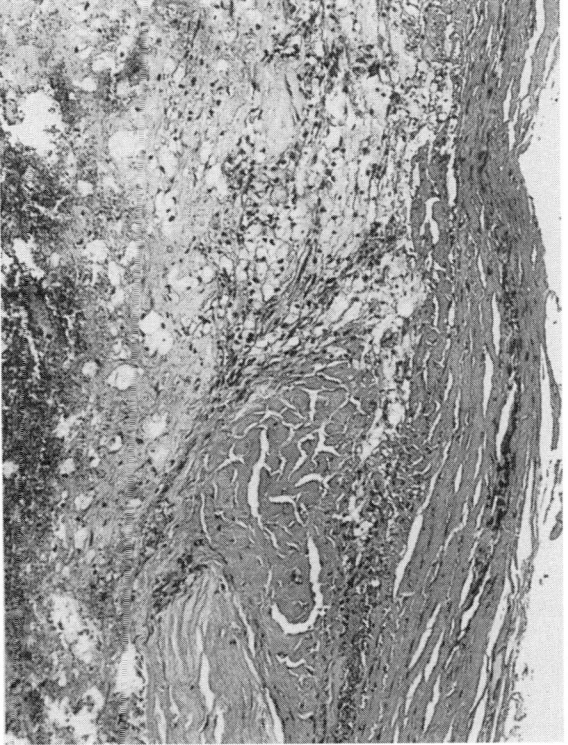

Fig. 7. Vascular effects of X-rays. Radiation-induced atherosclerotic plaque showing disruption and thrombosis. HES

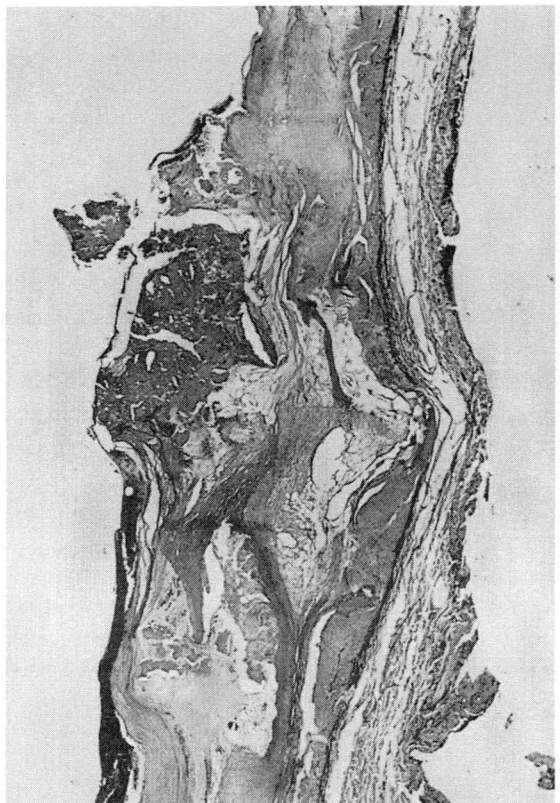

Fig. 8. Vascular effects of X-rays. Radiation-induced atherosclerotic calcified plaque. HES

Vascular changes caused by lasers

Energy carried by lasers, absorbed by living tissues, is transformed into heat. The target tissue undergoes coagulative necrosis resulting in evaporation and leaving a crater lined with coagulated and carbonised debris [36].

Experimental studies of various types have been carried out with different types of lasers; solid (ruby, YAG-neodyne) and gaseous (argon, carbon dioxide). They have been used in in vivo destruction of atheromatous plaques in animals, in in vitro destruction of atheromatous plaques taken from cadavers and exposed to the air, in destruction of in situ blood-immersed atheromatous plaques of occluded arteries in amputation specimens [37-39], in disintegration of occluding blood clots (clot-bursting) and in treatment of small superficial varicosities [40]. During la-

ser angioplasty, the beam vaporises the plaque or heats the tip of the catheter so that the plaque is burned or melted away. When the beam is shot into fluid, higher energies are needed because of partial absorption of energy by water and energy loss by cooling. The planar extent and volume of area destroyed depends on the direction of the beam. When the beam is co-axial, the destructive effect is localised. Depending on the quantity of energy released the intima and the innermost myocytes of the media may undergo coagulative necrosis (Fig. 9), leading to a genuine intimectomy with some loss of the internal elastic membrane [38]. When the beam is perpendicular to the arterial wall, complete rupture of the three arterial layers may occur. The damaged area is bordered by coagulative necrosis with carbonised tissue debris on the surface. These experimental data confirm that it is possible to destroy occlusive lesions, but with a non negligible risk of perforation (Fig. 10) [41-46]. Other experimental studies on the photochemical effects of lasers are also being conducted directed towards destruction of tumour vasculature [47, 48] labelling and disintegration of atherosclerotic plaques by means of fluorochrome pulsed-dye [49-54], sutureless vascular closure and anastomoses [55]. Some systems have been used in clinical trials to unblock arteries (AIS Excimer laser angioplasty system, Excimer laser-wire).

Complication rates (major and minor complications, 6% and perforation, 1%) with the Excimer laser are comparable to those expected with balloon angioplasty [56-63]. For other types of laser, laser angioplasty alone or combined with percutaneous balloon seems be a promising option to recanalize peripheral arteries. Bypass surgery is called for if severe ischemia persists (75% overall technical success, rare major complications) [64, 65].

Other radiations

Intravascular irradiation by both χ and β sources has been shown to prevent neointimal proliferation after balloon injury in the overstretched pig coronary model. Radiation may reduce smooth muscle cell proliferation at the adventitia and thus has a favorable effect on vessel remodelling. The use of vascular radiation in the presence of metallic stents is under investigation [66, 67], and shows promise.

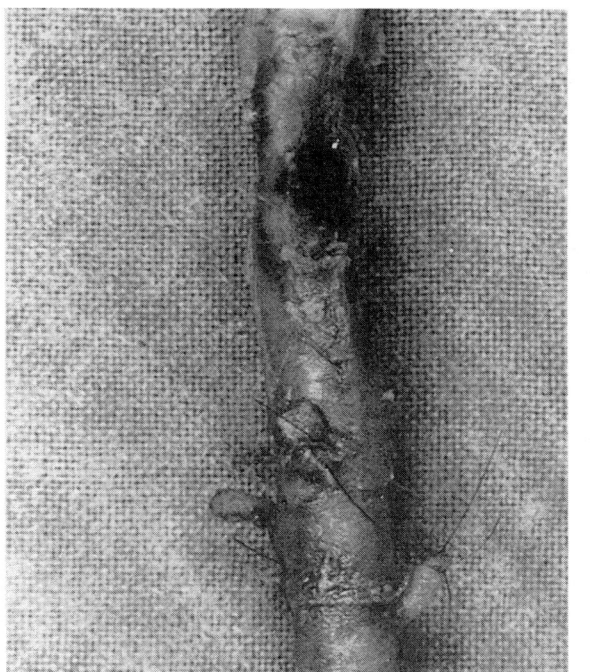
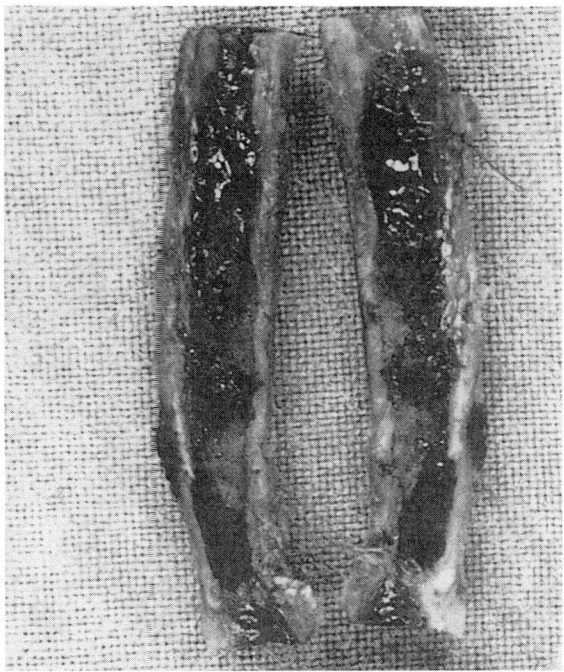

Fig. 9-10. Experimental Yag laser angioplasty. Transparietal coagulative necrosis with perforation and thrombosis of a cadaver's femoral artery

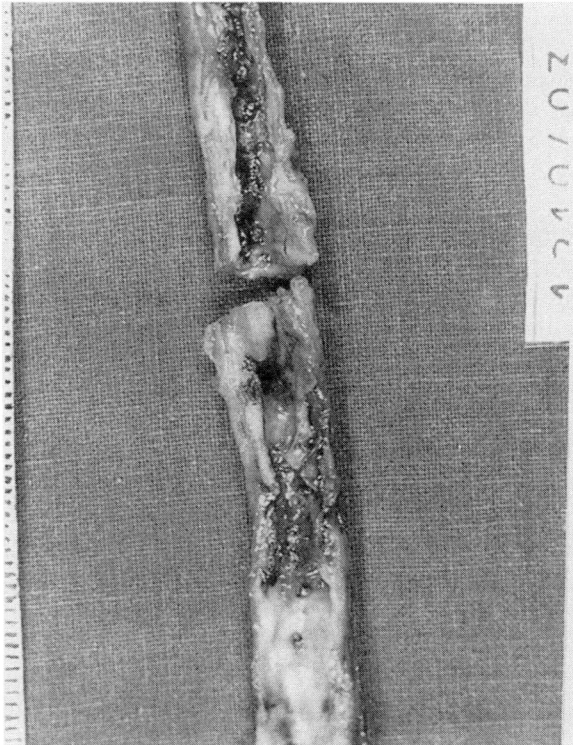
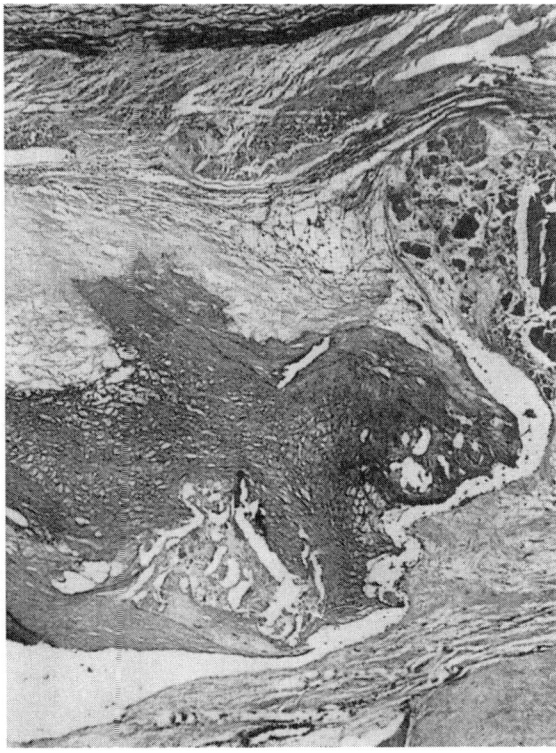

Fig. 11. Ultrasound angioplasty. Calcified atherosclerotic plaque (Courtesy Dr J. Marzelle)

Fig. 12. Ultrasound angioplasty. Calcified atherosclerotic plaque showing multiple cracks. HES

Ultrasound injuries

Ultrasonic energy, in continuous and pulsed modes, has been used to destroy atherosclerotic plaques in man. The feasibility of percutaneous intra-arterial ultrasonic recanalization was demonstrated in a preliminary in vivo study in dogs [46]. With a prototype ultrasonic wire probe, fibrous and calcified plaques are disrupted while normal portions of vessels appear unaffected. In our personal experience, calcified carotid plaques submitted to external ultrasonic angioplasty immediately before endaterectomy are shaken loose by multiple cracks (Fig. 11-12).

Hyperthermic injuries

Burns

Two types are distinguished according to the depth: partial-thickness and full-thickness burns. Pathophysiologic events following local thermal trauma are complex and involve a variety of mediator pathways [68].

Partial-thickness burns

The dermis with its skin appendages is spared. The epidermis is devitalised. Epidermal cells reveal evidence of deranged membrane permeability, with nuclear and cellular swelling or nuclear pyknosis and granular coagulation of the cytoplasm. Endothelial injury leads to vascular dilatation, proteinaceous fluid exudation, and a mild inflammatory reaction resulting in blisters. The regeneration of the epidermis results from preserved islands or dermal appendages.

Full-thickness burn

Here there is total destruction of the epidermis, extending into the dermis and sometimes even deeper. The epidermis is incinerated. The dermal collagen becomes a homogeneous gel, and the cytologic changes described for the partial-thickness burn may occur in the deeper fibroblasts, and deeper subcutaneous structures, including vessels. In vessels, the endothelium has large intercellular gaps 24 hours after the burn, with erythrocyte sludging, platelet and leukocyte-endothelial adherence, fibrin deposit, and release of circulating Factor VIII antigen [69-72]. These changes lead to endothelial detachment, disseminated intravascular coagulation, progressive ischaemia and necrosis in the tissue beneath and surrounding the burn [73, 74]. The systemic consequences of a burn are often more devastating than the local injury: neurogenic shock and hypovolemic shock resulting from copious loss of exudate from the burn surface and sepsis. Wound infections, mostly caused by *Pseudomonas aeruginosa*, *Staphylococcus aureus*, and *Candida* species, cause cellulitis, thrombophlebitis, infective endocarditis and pneumonia. All of these complications belong to the postburn multiple organ failure (PBMOF) syndrome [75-78]. Humoral and cellular immunity is also concerned with depressed lymphocyte and phagocyte function [79-81]. Associated pulmonary injuries from inhalation of hot gases and fumes may worsen the prognosis.

Systemic hyperthermia or Heat stroke

Abnormal elevation of the core body temperature above 40°C occurs in two clinical patterns: exertional heat stroke and classic heat stroke. Exertional heat stroke is seen mostly in marathon runners, football players, labourers, military recruits, and workers in foundries and boiler rooms. It is typically associated with hot, dry skin and cessation of sweating and a lactic acidosis. About one-third of the patients present with rhabdomyolysis, myoglobinaemia, myoglobinuria, and acute tubular necrosis. Classic heat stroke mostly occurs in the very young and the elderly, the chronically ill, alcoholics, and the morbidly obese. Classic heat stroke is sometimes precipitated by drugs that depress sweating (anticholinergics and phenothiazines). Disseminated intravascular coagulation (DIC) may occur in both types of heat injury.

Erythromelalgia

This rare syndrome is characterised by a burning distress in the skin of the extremities when exposed to a precise increase in temperature. It may be idiopathic or represent vascular symptom in various conditions including myeloproliferative disorders, and polycythemia vera, Fabry's disease, arterial hypertension, venous insufficiency, diabetes mellitus, systemic lupus erythematosus and rheumatoid arthritis, and influenza vaccination [82-90]. This condition affects men more often than women, begins mostly in adult life and may occur in an hereditary form [91, 92]. Clinically, burning distress involves the hands and feet while the patient is walking or in bed at night. This feeling, aggravated by warmth or fever, lasts from a few minutes to several hours and may be triggered by emotional disturbance. Relief can be obtained when the extremities are exposed to cool air or immersed into cold or icy water or by direct pressure on the skin. The burning areas are reddish or cyanotic, hot to the touch, and may be swollen.

Trophic changes, ulceration and gangrene can occur. The temperature at which symptoms appear varies with different individuals and different parts of the extremity within the range of 32 to 36°C. Clinical symptoms regress with temperatures lower or higher than the critical point. Burning distress is caused by local heating and not by increased blood flow. There is no satisfactory treatment. The treatment of underlying disease relieves secondary erythromelalgia. Symptomatic relief of primary erytheromelalgia may be obtained by avoidance of all causes giving rise to vasodilatation. Acetylsalicylic acid, phenoxybenzamine hydrochloride, serotonin-blocking agent and nitroprusside may produce some relief [93, 94].

Pathology and differential diagnosis

Examination of peripheral vessels reveals no evidence of occlusive arterial disease; however, this may be found in secondary enythromelalgia associated with polycythaemia vera. Sensations of burning in the extremities noted by patients with arteriosclerosis and peripheral neuritis is not indicative of this disease.

Hypothermic injuries

Hypothermic or cold injuries include chilblains, trench foot or immersion foot syndrome, and frostbite.

Chilblain (Erythema pernio, Perniosis)

This condition is characterised by erythema, itching, and burning, especially of the dorsum of the fingers and toes, and of the heels, nose, and ears. It occurs on exposure to progressive extreme cold (slow freeze) usually associated with high humidity. Lesions can be single or multiple, and may become blistered and ulcerated.

Erythema pernio may be part of a hypersensitive reaction to cold. It is probable that repeated vasospasm gives rise to vascular changes with tissue anoxia and secondary inflammatory reaction of varying extent and degree. The syndrome may have an underlying organic cause, including leukocytoclastic vasculitis, rheumatoid arthritis, Crohn's disease, systemic lupus erythematosus (SLE-Rowell's syndrome), primary antiphospholipid antibody syndrome, hypergammaglobulinaemia, chronic myelomonocytic leukaemia, and vibration-induced white finger. Cryoglobulinaemia and cold agglutinins may give rise to this symptomatology [95-101]. When exposure to

cold is repeated, chronic lesions may develop with erythema, ulceration, or haemorrhage, with residual fibrosis and atrophy of the skin. Bilateral and commonly symmetrical digital cyanosis is likely to occur [102-105]

Pathology and differential diagnosis.

Histological changes are not specific, as they occur in other conditions such as livedo reticularis, acrocyanosis, advanced Raynaud's syndrome, and frostbite. They include angiitis with intimal proliferation, thickening of the arterial wall, periarterial and perivenous infiltration of lymphocytes, monocytes and neutrophilic leukocytes. There is necrosis of the adipose tissue with a chronic inflammatory reaction; giant cells may be present. Endothelial swelling is noted in the upper and lower dermal capillary plexus of the subcutaneous fat. When the disease is chronic, hyperpigmentation with deposits of iron is seen. Biopsies from patients with SLE, cryofibrinogenaemia, primary antiphospholipid antibody syndrome, and hypergammaglobulinaemia may present a similar morphology comprising an interface dermatitis, superficial and deep angiocentric and eccrinotropic lymphocytic infiltrates, vascular ectasia, and dermal mucinosis with prominent involvement of the eccrine coil. A granulomatous vasculitis and a granuloma annulare-like tissue reaction may be noted in patients with iritis, rhumatoid arthritis (RA), and Crohn's disease.

The clinical history allows us to differentiate pernio from trench foot and immersion foot syndrome. Chronic exposure to mild cold may induce vascular disorders similar to those of Raynaud's phenomenon [106]. Other conditions to be ruled out are erythema induratum, nodular vasculitis, erythema nodosum and livido reticularis. Lesions of pernio syndrome do not harbour acid-fast bacilli, as may those of erythema induratum. Lesions of nodular vasculitis and erythema nodosum simulate those of pernio syndrome, but lesions of the first two diseases are more active with much more evidence of intimal thickening and obliteration in both arteries and veins than is observed in the pernio syndrome. Ulcerative lesions in livido reticularis may simulate chronic pernio but clinically lesions of livido reticularis do not occur in waves or go through the typical cycle of change from erythema to blisters to superficial ulceration.

Trench foot and immersion foot

These conditions result from repeated exposure to moderate cold (0-4°C) and wet. At first the extremities are cold, pale and cyanotic. The arterial pulses are reduced and absent. Orthostatic oedema may appear. If the exposure is of long duration, petechiae, ulceration and paraesthesia may occur over the ischaemic region. These symptoms resemble those of the early stage of chronic pernio. During the vasospastic and ischaemic phase, there is direct vasoconstriction of the superficial vessels and reflex vasoconstriction general body chilling. The functional vascular changes are caused in part by lowering of the body temperature and cooling of the circulating blood. The hyperaemic phase results from extreme vasodilatation. If the patient is removed from the cold and placed in a warmer place for a few hours, the feet become hot and red. The peripheral pulsations become full and bounding. Unless the extremities are elevated and cooled, swelling increases rapidly. Blebs occur in the affected parts with ecchymosis. Intense burning paraesthesia begins one week later. During this phase, lymphangitis, thrombophlebitis and cellulitis may complicate the clinical picture. This hyperaemic stage lasts about 2 weeks, then subsides and the circulation becomes normal [107, 108]. If exposure to cold and dampness is prolonged or when treatment is inadequate, vasospastic disorders and ischaemia may become chronic. Recovery is slow; coldness, pain stiffness and paraesthesia of the lower extremities persist, even in warm temperatures. Sensitivity to cold has been observed several years after the initial exposure.

Pathology and differential diagnosis.

Histopathological changes have mostly been recorded in chronic cases where the major changes consist of perivenous fibrosis with thrombosis; the veins become narrowed. Small arteries display mild fibrosis of the media and intimal thickening. In the surrounding tissues, haemosiderin deposits may be seen and striated muscle undergoes atrophy [109].

Frostbite

This condition is characterised by localised freezing of tissues caused by exposure to cold. Peripheral vasoconstriction occurs immediately on exposure and may persist for 24 hours or longer. Hyperaemia is caused by reactive vasodilatation. Many studies have been carried out to determine the mechanism of frostbite; direct action of cold, arterial spasm, thrombosis and anoxia all play a part [111]. Inexperienced mountain hikers in winter are frequently affected; those adequately informed of the danger and well-prepared can usually avoid injury. In mild frostbite, the affected area presents a dull yellow colour with numbness and an itching sensation. Ice crystals may be present in the tissues, within the extracellular fluid

and in the blood [112]. In severe frostbite, paraesthesia and digital stiffness become apparent; the affected extremity is frozen. When the affected area thaws, reactive hyperaemia develops with tenderness, burning pain and paraesthesia. Blisters and oedema occur and the skin may undergo superficial necrosis with gangrene. Frostbite may be superficial (involving the skin and superficial subcutaneous tissue) or deep, affecting subcutaneous tissue, muscle and even bone [113, 114]. Sequelae may include permanent colour changes, cold sensitivity, hyperhydrosis and occlusive arterial disease with Raynaud's phenomenon, hypoaesthesia and pain. Sympathectomy may be helpful.

Pathology and differential diagnosis

The histological changes of mild frostbite are similar to those of pernio. They consist of vasculitis, panniculitis and inflammatory reaction in affected tissues, but to a lesser degree. In severe frostbite, with prolonged vasoconstriction, small arteries and arterioles show intimal thickening. Thrombosis may occur by sludging or the action of cold haemagglutinins. In capillaries, endothelial damage leads to increased permeability. Underlying occlusive arterial disease may compromise the prognosis.

Effects of cold and heat of the lymphatic vessels

Changes in small lymphatics due to thermal injuries are difficult to detect clinically. They are compensated by collaterals or by regeneration. In the skin, gaping of the endothelial intercellular junctions in lymph vessels was noted after experimental injury by Casley-Smith [115].

Vibration-induced vascular diseases

Repeated and long-term occupational injury by vibration may cause excessive muscular contractions, decrease hand sensitivity and produce vasomotor disturbances leading to chronic occlusive arterial disease of the hands and fingers [116-120]. Usually, patients are manual workers (mean age 46.9 years, range 22-66) using pneumatic hammers to break up pavements, drill rocks, chip stone, or to ram sand, or are operatives of high-frequency percussive or vibrating tools (chain-saw operators, riveters, large polishing machines). Pianists, guitar player, typists and dentists may also be affected [121-123]. The pathogenesis is disputed. All studies suggest an abnormal spasm of small digital arteries. Vibrations may induce contraction of smooth muscle cells of the media of small arteries and arterioles, resulting in medial hyperplasia. Later on, these changes lead to thrombosis and inflammation with terminal trophic lesions. This process may be exacerbated by other variables, including poor physical condition, awkward working positions, concentration of excessive force on the fingers, temperature extremes, repetitive motions (typing, sewing) and underlying disease (diabetes mellitus) [124, 125].

This disorder is relatively rare. The mean duration of time between the start of regular use of the tool and onset of the clinical manifestations is 7.85 ± 5.16 years [126, 127]. Symptoms always occur in the working hand where, typically, there is unilateral Raynaud's phenomenon with discoloration of one or more fingers, anaesthesia, discomfort, and a decrease in warmth. Trophic changes, including painful ulcers, retracted scarring of the fingertip, and acro-osteolysis are rare [108, 122]. Examination reveals occlusion of the digital arteries or the ulnar portion of the palmar arch. The ulnar pulse may be lacking or decreased in amplitude. Capillaroscopy demonstrates a clear capillary dropout in 70% of patients and in 30% there is tortuosity of the capillary loops and elongation of their length [128]. Angiography reveals the presence of amputation-like appearances of the different digital, ulnar and radial arteries.

Pathology and differential diagnosis

Digital arteries are affected by changes resembling those seen in Raynaud's syndromes (see chapter XIII). The smooth muscle cells of the media hypertrophy (Fig. 13), leading to thickening of the media. Haemorrhages may be seen (Fig.14). Progressively, the smooth muscle cells present degenerative changes (cytoplasmic vacuolation, nuclear pyknosis) (Fig. 15). Fibrosis of the intima reduces the arterial lumen to a pinpoint (Fig. 16) and luminal thrombosis (Fig. 17) accelerates ischaemic changes, resulting in trophic disturbances. The differential diagnosis consists in ruling out occupational Raynaud's phenomenon, thromboangiitis obliterans, and scleroderma. Occupational Raynaud's phenomenon is not associated with organic arterial lesions. Thromboangiitis obliterans only exceptionally affects an isolated hand. Skin lesions caused by scleroderma present characteristic features.

Electric Shock or Lightning Injury

Sudden passage of a current of electricity through any portion of the body will damage the vascular system; blood-filled vessels are good conduits for electricity. When electrical current is routed through tissues, electrical is converted into thermal energy [129] and the heat produced causes coagulative necrosis, leading

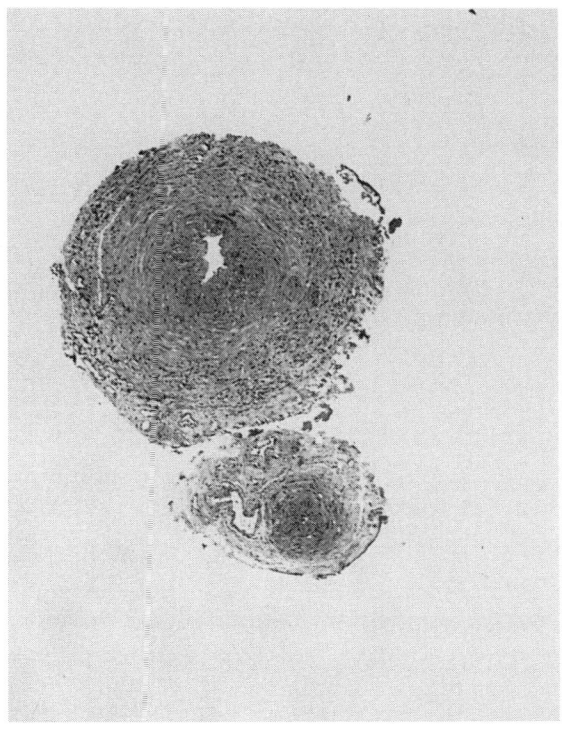

Fig. 13. Vibration disease. Marked medial hypertrophy of a digital arteriole. HES

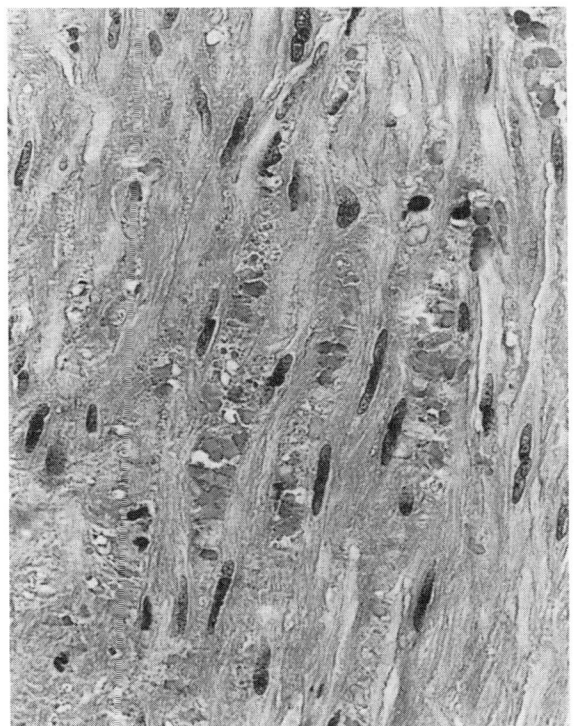

Fig. 14. Vibration disease. Intramedial haemorrhage. HES

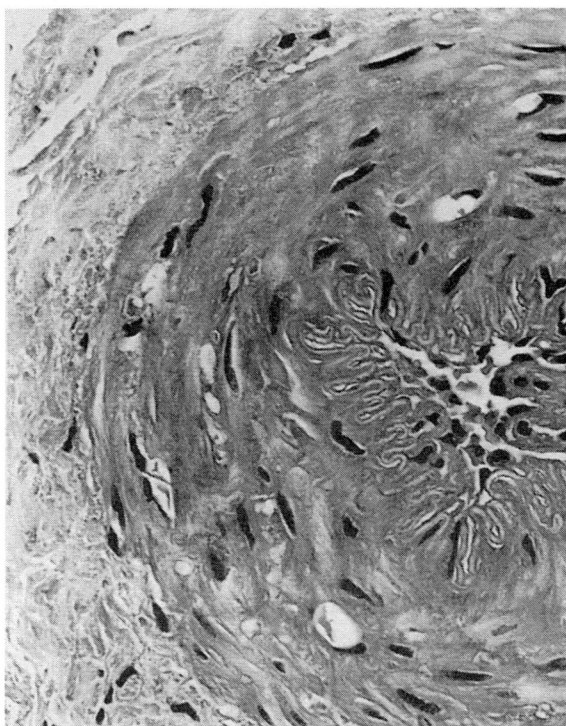

Fig. 15. Vibration disease. Degenerative changes of medial myocytes with cytoplasmic vacuolisation, nuclear pyknosis. HES

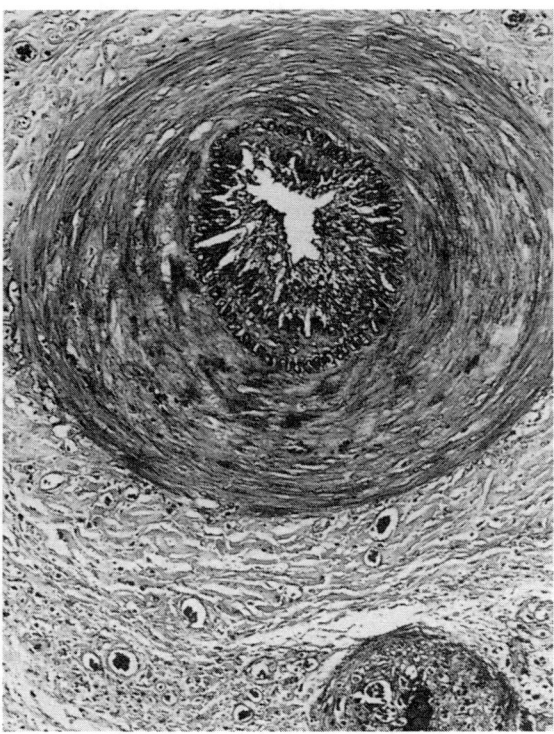

Fig. 16. Vibration disease. Associated intimal thickening reducing the vascular lumen. Orcein

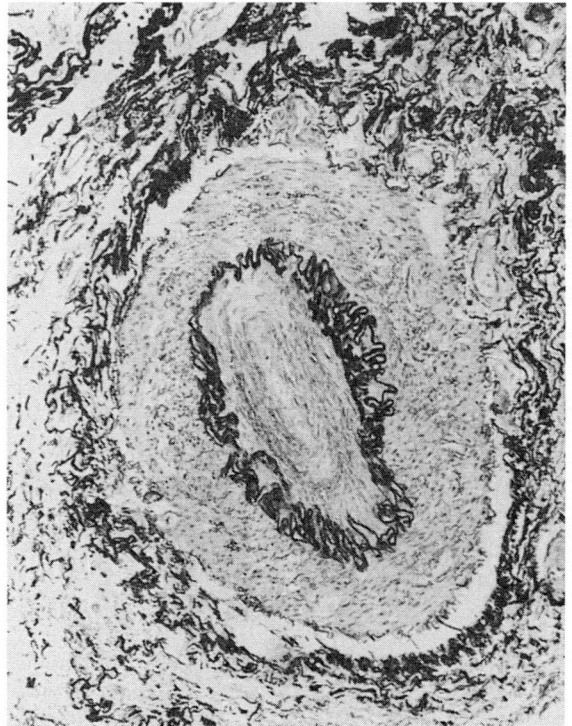

Fig. 17. Vibration disease. Occlusive organised thombus accelerating the distal ischaemic process. Orcein

to burns and tissue carbonisation (Fig. 18) [130, 131]. Although Joule's equivalent explains the heat exchange (often in thousands of degrees centigrade) with many variables to be considered, it is usually the voltage that can be determined and this is probably the most important factor. If the contact time is brief, nonthermal mechanisms of cell damage will be most important and the damage is mainly restricted to the cell membrane. When contact time is longer, however, heat damage predominates and the whole cell is directly affected [132]. Electrical injury can affect many viscera, depending on the path of the current. The volume conductor theory explains why extremity burns are much worse than torso burns and why extensive debridement is usually necessary. Experimental studies demonstrate that nerves and arteries are damaged when generated heat reaches 45°C. The subsequent progressive destruction of tissue is probably best explained by small vessel occlusion and possibly also by elevated levels of arachidonic acid in areas of greatest heat production [133]. Clinical manifestations include muscle spasms, seizures, interrupted breathing, irregular heartbeats and loss of consciousness [134]. In the majority of cases, the lesion is re-

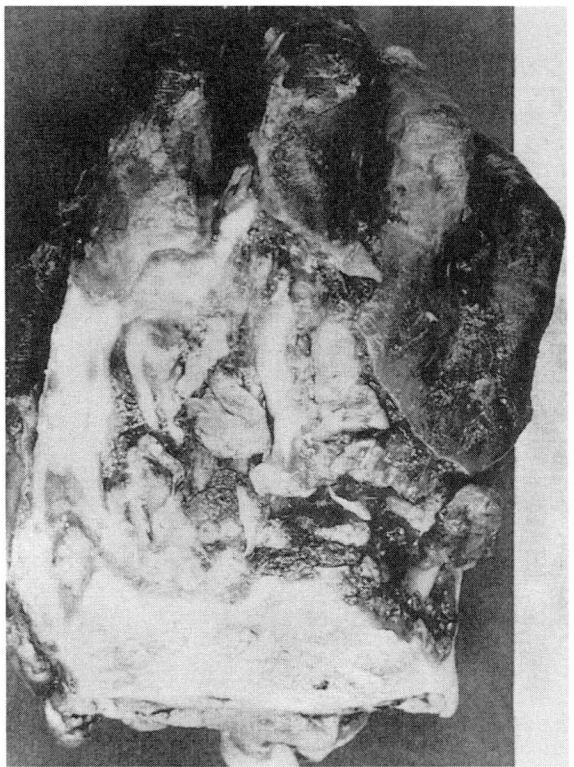

Fig. 18. Electric shock. Total carbonisation of the left hand imposing an amputation (Courtesy Dr P. Lagneau)

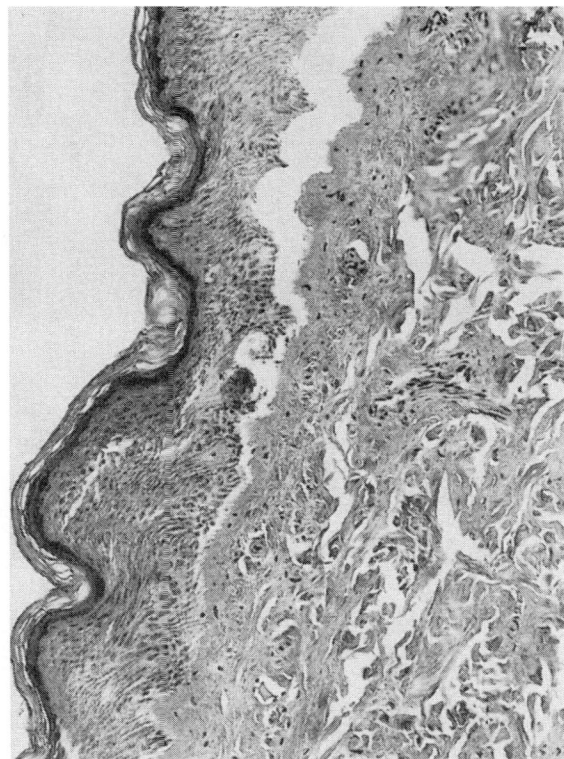

Fig. 19. Electric shock. Coagulative necrosis of dermis and epidermis. HES

presented by a third degree burn at the spots where the electricity enters and exits the body. In victims injured by lightning, the discrete external findings (arborescent skin marks) sometimes contrast markedly with the severe underlying thermal damage [135]. Fasciotomy permits evaluation of the severity of the underlying tissue and muscle necrosis [136, 137].

Pathology and differential diagnosis.

Lesions caused by low-voltage electrical burns present a rosette pattern with three zones; a central zone of carbonization, a pale ischaemic intermediate zone, and an erythematous peripheral zone. Histologically, coagulative necrosis involves the central zone (Fig. 19); vascular damage with thrombosis (Fig. 20) occurs in the intermediate and peripheral zones. In high-voltage electrical injury the great vessels, with their high blood flow, do not often show significant changes. Dissipation of heat by the blood flow prevents coagulative necrosis. Conversely, small vessels display endothelial necrosis and detachment (Fig. 21-22), thrombosis and a decreased number of smooth-muscle cells [138]. In the heart, the coronary arteries

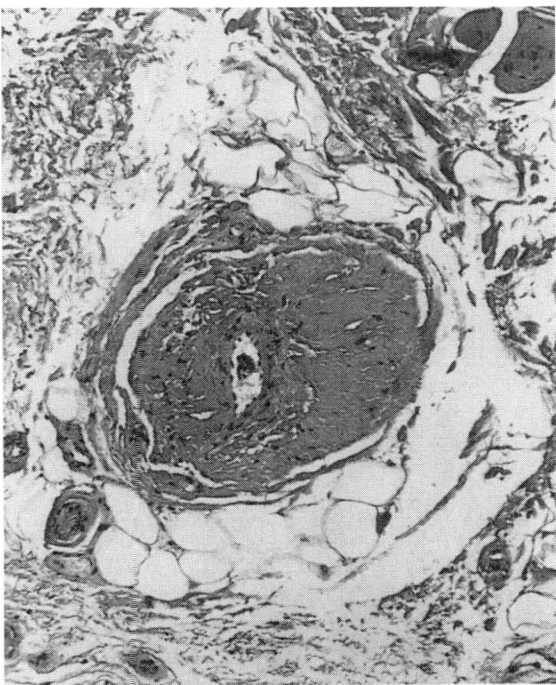

Fig. 20. Low-voltage electrical burn. Coagulative necrosis of a neighbouring vessel. HES

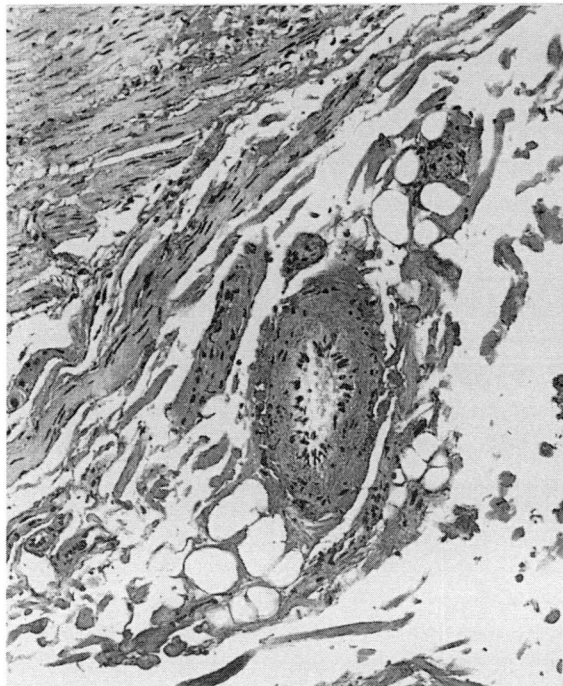

Fig. 21. High-voltage electrical injury. Endothelial necrosis in a small artery. HES

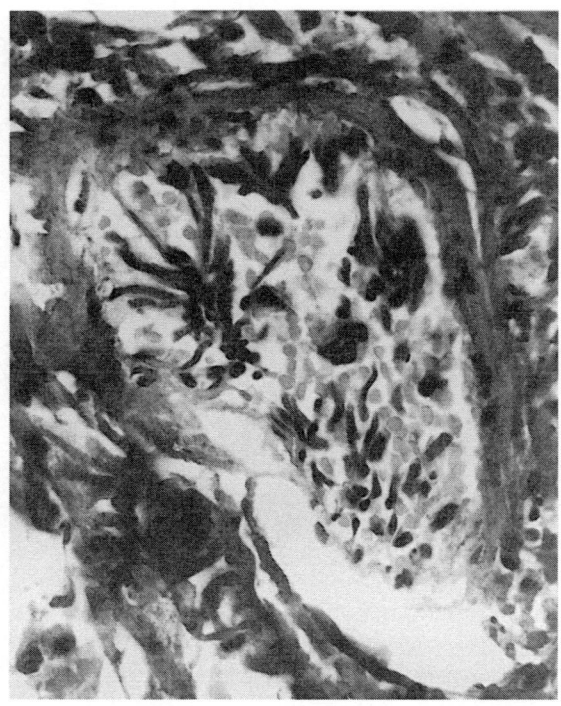

Fig. 22. High-voltage electrical injury. Coagulative necrosis of a small vessel with endothelial detachment. HES

show contraction band necrosis of smooth muscle cells in the media, leading to focal myocardial necrosis [139, 140].

High pressure impact damage and compression

This is one of the most frequently hazards affecting workers or do-it-yourselfers using high pressure guns (airless paint guns, grease guns, spray guns) (Fig. 23) [141-143], tear gas or air guns [144, 145], high pressure hydraulic cleansing tools or autoinjectors [146]. The nature of injected material varies but high temperature fluids [147], anticorrosive paint, grease and paint solvent [148, 149] inert gases such as freon [150, 151], diesel or fuel oil, plastic, and lead [152] have all been injected. Many variables are implicated in the pathogenesis of this complex injury; sudden compression of the nervous and vascular pedicles caused by space-occupying material in narrow anatomical areas, temporary or prolonged vascular spasm, direct trauma afflicting the vessels caused by the jet impact or the irritating action of injected material [149].

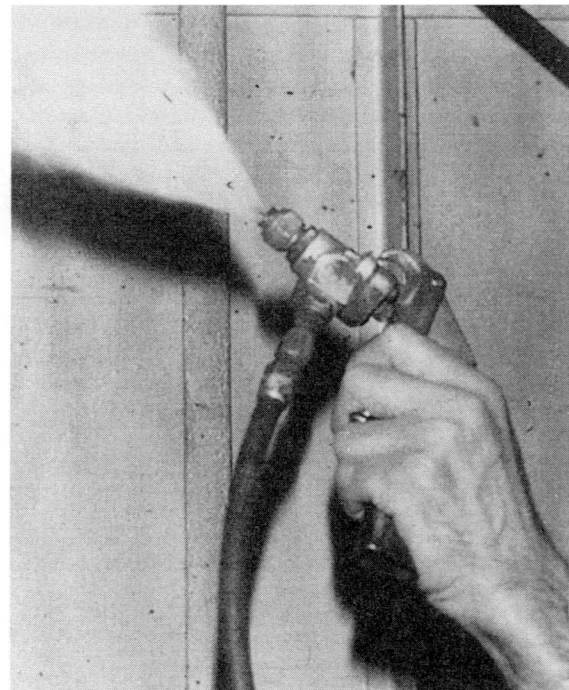

Fig. 23. Pressure paint gun

There is obstruction of the blood flow by thrombosis, superimposed infection and gangrene. Systemic manifestations (embolism, poisoning) may occur depending mostly on the nature of the foreign material. The palmar faces of the left digits, especially the distal phalanges, are commonly involved. Frequently, the jet impact appears as a pinpoint. A couple of hours later, other symptoms become manifest; exquisite pain involving the whole digit, swelling, digital stiffness, hypoesthesia, and occasional subcutaneous emphysema. Radiological examination may help identify injected material. Without treatment, the digit undergoes necrosis with gangrene (Fig. 24). Generally, the underlying lesion is more extensive [153]. Surgical debridement must avoid exposure of fragile anatomic structures once the necrotic tissue is resected; especially when immediate constructive surgery is contraindicated [154].

Pathology and differential diagnosis

Fingers and palms are mostly affected (Fig. 25). The vascular lesions include partial or complete rupture of the wall, compression, thrombosis and acute vasculitis caused by direct effect of injected material (Fig. 26). The surrounding tissues display acute inflammation with oedema and necrosis. Foreign material may be identified among collections of leukocytes and histiocytes. These cells may accumulate around empty cavities carved in the subcutaneous adipose tissue when emphysema develops. Oleomas, made up of large infiltrates of lipophages, may develop around injected oily material.

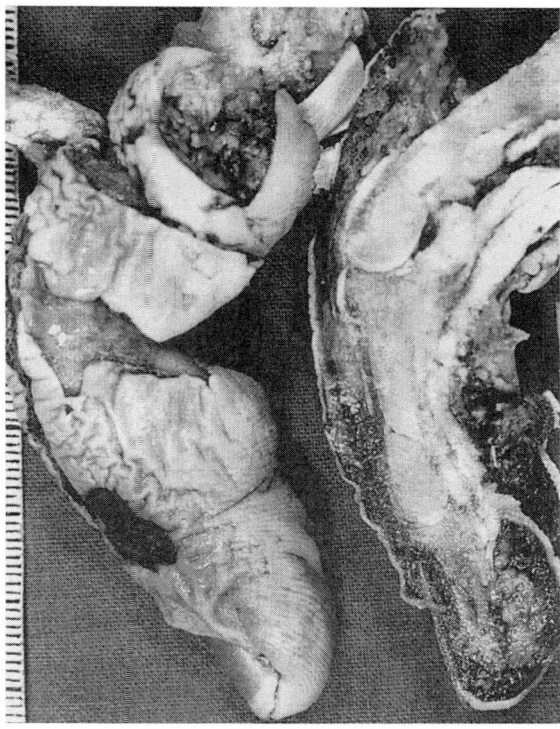

Fig. 25. Pressure paint gun. Index amputation specimen showing diffuse necrosis with oil and painting material in subcutaneous and soft tissues, far away from the point of impact located on the finger's dorsal face (Courtesy Dr E. Hautefort)

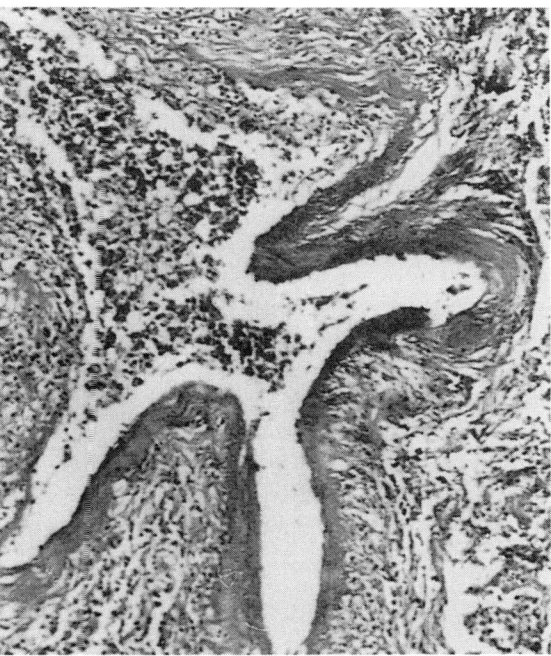

Fig. 26. Pressure paint gun. Vascular lesions include rupture, thrombosis and inflammation. HES

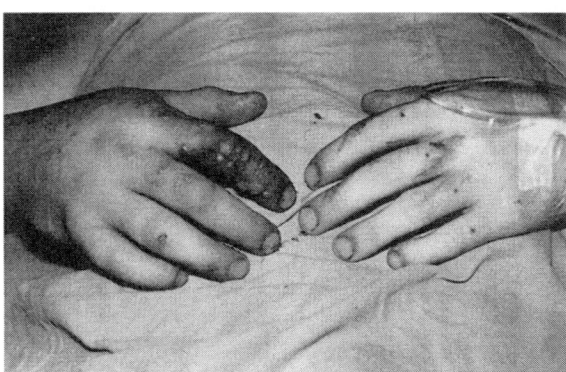

Fig. 24. Man, 30 yo, do-it-yourselfer using a pressure paint gun. Necrosis of the right index 24 hours after inadvertent paint injection (Courtesy Dr E. Hautefort)

2 – Chemical agents and drugs

Caustic agents (acids, bases) causing chemical burns [155] may directly attack vessels, leading to necrosis with inflammation and secondary vascular damage. Several drugs and chemical agents can produce vaso-motor impairments, including Raynaud's phenomenon (See chapter XIII), erythromelalgia, livedo reticularis, acrocyanosis, vasculitis and aortic dissection [156]. The role of the lymphatics in the transport of particulates is well documented, but pathological changes occur with relatively few elements or compounds. Symptoms may develop a few weeks or more after drug initiation, especially when other drugs are associated [157]. This review is limited to agents or drugs whose effect is manifest directly on the vascular wall.

Hypertonic solutions

These solutions may cause endothelial cells to shrink and cause intimal damage with increased permeability.

Ergotamine

Ergotamine and its derivatives produce adrenergic blockade (chiefly of the alpha-receptors) and persistent vasoconstriction produces stasis, and endothelial damage with oedema and thrombosis [158, 159]. Ergot poisoning gives rise to a feeling of intense heat and cold, burning pain (St Anthony's fire) [121, 160, 161], coldness and cyanosis of the extremities. In its severe form, gangrene may occur. Although this disease seems to be one associated with the Middle Ages in most peoples minds, acute poisoning with digital and visual changes has occurred in Europe in recent years, associated with small scale domestic farming and avoidance of the use of fungicides [162, 163]. Neurological symptoms consist of psychic derangement, paraesthesia, muscular spasms and convulsions. Raynaud's phenomenon and severe arteriospasm leading to gangrene have been reported in patients receiving excessive doses of ergotamine tartrate by injection or suppository for migraine headache [164, 165]. Arterial fibromuscular dysplasia and aortic dissection have also been reported in these patients [166-168].

Silicosis

Scar formation in silicosis involves the transporting lymphatic vessels. Obliterative changes develop with desquamation of the endothelium, stasis of macro-phages and precipitation of fibrin within the lymphatic vessels, followed by organisation and obliteration of the lumina. Lymphatic obstruction then increases the tissue deposition of mineral by reducing clearance. A similar pathogenic mechanism operates in non-inhalational forms of silicosis, and in a form of elephantiasis frequently found in Ethiopia – elephantiasis without filariasis. This entity develops after transcutaneous absorption of aluminium silicates through the skin of the feet, with fibrous obliteration of the lymph nodes and the lymph vessels and subsequent lymphostatic oedema. Silica and aluminium are found in the filtering lymph nodes of the affected legs [169-171].

Vinyl chloride (chloroethylene)

This substance is used as a polymerising agent in the plastics industry and is an established carcinogen in man. It also produces vascular and bony changes. Chronic exposure to fluorine-containing plastics and epoxy resins produces similar effects [172, 173]. Personal idiosyncrasy may play a role in the genesis of vinyl chloride intoxication. Susceptibility to this condition is increased in the presence of HLA-DR5 or of a gene in linkage disequilibrium with it and an antigen associated with the haplotype A1 B8, while DR3 favours progression of the disease [174]. Three percent of workmen involved with the polymerization process of vinyl chloride in the plastics industry develop Raynaud's syndrome of the fingers with scleroderma-like changes in the skin. Clubbing of the fingers caused by acro-osteolysis may occur [175].

Amantadine hydrochloride (1-Adamantanamine)

This is an antiviral agent used for influenza, also used to treat Parkinson's disease, where it increases dopamine release and reduces its reuptake into dopaminergic nerve terminals of substantia nigra neurons. Local release of catecholamines from a storage site in the peripheral nerves by amantadine may lead to vasospasm, oedema and livedo reticularis [176, 177].

Corrosive and freezing agents

Many different chemical entities are corrosive; acids (hydrofluoric, hydrochloric, methacrylic, sulfuric), alkalies, phenols and hot cooking oils are examples. Most accidental contacts are occupational (painters, drain and stone cleaners, workers preparing food, cooks) (Fig. 27). Topical effects are represented by severe full-thickness cutaneous burns. Deep tissue injury damages nerves, muscles, tendons, bones and blood vessels. Vascular lesions are non specific and there is infiltration of leukocytes, haemorrhage, thrombosis and necrosis, similar to what is seen in any necrotic lesion (Fig. 28-29) [178-182]. An associated metabolic disorder and coagulapathy may affect the prognosis [183, 184]. Accidental ingestion or self poisoning mostly involves the digestive mucosa (oesophagal and gastric) [185]. The regenerative process in the vascular system depends on the organ involved. In the gastric mucosa it starts, together with functional improvement, after 3 days. Normalization of the circulation in the injured stomach wall comes about after 14 days [186]. Gasoline immersion accidents are dominated by chemical burns and pulmonary damage. Hydrocarbon hepatitis with vascular endothelial damage is a reversible lesion with no reported long-term sequelae [187].

Freezing agents (liquid nitrogen, freon gas or monochlorodifluoromethane, propane and butane are widely used as refrigerants, propellants and industrial solvents. Direct contact causes deep frostbite with full-thickness skin necrosis [188-190].

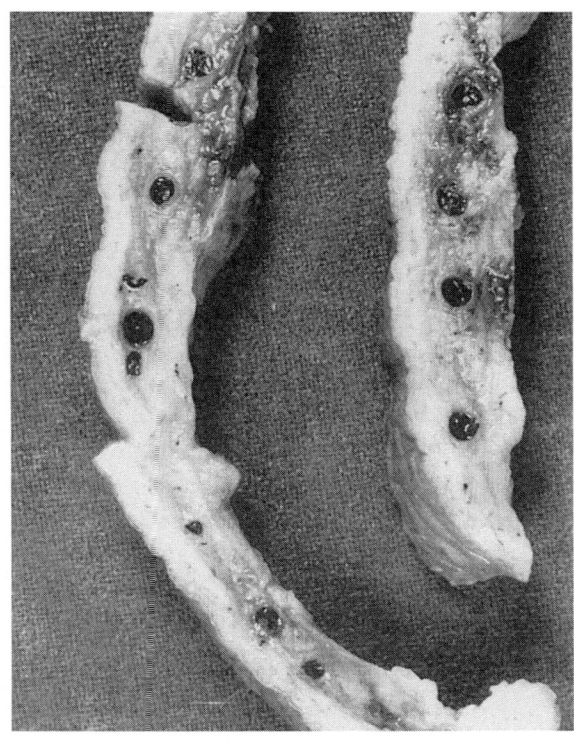

Fig. 27. Woman, 35 year-old painter using hydrofluoric acid. Inadvertent hydrofluoric acid burn causing necrosis of the palmar skin (Courtesy Dr O.Gouet)a

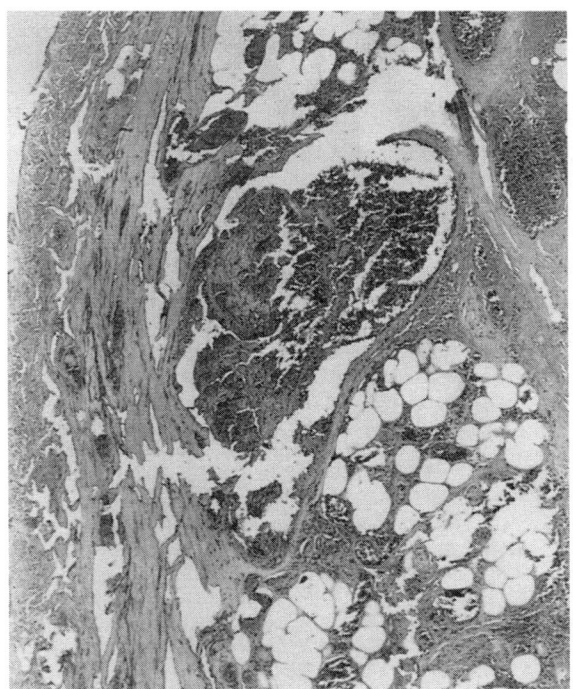

Fig. 28. Same patient. Severe chemical burn involving subcutaneous tissues, nerves and vessels. HES

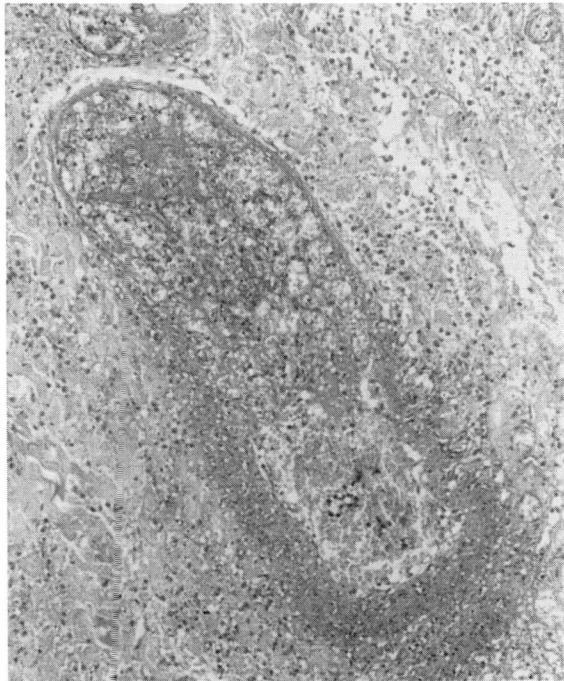

Fig. 29. Same patient. Diffuse vascular thrombosis with necrosis and acute inflammation in the damaged area. HES

Cocaine

Cardiovascular damage is common in young cocaine addicts. In the kidney, arteriolar sclerosis, medial thickening and luminal narrowing have been reported by Di Paolo 1997 [191].

Contrast media

The endothelial lining of lymphatics and lymph node sinus perfused with drugs or contrast media for lymphangiography become foamy and giant cells appear around the drops of contrast media (Fig. 30-31) [192]. These changes may be followed by fibrous obliteration of vessels and sinuses. Some cases of lymphostatic oedema become evident only after lymphangiography.

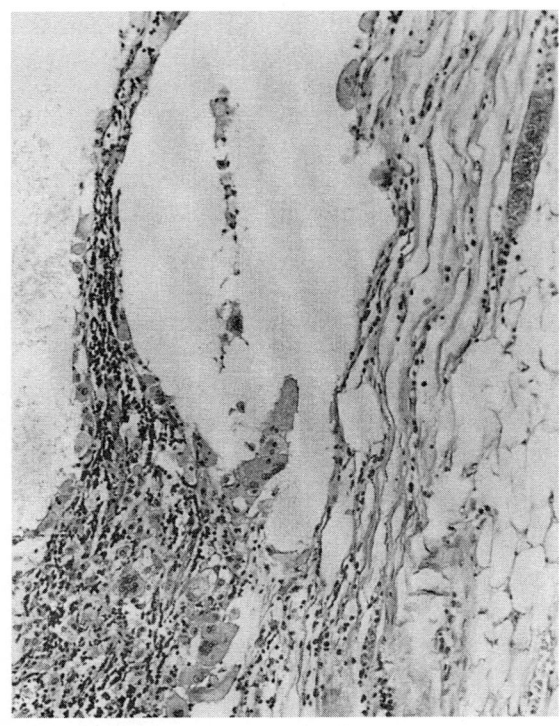

Fig. 31. Post-lymphography changes in a lymph node. Infiltration of foamy and giant cells next to the perfused contrast material accumulated in the marginal sinus. HES

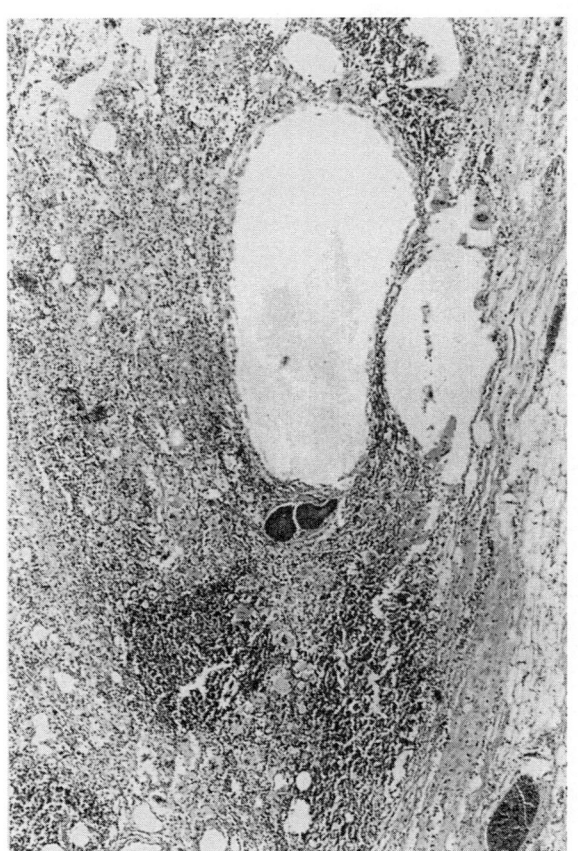

Fig. 30. Post-lymphography changes in a lymph node. Marked dilatation of the marginal sinus surrounding the lymph node cortex. HES

Bibliography

1. Prionas SD, Kowalski J, Fajardo LF, Kaplan I, Kwan HH, Allison AC (1990) Effects of X irradiation on angiogenesis. Radiat Res 124: 43-9
2. Okunieff P, Wang X, Rubin P, Finkelstein JN, Constine LS, Ding I (1998) Radiation-induced changes in bone perfusion and angiogenesis. Int J Radiat Oncol Biol Phys 42: 885-9
3. El-Naggar AM, El-Baz LM, Carsten AL, Chanana AD, Cronkite EP (1978) Radiation-induced damage to blood vessels: a study of dose-effect relationship with time after X-irradiation. Int J Radiat Biol Stud Phys Chem Med 34: 359-66
4. McCready RA, Hyde GL, Bivins BA, Mattingly SS, Griffen WO Jr (1983) Radiation-induced arterial injuries. Surgery 93: 306-12
5. Steiner H, Hackl A, Lammer J (1984) Radiation-induced vasculopathy of the carotid artery and vertebral artery. Rontgenblatter 37: 320-21
6. Murros KE, Toole JF (1989) The effect of radiation on carotid arteries. A review article. Arch Neurol 46: 449-55
7. Mathes SJ, Alexander J (1996) Radiation injury. Surg Oncol Clin N Am 5: 809-24
8. Goldstein I, Feldman MI, Deckers PJ, Babayan RK, Krane RJ (1984) Radiation-associated impotence. A clinical study of its mechanism. JAMA 251: 903-10

9. Rotman M, Seidenberg B, Rubin I, Botstein C, Bosniak M (1969) Aortic arch syndrome secondary to radiation in childhood. Arch Intern Med 124: 87-90

10. Fajardo LF, Colby TV (1980) Pathogenesis of veno-occlusive liver disease after radiation. Arch Pathol Lab Med 104: 584-8

11. Fajardo LF, Lee A (1975) Rupture of major vessels after radiation. Cancer 36: 904-13

12. Rajakulasingam K, Cerullo LJ, Raimondi AJ (1979) Childhood moyamoya syndrome. Postradiation pathogenesis. Childs Brain 5: 467-75

13. Baker DG, Krochak RJ (1989) The response of the microvascular system to radiation: a review. Cancer Invest 7: 287-94

14. Weidner N, Askin FB, Berthrong M, Hopkins MB, Kute TE, McGuirt FW (1987) Bizarre (pseudomalignant) granulation-tissue reactions following ionizing-radiation exposure. A microscopic, immunohistochemical, and flow-cytometric study. Cancer 59: 1509-14

15. Hasleton PS, Carr N, Schofield PF (1985) Vascular changes in radiation bowel disease. Histopathology 9: 517-34

16. Fajardo LF, Berthrong M (1988) Vascular lesions following radiation. Pathol Annu 23: 297-330

17. Engeset A (1970) Some observations on lymphatics in the rat thymus after irradiation. In Viamonte et al: Progress in lymphology II. Thieme, Stuttgart, pp 20-1

18. Tsyb AF, Bardychev MS, Guseva LI (1980) Secondary (radiation) oedemas of the extremities. Vestn Khir 125: 53-9

19. Brocheriou C, Verola O (1990) Consequences of radiation on tissues. Acta Chir Belg 90: 73-8

20. Kallfass E, Kramling HJ, Schultz-Hector S (1996) Early inflammatory reaction of the rabbit coeliac artery wall after combined intraoperative (IORT) and external (ERT) irradiation. Radiother Oncol 39: 167-78

21. Hallahan DE, Kuchibhotla J, Wyble C (1997) Sialyl Lewis X mimetics attenuate E-selectin-mediated adhesion of leukocytes to irradiated human endothelial cells. Radiat Res 147: 41-7

22. Sheehan JF (1944) Foam cell plaques in the intima of irradiated small arteries. Arch Pathology (Chicago) 37: 297-308

23. Schwartz RS, Koval TM, Edwards WD, Camrud AR, Bailey KR, Browne K, Vlietstra RE, Holmes DR Jr (1992) Effect of external beam irradiation on neointimal hyperplasia after experimental coronary artery injury. J Am Coll Cardiol 19: 1106-13

24. Schultz-Hector S, Kallfass E, Sund M (1995) Radiation sequelae in the large arteries. A review of clinical and experimental data. Strahlenther Onkol 171: 427-36

25. Zidar N, Ferluga D, Hvala A, Popovic M, Soba E (1997) Contribution to the pathogenesis of radiation-induced injury to large arteries. J Laryngol Otol 111: 988-90

26. Hayward RH (1972) Arteriosclerosis induced by radiation. Surg Clin North Am 52: 359-66

27. Mitomo M, Kawai R, Miura T, Kozuka T (1986) Radiation necrosis of the brain and radiation-induced cerebrovasculopathy. Acta Radiol Suppl (Stockh) 369: 227-30

28. Scodary DJ, Tew JM Jr, Thomas GM, Tomsick T, Liwnicz BH (1990) Radiation-induced cerebral aneurysms. Acta Neurochir (Wien) 102: 141-4

29. Casey AT, Marsh HT, Uttley D (1993) Intracranial aneurysm formation following radiotherapy. Br J Neurosurg 7: 575-9

30. Mellière D, Becquemin JP, Hoehne M, Dermer J, Carlier R (1983) True and false radiation arteritis. J Mal Vasc 8: 321-7

31. Himmel PD, Hassett JM (1986) Radiation-induced chronic arterial injury. Semin Surg Oncol 2: 225-47

32. Bole PV, Hintz G, Chander P, Chan YS, Clauss RH (1975) Bilateral carotid aneurysms secondary to radiation therapy. Ann Surg 181: 888-92

33. Fonkalsrud EW, Sanchez M, Zerubavel R, Mahoney A (1977) Serial changes in arterial structure following radiation therapy. Surg Gynecol Obstet 145: 395-400

34. Silverberg GD, Britt RH, Don Giffinet R (1978) Radiation-induced carotid artery disease. Cancer 39: 130-7

35. Elerding SC, Fernandez RN, Grotta JC, Lindberg RD, Causay LC, McMurtrey MJ (1981) Carotid artery disease following external cervical irradiation. Ann Surg 194: 609-15

36. Vuong NP, Baviera E, Houissa-Vuong S, Malier P, Piquet P, Lebrun-L'Allinec MC (1984) Conisation du col utérin au Laser CO2. Une étude anatomo-pathologique des altérations tissulaires et du processus de réparation à propos de huit observations. Arch Anat Cytol Path 32: 26-9

37. Abela GS, Normann S, Cohen D, Feldman RL, Geiser EA, Conti CR (1982) Effects of carbon dioxide, Nd-YAG, and argon laser radiation on coronary atheromatous plaques. Am J Cardiol 50: 1199-205

38. Choy DS, Stertzer S, Rotterdam HZ, Sharrock N, Kaminow IP (1982) Transluminal laser catheter angioplasty. Am J Cardiol 50: 1206-8

39. Becquemin JP, Benhaim-Sigaux N, Mellière D (1986) Effets du laser sur les plaques d'athérome: aspects actuels et perspectives d'avenir In Meyet Ph, Gilbert JC: Les médicaments de l'athérosclerose. Masson, Paris pp 188-98

40. Hohenleutner U, Wenig M, Walther T, Baumler W, Landthaler M (1998) Treatment of superficial varicosities with a flashlamp-pumped pulsed dye laser with 1.5 ms impulse time. Hautarzt 49: 560-5

41. Choy DS, Stertzer SH, Rotterdam HZ, Bruno MS (1982) Laser coronary angioplasty: experience with 9 cadaver hearts. Am J Cardiol 50: 1209-11

42. Pernes JM, Angel CY, Brenot P, Bruneval P, Camilleri JP, Gaux JC (1985) Effects of the argon laser on atheromas. Preliminary study on post-mortem arterial samples. J Radiol 66: 225-31

43. Abela GS, Seeger JM, Barbieri E, Franzini D, Fenech A, Pepine CJ, Conti CR (1986) Laser angioplasty with angioscopic guidance in humans. J Am Coll Cardiol 8: 184-92

44. Geschwind H, Fabre M, Chaitman BR, Lefebvre-Villardebo M, Ladouch A, Boussignac G, Blair JD, Kennedy HL (1986) Histopathology after Nd-YAG laser percutaneous transluminal angioplasty of peripheral arteries. J Am Coll Cardiol 8: 1089-95

45. Wollenek G, Laufer G, Fasol R, Zilla P, Wolner E (1986) Laser-induced vascular lesions by cw-NdYAG or pulsed UV lasers during angioplastic procedures. Thorac Cardiovasc Surg 34: 63-5

46. Siegel RJ, Fishbein MC, Forrester J, Moore K, DeCastro E, Daykhovsky L, DonMichael TA (1988) Ultrasonic plaque ablation. A new method for recanalization of partially or totally occluded arteries. Circulation 78: 1443-8

47. Paul BS, Anderson RR, Jarve J, Parrish JA (1983) The effect of temperature and other factors on selective microvascular damage caused by pulsed dye laser. Invest Dermatol 81: 333-6

48. Liu DL, Andersson-Engels S, Sturesson C, Svanberg K, Hakansson CH, Svanberg S (1997) Tumour vessel damage resulting from laser-induced hyperthermia alone and in combination with photodynamic therapy. Cancer Lett 111: 157-65

49. Spears JR, Serur J, Shropshire D, Paulin S (1983) Fluorescence of experimental atheromatous plaques with hematoporphyrin derivative. J Clin Invest 71: 395-9

50. Spears JR (1986) Percutaneous laser treatment of atherosclerosis: an overview of emerging techniques. Cardiovasc Intervent Radiol 9: 303-12

51. Prince MR, LaMuraglia GM, Seidlitz CE, Prahl SA, Athanasoulis CA, and Birngruber R (1990): Ball-tipped fibers for laser angioplasty with the pulsed-dye laser IEEE. J Quantum Electron 26: 2297-304

52. Gregory KW, Prince MR, LaMuraglia GM, Flotte TJ, Buckley L, J. Tobin JM, Ziskind AA, Caplin J, Anderson RR (1990) Effect of blood upon the selective ablation of atherosclerotic plaque with a pulsed dye laser. Lasers in Surgery & Medicine 10: 533-43

53. Delettre E, Brault D, Bruneval P, Vever-Bizet C, Dellinger M, Delgado O, Camilleri JP, Gaux JC, Peronneau P (1991) In vitro uptake of dicarboxylic porphyrins by human atheroma. Kinetic and analytical studies. Photochem Photobiol 54: 239-46

54. Garrand TJ, Stetz ML, O'Brien KM, Gindi GR, Sumpio BE, Deckelbaum LI (1991) Design and evaluation of a fiberoptic fluorescence guided laser recanalization system. Lasers Surg Med 11: 106-16

55. Dennis MB, Silverstein FE, Gilbert DA, Peoples JE (1981) Evaluation of Nd: YAG photocoagulation using a new experimental ulcer model with a single bleeding artery. Gastroenterology 80: 1522-7

56. Livesay JJ, Hogan PJ, McAllister HA (1985) The development of laser angioplasty. Herz 10: 343-50

57. Duda SH, Karsch KR, Haase KK, Huppert PE, Claussen CD (1990) Laser ring catheters in excimer laser angioplasty. Radiology 175: 269-70

58. Sanborn TA, Torre SR, Sharma SK, Hershman RA, Cohen M, Sherman W, Ambrose JA (1991) Percutaneous coronary excimer laser-assisted balloon angioplasty: initial clinical and quantitative angiographic results in 50 patients. J Am Coll Cardiol 17: 94-9

59. Bittl JA (1996) Clinical results with excimer laser coronary angioplasty. Semin Interv Cardiol 1: 129-34

60. Gijsbers GH, Hamburger JN, Serruys PW (1996) Homogeneous light distribution to reduce vessel trauma during excimer laser angioplasty. Semin Interv Cardiol 1: 143-8

61. Tcheng JE (1996) Saline infusion in excimer laser coronary angioplasty. Semin Interv Cardiol 1: 135-41

62. Safian RD, Freed M, Reddy V, Kuntz RE, Baim DS, Grines CL, O'Neill WW (1996) Do Excimer Laser angioplasty and rotational atherectomy facilitate balloon angioplasty? Implications for Lesion-Specific Coronary Intervention. J Am Coll Cardiol 27: 552-9

63. Holmes DR Jr, Mehta S, George CJ, Margolis JR, Leon MB, Isner JM, Bittl JA, King SB 3rd, Siegel RM, Sketch MH, Cowley MJ, Roubin GS, Brinker JA, Overlie PA, Tcheng J, Sanborn TA, Litvack F (1997) Excimer laser coronary angioplasty: the New Approaches to Coronary Intervention (NACI) experience. Am J Cardiol 80: 99K-105K

64. Jenkins RD, Sinclair IN, Leonard BM, Sandor T, Schoen FJ, Spears JR (1989) Laser balloon angioplasty versus balloon angioplasty in normal rabbit iliac arteries. Lasers Surg Med 9: 237-47

65. Barbeau GR, Seeger JM, Jablonski S, Kaelin LD, Friedl SE, Abela GS (1996) Peripheral artery recanalization in humans using balloon and laser angioplasty. Clin Cardiol 19: 232-8

66. Waksman R (1997) Response to radiation therapy in animal restenosis models. Semin Interv Cardiol 2: 95-101

67. Weinberger J (1997) Irradiation and stenting. Semin Interv Cardiol 2: 103-8

68. Ward PA, Till GO (1990) Pathophysiologic events related to thermal injury of skin. J Trauma 30: S75-S79

69. Boykin JV, Eriksson E, Pittman RN (1980) In vivo microcirculation of a scald burn and the progression of postburn dermal ischemia. Plast Reconstr Surg 66: 191-98

70. Nanney LB (1982) Changes in the microvasculature of skin subjected to thermal injury. Burns Incl Therm Inj 8: 321-7

71. Gross MA, Viders DE, Brown JM, Mulvin DW, Miles RH, Brentlinger ER, Velasco SE, Crawford TS, Burton LK, Repine JE, et al (1989) Local skin burn causes systemic (lung and kidney) endothelial cell injury reflected by increased circulating and decreased tissue factor VIII-related antigen. Surgery 106: 310-6

72. Choi M, Ehrlich HP (1993) U75412E, a lazaroid, prevents progressive burn ischemia in a rat burn model. Am J Pathol 142: 519-28

73. Raso SM, Gliori A, Lavagnino G, Bersini M, Ponzio E (1981) Platelet anti-aggregants in the prevention of disseminated intravascular coagulation in severe burns. Minerva Chir 36: 683-90

74. Regas FC, Ehrlich HP (1992) Elucidating the vascular response to burns with a new rat model. J Trauma 32: 557-63

75. Feng GZ (1992) Multiple organ failure after severe burns. Chung Hua Cheng Hsing Shao Shang Wai Ko Tsa Chih 8: 13-5

76. Iliopoulou E, Markaki S, Poulikakos L (1993) Autopsy findings in burn injuries. Arch Anat Cytol Pathol 41: 5-8

77. Zhou YP, Zhou ZH, Xue JZ (1993) Burns complicated with gastrointestinal haemorrhage—an analysis of 70 cases. Burns 19: 150-52

78. Garcia NM, Horton JW (1996) Burn injury alters coronary endothelial function. J Surg Res 60: 74-8

79. Loose LD, Megirian R, Turinsky J (1984) Biochemical and functional alterations in macrophages after thermal injury. Infect Immun 44: 554-8

80. Dong YL, Abdullah K, Yan TZ, Rutan T, Broemeling L, Robson M, Herndon DN, Waymack JP (1993) Effect of thermal injury and sepsis on neutrophil function. J Trauma 34: 417-21

81. Sparkes BG (1993) Mechanisms of immune failure in burn injury. Vaccine 11: 504-10

82. Michiels JJ, van Joost T, Vuzevski VD (1989) Idiopathic erythermalgia: a congenital disorder. J Am Acad Dermatol 21: 1128-30

83. Drenth JP, Michiels JJ, van Joost T, Vuzevski VD (1993) Secondary erythermalgia in systemic lupus erythematosus; comment. Rheumatol 20: 144-6

84. Cailleux N, Levesque H, Joly P, Thomine E, Courtois H (1995) Childhood acromelalgia apropos of a case revealing Fabry's disease. J Mal Vasc 20: 142-5

85. Cailleux N, Levesque H, Courtois H (1996) Erythermalgia and systemic lupus erythematosus. J Mal Vasc 21: 88-91

86. Levesque H (1996) Classification of erythermalgia. J Mal Vasc 21: 80-3

87. Ongenae K, Janssens A, Noens L, Wieme N, Geerts ML, Beele H, Naeyaert JM (1996) Erythromelalgia: a clue to

the diagnosis of polycythemia vera. Dermatology 192: 408-10

88. Confino I, Passwell JH, Padeh S (1997) Erythromelalgia following influenza vaccine in a child. Clin Exp Rheumatol 15: 111-3

89. Michiels JJ (1997) Erythromelalgia and vascular complications in polycythemia vera. Semin Thromb Hemost 23: 441-54

90. Kasapcopur O, Akkus S, Erdem A, Caliskan S, Tasdan Y, Demirkezen C, Peket F, Sever L, Arisoy N (1998) Erythromelalgia associated with hypertension and leukocytoclastic vasculitis in a child. Clin Exp Rheumatol 16: 184-6

91. Finley WH, Lindsey JR Jr, Fine JD, Dixon GA, Burbank MK (1992) Autosomal dominant erythromelalgia. Am J Med Genet 42: 310-15.

92. Guillet MH, Le Noach E, Milochau P, Sassolas B, Guillet G (1995) Familial erythermalgia treated with pizotifen. Ann Dermatol Venereol 122: 777-9

93. Lazareth I, Fiessinger JN, Priollet P (1988) Erythermalgia, rare acrosyndrome. 13 cases. Presse Med 17: 2235-9

94. Stone JD, Rivey MP, Allington DR (1997) Nitroprusside treatment of erythromelalgia in an adolescent female. Ann Pharmacother 31: 590-2

95. Kelly JW, Dowling JP (1985) Pernio. A possible association with chronic myelomonocytic leukemia. Arch Dermatol 121: 1048-52

96. Parodi A, Drago EF, Varaldo G, Rebora A (1989) Rowell's syndrome. Report of a case. J Am Acad Dermatol 21: 374-7

97. Morioka N, Tsuchida T, Ueda Y, Ishibashi Y (1991) Evaluation of the past history of chilblain in cases of systemic lupus erythematosus (SLE) and its similar diseases. Nippon Hifuka Gakkai Zasshi 101: 615-22

98. Klapman MH, Johnston WH (1991) Localized recurrent postoperative pernio associated with leukocytoclastic vasculitis. J Am Acad Dermatol 24: 811-3

99. Virokannas H, Anttonen H (1993) Risk of frostbite in vibration-induced white finger cases. Arctic Med Res 52: 69-72

100. Su WP, Perniciaro C, Rogers RS 3rd, White JW Jr (1994) Chilblain lupus erythematosus (lupus pernio): clinical review of the Mayo Clinic experience and proposal of diagnostic criteria. Cutis 54: 395-9

101. Crowson AN, Magro CM (1997) Idiopathic perniosis and its mimics: a clinical and histological study of 38 cases. Hum Pathol 28: 478-84

102. Jacob JR, Weisman MH, Rosenblatt SI, Bookstein JJ (1986) Chronic pernio. A historical perspective of cold-induced vascular disease. Arch Intern Med 146: 1589-92

103. Goette DK (1990) Chilblains (perniosis). J Am Acad Dermatol 23: 257-62

104. Spittell JA Jr, Spittell PC (1992) Chronic pernio: another cause of blue toes. Int Angiol 11: 46-50

105. Vayssairat M (1992) Chilblains. J Mal Vasc 17: 229-31

106. Mackiewicz Z, Piskorz A (1977) Raynaud's phenomenon following long-term repeated action of great differences of temperature. J Cardiovasc Surg 18: 151-4

107. Ishitake T, Kihara T, Matoba T (1996) A revised cold water immersion test for assessing peripheral circulatory function. Kurume Med J 43: 11-15

108. Falkenbach A, Watanabe I, Hartmann B, Agishi Y (1997) Raynaud's phenomenon in vibration syndrome: the impact of cold feet on skin temperature and vasomotion of the hand after immersion in cold water. Angiology 48: 1037-44

109. Blackwood W (1944) Studies in the pathology of "immersion foot". Br J Surg 31: 329-50

110. Vuong PN, Lagneau P (1987): Pathologie artérielle traumatique In Camilleri JP, Berry CL, Fiessinger J-N, Bariety J: Les maladies de la paroi artérielle, Flammarion, Paris 579-590

111. Wusteman M, Boylan S, Pegg DE (1996) The effect of cooling rate and temperature on the toxicity of ethylene glycol in the rabbit internal carotid artery. Cryobiology 33 :423-9

112. Strohecker B, Parulski CJ (1997) Frostbite injuries of the hand. Plast Surg Nurs 17(4) :212-6

113. Pulla RJ, Pickard LJ, Carnett TS (1994) Frostbite: an overview with case presentations. Foot Ankle Surg 33: 53-63

114. Reamy BV (1998) Frostbite: review and current concepts. J Am Board Fam Pract 11: 34-40

115. Casley-Smith JR, Bolton T (1973) Electron microscopy of the effects of histamine and thermal injury on the blood and lymphatic endothelium, and the mesothelium of the mouse's diaphragm, together with the influence of coumarin and rutin. Experientia 29: 1386-8

116. Laroche FG (1976) Traumatic vasospastic disease in chain-saw operators. Can Med Assoc J 115: 1217-20

117. Gemne G (1994) Pathophysiology of white fingers in workers using hand-held vibrating tools. Nagoya J Med Sci 57: S87-97

118. Bovenzi M (1998) Exposure-response relationship in the hand-arm vibration syndrome: an overview of current epidemiology research. Int Arch Occup Environ Health 71: 509-19

119. Chetter IC, Kent PJ, Kester RC (1998) The hand arm vibration syndrome: a review. Cardiovasc Surg 6: 1-9

120. Ikeda K, Ishizuka H, Sawada A, Urushiyama K (1998) Vibration acceleration magnitudes of hand-held tools and workpieces. Ind Health 36: 197-208

121. Spittell JA (1980) Raynaud's phenomenon and allied vasospastic disorders In Juergens JL, Spittell JA, Fairbairn II JF (ed) Peripheral vascular diseases. Saunders, Philadelphia, London, Toronto pp 555-83

122. Baran R, Tosti A (1993) Occupational acrosteolysis in a guitar player. Acta Derm Venereol 73: 64-5

123. Greenstein D, Kester RC (1998) The role of leukocytes in the pathogenesis of vibration-induced white finger. Angiology 49: 915-22

124. Maser RE, Lenhard MJ, DeCherney GS (1997) Vibratory thresholds correlation with systolic blood pressure in diabetic women. Am J Hypertens 10: 1044-8

125. Bovenzi M (1998) Vibration-induced white finger and cold response of digital arterial vessels in occupational groups with various patterns of exposure to hand-transmitted vibration. Scand J Work Environ Health 24: 138-44

126. Vayssairat M, Patri B, Guilmot JL, Housset E, Dubrisay J (1982) Capillaroscopy in vibration disease. Nouv Presse Med 11: 3111-5

127. Vayssairat M, Debure C, Cormier JM, Bruneval P, Lauriat C, Juillet Y (1987) Hypothenar hammer syndrome: seventeen cases with long-term follow-up. J Vasc Surg 5: 838-43

128. Littleford RC, Khan F, Hindley MO, Ho M, Belch JJ (1997) Microvascular abnormalities in patients with vibration white finger. QJM 90: 525-9

129. Hunt JL, McManus WF, Haney WP, Pruitt BA Jr (1974) Vascular lesions in acute electric injuries. J Trauma 14: 461-73

130. Fish R (1993) Electric shock, Part II: Nature and mechanisms of injury. J Emerg Med 11: 457-62

131. ten Duis HJ (1995) Acute electrical burns. Semin Neurol 15: 381-6

132. Lee RC (1997) Injury by electrical forces: pathophysiology, manifestations, and therapy. Curr Probl Surg 34: 677-764

133. Bingham H (1986) Electrical burns. Clin Plast Surg 13: 75-85

134. Baubion N, Metzger JP, Heulin A, Grosdemouge A, De Vernejoul P, Vacheron A (1985) Myocardial infarction caused by electric injury. Value of coronarography. Ann Med Interne (Paris) 136: 659-62

135. Zack F, Hammer U, Klett I, Wegener R (1997) Myocardial injury due to lightning. Int J Legal Med 110: 326-8

136. Solem L, Fischer RP, Strate RG (1977) The natural history of electrical injury. J Trauma 17: 487-91

137. Zelt RG, Daniel RK, Ballard PA, Brissette Y, Heroux P (1988) High-voltage electrical injury: chronic wound evolution. Plast Reconstr Surg 82: 1027-41

138. Koshima I, Moriguchi T, Soeda S, Murashita T (1991) High-voltage electrical injury: electron microscopic findings of injured vessel, nerve, and muscle. Ann Plast Surg 26: 587-91

139. James TN, Riddick L, Embry JH (1990) Cardiac abnormalities demonstrated postmortem in four cases of accidental electrocution and their potential significance relative to nonfatal electrical injuries of the heart. Am Heart J 120: 143-57

140. Vianello F (1997) A man in the thunderstorm: coronary injuries and electric shock (Letter) Cardiology 88: 486

141. Dickson RA (1976) High pressure injection injuries of the hand: a clinical, chemical and histological study. HAND 8: 189-93

142. Curka PA, Chisholm CD (1989) High pressure water injection injury to the hand. Am J Emerg Med 7: 165-7

143. Jebson PJL, Sanderson M, Rao VK, Engber WD (1993) High pressure injection injuries of the hand. Wis Med J 1: 13-6

144. Symonds FC, Garnes AL (1967) Tear gas gun injury of the hand. Plast Reconstr Surg 39: 175-7

145. Beguin JM, Poilvache G, Van Meerbeeck J, de Coninck A (1985) Hand injuries caused by high pressure injection. Contribution of loco-regional anaesthesia. Ann Chir Main 4: 37-42

146. Combs J, Hise L, Copeland R (1992) High pressure injection injury involving a 2 PAM Chloride autoinjector. Military Medicine 157: 434-5

147. Almind M, Broeng L (1993) A high velocity, high temperature injection injury. J Hand Surg [Br] 18: 249-50

148. Walton S (1971) Injection gun injury of the hand with anticorrosive paint and paint solvent. Clin Orthop 74: 141-5

149. Booth CM (1977) High pressure paint gun injuries. Br Med J 2: 1333-5

150. Caspi MD, Lin MD, Nerubay J, Ezra MD, Horoszowski H (1987) Subcutaneous emphysema following high pressure injection injury of inert gas. J Trauma 27: 1305-6

151. Goetting AT, Carson J, Burton BT (1992) Freon injection injury to the hand: a report of 4 cases. J Occup Med 34: 775-8

152. Lilis R, Green SM, Field J, Fischbein A (1981) Paint spray gun injury of the hand: report of an unusual source of lead poisoning. J A M A 246: 1233-5

153. O'Reilly RJ, Blatt G (1975) Accidental high pressure injection gun injuries of the hand: the role of the emergency radiologic examination. J Trauma 15: 24-31

154. Fery A, Basora J, Sommelet J (1977) Les blessures de la main par injection de fluides sous haute pression. J Chir Paris 113: 367-82

155. Wang CY, Su MJ, Chen HC, Ou SY, Liu KW, Hsiao HT (1992) Going deep into chemical burns. Ann Acad Med Singapore 21: 677-81

156. Golden MA, Vaughn DJ, Crooks GW, Holland GA, Bavaria JE (1997) Aortic dissection in a patient receiving chemotherapy for Hodgkin's disease—a case report. Angiology 48: 1063-5

157. Cacoub P, De Lacroix I, Tazi Z, Piette JC, Godeau P (1995) Drug-induced iatrogenic arterial diseases. Rev Med Interne 16: 827-32

158. Piquemal R, Emmerich J, Guilmot JL, Fiessinger JN (1998) Successful treatment of ergotism with Iloprost—a case report. Angiology 49: 493-7

159. Tay JC, Chee YC (1998) Ergotism and vascular insufficiency: a case report and review of literature. Ann Acad Med Singapore 27: 285-8

160. Aronson SM (1997) The fires of Saint Anthony. Med Health RI 80: 140-1

161. Kahn MF (1998) St Anthony's plight (Letter) Lancet 352(9138): 1478

162. Weaver R, Phillips M, Vacek JL (1989) St. Anthony's fire: a medieval disease in modern times: case history. Angiology 40: 929-32

163. Packer S (1998) Jewish mystical movements and the European ergot epidemics. Isr J Psychiatry Relat Sci 35: 227-39

164. Lamesch P, Raab R, Meyer HJ (1995) Ergotamine-induced anorectal lesions. Chirurg 66: 826-8

165. Brandt O, Abeck D, Breitbart E, Ring J (1997) Perianal ergotismus gangraenosus. Hautarzt 48: 199-202

166. Fievez M, Koerperich G, Dulieu J (1975) Arterial fibromuscular dysplasia and ergotism. Ann Anat Pathol (Paris) 20: 357-66

167. Paulson GW (1978) Fibromuscular dysplasia, antiovulent drugs, and ergot preparations (Letter). Stroke 9(2): 172

168. Honma Y, Ueta K, Nishimoto A, Satoh K, Tsutsui T (1983) Fibromuscular dysplasia (FMD) of the internal carotid artery—2 cases with suspected involvement of an estrogen or ergot preparation. Rinsho Shinkeigaku 23: 694-9

169. Price EW, Henderson WJ (1979) Silica and silicates in femoral lymph nodes of barefooted people in Ethiopia with special reference to elephantiasis of the lower legs. Trans R Soc Trop Med Hyg 73: 640-7

170. Spooner NT, Davies JE (1986) The possible role of soil particles in the aetiology of non-filarial (endemic) elephantiasis: a macrophage cytotoxicity assay. Trans R Soc Trop Med Hyg 80: 222-5

171. Kloos H, Bedri Kello A, Addus A (1992) Podoconiosis (endemic non-filarial elephantiasis) in two resettlement schemes in western Ethiopia. Trop Doct 22: 109-12

172. Yamakage A, Ishikawa H, Saito Y, Hattori A (1980) Occupational scleroderma-like disorder occurring in men engaged in the polymerization of epoxy resins. Dermatologica 161: 33-44

173. Rhomberg W, Bohler F, Vith A, Breitfellner G (1995) Generalized osteopathy with pathological fractures in a patient with long-term exposure to fluorine-containing plastics. Schweiz Med Wochenschr 125: 2330-7

174. Black C, Pereira S, McWhirter A, Welsh K, Laurent R (1986) Genetic susceptibility to scleroderma-like syndrome in symptomatic and asymptomatic workers exposed to vinyl chloride. J Rheumatol 13: 1059-62

175. Gama C, Meira JB (1978) Occupational acro-osteolysis. J Bone Joint Surg [Am] 60: 86-90

176. Grelak RP, Clark R, Stump JM, Vernier VG (1970) Amantadine-dopamine interaction: possible mode of action in Parkinsonism. Science 169: 203-4

177. Loffler H, Habermann B, Effendy I (1998) Amantadine-induced livedo reticularis. Hautarzt 49: 224-7

178. Kirkpatrick JJ, Burd DA (1995) An algorithmic approach to the treatment of hydrofluoric acid burns. Burns 21: 495-9

179. Roblin P, Richards A, Cole R (1997) Liquid nitrogen injury: a case report. Burns 23: 638-40

180. Linden CH, Scudder DW, Dowsett RP, Liebelt EL, Woolf AD (1998) Corrosive injury from methacrylic acid in artificial nail primers: another hazard fingernail products. Pediatrics 102: 979-84

181. Paulsen SM, Nanney LB, Lynch JB (1998) Titanium tetrachloride: an unusual agent with the potential to create severe burns. J Burn Care Rehabil 19: 377-81

182. McCullough JE, Henderson AK, Kaufman JD (1998) Occupational burns in Washington State, 1989-1993. J Occup Environ Med 40: 1083-9

183. Ferrandière M, Dequin PF, Legras A, Hazouard E, Benchellal Z, Perrotin D (1998) Severe self-poisoning with formol. Ann Fr Anesth Reanim 17: 254-6

184. Gallerani M, Bettoli V, Peron L, Manfredini R (1998) Systemic and topical effects of intradermal hydrofluoric acid. Am J Emerg Med 16: 521-2

185. Munoz Munoz E, Bretcha Boix P, Collera Ormazabal P, Rodriguez Santiago J, Gonzalez Pons G, Veloso Veloso E, Marco Molina C (1998) Swallowing of hydrochloric acid: study of 25 cases. Rev Esp Enferm Dig 90: 701-7

186. Filippov EM (1977) Changes in the intragastric vessels after a chemical burn. Vestn Khir 119: 121-5

187. Simpson LA, Cruse CW (1981) Gasoline immersion injury. Plast Reconstr Surg 67: 54-7

188. Corn CC, Malone JM, Wachtel TL, Robson MC, Hayward FG, Chou LS, Ko F (1991) The protection against and treatment of a liquid propane freeze injury: an experimental model. J Burn Care Rehabil 12: 516-20

189. Lacour M, Le Coultre C (1991) Spray-induced frostbite in a child: a new hazard with novel aerosol propellants. Pediatr Dermatol 8: 207-9

190. Wegener EE, Barraza KR, Das SK (1991) Severe frostbite caused by Freon gas. South Med J 84: 1143-6

191. Di Paolo N, Fineschi V, Di Paolo M, Wetly CV, Garosi G, Del Vecchio MT, Bianciardi G (1997) Kidney vascular damage and cocaine. Clin Nephrol 47: 298-303

192. Robb-Smith AHT, Taylor CR (1981) Lymph node biopsy. Oxford University Press, NewYork 308 p

VIII
Vessels and infectious diseases

Blood vessels and lymphatics play a central role in many infections or infestations. Viruses, bacteria fungi and parasites may all disseminate through vessels or demonstrate a tropism for vessel walls or a capacity to parasitise vessels in the long term, with mechanical complications. Vasculitis (see chapter XI), disseminated intravascular coagulation and thrombosis may occur [1, 2]. There is direct and indirect evidence establishing links between infection and vasculopathy, including aortitis, atherosclerosis, Wegener's granulomatosis and various vasculitic syndromes [3]. However, most complications are caused by the infectious disease itself (via toxins, haemolysis or cross-reacting antigens) or are facilitated by changes in the response of the immune system [4, 5].

1 – Diseases caused by viruses

Vascular changes in viral infections are mostly non-specific. Petechiae and ecchymoses may involve the skin, mucosae, viscera, and serosal cavities. Thrombosis may be part of disseminated intravascular coagulation (DIC) or result from infection of the endothelium. Viruses may cause vasculitis by a number of mechanisms [6-8].

Haemorrhagic fever

Viruses of the families *Arena-*, *Bunya-*, *Flavi-*, *Filo-*, *Toga-*, *Rhabdo-* and *Reoviridea* cause this syndrome. Some are tick- or mosquito-borne; others transmitted by mammals (bats, rodents). In most instances, haemorrhages are trivial [9]. Severe forms present with severe systemic disturbance and diffuse scattered petechiae, with visceral bleeding leading to shock, kidney damage with acute tubular necrosis, jaundice and neurological symptoms.

In patients suffering from dengue haemorrhagic fever (DHF), the abnormal haemostasis results from a complex mechanism combining a vasculopathy with thrombocytopaenia and platelet aggregation [10, 11]. Deficiency of prothrombin complex caused by liver damage, together with activation by mononuclear phagocytes, leads to coagulopathy.

In the skin eruptions, capillaries and small vessels of the papillary dermis display marked distortion with swelling of the endothelial cells, diapedesis of neutrophils, extravasation of erythrocytes and perivascular mononuclear cell infiltration. Ultra-structural observation reveals degeneration of neutrophils and endothelial cells with cytoplasmic vacuolisation, and formation of plasma membrane extruding into the lumen and narrowing it. In many of the vessels examined, these blebs may detach from the endothelium and are found free within the capillary lumen. Gap formations develop. Granular deposits of IgM and complement (β1C) appear in the blood vessel walls while fibrinogen is located within or about the blood vessels. Kidney percutaneous needle biopsies show focal thickening of the glomerular basement membrane, with hypertrophy of mesangial cells and deposit of IgG or IgM, or both, and C3. These findings suggest that an immunopathological process [12-15] causes the cutaneous rashes and renal changes occurring in DHF.

Rubella

Retinal vasculitis with optic neuritis and vascular changes in the fundi have been reported after rubella vaccination [16].

Measles

Measles virus infection of microvascular endothelium may lead to thrombotic vasculopathy with disseminated intravascular coagulation, ensuing endothelial cell activation, and gangrene [17]. Measles virus can induce endothelial tissue factor production *in vitro* [18].

Influenza

An association between influenza vaccination and small-vessel vasculitis has been suggested [19] but not confirmed.

Coxsackie virus infection

Henoch-Schonlein purpura has been reported to be associated with type B *coxsackie* viruses [20].

Papova virus infection

The coincidence of polyarteritis nodosa with serological conversion to parvovirus B19 has been reported [21].

Viral hepatitis

Viral hepatitis may lead to diffuse haemorrhage by impairing the synthesis of liver clotting factors. Leukocytoclastic vasculitis has been reported, together with cryoglobulinaemia, Henoch-Schonlein purpura, distal gangrene and membranous nephropathy in patients having HAV, HBV, HCV infections [22-29]. Angiographic investigation may disclose microaneurysms secondary to polyarteritis nodosa (PAN) associated with hepatitis B virus. It is possible that the vasculitic syndromes are immune complex-mediated and independent of cryoglobulins and hepatic involvement. There is a temporal relationship between the long-lasting regression of the vasculitic lesions and the decline in the levels of circulating immune complexes (CICs) and cryoglobulins (CICs/cryoglobulins) under antiviral therapy and interferon-alpha administration [30-35].

Herpes virus infections

Varicella-zoster virus

Granulomatous vasculitis with thrombosis and leukoencephalitis of the central nervous system may be a complication of herpes zoster ophthalmicus [36, 37].

Cytomegalovirus infection

CMV-associated vasculitis primarily affects vascular endothelial cells. In capillaries and small vessels, these cells swell and contain inclusion bodies in the nucleus or the cytoplasm (Fig. 1). When present the intracytoplasmic inclusions consist of clustered, small, granular, basophilic bodies of various sizes, staining positively with the periodic acid-Schiff (PAS) technique. The nuclear inclusion, eosinophilic in haematoxylineosin stained sections, is sharply demarcated inside the enlarged nucleus, whose chromatin is marginated (Fig. 2). Persistence of the nucleolus permits differentiation of *Cytomegalovirus* inclusion bodies from those of *Herpes*. Associated thrombi occlude blood vessels while mononuclear cells mostly CD3 +, CD4 +, and CD8 + lymphocytes, infiltrate the vascular wall leading to a local vasculitis ischaemia, necrosis and ulceration. The inflammatory cells often accumulate in the adventitia and invade the media. The intimal layer contains more macrophages and fewer lymphocytes than do the adventitial infiltrates. Similar findings have been produced experimentally [38]. Alternatively, the host immune response to cells ex-pressing viral antigen may be the stimulus for vasculitis. The CMV-associated vasculitides present a broad spectrum of disease: gastrointestinal vasculitis in nontransplant recipients has the best prognosis; cutaneous vasculitis seems to be a more fulminant disease, with a fatal outcome in the majority of cases. These differences most likely reflect the degree of viral burden and the state of immune competence. Additionally, since the virus itself is immunosuppressive, host defences may be further compromised by the infection [39].

CMV is a possible cause of accelerated allograft vasculopathy in human cardiac allografts [40]. Acute cytomegalovirus infection induces a subendothelial inflammation (endothelialitis) in the allograft vascular wall. Inflammatory infiltrates, made up mostly of T small lymphocytes (UCHL1 +), distort the subendothelium, increasing the intimal thickness in intramyocardial vessels of endomyocardial biopsy specimens when compared with cytomegalovirus-free recipients at one year. After the second year, the cytomegalovirus-associated endothelial cell response subsides, but the thickening of intima persists when compared with that of cytomegalovirus-free patients. Thereafter, the cytomegalovirus-associated changes reach a plateau [41-43] but may enhance allograft arteriosclerosis.

In non transplant recipients, the finding of CMV antigen and nucleic acid sequences in vascular smooth muscle cells (SMCs) suggests that cytomegalovirus (CMV) infection of the arterial wall may be common in the general population [44]. Recent studies on CMV immediate early gene (CMV-IE) have shown that transfection is capable of stimulating proliferation of vascular smooth muscle cells (SMCs) *in vitro* [45]. Since the viral genome (but not infectious virus) is found in arterial cells, the artery itself may be the site of CMV latency. Immuno-compromised patients actively infected with CMV are prone to develop accelerated atherosclerosis [46-51].

Human herpesviruses 8 (HHV8)

HHV8 is implicated in the aetiology of both Kaposi's sarcoma (KS) and primary effusion (body cavity-based) lymphoma (PEL) [52, 53] and resembles Epstein-Barr virus in its transforming properties [54]. Recently partial genomic DNA sequences of human herpesvirus 8 (HHV8) have been identified in AIDS-associated Kaposi sarcoma lesions; however, this was not confirmed in different series [55]. The presence of HHV8 in a very large fraction of KS indicates that detection of HHV8 by PCR is a useful tool in differen-

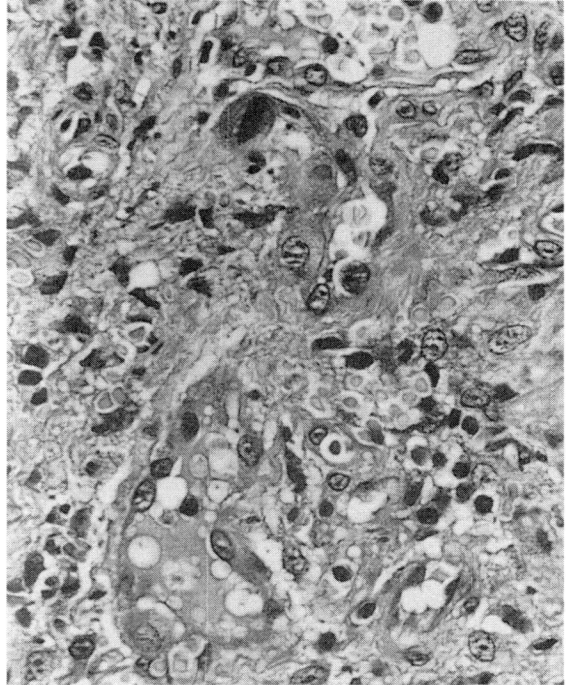

Fig. 1. Cytomegalovirus infection. Swollen endothelial cells in a blood capillary affected by CMV. Haematoxylin, eosin and saffron stain (HES)

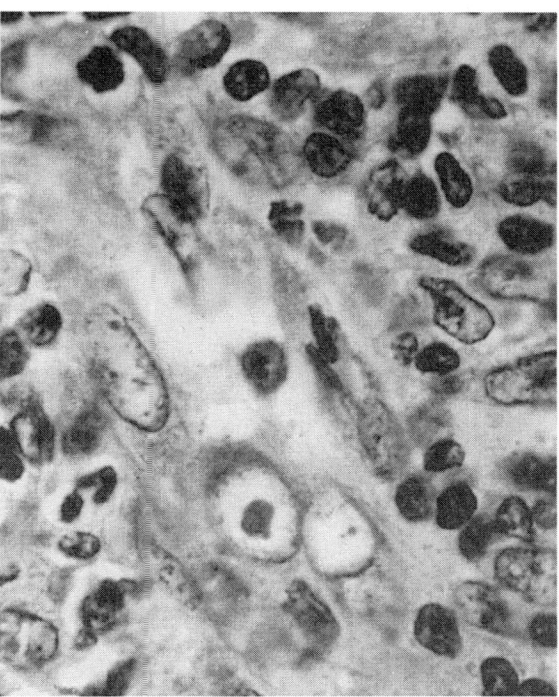

Fig. 2. Cytomegalovirus infection. CMV inclusion bodies in the nucleus of an endothelial cell. HES

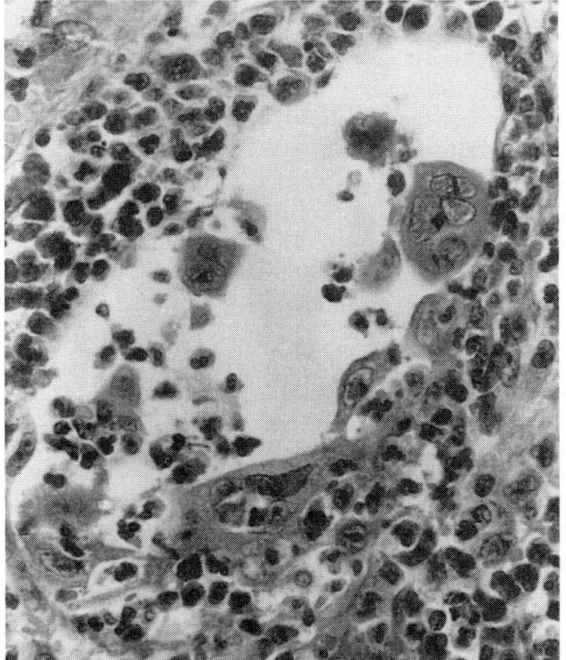

Fig. 3. Human herpesviruses 8 infection. Multinucleated endothelial cells affected by Herpesvirus. HES

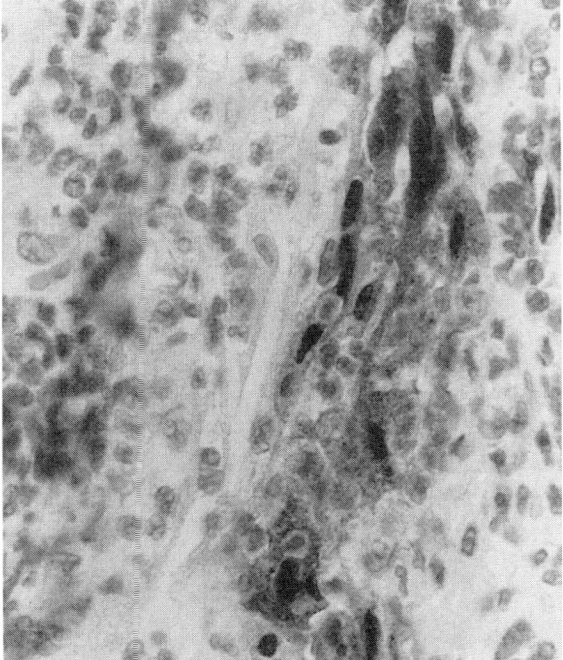

Fig. 4. Human herpesviruses 8 infection. Anti-herpes antibody helps identify infected endothelial cells. Per-oxidase antiperoxidase immunohistochemical technique (PAP)

tiating KS from other KS-mimicking vascular tumours [56]. Infected endothelial cells show nultinucleation (Fig. 3). Immunohistochemistry may help to confirm Herpesvirus vasculitis (Fig. 4).

HIV infection

Vasculitic syndromes associated with the human immunodeficiency virus (HIV) infection are protean and include polyarteritis nodosa, granulomatous giant cell arteritis, hypersensitivity vasculitis, Henoch-Schonlein purpura, lymphomatoid granulomatosis, primary angiitis of the central nervous system [5, 57-61], and a number of miscellaneous disorders, including veno-occlusive disease, pulmonary hypertension, disseminated intravascular coagulation (DIC), amyloid angiopathy, bacillary angiomatosis and bacillary peliosis, and accelerated atherosclerosis [62-67]. However, evidence of a direct pathogenic role of HIV in vasculitis has not been demonstrated [68]. Experimental infection in transgenic mice with HIV-1 provirus showed restricted expression of HIV non-structural genes in smooth muscle cells leading to migration and proliferation of these cells in blood vessels of all sizes and at different body sites. The vessel wall thickens and is invaded by T cells, occasionally by plasma cells. The intimal proliferation generates significant luminal narrowing in some vessels, and causes ischaemia in the affected tissues [69].

2 – Diseases caused by rickettsiae

Rickettsiae develop intracytoplasmically in lice (epidemic typhus), fleas (murine endemic typhus), mites (*Tsutsugamushi* scrub fever) and ticks (spotted fevers, Q fever) but do not grow in cell-free media. They invade the skin via bites or by the scratching of skin that is covered with insect faeces. The heart and vessels are involved in four major disease groups; Epidemic (*R. prowazekii*) and murine (*R.mooser*) typhus [70], Spotted fever (*R. rickettsii, R.sibirica, R.conorii, R.australis*) [71-73], *Tsusugamushi* scrub fever (*R.tsutsugamushi*) and Q fever (*Coxiella burnetii*) [74, 75].

Q fever (Q, for "query", so named because the aetiological agent was unknown) is propagated in sheep and cattle, where it produces no symptoms. Human infections result from contact with animals and with infected human beings and from air, dust and othesources. Immunofluorescence techniques are used in tissue diagnosis (*R. rickettsii, R. prowazekii*) [73, 76].

Regardless of the route of infection, rickettsiae infect host endothelial, vascular smooth muscle cells, fibroblasts, and macrophages and/or leukocytes [70]. In endothelial cells, rickettsiae bind to cholesterol-containing receptors, are endocytosed into phagolysosomes, escape into cytosol, and multiply until they burst the cells. These organisms generate an endotoxin and some *Rickettsiae* (*R. rickettsii, R. conorii*) can activate cytokines on endothelial cells, promoting production of platelet-activating factor (PAF) leading to rickettsiotic endothelialitis and local clotting [77-80]. These mechanisms result in widespread lymphohistiocytic capillaritis; venulitis and possible disseminated intravascular coagulation (DIC).

The capillaries, arterioles and venules of the skin, subcutaneous tissues, brain, lungs, heart, kidneys, liver and spleen are the most frequently involved. Infected endothelial cells swell, proliferate and cause luminal narrowing while a cuff of macrophages, lymphocytes and smaller numbers of plasma cells, PMNs and eosinophils surround the vessel. In spotted fever and scrub fever, these vascular changes give rise to leukocytoclastic vasculitis (LCV), which is most frequent in Rocky Mountain spotted fever. Vascular thromboses lead to gangrenous necrosis of peripheral structures and infarction of internal organs with "tâches noires" in the skin (*Rickettsia conorii*) [81].

3 – Diseases caused by treponema

Four diseases may involve vessels: pinta caused by *Treponema carateum*; yaws caused by *Treponema pertenue*; bejel, closely related to yaws, caused by a spirochete indistinguishable from *Treponema pertenue* and syphilis, caused by *Treponema pallidum*. The differences among these species are based on their distinct clinical syndromes and not on microbiologic characteristics. Pinta, yaws and bejel are transmitted by personal contact and/or arthropods [82].

Vasculitis caused by Pinta, Yaws and Bejel

In these conditions, plasma cell vasculitis often develops in the dermis. Dermal blood vessels with slight endothelial cell proliferation are surrounded by a chronic inflammatory infiltrate containing numerous plasma cells. The epidermis shows parakeratosis with marked acanthosis, widening and elongation of the rete ridges or pseudo-carcinomatous hyperplasia and spongiosis. Intraepidermal microabscesses are frequently encountered. Clusters of treponemes may be seen in the papillary dermis [83].

Syphilitic vasculitis

Cutaneous vessels are involved by syphilis in all stages. Whatever the stage of the disease, cutaneous syphilis is characterised by involvement of dermal vessels with endothelialitis, and dermohypodermic lymphoplasmocytic granulomata devoid of necrosis and having a perivascular coat-sleeve-like arrangement [84].

Multifocal superficial thrombophlebitis has been reported in secondary syphilis [85] though the affected veins do not harbour *Treponema pallidum*. Involvement of the heart and great vessels in classical cardiovascular syphilis is now exceptional but still more prevalent (14.9% in males and 8% in females) than neurosyphylis (9.4% in males and 5% in females). Involvement of arteries occurs during the tertiary stage of syphilis. In the aorta, the pathogenic mechanism is a direct invasion of the *Treponema pallidum* into the vasa vasora and the adventitia of the aorta from the periaortic lymphatic structures. A chronic inflammatory reaction develops within the media, adventitia and around the vasa vasora (Fig. 5-6). Obstruction of the vasa vasora leads to atrophy of myocytes in the media, disruption and weakening of the scleroprotein structure and dilatation with reactive thickening of the intimal surface. Syphilitic aortitis may progress to aortic valvulitis with aortic regur-

gitation, coronary ostial stenosis and aneurysm formation. Typically syphilitic aortitis begins at the root of the aorta, just above the aortic ring. The majority of syphilitic aneurysms are located in the thoracic aorta. According to Kampmeier, the frequency of occurrence at various sites is less than 1% at the sinus of Valsalva, 36% at the ascending aorta, 24% at the transverse arch, 5% at the descending aorta, and 4% at multiple sites [86]. The abdominal aorta and peripheral arteries are rarely affected.

On opening, the intima of affected vessels appears wrinkled and contains numerous small longitudinal striations ("tree-bark"). Histologically, the vasa vasora are infiltrated by lymphocytes and plasma cells; there are more T (CD3 positive) than B (CD22 positive) cells [87]. In the aorta, inflammatory infiltrates disrupt the elastic framework, giving rise to small stellate fibrotic scars. Elastin staining helps to demonstrate the so-called "mite-bite" pattern. Fibrosis and infiltrates of lymphocytes and plasma cells also thicken the adventitia.

Neurosyphilitic arteritis, responsible for ischaemic stroke, mostly involves the carotid arteries, the basilar and posterior cerebral arteries and the meningeal vessels. Intracranial arteries show marked intimal fibrosis or endarteritis [88-90].

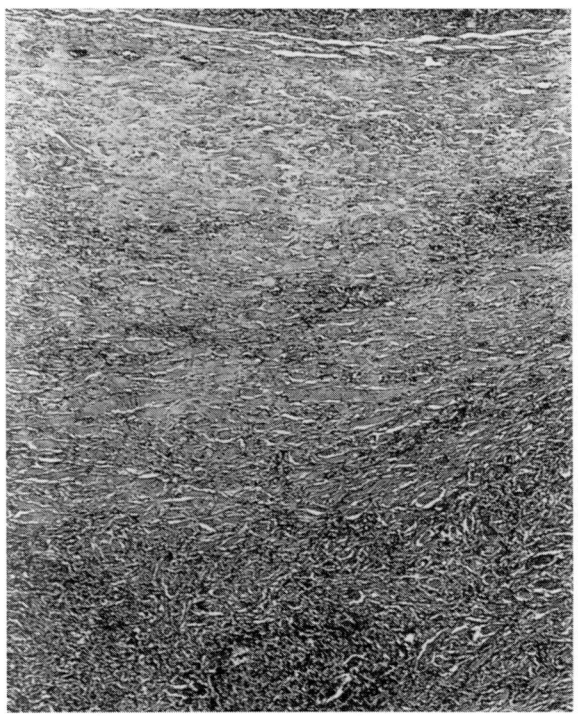

Fig. 5. Syphilitic aortitis. Note marked chronic inflammation of the adventitia. HES

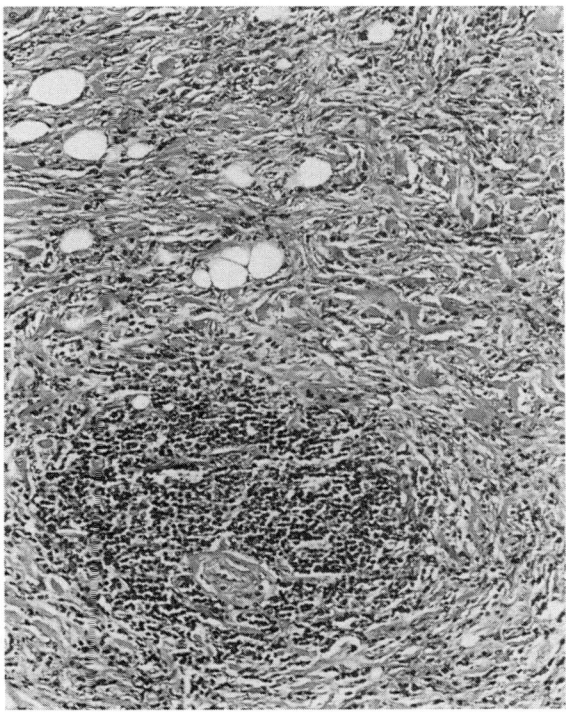

Fig. 6. Syphilitic aortitis. Lymphocytic vasculitis involving an adventitial vasa vasorum. HES

Diagnostic criteria are based on the characteristic vascular lesion, the presence of treponema, and positive staining with the Warthin-Starry method (Fig. 7) associated with positive serological tests. Immunofluorescence with polyclonal or specific monoclonal antibodies directed against *Treponema pallidum* is of great value. The differential diagnosis consists of ruling out any other inflammatory vasculitis that develops in a different clinical context, such as Takayasu's aortitis, giant cell arteritis, and systemic lupus erythematosus [91, 92].

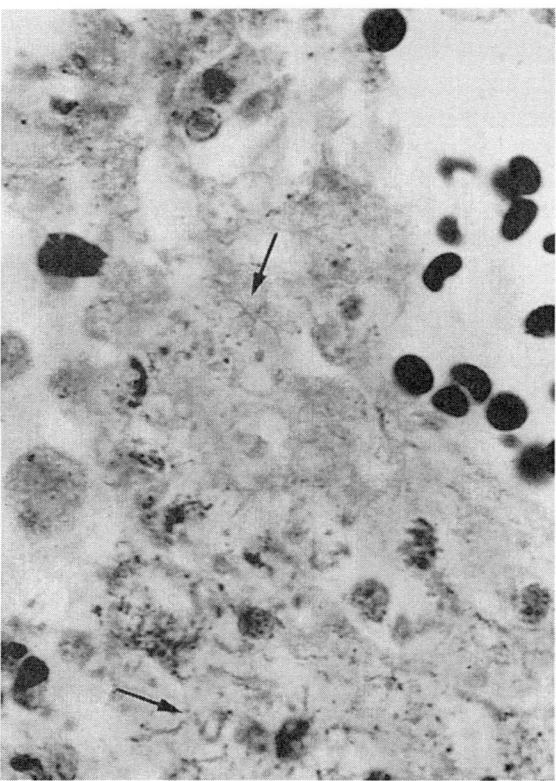

Fig. 7. Syphilitic aortitis. Treponema pallidum (arrows). Warthin-Starry stain. (Courtesy Dr M. Huerre)

4 – Diseases caused by bacteria

Bacterial vascular infections occur by direct or indirect routes of infection. Predisposing factors include infectious endocarditis, drug abuse, conditions in which immune function is compromised, and diabetes mellitus. The organisms most frequently invol-

ved in infectious vasculitis are *Salmonella, Staphylococcus*, and *Streptococcus* but causative agents include *H influenzae, Serratia, E. coli, Bactercides fragilis, Yersinia enterocolitica, Pseudomona aeruginosa, Clostridium septicum*, and diphtheroids [93-102]; however, this list is not exhaustive. Furthermore, the source of the infection cannot be identified in 50% of cases. Infectious vasculitis should be differentiated from immune-mediated infection-related vasculitides. Staphylococcal enterotoxin B and toxic shock syndrome toxin-1 also give rise to arteritis with lesions similar to those of Kawasaki disease, Wegener's granulomatosis and vasculitic neuropathy [4, 103-109]. Infective aneurysms may result from an abscess developing in the vascular wall. The main clinical feature of infective aneurysms is haemorrhage; early diagnosis is rarely made and these aneurysms have a high mortality.

Bartonellosis

This disease is endemic in certain valleys of the Andes in Peru, Chile, Ecuador, Bolivia, and Colombia. It is caused by *Bartonella bacilliformis* and transmitted by the bite of the nocturnally biting sandfly, *Lutzomyia* or *Phlebotomus verrucarum*. It is sometimes known as Carrion's disease, after a Peruvian medical student who, in 1885, through self-experimentation, died of bartonellosis [110].

Bartonella bacilliformis infection

There are two phases, an acute phase with non-specific manifestations including high fever, headache, muscle and joint pain and with profound anaemia secondary to parasitization of almost 100% of circulating red blood cells. A chronic or convalescent phase follows, characterised by red or purple skin lesions called *verruga peruana*, hepatosplenomegaly and lymphadenopathy [111]. Superficial lesions generally evolve over a period of 4-6 weeks, whereas deeper lesions persist for some months. In endemic areas (Peru, Ecuador and Colombia) "asymptomatic" patients, having an abbreviated course of the disease, may develop antibodies to *B. bacilliformis*. Healthy persons harbouring the organism may become the natural reservoir for the infection.

Bartonella bacilliformis produces an angiogenesis factor *in vitro* [112], which may be important in the production of the superficial lesions, *verruga peruana*, involving both the skin and subcutaneous tissue. The lesions are characterised by an exuberant, vaguely lobulated proliferation of either well-differentiated capillaries or solid angioblastic slits containing abundant *Bartonella bacilliformis*. These vessels are lined with plump atypical endothelial (verruga) cells. Electron-microscopic studies have shown that the characteristic cytoplasmic Rocha-Lima's inclusions, previously described as "chlamydozoa", correspond to phagocytic endothelial cells in which complex invaginations of the cell surface produced a labyrinth of interconnected channels and vacuoles containing degraded bacteria, extracellular matrix components, or both. Lymphocytes, plasma cells and neutrophils may form microabscesses. The lesion is surrounded by fibrosis. The differential diagnosis includes pyogenic granuloma, bacillary angiomatosis, cat-scratch-associated epithelioid haemangiomas in patients with AIDS and Kaposi sarcoma, and a variety of tumours (epithelioid haemangioendothelioma, epithelioid sarcoma, melanoma and metastatic carcinoma, fibrosarcoma, melanoma and leiomyosarcoma) [113-115].

Trench fever and bacillary (epithelioid) angiomatosis

These conditions, caused by *Bartonella quintana*, have now been classified with bartonellosis. Taxonomically, *Bartonella species* are relatively close to Rickettsiae.

The conditions were observed mainly in military populations during World Wars I and II, but have recently re-appeared in patients suffering from acquired immunodeficiency syndrome (AIDS) and other immunocompromised states [116]. Bacillary (epithelioid) angiomatosis develops as a reactive proliferation of vessels in various organs, often with hepatic peliosis [117] (See chaper XVII). First reported by Stoler et al in 1983 [118], bacillary (epithelioid) angiomatosis is caused by an opportunistic agent related to Bartonella species, most often *B. hanselae* and, in some patients, *B. quintana* [119, 120]. These agents were formerly included in the order Rickettsiales (*Rochalimaea hanselae*). An angiogenic factor may be secreted by the causative agent [121] and virus infections may act as cofactors in causation. Clinically, this condition mainly involves the skin and, rarely, mucosal surfaces, the lymph nodes, liver, spleen, bones and soft tissues. Skin lesions are characterised by multiple angiomatous or erythematous papules with or without crusts and papular angiokeratoma (Fig. 8). Bone involvement is manifest as osteomyelitis or osteolytic lesions. Common systemic symptoms include fever, chills, night sweats and weight loss. Bacillary angiomatosis is a potentially fatal disease in patients with HIV infection.

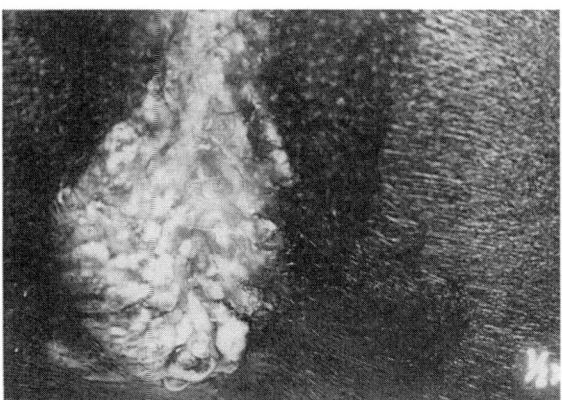

Fig. 8. Bacillary (epithelioid) angiomatosis. Male AIDS patient seeking medical assistance for multiple ulcerated angiomatous papules of the perianal skin (Courtesy Dr Th. du Puy Montbrun)

Pathology and differential diagnosis

Grossly, there are red papules or nodular subcutaneous masses. Histologically, the lesion consists of a lobular proliferation of round capillaries, having protuberant activated plump epithelioid endothelial cells, which may display nuclear atypia and mitoses (Fig. 9). Fibrous strands separate these capillaries. Scattered dense infiltrates of pycknotic neutrophils, eosinophils, histiocytes, and clumps of characteristic amphophilic, granular necrotic material are seen around the vessels. The Warthin-Starry staining technique (pH 4.0) and the Grocott-methenamine silver stain demonstrate clusters of diagnostic bacilli, which can also be seen in haematoxylin and eosin (H & E), Giemsa stains, periodic acid-Schiff and alcian blue stains. The bacteria (mostly extracellular) are either curved rods approximately 0.5-1.0 mm in length, isolated or arranged in short chains, or clumps intermingled with fibrin (Fig. 10) [122, 123]. In some cases electron microscopy and in situ hybridization permit detection of associated cytomegalovirus inclusions [124, 125] and Epstein-Barr virus genome [126] in capillary endothelial cells. A distinct ultrastructural form of collagen, fibrous long-spacing (FLS) collagen, may also be seen intermixed with subendothelial collagen or in close association with the organisms of bacillary angiomatosis [127].
Bacillary angiomatosis should be considered in the differential diagnosis of any vascular tumour in a patient with AIDS. The differential diagnosis includes Carrion's disease, pyogenic granuloma or lobular capillary haemangioma, and other variants of capillary haemangioma (lobular, histiocytoid or epithelioid,

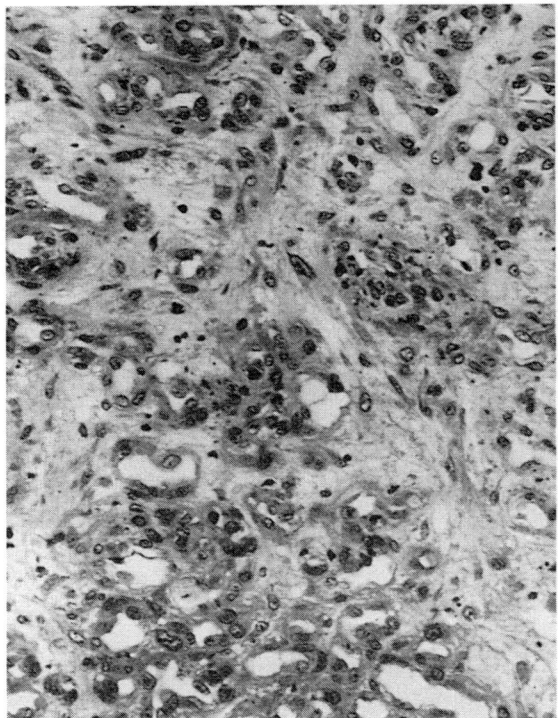

Fig. 9. Bacillary (epithelioid) angiomatosis. Lobular proliferation of blood capillaries mimicking Kaposi's sarcoma. HES

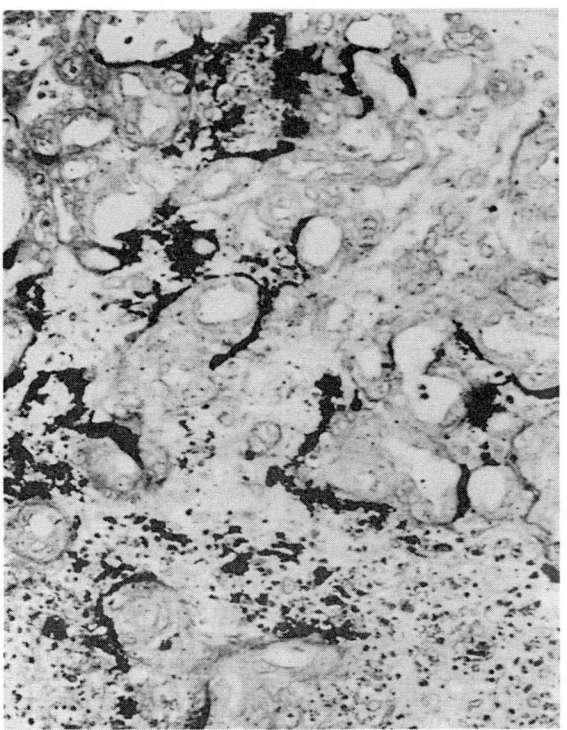

Fig. 10. Bacillary (epithelioid) angiomatosis. Clusters of Bartonella bacteria intermingled with fibrin. Grocott-methenamine silver stain. (Courtesy Dr M. Huerre)

glomeruloid) and the nodular stage of Kaposi's sarcoma (KS) – the two diseases may coexist in the same patient. The key differential features of BA include numerous neutrophils, nuclear dust, and purplish granular masses that consist of the rickettsia-like bacteria, the underlying cause of bacillary angiomatosis. However, in BA, the granulation tissue may contain some myofibroblasts but the tight streaming bundles of KS spindle cells are never seen. Moreover, the immunomorphological profile of KS is distinct.

Cat-scratch disease (cat-scratch fever, regional granulomatous lymphadenitis)

The cause of cat-scratch disease (CSD) is a *Bartonella* (formerly *Rochalimaea henselae),* an organism that is found in 30 to 50%of healthy cats. Healthy humans are infected by this gram-negative alpha-2-proteobacterium after a cat scratch or bite. *Afipia felis* is found in some patients suffering from CSD and *Rothia dentocariosa* was isolated in lymph nodes of CSD patients; other gram-positive rods may play a role together with *B. henselae* [128]. There is regional lymphadenitis, an indolent reaction, and symptoms

of a benign low-grade infection. CSD is diagnosed by the clinical symptoms, epidemiological data, and the intracutaneous test of Hanger and Rose. Serious complications may occur with uveitis, retinal vasculitis [129] or cerebral arteritis [130]. Patients suffering from AIDS develop bacillary angiomatosis, bacillary peliosis hepatis, endocarditis, and septicaemia.

Bovine brucellosis (Undulant fever, Malta fever, Mediterranean fever)

Involvement of the cardiovascular system leads to acute myocarditis with abscesses, granulomatous endocarditis and aortitis leading to mycotic aneurysm [131]. Several skin manifestations (purpuric maculonodules and papules on the limbs) arthritis and renal involvement (haematuria, proteinuria) have been reported. Skin biopsies show granulomatous vasculitis with no deposition of immunoglobulins or complement [132]. Rarely, allergic vasculitis develops with fibrinoid and leukocytoclastic vasculitis of the small veinules [133]. Renal biopsy may reveal glomerulonephritis with moderate diffuse hypercellularity involving the mesangium as well as capillary loops; immunoflurescence has revealed no staining for IgG, IgM, IgA, C3, or fibrinogen [134-137].

Chlamydia pneumoniae infection

The genus *Chlamydia* is one of small, coccoid, Gram-negative bacteria that resemble rickettsiae but which differ from them significantly by possessing a unique, obligately intracellular developmental cycle; intracytoplasmic microcolonies give rise to infectious forms by division. *Chlamydia pneumoniae* is a common human respiratory pathogen. Recently, this agent has been associated with atherosclerosis (see chapter IV) in several sero-epidemiological studies. Its presence in lesions has been demonstrated by culture, immunohistochemistry, PCR, and electron microscopy [138-144]. Experimentally, *C. pneumoniae* infection is capable of producing inflammatory atherosclerotic-like changes in the aortas of infected New Zealand White rabbits [145]. Reinfection with *Chlamydia pneumoniae* may induce isolated and systemic vasculitis (cerebral arteritis, giant cell arteritis, erythema nodosum, Cogan's syndrome) in virtually any organ of the body [146, 147].

Leprosy

There are few reports of cardiovascular changes accompanying leprosy. In the lepromatous form, blood vessels display swelling of endothelial cells and thickening of the basement membrane of endothelial and smooth cells. Hypertrophy of endothelial cells, with increased pinocytotic vesicles, is more often encountered in lepromatous leprosy than in other types. Bacilli are present in endothelial lining cells (Fig. 11) or smooth muscle cells in large masses (globi) in capillaries, venules, or arterioles [148, 149]. In tuberculoid leprosy extensive rough endoplasmic reticulum, suggesting protein synthesis, has been observed in endothelial cells [150]. Arteriographic abnormalities consist of tortuosity, stenosis, occlusion, and dilatation of peripheral vessels [151-154]. In the distal part of the limb, decreased blood flow and ischaemia leads to secondary ulceration, amputations and deformity. There is lymphocytic lymphangitis with hypertrophy of endothelial cells, which rarely harbour bacilli [155].

The role of vascular lesions on the degenerative changes in peripheral nerve fibers and loss of reflex vasodilatation is questionable [156, 157]. Secondary systemic amyloidosis involving the cardiovascular sys-

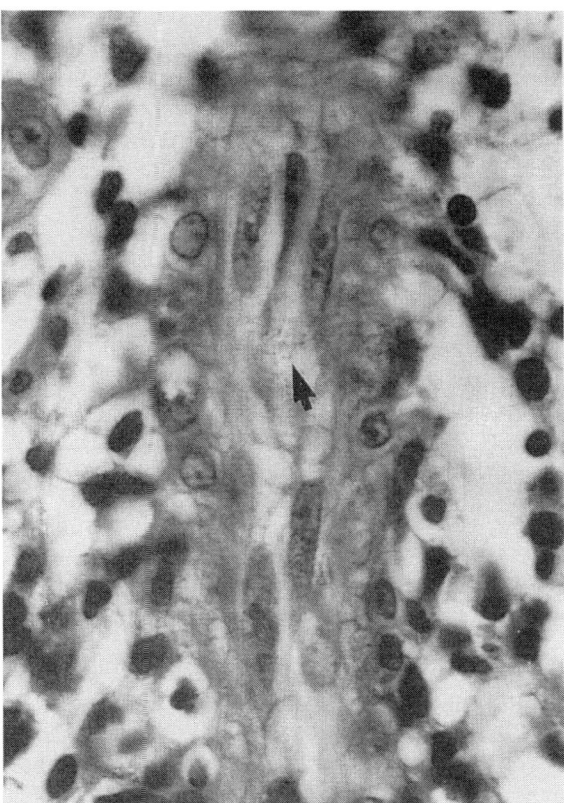

Fig. 11. Infected endothelial cells containing *Mycobacterium leprae* (arrow). HES. (Courtesy Dr M. Huerre)

tem and the kidneys may represent a serious complication of leprosy [158].

Uncommonly the immunological changes occurring in leprosy may be responsible for the genesis of a life-threatening vasculitis. Patients with lepromatous leprosy lack T cell-mediated immunity, and are anergic to lepromin. They develop diffuse lesions containing foamy macrophages stuffed with large numbers of mycobacteria. Lepromatous leprosy lesions do not contain CD4 + type 1 T cells at their margins but contain many CD8 + suppressor T cells instead. These cells inhibit helper T cells and induce antibody production by B cells. The antibody is not protective, and the formation of antigen-antibody complexes (Type II reaction) leads to an erythema nodosum leprosum (ENL) and glomerulonephritis.

Superficial and mid-dermal vessels show fibrin clots, fibrinoid necrosis, and infiltration of leukocytes and deposition of complement (C1q, C3) and fibrinogen. These changes lead to epidermal necrosis, bulla formation and ulceration [159]. Infiltrating cells and alteration of the ground substance are constant ultrastructural features [160]. Lepra bacilli are abundant around nerves and blood vessels, and many have been noted in vessel walls and endothelium [161]. ENL plays an essential role in a peculiar type of lepra reaction, named Lucio's phenomenon or necrotic erythema, one of the complications of diffuse lepromatous leprosy [162-164].

Leptospirosis

Vasculitis may be the most important factor in the pathogenesis of the bleeding disturbances in Leptospirosis [165] but we consider that thrombocytopaenia and hepato-renal failure are major contributing factors.

Listeriosis

Lesions produced by *Listeria monocytogenes* are characterised by focal necrosis with abscess formation and dense infiltration of neutrophils. The organisms can be demonstrated in tissue by Gram stain as gram-positive pleomorphic rods, 0,5 to 2 microns, and by silver methods, such as the Gomori-methanamine silver, Warthin-Starry, or Levaditi stains. Some patients dying from listerial meningoencephalitis may have a necrotizing vasculitis [166]. Subacute listerial endocarditis does not differ significantly from that caused by other bacteria.

Tuberculosis

Vascular tuberculosis results from contiguous extension of the tuberculous process. Haematogenous and lymphatic spread of tuberculosis to vessels is rare. Lung vessels and the thoracic and abdominal aorta are usually involved [167-169]. Histologically, the vascular walls are distorted by granulomata (Fig. 12) made up of aggregated or palisaded histiocytes and multinucleated giant cells (Fig. 13). These changes may cause an aneurysm to develop [170]. A tuberculous aneurysm is usually associated with miliary or cavitary tuberculosis. Smaller vessels are cuffed by infiltrate of lymphocytes and display obliterative lymphocytic vasculitis. Coarctation-like stenoses caused by perivascular fibrosis are rare [171]. Tuberculosis may rarely present as a cutaneous leucocytoclastic vasculitis [172].

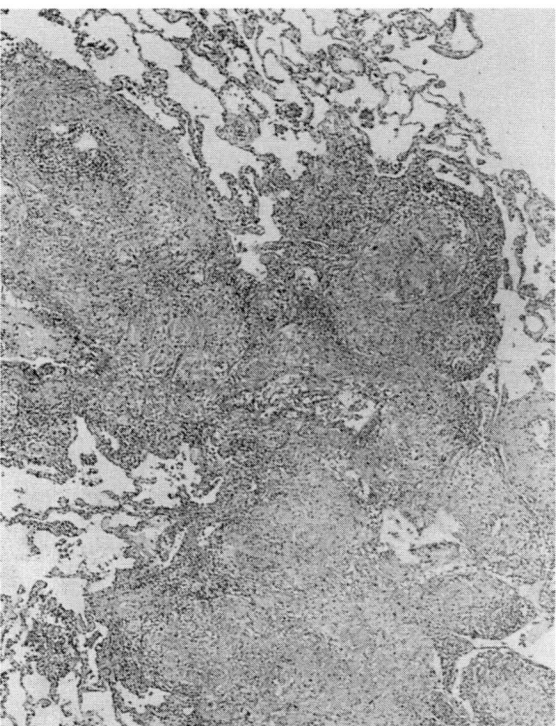

Fig. 12. Pulmonary tuberculosis showing clusters of granulomata made up of palisaded histiocytes and multinucleated giant cells. HES

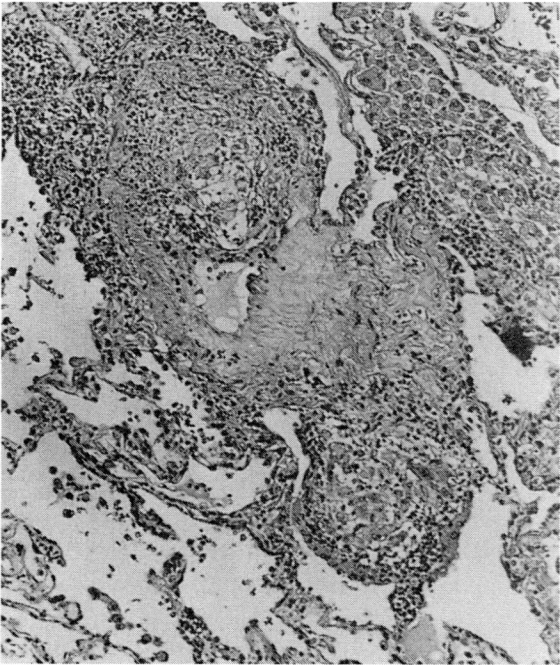

Fig. 13. Pulmonary tuberculosis. Associated granulomatous vasculitis may be a starting point for an aneurysm to develop. HES

5 – Diseases caused by parasites

Protozoa

Very few of the numerous protozoan species affect the cardiovascular system or spread through the blood or lymphatic vessels [173]. Those that do are of considerable clinical significance in some countries.

American trypanosomiasis (Chagas disease).

This condition, caused by *Trypanosoma cruzi*, affects millions of people in Central and South America. Dogs, rodents, and Man can act as reservoir hosts. In the acute form of infection, transmission of *T. cruzi* occurs from man to man or animal to man via insects. The reduviid bug defecates as it feeds, and scratching after bites results in infection. More rarely infection occurs through blood transfusions or occasionally through the placenta [174]. From experimental data it appears that the lymphatic system may be the main route of *T. cruzi* dissemination from the site of inoculation [175]. The trypomastigote (flagellate form) of *T. cruzi* in the blood is 3 µ wide and 16-22 µ long, including the flagellum. Its central oval-shaped nucleus is reddish pink with Giemsa stain. When the trypomastigotes enter tissue cells (muscle fibres and glia), they duplicate, lose the flagellum and become amastigotes. In *Trypanosoma cruzi* infection in mice, heightened platelet reactivity and evidence of endothelial cell dysfunction are found and these data suggest that the coronary microvascular spasm and/or occlusion associated with acute Chagas' disease may be mediated by these effects [176]. Blood vessels are also invaded by parasites, resulting in thrombosis and necrotizing arteritis [177]. In dogs [178], myocardial changes in acute *Trypanosoma cruzi* infection include invasion of myocytes with formation of compact or loose amastigote nests, interstitial infiltration by mononuclear cells and damage with necrosis of nonparasitized myocytes. Rupture of the amastigote nests induces an acute inflammatory process followed by a deposition of a fibrin network, proliferation of collagen, mastocytosis and fibrosis in the chronic stage. Alterations of nonparasitized myocytes range from mild oedema to severe myocytolysis. These changes are often accompanied by lymphocyte and macrophage infiltration around myocytes that have lost their basement membrane. Lymphocytes adhere to capillary endothelial cells. Platelet aggregates and fibrin microthrombi may develop in some capillaries

leading to diffuse bleeding with profound anaemia. These changes have also been reported in *Trypanosoma vivax* infection in Ayrshire cattle [179]. In Man, involvement of myocardial fibres results in an acute diffuse myocarditis.

Grossly, the heart undergoes hypertrophy and dilatation, and presents a fresh fish or cooked-meat like aspect. The myocardium displays a marked infiltration of lymphocytes, plasma cells and histiocytes replacing infected myocardial fibres. In the central nervous system the inflammatory process is disseminated in the white and grey matter with diffuse gliosis. Vessels are cuffed by marked infiltrates formed by lymphocytes, plasma cells and histiocytes.

In the chronic form, the pathogenesis of Chagas myocarditis is disputed; the two favored hypotheses are an antiheart immune or autoimmune reaction [178] and a neurogenic theory of damage to the autonomous nervous system with the presence of amastigote nests, ganglionitis, plexulitis and inflammation in some areas [177, 180]. Coronary vascular reactivity appears to be abnormal [181]. Repeated exogenous and/or endogenous re-infections may play a role as may anomalies of coronary microcirculation [182] where spasm and thrombosis have been implicated [176]. In this form of the disease hypertrophy and dilatation mainly affect the left ventricle. Myocardial infarction with rupture, tamponade, thrombosis and arterial embolism, leading to multiple visceral infarctions may occur [183]. The frequency of myocardial infarction caused by coronary arteriosclerosis seems to be higher in chagasics than in nonchagasics [184].

White nodules are seen on the surface of the heart with aneurysms mainly located at the apex of the ventricle. Histologically the myocardium is distorted by diffuse interstitial fibrosis. Thick collagen strands surround bundles of myocardial fibers and the intramyocardial coronary vessels [185]. Some inflammatory infiltrates of lymphocytes, plasma cells and histiocytes may be present. Immunohistochemical analyses reveal predominance of CD8 + cytolytic lymphocytes. Most of the lymphocytes in these lesions express lymphocyte function antigen-1 (LFA-1), CD44, and very late antigen-4, and a few display weak expression of LFA-3. HLA-DR antigens are not observed on myocardial cells, but are consistently upregulated on the endothelial cells in the hearts of patients with chronic chagasic cardiomyopathy. Intercellular adhesion molecule is expressed by endothelial cells of both chagasic and nonchagasic individuals, but E-selectin has been detected only on vessels of hearts from chagasic patients who had chronic cardiomyopathy [186].

Leishmaniasis (Leishmaniosis)

Infection with species of *Leishmania* results in a clinically ill-defined group of diseases traditionally divided into four major types: – visceral leishmaniasis (kala azar), Old World cutaneous leishmaniasis, New World cutaneous leishmaniasis and mucocutaneous leishmaniasis. Each is clinically and geographically distinct and each has in recent years been further subdivided into clinical and epidemiological subdivisions to give a more natural breakdown. Transmission is by various sandfly species of the genus *Phlebotomus* or *Lutzomyia*. Vascular changes involving both arteries and veins may develop in cutaneous leishmaniasis where fibrinoid necrosis, fibrin thrombi, hyalinosis and intimal proliferation may all be found. IgG and IgA are found within endothelial cells, in the media and the perivascular space by immunoperoxidase staining and the formation of immune complexes in the infected skin is apparently responsible for these alterations [187, 188]. Mesenteric vasculitis leading to colonic pseudotumoural stenosis has been reported in immunocompromised patients with disseminated visceral leishmaniasis [189].

Malaria

Detailed accounts of Malaria are given elswhere [190] but vascular involvement is common in many forms and stages of the disease. In malignant cerebral malaria caused by *P. falciparum*, the brain vessels are plugged with parasitized red blood cells, each cell containing dots of haemozoin pigment (Fig. 14). Vascular stasis induces local hypoxia leading to ring haemorrhages (Fig. 15) with small focal inflammatory reactions (called malarial or Dürck's granulomata).

Immunofluorescence reveals extravascular deposits of *P. falciparum* granular antigen associated with acute inflammatory lesions in cerebral tissue [191]. Progressive anaemia and circulatory stasis in chronically infected patients may induce non-specific focal hypoxic lesions in the heart.

In some patients, the myocardium shows focal interstitial neovascularisation with infiltrates (Fig. 16). Van der Wall et al [192] reported a case of acute myocardial infarction caused by a thrombosed aneurysm of a coronary artery in a 29-year-old male. The patient had no risk factors for atherosclerosis and his medical history revealed only repeated episodes of quartian malaria three years before. Pulmonary oedema or shock with DIC may cause death in nonimmune patients, sometimes in the absence of other characteristic lesions. Interstitial pneumonitis, eosinophil-rich, granulomatous hepatitis with severe liver cell necrosis,

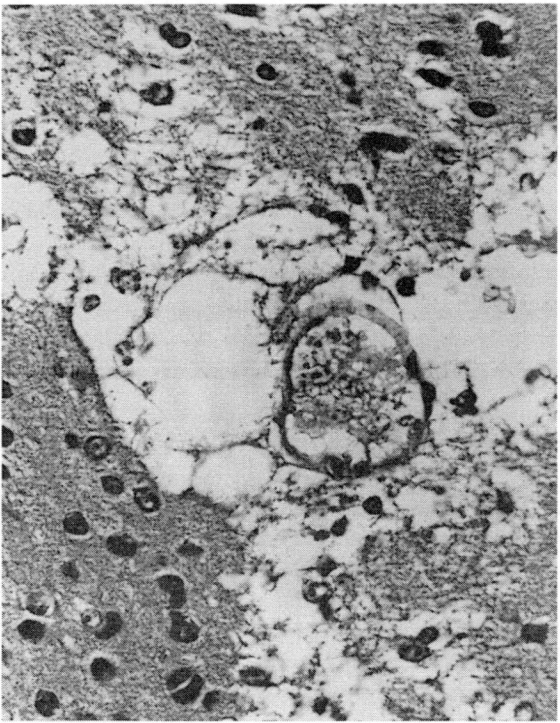

Fig. 14. Malaria. Parasitised red blood cells plugging brain vessels in malignant cerebral malaria caused by *P. falciparum.* HES

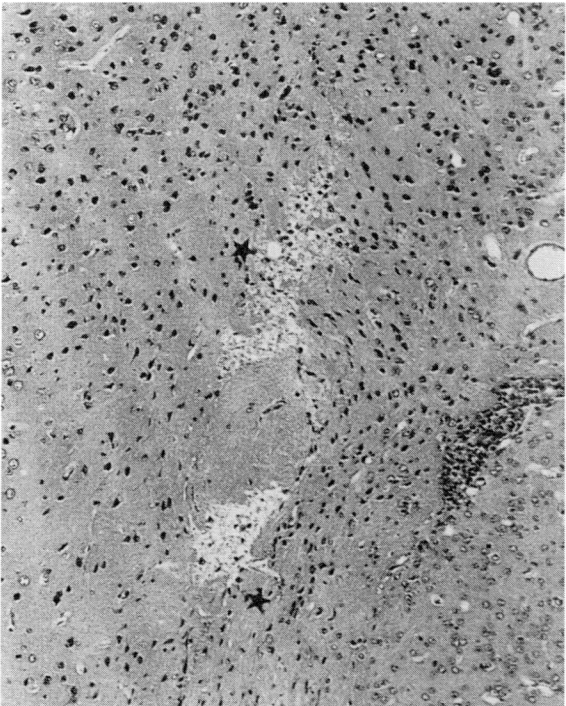

Fig. 15. Malaria. Cerebral haemorrhages (stars) neighbouring clogged vessels. HES

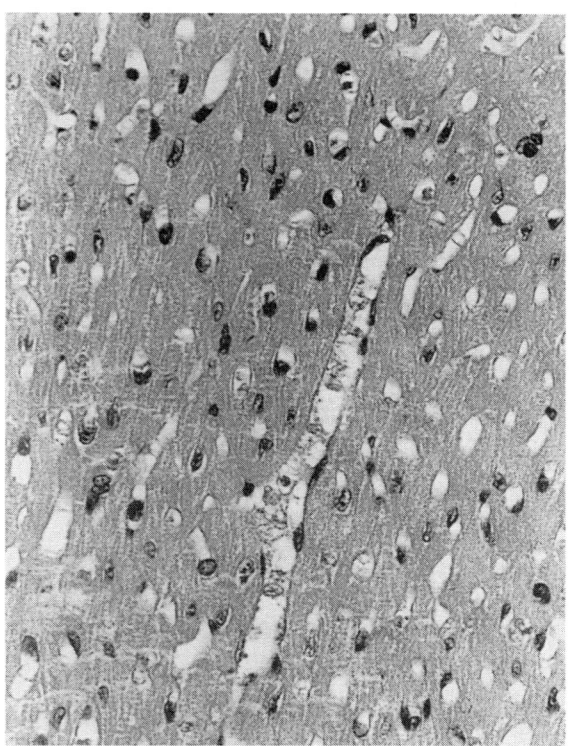

Fig. 16. Malaria. Interstitial neovascularisation in the myocardium. HES

glomerulonephritis, and kidney tubular necrosis, as well as the regional parasite sequestration and the role of immune complex in cerebral malaria, have been investigated in experimental models [193- 200].

Amoebic infections

Amoeba histolytica may occasionally be identified inside vessels without signs of vasculitis in intestinal, hepatic and extraintestinal amoebiasis [201]. The hepatic establishment of amoebae (in abscesses, for example) implies invasion of blood vessels and contact with endothelium. *In vitro, Entamoeba histolytica* adhesion to human endothelium is a marker of strain virulence [202]. Free-living soil or water amoebae may cause severe diseases of the central nervous system. *Naegleria* and *Acanthamoeba* are recognized causes of amoebic meningo-encephalitis in humans.

Infection by *Naegleria fowleri*, a thermophilic amoeba that grows well in tropical and subtropical climates is acquired by exposure to polluted water in ponds, swimming pools and man-made lakes. Victims are generally young healthy individuals with a history of recent water-related sport activities. Raised temperatures during the hot summer months or warm water

from power plants facilitate the growth of *N. fowleri*. The central nervous system infection, called Primary Amoebic Meningoencephalitis (PAM) is characterised by an acute fulminant meningoencephalitis leading to death 3-7 days after exposure. The portal of entry of the parasites is probably the nasal olfactory neuroepithelium. The amoebae penetrate the mucosa, migrate along and inside the blood vessels and nerve fibres centripetally, through the cribriform plate of the ethmoid into the subarachnoid space and from there into the brain. The changes produced are an acute haemorrhagic necrotizing meningoencephalitis with modest purulent exudate, mainly at the base of the brain, brain-stem and cerebellum. The protozoa may reach other internal viscera (lungs, kidneys, liver, pancreas and lymph nodes) by haematogenous dissemination.

The portal of entry of the *Acanthamoeba* species is the upper respiratory tract. The central nervous system is probably secondarily affected from another active focus, such as the lungs, the skin or the cornea [203].

Histologically in all these conditions the amoebae in the tissues are almost solely trophozoites. A few large cysts may be seen. The cytoplasm is clear but non-homogenous. The amoebae stain weakly with the iron haematoxylin-eosin and Goldner stains and are mostly gathered into clusters without focal destruction. The walls of large blood vessels are frequently invaded by amoebae and parasites are seen interspersed with dense inflammatory cell infiltrates. Thrombotic occlusion of vessels leads to ischaemic necrosis and perforation of the bowel, the final and most serious manifestation of transmural amoebic colitis [204].

A granulomatous reaction with giant cells has been described in granulomatous amoebic encephalitis. The small and medium blood vessels involved show fibrinoid necrosis of their walls, thrombosis, aneurysm, and extensive haemorrhages. Large numbers of amoebic trophozoites and few cysts are present in perivascular spaces and within necrotic CNS tissue [205]. Perivascular infiltrates with leukocytes, lymphocytes and plasma cells develop in the parenchyma. Similar lesions have been noted in animals [206]. In isolated cutaneous infection with Acanthamoeba, the purpuric lesions display prominent leukocytoclastic vasculitis as well as myriads of organisms [203].

NEMATODES

FILARIAL NEMATODES

Most filarial nematodes infest the lymphatic system; some affect blood vessels and some involve both.

Bancroftian and Malayan filariasis

Two closely related nematodes, *Wuchereria bancrofti* and *Brugia malayi*, are responsible for 90% and 10%, respectively, of the 90 million infections by filaria worldwide. The filariae, measuring from 4 (male) to 20 (female) cm in length, dwell in the lymphatic vessels during their entire lifetime (at least 15 years), and release microfilariae that can be found in the peripheral blood. Microfilariae are transmitted by female mosquitoes belonging to the species *Aedes, Anopheles, Culex* or *Mansonioides,* according to the type of filariae. In endemic areas, which include parts of Latin America, sub-Saharan Africa, and Southeast Asia, filariasis causes a spectrum of diseases, including asymptomatic microfilaremia, tropical pulmonary eosinophilia, and chronic lymphangitis with swelling of the dependent limb or scrotum (elephantiasis) [207]. In chronic lymphatic filariasis, damage to the lymphatics is caused directly by the adult parasites and mediated by cytokines produced TH1 helper T cells. Granulomata develop around the adult parasites and fibrosis leads to occlusion of the vessels. Immune responses to both adults and microfilariae normally eliminate microfilariae from the bloodstream and parasiteamia may persist in the immunosuppressed host. IgE-mediated hypersensitivity to microfilariae produces tropical pulmonary eosinophilia.

General symptoms of filariasis include fever, headaches, malaise, asthenia, arthralgia, and allergic respiratory manifestations. Very rapidly, the symptoms focus on the lymphatic system; recurrent acute lymphangitis develops with painful peripheral lymphoedema, fibrosing mediastinitis caused by involvement of the deep lymphatic trunks in the chest [208], acute orchitis leading to chylous hydrocele [209] and lymphadenopathy. Asymptomatic individuals infected with *W. bancrofti* have subclinical lymphatic disease with a marked increase in the calibre of lymphatic vessels, and diffuse distribution of collateral vessels revealed by specialised imaging techniques [210, 211].

Adult filariae, live, dead or calcified are present in the draining lymphatics or nodes, surrounded by eosinophilic and lymphocytic infiltrates. Organization of the endolymphatic exudate results in polypoid infoldings of the vessels. Severe, long-lasting lymphatic infection lead to a tough subcutaneous lymphoedema and fibrosis with epithelial hyperkeratosis [212-214]. Elephantoid skin displays dilatation of the dermal lymphatics, focal cholesterol deposits, and widespread lymphocytic infiltrates with accumulation of CD3 + and CD8 + T cells; the epidermis is thickened and hyperkeratotic. Patients with HLA-DR and -DQ alleles seem resistant to development of elephantiasis [215]. Pulmonary involvement by microfilariae is marked by eosinophilia caused by circulating antimicrofilarial IgEs that trigger degranulation of mast cells (tropical eosinophilia). Dead microfilariae are surrounded by stellate, hyaline, and eosinophilic necrotic material embedded in small epithelioid granulomata (Meyers-Kouvenaar bodies).

Dipetalonemiasis

This infection is caused by two among the 40 known species of the genus *Dipetalonema: D. perstans* and *D. streptocerca.* Streptocarciasis, a zoonosis caused by *Dipetalonema streptocerca*, affects man, the chimpanzee and the gorilla [216]. The vector is *Culicoides grahami.*

Adult worms and microfilariae dwell in the skin. Some patients may be asymptomatic but the most consistent feature of streptocerciasis is a chronic itching dermatitis with dermal thickening, and hypopigmented macules associated with rubbery, enlarged lymph nodes. Eosinophilia may be present.

In the skin, dermal lymphatics are dilated with oedema, fibrosis, infiltration of lymphocytes, histiocytes and eosinophils. Live adult worms are well adapted to man and produce no inflammatory reaction. Dead worms are cordoned by an intense inflammatory reaction with giant cell granulomata. Microfilariae of *D. streptocerca* may be found inside dilated lymphatics and sinuses of enlarged regional lymph nodes. Diagnosis is made by demonstrating microfilariae in wet mounts of fresh skin snips.

Mansonelliasis (Ozzardi's filariasis, mansonelliasis ozzardi)

This infestation by *Mansonella ozzardi* is spread by *Culicoides* and *Simulium amazonicum.* Man is the definitive host. Adult worms live in the serosal cavities (pericardium, pleura, peritoneum) and may dwell in the lymphatic vessels. Microfilariae are found in the peripheral blood with no significant periodicity. Clinical manifestations vary. Live organisms cause few or no symptoms but dead ones cause fever, pain, erythematous and itching skin plaques, and "varices" in the lower extremities with lymphadenopathy. The microfilariae circulate in the peripheral blood and lymphatic capillaries of the papillary and superficial reticular dermis with no significant periodicity. These vessels are surrounded by a perivascular infiltrate of lymphocytes and plasma cells [217]. Some microfilariae may be present in perivascular spaces and in the dermal interstitium. The diagnosis is based on identification of the microfilariae in peripheral blood smears.

Onchocerciasis

Onchocerca volvulus, a filarial nematode transmitted by blackflies, was, until major campaigns in recent years, a main cause of blindness in equatorial Africa, where the parasite has infected 20 million people.

Adult *O. volvulus* parasites mate in the dermis, where they are surrounded by a mixed infiltrate of host cells that produces a characteristic subcutaneous nodule (onchocercoma). The major pathology, however, which includes blindness and chronic pruritic dermatitis with "peau-d'orange" pattern, is caused by large numbers of microfilariae, released by females, which accumulate in the skin and in the eye chambers. Lymphadenitis and lymphangitis, with subsequent elephantiasis, involve the skin of the limbs (Fig. 17-18) and genitalia. Vascular perfusion of *Onchocerca volvulus* nodules by India ink, Microfil polymer, or acrylate perfusates and other special techniques reveal a proliferation of capillaries around the worms and communication between small vessels and the spaces around the worms. These findings suggest that *O. volvulus* may control blood vessel proliferation by release of angiogenesis factors, analogous to rapidly growing solid tumours [218, 219]. Microfilariae circulate in lymphatic capillaries and penetration into the extra-vascular tissues causes vascular change with inflammatory cell infiltration, granulomata and fibrosis [220-223]. *Onchocerca volvulus* can be found in dilated lymph vessels (Fig. 19).

These vessels may show dystrophic changes and thrombo-lymphangitis (Fig. 20). Microfilariae dwell in superficial dermal lymphatics running alongside blood capillaries (Fig. 21) [224]. In lymph nodes involved by onchocercal lymphadenitis, microfilariae are most numerous in the capsule and in the fibrous tissue of the medulla, but smaller numbers are also found within lymphoid tissue, in dilated lymphatics and in blood vessels [225].

Dirofilariasis

This infection is caused by filarial nematodes of the genus Dirofilaria. There are two forms: subcutaneous dirofilariais caused by *D. tenuis (D. conjunctivae)* and

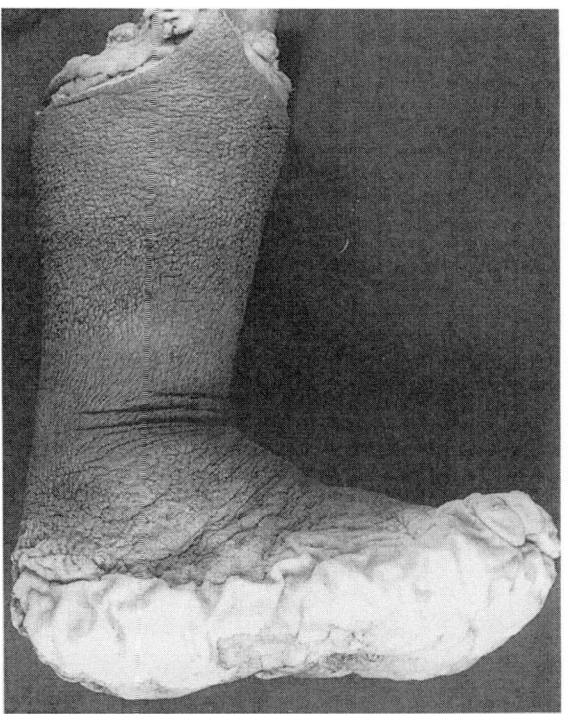

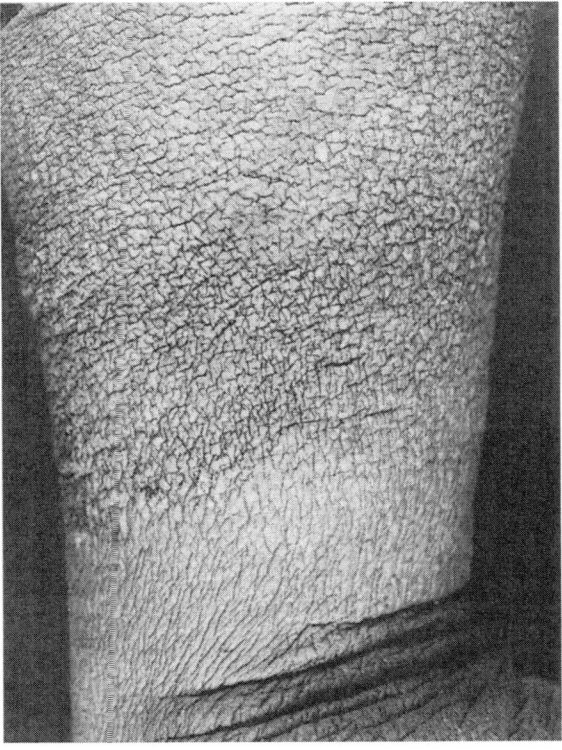

Fig. 17-18. Onchocerciasis. Elephantiasis of the leg with "peau d'orange" pattern

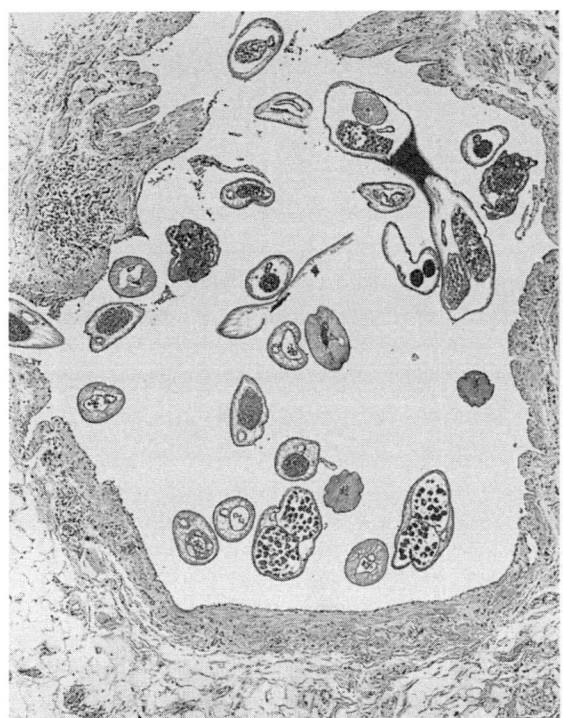

Fig. 19. Onchocerciasis. Sections of an *Onchocerca volvulus* in a lumen of a dilated lymphatic. HES

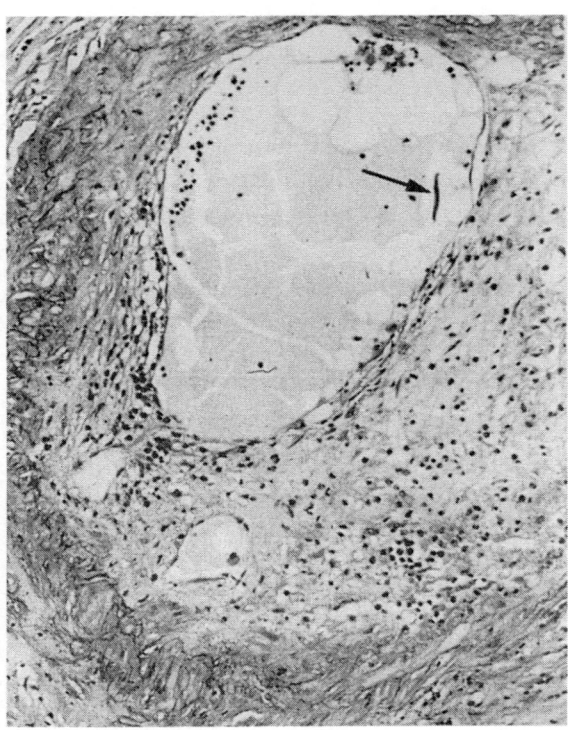

Fig. 20. Onchocerciasis. Thrombo-lymphangitis with thickened intima and infiltration of foam cells. Note an *Onchocerca volvulus* microfilaria (arrow) in the lumen. HES

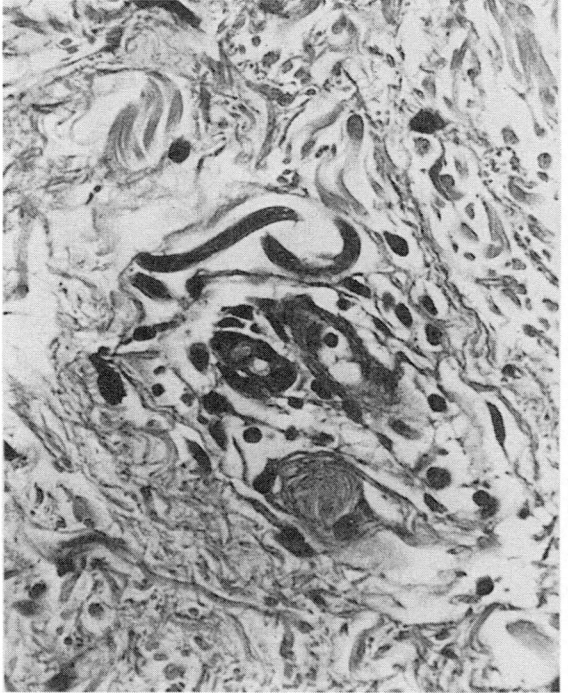

Fig. 21. Onchocerciasis. Skin snip displaying an *Onchocerca volvulus* microfilaria inside dilated lymphatic capillaries, running alongside a superficial dermal blood capilary. HES. (Courtesy Dr O. Bain)

D. repens, and pulmonary dirofilariasis, caused by *Dirofilaria immitis,* the dog heartworm. *D.immitis* is a common parasite of dogs, cats, rabbits, foxes, muskrats, wolves, sea lions, and other beasts [226-228]. The parasite is transmitted from animal to animal by many species of mosquitoes and Man is an accidental host. Adult worms coil and develop tangled masses in the right ventricle, inferior vena cava [229], and portal vein [230] of the definitive host. Immature worms dwell in human lungs and microfilariae circulate in the blood. Clinical manifestations vary; chest pain, cough, haemoptysis, fever, chills and malaise are common. Some patients develop asymptomatic peripheral "coin lesions" on chest X-rays; these may be multiple and simulate lung cancer [231]. The lesions have a necrotic area surrounded by granulomata. Small arteries often contain dead, fragmented and partially calcified single worms [232] and display varying degrees of endarteritis [233].

Loiasis (Calabar swelling, fugitive swelling)

This is a chronic disease caused by Loa loa, the African eye worm, a species of the family *Onchocercidae* (superfamily *Filarioidea*) which is indigenous to the western part of equatorial Africa, especially in the region of the Congo River.

Adult worms are white or gray-white, and thread-like, the males averaging 25 to 35 by 0.3 to 0.4 mm (with a curved tail) and the females ranging from 50 to 60 by 0.4 to 0.6 mm; microfilariae, measuring 275 by 7 microns, are ensheathed, with nuclei extending to the tip of the tail. The life cycle is somewhat similar to that of the *Wuchereria* species; man is the only known definitive host, and parasites are transmitted by Chrysops or mango flies (family Tabanidae).

Symptoms manifest approximately three to four years after a bite by an infected tabanid fly. When the infective larvae mature (3 years or more), the adult worms may persist in man for as long as 17 years. They move about in an irregular course through the connective tissue of the body (as rapidly as 1 cm per minute), frequently becoming visible beneath the skin and mucous membranes. Lymphadenitis may develop.

Histologically the live worms cause nonspecific inflammation with a few giant cells and fibrosis. Dead worms induce marked tissue reaction with chronic abscesses. Atrophy of lymphoid follicles, distention of sinuses filled with histiocytes and eosinophils, fibrosis of capsule and trabeculae, dilatation of lymphatic vessels of capsule and medulla, and inflammatory cell infiltrates [234] are seen in affected lymph nodes. Microfilariae may be found occasionally at numerous sites: the central nervous system, chroid and retina, lungs, myocardium and blood vessels. Usually the eosinophilic granulomata are similar to those in visceral larva migrans.

NON-FILARIAL NEMATODES

Apart from typical filariasis, other parasitic diseases may occasionally involve vessels. Lymphatic extensions with subsequent blockades of lymph flow have been reported in ascariasis, taeniasis and echinococcosis. Females of trichinella sp. may be transported via lacteals after penetration of the intestinal mucosa.

Visceral larva migrans (Toxocariasis)

Visceral larva migrans is caused by migrating larvae of *Toxocara canis* and *cati*. Man becomes infected after ingestion of eggs in contaminated soil or food. Experimentally, larvae are seen entering and within lymphatic vessels and the peritoneal cavity [235]. They enter the circulatory system and may locate in any organ in the body [236]. Larvae may lodge in the wall of a vein or an artery inducing a focal granulomatous vasculitis, seen in cats experimentally infected with ova of *Toxocara cati* [237].

Angiostrongyliasis

Two species, *Angiostrongylus cantonensis* (rat lung-worms) and *A. costaricensis* cause two distinct diseases in man.

1. *Angiostrongylus cantonensis* infection (Eosinophilic meningitis). This infection, prevalent in Asia, New Caledonia, Tahiti, Hawaii and in some islands of Oceania, is caused by *Angiostrongylus cantonensis*, Gnathostoma spp. The rat is the definitive host of *A. cantonensis*, which dwells in the pulmonary arteries. Eggs are laid within the vessels, swept to alveolar capillaries, hatch, penetrate the alveolar spaces, migrate up to the trachea, and are swallowed. First stage larvae are excreted in the faeces and may survive two weeks or more in a moist milieu. Intermediate hosts (aquatic snails or terrestrial slugs) are infected either through the integument or by ingestion. Rats become infected by eating the intermediate hosts. Man acquires the disease by ingesting raw or insufficiently cooked invertebrates containing third stage larvae. About one-third of the patients present meningoencephalitis with fever. Four to thirty percent of deaths are attributed to cerebral haemorrhage. However, death is uncommon, sequelae are infrequent and seldom severe [238, 239]. Grossly, the meninges and brain tissue show focal necroses and haemorrhages. These lesions correspond to tracks caused by the worms that are frequently recovered from the subdural and subarachnoid spaces. Samples of brain freshly teased between glass slides may yield fragments of worms. Histologically, areas of necrosis are infiltrated with eosinophils, lymphocytes, histiocytes and foreign body giant cells. These are centered by vessels containing dead or degenerated meandering worms. Thrombosis may be present. Multiple small aneurysms may appear. When no worm is identified, glial scars containing eosinophils, Charcot-Leyden crystals and haemosiderin are highly suggestive of the diagnosis. In the lungs, a reaction to the parasite and/or its metabolic products causes fatal necrotizing angiitis to develop, mimicking Wegener's granulomatosis [240]. Angiostrongyliasis cannot be distinguished from other parasitic encephalitides, including visceral larva migrans, cysticercosis, coenurosis, trichinosis, schistosomiasis, gnathostomiasis and paragonimiasis.

2. *Angiostrongylus costaricensis* infection. *Angiostrongylus costaricensis*, discovered by Morera and Cespedes in 1971 has wide geographical distribution, occurring from the United States to

Argentina [241, 242]. *Angiostrongylus costariensis* normally live in the mesenteric arteries near the caecum in rats. Eggs laid in either the tissue or the capillaries of the intestinal wall embryonate. The first stage larvae leave the egg, migrate into the intestinal lumen and are excreted. Man is infected by eating unwashed vegetables contaminated by infective larvae. These penetrate the intestinal wall and mature in the lymphatics and lymph nodes; the young adults migrate to the arterioles of the gastro-intesinal tract causing gastrointestinal haemorrhage, ischaemic enterocolitis and abdominal mass [243-245]. The condition is characterised by prolonged fever, pain in the right iliac fossa, anorexia and, sometimes, vomiting, and acute abdomenal pain [246]. The intra-abdominal mass is characterised by transmural inflammatory granulomatous reaction, extensive eosinophilic infiltration, eosinophilic vasculitis and the presence of worms in the lumen of many arterial branches associated with thrombosis leading to severe ischaemic lesions. Degenerated eggs and dead worms are surrounded by giant cell granulomata.

Ascariasis

Ascaris lumbricoides, has a complex life cycle. In Man, larvae penetrate the intestinal wall, enter the lymphatic vessels and the portal vein, migrate through the liver to the heart and are then pumped through the pulmonary arteries to the lungs. There, the larvae break out of the alveolar capillaries and invade the air spaces. These larvae migrate up the bronchi to the trachea and are swallowed. Erratic migration of larvae in the circulatory system may produce thrombosis. Allergic granulomatous angiitis with fibrinoid necrosis and eosinophilia may also develop in patients with various parasite antigens, including Ascaris suum antigen [247]. These lesions are similar to those observed experimentally in mice [248].

Trematodes

Schistosomiasis (Bilharziasis)

Mesenteric, colonic and pancreatic veins become the permanent residence of this parasite. Worms can invade the vena cava, and the lungs via the pulmonary arteries [249, 250]. Experimental studies with S. mansoni demonstrate that murine endothelial cells, activated by cytokines are capable of killing schistosomula through an arginine-depen-

dent mechanism involving production of nitric oxide (NO). These observations indicate that endothelial cells play an important role in immunity to *S. mansoni* [251]. Females produce hundreds of eggs per day, around which granulomata and fibrosis develop, the major pathological manifestation in schistosomiasis. In veins, these granulomata induce granulomatous phlebitis (Fig. 22-23) with thrombosis and perivascular fibrosis giving rise to "pipestem" fibrosis (Fig. 24-25) and oesophageal varices [252]. Schistosome eggs, diverted to the lung via portal collaterals, may produce granulomatous pulmonary arteritis with intimal hyperplasia, progressive arterial obstruction, angiomatoid lesions similar to those of idiopathic pulmonary hypertension, and, ultimately, heart failure. In the colon, the mucosa displays ischaemic colitis with tortuous, focally dilated and narrowed mucosal and submucosal veins [253].

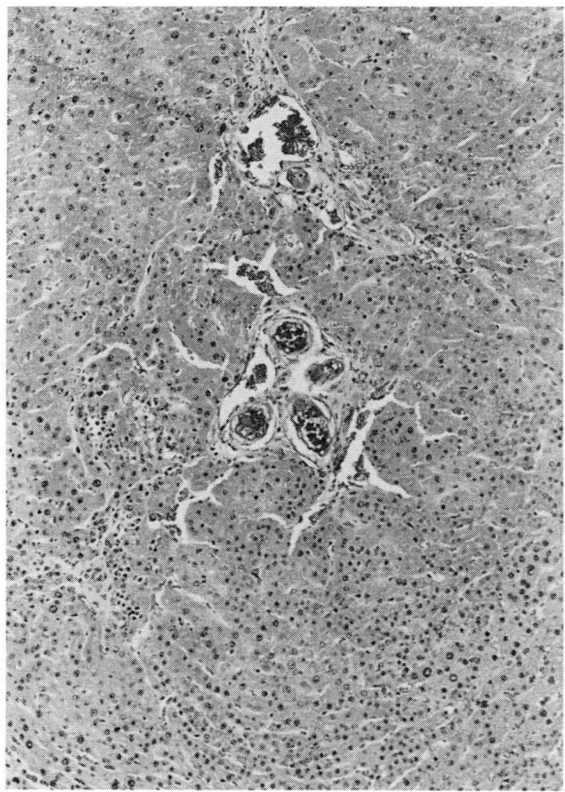

Fig. 22. Schistosomiasis. *Schistosoma haematobium* eggs clogging a portal vein. HES

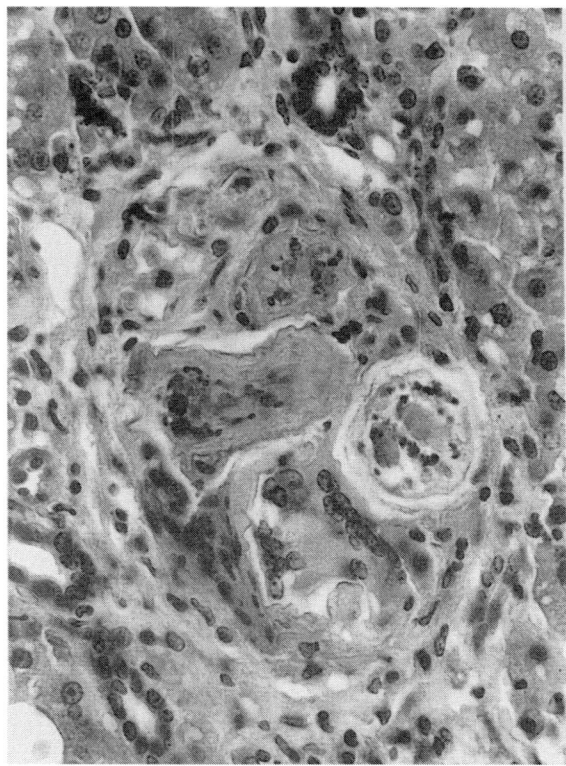

Fig. 23. Schistosomiasis. Granulomatous phlebitis involving a portal vein. Note a well preserved *Schistosoma haematobium* egg surrounded by multinucleated giant cells. HES

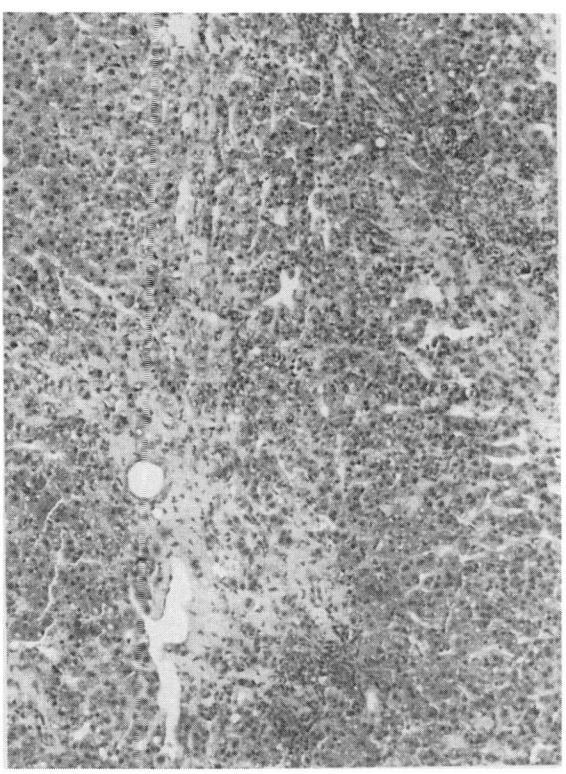

Fig. 24. Schistosomiasis. Liver pipestem fibrosis. Masson's trichrome

Cestodes

Coenurosis (Cenurosis, Cenuriasis)

This disease is produced by the presence of a cenuris cyst that, in sheep, causes a brain infection known as "gid" for the giddy gait induced in the infected animal. In contrast with hydatid disease, cerebral coenurosis is very unusual in man. Symptoms consist of repeated attacks of transient hemiparesis. The CSF shows lymphocytosis and increased immunoglobulins. Angiographic studies have shown an intracranial arteritis, probably secondary to the inflammatory reaction of the leptomeninges [254].

Aberrant sparganosis

This condition, caused by *Sparganum proliferum*, affects immuno-suppressed patients. The worm

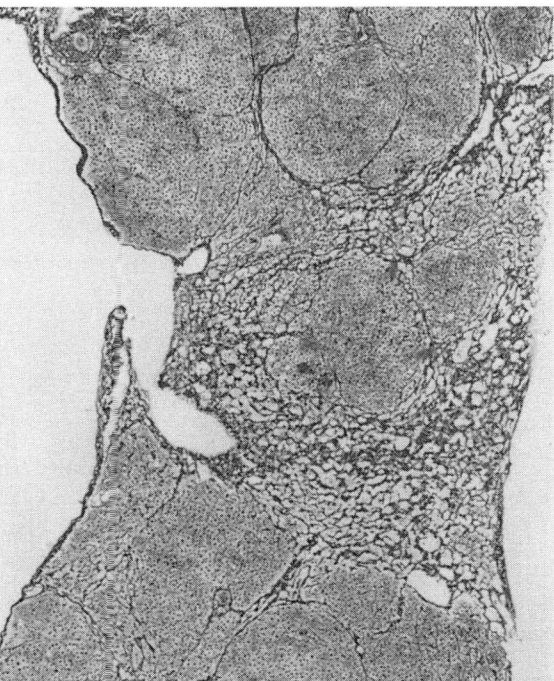

Fig. 25. Schistosomiasis. Liver pipestem fibrosis. Gordon-Sweet reticulin stain

grows by continuous branching and budding, and penetrates the blood vessels to spread to the body organs and lymph nodes through lymphatic vessels. Micro-abscesses formed around the parasite consist of granulation tissue, fibrosis and variable numbers of inflammatory cells, including lymphocytes, plasma cells, and neutrophils. Eosinophils, Charcot-Leyden crystals and non-destructive vasculitis may be present [255].

6 – Vascular diseases caused by fungi

Schematically, mycoses encompass two groups: the superficial, involving the skin, hair, nails and the mucosae only without systemic dissemination, and the deep mycoses, which invade and may disseminate by way of the blood stream and lymphatics to all parts of the body, giving rise to localized abscesses. Deep my-

Table 1. Staining techniques, results and limitations for diagnosis of fungi and actinomycotic infections (see Chandler 1980) (257)

MATERIAL	STAINING TECHNIQUES	RESULTS	COMMENTS
Smear	Giemsa, Wright, May-Grunwald	Blue fungi	Small yeasts, occasionally partially stained
	Grocott-Gomori methenamine-silver (GMS)	Black-brown fungi against a pale green background	*P. carinii, E. histolytica, Trichomonas, Giardia* also black
	India ink	*C.neoformans* (halos and cells) whitish on black background	
	Fluorescent antibody with fluresceine-isothiocyanate	Green-yellow fungi	
Histological section	Haematoxylin-eosin-saffron (HES)	Many fungi are blue	Not all fungi stain; some stain poorly
	Grocott-Gomori methenamine-silver (GMS)	Fungi are black-brown	Actinomycete filaments positive
	Periodic acid-Schiff (PAS)	Fungi reddish	
	Gridley	Hyphae, conidia, yeast capsules, elastin, and mucin appear in different shades of blue to purple	
	Mucicarmine (Mayer)	Specific stain for *C. neoformans*, mucoid capsule stains red	Some strains of *C. neoformans* without mucoid capsules are not stained
	Gram	Fungi partially stained	Actinomycetes and other bacteria positive
	Zeil -Nielsen	*Nocardia* mostly positive	Fungi not acid-fast

coses are frequent in patients whose immune function is depressed by severe debilitating diseases, including diabetes mellitus, leukaemia or lymphoma [256], and in individuals receiving immuno-suppressive drugs, broad spectrum antibiotics, corticosteroids, or a combination of these medicines. Several histological stains can be used to demonstrate fungi in tissue sections. With haematoxylin-eosin-saffron (HES) some fungi appear hyaline, others are unstained or poorly stained. The Grocott-Gomori methenamine silver (GMS), the Gridley and the periodic acid-Schiff (PAS) procedures help to identify fungi and their morphology. Table 1 indicates the staining techniques, their results and limitations in the diagnosis of fungal and actinomycotic infections.

Candidiasis (Candidosis, Moniliasis, Thrush)

Systemic candidiasis develops in debilitated patients, chiefly those suffering from immunodeficiency, or in drug addicts using intravenous injections [258]. A generalized fungaemia develops when blood vessels are invaded. Almost all organs may be involved. The most frequent species, apart from *C. albicans*, are *C. glabrata, C. guilliermondii, C krusei, C parapsilosis* and *C tropicalis* [259, 260]. Lesions in patients with systemic candidiasis are generally characterised by suppuration and necrosis especially in infection with *Candida albicans* [261]. Iatrogenic valvular endocarditis, and aortic rupture with large mycotic balls (candidomas) containing numerous *Candida sp.* (Fig. 26-27) may follow cardiac catheterisation or heart surgery [262, 263]. Fungal emboli from these candidomas lead to pulmonary and then to systemic candidiasis, distal embolism and acrocyanosis.

Lesions of angiitis and necrotising capillaritis (*Candida* vasculitis) associated with purpuric maculo-papular eruption and transitory presence of circulating immune complexes, may caused by Candidiasis. These symptoms and lesions may be induced by an intradermal test with candidine [264] and may unveil deep location of the disease. Associated fungal infections (aspergillosis, cryptococcosis) or synchronous septicemia are common.

Aspergillosis

There are four main pathogenic species of Aspergillus that cannot be distinguished histologically: *A. fumigatus, A. flavus, A.niger and A.terreus,* but more than 130 species are recognized.

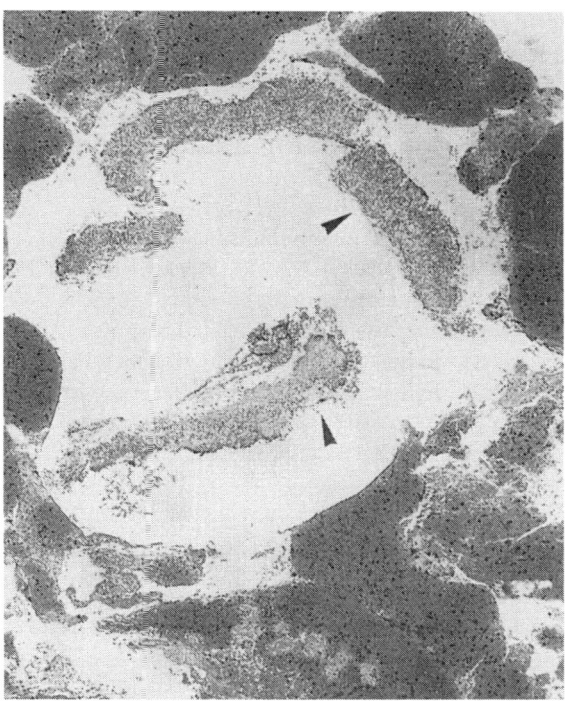

Fig. 26. Candiasis. Systemic candiasis with valvular endocarditis and candidoma embolism. (arrow heads: candidoma emboli). HES. (Courtesy Dr M. Romano)

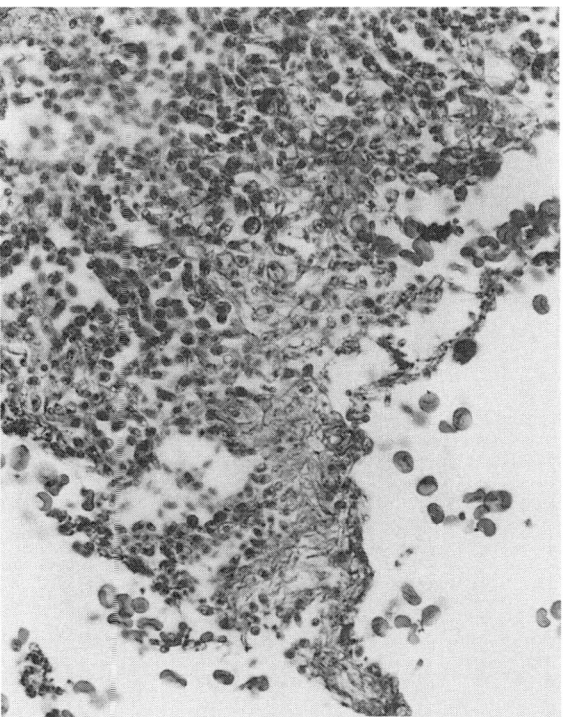

Fig. 27. Candiasis. Candida yeasts, filaments and leukocytes in a candidoma. Periodic acid-Schiff stain (PAS)

In the disseminated form, many organs, including the central nervous system, may be involved because of the propensity of the mycelium to invade blood vessels [265]. Hyphae penetrate walls of vessels directly, even those of the large muscular arteries without elastolysis [266] (Fig. 28-29). Multiple complications may appear, including aneurysms, occlusion, thrombosis, peripheral embolism (Fig.30), infarction and fatal haemorrhage [267-273]. Granulomatous lesions and abscesses may occur in many organs, especially the brain, meninges, and endocardium [274, 275].Calcium oxalate crystals, refractive to polarized light, are often associated with *A. niger* infection and their presence in biopsy and cytology specimens can be regarded as an important diagnostic aid [276, 277].

Zygomycosis (Phycomycosis, Mucormycosis)

This is a polymorphic disease entity caused by the various zygomycetes: fungi characterised by broad hyphae in tissues. In man there are two main types – the group *Mucorales* giving rise to mucormycosis, and the *Entomophthorales* responsible for entomophthoramycosis.

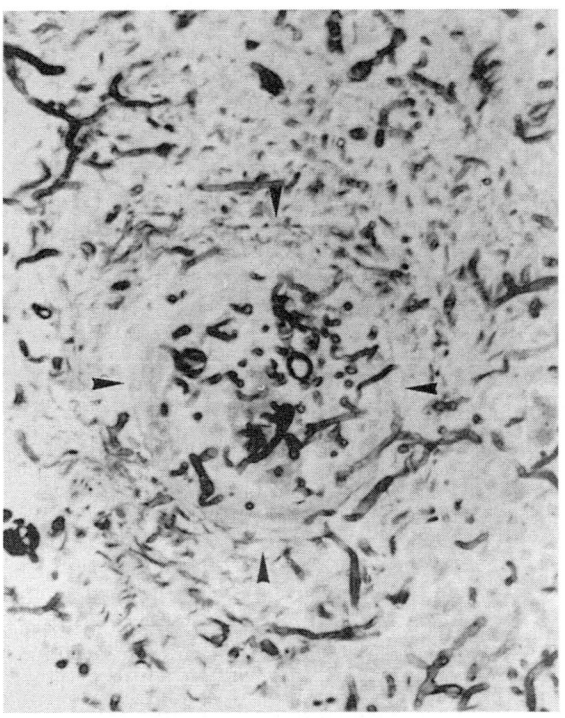

Fig. 28. Aspergillosis. *Aspergillus* hyphae invading an arterial wall (arrow heads). HES (Courtesy Dr M. Huerre)

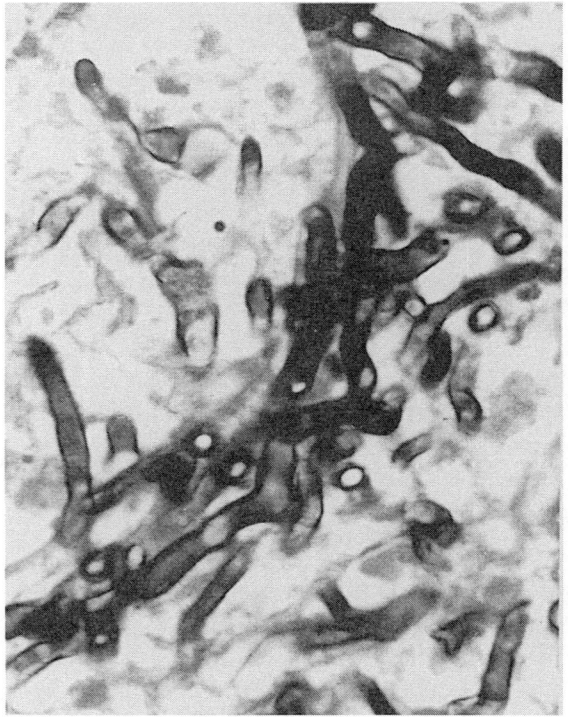

Fig. 29. Aspergillosis. *Aspergillus* hyphae. Grocott-Gomori methenamine-silver

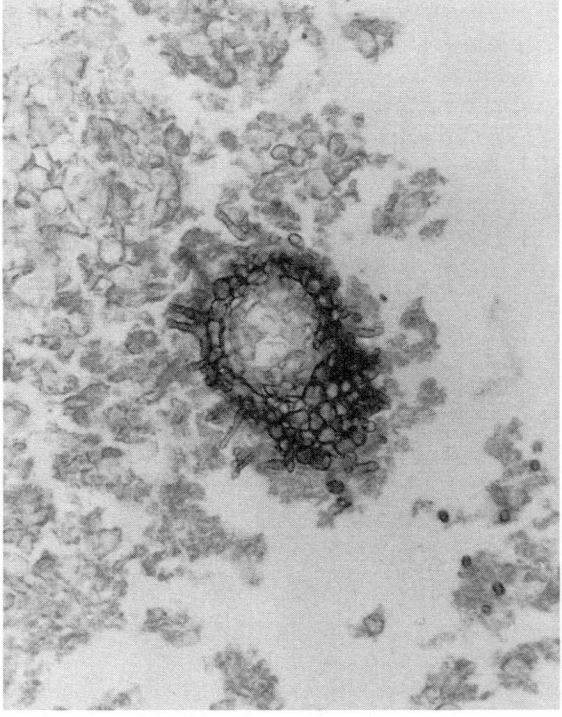

Fig. 30. Aspergillosis. An *Aspergillus* ball embolus among necrotic debris. Grocott-Gomori methenamine-silver

In Man, infection with the *Mucorales* mostly occurs in debilitated, immunocompromised, or acidotic patients (diabetus mellitus, malnutrition, severe burns, leukaemia and lymphoma, neoplasia, organ transplantation and immunosupression) [278-280]. Infections are usually fulminant, with the causative fungus exhibiting predilection for invasion of blood vessels with resultant infarction and necrosis. Nosocomial and iatrogenic infections have also been reported in healthy people and generally also present a fulminant course.

The portal of entry varies but may be via the skin, nose, lungs and the digestive tract. The *Mucorales* are peculiar for their great propensity to invade large and small arteries and, less frequently, veins (Fig. 31). Necrosis of vessel walls and mycotic thrombi (Fig. 32) lead to multiple fungal aneurysms, gangrene and fatal myocardial infarction with subsequent hematogenous or lymphatic dissemination [281-284]. Paradoxical thrombosis typifies the mucormycoses, the thromboses occurring simultaneously with massive haemorrhages in the vicinity of the thrombotic vessels. Secondary cutaneous and subcutaneous mucormycosis may be a source of obstructive lymphangitis when hyphae invade lymphatic vessels. Rhinocerebral mucormycosis results from pseudoaneurysm of the pulmonary artery and embolic spread to the brain, leading to fatal haemorrhage [285]. In areas of ischaemic necrosis, inflammation is sometimes minimal, despite the presence of numerous broad hyphae 10-20 microns, readily seen with the H & E stain [286]. These hyphae are wider than those of *Conidiobolus* and *Basidiobolus*, two genera of the group *Entomophthorales*. *Conidiobolus* infection mostly develops in the nasal mucosa after traumatic erosion and rarely becomes systemic. The *Basidiobolus* infection occurs anywhere on the skin with the formation of a subcutaneous nodule.

Paracoccidioidomycosis (Luzt-Splendore-Almeida's disease)

This condition is caused by *Paracoccidioides brasiliensis*. Paracoccidioidomycosis and blastomycosis have many similarities. Cardiovascular involvement consists of myocarditis with miliary epithelioid granulomata made up of macrophages. Hypertrophy of the right ventricle is caused by long-standing, chronic and fibrotic pulmonary lesions. Occasionally, fungal arteritis, with formation of thrombi containing fungi, develops in large vessels. Infection of arterial walls takes place by direct spread from lymph nodes and

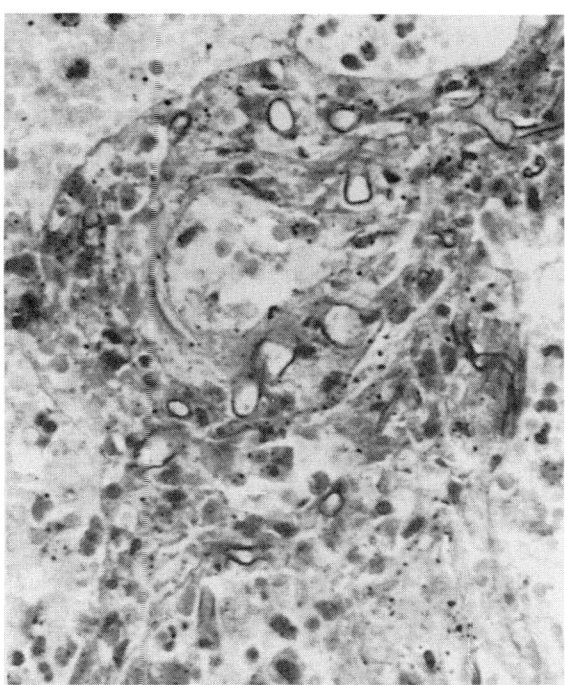

Fig. 31. Zygomycosis. *Mucor* mycotic ball. Grocott-Gomori methenamine-silver

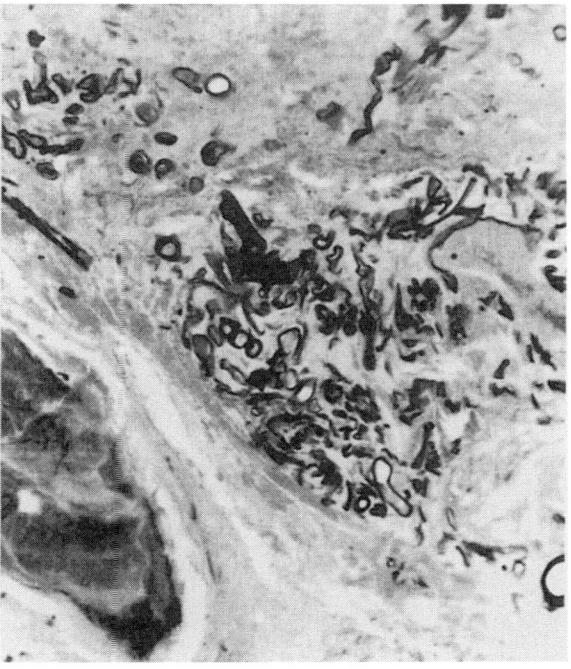

Fig. 32. Zygomycosis. Venous mycotic thrombosis. Grocott-Gomori methenamine-silver. (Courtesy Dr M. Huerre)

the lymphatic channels that become pseudotumours in later stages [287, 288]. Exceptionally, a granulomatous vasculitis may be noted with c-ANCA positivity [289]. Experimentally, these changes are correlated with the immune response of the infected animals [290-292].

Blastomycosis (North American blastomycosis, Gilchrist's disease)

This chronic granulomatous and suppurative disease of man and lower animals is caused by *Blastomyces dermitis*. In the systemic form, the infection may be confined to the lungs or may spread to other viscera and tissues of the body. When the skin is involved, the fungus produces an ulcerated or verrucous lesion, generally located on exposed body surfaces. Lymphangitis may develop with the formation of blastomycotic nodules along the lymph vessels [293, 294]. A positive culture is the gold standard of diagnosis; occasionally, the organism can be identified by its typical "shoe print" morphology with periodic acid-Schiff (PAS) stain. More sensitive serologic techniques (sandwich enzyme immunoassay and 120-kd antigen radioimmunoassay) and DNA probes have significantly improved the sensitivity of laboratory diagnosis [295, 296].

Histoplasmosis

Histoplasmosis is a localised or systemic mycotic disease of man and lower animals. There are two types of the organism, *Histoplasma capsulatum var. duboisii* causes a clinically distinct disease, African histoplasmosis, in which large yeast cells with thicker walls are found in tissues, in contrast to the better studied small celled *Histoplasma capsulatum var. farciminosum*, which typically causes pulmonary infections and epizootic lymphangitis. Histoplasmosis is a mainly pulmonary infection contracted by inhaling airborne fungi from soil contaminated by chicken or bat faeces (for example). Benign primary infection (common in the midwestwern United States) leads first to a solitary pulmonary subpleural lesion then involves the lymphatic vessels to disseminate towards regional lymph nodes, giving rise to the classical primary complex. The lymphatic vessels display lymphangitis. Active primary infection frequently produces a self-limiting hematogenous dissemination with small miliary lesions in the liver and spleen; however, the disseminated form is progressive and fatal if untreated.

Extended primary infection leads to multiple primary foci in both lungs. The spores are disseminated throughout the body by way of the blood vessels and set up early foci of infection within abundant histiocytes (lymph nodes, bone marrow, liver, spleen and lymphatic system of the digestive tract). In the immunosuppresed or poorly nourished, widespread involvement of all vital organs and tissues occurs with death a few weeks after the onset of the disease [297, 298]. This form of the disease was first recognised in the workers digging the Panama canal.

Disseminated histoplasmosis has been reported to cause enodocarditis and mycotic aneurysm of the thoracic aorta [299]. *Histoplasma capsulatum* can be found in the thrombi of cardiac valves and vascular emboli. Tissue reaction consists of a granulomatous inflammation with great numbers of yeast cells within the cytoplasm of histiocytes and monocytes (Fig. 33). Langhans' cells, epithelioid cells, and lymphocytes may be present. Fibrosis occurs in the chronic form. Prominent leukocytoclasia and associated dermal necrosis may be seen around the superficial blood vessels of the dermis in skin infections in patients with AIDS. These lesions should not be misinterpreted as atypical leukocytoclastic vasculitis [300].

Sporotrichosis

This disease, caused by *Sporothrix schenckii*, is usually limited to the skin and subcutaneous tissues. The portals of entry are injuries and scratches of the skin with single or multiple primary skin lesions. In the skin, the initial lesion usually develops on an exposed part of the body [301, 302]. From this site, the disease spreads along the path of lymphatic drainage and the lymphatic vessel becomes an indurated cord (Fig. 34).A series of secondary nodules or ulcerated lesions develop with adjacent osteoarticular involvement. Each nodule breaks down, ulcerates and discharges pus. Typical granulomata are often centered by microabcesses made up of polymorphonuclear leukocytes, cellular debris, caseous material and yeast-form cells of *S. schenckii*. Yeast cells are either free or surrounded by Splendore-Hoeppli material (the asteroid body) (Fig. 35). Exceptionally haematogenous dissemination may occur with subsequent systemic disease in bones, viscera and brain in AIDS patients [303, 304].

Scedosporium apiospermum infection

Also called *Monosporium apiospermum*, this imperfect state of the fungus *Pseudallescheria boydii* is one of the

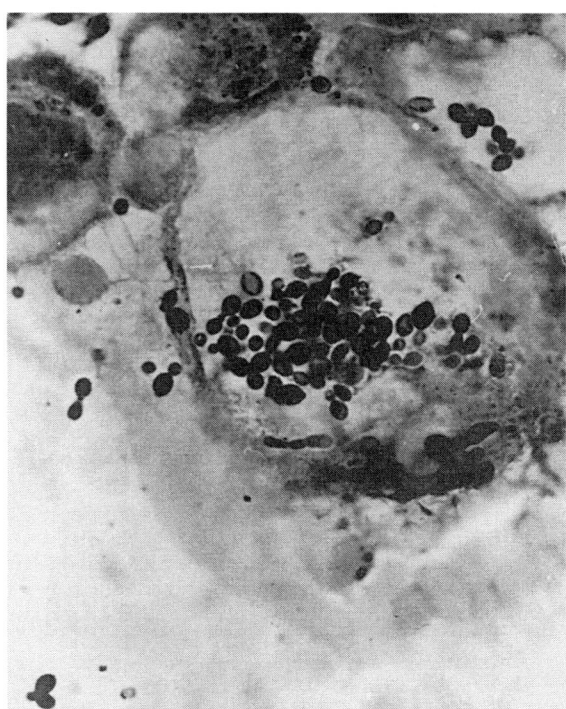

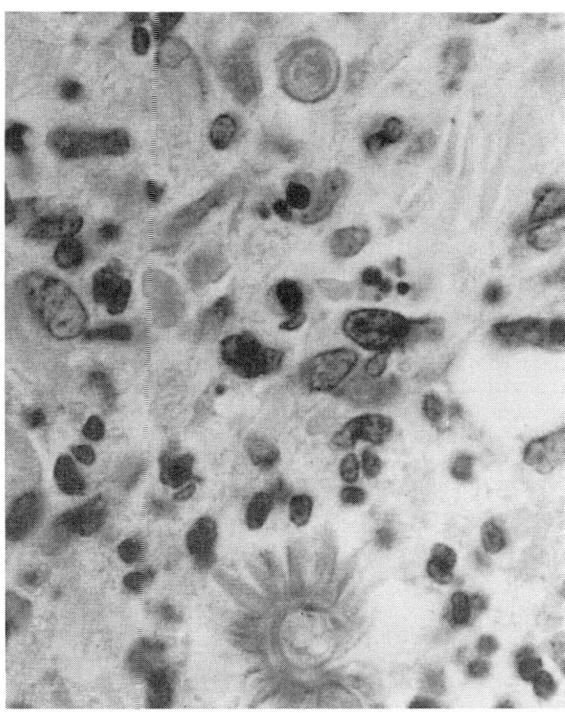

Fig. 33. Histoplasmosis. *Histoplasma capsulatum* yeast cells within the cytoplasm of histiocytes. Grocott-Gomori methenamine-silver

Fig. 35. Sporotrichosis. *Sporothrix schenckii* yeasts with Splendor-Hoepli phenomenon. HES. (Courtesy Dr M. Huerre)

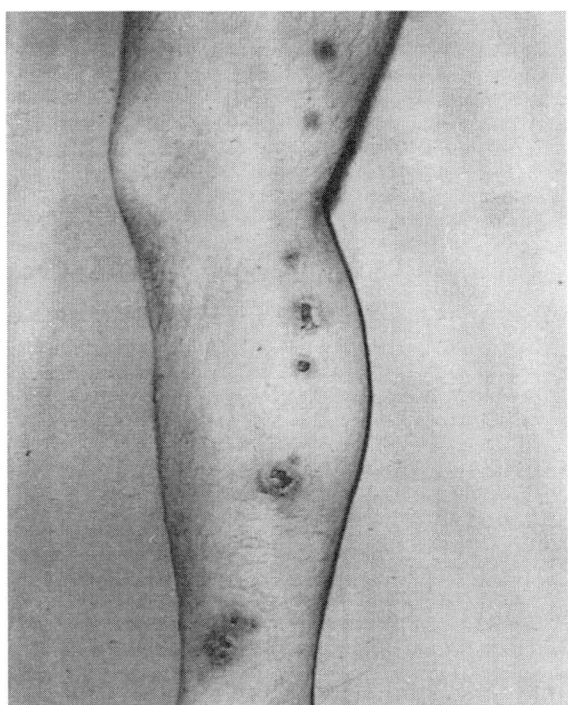

Fig. 34. Sporotrichosis. Nodular abcesses developed along a lymphatic drainage path of the leg (Courtesy Dr M. Huerre)

16 species of true fungi that may cause mycetoma in man. Disseminated infection may be fatal in immunocompromised hosts. Numerous fungal colonies develop in the lungs, heart, brain, kidney, spleen and liver. Involvement of vessels give rise to fungal mycotic aneurysms with secondary multiple abscesses [125, 305]. Lymphocutaneous infection produces suppurating cutaneous nodules spreading in a linear fashion up the limb, following the line of the lymphatic drainage, mimicking sporotrichosis [306, 307].

Bibliography

1. Lie JT (1996) Vasculitis associated with infectious agents. Curr Opin Rheumatol 8: 26-9
2. Coyle PK, Gerber O, Roque C (1997) Vasculitis owing to infection. Neurol Clin 15: 903-25
3. Mandell BF, Calabrese LH (1998) Infections and systemic vasculitis. Curr Opin Rheumatol 10: 51-7
4. Leung DY, Meissner C, Fulton D, Schlievert PM (1995) The potential role of bacterial superantigens in the pathogenesis of Kawasaki syndrome. J Clin Immunol 15: S11-S17
5. Gluck T, Straub RH, Scholmerich J, Lang B (1997) Infections and vasculitis. Z Rheumatol 56: 105-13
6. Genereau T, Tri Nguyen Q, Lortholary O, Cohen P, Guillevin L (1995) Vasculitis of viral origin. Pathogenesis and therapeutic implications. J Mal Vasc 20: 1-7

7. Guillevin L, Lhote F, Gherardi R (1997) The spectrum and treatment of virus-associated vasculitides. Curr Opin Rheumatol 9: 31-6

8. Martinez Aguilar NE, Guido Bayardo R, Vargas Camano ME, Compan Gonzalez D, Miranda Feria AJ (1997) Vasculitis and viral infection. Rev Alerg Mex 44: 23-30

9. Child PL (1976) Viral hemorrhagic fevers *In* Binford CH, Connor DH (Eds.) Pathology of tropical and extraordinary diseases, AFIP, Washington DC, p5-11

10. Butthep P, Bunyaratvej A, Bhamarapravati N (1993) Dengue virus and endothelial cell: a related phenomenon to thrombocytopenia and granulocytopenia in dengue haemorrhagic fever. Southeast Asian J Trop Med Public Health 24: 246S-249S

11. Hathirat P, Isarangkura P, Srichaikul T, Suvatte V, Mitrakul C (1993) Abnormal hemostasis in dengue haemorrhagic fever. Southeast Asian J Trop Med Public Health 24: S80-S85

12. Boonpucknavig V, Bhamarapravati N, Boonpucknavig S, Futrakul P, Tanpaichitr P (1976) Glomerular changes in dengue haemorrhagic fever. Arch Pathol Lab Med 100: 206-12

13. Boonpucknavig S, Boonpucknavig V, Bhamarapravati N, Nimmannitya S (1979) Immunofluorescence study of skin rash in patients with dengue haemorrhagic fever. Arch Pathol Lab Med 103: 463-6

14. Sahaphong S, Riengrojpitak S, Bhamarapravati N, Chirachariyavej T (1980) Electron microscopic study of the vascular endothelial cell in dengue haemorrhagic fever. Southeast Asian J Trop Med Public Health 11: 194-204

15. Yu HS, Wang MT, Tai CL, Yang SA, Chien CH (1989) Skin eruption and histopathological changes in dengue fever. Kao Hsiung I Hsueh Ko Hsueh Tsa Chih 5: 17-23

16. Riikonen RS (1995) Retinal vasculitis caused by rubella. Neuropediatrics 26: 174-6

17. Wynne JM, Williams GL, Ellman BA (1977) Gangrene of the extremities in measles. S Afr Med J 52: 117-21

18. Mazure G, Grundy JE, Nygard G, Hudson M, Khan K, Srai K, Dhillon AP, Pounder RE, Wakefield AJ (1994) Measles virus induction of human endothelial cell tissue factor procoagulant activity *in vitro*. J Gen Virol 75: 2863-71

19. Blumberg S, Bienfang D, Kantrowitz FG (1980) A possible association between influenza vaccination and small-vessel vasculitis. Arch Intern Med 140: 847-8

20. Costa MM, Lisboa M, Romeu JC, Caldeira J, De Queiroz V (1995) Henoch-Schonlein purpura associated with coxsackie-virus B1 infection. Clin Rheumatol 14: 488-90

21. Gaches F, Loustaud V, Vidal E, Delaire L, Guiard-Schmid JB, Lavoine E, Negrier P, Liozon F (1993) Periarteritis nodosa and *parvovirus B19* infection. Rev Med Interne 14: 323-5

22. Ilan Y, Hillman M, Oren R, Zlotogorski A, Shouval D (1990) Vasculitis and cryoglobulinemia associated with persisting cholestatic hepatitis A virus infection. Am J Gastroenterol 85: 586-7

23. Dumoulin FL, Klein P, Fischer HP, Spengler U, Sauerbruch T (1994) Chronic hepatitis C in type-II cryoglobulinemia and cutaneous vasculitis. Dtsch Med Wochenschr 119: 1239-42

24. Bonkovsky HL, Liang TJ, Hasegawa K, Banner B (1995) Chronic leukocytoclastic vasculitis complicating HBV infection. Possible role of mutant forms of HBV in pathogenesis and persistence of disease. J Clin Gastroenterol 21: 42-7

25. Mouthon L, Deblois P, Sauvaget F, Meyrier A, Callard P, Guillevin L (1995) Hepatitis B virus-related polyarteritis nodosa and membranous nephropathy. Am J Nephrol 15: 266-9

26. Buezo GF, Garcia-Buey M, Rios-Buceta L, Borque MJ, Aragues M, Dauden E (1996) Cryoglobulinemia and cutaneous leukocytoclastic vasculitis with hepatitis C virus infection. Int J Dermatol 35: 112-5

27. Daoud MS, el-Azhary RA, Gibson LE, Lutz ME, Daoud S (1996) Chronic hepatitis C, cryoglobulinemia, and cutaneous necrotizing vasculitis. Clinical, pathologic, and immunopathologic study of twelve patients. J Am Acad Dermatol 34: 219-23

28. Jacq F, Emmerich J, Heron E, Lortholary O, Bruneval P, Fiessinger JN (1997) Distal gangrene and cryoglobulinemia related to hepatitis C virus infection with presence of anticardiolipin antibodies. Rev Med Interne 18: 324-7

29. Press J, Maslovitz S, Avinoach I (1997) Cutaneous necrotizing vasculitis associated with hepatitis A virus infection. J Rheumatol 24: 965-7

30. Turki S, Guillevin L, Dallot A, Jarrousse B, Vernier I, Laroche L, Pourrat J, Amouroux J (1994) Nodular and granulomatous form of periarteritis nodosa caused by the hepatitis B virus. Ann Dermatol Venereol 121: 325-7

31. Darras-Joly C, Lortholary O, Cohen P, Brauner M, Guillevin L (1995) Regressing microaneurysms in 5 cases of hepatitis B virus related polyarteritis nodosa. J Rheumatol 22: 876-80

32. Sepp NT, Umlauft F, Illersperger B, Grunewald K, Schuler G, Greil R, Vogel W (1995) Necrotizing vasculitis associated with hepatitis C virus infection: successful treatment of vasculitis with interferon-alpha despite persistence of mixed cryoglobulinemia. Dermatology 191: 43-5

33. Schirren CA, Zachoval R, Schirren CG, Gerbes AL, Pape GR (1995) A role for chronic hepatitis C virus infection in a patient with cutaneous vasculitis, cryoglobulinemia, and chronic liver disease. Effective therapy with interferon-alpha. Dig Dis Sci 40: 1221-5

34. Manna R, Todaro L, Latteri M, Gambassi G, Massi G, Grillo MR, Romito A, Caputo S, Gasbarrini GB (1997) Leucocytoclastic vasculitis associated with hepatitis C virus antibodies. Br J Rheumatol 36: 124-5

35. Nityanand S, Holm G, Lefvert AK (1997) Immune complex mediated vasculitis in hepatitis B and C infections and the effect of antiviral therapy. Clin Immunol Immunopathol 82: 250-7

36. Munoz A, Vinuela F, Mesa A, Fernandez JM, Garcia Moreno JM, Izquierdo G (1995) CNS vasculitis after ophthalmic *herpes zoster* infection. Rev Neurol 23: 1063-6

37. Terborg C, Busse O (1995) Granulomatous vasculitis of the CNS as a complication of herpes zoster ophthalmicus. Fortschr Neurol Psychiatr 63: 383-7

38. Dangler CA, Baker SE, Kariuki Njenga M, Chia SH (1995) Murine *cytomegalovirus*-associated arteritis. Vet Pathol 32: 127-33

39. Golden MP, Hammer SM, Wanke CA, Albrecht MA (1994) *Cytomegalovirus* vasculitis. Case reports and review of the literature. Medicine (Baltimore) 73: 246-55

40. Pouria S, State OI, Wong W, Hendry BM (1998) CMV infection is associated with transplant renal artery stenosis. QJM 91: 185-9

41. Koskinen PK, Nieminen MS, Krogerus LA, Lemstrom KB, Mattila SP, Hayry PJ, Lautenschlager IT (1993) *Cytomegalovirus* infection and accelerated cardiac allograft vasculopathy in human cardiac allografts. J Heart Lung Transplant 12: 724-9

42. Koskinen P, Lemstrom K, Bruggeman C, Lautenschlager I, Hayry P (1994) Acute cytomegalovirus infection induces a subendothelial inflammation (endothelialitis) in the allograft vascular wall. A possible linkage with enhanced allograft arteriosclerosis. Am J Pathol 144: 41-50

43. Manito N, Perez JL, Roca J, Niubo J, Gausi C, Castells E (1995) The significance of *cytomegalovirus* infection in the period after a heart transplant. Rev Esp Cardiol 48: S108-S114

44. Melnick JL, Adam E, Debakey ME (1993) *Cytomegalovirus* and atherosclerosis. Eur Heart J 14: S30-S38

45. Yonemitsu Y, Komori K, Sueishi K, Sugimachi K (1998) Possible role of *cytomegalovirus* infection in the pathogenesis of human vascular diseases. Nippon Rinsho 56: 102-8

46. Hendrix MGR, Daemen M, Bruggeman CA (1991) Cytomegalovirus nucleic acid distribution within the human vascular tree. Am J Pathol 138: 563-7

47. Paton P, Tabib A, Loire R, Tete R (1993) Coronary artery lesions and human immunodeficiency virus infection. Res Virol 144: 225-31

48. Capron L, Kim YU, Laurian C, Bruneval P, Fiessinger JN (1992) Atheroembolism in HIV-positive individuals (Letter). Lancet 340: 1039-40

49. Bayad J, Galteau MM, Siest G (1993) Viral theory of atherosclerosis. Role of cytomegalovirus. Ann Biol Clin (Paris) 51: 101-7

50. Kol A, Sperti G, Maseri A (1997) Association between prior cytomegalovirus infection and the risk of restenosis after coronary atherectomy. N Engl J Med 336: 587-8

51. Adler SP, Hur JK, Wang JB, Vetrovec GW (1998) Prior infection with cytomegalovirus is not a major risk factor for angiographically demonstrated coronary artery atherosclerosis. J Infect Dis 177: 209-12

52. Kennedy MM, Cooper K, Howells DD, Picton S, Biddolph S, Lucas SB, McGee JO, O'Leary JJ (1998) Identification of HHV8 in early Kaposi's sarcoma: implications for Kaposi's sarcoma pathogenesis. Mol Pathol 51: 14-20

53. Muralidhar S, Pumfery AM, Hassani M, Sadaie MR, Azumi N, Kishishita M, Brady JN, Doniger J, Medveczky P, Rosenthal LJ (1998) Identification of kaposin (open reading frame K12) as a human *herpesvirus 8* (Kaposi's sarcoma-associated herpesvirus) transforming gene. J Virol 72: 4980-8

54. Cathomas G (2000) Human herpes virus 8: a new virus discloses its face.Virchow Arch 436: 195-206

55. Lasota J, Miettinen M (1999) Absence of Kaposi's sarcoma-associated virus (human herpesvirus-8) sequences in angiosarcoma. Virchows Arch 434: 51-6

56. Kang GH, Kwon GY, Kim CW (1998) Human *herpesvirus 8* in Kaposi's sarcoma and Kaposi's sarcoma-mimicking vascular tumors. J Korean Med Sci 13: 54-9

57. Chamouard JM, Smadja D, Chaunu MP, Bouche P (1993) Neuropathy caused by necrotizing vasculitis in HIV-1 infection. Rev Neurol (Paris) 149: 358-61

58. Gherardi R, Belec L, Mhiri C, Gray F, Lescs MC, Sobel A, Guillevin L, Wechsler J (1993) The spectrum of vasculitis in human immunodeficiency virus-infected patients. A clinicopathologic evaluation. Arthritis Rheum 36: 1164-74

59. Boggian K, Leu HJ, Schneider J, Turina M, Oertle D (1994) True aneurysm of the ascending aorta in HIV disease. Schweiz Med Wochenschr 124: 2083-7

60. Dronda F, Gonzalez-Lopez A, Lecona M, Barros C (1996) Erythema elevatum diutinum in human immunodeficiency virus-infected patients—report of a case and review of the literature. Clin Exp Dermatol 21: 222-5

61. Brannagan III TH (1997) Retroviral-associated vasculitis of the nervous system. Neurol Clin 15: 927-44

62. Calabrese LH (1991) Vasculitis and infection with the human immunodeficiency virus. Rheum Dis Clin North Am 17: 131-47

63. Gray F, Geny C, Lionnet F, Dournon E, Fenelon G, Gherardi F., Poirier J (1991) Neuropathologic study of 135 adult cases of acquired immunodeficiency syndrome. Ann Pathol 11: 236-47

64. Ruchelli ED, Nojadera G, Rutstein RM, Rudy B (1994) Pulmonary veno-occlusive disease. Another vascular disorder associated with human immunodeficiency virus infection? Arch Pathol Lab Med 118: 664-6

65. Escamilla R, Hermant C, Berjaud J, Mazerolles C, Daussy X (1995) Pulmonary veno-occlusive disease in a HIV-infected intravenous drug abuser. Eur Respir J 8: 1982-4

66. Roh SS, Gertner E (1997) Digital necrosis in acquired immune deficiency syndrome vasculopathy treated with recombinant tissue plasminogen activator. J Rheumatol 24: 2258-61

67. Mesa RA, Edell ES, Dunn WF, Edwards WD (1998) Human immunodeficiency virus infection and pulmonary hypertension: two new cases and a review of 86 reported cases. Mayo Clin Proc 73: 37-45

68. Massari M, Salvarani C, Portioli I, Ramazzotti E, Gabbi E, Bonazzi L (1996) Polyarteritis nodosa and HIV infection: no evidence of a direct pathogenic role of HIV. Infection 24: 159-61

69. Tinkle BT, Ngo L, Luciw PA, Maciag T, Jay G (1997) Human immunodeficiency virus-associated vasculopathy in transgenic mice. J Virol 71: 4809-14

70. Wisseman CL Jr, Waddell A (1983) Interferonlike factors from antigen– and mitogen-stimulated human leukocytes with antirickettsial and cytolytic actions on *Rickettsia prowazekii*. Infected human endothelial cells, fibroblasts, and macrophages. J Exp Med 157: 1780-93

71. Feng HM, Wen J, Walker DH (1993) Rickettsia australis infection: a murine model of a highly invasive vasculopathic rickettsiosis. Am J Pathol 142: 1471-82

72. Davi G, Giammarresi C, Vigneri S, Ganci A, Ferri C, Di Francesco L, Vitale G, Mansueto S (1995) Demonstration of Rickettsia Conorii -induced coagulative and platelet activation *in vivo* in patients with Mediterranean spotted fever. Thromb Haemost 74: 631-4

73. Kao GF, Evancho CD, Ioffe O, Lowitt MH, Dumler JS (1997) Cutaneous histopathology of Rocky Mountain spotted fever. J Cutan Pathol 24: 604-10

74. Ng FK, Oaks SC Jr, Lee M, Groves MG, Lewis GE Jr (1985) A scanning and transmission electron microscopic examination of *Rickettsia tsutsugamushi* -infected human endothelial, MRC-5, and L-929 cells. Jpn J Med Sci Biol 38: 125-39

75. Fournier PE, Casalta JP, Piquet P, Tournigand P, Branchereau A, Raoult D (1998) *Coxiella burnetii* infection of aneurysms or vascular grafts: report of seven cases and review. Clin Infect Dis 26: 116-21

76. Hall WC, Bagley LR (1978) Identification of Rickettsia rickettsii in formalin-fixed, paraffin-embedded tissues by immunofluorescence. J Clin Microbiol 8: 242-5

77. Scaffidi L, Scaffidi A (1981) Characteristics of the rash in Mediterranean boutonneuse fever. Minerva Med 72: 2085-96

78. Walker TS (1984) Rickettsial interactions with human endothelial cells *in vitro*: adherence and entry. Infect Immun 44: 205-10

79. Walker TS, Mellott GE (1993) Rickettsial stimulation of endothelial platelet-activating factor synthesis. Infect Immun 61: 2024-9

80. Kaplanski G, Teysseire N, Farnarier C, Kaplanski S, Lissitzky JC, Durand JM, Soubeyrand J, Dinarello CA, Bongrand P (1995) IL-6 and IL-8 production from cultured human endothelial cells stimulated by infection with *Rickettsia conorii* via a cell-associated IL-1 alpha-dependent pathway. J Clin Invest 96: 2839-44

81. Montenegro MR, Mansueto S, Hegarty BC, Walker DH (1983) The histology of "taches noires" of boutonneuse fever and demonstration of *Rickettsia conorii* in them by immunofluorescence. Virchows Arch A Pathol Anat Histopathol 400: 309-17

82. Gip LS (1989) Yaws revisited. Med J Malaysia 44: 307-11

83. Engelkens HJ, Vuzevski VD, Judanarso J, van Lier JB, van der Stek J, van der Sluis JJ, Stolz E (1990) Early yaws: a light microscopic study. Genitourin Med 66: 264-6

84. Drobacheff C, Moulin T, Van Landuyt H, Merle C, Vigan M, Laurent R (1994) Cutaneous tertiary syphilis with neurological symptoms. Ann Dermatol Venereol 121: 34-6

85. Jordaan HF (1986) Widespread superficial thrombophlebitis as a manifestation of secondary syphilis—a new sign. A report of 2 cases. S Afr Med J 70: 493-4

86. Berkmen YM (1986) Medical aspects of infectious aortitis *In* Lande A, Berkmen YM and McAllister HA (ed) Aortitis: Clinical, Pathologic and Radiographic aspects. Raven Press, New York p: 161-72

87. Engelkens HJ, ten Kate FJ, Judanarso J, Vuzevski VD, van Lier JB, Godschalk JC, van der Sluis JJ, Stolz E (1993) The localisation of treponemes and characterisation of the inflammatory infiltrate in skin biopsies from patients with primary or secondary syphilis, or early infectious yaws. Genitourin Med 69: 102-7

88. Molin A, Alvarez Sabin J, Malagelada A, Codina A (1992) Hemiparesis-ataxia in meningovascular syphilis. Neurologia 7: 190-3

89. Peters M, Gottschalk D, Boit R, Pohle HD, Ruf B (1993) Meningovascular neurosyphilis in human immunodeficiency virus infection as a differential diagnosis of focal CNS lesions: a clinicopathological study. J Infect 27: 57-62

90. Fedotov VV, Aminev KhK, Shcheglov AG, Saprykina GD (1995) The involvement of the cardiovascular system in syphilis. Klin Med (Mosk) 73: 27-30

91. Johansson EA, Niemi KM, Mustakallio KK (1977) A peripheral vascular syndrome overlapping with systemic lupus erythematosus. Recurrent venous thrombosis and haemorrhagic capillary proliferation with circulating anticoagulants and false-positive seroreactions for syphilis. Dermatologica 155: 257-67

92. MacLeod CB, Johnson D, Frable WJ (1992) «Tree-barking» of the ascending aorta. Syphilis or systemic lupus erythematosus? Am J Clin Pathol 97: 58-62

93. O'Brien TJ, Mcdonald MI, Reid BF, Trethewie D (1995) Streptococcal septic vasculitis. Australas J Dermatol 36: 211-3

94. Escamilla Y, Gutierrez M, Martinez T, Bodoque M, Gomez JM, Moreno A (1996) Vasculitis caused by *Pseudomonas*: a case report. Acta Otorrinolaringol Esp 47: 404-6

95. Jones R, Kirton OC (1996) Lung microvessel injury from peritoneal abscesses and gram-negative bacteremia. Microvasc Res 52: 84-100

96. Sailors DM, Eidt JF, Gagne PJ, Barnes RW, Barone GW, McFarland DR (1996) Primary *Clostridium septicum* aortitis: a rare cause of necrotizing suprarenal aortic infection. A case report and review of the literature. J Vasc Surg 23: 714-8

97. Carreras M, Larena JA, Tabernero G, Langara E, Pena JM (1997) Evolution of *salmonella* aortitis towards the formation of abdominal aneurysm Eur Radiol 7: 54-6

98. Gauthier T, So AK (1997) Vasculitis and bacteraemia with *Yersinia enterocolitica* in late-onset systemic lupus erythematosus. Br J Rheumatol 36: 1122-4

99. La Scola B, Musso D, Carta A, Piquet P, Casalta JP (1997) Aortoabdominal aneurysm infected by *Yersinia enterocolitica* serotype O: 9. J Infect 35: 314-5

100. Resche S, Karacatsanis C, Minet J, Lestrat A, Jego P, Grosbois B (1997) *Yersinia enterocolitica* suppurated phlebitis (Letter). Presse Med 26: 1238

101. Grotemeyer D, Graupe F, Mackrodt HG, Stock W (1998) *Salmonella enteritidis* infected false aneurysm of the superficial femoral artery in an HIV seropositive patient. Chirurg 69: 204-6

102. Semba CP, Sakai T, Slonim SM, Razavi MK, Kee ST, Jorgensen MJ, Hagberg RC, Lee GK, Mitchell RS, Miller DC, Dake MD (1998) Mycotic aneurysms of the thoracic aorta: repair with use of endovascular stent-grafts. J Vasc Interv Radiol 9: 33-40

103. Smail A, Ducroix JP, Tondriaux A, Sevestre H, Yzet T, Baillet J (1988) The role of infection in the precipitation of periarteritis nodosa. Ann Med Interne (Paris) 139: 324-30

104. Anderson DG, Warner G, Barlow E (1995) Kawasaki disease associated with streptococcal infection within a family. J Paediatr Child Health 31: 355-7

105. Ekman-Joelsson BM, Kjellman B, Hattevig G (1995) Tongue necrosis due to vasculitis. Acta Paediatr 84: 1333-6

106. Malcic I, Buljevic AD, Vucinic D, Carin R (1996) Polyarteritis nodosa—cutaneous or systemic form? Possible role of bacterial superantigens in the onset of systemic disease. Reumatizam 43: 16-24

107. van Putten JW, van Haren EH, Lammers JW (1996) Association between Wegener's granulomatosis and *Staphylococcus aureus* infection? Eur Respir J 9: 1955-7

108. Leung DY, Sullivan KE, Brown-Whitehorn TF, Fehringer AP, Allen S, Finkel TH, Washington RL, Makida R, Schlievert PM (1997) Association of toxic shock syndrome toxin-secreting and exfoliative toxin-secreting *Staphylococcus aureus* with Kawasaki syndrome complicated by coronary artery disease. Pediatr Res 42: 268-72

109. Abe Y, Nakano S, Aita K, Sagishima M (1998) Streptococcal and staphylococcal superantigen-induced lymphocytic arteritis in a local type experimental model: comparison with acute vasculitis in the Arthus reaction. J Lab Clin Med 131: 93-102

110. Garcia-Caceres U, Garcia FU (1991) Bartonellosis. An immunodepressive disease and the life of Daniel Alcides Carrion. Am J Clin Pathol 95: S58-S66

111. Arias-Stella J, Lieberman PH, Erlandson RA, Arias-Stella J Jr (1986) Histology, immunohistochemistry, and ultrastructure of the verruga in Carrion's disease. Am J Surg Pathol 10: 595-610

112. Garcia FU, Wojta J, Broadley KN, Davidson JM, Hoover RL (1990) *Bartonella bacilliformis* stimulates endothelial cells *in vitro* and is angiogenic *in vivo*. Am J Pathol 136: 1125-35

113. Arias-Stella J, Lieberman PH, Garcia-Caceres U, Erlandson RA, Kruger H, Arias-Stella J Jr (1987) Verruga peruana mimicking malignant neoplasms. Am J Dermatopathol 9: 279-91

114. Arrese Estrada J, Pierard GE (1992) Dendrocytes in verruga peruana and bacillary angiomatosis. Dermatology 184: 22-5

115. Caceres-Rios H, Rodriguez-Tafur J, Bravo-Puccio F, Maguina-Vargas C, Diaz CS, Ramos DC, Patarca R (1995) Verruga peruana: an infectious endemic angiomatosis. Crit Rev Oncog 6: 47-56

116.– Cockerell CJ, Tierno PM, Friedman-Kien AE, Kim KS (1991) Clinical, histologic, microbiologic and biochemical characterization of the causative agent of bacillary (epithelioid) angiomatosis: a rickettsial illness with features of bartonellosis. J Invest Dermatol 97: 812-7

117. Slater LN, Welch DF, Min KW (1992) *Rochalimaea hanselae* causes bacillary angiomatosis and peliosis hepatis. Arch Intern Med 152: 602-6

118. Stoler MH, Bonfiglio TA, Steigbigel RT, Pereira M (1983) An atypical subcutaneous infection associated with acquired immunodeficiency syndrome. Am J Clin Pathol 80: 714-8

119. Relman DA, Loutit JS, Schmidt TM, Falkow S, Tompkins LS (1990) The agent of bacillary angiomatosis. An approach to the identification of uncultured pathogens. N Engl J Med 323: 1573-80

120. Schwartz RA, Nychay SG, Janniger CK, Lambert WC (1997) Bacillary angiomatosis: presentation of six patients, some with unusual features. Br J Dermatol 136: 60-5

121. LeBoit PE, Berger TG, Egbert BM, Beckstead JH, Yent TSB, Stoler MH (1989) Bacillary angiomatosis. The histopathology and differential diagnosis of a pseudoneoplastic infection in patient with human immunodeficiency virus disease. Am J Surg Pathol 13: 909-20

122. Mainguene C, Moreau A, Hofman P, Milpied-Homsi B, Roulot D, Marullo S, Clauvel J-P, Lenne Y, Amouroux J (1993) Péliose bacillaire au cours du Sida. Etude anatomo-clinique de 2 observations. Ann Pathol 13: 341-5

123. Sanchez MA, Rorat E (1996) Fine needle aspiration diagnosis of intramuscular bacillary angiomatosis. A case report. Acta Cytol 40: 751-5

124. Lopez-Elzaurdia C, Fraga J, Sols M, Burgos E, Sanchez Garcia M, Garcia Diez A (1991) Bacillary angiomatosis associated with cytomegalovirus infection in a patient with AIDS. Br J Dermatol 125: 909-20

125. Hofman P, Lacour J Ph, Michiels JF, Saint-Paul MC, Perrin C (1993) Angiomatose bacillaire et infection à Cytomégalovirus cutanées au cours du SIDA: une association fortuite? Ann Pathol 13: 194-5

126. Guarner J, Unger ER (1990) Association of Epstein-Barr virus in epithelioid angiomatosis of AIDS patients. Am J Surg Pathol 14: 956-60

127. Borczuk AC, Niedt G, Sablay LB, Kress Y, Mannion CM, Factor SM, Tanaka KE (1998) Fibrous long-spacing collagen in bacillary angiomatosis. Ultrastruct Pathol 22: 127-33

128. Muller HE (1997) Cat-scratch disease: historical, clinical, phylogenetic and taxonomic aspects. Tierarztl Prax 25: 94-9

129. Soheilian M, Markomichelakis N, Foster CS (1996) Intermediate uveitis and retinal vasculitis as manifestations of cat scratch disease. Am J Ophthalmol 122: 582-4

130. Selby G, Walker GL (1979) Cerebral arteritis in cat-scratch disease. Neurology 29: 1413-8

131. Aguado JM, Barros C, Gomez Garces JL, Fernandez-Guerrero ML(1987) Infective aortitis due to *Brucella melitensis*. Scand J Infect Dis 19: 483-4

132. Franco Vicario R, Balparda J, Santamaria JM, Alvaro C, Arizaga C, de la Villa FM, Arrinda JM, Fernandez Moral R, Celada A (1985) Cutaneous vasculitis in a patient with acute brucellosis. Dermatologica 171: 126-8

133. Boudghene-Stambouli O, Merad-Boudia A, Ghernaout-Benchouk S (1994) Allergic vasculitis in brucellosis. Ann Dermatol Venereol 121: 240-1

134. Yrivarren JL, Lopez LR (1987) Cryoglobulinemia and cutaneous vasculitis in human brucellosis. J Clin Immunol 7: 471-4

135. Vazquez Doval FJ, Ruiz de Erenchun Lasa F, Sola Casas MA, Soto de Delas J, Quintanilla Gutierrez E (1991) Acute brucellosis presenting as leukocytoclastic vasculitis. J Investig Allergol Clin Immunol 1: 411-3

136. Hermida I Garcia F, Ramos C, Yus C, Losfablos F (1994) Necrotizing vasculitis as cutaneous manifestation of brucellosis. Enferm Infec Microbiol Clin 12: 515-6

137. Elzouki AY, Akthar M, Mirza K (1996) Brucella endocarditis associated with glomerulonephritis and renal vasculitis. Pediatr Nephrol 10: 748-51

138. Kuo CC, Shor A, Campbell LA, Fukushi H, Patton DL, Grayston T (1993) Demonstration of *Chlamydia pneumoniae* in atherosclerotic lesions of coronary arteries. J Infect Dis 167: 841-9

139. Blasi F, Denti F, Erba M, Cosentini R, Raccanelli R, Rinaldi A, Fagetti L, Esposito G, Ruberti U, Allegra L (1996) Detection of *Chlamydia pneumoniae* but not *Helicobacter pylori* in atherosclerotic plaques of aortic aneurysms. J Clin Microbiol 34: 2766-9

140. Miettinen H, Lehto S, Saikku P, Haffner SM, Ronnemaa T, Pyorala K, Laakso M (1996) Association of Chlamydia pneumoniae and acute coronary heart disease events in non-insulin dependent diabetic and non-diabetic subjects in Finland. Eur Heart J 17: 682-8

141. Ong G, Thomas BJ, Mansfield AO, Davidson BR, Taylor-Robinson D (1996) Detection and widespread distribution of Chlamydia pneumoniae in the vascular system and its possible implications. J Clin Pathol 49: 102-6

142. Andreasen JJ (1997) *Chlamydia* pneumoniae and atherosclerosis. Ugeskr Laeger 159: 5503-7

143. Chiu B, Viira E, Tucker W, Fong IW (1997) *Chlamydia pneumoniae, cytomegalovirus*, and *herpes simplex* virus in atherosclerosis of the carotid artery. Circulation 96: 2144-8

144. Jackson LA, Campbell LA, Kuo CC, Rodriguez DI, Lee A, Grayston JT (1997) Isolation of *Chlamydia pneumoniae* from a carotid endarterectomy specimen. J Infect Dis 176: 292-5

145. Laitinen K, Laurila A, Pyhala L, Leinonen M, Saikku P (1997) *Chlamydia pneumoniae* infection induces inflammatory changes in the aortas of rabbits. Infect Immun 65: 4832-5

146. Kousa M, Saikku P, Kanerva L (1980) Erythema nodosum in chlamydial infections. Acta Derm Venereol 60: 319-22

147. Ljungstrom L, Franzen C, Schlaug M, Elowson S, Viidas U (1997) Reinfection with *Chlamydia pneumoniae* may induce isolated and systemic vasculitis in small and large vessels. Scand J Infect Dis Suppl 104: 37-40

148. Coruh G, McDougall AC (1979) Untreated lepromatous leprosy: histopathological findings in cutaneous blood vessels. Int J Lepr Other Mycobact Dis 47: 500-11

149. Yajima M, Narita M (1997) Pathology of the heart and blood vessels in Hansen's disease. Nihon Hansenbyo Gakkai Zasshi 66: 109-18

150. Yajima M, Murata J, Yamada N, Asano G (1991) Ultrastructural observations of small blood vessels in leprosy patients. Nippon Rai Gakkai Zasshi 60: 121-7

151. Kaur S, Wahi PL, Chakravarti RN, Sodhi JS, Vadhwa MB, Khera AS (1976) Peripheral vascular deficit in leprosy. Int J Lepr Other Mycobact Dis 44: 332-9

152. Johnson AC, Reddy R, Johnson S, James AE Jr (1978) Lower limb angiography in leprosy. Radiology 126: 327-32

153. Yadav SS (1978) Arteriographic evaluation of vascular changes in leprosy. Angiology 29: 17-21

154. Agrawal BR, Agrawal RI (1985) Arteriography in leprosy. Indian J Lepr 57: 138-45

155. Mukherjee A, Misra RS, Meyers WM (1989) An electron microscopic study of lymphatics in the dermal lesions of human leprosy. Int J Lepr Other Mycobact Dis 57: 506-10

156. Chopra JS, Kaur S, Murthy JM, Kumar B, Radhakrishnan K, Suri S, Sawhney BB (1981) Vascular changes in leprosy and its role in the pathogenesis of leprous neuritis. Lepr India 53: 443-53

157. Kumar V, Narayanan RB, Malaviya GN (1989) An ultrastructural study of blood vessels in peripheral nerves of leprosy patients: blood vessels in peripheral nerves. Nippon Rai Gakkai Zasshi 58: 179-84

158. Looi LM, Jayalakshim P, Lim KJ, Rajagopalan K (1988) An immunohistochemical and morphological study of amyloidosis complicating leprosy in Malaysian patients. Ann Acad Med Singapore 17: 573-8

159. Giam YC, Ong BH, Tan T (1987) Erythema nodosum leprosum in Singapore. Ann Acad Med Singapore 16: 658-62

160. Anthony J, Vaidya MC, Dasgupta A (1983) Ultrastructure of skin in erythema nodosum leprosum. Cytobios 36: 17-23

161. Chimelli L, Freitas M, Nascimento O (1997) Value of nerve biopsy in the diagnosis and follow-up of leprosy: the role of vascular lesions and usefulness of nerve studies in the detection of persistent bacilli. J Neurol 244: 318-23

162. Rea TH, Ridley DS (1979) Lucio's phenomenon: a comparative histological study. Int J Lepr Other Mycobact Dis 47: 161-6

163. Pursley TV, Jacobson RR (1980) Lucio's phenomenon. Arch Dermatol 116: 201-4

164. Saul A, Novales J (1983) Lucio-Latapi leprosy and the Lucio phenomenon. Acta Leprol 1: 115-32

165. Nicodemo AC, Del Negro G, Amato Neto V (1990) Thrombocytopenia and leptospirosis. Rev Inst Med Trop Sao Paulo 32: 252-9

166. Tokonami F, Imamura S, Suga M, Tokunaga K, Fukuda Y (1993) A case of Listeria rhombencephalitis with a secondary vasculitis suggested by MRI. Rinsho Shinkeigaku 33: 637-41

167. Silbergleit A, Arbulu A, Defever BA, Nedwicki EG (1965) Tuberculous aortitis. Surgical resection of ruptured abdominal false aneurysm. JAMA 193: 333-5

168. Volini FI, Olfield RCJr, Thompson JR, Kent G (1962) Tuberculosis of the aorta. JAMA 181: 78-83

169. Sellers AL, Light JG, Friedman NB (1976) Acute anuric renal failure secondary to tuberculous aortitis of the thoracic aorta. JAMA 236: 1384-5

170. Felson B, Akers PV, Hall GS, Schrelber JT, Greene RE, Pedrosa CS (1977) Mycotic tuberculous aneurysm of the thoracic aorta. JAMA 237: 1104-8

171. Gajaraj A, Victor S (1981) Tuberculous aortitis. Clin Radiol 32: 461-6

172. Sais G, Vidaller A, Jucgla A, Peyri J (1996) Tuberculous lymphadenitis presenting with cutaneous leucocytoclastic vasculitis. Clin Exp Dermatol 21: 65-6

173. Huerre MR, Piens MA (1996) Protozoa histopathology. Arch Anat Cytol Path 44: 209-24

174. Fretes RE, de Fabro SP (1995) Human chagasic placenta: structural and cytochemical changes of blood vessels. Rev Fac Cien Med Univ Nac Cordoba 53: 11-5

175. Bijovsky AT, Milder RV, Abrahamsohn IA, Sinhorini IL, Mariano M (1984) The influence of lymphatic drainage in experimental Trypanosoma cruzi infection. Acta Trop 41: 207-14

176. Tanowitz HB, Burns ER, Sinha AK, Kahn NN, Morris SA, Factor SM, Hatcher VB, Bilezikian JP, Baum SG, Wittner M (1990) Enhanced platelet adherence and aggregation in Chagas' disease: a potential pathogenic mechanism for cardiomyopathy. Am J Trop Med Hyg 43: 274-81

177. Okumura M (1996) Pathogenesis of chagasic myocarditis: an experimental study. Rev Hosp Clin Fac Med Sao Paulo 51: 166-74

178. Andrade ZA, Andrade SG, Correa R, Sadigursky M, Ferrans VJ (1994) Myocardial changes in acute Trypanosoma cruzi infection. Ultrastructural evidence of immune damage and the role of microangiopathy. Am J Pathol 144: 1403-11

179. Gardiner PR, Assoku RK, Whitelaw DD, Murray M (1989) Haemorrhagic lesions resulting from Trypanosoma vivax infection in Ayrshire cattle. Vet Parasitol 31: 187-97

180. Machado CR, Ribeiro AL (1989) Experimental American trypanomiasis in rats: sympathetic denervation, parasitism and inflammatory process. Mem Inst Oswaldo Cruz 84: 549-56

181. Torres FW, Acquatella H, Condado JA, Dinsmore R, Palacios IF (1995) Coronary vascular reactivity is abnormal in patients with Chagas' heart disease. Am Heart J 129: 995-1001

182. Factor SM, Cho S, Wittner M, Tanowitz H (1985) Abnormalities of the coronary microcirculation in acute murine Chagas' disease. Am J Trop Med Hyg 34: 246-53

183. De Morais CF, Higuchi ML, Lage S (1989) Chagas' heart disease and myocardial infarct. Incidence and report of four necropsy cases. Ann Trop Med Parasitol 83: 207-14

184. Lopes ER, de Mesquita PM, de Mesquita LF, Chapadeiro E (1995) Coronary arteriosclerosis and myocardial infarction in chronic Chagas' disease. Arq Bras Cardiol 65: 143-5

185. Rossi MA (1991) The pattern of myocardial fibrosis in chronic Chagas' heart disease. Int J Cardiol 30: 335-40

186. Reis DD, Jones EM, Tostes S, Lopes ER, Chapadeiro E, Gazzinelli G, Colley DG, McCurley TL (1993) Expression of major histocompatibility complex antigens and adhesion molecules in hearts of patients with chronic Chagas' disease. Am J Trop Med Hyg 49: 192-200

187. Veress B, el Hassan AM (1986) Vascular changes in human leishmaniasis: a light microscope and immunohistological study. Ann Trop Med Parasitol 80: 183-8

188. Essa MH, Mangoud AM, Morsy TA, Aly MA, Salama MM (1989) Vascular changes in cutaneous leishmaniasis. J Egypt Soc Parasitol 19: 683-7

189. Lemaistre AI, Chapel F, Cie P, Jeantils V, Guettier C (1997) Unusual vascular lesions in the course of a colonic leishmaniasis in an HIV positive patient. Ann Pathol 17: 200-2

190. Connor DH, Neafie RC, Hockmeyer WT (1976) Malaria In Binford CH, Connor DH (Eds.) Pathology of tropical and extraordinary diseases, AFIP, Washington DC, p 273-283

191. Boonpucknavig V, Boonpucknavig S, Udomsangpetch R, Nitiyanant P (1990) An immunofluorescence study of ce-

rebral malaria. A correlation with histopathology. Arch Pathol Lab Med 114: 1028-34

192. van der Wall EE, Padmos I, Cats VM (1988) Coronary arterial aneurysm: possible relation with malaria? Int J Cardiol 21: 351-3

193. Wedderburn N, Davies DR, Mitchell GH, Desgranges C, de The G (1988) Glomerulonephritis in common marmosets infected with *Plasmodium brasilianum* and Epstein-Barr virus. J Infect Dis 158: 789-94

194. Andrade Junior HF, Corbett CE, Laurenti MD, Duarte MI (1991) Comparative and sequential histopathology of *Plasmodium chabaudi*-infected Balb/c mice. Braz J Med Biol Res 24: 1209-18

195. Khan ZM, Vanderberg JP (1991) Eosinophil-rich, granulomatous inflammatory response to Plasmodium berghei hepatic schizonts in nonimmunized rats is age-related. Am J Trop Med Hyg 45: 190-201

196. Kremsner PG, Neifer S, Chaves MF, Rudolph R, Bienzle U (1992) Interferon-gamma induced lethality in the late phase of *Plasmodium vinckei* malaria despite effective parasite clearance by chloroquine. Eur J Immunol 22: 2873-8

197. Boulard Y, Coquelin F, Mora Silvera E, Renia L, Gautret P, Deharo E, Snounou G, Vuong PN, Chabaud A, Landau I (1996) Dendritic leukocytes as possible carriers of murine *Plasmodium* merozoites. Preliminary notes. Parasite. 4: 383-6

198. Mora-Silvera E, Coquelin F, Vuong P, Deharo E, Gautert P, Renia L, Chabaud A, Landau I (1997) Role of macrophages as possible transporters of *Plasmodium Yoeli Nigerinesis* mezoroites through the lymphatic system. Preliminary note. Parasite 4: 83-5

199. Udomsangpetch R, Chivapat S, Viriyavejakul P, Riganti M, Wilairatana P, Pongponratin E, Looareesuwan S (1997) Involvement of cytokines in the histopathology of cerebral malaria. Am J Trop Med Hyg 57: 501-6

200. Vuong PN, Richard F, Snounou G, Coquelin F, Renia L, Gonnet F, Chabaud AG, Landau I (1999) Development of irreversible lesions in the brain, heart and kidney following acute and chronic murine malaria infection. Parasitology 119: 543-53

201. Bourdeix O, Andreu JM, Sartelet H, Diallo B, Brissiaud JC, Vicq P, Michel G (1996) Post-partum malignant amoebic colitis. Apropos of a case. Ann Chir 50: 566-9

202. Flores-Romo L, Estrada-Garcia T, Shibayama-Salas M, Campos-Rodriguez R, Bacon K, Martinez-Palomo A, Tsutsumi V (1997) *In vitro Entamoeba histolytica* adhesion to human endothelium: a comparison using two strains of different virulence. Parasitol Res 83: 397-400

203. Helton J, Loveless M, White CR Jr (1993) Cutaneous *acanthamoeba* infection associated with leukocytoclastic vasculitis in an AIDS patient. Am J Dermatopathol 15: 146-9

204. Luvuno FM, Mtshali Z, Baker LW (1985) Vascular occlusion in the pathogenesis of complicated amoebic colitis: evidence for an hypothesis. Br J Surg 72: 123-7

205. Martinez AJ, Guerra AE, Garcia-Tamayo J, Cespedes G, Gonzalez-Alfonzo JE, Visvesvara GS (1994) Granulomatous amoebic encephalitis: a review and report of a spontaneous case from Venezuela. Acta Neuropathol (Berl) 87: 430-4

206. van der Lugt JJ, Van der Merwe HE (1990) Amoebic meningoencephalitis in a sheep. J S Afr Vet Assoc 61: 33-6

207. Myung K, Massougbodji A, Ekoue S, Atchade P, Kiki-Fagla V, Klion AD (1998) Lymphatic filariasis in a hyperendemic region: a ten-year, follow-up panel survey. Am J Trop Med Hyg 59: 222-6

208. Gilbert HM, Hartman BJ (1996) Short report: a case of fibrosing mediastinitis caused by Wuchereria bancrofti. Am J Trop Med Hyg 54: 596-9

209. Noroes J, Addiss D, Amaral F, Coutinho A, Medeiros Z, Dreyer G (1996) Occurrence of living adult Wuchereria bancrofti in the scrotal area of men with microfilaraemia. Trans R Soc Trop Med Hyg 90: 55-6

210. Dissanayake S, Watawana L, Piessens WF (1995) Lymphatic pathology in *Wuchereria bancrofti* microfilaraemic infections. Trans R Soc Trop Med Hyg 89: 517-21

211. Freedman DO, Horn TD, Maia e Silva CM, Braga C, Maciel A (1995) Predominant CD8+ infiltrate in limb biopsies of individuals with filarial lymphoedema and elephantiasis. Am J Trop Med Hyg 53: 633-8

212. Dresden MH, Ewert A (1984) Collagen metabolism in experimental filariasis. J Parasitol 70: 208-12

213. Sakamoto M, Meier JL, Folse DS, Ewert A (1985) Perturbation of lymphatic endothelial cells in experimental *Brugia malayi* infections. Microcirc Endothelium Lymphatics 2: 487-98

214. Kaiser L, Mupanomunda M, Williams JF (1996) *Brugia pahangi*-induced contractility of bovine mesenteric lymphatics studied *in vitro*: a role for filarial factors in the development of lymphoedema? Am J Trop Med Hyg 54: 386-90

215. Yazdanbakash M, Abadi K, de Roo M, van Wouwe L, Denham D, Medeiros F, Verduijn W, Schreuder GM, Schipper R, Giphart MJ, de Vries RR (1997) HLA and elephantiasis revisited. Eur J Immunogenet 24: 439-42

216. Meyers WM, Neafie RC, Moris R, Bourland J (1977) Streptocerciasis: observation of adult male *Dipetalonema streptocerca* in man. Am J Trop Med Hyg 26: 1153-5

217. Ewert A, Smith JH, Corredor A (1981) Microfilariae of *Mansonella ozzardi* in human skin biopsies. Am J Trop Med Hyg 30: 988-91

218. George GH, Palmieri JR, Connor DH (1985) The onchocercal nodule: interrelationship of adult worms and blood vessels. Am J Trop Med Hyg 34: 1144-8

219. Smith RJ, Cotter TP, Williams JF, Guderian RH (1988) Vascular perfusion of *Onchocerca volvulus* nodules. Trop Med Parasitol 39: S418-S421

220. Vuong-Ngoc P, Bain O, Petit G, Chabaud AG (1986) Anatomo-pathologic study of skin and ocular lesions in rodents infested by *Monanema* spp.: significance for the study of human onchocerciasis. Ann Parasitol Hum Comp 61: 311-20

221. Vuong PN, Spratt D, Wanji S, Aimard L, Bain O (1993) *Onchocerca*-like lesions induced by the filarioid nematode Cercopithifilaria johnstoni, in its natural hosts and in the laboratory rat. Ann Parasitol Hum Comp 68: 176-81

222. Vuong PN, Wanji S, Prod'Hon J, Bain O (1994) Subcutaneous nodules and cutaneous lesions caused by different Onchocerca in African cattle. Rev Elev Med Vet Pays Trop 47: 47-51

223. Bain O, Wanji S, Vuong PN, Marechal P, Le Goff L, Petit G (1994) Larval biology of six filariae of the sub-family Onchocercinae in a vertebrate host. Parasite 1: 241-54

224. Vuong PN, Traoré S, Wanji S, Diarrassouba S, Balaton A, Bain O (1992) Ivermectin in human onchocerciasis: A clinical-pathological study of skin lesions before and three days after the treatment. Ann Parasitol Hum Comp 67: 194-6

225. Gibson DW, Connor DH (1978) Onchocercal lymphadenitis: Clinicopathologic study of 34 patients. Trans R Soc Trop Med Hyg 72: 137-54

226. Tada Y (1992) Analysis of body-length distribution of *Dirofilaria immitis* in the cardio– pulmonary blood vessel of naturally infected dogs in Shiga Prefecture, Japan. J Vet Med Sci 54: 53-6

227. McCracken MD, Patton S (1993) Pulmonary arterial changes in feline dirofilariasis. Vet Pathol 30: 64-9

228. Sato T, Nogami S, Nakagaki K, Inoue I, Shirai W, Araki K (1994) Histopathology of the lungs of rabbits experimentally infected with *Dirofilaria immitis*. J Comp Pathol 110: 403-6

229. Matsukura Y, Washizu M, Kondo M, Motoyoshi S, Itoh A, Nakajyo S, Shimizu K, Urakawa N (1997) Decreased pulmonary arterial endothelium-dependent relaxation in heartworm-infected dogs with pulmonary hypertension. Am J Vet Res 58: 171-4

230. Badhe BP, Sane SY (1989) Human pulmonary dirofilariasis in India: a case report. J Trop Med Hyg 92: 425-6

231. Saida Y, Miyakawa E, Kon Y, Tsunoda HS, Matsueda K, Tanaka Y, Nozawa K, Kurosaki Y, Itai Y (1992) CT of pulmonary dirofilariasis—differential diagnosis from lung cancer. Nippon Igaku Hoshasen Gakkai Zasshi 52: 1273-80

232. Kawamura S, Yasuoka C, Koga H, Tashiro T, Etoh H, Ashida M, Araki J, Asai S, Izumikawa KI, Ayabe H, Kohno S (1996) Two cases of pulmonary dirofilariasis in Nagasaki Prefecture. Kansenshogaku Zasshi 70: 746-51

233. Milanez de Campos JR, Barbas CS, Filomeno LT, Fernandez A, Minamoto H, Filho JV, Jatene FB (1997) Human pulmonary dirofilariasis: analysis of 24 cases from Sao Paulo, Brazil. Chest 112: 729-33

234. Paleologo FP, Neafie RC, Connor DH (1984) Lymphadenitis caused by Loaloa. Am J Trop Med Hyg 33: 395-402

235. Abo-Shehada MN, Al-Zubaidy BA, Herbert IV (1984) The migration of larval *Toxocara canis* in mice. I. Migration through the intestine in primary infections. Vet Parasitol 17: 65-73

236. Grunebaum M, Ziv N, Kornreich L (1986) The sonographic evaluation of the great vessels' interspace in the pediatric retroperitoneum. Pediatr Radiol 16: 384-7

237. Weatherley AJ, Hamilton JM (1984) Possible role of histamine in the genesis of pulmonary arterial disease in cats infected with *Toxocara cati*. Vet Rec 114: 347-9

238. Koo J, Pien F, Kliks MM (1988) *Angiostrongylus (Parastrongylus)* eosinophilic meningitis. Rev Infect Dis 10: 1155-62

239. Hwang KP, Chen ER (1991) Clinical studies on *angiostrongyliasis cantonensis* among children in Taiwan. Southeast Asian J Trop Med Public Health 22: S194-S199

240. Pirisi M, Gutierrez Y, Minini C, Dolcet F, Beltrami CA, Pizzolito S, Pitzus E, Bartoli E (1995) Fatal human pulmonary infection caused by an *Angiostrongylus*-like nematode. Clin Infect Dis 20: 59-65

241. Mojon M (1994) Human angiostrongyliasis caused by *Angiostrongylus costaricensis*. Bull Acad Natl Med 178: 625-31

242. Pena GP, Andrade Filho J, de Assis SC (1995) *Angiostrongylus costaricensis*: first record of its occurrence in the State of Espirito Santo, Brazil, and a review of its geographic distribution. Rev Inst Med Trop Sao Paulo 37: 369-74

243. Silvera CT, Ghali VS, Roven S, Heimann J, Gelb A (1989) Angiostrongyliasis: a rare cause of gastrointestinal haemorrhage. Am J Gastroenterol 84: 329-32

244. Duarte Z, Morera P, Vuong PN (1991) Abdominal angiostrongyliasis in Nicaragua: a clinico-pathological study on Ann Parasitol Hum Comp 66: 259-62

245. Vazquez JJ, Boils PL, Sola JJ, Carbonell F, de Juan Burgueno M, Giner V, Berenguer-Lapuerta J (1993) Angiostrongyliasis in a European patient: a rare cause of gangrenous ischaemic enterocolitis. Gastroenterology 105: 1544-9

246. Fauza D de O, Maksoud Filho JG, el Ibrahim R (1990) Acute abdomen in childhood caused by intestinal *angiostrongylus* infection: a case report. AMB Rev Assoc Med Bras 36: 150-2

247. Kobayashi A, Maeda K, Fu A, Hamada K, Chou S, Kunimatsu M, Narita N (1996) Allergic granulomatous angiitis in a patient with positive reactions on serological tests for parasite antigens. Nippon Kyobu Shikkan Gakkai Zasshi 34: 1130-5

248. Alwie ML, Wakaki K, Kurashige Y, Koizumi F (1995) Experimental granulomatous vasculitis induced by sensitization with Ascaris suum antigen in mice. Pathol Int 45: 914-24

249. Bayssade-Dufour C, Vuong PN, Farhati K, Picot H, Albaret J-L (1994) Experimental schistosomiasis: The speed of skin penetration of cercariae and the initial migration route of schistosomulae in *Schistosoma haematobium* infection of *Meriones unguiculatus*. CR Acad Sci, Paris.Sciences de la vie/Life Sciences 317: 529-33.

250. Vuong PN, Bayssade-Dufour Ch, Albaret JL, Farhati K (1996) Histo-pathological observations in new and classical models of experimental *Schistosoma haematobium* infections. Trop Med International Health 1: 348-58

251. Oswald IP, Eltoum I, Wynn TA, Schwartz B, Caspar P, Paulin D, Sher A, James SL (1994) Endothelial cells are activated by cytokine treatment to kill an intravascular parasite, *Schistosoma mansoni*, through the production of nitric oxide. Proc Natl Acad Sci U S A 91: 999-1003

252. Aboul-Enein A, Arafa S, Sakr M (1994) Pathogenesis of varices in schistosomal portal hypertension. Dig Dis Sci 39: 39-45

253. Geboes K, el-Deeb G, el-Haddad S, Amer G, el-Zayadi AR (1995) Vascular alterations of the colonic mucosa in schistosomiasis and portal colopathy. Hepatogastroenterology 42: 343-7

254. Michal A, Regli F, Campiche R, Cavallo RJ, de Crousaz G, Oberson R, Rabinowicz T (1977) Cerebral coenurosis. Report of a case with arteritis. J Neurol 216: 265-72

255. Aoshima M, Nakata K, Matsuoka M, Kawabata M, Nakamura T (1989) A case of proliferative sparganosis associated with PIE syndrome and pulmonary embolism. Nippon Kyobu Shikkan Gakkai Zasshi 27: 1521-7

256. Kuttin ES (1997) Fungal infections of the cardiovascular system—a review. Mycoses 40: 3-24

257. Chandler FW, Kaplan W, Ajello L (1980) A colour atlas and textbook of the histopathology of mycotic diseases. Wolfe Medical Publications Ltd, London p333

258. Hernandez Hernandez JA, Gonzalez-Moreno Portugal M, Casan Cava JM, Aloy Duch A, Llibre Codina JM, Capdevilla Morell JA (1993) Endocarditis due to *Candida albicans* with peripheral arterial embolism and a cerebral mycotic aneurysm in an IV drug addict. Rev Clin Esp 192: 223-5

259. Block CS, Young CN, Myers RAM (1977) *Torulopsis glabrata* fungaemia. S Afr Med J 51: 632-6

260. Klotz SA, Drutz DJ, Harrison JL, Huppert M (1983) Adherence and penetration of vascular endothelium by Candida yeasts. Infect Immun 42: 374-84

261. Ruchel R (1983) On the role of proteinases from *Candida albicans* in the pathogenesis of acronecrosis. Zentralbl Bakteriol Mikrobiol Hyg [A] 255: 524-36

262. Robboy SJ, Kaiser J (1975) Pathogenesis of fungal infection on heart valve prostheses. Human Pathol 6: 711-5

263. Albes J, Haverich A, Freihorst J, von der Hardt H, Manthey-Stiers F (1990) Management of mycotic rupture of the ascending aorta after heart-lung transplantation. Ann Thorac Surg 50: 982-3

264. Bourrain JL, Beani JC, Amblard P (1995) *Candida* vasculitis. Allerg Immunol (Paris) 27: 375-6

265. Bodey GP, Vartivarian S (1989) Aspergillosis. Eur J Clin Microbiol Infect Dis 8: 413-37

266. Denning DW, Ward PN, Fenelon LE, Benbow EW (1992) Lack of vessel wall elastolysis in human invasive pulmonary aspergillosis. Infect Immun 60: 5153-6

267. Fernando SS, Lauer CS (1982) Aspergillus fumigatus infection of the optic nerve with mycotic arteritis of cerebral vessels. Histopathology 6: 227-34

268. Caulet S, Capron F, Laaban JP, Prudent J, Rochemaure J, Diebold J (1990) Fatal hemoptysis during bronchial aspergillosis with multiple pulmonary artery aneurysms. Ann Pathol 10: 177-80

269. Hori MK, Knight LL, Carvalho PG, Stevens DL (1991) Aspergillar myocarditis and acute coronary artery occlusion in an immunocompromised patient. West J Med 155: 525-7

270. Hayashi H, Takagi R, Onda M, Kumazaki T (1994) Invasive pulmonary aspergillosis occluding the descending aorta and left pulmonary artery: CT features. J Comput Assist Tomogr 18: 492-4

271. Radhakrishnan VV, Saraswathy A, Rout D, Mohan PK (1994) Mycotic aneurysms of the intracranial vessels. Indian J Med Res 100: 228-31

272. Heussel CP, Kauczor HU, Heussel G, Mildenberger P, Dueber C (1997) Aneurysms complicating inflammatory diseases in immunocompromised hosts: value of contrast-enhanced CT. Eur Radiol 7: 316-9

273. Gavilan F, Torre-Cisneros J, Delgado M, Briceno J, Herrero C, Martinez L, de la Mata M, Mino G (1998) Thrombosis of the hepatic artery and portal vein secondary to invasive aspergillosis following liver transplantation. Enferm Infecc Microbiol Clin 16: 127-9

274. Kitakami A, Nishizawa Y, Yamamoto S, Chiba M, Tuiki K, Hasegawa H, Saiki I, Kanaya H (1988) Two cases of cerebral aspergillosis with intracerebral haemorrhage. No Shinkei Geka 16: 863-8

275. Kurino M, Kuratsu J, Yamaguchi T, Ushio Y (1994) Mycotic aneurysm accompanied by aspergillotic granuloma: a case report. Surg Neurol 42: 160-4

276. Lee SH, Barnes WG, Schaetzel WP (1986) Pulmonary aspergillosis and the importance of oxalate crystal recognition in cytology specimens. Arch Pathol Lab Med 110: 1176-9

277. Kimmerling EA, Fedrick JA, Tenholder MF (1992) Invasive *Aspergillus niger* with fatal pulmonary oxalosis in chronic obstructive pulmonary disease. Chest 101: 870-2

278. Marisavljevic D, Suvajdzic N, Jovanovic V, Kranjcic-Zec I, Boskovic D, Colovic M (1992) Disseminated zygomycosis in patients with acute leukaemia. Srp Arh Celok Lek 120: 65-9

279. Sugar AM (1992) Mucormycosis. Clin Infect Dis 14: S126-S129

280. Muhm M, Zuckermann A, Prokesch R, Pammer J, Hiesmayr M, Haider W (1996) Early onset of pulmonary mucormycosis with pulmonary vein thrombosis in a heart transplant recipient. Transplantation 62: 1185-7

281. Kikuchi K, Watanabe K, Sugawara A, Kowada M (1985) Multiple fungal aneurysms: report of a rare case implicating steroid as predisposing factor. Surg Neurol 24: 253-9

282. Benbow EW, McMahon RF (1987) Myocardial infarction caused by cardiac disease in disseminated zygomycosis. J Clin Pathol 40: 70-4

283. Grothey A, Donhuijsen K (1991) Mucoraceae mycoses: clinical aspects and pathology in ten patients. Mycoses 34: S29-S32

284. Liao WQ, Yao ZR, Li ZQ, Xu H, Zhao J (1995) Pyoderma gangrenosum caused by *Rhizopus arrhizus*. Mycoses 38: 75-7

285. Coffey MJ, Fantone J 3d, Stirling MC, Lynch JP 3d (1992) Pseudoaneurysm of pulmonary artery in mucormycosis. Radiographic characteristics and management. Am Rev Respir Dis 145: 1487-90

286. Baker RD (1971). Mucormycosis *In* Baker RD (ed.): The pathologic anatomy of mycoses, Springer-Verlag, Berlin 832-918

287. Bowler S, Woodcock A, Da Costa P, Turner-Warwick M (1986) Chronic pulmonary paracoccidioidomycosis masquerading as lymphangitis carcinomatosa. Thorax 41: 72-3

288. Manns BJ, Baylis BW, Urbanski SJ, Gibb AP, Rabin HR (1996) Paracoccidioidomycosis: case report and review. Clin Infect Dis 23: 1026-32

289. Stappaerts I, Bogers J, Ebo D, Vanden Broecke E, Stevens WJ, Van Marck E, Vermeire P (1997) c-ANCA positivity in a Belgian patient with pulmonary paracoccidioidomycosis. Eur Respir J 10: 2419-22

290. Tani EM, Franco M, Peracoli MT, Montenegro MR (1987) Experimental pulmonary paracoccidioidomycosis in the Syrian hamster: morphology and correlation of lesions with the immune response. J Med Vet Mycol 25: 291-300

291. Defaveri J, Martin LC, Franco M (1989) Histological and ultrastructural study of the inflammation evoked by Paracoccidioides brasiliensis antigen in previously immunized mice. Mycopathologia 105: 53-8

292. Singer-Vermes LM, Caldeira CB, Burger E, Calich LG (1993) Experimental murine paracoccidioidomycosis: relationship among the dissemination of the infection, humoral and cellular immune responses. Clin Exp Immunol 94: 75-9

293. Lima NS, Teixeira G, Miranda J, do Valle AC (1977) Treatment of South American blastomycosis (paracoccidioidomycosis) with miconazole by the oral route: an ongoing study. Proc R Soc Med 70: S35-S39

294. Bradsher RW (1997) Clinical features of blastomycosis. Semin Respir Infect 12: 229-34

295. Areno JP 4th, Campbell GD Jr, George RB (1997) Diagnosis of blastomycosis. Semin Respir Infect 12: 252-62

296. Chao D, Steier KJ, Gomila R (1997) Update and review of blastomycosis. J Am Osteopath Assoc 97: 525-32

297. Schwarz J, Salfelder K, Viloria JE (1977) *Histoplasma capsulatum* in vessels of the choroid. Ann Ophthalmol 9: 633-6

298. Bednar B, Schwarz J, Kaplan W (1978) Acute pulmonary histoplasmosis. 1st findings in Czechoslovakia. Cesk Patol 14: 51-6

299. Matthay RA, Levin DC, Wicks AB, Ellis JH (1976) Disseminated histoplasmosis involving an aortofemoral prosthetic graft. JAMA 235: 1478-9

300. Eidbo J, Sanchez RL, Tschen JA, Ellner KM (1993) Cutaneous manifestations of histoplasmosis in the acquired immune deficiency syndrome. Am J Surg Pathol 17: 110-6

301. Frankel EH, Frankel DF (1982) Sporotrichosis of the abdomen. Cutis 29: 189-90

302. Barbee WC, Ewert A, Folse D (1977) The combined effect of a cutaneo-lymphatic fungus, *Sporothrix schenckii* and a lymphatic-dwelling nematode, *Brugia Malayi*. Trop Geogr Med 29: 65-73

303. Anandi V, Kurien T, Jacob M, Koshi G (1994) Cutaneous lymphatic sporotrichosis. Indian J Pathol Microbiol 37: 97-100

304. Donabedian H, O'Donnell E, Olszewski C, MacArthur RD, Budd N (1994) Disseminated cutaneous and meningeal sporotrichosis in an AIDS patient. Diagn Microbiol Infect Dis 18: 111-5

305. Baudrillard JC, Rousseaux P, Lerais JM, Toubas O, Scherpereel B, Gari M, Comte P (1985) Fungal mycotic aneurysms and multiple cerebral abscesses caused by *Scedosporium apiospermum*. Apropos of a case with review of the literature. J Radiol 66: 321-6

306. Torok L, Simon G, Csornai A, Tapai M, Torok I (1995) *Scedosporium apiospermum* infection imitating lympho-cutaneous sporotrichosis in a patient with myeloblastic-monocytic leukaemia. Br J Dermatol 133: 805-9

307. Kusuhara M, Hachisuka H (1997) Lymphocutaneous infection due to *Scedosporium apiospermum*. Int J Dermatol 36: 684-8

IX
Thrombosis and embolism

1 – Thrombosis

Thrombosis is the formation of a solid mass, derived from the consituents of the blood, within the vascular system during life. As an important part of haemostasis, it depends on a normally functioning endothelium and underlying subendothelial layer, platelets, and the coagulation cascade.

Variables predisposing to thrombosis

There are three major variables: Injury to the endothelium, alteration of the normal blood flow and alteration in the blood (hypercoagubility).

Endothelial injury

This is particularly important in the development of thrombosis. Any damage to the endothelium may allow the process of thrombosis to begin and advanced atherosclerotic disease, infection, myocardial infarction, radiation injury, chemical agents of exogenous (derivatives of cigarette smoke) or endogenous origin (in abnormal lipid metabolism) [1, 2], bacterial toxins, and immunological injury (immune complex deposits) are part of the wide spectrum of initiating factors.

Alteration of the normal blood flow

Stasis and turbulence contribute to the development of thrombosis. In normal laminar flow, the formed elements of the blood circulate in an axial stream (this is true of vessels over 100 μm). Turbulence and stasis disrupt laminar flow and bring platelets in contact with the endothelium, preventing dilution of activated coagulation factors, delaying the inflow of inhibitors of clotting factors, and contributing to dysfunction or damage in the endothelium. All of these factors favour the formation of thrombi.

Alteration in the blood (hypercoagubility)

This is not a common cause of thrombosis and, although with advancing age a number of variables are changed in a way which predisposes to thrombus formation (increased aggregability of platelets, reduced relasease of PGI2 and reduced fibrinolytic response), these alone are seldom of significance. Hypercoagulability may be primary or secondary [3-5] (see Table 1). There are a number of predisposing factors which affect large segments of the population ; smoking increases the risk of thrombosis and users of oral contraceptives who are smokers have a greater risk of developing venous thrombosis. Obesity also increases the predisposition. Some patients with high titers of autoantibodies directed against anionic phospholipids (cardiolipin) have a high frequency of arterial and venous thrombosis [6-8]. Concomitant infections may increase the risk of thrombosis [9]. Oral contraceptive and hormone replacement therapy do not increase the susceptibility of the artery wall to develop an occlusive thrombus following injury and stenosis [10].

Morphology of thrombosis

Thrombosis may occur in arteries or veins, and in the microcirculatory bed. The clinical features depend on the types of vessels involved.

Arterial thrombosis

An arterial thrombus is made up of platelet aggregates trapped in fibrin strands with only a few red blood cells. This clot is adherent to the intima, unlike an embolus. In material obtained from unblocking procedures, serial sections are called for to identify the adherence zone. The differential diagnosis is quite impossible when organization occurs, whatever the type of the occluding thrombus. The diagnosis depends on the clinical context.

Venous thrombosis

Two main types are often described, phlebothrombosis and thrombophlebitis [11, 12]. Theoretically, inflammatory signs are lacking in the first type but manifest in the second. In reality, this is an artificial distinction and it is difficult to separate the processes, which may develop before or after one another. But the outcome is affected by the process which occurs, since thrombo-phlebitis minimizes the risk of a thrombo-embolism, the inflammatory process facilitating acherence of the thrombus to the venous wall. In phlebo-thrombosis, the thrombus is non adherent and does not organise; thus the risk of embolism is high. Victims of thrombophlebitis are primarily females, but young adults with no known risk factors may be involved. Fifty to eighty percent of patients

Table 1. Hypercoagulable states

HYPERCOAGULABLE STATES	CAUSES
Primary (genetic) states	Antithrombin III deficiency Defects in fibrinolysis Protein C and/or S deficiencies
High risk, secondary (acquired) states	Prolonged bed rest and immobilisation Cardiac failure and ischaemia Prosthetic valves Homocystinuria Neoplasia Tissue damage (fracture, burn, surgery) Thombotic thrombocytopenia Disseminated intravascular coagulation
Low risk, secondary (acquired) states	Atrial fibrillation, Cardiomyopathy Hyperlipidaemia Nephrotic syndrome Lupus anticoagulant Oral contraceptives Pregnancy (late term) and post-partum period Sickle cell anaemia Thrombocytosis

are treated conservatively, but early thrombectomy dramatically reduces the incidence of late symptoms. Stent placement may be called for after failed lytic treatment [13].

Pathology and differential diagnosis

Thrombosis usually starts in the venous sinuses and in the valve cusps where blood flow is slow and activated clotting factors accumulate. It consists of a fibrin mesh harbouring red blood cells, some leukocytes and a few platelets (Fig. 1-2). Generally, the venous wall does not show an inflammatory infiltrate in deep venous thrombosis and in thrombosis of varicosities; however, during organization of the thrombus, some lymphocytes and plasma cells can be seen in the adventitia and the media. In a vein affected by thrombo-phlebitis, the venous wall is infiltrated by oedema and inflammatory cells (Fig. 3-4). This process includes the peri-venous tissues and usually takes between 2 and 6 weeks to regress. The thrombus adheres to the venous wall and extends proximally or distally without inflammatory features.

All types of venous thrombosis undergo rapid organization. Unlike arterial thromboses, organized venous thromboses tend to undergo recanalization until the venous flow tends towards normal. However, complete return to normal venous function is prevented by factors such as parietal thickening with concentric or eccentric myointimal hyperplasia, deformation and valvular insufficiency leading to phlebosclerosis. These factors are of no importance in superficial veins because of the abundance of collaterals. In deep veins, however, these factors may lead to a stasis syndrome that results in chronic venous insufficiency. In great veins, such as the vena cava, occlusive thrombus is rare, but even partial thrombosis can produce downstream effects. Calcification may be seen (Fig. 5). Retro-extension of a large thrombus into venous collaterals can occur.

Clinical syndromes

1. **Superficial venous thrombosis.** The affected vein appears as a tender and indurated cord. Thrombophlebitis migrans is characterized by intermittent episodes of thrombosis of short segments of superficial veins in the arm or leg. Involvement of the veins of the upper extremities and the chest wall typify Mondor's disease. Mild fever and an in-

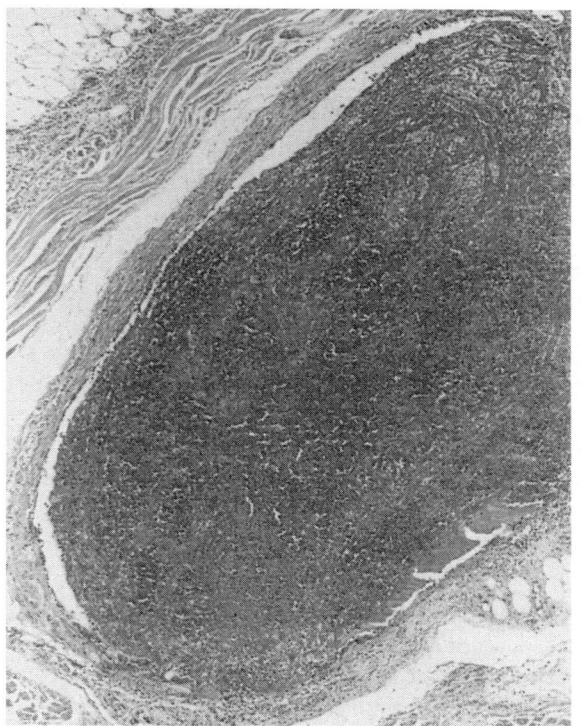

Fig. 1. Fresh venous thrombus. Haematoxylin, eosin and saffron stain. (HES)

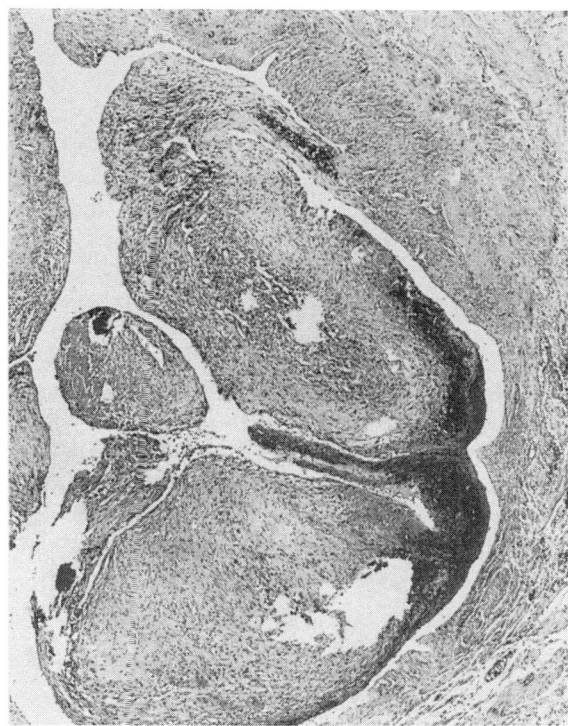

Fig. 2. Organising venous thrombus. HES

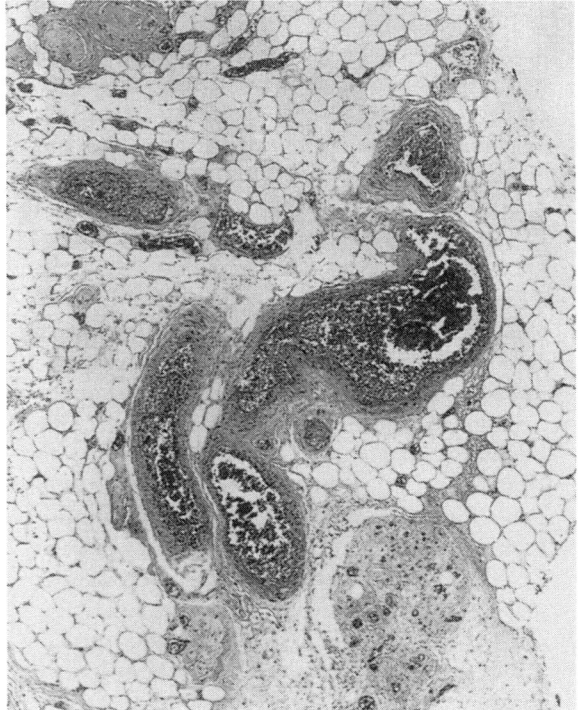

Fig. 3. Diffuse thrombo-phlebitis. HES

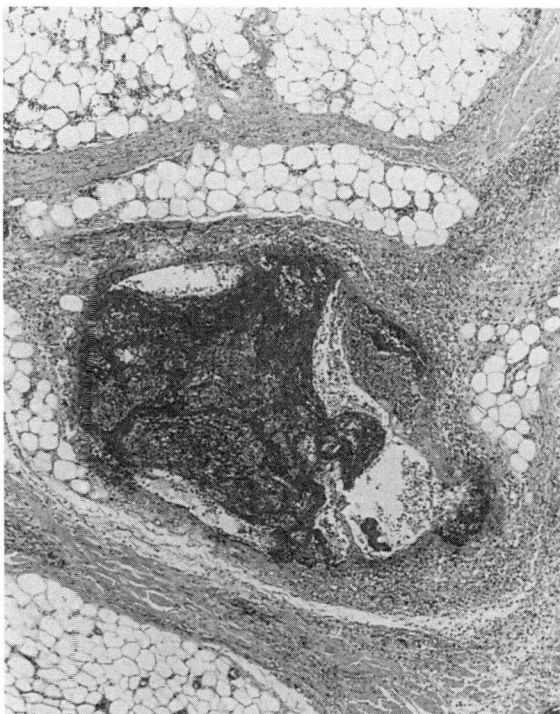

Fig. 4. Thrombophlebitis. Note marked infiltration of leukocytes in the venous wall. HES

creased white cell count are present in 35% of patients. Most attacks resolve spontaneously but deep venous thrombosis may follow and pulmonary embolism may occur. Recurrence is possible in the same vein or in other superficial areas.

Thrombosis of the subclavian and axillary veins produces swelling, pain in the entire arm and distension of collateral veins over the anterior chest wall. Imaging procedures may identify the occluded proximal vein at the thoracic outlet. Effective and early thrombectomy permits rapid recovery within 1 to 3 weeks and reduces the incidence of late symptoms. In acute iliofemoral venous thrombosis, aggressive regional therapy with contemporary venous thrombectomy or catheter-directed thrombolysis [14] should be carried out. In general, causes of superficial thrombophlebitis are similar to those of deep thrombophlebitis: any hypercoagulable state and trauma, indwelling catheters, therapeutic devices [15, 16], intravenous self-administration of drugs and external compression (adjacent fractures, the thoracic outlet syndrome, congenital abnomalities of muscle insertion) are all implicated [17].

2. **Deep venous thrombosis in large veins.**

   Thrombosis of the inferior vena cava is discussed in Budd-Chiari syndrome (see chapter XIII). Causes include Behçet's disease, lung cancer, and tuberculosis [18].

   More than two-thirds of cases of thrombosis of the renal veins are seen in newborns of less than a month of age [19]. In adults, thrombosis at this site is usually secondary to renal infection, ascending caval thrombosis or caval occlusion by tumour. This condition is usually unilateral, rarely bilateral, and often leads to necrosis of the renal parenchyma resulting in atrophy with chronic renal failure and hypertension. Mesenteric or colonic inflammatory veno-occlusive disease, a recently reported entity, may be a cause of digestive tract ischaemia [20, 21]. This condition occurs twice as often in men as in women. None of the patients has had an underlying systemic vasculitis, connective tissue disease, inflammatory bowel disease, infection, drug allergy, or history of ingestion of food contaminants or toxins.

3. **Phlegmasia cerulea dolens.** Phlegmasia cerulea dolens (PCD) is a potentially devastating complication of extensive deep venous thrombosis with total or near-total occlusion of the venous drainage of the limb (Fig. 6), including the microvascular collaterals (Fig. 7-8). It can lead to venous

gangrene and ultimate limb loss [22]. Clinical manifestations include severe pain, pathognomonic cyanosis and characteristic oedema. Pain is always severe, and the oedema is of a woody or rubbery consistency. Cutaneous blebs or bullae may appear after a few days. Motion of, and sensation in, the foot and hand of affected limbs are within normal limits or only slightly impaired. At the onset, the arterial pulse may be felt in only 50% of the patients and be undetectable in 25%. However, arteriography and noninvasive tests help to demonstrate patency of the arterial tree [23]. Circulatory collapse or hypovolaemic shock occurs in most patients, caused by excessive fluid loss in the extremity involved, ranging from 3 to 5 litres [24]. The subsequent rise of the tissue pressure is frequently responsible for a compartment syndrome with associated interruption of the arterial circulation and subsequent ischaemia [25, 26].

Phlegmasia alba dolens (PAD) is a variant of PCD. This syndrome is characterised by arterial spasm or compression because of massive oedema ; the leg is pale and cool with diminished or absent pulses. Irreversible ischaemia may also develop. In some cases, PAD fails to appear or may be unnoticed.

4. **Venous gangrene.** This usually occurs within 4 to 8 days after the onset of ischaemic signs. The extent of the gangrene varies ; however, the majority of patients display limited lesions, of either the toes or the foot [24]. Differential diagnoses include acute infectious diabetic gangrene, gangrene complicating acute prolonged vascular collapse, embolic gangrene, concomitant acute arterial and venous occlusions, and skin necrosis associated with anticoagulant therapy [27-30]. The haemodynamic effects of total venous occlusion result in an immediate rise in venous pressure and arterial blood flow decreases. Arterial blood pressure and visible arterial pulsations remain normal for a number of hours but after around 12 hours of occlusion, the distal pulse usually disappears. Several factors participate in the pathogenic mechanisms of PCD and VG. Venous thrombosis is usually massive and sudden. This "malignant" thrombosis is virtually unaffected by anticoagulant treatment. Experimental and clinical pathological data have shown that massive or complete blockage of the venous return is a prerequisite for the occurrence of either PCD or gangrene. The significant fact emerging from these experimental data is that potential reversibility of the ischaemia is possible, at least within a 6-hour period. Irreversible changes

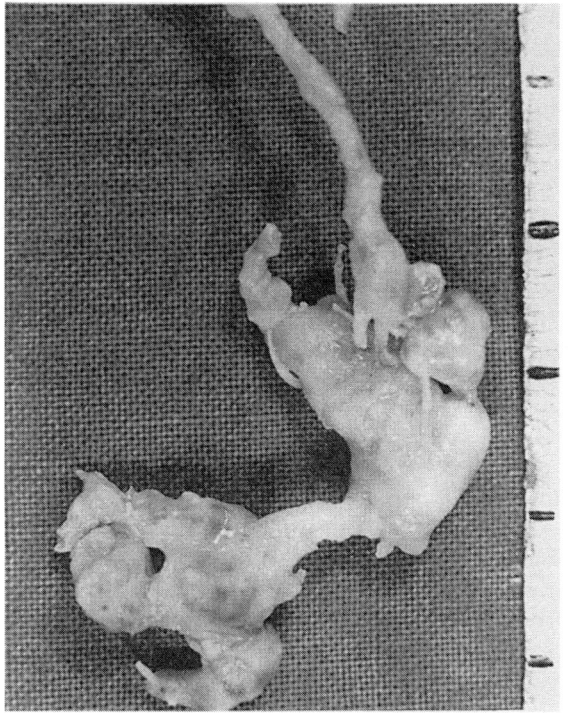

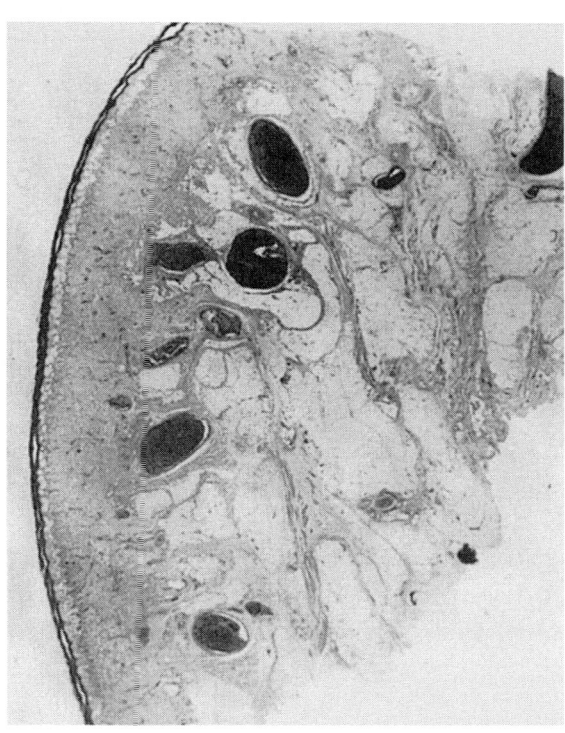

Fig. 5. Organised coralline thrombus of the vena cava (Courtesy Pr J-M Cormier)

Fig. 6. Phlegmasia cerulea dolens with extensive venous thrombosis involving subcutaneous and deep veins. HES

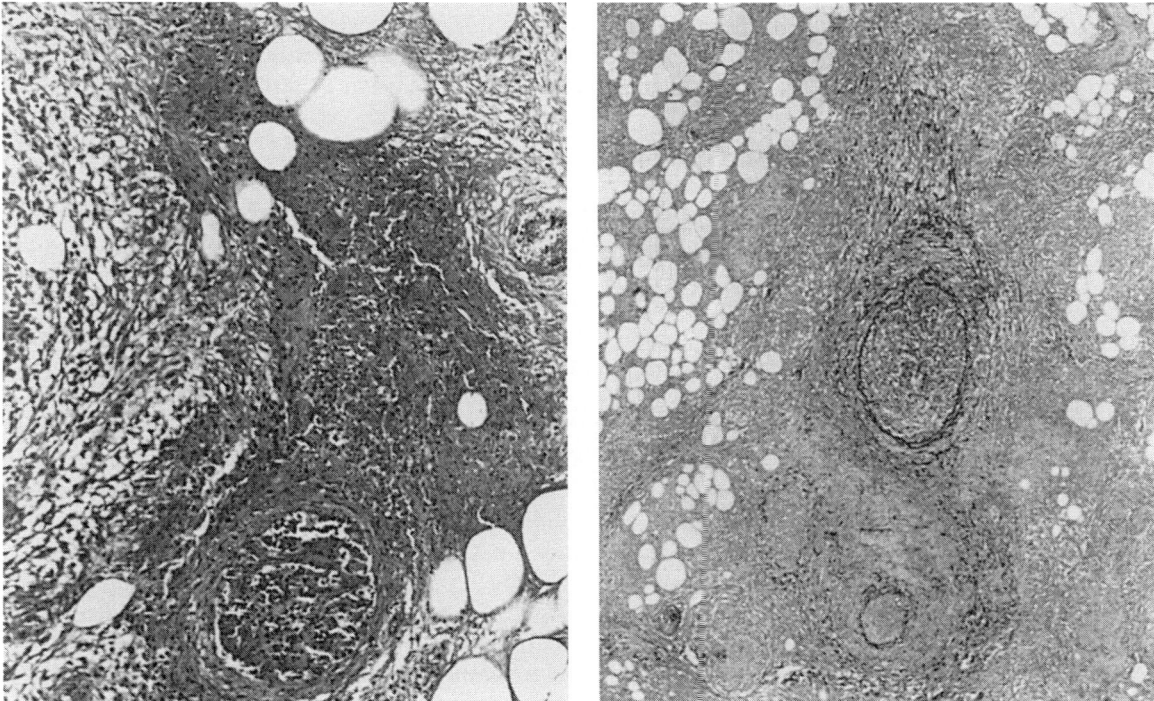

Fig. 7-8. Occlusion of microvascular collaterals associated with diffuse inflammation and gangrene. HES

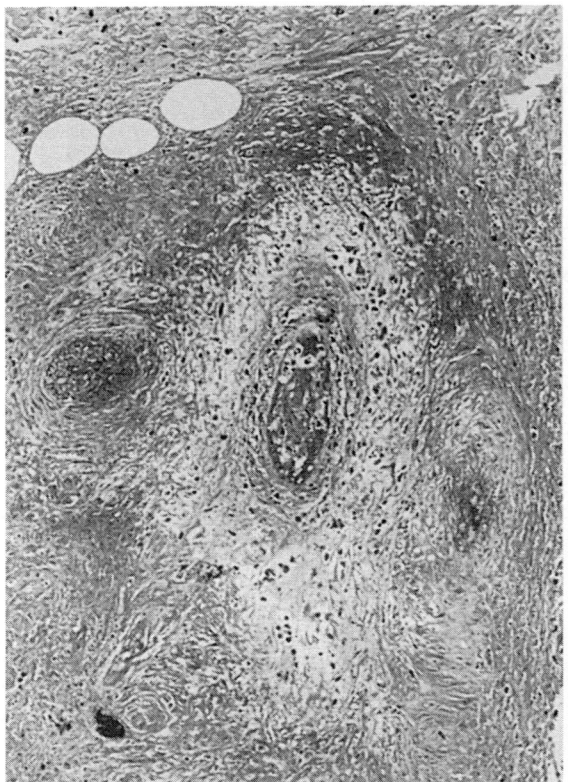

Fig. 9. Irreversible venous extensive thrombosis in venous gangrene. HES

occur within a 12-hour period [24] (Fig. 9). The factors that determine the prognosis of PCD and VG are local (presence or absence of gangrene) and systemic (shock, pulmonary embolism and the underlying diseases). In the two conditions, circulatory collapse affects 21.5–28% of the patients. Fatal pulmonary embolism occurs in 3.4% of the patients suffering from venous gangrene. Predisposing conditions include malignancy [31], postoperative state, diabetes mellitus, previous deep venous thrombosis, hypercoagulation, thrombocytopaenia, and some auto-immune diseases [32-35]. Little advance in management, or in life and limb salvage, has been made in the past 30 years. Associated mortality (42%) and morbidity rates are high, especially when progression to venous gangrene has occurred [24, 36].

Lymphatic thrombosis

Lymphatic thrombosis is an exceptional phenomenon and is frequently secondary to lesions of the blood vessels. Secondary thrombolymphangitis usually occurs in association with thromboses of the limbs, ra-

rely in the cervical segment of the thoracic duct. Following organization of these thrombi newly-formed capillaries in the peri-lymphatic tissue crisscross the thrombus. The presence of red blood cells in these capillaries may make the diagnosis difficult [37].

Concomitant arterial, venous and lymphatic thrombosis

This condition occurs in some hematological disorders and infections. Gangrene may develop if there is lymphoedema.

Disseminated intravascular coagulation (DIC)

This is a pernicious clinical event in which the balance between coagulation and fibrinolysis tips toward coagulation. This condition is characterized by formation of multiple thrombi in the microcirculatory bed. DIC produces changes in all consituents of the blood, including red cells.There are two main anatomo-clinical syndromes: fast and slow DIC.

Fast DIC presents as an acute, fulminant, uncompensated consumptive coagulopathy with multifocal bleeding, shock, acute renal insufficiency and cutaneous necrosis. Replacement of deficient or consumed factors is the main treatment.

Slow DIC is less apparent, and sometimes difficult to detect. It occurs in chronic, indolent and compensated diseases that present little overt manifestation of bleeding: recurrent epistaxis, haemorrhage at injection sites, thrombosis, microcirculatory ischaemia and end organ infarction. This condition may respond to heparinization.

Two mechanisms are implicated. Firstly, with the development of multiple and diffuse micro-thrombi in the microcirculatory bed, there is rapid consumption of platelets and depletion of coagulation factors. Secondly, micro-thrombi release tissue thromboplastin activator (thromboplastin III). This factor triggers the fibrinolytic system, which destroys micro-thrombi and promotes the extrinsic pathway of coagulation, thus worsening the condition. Laboratory findings reflect the mechanism. The first step includes transient hyper-fibrinogenaemia and hyperactivity of factors V and VIII; depletion of normally consumed coagulation factors (decrease in platelet level, hypofibrinogenaemia, hypoactivity of factors II, V, VIII and XIII). The second step is characterized by the appearance of soluble fibrinolytic complexes, such as fibrin split products (FSP) and non-transformed fibrin monomers in the plasma [38].

Pathology and differential diagnosis

Micro-thrombi are not visible to the naked eye; however, their consequences may be apparent in superficial (muco-cutaneous purpura) or deep-seated haemorrhage; intestinal submucosa, lungs, retroperitoneum, adrenals, brain and meninges, myocardium, uterus and ovaries, and sub-pleural space may all be affected. Necrosis may affect the renal cortex, brain and liver (periportal areas in eclampsia, the entire liver in fulminating hepatitis, and the pituitary (Sheehan's syndrome). Massive pulmonary oedema may be associated with visible venous and arterial thrombosis. Histologically, micro-thrombi are present in small vessels and may be difficult to find because of fibrinolysis. They appear as fibrinous or hyaline masses containing fibrin and platelet debris (Fig. 10) most abundant in the kidneys, occluding the afferent arteries and capillaries of glomeruli (Fig. 11). They are frequently found in the spleen, liver, lungs (Fig. 12), uterus, brain, adrenals, skin, digestive tract testes, hypophysis and heart. In autopsy material, DIC should be considered as a diagnosis when ten micro-thrombi are seen in more than three viscera.

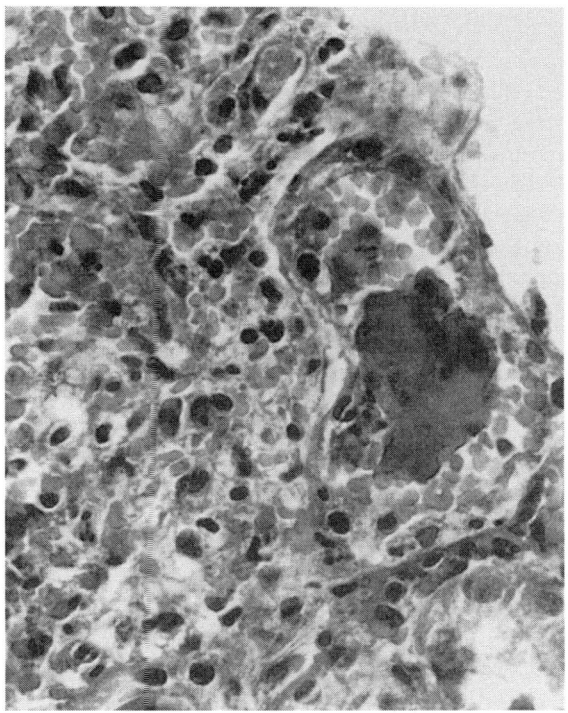

Fig. 11. A glomerular capillary clogged by an hyaline micro-thrombus. HES

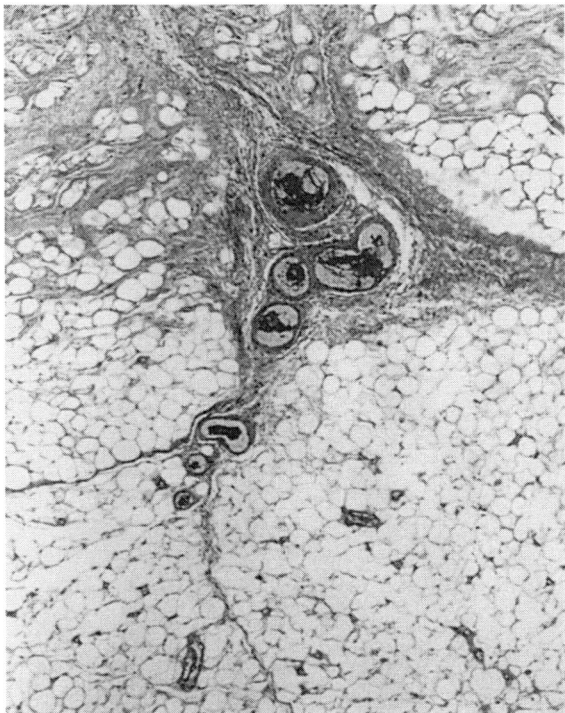

Fig. 10. Hyaline micro-thrombi made up of fibrin and platelet debris in small vessels. HES

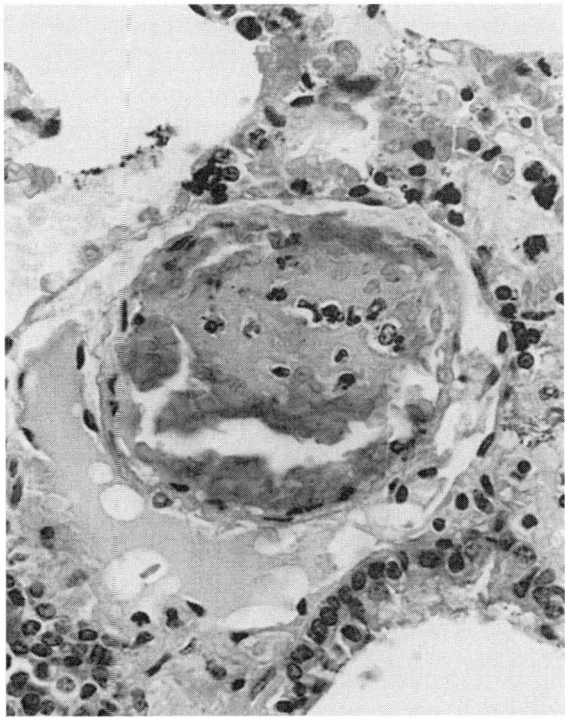

Fig. 12. Micro-thrombi occluding a bronchial capillary. HES

2 – Embolism

The effects of embolism depend on the vessels involved and the nature of the embolus. Direct consequences include acute ischaemia with tissue necrosis if a terminal vessel is involved; other changes depend on the nature of the embolus. Endothelial damage may initiate formation of more thrombi resulting in complete occlusion of the vessel.

Vascular classification of embolism

Peripheral arterial embolism

An embolus may detach from a lesion in the left side of the heart or from an artery. Paradoxical embolism occurs when a venous embolus enters the systemic circulation through a shunt (septal defects or arteriovenous fistulae). The real frequency is unknown [39-41], but it is considered to be a rare mechanism of cerebral embolism.

Pulmonary thrombo-embolic syndrome

Elderly, immobilized patients are the most frequent victims. A history of deep venous thrombosis is found in 33% of patients, but the initial thrombosis is often only discovered some days after the embolic event. In young patients, men are more often affected than women.

Clinical manifestations of pulmonary embolism are related both to the pre-embolic state of the cardiovascular system and to arterial obstruction. When there is no pre-existing cardiovascular disorder, the degree of cardiovascular impairment is proportional to the extension of arterial obstruction. Sudden death can occur caused by pulmonary or coronary vessel spasm or circulatory disturbance secondary to a cardio-inhibitory reflex. Less than 10% of pulmonary emboli produce infarction, usually peripherally in the lower lobes. Infarcts occur only when there is a predisposing clinical condition (usually congestive heart failure) [19].

Causes are multiple. Deep venous thrombosis in the lower limbs is usually the source of pulmonary embolism but thrombi can also originate in other systemic veins [42]. Emboli may be produced by tumours, including renal cell carcinoma and myxomas of the right atrium or ventricle. Fifty percent of patients suffering from congestive heart failure will have a pulmonary embolism and 15% of patients having right heart failure suffer from emboli originating in the pelvic veins or the right side of the heart. There is an increased risk of pulmonary embolism during pregnancy and the puerperium. Five percent of all postoperative deaths are caused by pulmonary thromboembolism [43].

Pathology and differential diagnosis

Generally, the thrombus is small and blocks a lobar or segmental branch of the pulmonary artery; large emboli are rarer although over-represented in autopsy material. After pulmonary embolism, progressive lysis of the clot is usually apparent within 4 to 6 weeks, but the injured area can be detected by lung scanning or arteriography. In the pulmonary artery, localized thickening of the intima may represent an incorporated embolus. Organizing thrombi or emboli contain remnants of laminated fibrin and multiple newly-formed capillaries. Affected vessels show extensive elastosis at the intimal-medial interface, often with an eccentric lumen. This condition should be distinguished from occlusive intimal fibroelastosis (Grade 3 pulmonary hypertension). Concentric intimal fibroelastosis has a single central lumen, if any lumen remains. Elastic tissue stains are of great help in the differential diagnosis.

Classification of the embolus by composition

Detached thrombus

The clinical history may suggest the diagnosis; Green [44] found atrial fibrillation in 49% of cases, congestive heart failure in 17%, myocardial infarction in 17%, a history of cardiovascular surgery in 8%, with infectious endocarditis, aortic valve prosthesis, thoracic outlet syndrome, aneurysm, deep venous thrombosis and miscellaneous causes making up a further 9%. Histologically, it may be difficult to distinguish a fresh embolus from a thrombus. The adherence of the mass to the intima favors the diagnosis of thrombus. The presence of cholesterol crystals and lipophages within the clot suggest detachment from an atherosclerotic proximal vessel.

Air and gas

1. **Air embolism.** This occurs when a large amount (more than 35 mls) of air invades the circulatory system, giving rise to multiple bubbles distending a vessel or scattered in the capillary network. Venous embolism results from aspiration of air or gas into negative-pressure veins, including the jugular veins, and the intracranial dural sinuses, following rupture of the vena cava, in blunt chest trauma with rupture of the lungs and into the uterine veins after difficult labour. Arterial embolism appears when air or gas bubbles pass through the pulmonary veins and reach the left side of the heart, the aorta and its branches. As air accumulates in the cardiac cavities a froth forms and the victim dies rapidly of cardiac failure as pumping ceases to be effective. Diagnosis of air embolism is not always possible macroscopically although it can be made if the heart is opened under water. Histologically, air embolism is not readily identifiable but the diagnosis is suggested when small foci of ischaemic necrosis are found in bone and central nervous system.

2. **Gas embolism.** This complication results from the presence in the blood of normally dissolved gases forced out of solution by a rapid decrease in atmospheric pressure [45]. Bubbles in the blood vessels migrate and block the microcirculatory bed. Oxygen and carbon dioxide are readily reabsorbed and nitrogen is the chief offender. Decompression sickness, also known as caisson disease, diver's disease and the bends [46], also affects aviators who climb rapidly to more than 9000 m (about 30,000 ft), where the atmospheric pressure is less than one-third the normal. The effects of gas embolism are most evident in tissues having a dense capillary network, including the epiphyseal spongy bones and the central nervous system. These tissues undergo focal ischaemia and demyelinization [47]. Lipid droplets, released from disintegrated adipocytes, pass into the blood flow and lead to a combined fat and gas embolism. Blood clotting may be triggered by contact of blood with air, and disseminated intravascular coagulation (DIC) may occur.

Foreign bodies

Various particles (starch, talc, or excipients) may be introduced into the blood flow by intravascular injection, perfusion, haemodialysis (Fig. 13) or other manœuvers (invasive roentgenographic techniques, pro-cedures to restore vascular continuity or drug abuse). Exceptionally, bullets, shrapnel or metallic mercury embolism have been reported. Silicone embolism secondary to intramammary injections of a silicone fluid mixture may induce acute pneumonitis [48]. Controlled embolisation using Gelfoam particles, blood clots, glass beads and autologous muscle tissue (Fig. 14) may be helpful in treating angiomas, arteriovenous fistulae or in preventing haemorrhage and tumour cell migration in hypervascular malignant tumours. Liquid embolisation with ethanol provokes direct cellular toxic necrosis, comparable with a true mummification and is used in palliative medical nephrectomy for renal cancer [49]. Lipiodol-containing material produces rapid thrombosis with myospherulosis associated with inflammation [50] (Fig. 15).

Tumour cells

Many cancers tend to shed cells into the bloodstream early in their course and the site of vascular invasion determines the pathway of the embolisation and the location of the metastases. Systematic study of end products of material obtained in the restoration of the vascular lumen can help detect detached tumour fragments (Fig. 16) and identify their nature [51]. A case of livedo racemosa generalisata has been reported in arterial embolism of a myxoma [52].

Fat

Aggregates of adipocytes, and fragments of bone may be found in the pulmonary arteries and fat globules in small vessels of the brain, kidney, skin or eye of trauma victims. Fat embolism may be part of two phenomena: latent fat embolism, devoid of functional or organic consequences, and fat embolism syndrome (FES), which encompasses disseminated tissue lesions, biological alterations and complex disorders of the lipid metabolism.

The patient usually has a lucid interval of several hours to several days after the trauma, then symptoms become manifest: fever, cardio-respiratory distress (adult respiratory distress syndrome) purpura and psycho-neurological disorders [53-55]. The presence of an interval between the initiating cause and the symptoms may suggest that fat emboli appear in the circulating blood as a result of metabolic changes.

Fat embolism may occur after fractures of the long bones, orthopedic surgery, severe burns involving the subcutis, liposuction, inadvertent or accidental intravenous injection of oily material during the course of an abortion, lymphography or the treatment of impotence [56, 57]. A fat embolus is made of triglycerides

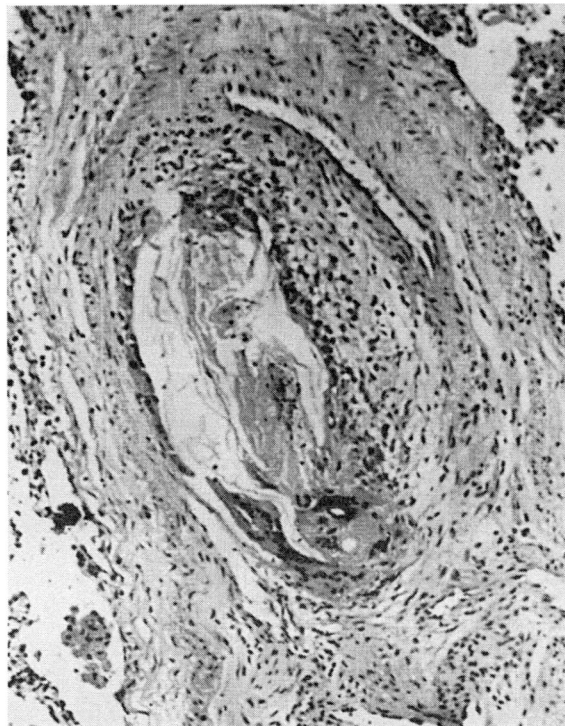

Fig. 13. Contaminant membrane embolus occluding a pulmonary vein after haemodialysis. Note surrounding foreign body granuloma around. HES

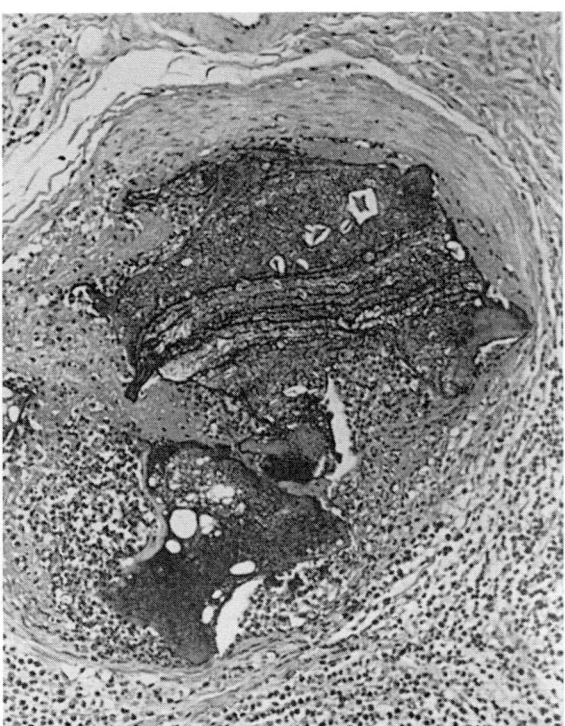

Fig. 14. Preoperative gel-foam particle embolus with secondary thrombosis. HES

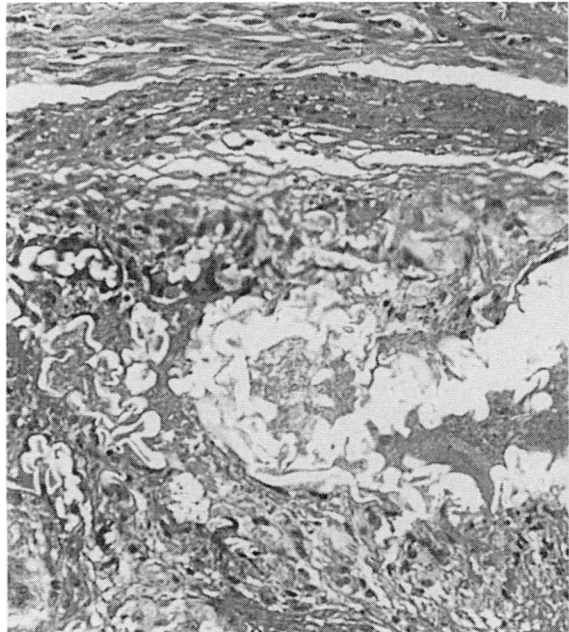

Fig. 15. Preoperative embolisation of a congenital arterio-venous malformation with lipiodol. Note saccular formations containing red blood cells characteristic of myospherulosis surrounded by foreign body granulomata distorting the vascular wall. HES. (Courtesy Dr F. Cormier)

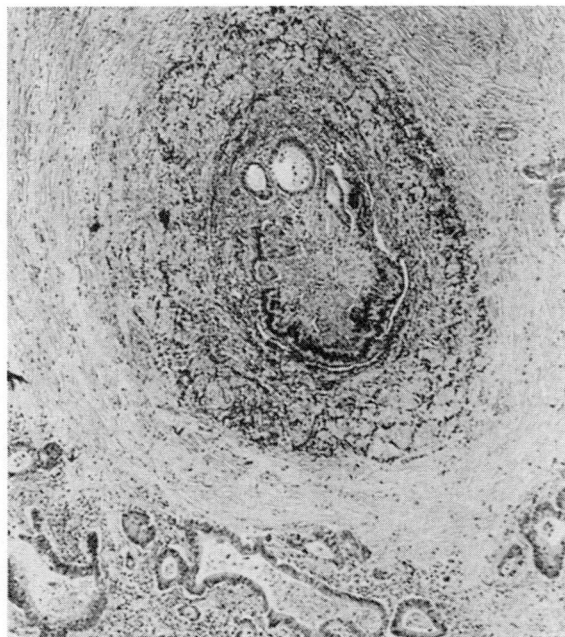

Fig. 16. Venous thrombosis caused by a colonic adenocarcinoma embolus. Orcein

liberated from adipose tissue. Fat emboli can deform and pass through the lungs, resulting in systemic embolisation, most commonly to the brain and kidneys [58]. Migration of triglyceride globules into the pulmonary microcirculatory bed produces a decrease in the arterial pressure of O_2. Enzymatic lysis of triglycerides and breakdown of plasma lipoproteins liberate free fatty acids, which damage the endothelial lining. The endothelial lesions cause pulmonary oedema, microscopic haemorrhages and thromboses with focal ischaemia.

Grossly, fat embolism does not produce specific lesions. In the course of an autopsy, scattered haemorrhages are found in tissues and viscera. Living patients display highly suggestive lesions, such as petechiae in the conjunctiva with retinal haemorrhage. Histologically, a fat embolism can be detected in a renal or cutaneous biopsy. Adipocyte aggregates or bone marrow fragments are easily recognizable within the vascular lumen. In contrast, fat globules do not have a typical structure appearing as empty round or elongated spaces within the lumen of an artery or a capillary. These spaces are often at the branching site of a vessel, compressing the red blood cells against the degenerated endothelium. Oedema, haemorrhage, and infiltrates of histiocytes are seen in the surrounding tissues. Association with disseminated intravascular coagulation (DIC) occurs. The site of visceral lesions depends on the distribution of the emboli: foci or coalescent areas of exudative and haemorrhagic alveolitis are seen in the lungs, and occlusion of glomerular capillaries and degenerative changes with fatty infiltration of the epithelium of the proximal convoluted tubules in the kidney, the latter responsible for the presence of fat globules in the urine. Foci of demyelinization occur in the brain and retina.

Bone marrow

The embolus is of bone marrow originating in fractured spongy bone. Bone marrow embolism does not cause clinical manifestations. This condition occurs in patients having rib, pelvic or vertebral fractures and may follow cardiac massage.

Amniotic fluid and placental material

During pregnancy, or ceasarean section, trophoblast fragments released in intervillous spaces may penetrate the maternal blood flow via marginal sinuses and migrate into the pulmonary arteries (Fig. 17). They most often disappear rapidly after delivery.

Amniotic fluid embolism is the most unpredictable and catastrophic complication of pregnancy, ac-

counting for 10% to 20% of maternal deaths [59, 60]. The pathogenesis may include entry of amniotic fluid through lacerations or ruptures of the uterus or cervix, through endocervical veins and through abnormal uteroplacental sites, as in placental abruption, placenta previa, or placenta accreta [61]. Leucotrienes, prostaglandins and other vasoactive substances contained in amniotic fluid are thought to cause severe haemodynamic disturbance with respiratory distress, shock, and possibly tonic-clonic seizures. DIC occurs; amniotic fluid is thought to possess thromboplastin-like properties. The pulmonary oedema probably results from alveolar capillary leakage and may be potentiated by high maternal extracellular volume, and, in some patients, by depressed myocardial function.

Autopsy demonstrates moderate to severe pulmonary oedema with haemorrhage. The embolus is made up of large numbers of fetal squames, amniotic cells, and lanugo. Other histological features are focal myocardial and hepatocellular necrosis with secondary interstitial inflammation [60]. In post-mortem tissues, detachment of endothelial cells from the intima may simulate an amniotic embolus. In well-pre-

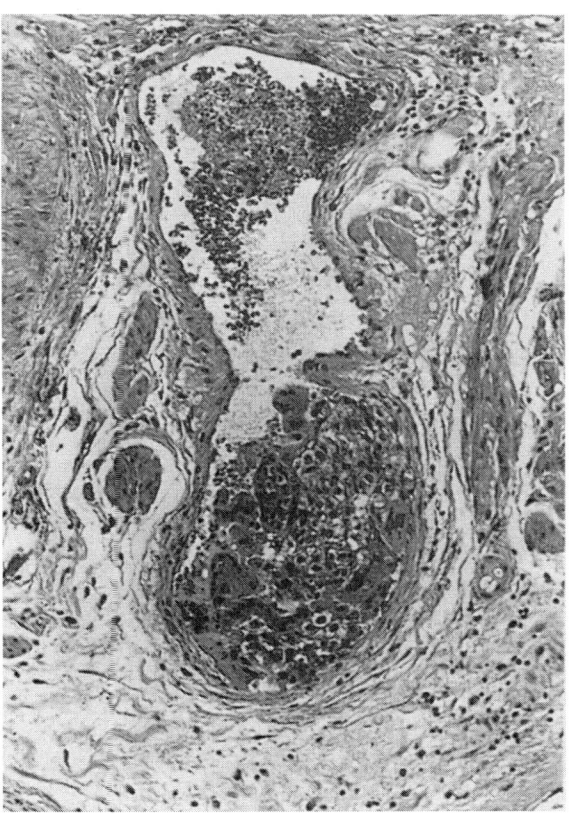

Fig. 17. Embolism of trophoblasts in an uterine vein. HES

served tissues, immunohistochemical techniques help rule out this artifact.

Microbial and Parasitic Pathogens

An infectious embolus disseminates the pathogen by the blood or lymph with septic pyaemia, vasculitis, lymphangitis and metastatic abscesses in the viscera, skin, and limbs. The most frequent cause is infectious endocarditis developed on deformed valves, prostheses, or shunts. Diagnostically, the common post-mortem collections of bacteria or *Candida albicans* developed inside the vascular lumen are never associated with inflammation. Some bacteria may produce gases (methane, ethylene, carbon dioxide) causing post-mortem thrombus or fatty material to migrate [62]. A hydatid cyst may erode a venous wall, producing massive pulmonary embolism of cystic material and offspring vesicles [63, 64] with fatal anaphylactic shock. In patients with schistosomiasis, mature worms dwelling in the venous pelvic plexuses may release egg emboli into tributaries of the portal veins [65, 66].

Bibliography

1. Cattaneo M (1997) Hyperhomocysteinemia : a risk factor for arterial and venous thrombotic disease. Int J Clin Lab Res 27: 139-44
2. D'Angelo A, Mazzola G, Crippa L, Fermo I, Vigano D'Angelo S (1997) Hyperhomocysteinemia and venous thromboembolic disease. Haematologica 82: 211-9
3. Moake JL (1990) Hypercoagulable states. Adv Intern Med 35: 235-47
4. Schenk S, Goodnight SH (1992) Inherited hypercoagulable states: questions and controversies. Nurse Pract Forum 3: 82-5
5. Eby CS (1993) A review of the hypercoagulable state. Hematol Oncol Clin North Am 7: 1121-42
6. Oeffinger KC, Roaten SP Jr (1994) Antiphospholipid syndrome. J Fam Pract 38: 611-9
7. Atterbury JL, Munn MB, Groome LJ, Yarnell JA (1997) The antiphospholipid antibody syndrome: an overview. J Obstet Gynecol Neonatal Nurs 26: 522-30
8. Disdier P, Weiller PJ (1998) Antiphospholipid antibodies syndrome. Rev Prat 48: 626-31
9. Suarez Ortega S, Artiles Vizcaino J, Balda Aguirre I, Melado Sanchez P, Arkuch Saade ME, Ayala Galan E, Betancor Leon P (1993) Tuberculosis as risk factor for venous thrombosis. An Med Interna 10: 398-400
10. Bellinger DA, Williams JK, Adams MR, Honore EK, Bender DE (1998) Oral contraceptives and hormone replacement therapy do not increase the incidence of arterial thrombosis in a nonhuman primate model. Arterioscler Thromb Vasc Biol 18: 92-9
11. Hirsh J, Buchanan MR, Ofosu FA, Weitz J (1987) Evolution of thrombosis. Ann N Y Acad Sci 516 :586-604
12. Moser KM (1990) Venous thromboembolism. Am Rev Respir Dis 141: 235-49
13. Koizumi J, Kusano S, Akima T, Isoda K, Hikita H, Kurita A, Nakamura H (1998) Emergent Z stent placement for treatment of cor pulmonale due to pulmonary emboli after failed lytic treatment: technical considerations. Cardiovasc Intervent Radiol 21: 254-5
14. Comerota AJ, Aldridge SC, Cohen G, Ball DS, Pliskin M, White JV (1994) A strategy of aggressive regional therapy for acute iliofemoral venous thrombosis with contemporary venous thrombectomy or catheter-directed thrombolysis. J Vasc Surg 20: 244-54
15. Gould JR, Carloss HW, Skinner WL (1993) Groshong catheter-associated subclavian venous thrombosis. Am J Med 95: 419-23
16. Lajvardi A, Trerotola SO, Strandberg JD, Samphilipo MA, Magee C (1995) Evaluation of venous injury caused by a percutaneous mechanical thrombolytic device. Cardiovasc Intervent Radiol 18: 172-8
17. Cavatorta F, Campisi S, Zollo A (1997) Subclavian vein stenosis : a potentially serious complication in chronic hemodialysis patients with permanent cardiac pacemakers. Int J Artif Organs 20: 316-8
18. Ousehal A, Essadki O, Abdelouafi A, Kadiri R (1993) Superior vena cava thrombosis. Radiological aspects. Apropos of 28 cases. Ann Radiol (Paris) 36: 303-9
19. Belcaro G, Nicolaides AN, Veller M (1995) Venous disorders. A manual of diagnosis and treatment. Saunders, London, Philadelphia, Toronto, Sydney, Tokyo
20. Matsunaga I, Oka H, Ueda M, Arakawa T, Kobayashi K (1995) Idiopathic colonic phlebitis with massive ascites. Intern Med 34: 776-81
21. Lie JT (1997) Mesenteric inflammatory veno-occlusive disease (MIVOD) : an emerging and unsuspected cause of digestive tract ischaemia. Vasa 26: 91-6
22. Sennewald K, Fajman WA (1991) Evaluation of phlegmasia cerulea dolens using radionuclide venography. Clin Nucl Med 16: 737-40
23. Wulff C, Lorentzen T, Christensen E, Pedersen EB (1996) Phlegmasia alba dolens diagnosed with Doppler ultrasonography. Ugeskr Laeger 158: 6623-4
24. Haimovici H (1984) Ischaemic venous thrombosis : phlegmasia cerulea dolens and venous gangrene In Haimovici H (Ed) Vascular surgery. Appleton-Century-Crofts, Northwalk, 1019-33
25. Saffle JR, Maxwell JG, Warden GD, Jolley SG, Lawrence PF (1981) Measurement of intramuscular pressure in the management of massive venous occlusion. Surgery 89: 394-7
26. Qvarfordt P, Eklof B, Ohlin P (1983) Intramuscular pressure in the lower leg in deep vein thrombosis and phlegmasia ceruleae dolens. Ann Surg 197: 450-3
27. Humphries JE, Gardner JH, Connelly JE (1991) Warfarin skin necrosis : recurrence in the absence of anticoagulant therapy. Am J Hematol 37: 197-200
28. Comp PC (1993) Coumarin-induced skin necrosis. Incidence, mechanisms, management and avoidance. Drug Saf 8: 128-35
29. Shahak A, Posan E, Szucs G, Rigo J, Boda Z (1996) Coumarin-induced skin necrosis following heparin-induced thrombocytopenia and thrombosis. A case report. Angiology 47: 725-7
30. Harenberg J, Huhle G, Wang L, Hoffmann U, Bayerl C, Kerowgan M (1999) Association of heparin-induced skin lesions, intracutaneous tests, and heparin-induced IgG. Allergy 54: 473-7
31. Naschitz JE, Yeshurun D, Eldar S, Lev LM (1996) Diagnosis of cancer-associated vascular disorders. Cancer 77: 1759-67

32. Goldammer R (1981) Phlegmasia coerulea dolens, a paraneoplastic syndrome. Med Welt 32: 358-9

33. Battey PM, Salam AA (1985) Venous gangrene associated with heparin-induced thrombocytopenia. Surgery 97: 618-20

34. Feinman LJ, Meltzer AJ (1989) Phlegmasia cerulea dolens as a complication of percutaneous insertion of a vena caval filter. J Am Osteopath Assoc 89: 63-8

35. Hood DB, Weaver FA, Modrall JG, Yellin AE (1993) Advances in the treatment of phlegmasia cerulea dolens. Am J Surg 166: 206-10

36. Perkins JM, Magee TR, Galland RB (1996) Phlegmasia caerulea dolens and venous gangrene. Br J Surg 83: 19-23

37. Vuong PN, Wanji S, Sakka L, Klager S, Bain O (1991) The murid filaria Monanema martini: A model for onchocerciasis. Part I.– Description of lesions. Ann Parasitol Hum Comp 66: 109-20

38. Muller-Berghaus G, Hasegawa H (1983) Pathogenesis of disseminated intravascular coagulation. Bibl Haematol 49: 3-13

39. Gautier JC, Durr A, Koussa S, Lascault G, Grosgogeat Y (1990) Paradoxal cerebral embolism: role of patent oval foramen. Bull Acad Natl Med 174: 1031-8

40. Andres del Barrio MT, Pardo Moreno J, Egido Herrero JA, Gonzalez Gutierrez JL, Rodrigo JL (1997) Transient paradoxical embolism. Importance of early ultrasonography diagnosis. Med Clin (Barc) 108: 618-20

41. Elejalde Guerra JI, Alonso Martinez JL, Lezaun Burgui R, Garcia Mouriz ME (1998) Paradoxal air embolism caused by a central venous catheter. An Med Interna 15: 562-3

42. Lang E, Bouwman O, Faiss J (1993) Recurrent lung embolisms in aneurysm of the popliteal vein. Chirurg 64: 503-4

43. Zerbino DD, Lukasevich LL, Servetnik MI (1994) Thrombosis and embolism as paraneoplastic syndrome. Arkh Patol 56: 77-80

44. Green RM, DeWeese JA, Rob CG (1975) Arterial embolectomy before and after the Fogarty catheter. Surgery 77: 24-33

45. Ghimouz A, Loisel B, Kheyar M, Fried D, Bouret JM (1996) Carbon dioxide embolism during hysteroscopy followed by transient blindness. Ann Fr Anesth Reanim 15: 192-5

46. Gregg PJ, Walder DN (1986) Caisson disease of bone. Clin Orthop (210): 43-54

47. Davidson JK (1989) Dysbaric disorders : aseptic bone necrosis in tunnel workers and divers. Baillieres Clin Rheumatol 3: 1-23

48. Matsuba T, Sujiura T, Irei M, Kyan Y, Kunishima N, Uchima H, Miyagi S, Iwata Y, Matsuba K (1994) Acute pneumonitis presumed to be silicone embolism. Intern Med 33: 481-3

49. Nadalini VF, Zambelli S, Bruttini GP, Pacella M, Giglio C (1984) Liquid embolization of the renal artery with absolute ethanol. J Radiol 65: 301-5

50. Vuong PN, Melki JP, Cormier F, Cormier JM (1996) Myosphérulose intra-vasculaire induite par une embolisation d'une fistule artério-veineuse : deux cas. Sem Hôp Paris 72: 565-6

51. Vuong PN, Cogan M, Nguyen PC, Colin JP, Piriou L (1995) Myxome de l'oreillette gauche révélé par une embolie fémorale : Intérêt de l'étude anatomo-pathologique du produit de désobstruction vasculaire (Lettre) Press Med 24: 1222

52. Rambusch EG, Musholt P, Weissenborn K, Kiehl P, Deicher H (1996) Livedo racemosa generalisata in atrial myxoma. Z Rheumatol 55: 58-62

53. Fleischer E, LeBel LA (1993) Fat embolism syndrome. Nurse Anesth 4: 18-27

54. Johnson MJ, Lucas GL (1996) Fat embolism syndrome. Orthopedics 19: 41-8

55. Bardana D, Rudan J, Cervenko F, Smith R (1998) Fat embolism syndrome in a patient demonstrating only neurologic symptoms. Can J Surg 41: 398-402

56. Laub DR Jr, Laub DR (1990) Fat embolism syndrome after liposuction: a case report and review of the literature. Ann Plast Surg 25: 48-52

57. Thomas P, Boussuges A, Gainnier M, Quenee V, Donati S, Ayem ML, Barthelemy A, Sainty JM (1998) Fat embolism after intrapenile injection of sweet almond oil Rev Mal Respir 15: 307-8

58. Richards ER (1997) Fat embolism syndrome. Can J Surg 40: 334-9

59. Masson RG (1992) Amniotic fluid embolism. Clin Chest Med 13: 657-65

60. Lau G, Chui PP (1994) Amniotic fluid embolism: a review of 10 fatal cases. Singapore Med J 35: 180-3

61. Price TM, Baker VV, Cefalo RC (1985) Amniotic fluid embolism. Three case reports with a review of the literature. Obstet Gynecol Surv 40: 462-75

62. Durigon M, Barbet JP, Barres D, Gherardi R, Guillon F, Paraire F, Polivka (1988) Pathologie médico-légale. Masson, Paris, Milan, Barcelone, Mexico 171 p

63. Ege E, Soysal O, Gulculer M, Ozdemir H, Pac M (1997) Cardiac hydatid cyst causing massive pulmonary embolism. Thorac Cardiovasc Surg 45: 249-50

64. Kammoun S, Zayene M, Fendri S, Fourati S, Marouene M, Ben Youssef S, Guermazi F, Daoud M (1997) Chronic cor pulmonale caused by hydatid embolism complicating hepatic hydatid cyst. Ann Cardiol Angeiol (Paris) 46: 317-20

65. Luchtrath H, Seitz HM (1990) Embolized Schistosoma ova in the lung. Pathologe 11: 304-6

66. Vuong PN, Bayssade-Dufour Ch, Albaret JL, Farhati K (1996) Histo-pathological observations in new and classical models of experimental Schistosoma haematobium infections. Trop Med International Health 1: 348-58

X
Aneuryms and other changes in vascular dimensions

1 – Aneurysms

An aneurysm is a localised dilatation of a vessel wall involving all of its coats. Arteries most often become aneurysmal but aneurysms are also found in the microcirculation and, rarely, in veins.

Arterial aneurysms

The fundamental cause of aneurysmal dilatation of a vessel is a mechanical failure of the wall, such that it is unable to provide a functionally appropriate response to applied loads. Any disease process that destroys the mechanical function of the media, focally or over an extended segment, will predispose to aneurysm formation. Although the so-called "berry" aneurysms are said to be congenital they are not; these lesions are not present at birth. What is true, however, is that the wall of some cerebral vessels is defective in a way which permits subsequent aneurysm formation [1, 2] It is interesting to note that new aneurysms may occur after repair of documented lesions [3]. A number of hereditary diseases in which scleroprotein structure is affected and some acquired diseases, together with trauma, may all produce aneurysms [4-6]. Changes in vessels with age will tend to produce a uniform increase in vessel diameter due to loss of elastic function (a change which can be distinguished from aneurysm formation by its uniformity). The physical laws underlying aneurysm formation are simple; as the diameter of a vessel increases so the tension in its wall increases; assuming the pressure within it remains constant any increase in pressure will accelerate the change. Any artery can develop an aneurysm and the clinical manifestations depend on the location and size. Progression is inevitable [7-12]. The natural course of an aneurysm is of progressive growth leading to rupture; in the aorta, the growth rate of aneurysms averages approximately 1.5 mm in diameter in the thoracic, and 4 mm in the abdominal aorta, per year [13]. In the aorta three factors have been shown to affect growth rate: the initial size of the aneurysm, the presence of hypertension and the presence of (-adrenergic blockade. The latter factor has an independent effect on aneurysm growth rate [14].

"Congenital" cerebral aneurysms (berry aneurysms, micro aneurysms of Charcot Bouchard)

The nature of the development of the cerebral circulation with the rapid expansion of the cerebrum in vertebrates produces bifurcations which are often muscle deficient. At these sites aneurysms develop with time and with disease processes which raise blood pressure, or further damage the wall. Increasing age and hypertension, and much less commonly, disorders of scleroprotein synthesis (Ehlers Danlos syndrome, pseudoxanthoma elasticum, Marfan syndrome) may facilitate formation of berry aneurysms. Statistical information has been collected in a number of ways; the frequency of berry aneurysms is 0.8% of patients coming to autopsy in an unselected Japanese series [15], the incidence of multiple berry aneurysms in a Thai population is 6.5% [16], and familial intracranial aneurysms have been documented by large epidemiological studies in Sweden and Finland, with a frequency as high as 6.7 to 10%. [1]. There is an increased risk among patients with adult onset polycystic kidney and liver disease [17-21]. Schievink and his co-workers have documented dissection and aneurysm rupture in alpha 1-antitrypsin deficiency [22, 23]. Berry aneurysms are an important cause of fatal intracranial bleeding in young patients [24]; however rupture is commoner in the elderly. Over half of the deaths caused by ruptured berry aneurysm occur in the 50-80 year age group, the overall male/female ratio being 2: 3 [25].

Pathology and differential diagnosis

The circle of Willis is the major site of occurrence and most develop in the anterior circulation (Fig. 1). Major sites of involvement are the internal carotid posterior communicating artery junction (42%), the anterior communicating artery (34%), and the middle cerebral artery (20%) [26]. More than 70% of the anterior communicating artery aneurysms occurred as single aneurysms; less than 30% of the middle cerebral artery aneurysms were single. Anterior communicating artery aneurysms showed a right side predominance in males but not in females [27]. Berry aneurysms are saccular out pouchings, measuring from a few mm to 2 or 3 cm having a bright, red, shiny surface with a thin translucent wall (Fig. 2). Most of them occur at arterial bifurcations (Fig. 3).

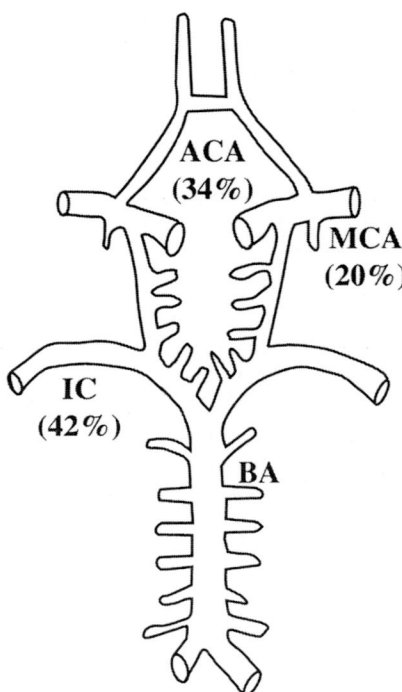

Fig. 1. Major sites of congenital intracranial aneurysms according to Escourolle and Poirier (26). ACA: anterior communicating artery; BA: basilar artery; IC: internal carotid artery; MCA: middle cerebral artery

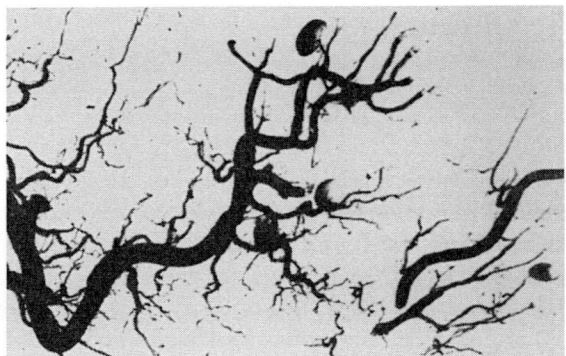

Fig. 2. Angiographic pattern of intracranial berry aneurysms. Post-mortem preparation. (Document of Pr G. Salamon. Courtesy Dr JP. Véron)

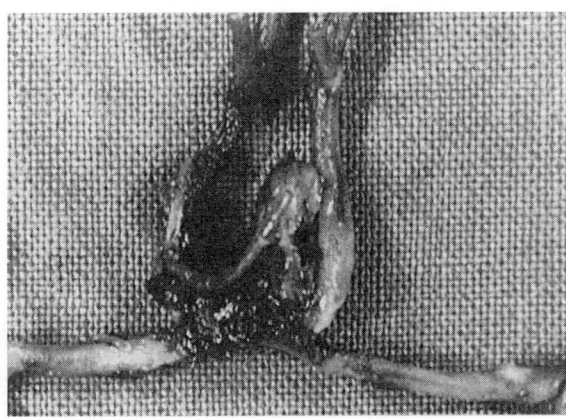

Fig. 3. Berry aneurysm developed at the anterior communicating artery. (Courtesy Pr D. Hénin)

Histologically, the arterial wall adjacent to the neck of the aneurysm often shows some intimal thickening and gradual attenuation of the media as it approaches the neck. At the neck of the aneurysm, the muscular wall and intimal elastic lamina are usually absent or fragmentary, and the wall of the sac is made up of thickened and hyalinized intima (Fig. 4). The adventitia covering the sac is continuous with that of the parent artery [28]. Usually, the site of rupture is not readily visible and, for this reason, surgical specimens should be submitted to serial sections in order to identify the rupture zone. Atheromatous plaques, calcification, or thrombotic occlusion of the aneurysm may be found.

Acquired aneurysms

Atherosclerotic aneurysms

Atherosclerosis is by far the commonest cause of aneurysm formation in the developed world, aneurysms resulting from destruction and weakening of the media by atheroma or by the effects of compression of the complex load bearing structure of the media by the atheromatous mass [29]. The abdominal aorta, from below the renal arteries to the iliac bifurcation, is the most frequently affected site [13, 30-32]. The common iliac vessels and the cervical portion of carotid arteries are commonly involved [33, 34]. The coeliac trunk and mesenteric arteries may be aneurysmal [35]. Aneurysms of the coronary arteries occur in 1.5-4.9% of coronary angiograms [36].

Pathology and differential diagnosis

Atherosclerotic aneurysms are generally fusiform and often involve a long segment of the vessel. They generally contain laminated mural thrombus. Histologically, the luminal aspect is composed of plaque or thrombus overlying ulcerated plaque or a fibrous intimal surface. Acute complete thrombotic occlusion may occur.

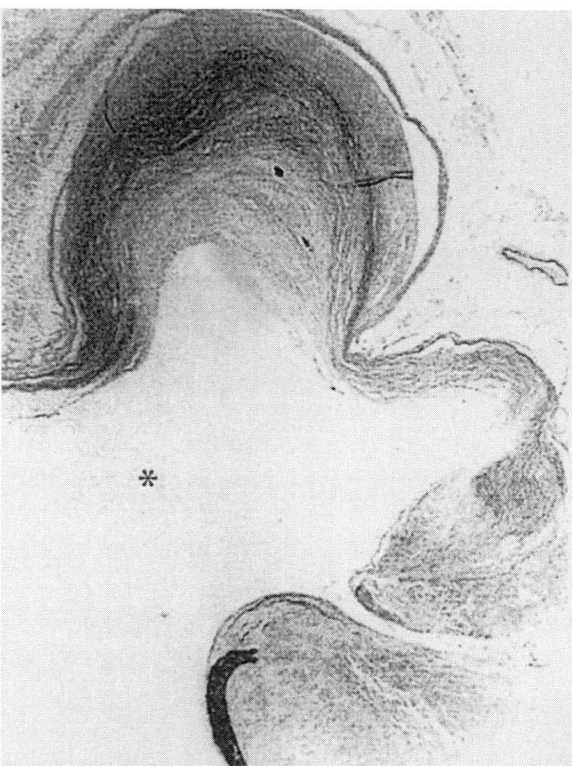

Fig. 4. Rather collapsed berry aneurysm of the circle of Willis. Elastic membrane (black line) curled over its neck (asterisk). Orcein elastic stain (Orcein)

Inflammatory aneurysms

It is not clear whether an inflammatory aneurysm is a separate entity or an early stage in the evolution of an underlying disease with inflammation of the aorta and fibrosis. Inflammatory changes in an atherosclerotic aneurysm are presumed to be a consequence of microscopic ruptures in the wall. Leakage of atherosclerotic material into the peri-aneurysmal tissue is associated with chronic inflammation (Fig. 5) or autoimmune response to antigens coming from the atheromatous plaque [37-39]. In Takayasu's disease, temporal arteritis (Fig. 6-7), classic polyarteritis nodosa, Kawasaki's disease, sarcoidosis and Behçet's disease, inflammation may produce destructive changes which give rise to aneurysms. Aneurysms with marked inflammation occur in the aorta and its major branches, the cerebral and coronary arteries and other medium sized arteries [40-43].

Pathology and differential diagnosis

Grossly, the wall is considerably thickened without clear demarcation between the arterial layers and the

peri adventitial tissues. Histologically, the luminal aspect is covered by laminated thrombus beneath which complete or ulcerated atheromatous plaques may be found. The underlying media shows loss of the normal lamellar pattern and there is extensive fibrosis extending to the adventitia and entrapping periaortic tissue [44]. The cells in the infiltrate are made up of similar numbers of CD3+/CD4+ and CD3+/CD8+ T lymphocytes [38, 45]. Focal or diffuse heavy infiltrates of lymphocytes and plasma cells and granulomas are present. However, some histological characteristics may suggest a specific diagnosis.

Syphilitic aneurysm

Syphilis is now an exceptional cause of isolated aneurysms, usually affecting the ascending aorta and arch and more rarely the proximal branches of the arch vessels [46, 47].

Pathology and differential diagnosis

Syphilitic aneurysm may be fusiform or saccular. They typically enlarge slowly compressing contiguous

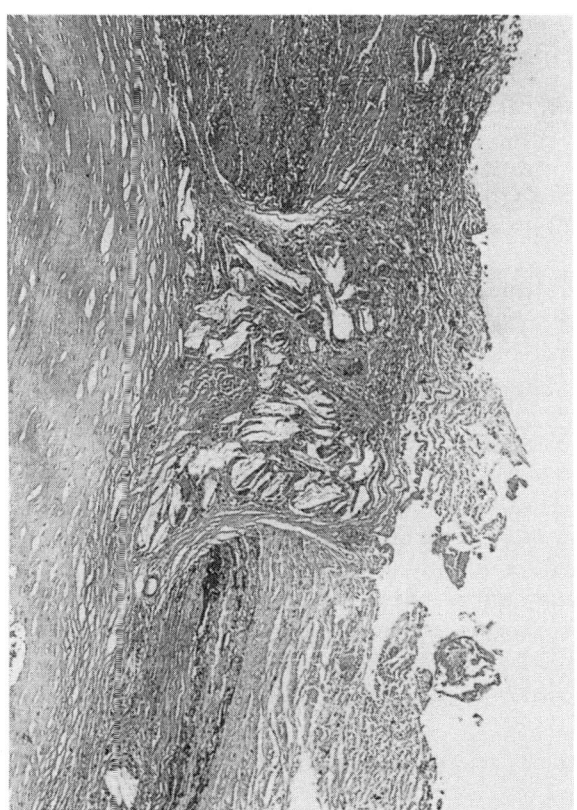

Fig. 5. Inflammatory atherosclerotic aneurysm. Note leakage of atherosclerotic material containing cholesterol crystals into the adventitia. Haematoxylin, eosin and saffron stain. (HES)

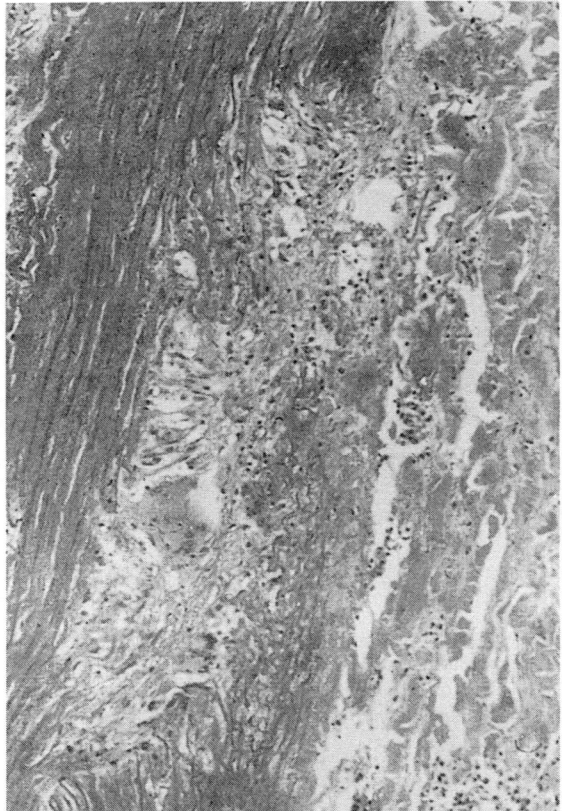

Fig. 6. Inflammatory aneurysm of the aorta caused by giant cell arteritis. Note distortion of the media by granulomas. HES

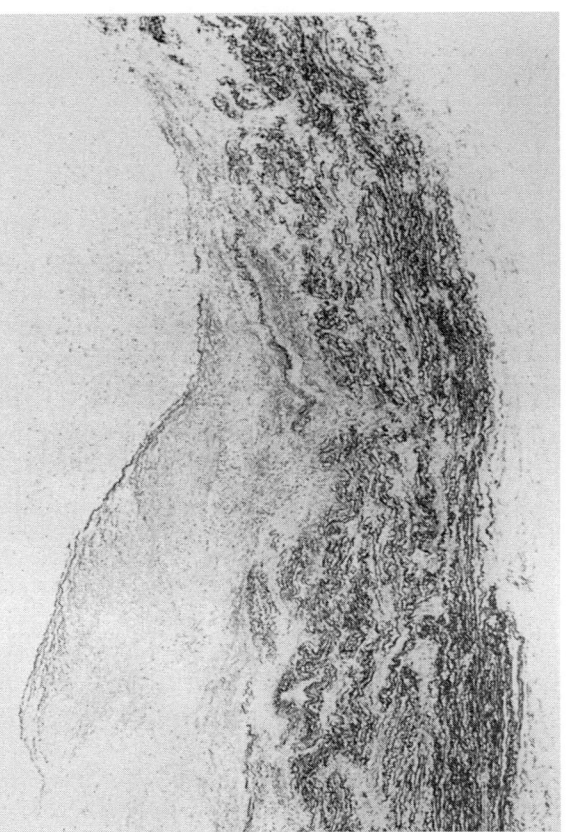

Fig. 7. Inflammatory aneurysm of the aorta caused by giant cell arteritis. "Tiger skin" pattern of the medial elastic frame. Orcein

structures and erode them [48, 49]. Microscopically, there is endarteritis and periarteritis of the vasa vasora, with obliterative changes, leading to focal necrosis and scarring of the media, with disruption of the elastic lamellae and weakening of the wall. There is an inflammatory infiltrate containing plasma cells, lymphocytes, and histiocytes. Fine calcification may develop within the wall of the vessel. Dissection is infrequent, probably because of the relatively intact intima and because of the extensive fibrosis in the media, but fatal rupture into the thoracic cavity, oesophagus or vena cava is a common cause of death.

Aneurysms caused by fibromuscular dysplasia

Aneurysms occur in any artery involved by the extensive medial subtype of fibromuscular dysplasia. They may be a source of fatal intracranial haemorrhage (Fig. 8). They develop in a fragile area of the arterial wall or in a post-stenotic segment of the affected artery and may be multiple [50, 51].

Pathology and differential diagnosis

Grossly, these aneurysms may be single or multiple. They are mostly sack-like (Fig. 9-10) and are variable in size. Their histological appearance is unremarkable, the aneurysmal wall being mainly composed of fibrotic tissue. Some atherosclerotic plaques may thicken the luminal aspect (Fig. 11). Identification of the primary lesion is possible only in operative specimens including a non-aneurysmal area. In the renal artery, an exceptional complication of this type of aneurysm is rupture into the corresponding vein, giving rise to a fistula [52, 53].

Posttraumatic or false aneurysm (pulsating haematoma)

False aneurysms may develop after trauma of any type. Metastatic tumours may rarely be the initiating factor, causing rupture of the intima and media with formation of a haematoma within the wall of the ves-

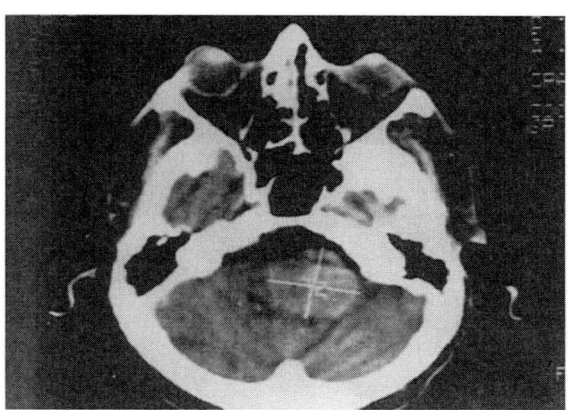

Fig. 8. Computed tomography pattern of a single sacciform aneurysm compressing the left cerebellum. (Courtesy Dr E. Meary)

sel [54]. Clinically, the lesion is evident as a pulsatile mass of variable size.

Pathology and differential diagnosis

Histological examination reveals remnants of the vascular coats within an organised haematoma.

Elastin stains help identify the fragmented internal elastic lamina; the external elastic lamella is often unaffected.

Poststenotic aneurysms

Any vascular stenotic lesion (compression, stenosis or coarctation) will be accompanied by post stenotic dilatation, which may become aneurysmal [55-58]. When the stenosis is removed in its early stage, the dilated segment may recover its normal size.

Pathology and differential diagnosis

Poststenotic aneurysms are characterised by jet lesions resulting from the jet of blood striking the wall after passing through the narrowed lumen. Grossly, they appear as corrugated patches on the intima, distal to the stenosis. Histologically, the area shows localised fibrous intimal thickening; the underlying media may be distorted with loss of elastic tissue. Superimposed atherosclerotic plaques may develop. Intraluminal thrombosis leads to irreversible post stenotic dilatation and can be a source of distal embolism.

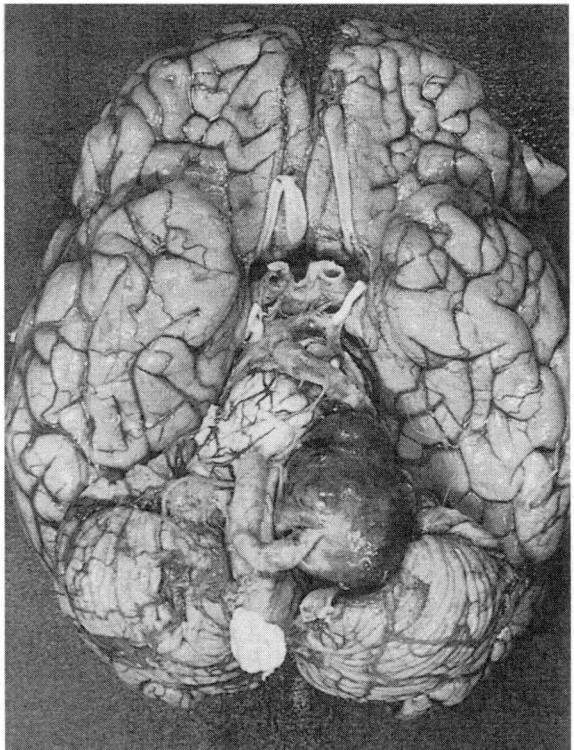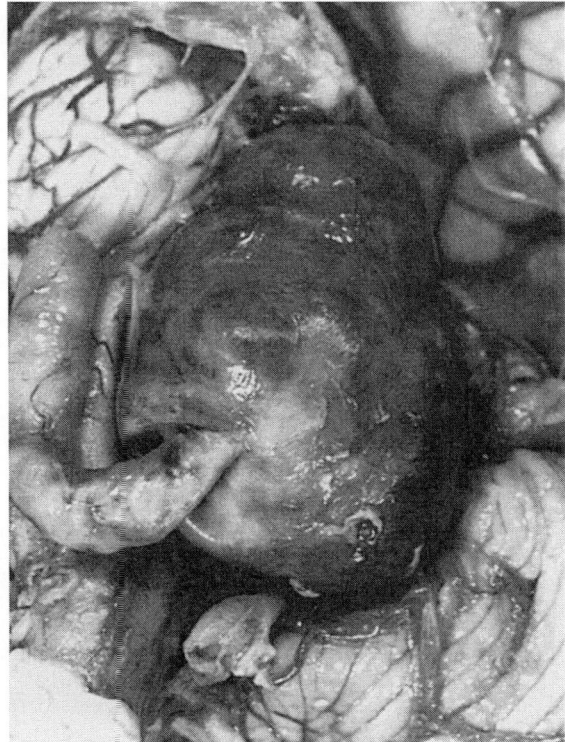

Fig. 9-10. Sacciform aneurysm of the basilar artery caused by fibromuscular dysplasia. (Courtesy Dr F. Beuvon)

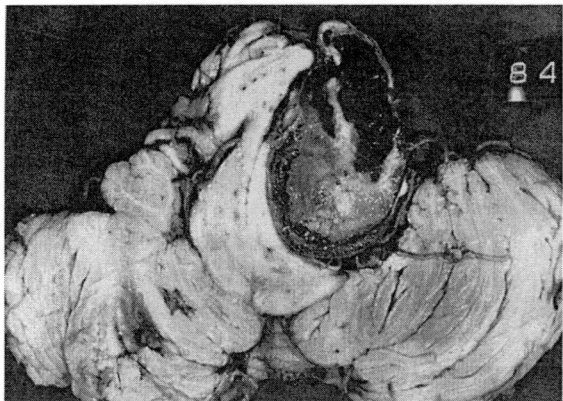

Fig. 11. Sacciform aneurysm of the basilar artery. Note occlusive luminal thrombosis. (Courtesy Dr F. Beuvon)

Venous aneurysms

Venous aneurysms are rare. Harris reported the first case of a jugular vein aneurysm in 1928 and around 600 cases of venous aneurysms have been recorded in the medical literature, 172 involving the lower limbs, 20 of them the popliteal veins (Fig. 12) [59, 60]. Some authors consider venous aneurysm to be the result of a localised dysplasia or malformation [61]; others contend that they are caused by parietal fibrosis secondary to incorporation of a thrombus [62] or varicosity. Most are asymptomatic; when patent they may present as a non expanding and non murmuring mass present in the standing position, which flattens when the patient lies down or when pressure is applied. Recurrent pulmonary embolism is characteristic of popliteal vein aneurysms [59, 63-65]. Fatal haemorrhage may result from a ruptured intracerebral venous aneurysm.

Pathology and differential diagnosis

A venous aneurysm may be sack like or funnel shaped. Histological findings have been described very rarely; some authors have reported hypoplasia of the media with or without valvular agenesis (Fig. 13-14), and thinning of elastic fibres, but preservation of the architecture of the venous wall (Fig. 15). Others have described fibrosis. Differential diagnosis includes false aneurysm caused by venous rupture or a thrombosed varicocele.

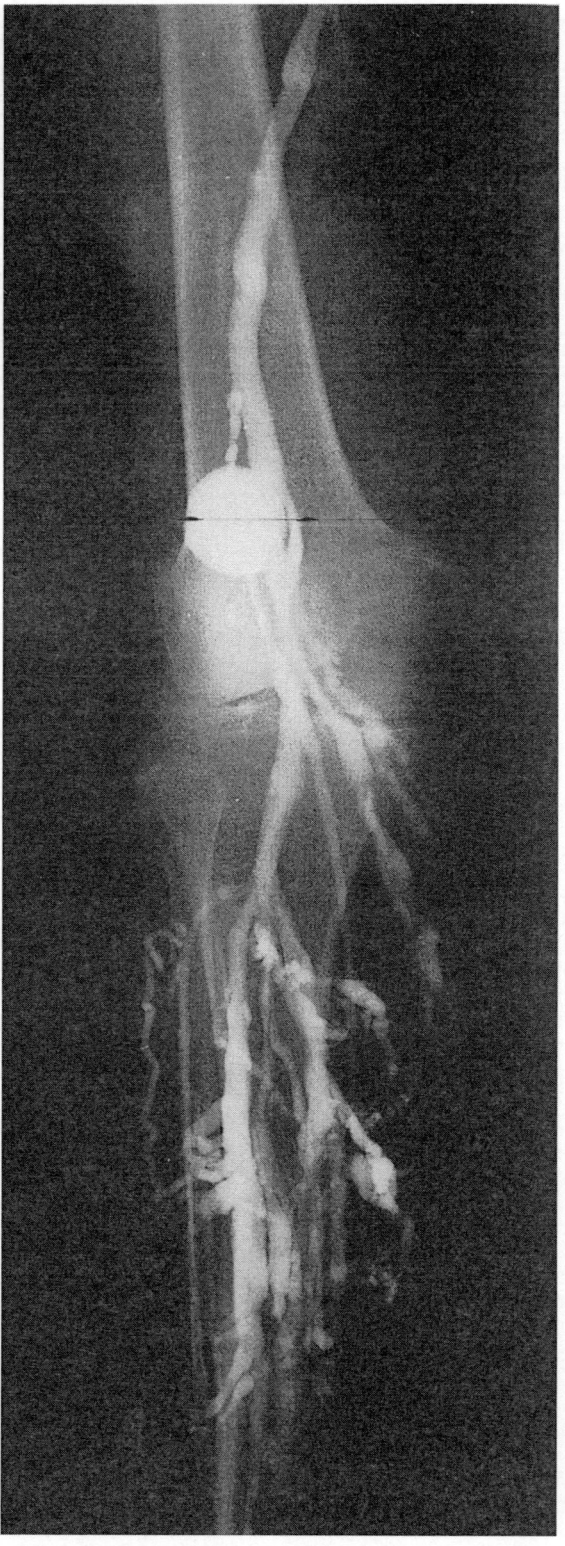

Fig. 12. Selective angiogram showing a large popliteal aneurysm. Note associated dystrophic changes of other venous collaterals (Courtesy Dr P. Lagneau)

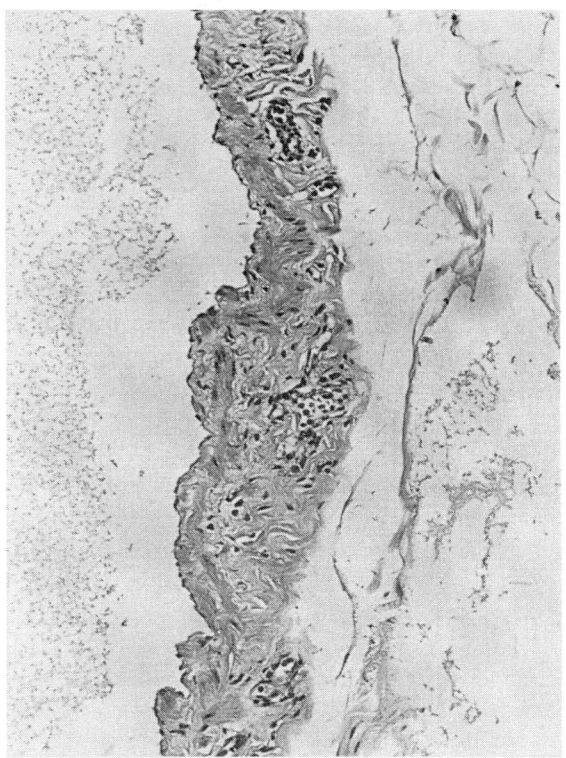

Fig. 13. Popliteal vein aneurysm. Note irregular thickness of the venous wall, devoid of valves. HES

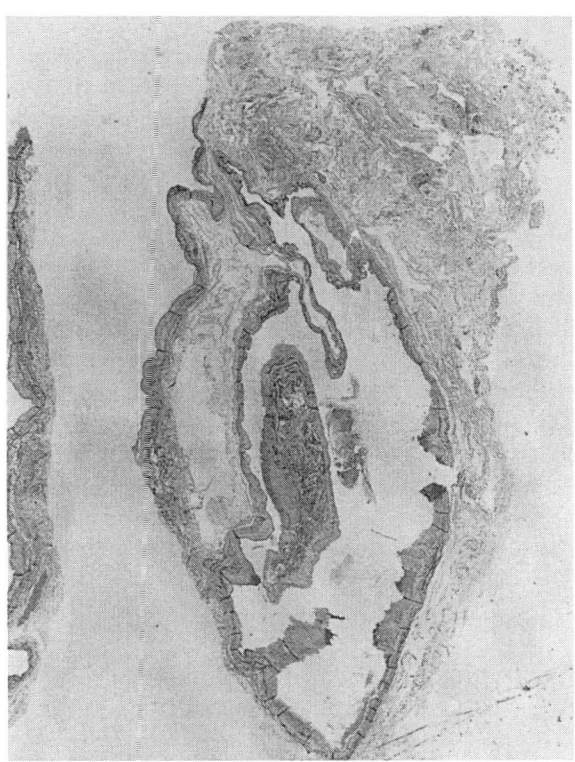

Fig. 14. Popliteal vein aneurysm showing hypoplasia of the media. Smooth muscle cells are lacking in some areas. HES

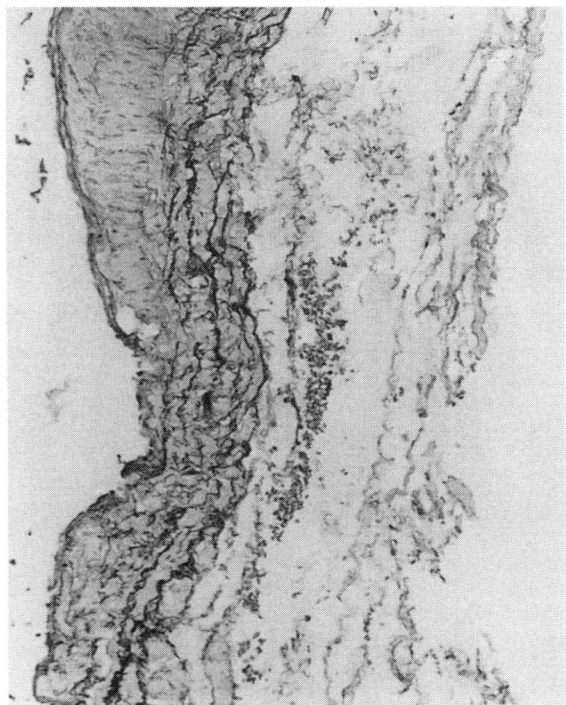

Fig. 15. Popliteal vein aneurysm. Area of generally well-preserved architecture. Orcein

2 – Dissecting aneurysm

Dissection is defined as a splitting of the vascular wall, with blood entering through an intimal tear or, less commonly, by primary intraparietal haemorrhage. It generally occurs without true arterial dilatation but may be part of a widespread atheromatous process. The term "dissecting haematoma" is a much more accurate designation for this lesion, which mostly involves the aorta but may occur in medium or small arteries.

Dissection of the aorta

This condition is relatively rare in clinical practise with a frequency of about 3.0/100,000/year admissions in a general hospital [66]. However, it accounts for 1 to 5% of sudden deaths.

Clinical presentation

In the authors' experience dissection may occur at any age, but patients younger than 40 yr. are generally suffering from a metabolic or endocrine defect [67].

From around 40 years, excluding those cases due to compression and laceration of the media due to road traffic accidents, there is a clear predominance in men (1.6 M/1F) [66]. The great arteries of the neck are involved in 20-40% of cases. Hypertension is also common (70%) and may contribute to the pathogenesis. Arterial and venous compression may occur and dissection may occlude the coronary ostia in this way, or may track back and rupture into the pericardium, with tamponade. Rupture into neighbouring viscera is common [68]. The course of a dissecting haematoma varies but it rarely remains circumscribed. In the first 48 hours, the mortality for Type A dissections (see table 1) approaches 1% per hour. Without treatment, mortality is 74% after two weeks and 93% after 1 year. In one study, the two-year mortality in surgically treated patients with Type A dissection approached 50%. Initial mortality was 40% in these patients. The long-term prognosis is still poor [69].

Aetiology

Various conditions favour dissection. Atherosclerosis, hypertension and congenital malformations (bicuspid aortic valve, coarctation, hypoplasia, stenosis of the aortic isthmus) can all accelerate age-related degeneration of the aortic wall. Changes in pregnancy and, most importantly, in the Marfan syndrome, Ehlers Danlos' disease, and Touraine's systemic elastorrhexis [70-73] all increase the risk of developing a dissection. The occurrence of isolated familial cases suggests an undefined underlying hereditary predisposition [74], but as genetic knowledge increases it seems that familial occurrence is almost always associated with genetic defects in scleroprotein assembly. Other causative conditions include vasculitis, mycotic aneurysms, blunt trauma and iatrogenic injury [75, 76].

Experimentally, poisoning with bêta-amminoproprionitrile and changes in collagen induced by copper deficiency weaken the wall in a manner which favours dissection [77].

Pathology and differential diagnosis

Three main classifications permit easy description of the aortic dissection, its extension and the site of the entry orifice. Table 1 summarises these.

1. **Houston classification (De Bakey 1965)** [78]. The extent of the dissection determines the classification. In Type 1 the dissection involves the ascending aorta from the aortic valve to the ostium of the left subclavian artery; it can extend to the whole aorta. In type 2 only the ascending aorta is involved. In type 3 the dissection starts at the left sub clavicular ostium and extends to the descending aorta (Fig. 16). Types 1 and 3 are frequent, type 2 rare. Type 3 may have a "retrograde" course.

2. **Stanford classification (Daily 1970)** [79]. This simplified classification describes two types. Type A describes dissection involving the ascending aorta, whatever the starting point and type B dissection involving only the descending aorta (Fig. 16).

3. **Classification of Dubost-Guilmet (Guilmet 1990)** (80). A letter (A, B, C, and D) designates the site of entry; A ascending aorta, B aortic arch, C descending thoracic aorta and D abdominal aorta. Additional roman numerals II III IV) and (I indicate the extension of the cleavage plane; I ascending aorta, II aortic arch, III descending thoracic aorta, IV abdominal aorta. The letter R precedes this number when a "retrograde" course exists (Fig. 16).

Table 1: Houston (De Bakey) classification of aortic dissection and equivalencies (eo: entry orifice; dp: dissecting plane)

HOUSTON (DE BAKEY)	STANFORD (DAILY)	DUBOST-GUILMET
Type 1: Ascending aorta from aortic valves to left subclavian artery	A: Ascending aorta	Ascending aorta (A: eo; I: dp) Aortic arch (B: eo; II: dp)
Type 2: Ascending aorta	A: Ascending aorta	
Type 3: Left subclavian ostium to descending aorta	B: Descending aorta	Thoracic aorta (C: eo; III: dp) Abdominal aorta (D: eo; IV: dp)

Grossly, the dissected area is dilated. The entry orifice allows blood to penetrate into the outermost part of the media, where the pattern of distribution of the intercellular contacts, the loads in the wall and alteration in the relative strengths of different parts of the media ensure that the cleavage plane occurs at the junction of the inner two thirds and the outer third of the wall [81]. On section, there are two lumina, the primary lumen, often partially collapsed, the second one at the cleavage line. In the aorta, the entry orifice is generally located in the ascending aorta, 1 to 2 cm from the aortic valves [82] more rarely in the isthmus and the descending aorta. It is frequently linear, transverse and between 1 to 2 cm in length. Extension downstream or into the main aortic branches is the rule.

Longitudinal and spiral aortic dissection preferentially involves the right coronary and cervical arteries, the left renal artery and ilio-femoral axis. In 10 to 35% of cases, there is a re entry orifice in the downstream aorta or in the iliac arteries. In retrograde ex-

tension, the haematoma may tear the aortic ring and evert the valves, causing acute aortic insufficiency (8 to 10%). Myocardial infarction occurs in 5 to 10% of patients. Disruption of the auriculo– ventricular innervation occurs when the haematoma distorts the cardiac walls and septa (Fig. 17). Fatal external rupture of the haematoma into body cavities may occur (81.0% of patients in the series of Meszaros et al) [66] during the first 48 hours or in the first month. In the acute stage, the cleavage line is distended by an haematoma (Fig. 18). It is commonly located at the internal – external junction of the aortic wall (Fig. 19) with mural haemorrhage and neutrophil infiltration (Fig. 20). In later stages, organisation of the haematoma gives rise to granulation tissue made up of loose fibrotic tissue, and haemosiderin loaded macrophages among newly formed capillaries. In the chronic stage (Fig. 21-23) the cleavage plane is sealed by fibrous tissue which may give rise to stenosis; proliferating vessels grow in from the adventitia [83, 84]. Vasa vasora criss-crossing the adventita often display medial hyperplasia, mimicking leiomyoma (Fig. 24). Differential diagnosis should exclude peri medial or sub adventitial fibrodysplasia, the fibrotic chronic stage of Takayasu's aortitis, and changes related to the previous use of adhesive agents used to treat acute dissection.

Dissection of medium, small arteries and veins

Isolated dissection may involve arteries other than the aorta [85, 86] and veins. Causes include ageing, fibromuscular dysplasia, trauma (spontaneous or iatrogenic) or vasculitis. In veins the most frequent causes are medial degeneration associated with age and trauma.

3 – Arteriovenous fistulae

This term describes all conditions that give rise to abnormal communication between an artery and a vein. An arteriovenous fistula may be acquired or congenital.

Acquired arteriovenous fistulae

Most acquired arteriovenous fistulae are caused by penetrating wounds, blunt trauma (Fig. 25) or iatrogenic injury [87-92]. Other causes include sponta-

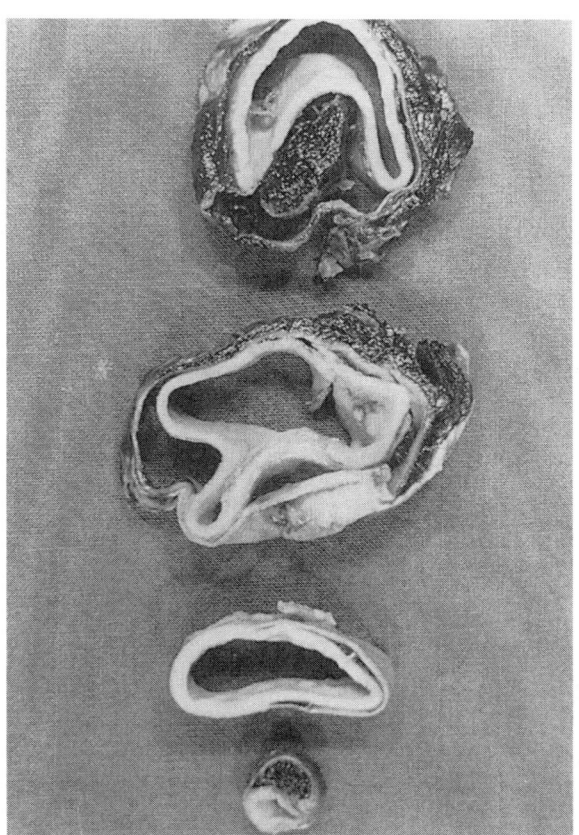

Fig. 16. Acute dissection of the aorta. Houston type 3 or Stanford type B or Dubost-Guilmet type CIII

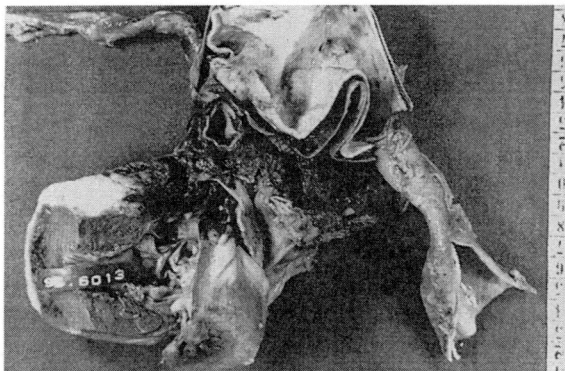

Fig. 17. Retrograde extension of acute dissection of the aorta. Houston type 3 or Dubost-Guilmet type CRIII

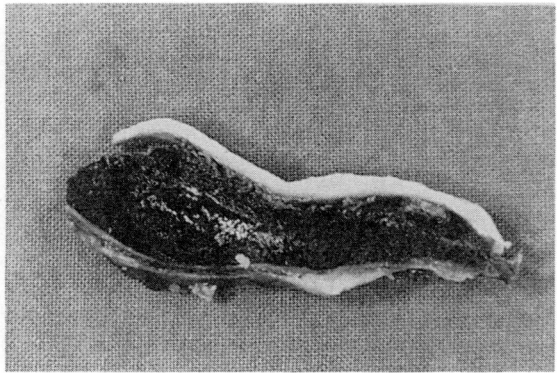

Fig. 18. Acute dissection of the aorta. Dissecting cleavage plane occluded by a fresh haematoma

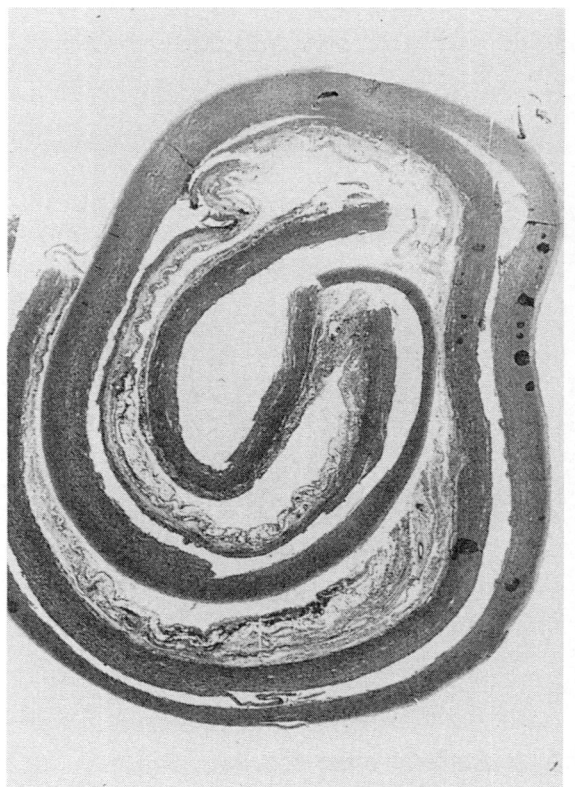

Fig. 19. Acute dissection of the aorta. Dissecting cleavage plane located at the internal 3/4-external 1/4 junction of the aortic wall. HES

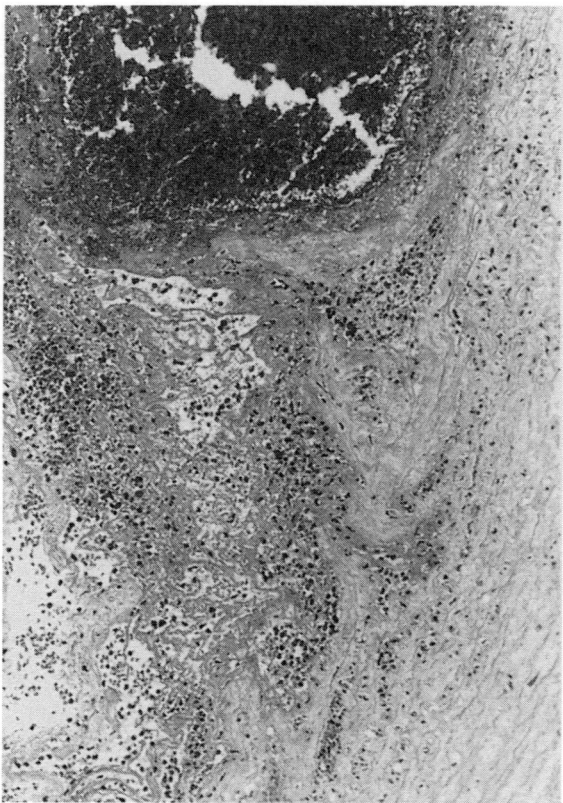

Fig. 20. Acute dissection of the aorta. Note parietal haemorrhage and neutrophil infiltration along the cleavage plane. HES

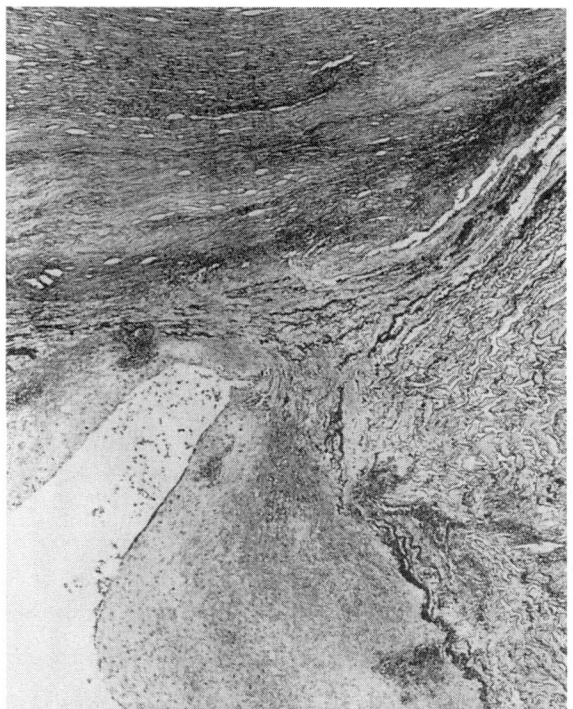

Fig. 21. Organised cleavage plane displaying a newly-formed internal elastic membrane. Orcein

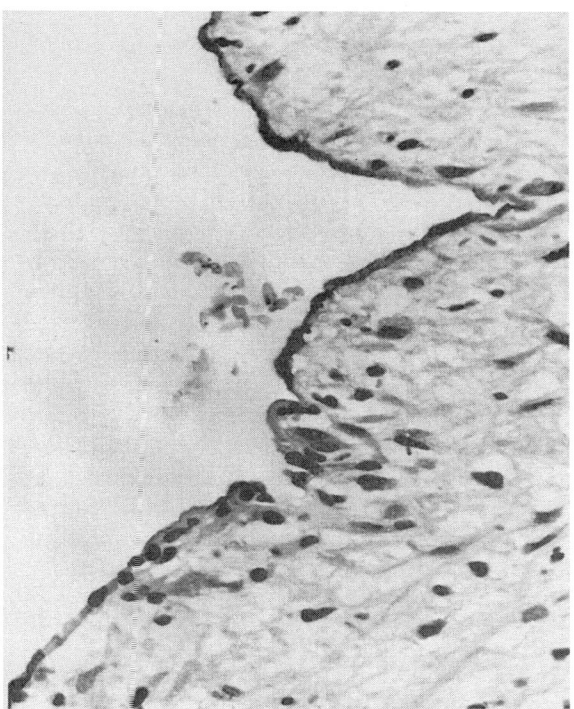

Fig. 22. Chronic dissection of the aorta. Organised cleavage plane invested by endothelial cells evidenced by CD34 antibody-labelling. Per-oxidase antiperoxidase immunohistochemical technique (PAP)

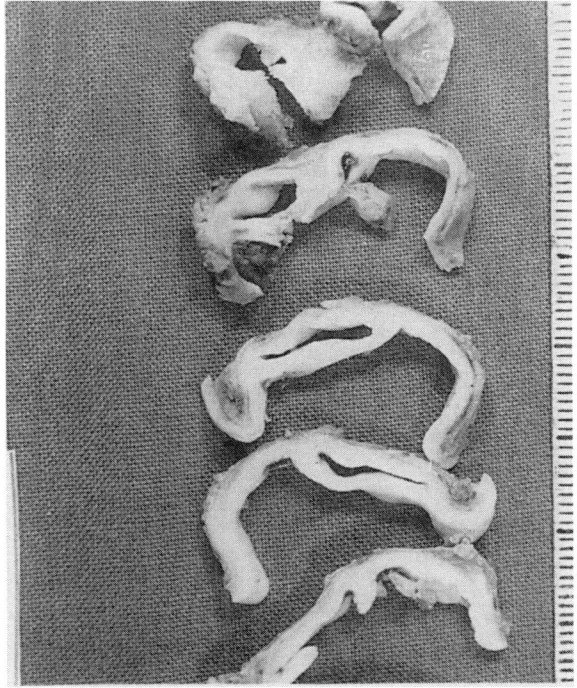

Fig. 23. Chronic dissection of the aorta. Specimen opened along the organised dissecting plane. Note partially collapsed primary lumen

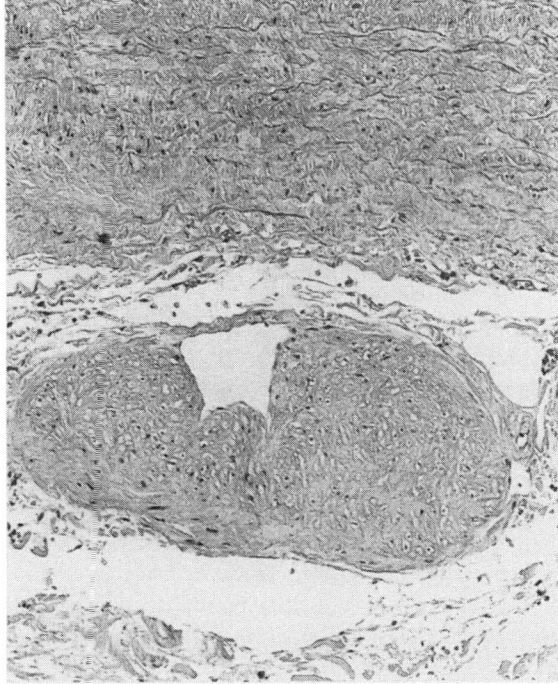

Fig. 24. Dissection of an aorta with medial cystic change. Note leiomyomatous hyperplasia of the media of an adventitial vasa vasorum. HES

neous rupture of an arterial aneurysm into neighbouring veins and infectious arteritis with spontaneous perforation [90, 93-97].

The clinical manifestations depend on the vessels affected and unusual presentations include pulsatile tinnitus, Jacksonian seizures, tracheal compression and stridor, ascites, abdominal pain, portal hypertension and the throbbing buttock syndrome [98-102]. Arteriovenous fistulae may give rise to unilateral varicose veins, limb hypertrophy [103] and, if a large shunt occurs, heart failure. Complications include thrombosis, rupture, haemorrhage and ischaemia [104]. Rarely, spontaneous thrombosis may close the fistula [105]. Bacterial endarteritis, alone or concomitant with bacterial endocarditis, is a rare complication. The abnormal haemodynamic strain on the venous walls leads to ischaemic changes with oedema, stasis pigmentation, chronic induration, skin ulceration of distal parts of the extremities and exceptional kaposiform angiodermatitis (Bluefarb-Stewart syndrome) [106]. Leiomyosarcoma has been reported in an arteriovenous fistula [107].

Pathology and differential diagnosis

There are three main types of acquired arteriovenous fistulae. There may be a direct connection between an artery and its accompanying vein, direct connection of an arterial aneurysm to a vein, or a fistula or an aneurysm is interposed between the artery and the vein.

Grossly, during the first few weeks after a fistula has developed, the vein is distended locally and its wall is thickened. When the fistula is large, the vein may become so distended that it mimics an aneurysm (Fig. 26). The artery proximal to the fistula dilates and undergoes aneurysmal dilatation [88]. In the healing state, the arterial wall proximal to or at the fistula becomes rigid and even stenosed because of fibrosis. Histological features are similar, whatever the cause. If the fistula is small, the vein progressively assumes the appearance of an artery until, at the end of 6 to 9 months, it may be impossible to distinguish the vein from the artery except by its anatomical position. When the fistula is large, the veins in the region of the fistula undergo major changes. The intima thickens and contains numerous newly formed elastic fibers arranged in a circular layer. The media also shows thickening by newly formed elastic fibers interspersed with thick, old, stretched ones, and hyperplastic smooth muscle cells merging with a fibrotic intima (Fig. 27). In the artery the media becomes thinned; this is caused partly by the disappearance of elastic tis-

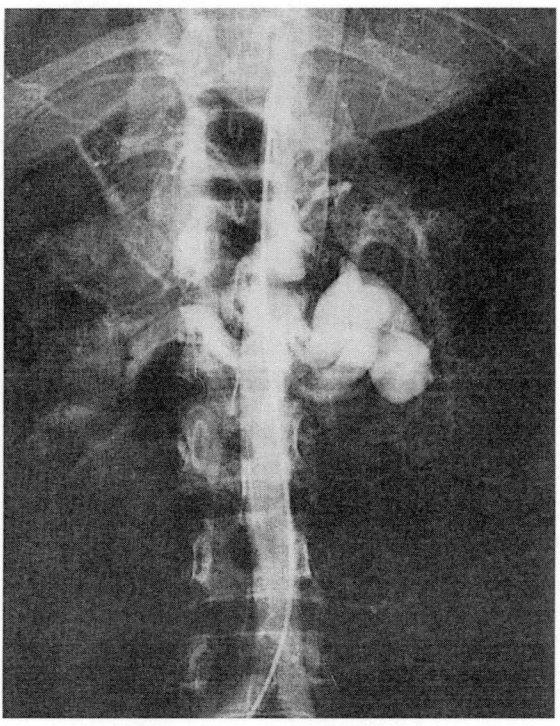

Fig. 25. Acquired arteriovenous fistula of the renal vessels caused by a blunt trauma. Angiographic aspect (Courtesy Dr P. Lagneau)

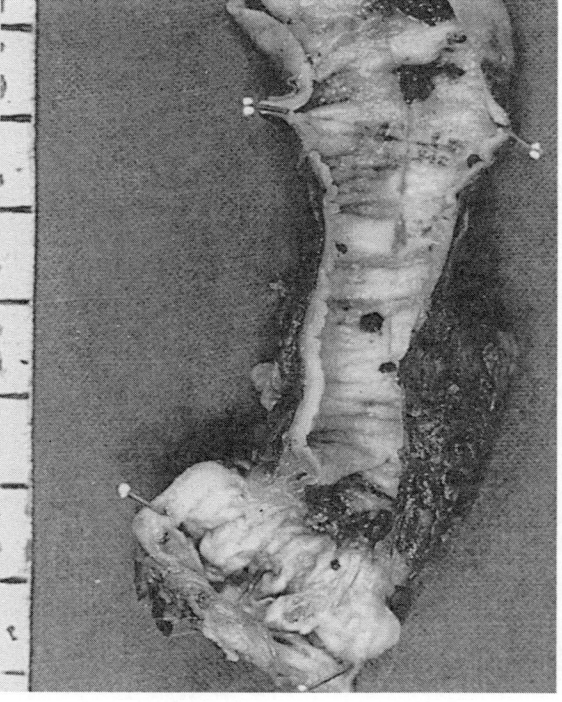

Fig. 26. Acquired arteriovenous fistula of the renal vessels. Marked dilatation of the venous side mimicking an aneurysm

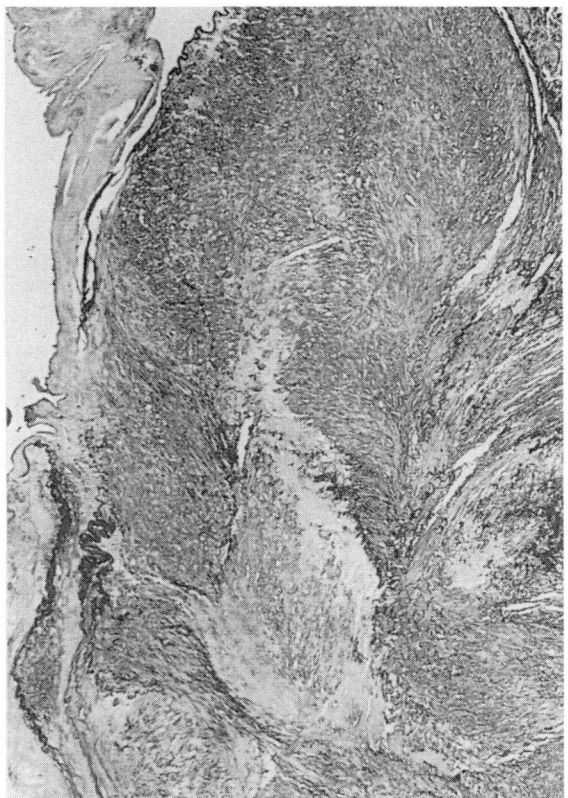

Fig. 27. Acquired arteriovenous fistula of the renal vessels. Arterialisation of the venous side with newly-formed internal elastic membrane and intimal thickening. Orcein

sue, partly by a loss of smooth muscle cells and partly by dilatation.

Congenital arteriovenous fistula

Many terms have been used to describe this condition [108]. Congenital arteriovenous fistulae can develop in any portion of the body, but most commonly affect the head, neck and lower extremities [109, 110]. Small superficial lesions occur as asymptomatic cutaneous nodules without thrill or bruit. Large fistulae involving an extremity may produce an increase in the muscle volume, bone length, and local temperature, with increased sweating and hair growth. Birthmarks or other vascular lesions may be present in 50% of cases. Varicose pulsatile veins, with ulceration and gangrene are almost invariably present.

Pulmonary arteriovenous fistula may be large and multifocal with a bloody cough, hypoxaemia with clubbing, cyanosis and reactive polycythaemia. There may be associated anomalous venous drainage to the

vena cava or to the right atrium [111, 112]. Gastrointestinal and renal lesions may give rise to fatal haemorrhage [113]. Concomitant pulmonary and cerebral arteriovenous fistulae have been reported [114]. Multiple, large, congenital arteriovenous fistulas are often associated with other vascular malformations and angiomatous complex syndromes including the Osler Weber Rendu, Parkes Weber, Sturge Weber, Klippel Trenaunay, Servelle Martorell and LEOPARD syndromes [115-120]. In the trunk, congenital arteriovenous fistulas may be associated with cutaneous and intradural spinal haemangiomas in the same metameric segment. Intraosseous arteriovenous fistulae of the extremities are rare malformations frequently associated with severe systemic haemodynamic alterations [121]. Some small fistulas may undergo thrombosis and regress; others grow slowly and reach only a small size. Congestive heart failure is rare, with intracerebral fistulae in the neonate an important group presenting in this way. Kaposiform angiodermatitis (Bluefarb-Stewart syndrome) may occur.

Pathology and differential diagnosis

There are collections of irregularly distributed vessels of variable size; some thrombosed, others patent. Histologically, there are collections of anomalous patulous vessels having a structure that is atypical for both arteries and veins. Serial sections hardly permit the identification of small precapillary arteriovenous communications and the fistula may be quite impossible to diagnose out of context. Local haemorrhages, haemosiderin deposits together with capillary proliferation and fibrosis may be seen. In the skin, these changes, mostly secondary to chronic ischaemia, may represent part of the Bluefarb-Stewart syndrome or kaposiform angiodermatitis (Fig. 28-32) [122]. This complication should be differentiated from Kaposi's sarcoma but cellular atypia and necrosis are lacking [123-125]. In the lungs, arteriovenous fistulas often develop away from the bronchial tree and must be distinguished from normal arteriovenous shunts, which are frequently found in the periphery. Confusion may occur when these physiological shunts are accentuated after embolism or in patients with pulmonary stenosis and sickle cell anemia.

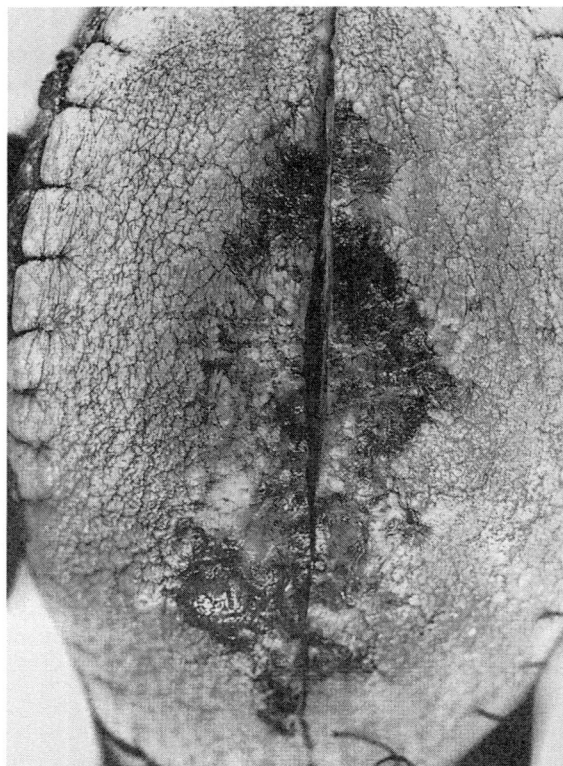

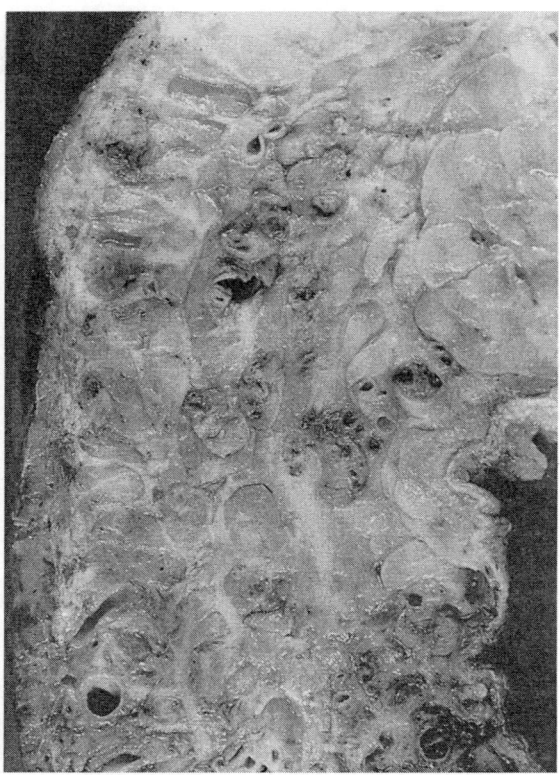

Fig. 28. Bluefarb-Stewart syndrome. A 28 year-old man having at birth a superficial arterio-venous malformation of the skin and sub-cutaneous tissue of the right greater trochanter. This lesion suddenly increased in size over a one-year period with thrill and skin erosion

Fig. 29. Bluefarb-Stewart syndrome. Operative specimen showing multiple patoulous vessels with surrounding haemorrhages on cut section

4 – Vasculomegaly, tortuosity, coiling and kinking

Vasculomegaly

Markedly ectatic, irregular blood vessels (arteries or veins) may be associated with reduced rates of blood flow [126, 127]. The change is often age dependent (Fig. 33-34) but occurs in the Beckwith Wiedemann syndrome and acromegaly; however, not all acromegalics are affected. Any vessel may be involved [128].

Tortuosity, coiling and kinking

Some authors have found it useful to classify arterial wall deformity as tortuosity, when the artery has a "C" or "S" shape; coiling, when the elongation is more evident and the artery forms one or more loops (Fig. 35-

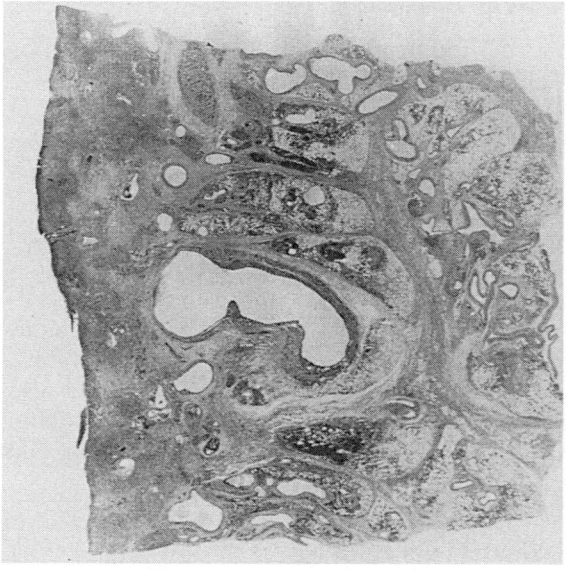

Fig. 30 Bluefarb-Stewart syndrome. Reactional proliferation of blood capillaries distorting the dermis. HES

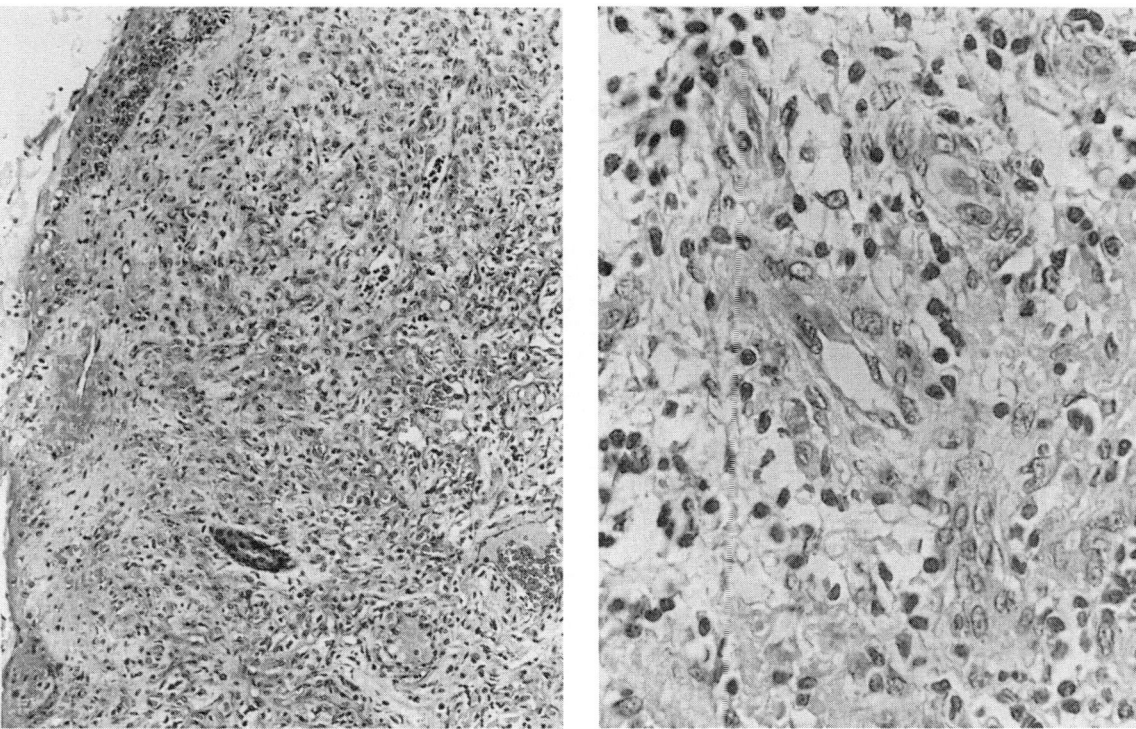

Fig. 31-32. Bluefarb-Stewart syndrome. Endothelial cells lining these capillaries are regular and devoid of atypia. HES

36, 37); and kinking, when there is a sharp angulation of the first portion of the internal carotid artery [129-131].

The incidence of coiling and kinking of the internal carotid artery is estimated to be from 10% to 16% in the general population [132]. Kinking and coiling of the internal carotid artery (ICA) may result in symptomatic cerebrovascular disease leading to fatal stroke [133, 134]. The condition may be acquired af-

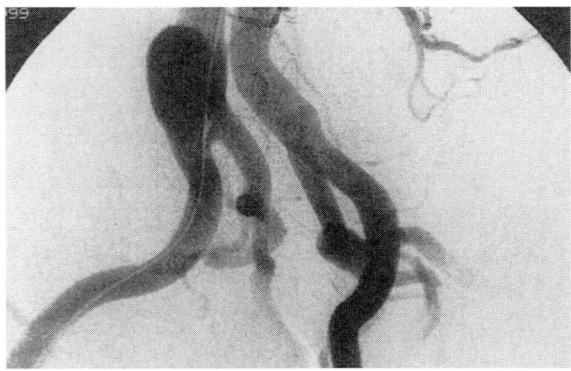

Fig. 33. Angiographic pattern of a mega-iliac artery in a 70 year-old man

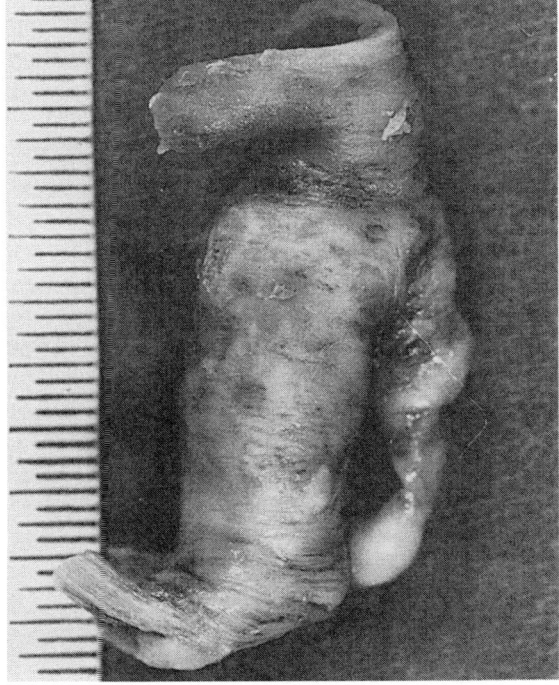

Fig. 34. Gross aspect of the same mega-iliac artery showing ectasia with an uneven calibre

ter an endarterectomy and caused by fibrosis [135]. Fibromuscular dysplasia has also been reported as a cause [136].

The aetiology of these changes is probably developmental. As in arteriomegaly, the significant changes are degenerative alterations in the arterial wall at the site of the loops and kinks, caused by the haemodynamic overload [137].

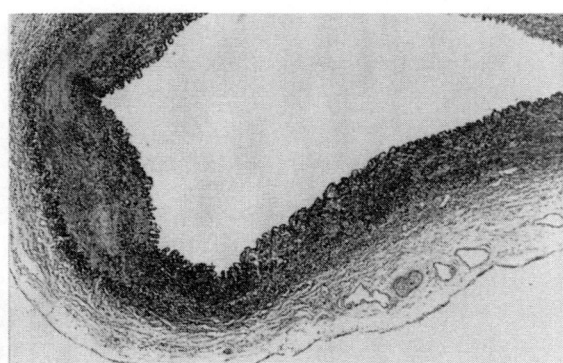

Fig. 37. C-coiling of the internal carotid artery. Note abnormally persistent elastic lamellae in the media. Orcein

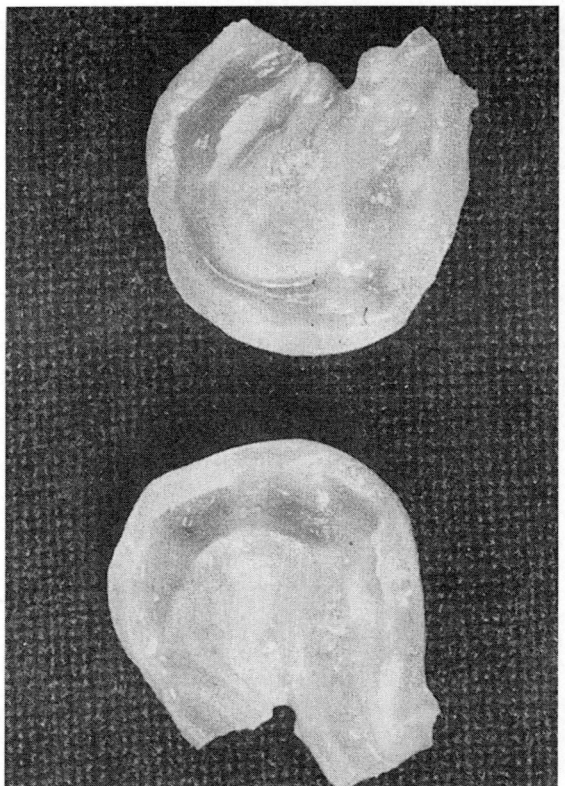

Fig. 35. C-coiling of the internal carotid artery

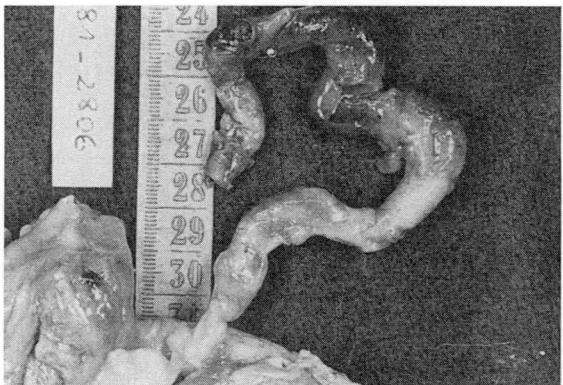

Fig. 36. Tortuosity and elongation of the right coronary artery causing thrombosis and fatal myocardial infarction in a young man

Bibliography

1. Lejeune JP (1997) Familial intracranial aneurysms. Review of the literature. Neurochirurgie 43: 292-8
2. Lee J, Berry CL (1978) Cerebral micro aneurysm formation in the hypertensive rat. J Pathol 124: 7-11
3. Rinne JK, Hernesniemi JA (1993) *De novo* aneurysms: special multiple intracranial aneurysms. Neurosurgery 33: 981-5
4. Tilson MD (1982) Decreased hepatic copper levels. A possible chemical marker for the pathogenesis of aortic aneurysms in man. Arch Surg 117: 1212-3
5. Nishikawa H, Miyakoshi S, Nishimura S, Seki A, Honda K (1989) A case of aortic intimal sarcoma manifested with acutely occurring hypertenesion and aortic occlusion. Heart Vessels 5: 54-8
6. Tamisier D, Goutiere F, Sidi D, Vaksmann G, Bruneval P, Vouhe P, Leca F (1997) Abdominal aortic aneurysm in a child with tuberous sclerosis. Ann Vasc Surg 11: 637-9
7. Anidjar S, Salzmann JL, Gentric D, Lagneau P, Camilleri JP, Michel JB (1990) Elastase induced experimental aneurysms in rats. Circulation 82: 973-81
8. Anderson LA (1994) An update on the cause of abdominal aortic aneurysms. J Vasc Nurs 12: 95-100
9. Halloran BG, Baxter BT (1995) Pathogenesis of aneurysms. Semin Vasc Surg 8: 85-92
10. Ghorpade A, Baxter BT (1996) Biochemistry and molecular regulation of matrix macromolecules in abdominal aortic aneurysms. Ann N Y Acad Sci 800: 138-50
11. Kondo S, Hashimoto N, Kikuchi H, Hazama F, Nagata I, Kataoka H (1998) Apoptosis of medial smooth muscle cells in the development of saccular cerebral aneurysms in rats. Stroke 29: 181-8
12. Thompson RW, Parks WC (1996) Role of matrix metalloproteinases in abdominal aortic aneurysms. Ann N Y Acad Sci 800: 157-74
13. Matsuo H (1993) Aortic aneurysm. Nippon Rinsho 51: 2153-9
14. Englund R, Hudson P, Hanel K, Stanton A (1998) Expansion rates of small abdominal aortic aneurysms. Aust N Z J Surg 68: 21-4
15. Inagawa T, Hirano A (1990) Autopsy study of unruptured incidental intracranial aneurysms. Surg Neurol 34: 361-5

16. Phuenpathom N, Ratanalert S, Sripairojkul B (1998) Multiple intracranial aneurysms in Songklanagarind Hospital. J Med Assoc Thai 81: 75-9
17. Istvan M (1981) Relation between polycystic kidney and intracranial aneurysm. Orv Hetil 122: 504-6
18. Schievink WI, Torres VE, Piepgras DG, Wiebers DO (1992) Saccular intracranial aneurysms in autosomal dominant polycystic kidney disease. J Am Soc Nephrol 3: 88-95
19. Schievink WI (1997) Genetics of intracranial aneurysms. Neurosurgery 40: 651-62
20. Schievink WI, Spetzler RF (1998) Screening for intracranial aneurysms in patients with isolated polycystic liver disease. J Neurosurg 89: 719-21
21. Schievink WI, Prendergast V, Zabramski JM (1998) Rupture of a previously documented small asymptomatic intracranial aneurysm in a patient with autosomal dominant polycystic kidney disease. Case report. J Neurosurg 89: 479-82
22. Schievink WI, Prakash UB, Piepgras DG, Mokri B (1994) Alpha 1 antitrypsin deficiency in intracranial aneurysms and cervical artery dissection. Lancet 343(8895): 452-53
23. Schievink WI, Parisi JE, Piepgras DG, Michels VV (1997) Intracranial aneurysms in Marfan's syndrome: an autopsy study. Neurosurgery 41: 866-70
24. Meldgaard K, Vesterby A, Ostergaard JR (1997) Sudden death due to rupture of a saccular intracranial aneurysm in a 13 year old boy. Am J Forensic Med Pathol 18: 342-4
25. Bowen DA (1984) Ruptured berry aneurysms: a clinical, pathological and forensic review. Forensic Sci Int 26: 227-34
26. Escourolle R, Poirier J (1971) Manuel élémentaire de neuropathologie. Masson Paris pp 109-12
27. Andrews RJ, Spiegel PK (1981) Intracranial aneurysms: characteristics of aneurysms by site, with special reference to anterior communicating artery aneurysms. Surg Neurol 16: 122-6
28. Scanarini M, Mingrino S, Giordano R, Baroni A (1978) Histological and ultrastructural study of intracranial saccular aneurysmal wall. Acta Neurochir (Wien) 43: 171-82
29. De Caro R, Parenti A, Munari PF (1996) Megalodolichobasilaris: the effect of atherosclerosis on a previously weakened arterial wall? Clin Neuropathol 15: 187-91
30. Cabellon S Jr, Moncrief CL, Pierre DR, Cavanaugh DG (1983) Incidence of abdominal aortic aneurysms in patients with atheromatous arterial disease. Am J Surg 146: 575-6
31. Shapira OM, Pasik S, Wassermann JP, Barzilai N, Mashiah A (1990) Ultrasound screening for abdominal aortic aneurysms in patients with atherosclerotic peripheral vascular disease. J Cardiovasc Surg (Torino) 31: 170-2
32. Vayssairat M, Gouny P, Nussaume O (1993) Atheromatous aneurysm of the sub renal aorta. Evolution of concepts for a current disease. Presse Med 22: 1431-3
33. Sekkal S, Cornu E, Christides C, Virot P, Laskar M, Serhal C, Bertin F, Ghossein Y, Gandara F, Rolle F, et al (1993) Isolated iliac aneurysms. Sixty seven cases in forty eight patients. J Mal Vasc 18: 13-7
34. Baudrimont M (1994) Cervico cerebral atheroma. Ann Radiol (Paris) 37: 17-23
35. Beh PS, Dickens P (1998) Fatal gastrointestinal haemorrhage due to coexisting primary aorto enteric and aorto colic fistulae. Complicating untreated atheromatous abdominal aortic aneurysm. Forensic Sci Int 96: 101-6

36. Vranckx P, Pirot L, Benit E (1997) Giant left main coronary artery aneurysm in association with severe atherosclerotic coronary disease. Cathet Cardiovasc Diagn 42: 54-7
37. Feiner HD, Raghavendra BH, Phelps R, Rooney L (1984) Inflammatory abdominal aortic aneurysm: Report of six cases. Hum Pathol 15: 454-9
38. Cavallini M, Uccini S, Luzi G, Murante G, Tagliacozzo S (1997) Arteriomegaly and inflammatory abdominal aortic aneurysm. Case report. J Cardiovasc Surg (Torino) 38: 37-41
39. Zdrojewski Z (1998) Retroperitoneal fibrosis and chronic peri aortitis new hypothesis. Pol Merkuriusz Lek 4: 50-3
40. Cormier JM, Vuong Ngoc P (1995) Un anévrysme inflammatoire inhabituel: maladie de Horton de l'aorte sous rénale. Cardinale 7: 22-5
41. Le Tourneau T, Agraou B, Beregi JP, Maurage CA, Asseman EP (1997) Cardiovascular manifestations of Horton disease: an underestimated disease in cardiology. Arch Mal Cœur Vaiss 90: 1403-7
42. Habon T, Toth K, Keltai M, Lengyel M, Palik I (1998) An adult case of Kawasaki disease with multiplex coronary aneurysms and myocardial infarction: the role of transesophageal echocardiography. Clin Cardiol 21: 529-32
43. Rothova A, Lardenoye C (1998) Arterial macroaneurysms in peripheral multifocal chorioretinitis associated with sarcoidosis. Ophthalmology 105: 1393-7
44. Amrani M, Dardenne B, Six C (1991) Inflammatory aortic aneurysm and retroperitoneal fibrosis. Report of 6 cases. J Mal Vasc 16: 13-7
45. Toure MK, Pasquier G, Herreman F, Bonnin A, Fouchard J, Houille F (1982) Aneurysms in Takayasu disease. Arch Mal Cœur Vaiss 75: 695-700
46. Boundy K, Bignold LP (1987) Syphilitic aneurysm of the right subclavian artery presenting with hemoptysis. Aust N Z J Med 17: 533-5
47. Nakane H, Okada Y, Ibayashi S, Sadoshima S, Fujishima M (1996) Brain infarction caused by syphilitic aortic aneurysm. A case report. Angiology 47: 911-7
48. Pessotto R, Santini F, Bertolini P, Faggian G, Chiominto B, Mazzucco A (1995) Surgical treatment of an aortopulmonary artery fistula complicating a syphilitic aortic aneurysm. Cardiovasc Surg 3: 707-10
49. Fulton JO, Zilla P, De Groot KM, Von Oppell UO (1996) Syphilitic aortic aneurysm eroding through the sternum. Eur J Cardiothorac Sur 10: 922-4
50. Kalyanaraman UP, Elwood PW (1980) Fibromuscular dysplasia of intracranial arteries causing multiple intracranial aneurysms. Hum Pathol 11: 481-4
51. Radhi JM, McKay R, Tyrrell MJ (1998) Fibromuscular dysplasia of the aorta presenting as multiple recurrent thoracic aneurysms. International journal of Angiology 7: 215-8
52. Poutasse EF (1975) Renal artery aneurysms. J Urol 13: 443-9
53. Castaneda Zuniga W, Zollikofer C, Valdez Davila O, Nath PH, Amplatz K (1979) Giant aneurysms of the renal arteries: an unusual manifestation of fibromuscular dysplasia. Radiology 133: 327-30
54. Kalafut M, Vinuela F, Saver JL, Martin N, Vespa P, Verity MA (1998) Multiple cerebral pseudoaneurysms and haemorrhages: the expanding spectrum of metastatic cerebral choriocarcinoma. J Neuroimaging 8: 44-7
55. Mitchell IM, Pollock JC (1990) Coarctation of the aorta and post stenotic aneurysm formation. Br Heart J 64: 332-3

56. Gyftokostas D, Koutsoumbelis C, Mattheou T, Bouhoutsos J (1991) Post stenotic aneurysm in popliteal artery entrapment syndrome. J Cardiovasc Surg (Torino) 32: 350-2

57. Desai Y, Robbs JV (1995) Arterial complications of the thoracic outlet syndrome. Eur J Vasc Endovasc Surg 10: 362-5

58. Raso AM, Rispoli P, Maggio D, Bellan A, Melloni CD (1996) Post stenotic aneurysm of the inferior mesenteric artery: case report and discussion. J Cardiovasc Surg (Torino) 37: 359-62

59. Vuong PN, Marotel M, Zuccarelli F, Lagneau P, Gautier C (1996) Anévrysme veineux poplité vrai : deux observations (Letter). Presse Med 25: 733

60. Fourneau I, Reynders Frederix V, Lacroix H, Nevelsteen A, Suy R (1998) Aneurysm of the iliofemoral vein. Ann Vasc Surg 12: 605-8

61. Raybaud CA, Strother CM, Hald JK (1989) Aneurysms of the vein of Galen: embryonic considerations and anatomical features relating to the pathogenesis of the malformation. Neuroradiology 31: 109-28

62. Langeron P, Gosselin J, Marin J (1990) Les anévrysmes de la veine poplitée. J Mal Vasc 15: 188-93

63. Grice GD, Smith RB, Robinson PH, Rheudasil JM (1990) Primary popliteal venous aneurysm with recurrent pulmonary emboli. J Vasc Surg 12: 316-8

64. Biessaux Y, Van Damme H, Raskinet B, Pierard LA (1994) Popliteal venous aneurysm: unusual source of pulmonary embolism. Acta Clin Belg 49: 92-4

65. Brunner U, Hauser M (1997) Hemodynamic assessment of venous aneurysm of the lower leg and therapeutic consequences. Zentralbl Chir 122: 809-12

66. Meszaros I, Morocz J, Szlavi J, Schmidt J, Nagy L, Somogyi J, Szep L, Papp A, Tornoczi J (1997) Incidence and mortality of aortic dissection. Orv Hetil 138: 2783-8

67. Shigeta O, Makuuchi H, Kaneko Y, Takuma S, Konishi T, Omura M (1994) A case of acute aortic dissection associated with myxedema. Nippon Kyobu Geka Gakkai Zasshi 42: 1096-100

68. Razavi M (1995) Acute dissection of the aorta: options for diagnostic imaging. Cleveland Clinic Journal of Medicine 62: 360-5

69. Vuong PN, Desoutter P, Guyot H, Mot JC, Romano M, Lessana A (1995) Mort subite par dissection aiguë (Anévrysme disséquant) de l'aorte au cours d'une fibroscopie gastrique : Une observation. Sem Hôp Paris 71: 94-7

70. Vuong PN, Janneau D, Jousse Hua D, Bensaïd P (1996) Anévrysme disséquant de l'aorte sous rénale de découverte fortuite : un cas (Letter). Sem Hôp Paris 72: 628

71. Bercau G, Castaigne V, Mihaileanu S, Couetil JP, Freund M, Sauvanet E (1997) Dissection of the ascending aorta in pregnancy. Apropos of a case and review of the literature. J Gynecol Obstet Biol Reprod (Paris) 26: 540-2

72. Cheng TO (1998) Aortic dissection during pregnancy. Ann Thorac Surg 65: 1511-2

73. Yamaguchi A, Adachi H, Kamio H, Murata S, Okada M, Adachi K, Ino T, Ichikawa T, Nagai J, Yamada S (1998) A combination of preductal aortic coarctation and type B dissection: report of a case. Surg Today 28: 435-7

74. Harada H, Ichimiya Y, Kamata K, Kazui T, Komatsu S (1990) Three cases of familial dissecting aortic aneurysm. Nippon Kyobu Geka Gakkai Zasshi 38: 1497-500

75. Alfonso F, Almeria C, Fernandez Ortiz A, Segovia J, Ferreiros J, Goicolea J, Hernandez R, Banuelos C, Gil Aguado M, Macaya C (1997) Aortic dissection occurring during coronary angioplasty: angiographic and transesophageal echocardiographic findings. Cathet Cardiovasc Diagn 42: 412 5

76. Hussain KM, Chandna H, Santhanam V, Sehgal S, Jain A, Denes P (1998) Aortic dissection in a young corticosteroid treated patient with systemic lupus erythematosus a case report. Angiology 49: 649-52

77. Berry CL, Greenwald SG, Menahem N (1981) Effect of beta amminoproprionitrile on the static elastic properties and blood pressure of spontaneously hypertensive rats. Cardiovascular Research 15: 373-81

78. De Bakey ME, Henly WS, Cooley DA (1965) Surgical management of dissecting aneurysms of the aorta. J Thorac Cardiovasc Surg 49: 130-49

79. Daily PO, Trueblood HW, Stinson B, Wuerflein RD, Shumway NE (1970) Management of acute aortic dissections. Ann Thorac Surg 10: 237-47

80. Guilmet D (1990) Chirurgie des dissections aiguës de l'aorte. Encycl Med Chir (Elsevier, Paris). Instantanés Médicaux 9: 1-12

81. Berry CL, Sosa Melgarejo JA, Greenwald SE (1993) The relationship between wall tension, lamellar thickness, and intercellular junctions in the fetal and adult aorta: its relevance to the pathology of dissecting aneurysm. J Pathol 169: 15-20

82. Stehbens WE (1995) Aneurysms In Stehbens WE and Lie JT: Vascular pathology. Chapman & Hall Medical pp 353-414

83. Schlatmann TJM, Becker AE (1977) Histologic changes in the normal aging aorta: implications for dissecting aortic aneurysms. Am J Cardiol 39: 13-20

84. Schlatmann TJM, Becker AE (1977) Pathogenesis of dissecting aneurysm of aorta. Comparative histopathologic study of significance of medial changes. Am J Cardiol 39: 21-6

85. Guthrie W, McLean H (1972) Dissecting aneuryms of arteries other than the aorta. J Pathol 223: 550-1

86. Basso C, Morgagni GL, Thiene G (1996) Spontaneous coronary artery dissection: a neglected cause of acute myocardial ischaemia and sudden death. Heart 75: 451-4

87. Meier DE, Ammons DH, Estrera AS (1981) Missile embolus to the lung associated with a corotid jugular arteriovenous fistula. J Trauma 21: 1048-9

88. Linder F (1985) Acquired arterio venous fistulas. Report of 223 operated cases. Ann Chir Gynaecol 74(1): 1-5

89. Serrano Hernando FJ, Paredero VM, Solis JV, Del Rio A, Lopez Parra JJ, Orgaz A, Aroca M, Tovar A, Paredero del Bosque V (1986) Iliac arteriovenous fistula as a complication of lumbar disc surgery. Report of two cases and review of literature. J Cardiovasc Surg (Torino) 27: 180-4

90. Khargi K, Bemelman WA, Voorwinde A, Keeman JN (1991) Aortocaval fistulas. Neth J Surg 43: 1-5

91. Sieunarine K, Ibach G, Prendergast FJ (1994) Femoral arteriovenous fistulas complicating percutaneous cardiac procedures. Cardiovasc Surg 2: 23-5

92. Ferrera PC (1997) Traumatic carotid cavernous sinus fistula with spontaneous resolution. Am J Emerg Med 15: 386-8

93. Bahar S, Chiras J, Carpena JP, Meder JF, Bories J (1984) Spontaneous vertebro vertebral arterio venous fistula associated with fibro muscular dysplasia. Report of two cases. Neuroradiology 26: 45-9

94. François G, Desveaux B, Garnier LF, Charbonnier B, Alison D, Brochier M (1986) Arteriovenous fistula disclosing a renal cancer. A propos of a case. Arch Mal Cœur Vaiss 79: 1632-5

95. Taki W, Nakahara I, Nishi S, Yamashita K, Sadatou A, Matsumoto K, Tanaka M, Kikuchi H (1994) Pathogenetic and therapeutic considerations of carotid cavernous sinus fistulas. Acta Neurochir (Wien) 127: 6-14

96. Vinchon M, Laurian C, George B, D'arrigo G, Reizine D, Aymard A, Riche MC, Merland JJ, Cormier JM (1994) Vertebral arteriovenous fistulas: a study of 49 cases and review of the literature. Cardiovasc Surg 2: 359-69

97. Vukobratov V, Damjanov D, Avramov S, Pfau J, Hadnadev L, Pasternak J (1998) Aorto enteric fistula as a rare manifestation of rupture of an abdominal aortic aneurysm case report. Med Pregl 51: 441-4

98. Bova VE (1982) Clinical picture and pathogenesis of Jacksonian seizures in cerebral arteriovenous aneurysms. Zh Nevropatol Psikhiatr 82: 57-62

99. Watson WD, Bonta MJ, Bush CR (1986) Splenic arteriovenous fistula causing massive ascites: a case report. Angiology 37: 36-40

100. Natali J, Jue Denis P, Kieffer E, Merland JJ (1989) Throbbing buttocks syndrome. J Mal Vasc 14: 183-9

101. Machini C, Kennel P, Hermann D, Piller P, Hemar P, Conraux C (1993) Pulsatile tinnitus and arteriovenous fistula. A propos of a case. Ann Otolaryngol Chir Cervicofac 110: 222-6

102. Dohlemann C, Hauser M, Nicolai T, Kreuzer E (1995) Innominate artery enlargement in congenital arteriovenous fistula with subsequent tracheal compression and stridor. Pediatr Cardiol 16: 287-90

103. Belcaro G, Nicolaides AN, Veller M (1995) Venous disorders. A manual of diagnosis and treatment. Saunders, London, Philadelphia, Toronto, Sidney, Tokyo

104. Reider Grosswasser I, Loewenstein A, Gaton DD, Lazar M (1993) Spontaneous thrombosis of a traumatic cavernous sinus fistula. Brain Inj 7: 547-50

105. Suchato C, Suwanraks C, Sukapanpotharam C, Sukumalanadana S (1976) Spontaneous closure of traumatic arteriovenous fistula. Radiology 118: 291-2

106. Kim TH, Kim KH, Kang JS, Kim JH, Hwang IY (1997) Pseudo Kaposi's sarcoma associated with acquired arteriovenous fistula. J Dermatol 24: 28-33

107. Weinreb W, Steinfeld A, Rodil J, Esparza A, Trebbin W (1983) Leiomyosarcoma arising in an arteriovenous fistula. Cancer 52: 390-2

108. Herbreteau D, Borsik M, Enjolras O, Riche M (1992) Arteriovenous malformations. Rev Prat 42: 2037-40

109. Leu HJ (1990) Pathomorphology of vascular malformations. Analysis of 310 cases. Int Angiol 9: 147-54

110. Kaplan SA, Brown W, Bixon R, O'Toole K, Benson MC (1992) Arteriovenous malformation of ureter. Urology 40: 450-2

111. Knight WB, Bush A, Busst CM, Haworth SG, Bowyer JJ, Shinebourne EA (1989) Multiple pulmonary arteriovenous fistulas in childhood. Int J Cardiol 23: 105-16

112. Camilleri L, Gabrillargues J, Lemaire JJ, Legault B, Brazzalotto I, Bailly P, Lusson JR, de Riberolles C (1995) Congenital pulmonary arteriovenous fistula. Apropos of 2 cases. Arch Mal Cœur Vaiss 88: 767-70

113. Beteta Chinchilla CE, Ramirez Mayans JA, Mora Tiscareno MA, Flores Calderon J, Casaubon Garcin P (1991) Intestinal arteriovenous malformations in children. Rev Gastroenterol Mex 56: 203-11

114. Blatchford JW 3d, Bolman RM 3d, Hunter DW, Amplatz K (1985) Concomitant pulmonary and cerebral arteriovenous fistulae. Chest 88: 782-4

115. Langer M, Langer R (1982) Radiologic aspects of the congenital arteriovenous malformations, Klippel Trenaunay type, and Servelle Martorell type. ROFO Fortschr Geb Rontgenstr Nuklearmed 136: 577-82

116. Jurecka W, Gebhart W, Knobler R, Schmoliner R, Moslacher H (1983) The leopard syndrome, a cardio cutaneous syndrome. Wien Klin Wochenschr 95: 652-6

117. Wu ZQ (1993) Parkes-Weber's syndrome: report of 5 cases. Chung Hua Wai Ko Tsa Chih 31: 749-51

118. Calzavara Pinton P, Carlino A, Manganoni AM, Donzelli C, Facchetti F (1990) Epidermal nevus syndrome with multiple vascular hamartomas and malformations. G Ital Dermatol Venereol 125: 251-4

119. Calzavara Pinton PG, Colombi M, Carlino A, Zane C, Gardella R, Clemente M, Facchetti F, Moro L, Zoppi N, Caimi L, et al (1995) Angiokeratoma corporis diffusum and arteriovenous fistulas with dominant transmission in the absence of metabolic disorders. Arch Dermatol 131: 57-62

120. Nomura M, Kitagawa K, Fujimura M, Matsuda T (1995) A case of Rendu Osler Weber syndrome and pulmonary arteriovenous fistula. Nippon Kyobu Shikkan Gakkai Zasshi 33: 1009-12

121. Perrelli L, Cina G, Cotroneo AR, Falappa P, Nanni L (1994) Treatment of intraosseous arteriovenous fistulas of the extremities. J Pediatr Surg 29: 1380-3

122. Bluefarb SM, Adams LA (1967) Arteriovenous malformation with angiodermatitis. Arch Dermatol 96: 176-81

123. Konig A, Brungger A, Schnyder UW (1990) Kaposiform acro-angiodermatitis with arteriovenous malformation (Stewart Bluefarb syndrome). Dermatologica 181: 254-7

124. Koppel RA, Marrogi AJ, Fishman SJ (1994) Unilateral pseudo Kaposi's sarcoma (Bluefarb Stewart type). Cutis 54: 257-60

125. Vuong PN, Laurian Cl, Houissa-Vuong S, Desoutter P (2000) Kaposiform angiodermatitis (Bluefarb-Stewart syndrome) caused by a superficial arterio-venous malformation of the trochanter area: apropos of a case. J Mal Vasc (Paris) 25: 280-3

126. Carlson DH, Gryska P, Seletz J, Armstrong S (1975) Arteriomegaly. Am J Roentgenol Radium Ther Nucl Med 125: 553-8

127. D'Andrea V, Malinovsky L, Cavallotti C, Benedetti Valentini F, Malinovska V, Bartolo M, Todini AR, Biancari F, Di Matteo FM, De Antoni E (1997) Angiomegaly. J Cardiovasc Surg (Torino) 38: 447-55

128. Elliott M, Bayly R, Cole T, Temple IK, Maher ER (1994) Clinical features and natural history of Beckwith Wiedemann syndrome: presentation of 74 new cases. Clin Genet 46: 168-74

129. Mascoli F, Mari C, Liboni A, Virgili T, Marcello D, Mari F, Donini I (1987) The elongation of the internal carotid artery. Diagnosis and surgical treatment. J Cardiovasc Surg (Torino) 28: 9-11

130. Dolmatov EA, Diuzhikov AA (1989) Surgical treatment of pathologic twisting of the internal carotid arteries. Kardiologiia 29: 45-7

131. Horsch S, Ktenidis K, Berg P (1994) Loops and folds of the carotid and vertebral arteries: indications for surgery. J Mal Vasc 19: S55-S9

132. Poulias GE, Skoutas B, Doundoulakis N, Haddad H, Karkanias G, Lyberiadis D (1996) Kinking and coiling of internal carotid artery with and without associated stenosis. Surgical considerations and long term follow up. Panminerva Med 38: 22-7

133. Desai B, Toole JF (1975) Kinks, coils, and carotids: a review. Stroke 6: 649-53

134. Barbour PJ, Castaldo JE, Rae Grant AD, Gee W, Reed JF 3rd, Jerny D, Longennecker J (1994) Internal carotid ar-

tery redundancy is significantly associated with dissection. Stroke 25: 1201-6

135. Collins PS, Orecchia P, Gomez E (1991) A technique for correction of carotid kinks and coils following endarterectomy. Ann Vasc Surg 5: 116-20

136. Danza R, Baldizan J, Navarro T (1983) Surgery of carotid kinking and fibromuscular dysplasia. J Cardiovasc Surg (Torino) 24: 628-33

137. Matskevichus ZK, Pauliukas PA (1990) The morphological changes in the wall of the carotid and vertebral arteries in pathological kinks and loops. Arkh Patol 52: 53-8

138. Vuong PN, Janzen J, Lanzer P (2001) Fatal myocardial infarction in a young man caused by a right megadolichocoronary artery with thrombosis: a case report. Z Kardiol 90: 203-7

XI
Vasculitis

Inflammation of blood vessels (vasculitis, angiitis) may involve arteries, veins or capillaries. The vasculitic syndromes discussed below generally affect either arteries alone, or a mixture of arteries, veins and lymphatics.

1 – Classification and pathogenesis

Classification

The pathogenesis of most systemic and/or isolated vasculitides is unknown, making a rational classification difficult. Most attempts are based on the size or location of vessels, the histological appearance of the lesions and the clinical features. The overlap among entities defined in this way is considerable [1-9]. Table 1 summarizes correspondences between some different classifications.

Pathogenesis

The two major pathogenetic mechanisms of vasculitis are direct injury to vessels by infectious pathogens and, more significantly, as a result of immunologically mediated inflammation [10, 11]. Immunologically mediated vasculitides are of four types: immune complex, direct antibody attack, anti-neutrophil cytoplasmic antibody (ANCA) associated, and cell-mediated.

Immune complex-mediated vasculitis

This condition is triggered by the deposition of antigen-antibody or antigen-antibody-complement complexes in the vascular wall, with subsequent involvement of breakdown products of complement, platelets, and polymorphonuclear leukocytes, and development of vasculitis. Nephritis is common. The Arthus phenomenon and serum sickness are classic examples, but many other disorders, including most of the connective tissue diseases, may belong to this category. Defects in immunoregulation predispose to the development of vasculitis produced by cytotoxic antibodies to normal endothelial cells, seen in patients with active SLE.

Direct antibody attack-mediated vasculitis

Deposition of antibodies on a particular structure, especially the basement membrane or endothelial cells "activated" by cytokines, results in binding of C^3 and other components of complement and triggers the inflammatory process. Goodpasture's syndrome and Kawasaki's disease are conditions in which this mechanism operates.

Antineutrophil cytoplasmic autoantibody (ANCA) associated vasculitis

Many patients with vasculitis have antineutrophil cytoplasmic autoantibodies (ANCA) [12-16]. The pathogenic mechanism whereby these antibodies produce vasculitis is not clear; they may activate neutrophils, stimulating the release of lytic enzymes and production of free radicals and tissue damage. A role for free radicals is supported by the fact that administration of antibodies against myeloperoxidase produces glomerulonephritis and granulomatous vasculitis of small vessels in the rat [17]. Immunohistochemistry confirms the presence of ANCA in neutrophils. There are two patterns of neutrophil immunofluorescence; cytoplasmic (C-ANCA) and perinuclear (P-ANCA). P-ANCA is directed largely toward myeloperoxidase in the primary granules of neutrophils; one of the neutrophil antigens involved in C-ANCA is a potentially tissue-destructive, neutral leukocyte protease (proteinase 3) [18, 19]. A C-ANCA pattern is present in most patients with active Wegener's granulomatosis and microscopic polyangiitis. P-ANCA is frequently observed in patients with polyarteritis nodosa (PAN) and primary glomerular disease. The ANCA's are useful diagnostic markers of vasculitis [20, 21]; their presence and titres usually correlate well with disease activity.

Cell-mediated vasculitis

Vasculitis in transplant rejection results from a complex process in which cell-mediated immunity predominates. Although there is little doubt that T cells are pivotal in this type of vasculitis, antibodies evoked against alloantigens can also mediate rejection. Moreover, in some vasculitides, the presence of T lymphocytes, monocytes and granulomata suggests a role of cell-mediated immunity directed against foreign antigens or endogenous components of the vascular wall. These mechanisms have been reviewed in terms of their involvement in the major organ transplantation fields in man in a recent volume [22].

Table 1. Classification of vasculitides according to their pathogenesis, histological features, sizes and types of vessels involved

PATHOGENESIS	TYPES	HIS	C	SA	MA	LA	SV	LV	LY
INFECTIOUS	Viral	L	+						
	Bacterial	N	+	+	+	+	+	+	
	Rickettsial	N	+						
	Spirochetal	G				+			
	Fungal	NG		+	+	+	+	+	
IMMUNOLOGIC • Immune complex-mediated (Hypersensivity vasculitis)	Henoch-Schonlein purpura	N	+						
	Essential mixed cryoglobulinaemic vasculitis	N	+	+					
	Leukocytoclastic angiitis	N	+	+	+				
	Leukocytoclastic angiitis subgroups (Urticarial vasculitis, HBC microscopic polyarteritis, Serum sickness/drug reactions)	LNE	+	+			+		
	Vasculitis and connective tissue diseases (SLE, RA)	NG	+	+	+	+	+		
	Vasculitis and sero-negative spondylarthropathies	G		+	+	+			
	Vasculitis associated with neoplasms, and other primary disorders	NG	+	+			+		
• Direct antibody attack-mediated (anti-basement membrane, endothelial antibodies)	Goodpasture's syndrome	NG		+	+	+	+		
	Kawasaki's disease	N		+	+	+			
• ANCA associated (possibly ANCA mediated)	Wegener's granulomatosis	GN	+	+	+				
	Microscopic polyangiitis	N	+	+					
	Churg-Strauss syndrome	N	+	+			+		
• Cell-mediated	Allograft rejection vasculitis	NG	+	+	+	+	+	+	
UNKNOWN	Giant cell arteritides	G				+			
	Takayasu's arteritis	G			+	+			
	Classic Polyarteritis nodosa	NL	+	+	+	+	+	+	
	Isolated visceral vasculitis	NG		+	+		+		
	Primary angiitis of the CNS	G		+			+		
	Behçet's syndrome	N			+	+	+	+	
	Thromboangiitis obliterans	NG		+	+	+	+	+	
	Cogan's syndrome	NL	+	+	+	+	+		
	Sarcoid vasculitis	G		+	+			+	
	Erythema nodosum	L	+	+			+		
	Erythema elevatum diutinum	N		+					
	Nodular vasculitis	L		+			+		+
	Weber-Christian disease	LG		+			+		
	Granuloma faciale	NL	+	+			+		
	Pyoderma gangrenosum	NL		+			+		

(ANCA: Antineutrophil cytoplasmic antibodies; C: blood capillaries; CNS: Central nervous system; E: eosinophilic vasculitis; G: granulomatous vasculitis; HBC: hepatitis B and C; HIS: Histological features; L: lymphocytic vasculitis; LA: large arteries; LV: large veins; LY: lymphatic vessels; MA: medium-sized arteries; N: necrotizing vasculitis; SA: small arteries; SNV: systemic necrotizing vasculitis; SV: small veins, SLE: systemic lupus erythematosus; RA: rheumatoid arthritis)

2 – Infectious vasculitis

Vessels may be directly attacked by infectious and parasitic agents. A number of infectious agents infecting vessels have produced septicaemia or metastatic abscesses by embolization from infective thrombosis or endocarditis. Others have an affinity for vascular targets including some fungi (aspergillosis, mucormycosis, actinomycosis) and viruses (cytomegalovirus, varicella zoster). Necrotizing, granulomatous, or lymphocytic vasculitis may be produced (see chapter VIII).

3 – Immunologic vasculitis or immune complex-mediated vasculitis (hypersensitivity vasculitis)

Leukocytoclastic angiitis

This vasculitis results from an immune complex-mediated process following exposure to foreign (infectious agent/drug) or endogenous (tumour) antigens. Deposits of immune complex containing a slight antigen excess induce activation of the complement cascade, triggering the inflammatory mechanism. This results in production of a leukocyte chemotactant, C5a, leading to infiltration of neutrophils, which release lysosomal enzymes, including elastase and collagenase. Damage to the vascular wall results in fibrin deposits, thrombosis and erythrodiapedesis into the surrounding connective tissue (purpura). Table 2 summarises diverse causes of leukocytoclastic angiitis [23-31].

Disseminated vascular lesions of hypersensitivity angiitis may also appear in a number of relatively distinct syndromes, including Henoch-Schönlein purpura, and essential mixed cryoglobulinaemia). The condition affects any age group without sex predilection and typically involves the skin, mucous membranes, lungs, brain, heart, gastrointestinal tract, kidneys, and muscle. The term "cutaneous leukocytoclastic angiitis" is restricted to vasculitis in the skin without involvement of vessels in any other organ [2]. Skin lesions (palpable purpura, erythematous papules, vesicles and bullae) occur on dependent areas. Subcutaneous nodules, ulcers, recurrent or chronic urticaria, and oedema may be found [32]. Systemic manifestations consist of fever, arthralgia, malaise, and gastro-intestinal pain. The most frequent laboratory abnormality was a high erythrocyte sedimentation rate in 30% of the patients tested. P-ANCA are present in 70% of patients. Hypocomplementaemia may be noted in cases associated with autoimmune diseases. The outcome of leukocytoclastic angiitis is variable, ranging from a mild, self-limiting disease to a severe fatal illness, especially when there is renal involvement. In general, lesions occur in episodes, lasting from 1 to 4 weeks, and resolve without treatment, leaving atrophic scars with hyperpigmentation in the skin.

Table 2. Causes of leukocytoclastic angiitis

PATHOLOGICAL ENTITIES	CAUSATIVE AGENTS
Infections	Hepatitis B and C virus, Influenza virus, Rickettsiae, Streptococcus, M. tuberculosis
Drugs	Penicillin, Sulfapyridine, Sulfonamides, Streptomycin, Imipenem-cilastatin, Thiouracil, Hydantoin compounds, Aspirin, Phenacetin, Iodides, Phenothiazines, Nonsteroidal anti-inflammatory agents
Chemicals	Insecticides, Petroleum products, Dye excipient
Foreign proteins	Serum sickness, Hyposensitization antigen, Staphylococcal protein A
Connective tissue and autoimmune diseases,	Systemic lupus erythematosus, Ulcerative colitis. Crohn's disease, Rheumatoid arthritis, Sjogren's disease, Primary biliary cirrhosis, Dermatomyositis, Progressive systemic sclerosis, Haemolytic anaemia
Neoplasia	Lymphoproliferative diseases (Hodgkin's disease, hairy cell leukaemia), Carcinomas

Pathology and differential diagnosis.

Leukocytoclastic angiitis affects smaller vessels than does PAN. In the early stages, the histological features are those of fibrinoid necrosis with endothelial cell swelling, and infiltration of the blood vessel walls by neutrophils and mononuclear cells, but in some lesions the change is limited to infiltration with neutrophils, which become fragmented as they penetrate the vessel wall (leukocytoclasis) (Fig. 1). Immunoglobulins (IgM, IgG), complement (C3), fibrinogen and albumin can be identified in vitro by immunoflourescence or immunoperoxidase techniques in biopsies from recent lesions (less than 24 hours old) in the blood vessel wall [33]. In advanced stages, the inflammatory cell infiltrate changes progressively from neutrophil to lymphocyte predominance over a 5-day period. Only neutrophilic dominance is associated with hypocomplementaemia.

Leukocytoclastic angiitis subgroups

Urticarial vasculitis (hypocomplementemic vasculitis)

This uncommon vasculitis encompasses a large spectrum of illnesses, ranging from mild idiopathic chronic urticaria to more serious systemic illness with leukocytoclastic venulitis [34,35]. This condition is most commonly an acquired idiopathic phenomenon but may occur in association with other disorders, such as systemic lupus erythematosus, Sjogren's syndrome and serum sickness. Urticarial vasculitis may occur at any age with a predilection for middle-aged women (2:1) with an incidence between 2% and 20%. Skin manifestations are characterised by urticaria with pruritus, pain and a burning sensation. Usually, the lesions last from 1 to 3 days and resolve, leaving areas of hyperpigmentation, scaling or purpura. The diagnosis is suggested clinically by more persistent (lasting > 24 hours) and more symptomatic weals than in ordinary urticaria and by the presence of residual bruising [36]. Extracutaneous symptoms include joint stiffness and articular pain. Proteinuria and haematuria, and nausea, vomiting and diarrhoea indicate renal and gastrointestinal involvement. Fever, lymphadenopathy, and neurological disturbances occur. There is a raised erythrocyte sedimentation rate with hypocomplementaemia (C1q, C4 and C2) in 50% of cases [37]. Circulating immune complexes are rarely found.

Pathology and differential diagnosis

The histological appearance of urticarial vasculitis is similar to that of necrotizing leukocytoclastic vasculi-

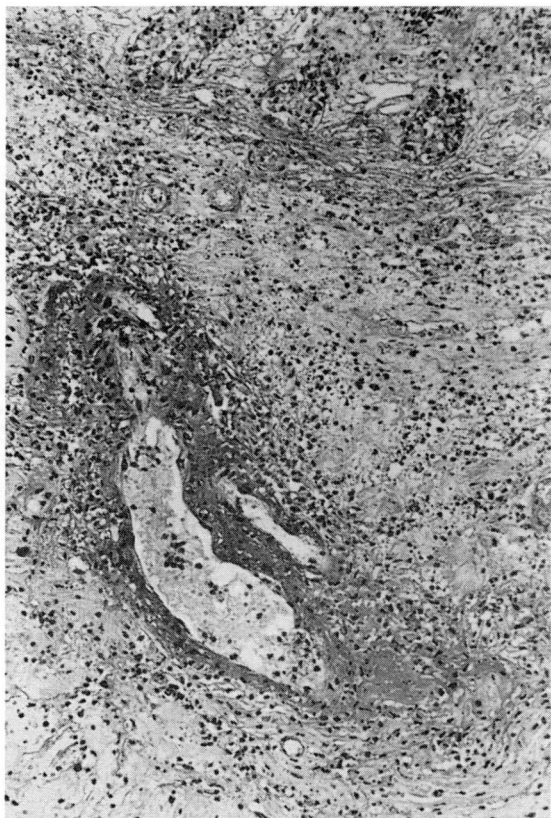

Fig. 1. Leukocytoclasic angiitis. Note infiltration of the arterial wall by neutrophils with fibrinoid necrosis. Haematoxylin, eosin and saffron stain. (HES)

tis (Fig. 2-3), although, occasionally, either eosinophils or lymphocytes (Fig. 4) may be present rather than neutrophils. It differs from ordinary urticaria, where vascular dilatation with oedema and a mild perivascular chronic cell infiltrate may be seen. In skin biopsies, immunofluorescence may reveal immunoglobulins (most often IgM) and complement in blood vessel walls and at the epidermo-dermal junction.

Hepatitis B and C microscopic polyarteritis

Approximately 30% of patients with microscopic polyarteritis have the hepatitis B antigen (HBsAg) and hepatitisB immune complexes in their serum [38]. Furthermore, the presence of chronic hepatitis B antigenemia predisposes patients to the development of vasculitis [39]. The demonstration of circulating immune complexes made up of hepatitis B surface antigen and antibody directed against this determinant strongly supports the hypothesis that immune complexes are involved in the pathogenesis of microscopic polyarteritis. However, patients with chronic aggres-

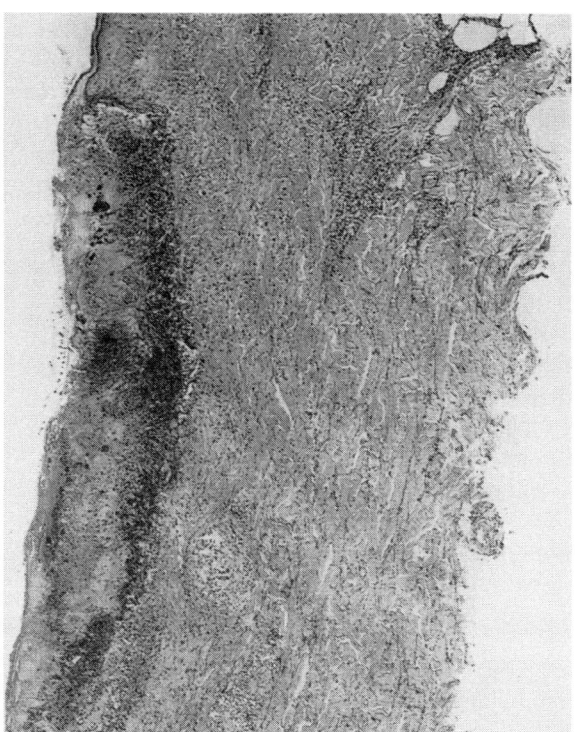

Fig. 2. Urticarial vasculitis. Skin biopsy showing involvement of dermic vessels. HES

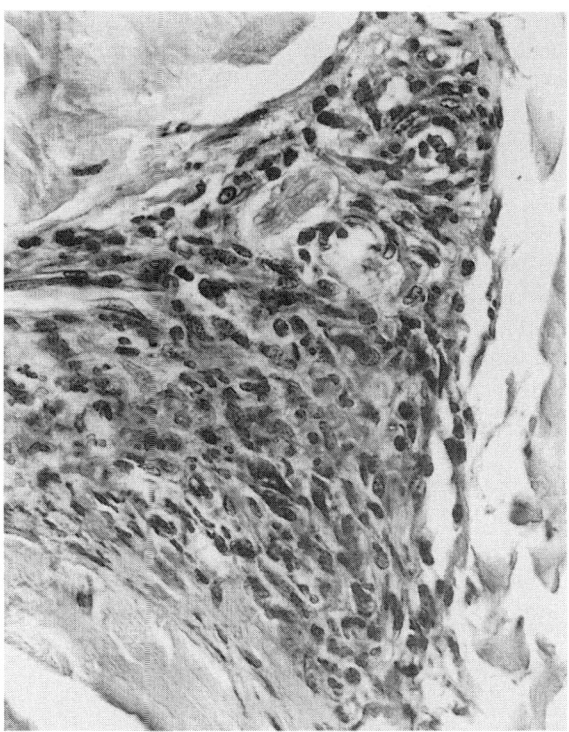

Fig. 3. Urticarial vasculitis. Vascular change may mimick necrotizing leukocytoclastic vasculitis. HES

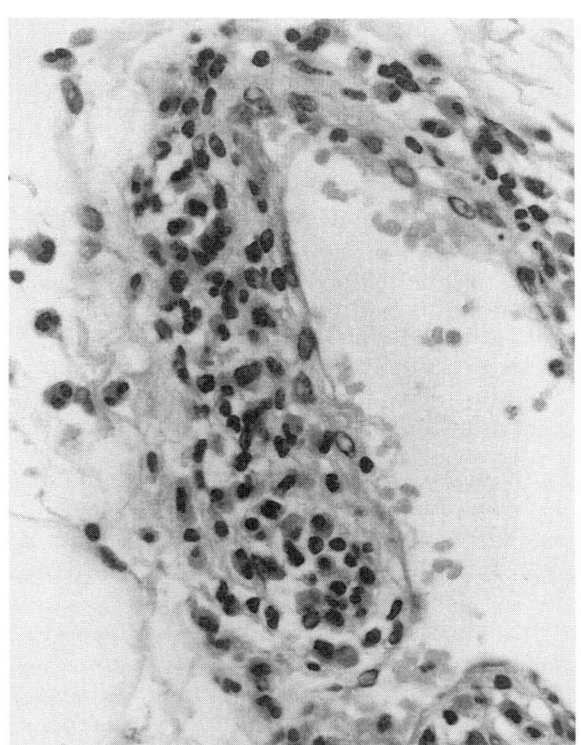

Fig. 4. Urticarial vasculitis. Eosinophils and lymphocytes predominating the inflammatory infiltrate. HES

sive hepatitis may have hepatitis B immune-complexes in their vessels without vasculitis. Recently, similar changes have been found in patients with chronic hepatitis C virus (HCV) hepatitis and glomerulonephritis. HCV-RNA was detected in their serum, and cryoprecipitates contained IgG anti-HCV antibodies within glomerular capillaries, suggesting that deposits of HCV-anti-HCV immune complexes are the starting mechanism [40-45].

Serum sickness and drug reactions

This immune complex disease appears some days after injection of foreign serums or heterologous serum proteins. There is local and systemic reaction, including urticaria, fever, general lymphadenopathy, oedema, joint pain, and, occasionally, albuminuria. Deposits of immune complex are responsible for the widespread vasculitis whose frequency and severity are directly related to the volume of foreign protein injected. The urticarial component of the cutaneous manifestations may be mediated by IgE with or without immune complex deposition. Serum sickness is now rarely seen but a syndrome, similar to serum sickness, may occur after administration of non-protein containing drugs, including penicillin, sulfapyridine, sulfonamides, streptomycin, thiouracil, hydantoin compounds, aspirin, phenacetin, iodides, and phenothiazines. Generally, a pruritic erythematous swelling occurs at the injection site 1 to 3 days before the classical clinical manifestations of fever, urticaria, arthralgias and lymphadenopathy become apparent. The full clinical syndrome occurs 7 to 10 days following primary exposure to the antigen. Laboratory findings include a mild leukocytosis and an elevated ESR. Hypergammaglobulinaemia, plasmacytosis, circulating light chains, and IgG antibodies against heterologous serum proteins may be present. The majority of serum sickness and serum sickness like reactions resolve spontaneously in from several days to 2 weeks after removal of the offending antigen.

Henoch-Schönlein purpura (Acute vascular purpura, Anaphylactoid purpura)

Henoch-Schonlein purpura (HSP), probably first described by Heberden and Willan in the early 1800's, is an acute or chronic vasculitis primarily affecting small vessels and characterised by an eruption of non-thrombocytopaenic purpuric lesions associated with joint pain and swelling, colic, and passage of bloody stools. Glomerulonephritis may occur during an initial episode or develop later. Numerous antigens resulting from infections (streptococcal throat infection, yersiniosis, Campylobacter jejuni enteritis, tuberculosis, chickenpox) [26, 46], drugs (ampicillin, penicillin, erythromycin), insect stings, foods, underlying connective tissue disease or malignancy [47-49], and immunisations have all been implicated in the pathogenesis of the lesions.

HSP mainly affects children between 3 and 10 years of age. Males are affected more often than females (1.5:1) and in about two thirds of children an upper respiratory tract infection precedes the onset of HSP by one to three weeks. The incidence shows a seasonal variation with the peak around November to January in the northern hemisphere. In general, the disease starts as a flu-like syndrome with fever and fatigue. A symmetrical erythematous macular rash initially develops on the skin around the malleoli of the ankle, but usually extends to the dorsal surface of the legs, the buttocks and ulnar surfaces of the arms. After 12-24 hours, the lesions become dusky red, have a diameter of 0.5-2cm, and may coalesce into larger palpable purpura. Oedema may occur in the scalp and the periorbital area [50, 51]. Systemic manifestations include arthralgia, colicky abdominal pain (50% of cases) with melena, or bloody diarrhoea. Renal involvement can be a prominent feature of HSP. There may be microscopic haematuria with mild or moderate proteinuria (50-70% of cases); however, glomerulonephritis becomes clinically manifest in only 20–30% of unselected children. Comparative clinical studies indicate that Henoch-Schonlein purpura and hypersensitivity vasculitis are similar but separate clinical syndromes [52].

This condition is generally benign, but fatal complications, such as necrosis of the digestive tract with massive gastrointestinal hemorrhage [53], respiratory insufficiency and renal failure may occur. The finding of diffuse glomerular involvement or of crescentic changes in most glomeruli in a renal biopsy predicts progressive renal failure.

High levels of circulating IgA containing immune complexes have been found during the initial phase of the disease and are simultaneously present in cutaneous vessel walls in 95% of the patients [54]. Deposition of IgA-containing immune complexes with consequent activation of complement is thought to represent the pathogenic mechanism of the vasculitis.

Pathology and differential diagnosis

A biopsy of an acute skin lesion reveals an aseptic vasculitis with fibrinoid necrosis of vessel walls and perivascular cuffing of vessels with polymorphonuclear leukocytes [55]. These changes are those of a leukocytoclastic vasculitis [52]. In the kidneys, the glomerular changes range from a normal pattern through mild mesangial proliferation, focal and segmental intracapillary and extra capillary proliferation with adhesions in small crescents, and diffuse proliferation with infiltration of polymorphonuclear leukocytes, circumferential crescents associated with tubular atrophy and interstitial infiltration with mononuclear cells. Immunofluorescence demonstrates the presence of granular deposits of Ig reactive for IgA in the walls of cutaneous capillaries and the mesangium of glomeruli. In addition to IgA, the deposits frequently contain IgG, fibrin, C3 and properdin.

Hypersensitivity vasculitis

This is a non-specific histological lesion of diverse origin [56]. Diagnostic criteria suggested by the American College of Rheumatology include an age greater than 16 at disease onset, history of taking a medication that may have been a precipitating factor, the presence of palpable purpura, the presence of maculopapular rash, and a biopsy demonstrating granulocytes around an arteriole or venule [57]. The diagnosis depends on the clinical context. Most patients who would have been given this diagnosis fall into the category of microscopic polyangiitis (microscopic polyarteritis) or cutaneous leukocytoclastic angiitis. In the predominantly cutaneous form (cutaneous leukocytoclastic angiitis), the main differential diagnosis is Sweet's syndrome (acute febrile neutrophilic dermatosis). In the latter syndrome, there is little or no nuclear dust, no fibrin in the walls of venules, and no prominent extravasation of red blood cells.

Vasculitis associated with connective tissue diseases

Vasculitis is common in systemic lupus erythematosus and often seen in rheumatoid arthritis [58-61].

Systemic lupus erythematosus

SLE is a complex and highly variable disease of multifactorial origin resulting from interactions of hormonal, environmental and genetic factors, which act together to activate helper T cells and B cells, leading to secretion of several types of autoantibodies. Antibodies are classified into two major classes based on their action against nuclear and cytoplasmic components of the cell, whatever the tissue type.

SLE is predominantly a disease of women with a female-to-male ratio of 9:1. The frequency is 1 in 700 among women between the ages of 20 and 64; however, it may become manifest at any age, even in early childhood. Black women are three times more often affected than white and their disease is generally more severe. The onset of SLE may be sudden or progressive. Table 3 lists the frequency of symptoms of SLE.

The clinical manifestations of vasculitis depend upon the tissues involved. In the skin petechiae and purpura occur; involvement of the brain gives rise to

headaches, behavioural disturbances, confusion, seizures, and strokes. Peripheral nerve involvement produces numbness, tingling, and loss of sensation or strength; in the digestive tract cramping abdominal pain and bloating are experienced and melaena and necrosis with perforation have been reported. Involvement of the heart (angina), lungs (pneumonia-like episodes, haemoptysis), kidney (hypertension), and eyes (visual blurring or partial loss of vision) are further signs of involvement. Table 4 summarises the eleven criteria used in the diagnosis of SLE [62], which is likely to be present when four or more are present.

The course of the disease is variable and unpredictable. Acute cases may die within weeks or months. More often, the disease presents with exacerbations and remissions. During acute exacerbations, increased formation of immune complexes and the accompanying complement activation often lead to hypocomplementaemia [63]. Disease flare-ups are usually treated by corticosteroids or other immunosuppressant drugs. In most cases, the disease runs a benign course with skin symptoms and mild haematuria for years, even without treatment. In the recent past, an approximately 70% 10-year survival could be expected. The most common causes of death are intercurrent infections, diffuse CNS disease, hypertension and renal failure.

Pathology and differential diagnosis

The most characteristic lesions result from the deposits of immune complexes found in the kidneys (Fig. 5-6), connective tissue, skin and the blood vessels. An acute necrotizing vasculitis involving small arteries and arterioles (Fig. 7-8) may be present in any tissue, although the skin, muscles, serosa and joint synovial membranes are most commonly affected. The arteritis is characterised by deposits of eosinophilic fibrinoid material under the endothelium and in the adventitia of these vessels. Lymphocytes infiltrate the media and adventitia. Endothelial proliferation narrows the vascular lumen and thrombosis may occur. In chronic stages, vessels undergo fibrous thickening with luminal narrowing. Occasionally, migratory phlebitis may occur. In the spleen, vascular lesions involve the central penicilliary arteries and are characterised by marked perivascular fibrosis, producing so-called onionskin lesions. In the extremities, recurrent venous and arterial thromboses involve small vessels. In the liver, acute vasculitis may occur in the portal system, accompanied by lymphocytic infiltrates, leading to nonspecific portal triaditis. In the heart, involvement is manifested primarily in the form of pericarditis and valvular nonbacterial verrucous

Table 3. Symptoms of systemic lupus erythematosus

SYMPTOMS	(%)
Arthralgia	95
Fever, Arthritis	90
Prolonged or extreme fatigue	81
Skin rashes	74
Anaemia	71
Kidney involvement	50
Serositis	45
Butterfly-shaped rash across the cheeks and nose	42
Hair loss	27
Raynaud's phenomenon	17
Seizures	15
Mouth or nose ulcers	12

Table 4. The eleven criteria used for the diagnosis of lupus

CRITERIA	DEFINITION
Malar rash	Rash over the cheeks
Discoid rash	Red raised patches
Photosensitivity	Reaction to sunlight, resulting in the development of or increase in skin rash
Oral ulcers	Ulcers in the nose or mouth, usually painless
Arthritis	Nonerosive arthritis involving two or more peripheral joints (arthritis in which the bones around the joints do not become destroyed)
Serositis	Pleuritis or pericarditis
Renal disease	Excessive protein in the urine (greater than 0.5 gm/day or 3+ on test sticks) and/or cellular casts (abnormal elements in the urine, derived from red and/or white cells and/or kidney tubule cells)
Neurological manifestations	Seizures (convulsions) and/or psychosis in the absence of drugs or metabolic disturbances that are known to cause such effects
Hematological disorder	Haemolytic anaemia or leukopaenia (white blood count below 4,000 cells per cubic millimetre) or lymphopaenia (fewer than 1,500 lymphocytes per cubic millimetre) or thrombocytopaenia (fewer than 100,000 platelets per cubic millimetre). The leukopaenia and lymphopaenia must be detected on two or more occasions. The thrombocytopaenia must be detected in the absence of drugs known to induce it.
Immunological disorder	Positive LE prep test, positive anti-DNA test, positive anti-Sm test or false positive syphilis test (VDRL).
Antinuclear antibody	Positive test for antinuclear antibodies (ANA) in the absence of drugs known to induce.

endocarditis (Libman-Sacks type). Active arteritis with fibrinoid necrosis and obliterative endarteritis of vasa vasorum may lead to dissection of the aorta [64, 65] and a "tree-bark" pattern [66]. However, an increasing number of young patients with long-standing disease, especially those who have been treated with corticosteroids, present with angina, and myocardial infarction caused by accelerated coronary atherosclerosis. The pathogenic mechanism of this condition remains unclear. In the brain, focal neurological symptoms have often been attributed to acute vasculitis [67, 68].

Systematic histological studies rarely demonstrate significant vasculitis [69] except for occasional intimal proliferation of small vessels, probably resulting from endothelial damage caused by antiphospholipid antibodies [70]. These antibodies and/or immune complexes may also favour development of atherosclerosis [71]. Some recent studies suggest that CNS symptoms are caused by antibodies against a synaptic membrane protein [72]. Renal glomeruli are involved in 60 to 70% of cases and changes may be classified into five major patterns; normal by light, electron, and immunofluorescent microscopy, which is uncommon, mesangial glomerulonephritis, focal proliferative glomerulonephritis, diffuse proliferative glomerulonephritis, and membranous glomerulonephritis. Mixtures of types may occur [73]. Glomerular arteries are rarely involved [74]. It should be noted, however, that none of these changes is specific for lupus. The main pathogenic mechanism is the deposition of DNA/anti-DNA complexes within the glomeruli but why the morphologic patterns differ is unclear. Immune complexes may be mesangial, intramembranous, subepithelial, or subendothelial in location. Subendothelial deposits frequently create a peculiar but non-specific thickening of the capillary wall, which can be seen by means of light microscopy as a "wireloop" lesion. They usually reflect active disease and generally indicate a poor prognosis. Differentiation of concurrent glomerular involvement secondary to some forms of small vessel vasculitis, such as microscopic polyangiitis (which is called hypersensitivity angiitis by some) versus lupus nephritis would be difficult, if not impossible. If a lupus patient does not have immune complex glomerulonephritis the presence of a pauci-immune necrotizing glomerulonephritis caused by a small vessel vasculitis may be

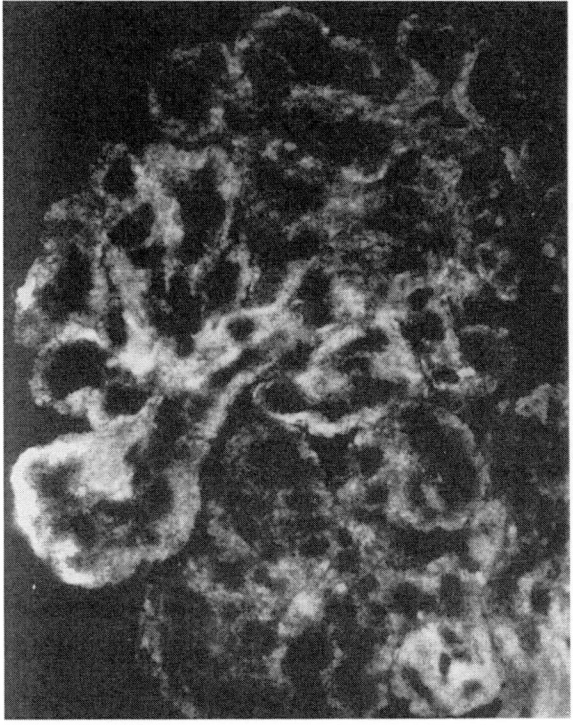

Fig. 5. Systemic lupus erythematosus. Deposition of immune complexes along the glomerular capillaries evidenced by immunofluorescence technique (Courtesy Dr D. Droz)

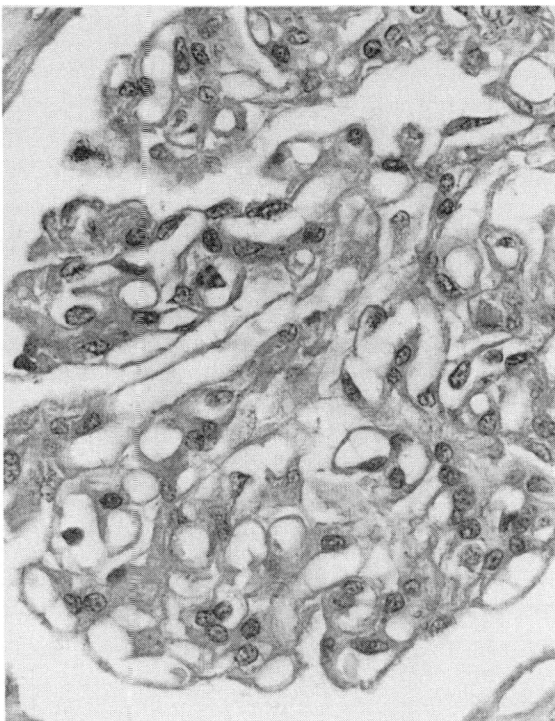

Fig. 6. Systemic lupus erythematosus. Corresponding "wire-loop" pattern of glomerular capillary wall. Masson's trichrome stain (Masson's trichrome). (Courtesy Dr D. Droz)

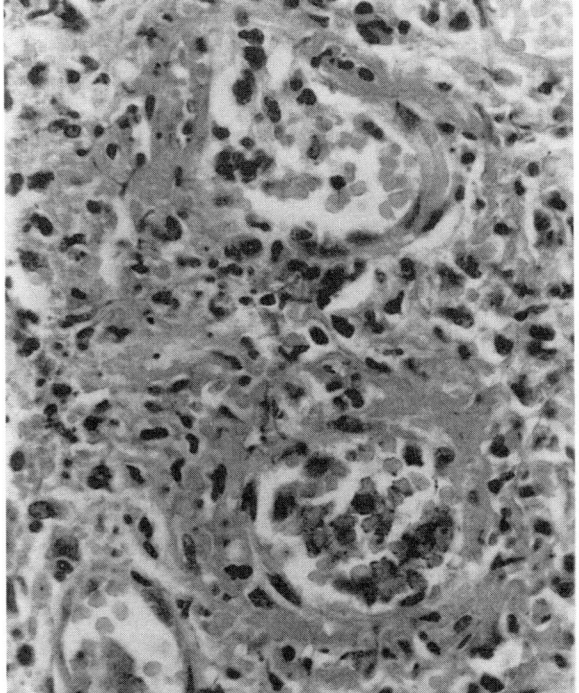

Fig. 7. Systemic lupus erythematosus. Acute necrotizing vasculitis involving renal arcuate arteries. HES

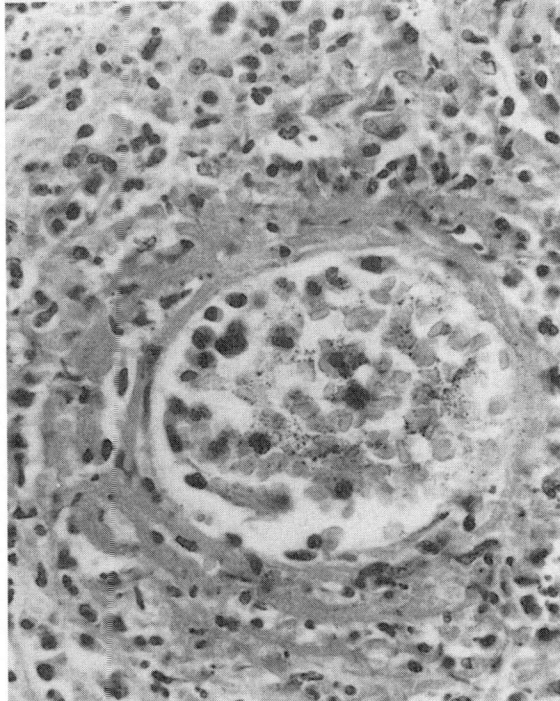

Fig. 8. Systemic lupus erythematosus. Acute necrotizing vasculitis. HES

considered. Comparison of the glomerular disease in ANCA-positive lupus glomerulonephritis patients with that in ANCA-negative lupus glomerulonephritis patients reveals no significant differences (there is no difference in the incidence of glomerular necrosis or crescent formation, or vasculitis in renal arteries).

Rheumatoid arthritis RA

It is possible to draw analogies between RA and a number of connective tissue syndromes in which vasculitis is significant. The disease may be triggered by exposure of an immunogenetically susceptible individual to an arthritogenic microbial antigen. Many facts support this hypothesis; 65 to 80% of patients with RA are HLA-DR4 or DR1 or both [75]. Among microbial agents, the potential offenders are Epstein-Barr virus (EBV), retroviruses, parvoviruses, mycobacteria, Borrelia, and Mycoplasma. Autoimmunity to type II collagen can be demonstrated in most patients with RA. EBV and type II collagen may share some cross-reactive antigenic determinant that can combine with antibodies or T cell receptors. Once an inflammatory synovitis has been initiated by a microbial agent the T cells may play a pivotal role with the local release of inflammatory mediators and lytic cytokines that ultimately destroy the joint.

The diagnosis, based primarily on the clinical features, requires the presence of four of the following criteria [76]: morning stiffness, arthritis in three or more joint areas, arthritis of hand joints, symmetrical arthritis, rheumatoid nodules, serum rheumatoid factor, and typical radiographic changes. The combined features of RA, splenomegaly, and neutropaenia are known as Felty's syndrome.

Death in this chronic illness usually results from vascular complications with multiple visceral infarctions, fatal gastrointestinal bleeding related to long-term therapy (aspirin or NSAID's) and infections associated with long-term steroid use. Complications of RA include systemic amyloidosis and lymphoedema [77, 78]. Vasculitic syndromes affect the prognosis and symptoms vary according to the types of vessels involved. The most common related findings are periungual infarcts, which are of no significance. Systemic vasculitis is more serious and may present with a wide range of symptoms, including fever, anaemia, hypersplenism, digital infarcts, palpable purpura, cutaneous ulcers, mononeuritis multiplex, pleurisy with pulmonary nodular fibrosis; pericarditis, myocarditis with cardiac valvular disease, and granulomatous aortitis [79]. This picture may mimic polyarteritis nodosa but digestive tract and renal involvement with

hypertension are very uncommon in rheumatoid arthritis, although they have been reported [80]. Obstruction of the lymphatics caused by fibrin and other degradation products of the coagulation system may result in lymphoedema.

Pathology and differential diagnosis

The morphological features of rheumatoid vasculitis (RV) are similar to those of polyarteritis nodosa. Small vessels, such as digital arteries, vasa nervorum, and venules are mostly affected. RV resembles classical leukocytoclastic vasculitis with medial necrosis, neutrophil infiltration and intimal thickening. The presence of immunoglobulin and complement deposits in the small vessels suggests that immune-complexes may play a pivotal role. The tissues most frequently involved are the heart, skeletal muscles and peripheral nerves [81]. In about 20% of patients, rheumatoid nodules may develop in great vessels [79, 82], including the aorta where they are found in the first 2 to 5 cm, rarely its whole length. The involvement may be continuous or segmentary with clear demarcated skip areas. In affected areas, rheumatoid nodules appear firm to the touch, greyish, and contain yellowish necrotic areas, which may undergo cavitation. Their size varies from some millimetres to several centimeters in diameter. Histologically, the nodules, centred by necrosis, are surrounded by palisading, closely-packed epithelioid cells, interspersed with some giant cells. A rim of lymphocytes, plasma cells, and fibroblasts surrounds the periphery. In early lesions, the granulomata may contain more acute inflammatory cells [83].

Seronegative spondyloarthropathies

These conditions are defined by the lack of rheumatoid factor. They include ankylosing spondylitis, Reiter's syndrome, psoriatic arthritis, and enteropathic arthritis. They all share overlapping clinical features, and many are associated with HLA-B27. The first three entities may manifest by a vasculitis [84].

Ankylosing spondylitis

The presence of the HLA-B27 antigen in 90% of patients and 50% of their first-degree relatives is highly suggestive of a hereditary factor predisposing to the development of autoantibodies directed at joint elements following infection [85]. It should be emphasised that HLA-B27 antigen association is also noted in patients with ulcerative colitis, Crohn's regional enteritis, Reiter's syndrome (Fiessinger-Leroy-Reiter syndrome), and psoriasis. The disease typically affects young males with a male/female ratio of 8:1. Chronic synovitis leads to destruction of articular cartilage with bony ankylosis, and lipping of vertebral margins. Involvement of the sacroiliac and apophyseal joints causes chronic low back pain. Other peripheral joints, such as the hips, knees, and shoulders, may also be involved. Extra-articular manifestations include iritis, prostatitis and systemic amyloidosis [86]. Aortic valvular disease occurs frequently in patients with ankylosing spondylitis, 1 to 10% of cases presenting with the consequences of involvement of the aorta [87-89]. Aortic dilatation and valvular incompetence occur and nodularities develop in the aortic cusps and the anterior mitral leaflet with fibrosis and calcification.

Pathology and differential diagnosis

In the aorta, lesions frequently affect the ascending part above the sinuses of Valsalva and do not tend to extend. In the active phase, the aortic wall is infiltrated with lymphocytes and plasma cells. Later, fibrosis distorts the three aortic layers and dilatation occurs. The coronary ostia may be affected with fibrotic narrowing. Thickening of the basal portion of the aortic cusps combined with aortic root dilatation causes valvular insufficiency.

Reiter's syndrome (Fiessinger-Leroy-Reiter Syndrome)

This autoimmune condition is thought to be initiated by previous infections (80% of patients express the HLA-B27 antigen) [90]. Possible offenders include Shigella, Salmonella, Yersinia, Campylobacter, and Chlamydia [91]. There is a predominance in men in their third to fourth decades. Extra-articular manifestations include urethritis (56.7%), ophthalmic-conjunctivitis (46.5%), and mucocutaneous-balanitis (12.3%) [92]. Cardiac conduction abnormalities, aortitis with aortic valve regurgitation, and coronary artery stenosis have all been reported, and thrombophlebitis may occur [93-95]. Systemic leukocytoclastic vasculitis with livedo reticularis has been described [91, 96].

Psoriatic arthritis

Vasculitis, when present in this arthropathy, is part of the synovial disease. Arthritis is usually transient, lasting for about a year and is rarely accompanied by ankylosing spondylitis. Remissions are frequent, and the joint destruction minimal.

Pathology and differential diagnosis

Synovial vessels commonly show transmural inflammatory infiltrates with swelling of endothelial cells.

Relapsing polychondritis

This degenerative disease of the cartilage presents with aseptic inflammation and destruction of the nasal or ear cartilages and symptoms due to similar damage in the tracheobronchial tree [97]. The two life threatening complications of relapsing polychondritis are the involvement of the cartilaginous structures of the respiratory tract and progressive aortic insufficiency caused by aortitis. Aortic regurgitation is caused by progressive dilatation of the aortic ring and, often, the ascending aorta, rather than by inflammation of the valve leaflets [98-100]. In about 10% of patients, destruction of the aortic medial structure may lead to aneurysm formation [101-104] and dissection with fatal rupture [105].

Pathology and differential diagnosis

Cartilage displays necrosis of chondrocytes with destruction of the matrix, loss of basophilia in the elastic cartilage, and infiltration by inflammatory cells. Segments of cartilage may be sequestrated by granulation tissue. In the aorta, the media is destroyed by large infiltrates of inflammatory mononuclear cells distorting the elastic frame of the media. These areas are then replaced by highly vascular granulation tissue and fibrosis. The differential diagnosis includes Marfan's syndrome, syphilitic aortitis, and giant cell aortitis.

Vasculitis associated with neoplasms

Systemic and cutaneous vasculitis may predate or follow appearance of malignant tumours. The incidence of this association is 4,95% [106]. The existence of distinct tumour-associated antigens may be accompanied by circulating immune complexes in approximately one third to one half of patients with both lymphoma and solid tumours. Cryoglobulins can be demonstrated in some patients with lymphoma or multiple myeloma. Isolated cases of neoplasms associated with vasculitis have been reported and table 5 lists some previously published examples. Generally, the vasculitic syndrome presents the clinical features of a leukocytoclastic vasculitis or mononeuritis multiplex. In the majority of cases, vasculitis reveals an underlying tumour or indicates a tumour recurrence. According to Naschitz et al [107], a cutaneous leukocytoclastic vasculitis presenting after the age of 50 years is frequently associated with an underlying cancer. Treatment of the underlying neoplasm may improve the vasculitis. Pathological changes vary according to the clinical syndrome and systemic PAN,

Table 5. Vasculitis and neoplasms

NEOPLASIAS	ASSOCIATED VASCULITIDES	REFERENCES
Haemopathies, primary myelofibrosis, acute myelomonocytic leukemia, hairy-cell leukaemia	LCV, PAN, LV, GV, PR	28, 108, 109, 110, 111, 112, 113
Chronic lymphocytic leukemia	LV	114
Cryoglobulinaemia (lymphocytic lymphoma or Waldenstrom's macro-globulinaemia)and multiple myeloma	LCV, PAN, HSP	28, 115, 116, 117
Hodgkin's disease	Wegener's granulomatosis	28
Non-Hodgkin lymphomas	LV, GV, HSP, and temporal arteritis	28, 109, 114
Solid tumours: non-secreting pheochromocytoma, cardiac myxoma, carcinomas (lung, colon, kidney, liver, prostate), malignant melanoma, liposarcoma	LCV, PAN, HSP, and allergic vasculitis	109, 115, 118, 119, 120, 121, 122

(HSP: Henoch-Schonlein purpura, GV: granulomatous vasculitis, LCV: leukocytoclastic vasculitis, LV: lymphocytic vasculitis, PAN: periarteritis nodosa, PR: purpura rheumatica)

leukocytoclastic vasculitis, or CNS granulomatous vasculitis may all occur.

Essential mixed cryoglobulinaemic vasculitis

Precipitation of circulating cryoglobulins as blood cools while flowing through the microvasculature of the skin and subcutaneous tissues of the extremities leads to small vessel damage with resultant purpura and gangrene. Most cryoprecipitates contain immunoglobulins (IgM and IgG antibodies) and complement components. There are three types of cryoglobulins. Table 6 summarises their major characteristics and the pathological entities with which they are associated [123]. Deposition of these immune complexes in the vessels of the skin and the kidneys produces a leukocytoclastic angiitis.

Clinical manifestations include either urticaria or pruritic vascular purpura with skin infarction, digital gangrene, livedo and Raynaud's phenomenon. Purpura may be precipitated by prolonged standing, or exposure to cold. Other symptoms include arthritis, polyneuritis, gastrointestinal haemorrhage, hepatosplenomegaly and generalised vasculitis. Renal involvement is uncommon, but some patients may present with haematuria, proteinuria (nephrotic syndrome) and, rarely, anuria. Cryoglobulinaemia can be recognised after clotting whole blood at 37° C, incubating the separated serum at 4° C for 24 h, and examining the serum for a gel or precipitate. Laboratory findings include leukocytosis, hypocomplementemia, presence of immune complex-like material or IgM and IgG cryoglobulins precipitable by C1q at low temperatures. The IgM cryoglobulin contains a rheumatoid factor-like monoclonal kappa component [124, 125]. In some patients, hepatitis B virus surface antigen or anti-hepatitis B antibodies may be found in either the serum or the cryoprecipitate.

Pathology and differential diagnosis

The characteristic lesions of monoclonal cryoglobulinaemia are those of vascular dilatation, endothelial swelling, and intraluminal deposits of hyaline material that is diastase-resistant periodic acid-Shiff positive. Patients with severe renal involvement may have membranoproliferative glomerulonephritis. Histological patterns of mixed cryglobulinemia are those of an immune complex-mediated acute hypersensitivity vasculitis involving small vessels. Immunofluorescence displays labelling of IgG and IgM in the vascu-

Table 6. Characteristics of cryoglobulins

TYPES	COMPOSITION	PATHOLOGICAL ENTITIES
1	Monoclonal immunoglobulins (either kappa or lambda)	Lympho-proliferative conditions (multiple myeloma, Waldelström's macroglobulinaemia, lymphoma and lympho-cytic leukaemia) Carcinoma (lung)
2	Monoclonal immunoglobulins (usually IgM) reacting against IgG	Connective tissue diseases: systemic lupus erythematosa, Sjogren's syndrome, rheumatoid arthritis. Infectious conditions: cytomegalovirus, infectious mononucleosis, subacute bacterial endocarditis, leprosy, syphilis, trypanosomiasis
3	Mixed polyclonal immunoglobulins (usually IgG-IgM)	-id- type 2

lar walls. Occasionally, hyaline thrombi may be seen in the lumen. Renal involvement leads to intracapillary thrombosis, vasculitis and membranoproliferative glomerulonephritis.

4 – Direct antibody attack-mediated vasculitis

Goodpasture's syndrome

This glomerulonephritis of the anti-basement membrane type is associated with or preceded by haemoptysis. The nephritis usually progresses rapidly leading to death from renal failure; the lungs at autopsy show extensive haemosiderosis or recent haemorrhage. First described by Ernest Goodpasture during the influenza pandemic of 1919 [126], this syndrome is an excellent example of anti-glomerular basement membrane disease which has a wide spectrum of clinical manifestations [127], including systemic vasculitis. Goodpasture's syndrome is mediated by anti-GBM antibodies and exhibits linear fluorescence of IgG, C3 and complement along the basement membranes of the glomerular capillary loops and the alveolar septal walls. The primary target antigen is the alpha 3 component of type IV collagen of basement membrane [128-131]. Many factors are thought to cause the production of anti-GBM antibody, including environmental exposure to hydrocarbon solvents, metal dusts, and chlorine. Other possible causes include influenza A2 virus infection and D-penicillamine therapy in Wilson's disease. Isolated cases of anti-GBM antibody-mediated disease have been reported in recipients of renal transplants for the Alport type of hereditary nephritis [132, 133].

Pathology and differential diagnosis.

In the kidney, the glomerular lesions, although not necessarily unique or specific, are often sufficiently distinct to suggest the diagnosis of Goodpasture's syndrome. In the early stage, glomeruli show local capsular epithelial proliferation (Fig. 9). With progression of the disease, the lesions advance into Bowman's urinary space, encroaching upon glomerular capillary tufts, which become compressed in the epithelial pannus. Silver staining reveals sites of perforation of capillary walls plugged with cellular elements and fibrin. Fibrosis develops in the epithelial crescents and in the collapsed glomerular tufts resulting in partially or completely fibrosed glomeruli. Glomerular fibrosis may become widespread and terminate in a pattern of end-stage severe fibrosis indistinguishable from other forms of chronic glomerulonephritis. Renal, systemic and intracranial vasculitides have been reported in several series of anti-GBM antibody-mediated disease (Fig. 10) [134-137]. Tubulointerstitial inflammation is frequently apparent with mononuclear cell infiltration.

The parenchyma of the lungs shows intra-alveolar haemorrhage interspersed with haemosiderin-laden macrophages. Vasculitis occurs in widened alveolar septa with infiltration of neutrophils, eosinophils and oedema [138, 139]. Immunofluorescence studies demonstrate characteristic linear constant ribbonlike deposits of IgG along the GBM in the kidneys. Less commonly IgA, IgM and C3 deposits have been also reported. Pulmonary biopsies evidence similar linear or segmental linear antibody deposits along alveolar capillary basement membranes. However, these findings are not specific [140] so renal biopsy remains the diagnostic procedure of choice in this condition.

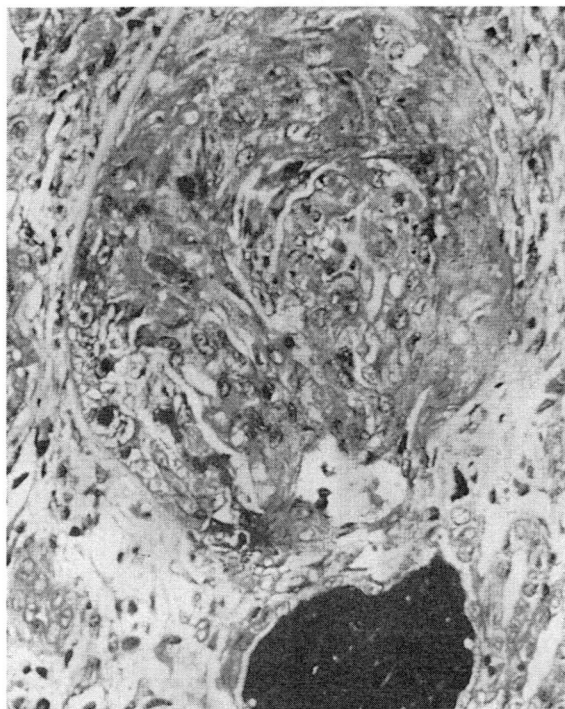

Fig. 9. Goodpasture's syndrome. Proliferative glomerulone-phritis. Masson's trichrome. (Courtesy Dr D. Droz)

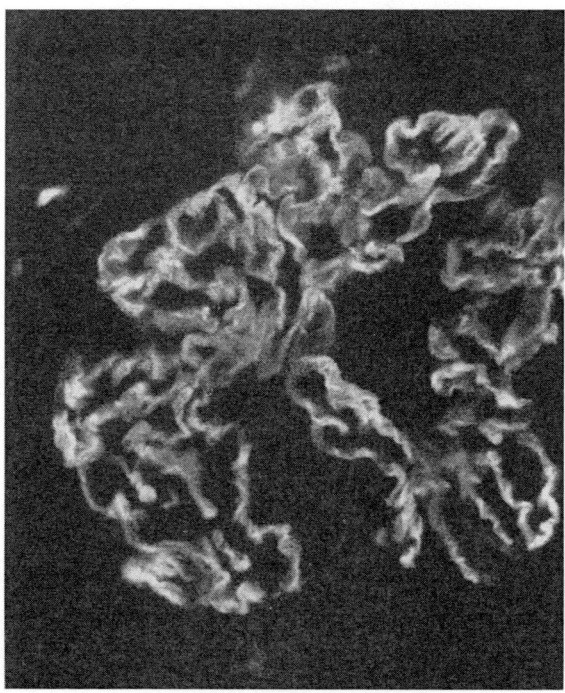

Fig. 10. Goodpasture's syndrome. Linear ribbonlike deposits of IgG along the glomerular basement membrane in Good-pasture's syndrome evidenced by immunofluorescence technique. (Courtesy Dr D. Droz)

Mucocutaneous lymph node syndrome (Kawasaki's disease)

This acute vasculitis of unknown aetiology typically affects young children who present with clinical symptoms and signs including fever, conjunctivitis, pharyngitis, cervical lymphadenopathy and an erythematous peripheral rash. Involvement of the cardio-vascular system is the most significant component of the illness and the coronary arteries are frequently affected [141, 142]. Eighty percent of the patients are under 4 yrs; after the age of 10 years Kawasaki's disease is extremely rare and the diagnosis should be regarded with suspicion [143, 144]. The male to female ratio is 1.6 to 1. The disease is commoner in Asian populations, especially of Japanese ancestry, but any ethnic group may be affected. The incidence is 67/100000 in Japan, and 6 to 9/100000 in the USA. There appears to be a seasonal predilection between December and May [145-149].

Clinically the acute illness usually begins with a fever of 5 or more days duration and the diagnosis is made when 4 out of the following 5 symptoms are present: bilateral conjunctival injection without exudate changes in the extremities (erythema and oedema of the hands and feet, or membranous desquamation of the fingertips), polymorphous exanthema, changes in the lips and oral cavity (erythema, cracked lips, strawberry tongue, diffuse injection of the oral and pharyngeal mucosa), and acute cervical lymphadenopathy [150]. Other clinical signs include arthralgia, arthritis, and cardiac involvement. Infections, toxic exposures, allergic and immunologically mediated origins have all been suggested but none has been generally accepted. The clinical and epidemiological characteristics favour an infectious aetiology [151] and retroviruses and parvo B19 virus have been discussed as possible causes. Associations of Kawasaki's disease with antecedent respiratory illness and rug shampoo exposure have been reported but remain unexplained [152]

Affected patients have some immunoregulatory disturbances, including T-cell activation, polyclonal B-cell activation, and circulating immune complexes. Lytic autoantibodies to cytokine-activated endothelial cells found during acute episodes and disappearing in convalescence may contribute to the vascular injury in this disorder [153-156].

Myocardial infarction secondary to coronary thrombosis accounts for most of the morbidity and mortality during the acute period or in the first year of the disease. Aneurysms, myocarditis, arrhythmias, valvulitis and, less commonly mitral insufficiency may all occur [157-161]. However, the prognosis is good with a mortality rate of approximately 0.4%. There is some concern that children with damaged coronary arteries will have problems later in life, but this seems to be very rare. Some case reports suggest that some severe coronary diseases in adults might be a consequence of childhood Kawasaki's disease [162].

Pathology and differential diagnosis

The vasculitis resembles that of PAN, with necrosis and severe inflammation affecting the entire vascular wall. The inflammatory infiltrate is made up of lymphocytes, and neutrophils; some eosinophils may be seen. In rare cases only the intima is affected, with swelling and proliferation of endothelial cells. Generally, the large and medium-sized extramural branches of the coronary arteries are much more severely involved than the small intramyocardial branches. As with PAN, severe lesions can lead to weakening of the vascular wall with thrombosis, formation of aneurysms, and rupture. These complications may cause fatal myocardial infarction or sudden death. The morphological changes of cardiac valves consist mainly of inflammatory infiltration, and proliferation of small capillaries and fibrosis. The difference between Kawasaki's disease and infantile periarteritis nodosa has been widely discussed [163, 164], but clear cut separation is not possible in either clinical or pathological findings. Aneurysm or thombosis of coronary arteries may occur in some cases of rheumatic fever [165]. The vascular changes in rheumatic fever resemble those of classical periarteritis nodosa and mostly involve the small arteries.

5 – ANCA associated vasculitis

Wegener's granulomatosis

This disease is characterised by necrotizing, destructive, granulomatous lesions in the upper and lower respiratory tracts [166]. There is focal necrotizing vasculitis affecting medium-sized to small vessels involving all organs of the body and renal damage in the form of focal or diffuse necrotizing glomerulitis [167]. There is a limited form with long survival when the disease is predominantly restricted to the lungs. Untreated Wegener's granulomatosis has a mean survival rate of 5 months with a mortality rate of 90% at 2 years.

The cause is unknown. The presence of granulomata and rapid response to cytotoxic immunosuppressive drugs suggests an immunologically mediated mechanism, perhaps of the cell-mediated type. Wegener's granulomatosis may represent a form of hypersensitivity, but attempts to demonstrate a causative agent have been unsuccessful.

This uncommon disease affects patients of all ages, from early childhood to an advanced age, but the peak incidence is in the fifth decade. There is a slight predominance in males, generally in the ratio of 3:2.

In the generalised form, the disease mostly affects the kidneys and, to a lesser extent, the joints, skin, nervous system and the digestive tract. Renal involvement (occurring in 80% of all cases) is manifested by proteinuria and abnormal urinary sediment. Cutaneous manifestations (40 to 50% of patients) consist of purpura, bruising, nodules, and pyoderma gangrenosum-like lesions leading to ulceration and necrosis [168]. Prominent neurologic symptoms (mononeuritis) are caused by focal arteritis with ischaemia.

A positive indirect immunofluorescent test for anti-neutrophil cytoplasm antibodies (ANCA) is present in 92% of patients and this appears to be a good marker for disease activity. During treatment, a rising titer of ANCA suggests a relapse; most patients in remission have a negative test or the titer falls significantly.

Two other limited forms of Wegener's granulomatosis have been described: patients with limited pulmonary granulomatosis present with respiratory symptoms, fever and weight loss [169-171]. There is no renal involvement and the prognosis is better than that of classical (generalised) Wegener's granulomatosis. "Pathergic" granulomatosis presents with mucosal and cutaneous lesions and may persist for long periods resulting in facial mutilation long before renal failure occurs [172].

Pathology and Differential diagnosis

Biopsy reveals characteristic granulomatous inflammation of tissue with vasculitis affecting small arteries and veins. Vasculitis has been described in virtually every vessel and organ of the body. Skin biopsies show leukocytoclastic vasculitis. The lung parenchyma shows infarct-like necrotic areas but with little haemorrhage (Fig. 11-12). Lesions have two main features; granulomata with dense infiltrates of chronic and acute inflammatory cells interspersed with multinucleated giant cells and areas of necrosis (Fig. 13), and necrotizing vasculitis involving arteries and veins with fibrinoid necrosis (Fig. 14). Infiltration of leukocytes and mononuclear cells and fibrosis (Fig. 15) are seen in the surrounding parenchyma [173]. Associations with marked eosinophilia in the granuloma, the

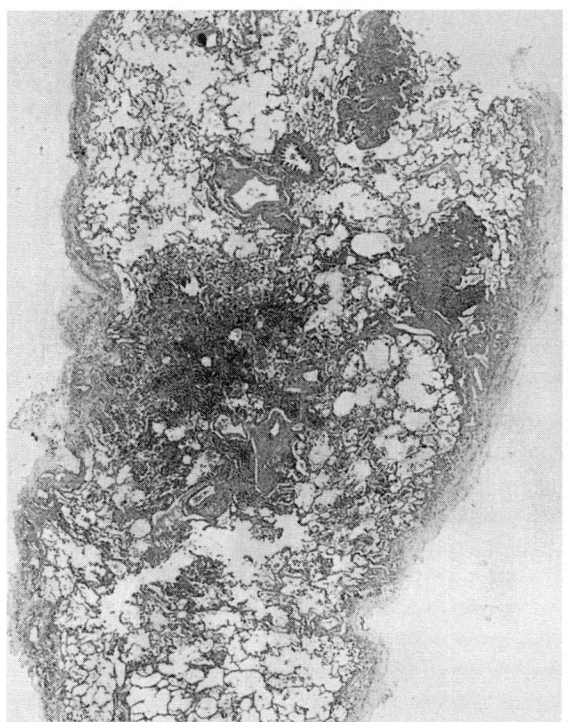

Fig. 11. Wegener's granulomatosis. Lung biopsy showing infarct-like necrotic areas. HES

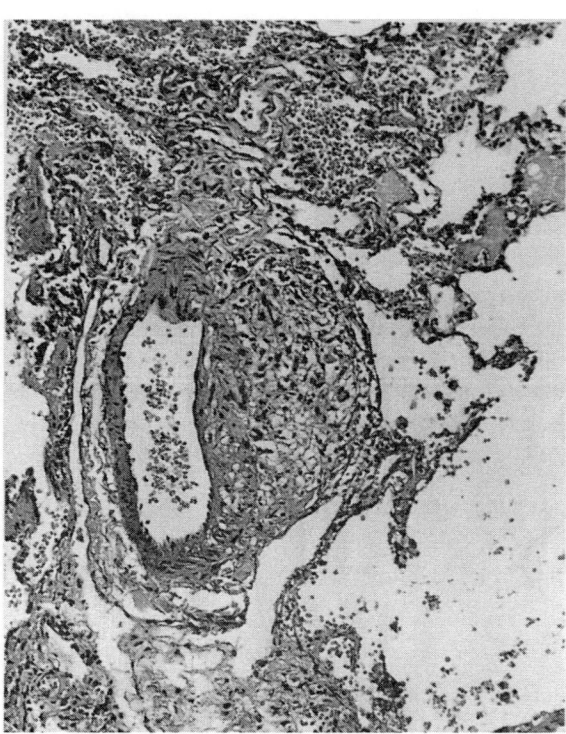

Fig. 13. Wegener's granulomatosis. Granulomatous vasculitis. HES

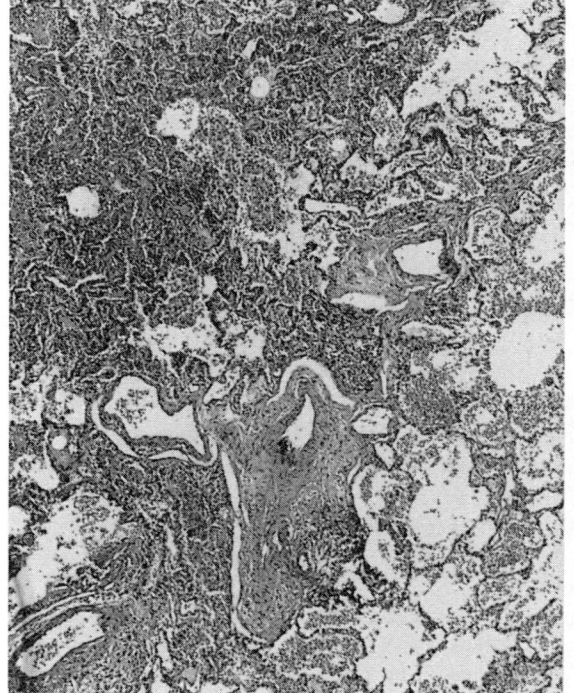

Fig. 12. Wegener's granulomatosis. Diffuse vascular involvement in the lesion. HES

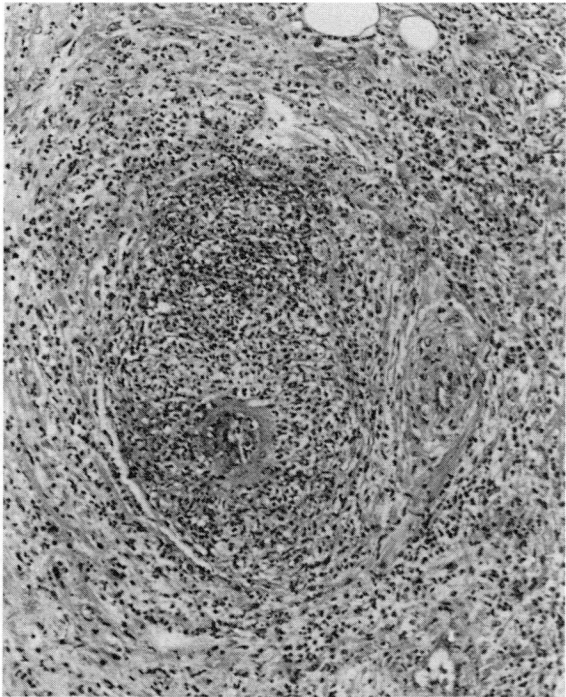

Fig. 14. Wegener's granulomatosis. Necrotizing vasculitis. HES

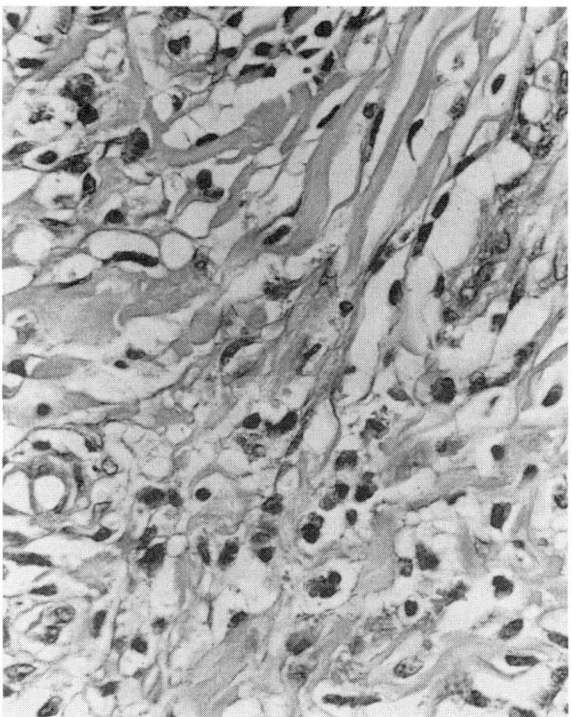

Fig. 15. Wegener's granulomatosis. Infiltration of leukocytes and fibrosis of the surrounding parenchyma. HES

peripheral blood and the pleural effusion have been reported [174].

In the kidneys, selective angiography reveals stenoses of interlobar and arcuate arteries. The parenchyma displays interstitial granulomata and glomerular changes. Segmental and focal necrotizing glomerulonephritis involves only a few glomeruli with crescent formation but eventually becomes widespread, leading to diffuse proliferative glomerulonephritis. Some glomerular capillaries have a thickened wall while electron microscopy demonstrates subepithelial densities in the basement membrane. Immunofluorescence demonstrates granular immunoglobulin deposits along the epithelial side of the glomerular basement membrane.

According to the 1994 International Consensus Conference on Nomenclature of systemic vasculitides, the name "Wegener's granulomatosis" is restricted to patients with granulomatous inflammation. Patients with exclusively nongranulomatous small vessel vasculitis involving the upper or lower respiratory tract (e.g., alveolar capillaritis) fall into the category of microscopic polyangiitis (microscopic polyarteritis) [2]. In the upper airways, Wegener's granulomatosis should also be distinguished from so-called idiopathic

midline granuloma (granuloma gangrenescens, or Stewart's malignant granuloma or idiopathic midline destructive syndrome), a progressive, necrotic and highly aggressive disease destroying and perforating the palate [175-177]. The majority of these lesions are T-cell lymphomas [178, 179], although some cases have shown natural killer cell immunohistochemistry [180]. Other differential diagnosis includes the Churg-Strauss syndrome.

Microscopic polyarteritis

This condition involves small arteries and/or arterioles [181] with or without involvement of medium-sized arteries. It is a necrotizing vasculitis with few or no immune deposits. Cryoglobulinemic vasculitis, Henoch-Schonlein purpura and other forms of immune complex-mediated small vessel vasculitis must be ruled out to make this diagnosis [182]. The distribution of vascular lesions, clinical manifestations and complications differ in microscopic and classic polyarteritis but the lesions are similar to those of classic polyarteritis nodosa. Renal changes are those of focal, segmental, proliferative or necrotizing glomerulonephritis.

Churg-Strauss syndrome (Allergic granulomatosis, Allergic granulomatous angiitis)

This condition is characterised by asthma, fever, eosinophilia, and various symptoms and signs of vasculitis, primarily affecting small arteries, with vascular and extravascular granulomata. The American College of Rheumatology 1990 criteria for the classification of the Churg-Strauss syndrome include asthma, eosinophilia greater than 10% on differential white blood cell count, mononeuropathy (including multiplex) or polyneuropathy, non-fixed pulmonary infiltrates on roentgenography, paranasal sinus abnormality, and biopsy containing a blood vessel with extravascular eosinophils. The presence of 4 or more of these 6 criteria yielded a sensitivity of 85% and a specificity of 99.7% [183]. The aetiology is unknown but the occasional finding of immunoglobulin and complement within the blood vessel wall favours the hypothesis of an immune complex-induced process. Some patients have a history of asthma, allergy rhinitis or drug sensitivity [184, 185]. P-ANCA are present in more than 60% of patients [11, 16].

Pathology and differential diagnosis

In the lungs, the parenchyma shows nodules, varying from a few to many hundreds of variable sized lesions measuring up to 1.5 cm in diameter; these nodules may coalesce. Histologically they show an area of central necrosis, surrounded by epithelioid cells. Some occasional giant cells may be present [186]. The adjacent parenchyma is infiltrated by a large number of eosinophils with neutrophils, histiocytes, lymphocytes and plasma cells. Small arteries and sometimes veins show vasculitis. In the skin, early lesions consist of areas of collagen degeneration in association with variable infiltration of sparse and numerous eosinophils, some neutrophils, histiocytes and lymphocytes. Leukocytoclasis may be frequent. In the advanced stage, mature extravascular granulomata may appear. Less commonly, the features of necrotizing vasculitis are evident in superficial small blood vessels; fibrinoid necrosis, infiltration of eosinophils and neutrophils, and leukocytoclasis are all seen. Occasionally, polyarteritis nodosa-like lesions involve the arteries of the dermis and subcutis. Although there are clinical and histological overlaps, Churg-Strauss syndrome, polyarteritis nodosa and Wegener's granulomatosis present sufficient differences to justify their separate classification (Table 7) [187]. Asthma may be manifest in both periarteritis nodosa and Churg-Strauss syndrome. However, polyarteritis nodosa characteristically affects medium-sized and small arteries while Churg-Strauss syndrome involves small arteries and veins. In polyarteritis nodosa, the inflammatory cell infiltrate contains numerous neutrophils, while in Churg-Strauss syndrome, eosinophils are the major cellular components. Necrotizing extravascular granulomata are not a feature of polyarteritis nodosa. Wegener's granulomatosis is characterised by necrotic and ulcero-proliferative lesions of the upper respiratory tract, chest pain, and haemoptysis rather than asthma. Renal involvement, common in Wegener's granulomatosis, is infrequent in Churg-Strauss syndrome as is granulomatous vasculitis.

6 – Rejection vasculitis

Rejection is a complex process in which both circulating antibodies and cell-mediated immunity play a role. The relative participation of these two mechanisms in rejection depends on the type of transplant and is reflected in the histological appearance. Vessels play a major role in the rejection phenomenon and undergo changes themselves – rejection vasculitis. A detailed account of the processes involved can be found in Berry [22].

Hyperacute rejection

This develops within minutes or hours after transplantation, immediately after the graft vasculature is anastomosed to the recipient's. The morphological changes typify a classic antibody-mediated reaction (Arthus phenomenon). Small vessels (arterioles, ca-

Table 7. Main differential characteristics of Churg-Strauss syndrome (C-SS), Periarteritis nodosa (PAN), Wegener's granulomatosis (WG)

	DIFFERENTIAL DIAGNOSIS	C-S S	PAN	WG
Visceral involvement	Upper respiratory tract: ulceration, proliferation	+		+
	Asthma	+	+	+
	Heamoptysis			+
	Renal involvement		+	+
Vascular involvement	Medium-sized arteries		+	+
	Small arteries	+	+	+
	Veins	+		+
Histological aspects	Vascular necrosis		+	+
	Neutrophils	+	+	+
	Eosinophils	+++		
	Extravascular granuloma	+		+

pillaries) display an accumulation of neutrophils and rapid deposition of immunoglobulins and complement, while fibrin-platelet thrombi occlude the vascular lumen and endothelial cells undergo early injury. These changes rapidly become diffuse and arterial walls are distorted by fibrinoid necrosis and diffuse infarction of the graft parenchyma may follow [22].

Acute rejection

This occurs within days of transplantation in the untreated recipient or may appear suddenly months or even years later, when immunosuppressive therapy is discontinued. Acute graft rejection results from both cellular and humorally-mediated reactions. Histologically, cellular-mediated rejection is marked by an interstitial infiltration of mononuclear cells (CD4+ and CD8+ lymphocytes) and humorally-mediated rejection is associated with "acute rejection" vasculitis. Vascular changes include necrotizing vasculitis with endothelial necrosis (Fig. 16-17), infiltration of neutrophils, deposition of immunoglobulins, complement, and fibrin and diffuse thrombosis (Fig. 18) [188].

Subacute rejection

Modern tissue matching techniques have ensured that this form of rejection is more often seen than acute forms. It occurs during the first few months after transplantation. Characteristic arterial lesions are seen in the intima with considerable thickening giving rise to a cushion of proliferating fibroblasts, myocytes, and foamy macrophages (Fig. 19-20) [189]. Scattered neutrophils and mononuclear cells, together with deposits of immunoglobulin and complement, may be present. The changes result in luminal narrowing or obliteration.

Chronic rejection

Generally, vascular changes of chronic rejection are not remarkable. They include endothelialitis, arteriosclerosis and atherosclerosis. Endothelialitis [190] is characterised by infiltration of small lymphocytes, mostly T cells (UCHL1+), in the subendothelial space with degenerative changes in endothelial cells (Fig. 21). However, this lesion is not specific to the rejection. Arteriosclerosis may be diffuse and mostly involves small arteries (Fig. 22-23-24). Atherosclerosis is seen later, but the plaques contain more lipid and are more diffuse than in typical disease (Fig. 25). Other morphological features of chronic rejection depend

mostly on the transplant itself. Parenchymal changes vary in severity but in all transplants vascular changes always occur.

7 – Vasculitis of unknown origin

Giant cell arteritis (Temporal arteritis, Cranial arteritis, Granulomatous arteritis, Horton's disease)

This panarteritis, with medial necrosis and multinucleated giant cells, typically affects the temporal, retinal, or intracerebral arteries of elderly patients (the incidence is 1.4/100,000 in patients of 50 yr but 26.9/100,000 in patients over 80) with a relative female predominance (1.5:1). It may present with constitutional symptoms including severe localised or bitemporal headache, temporal artery tenderness or decreased temporal artery pulse and ocular symptoms, with the danger of sudden loss of vision in one eye. There is a genetic predisposition; an increased prevalence of HLA-DR4 antigen is found in these patients, and occasional familial clusters occur. This form of vasculitis is now well documented in almost all large arteries and recent reports include cerebral, vertebral, internal carotid, brachial and pulmonary vessel involvement [191-194]. Thus, the clinical manifestations may be variable with aortic valve insufficiency [195], aneurysm [196] with fatal rupture [197], aortic dissection [198], aortic – gastrointestinal fistula [199, 200], reno vascular hypertension, and small intestine or scalp necrosis [201], all documented. Ostberg [202] reviewed a series of 16 autopsies and found that the aorta and large arteries were involved in 12 cases. Lesions affected either the whole aorta (6 cases) or parts of it (6 cases). In a series of 248 patients with giant cell temporal arteritis reported by Klein et al [203], 34 patients had evidence that the disease involved the aorta or its major branches.

Laboratory findings include marked elevation of the erythrocyte sedimentation rate, mild normochromic normocytic anaemia, moderate leukocytosis, red blood cell rouleaux in peripheral blood smears, and increased alpha 2-globulin. Patients may develop intravascular coagulation and fibrinolysis with prolonged prothrombin times, thrombocytosis, and increased levels of fibrinogen and fibrinogen split-products.

Generally, the disease runs a self-limited course, and active lesions gradually subside. Gonzalez-Gay et al [204] have documented the low long-term morta-

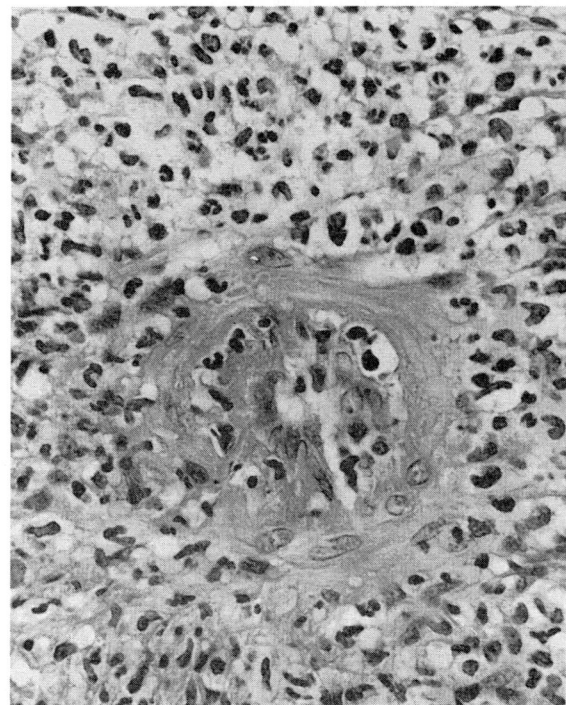

Fig. 16. Rejection vasculitis. Acute rejection of a renal graft. Necrotizing vasculitis with endothelial necrosis. HES

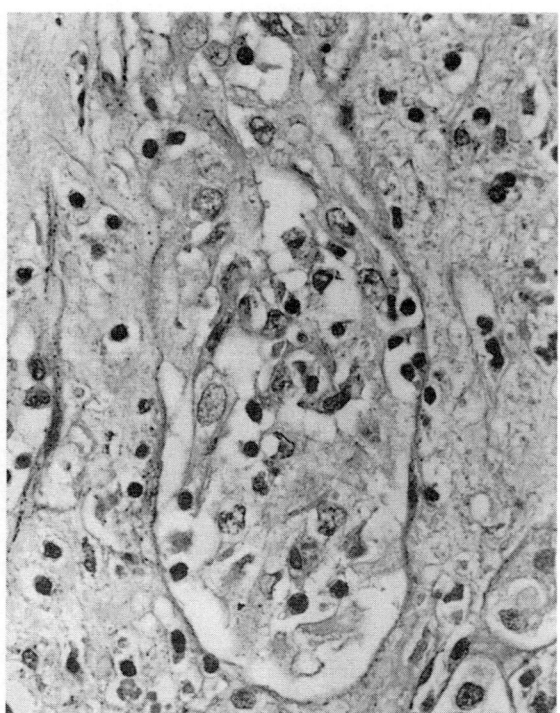

Fig. 17. Rejection vasculitis. Acute rejection of a renal graft. Necrotizing vasculitis with detachment of endothelial cells. HES

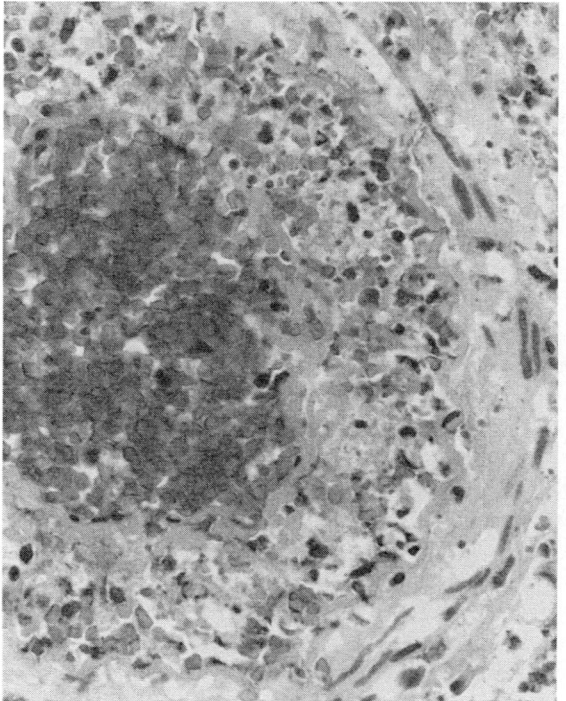

Fig. 18. Rejection vasculitis. Acute rejection of a renal graft. Necrotizing vasculitis with thrombosis. HES

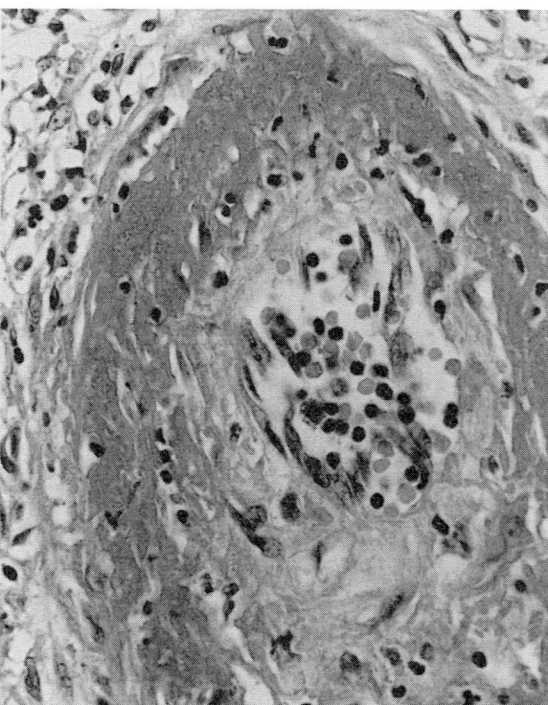

Fig. 19. Rejection vasculitis. Subacute rejection of a renal graft. Intimal thickening with inflammatory infiltrate in the vascular wall. HES

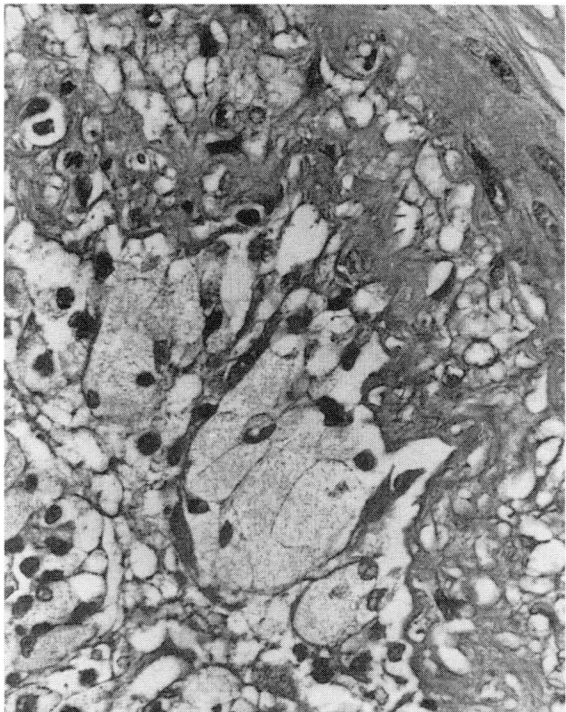

Fig. 20. Rejection vasculitis. Subacute rejection of a renal graft. Foam cell vasculitis. HES

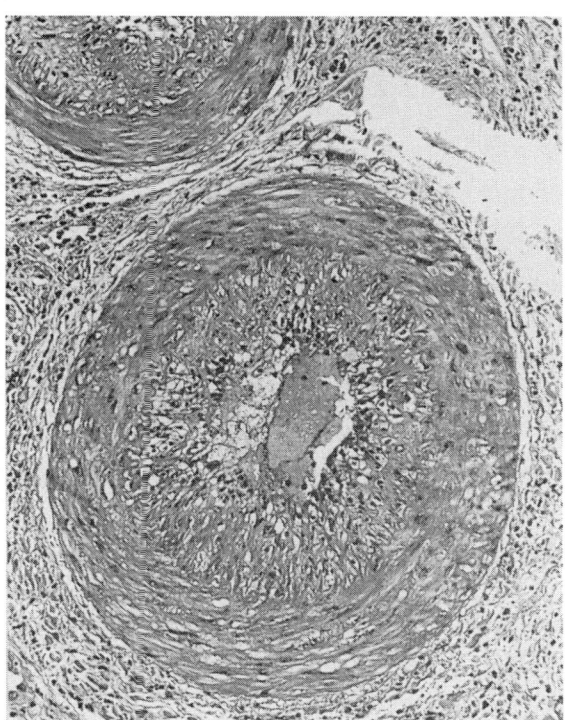

Fig. 21. Rejection vasculitis. Chronic rejection of a cardiac graft. Endothelialitis with infiltration of small lymphocytes and endothelial degenerative changes. HES

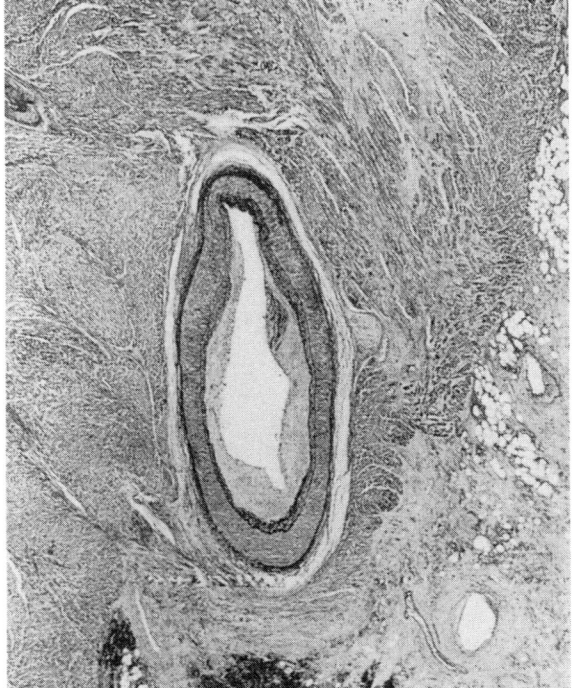

Fig. 22. Rejection vasculitis. Chronic rejection of a cardiac graft. Coronary artery displaying arteriosclerotic changes. Orcein elastic stain. (Orcein)

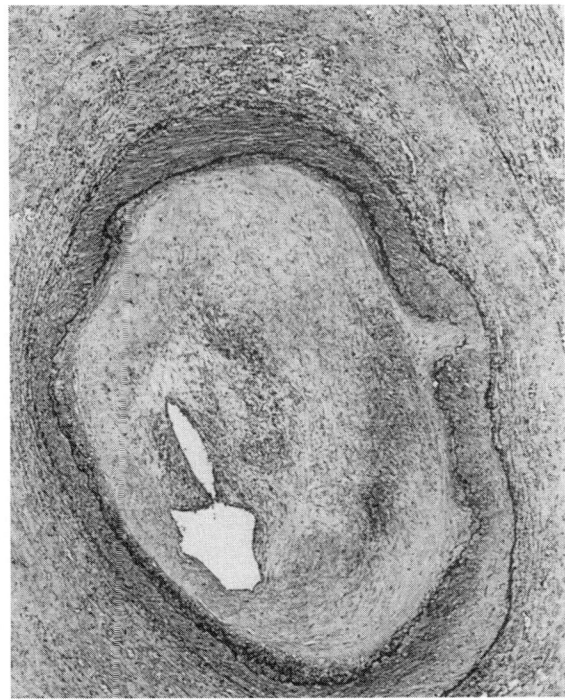

Fig. 23. Rejection vasculitis. Chronic rejection of a cardiac graft. Occlusive intimal thickening of a coronary artery. (Orcein)

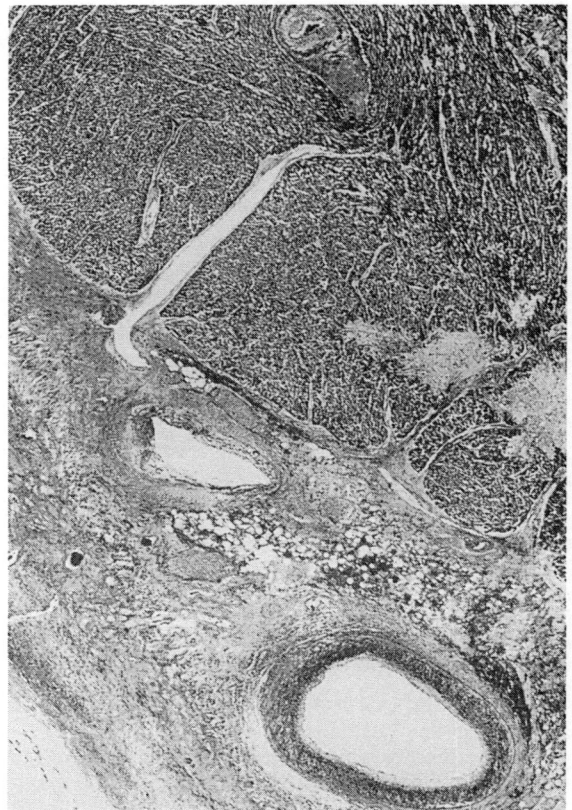

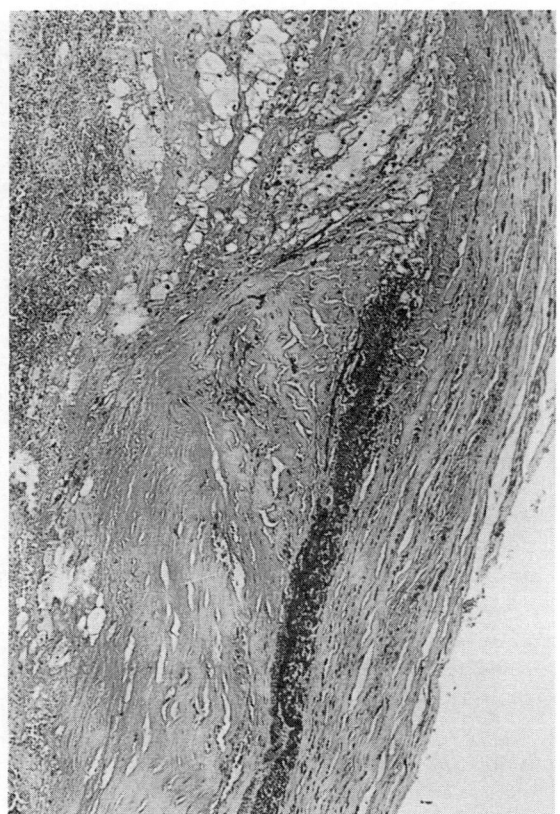

Fig. 24. Rejection vasculitis. Chronic rejection of a cardiac graft. Diffuse coronary arteriosclerosis with interstitial patchy fibrosis. Masson's trichrome

Fig. 25. Rejection vasculitis. Chronic rejection of a cardiac graft. Atherosclerotic-like lesion. HES

lity. Visual disturbance caused by involvement of the ophthalmic or retinal arteries makes this disease a true ophthalmic emergency.

The cause of this relatively common disease remains unknown. The morphological changes suggest an immunological reaction against a component of the arterial wall, such as elastin. Some support for this is provided by the finding of T cell-mediated immunity to local arterial antigens in some patients and by the clinical improvement that is almost always achieved by corticosteroids [205-210]. Active lesions may contain IgA, IgG, IgM, fibrinogen and C3 [211, 212]. Velvart et al [213] have found linear deposits of leukocyte elastase along the fragmented internal lamina. O'Brien and Regan [214] have suggested that actinic degeneration of elastin produces material sufficiently altered to induce the disease. Tomita and Imakawa [215] believe that imbalance between metalloproteinase activation and inhibition plays a role in the intimal hyperplasia seen.

Pathology and Differential diagnosis

The arteritis involves major branches of the external carotid artery selectively (temporal, occipital, facial, basilary vertebral and lingual) and the intra-petrous segment of the internal carotid artery (ophthalmic artery). In peripheral arteries, the lesions are fairly symmetrical on both sides of the body and are separated by normal arterial segments. The affected artery becomes a rigid cord harbouring nodular humps that can be palpated when they run superficially, as in the temporal artery.

The histological pattern depends on the extent and age of the lesions. Three criteria typify temporal arteritis; elastorrhexis involving the internal and/or the external elastic lamina (Fig. 26), phagocytosis of the disintegrated elastic membrane with foreign body granuloma, containing multinucleated giant cells (Fig. 27-28), mononuclear cell infiltrates and fibroblastic thickening of the intima with thrombosis (Fig. 29). There is a non-specific inflammatory infiltrate extending to the adventitia. Fibrinoid necrosis is rarely seen. After healing, the artery is distorted by fibrosis which may be difficult to distinguish from ageing changes, but may remain only as a fibrous cord. Characteristic lesions are present in only half of the cases, even when the symptoms are suggestive. The segmental character of the lesion explains why a temporal artery biopsy may be negative and why extensive biopsies (2-3 cm) sectioned at several sites, are necessary for tissue diagnosis. However, a negative or non-diagnostic temporal artery biopsy does not rule out the diagnosis [216, 217].

The interpretation of long-standing lesions may be difficult. The inflammatory infiltrate accompanying an organising intimal rupture may simulate a healed lesion, but usually does not contain giant cells (Fig. 30). Haemosiderin-loaded macrophages are numerous. In all instances, the external elastic membrane is preserved at any given point. In the aorta and elastic arteries, the lesions are primarily confined to the media with fragmentation of the elastic structure, loss of smooth muscle cells and fibrosis, depending on the stage of the disease. Active lesions contain gra-

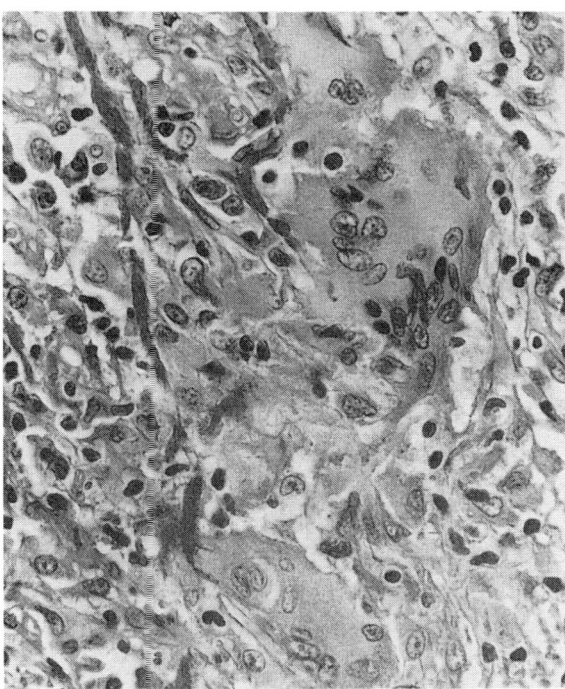

Fig. 27. Giant cell arteritis of temporal artery. Elastic membrane disintegration with foreign body granulomata. HES

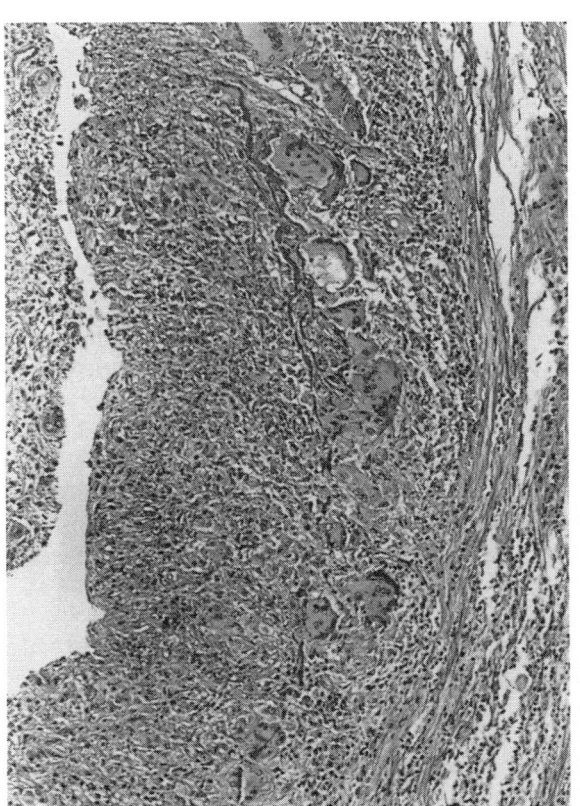

Fig. 26. Giant cell arteritis of temporal artery. Marked involvement of the internal elastic membrane. Masson's trichrome

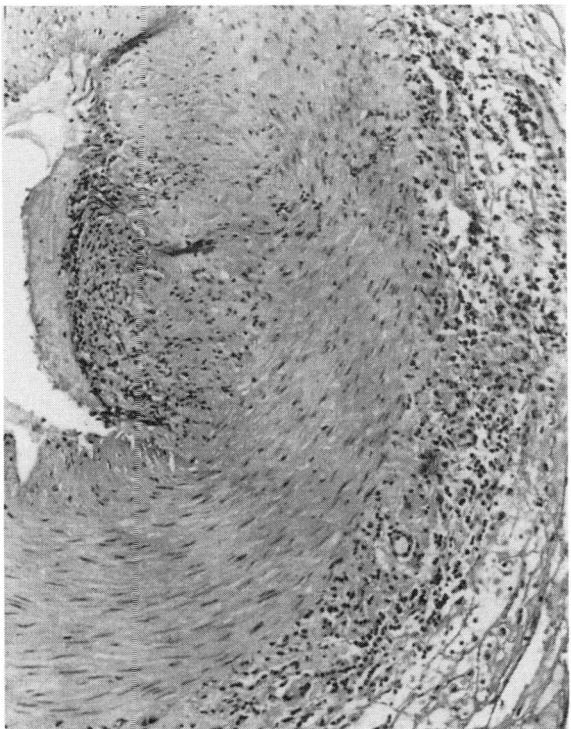

Fig. 28. Giant cell arteritis of temporal artery. Simultaneous involvement of both internal and external elastic membranes. HES

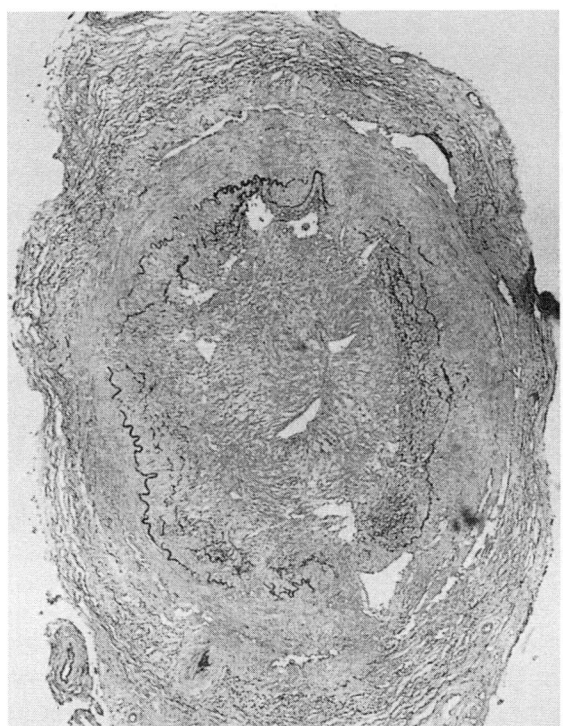

Fig. 29. Giant cell arteritis of temporal artery. Occlusive luminal thrombus giving a cord-like pattern to the artery. Orcein

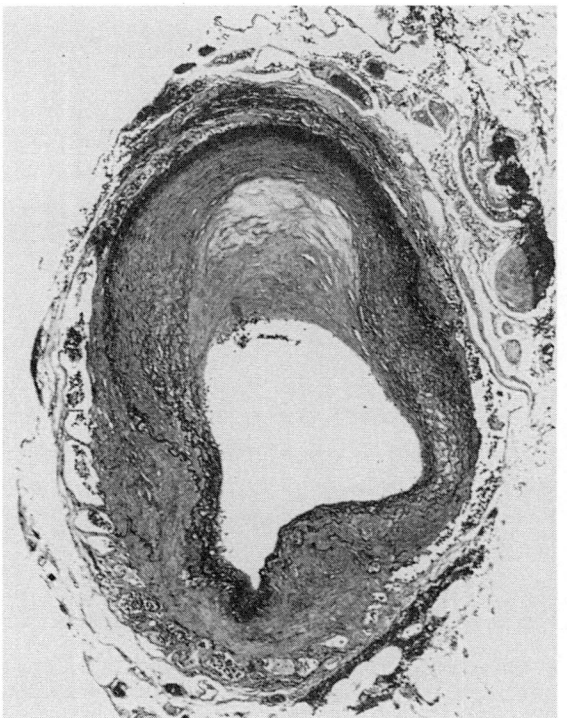

Fig. 30. Giant cell arteritis of temporal artery. Healed stage showing fibrosis engulfing disrupted internal elastic membrane. Orcein

nulomata with multinucleated giant cells phagocytizing elastic fibers, with histiocytes, lymphocytes and plasma cells. In old lesions, fibrosis predominates with increased vascularity in the media and some perivascular infiltrates of mononuclear cells. Focal areas of elastic tissue loss are best appreciated in elastic stains. In large muscular arteries, the morphological pattern is similar to that in the temporal arteries. Because of extensive destruction of the media with little or no adventitial involvement, giant cell aortitis is often associated with aortic dilatation, rupture and aneurysm. This pattern helps rule out Takayasu's arteritis, which predominantly involves the adventitia but where the inflammatory process extends to the outermost part of the media, disrupting the external elastic lamellae. Differential diagnosis becomes impossible when old trauma results in dense fibrosis, disruption of elastic membranes and calcification. In mediacalcosis, calcification accumulating on the medial aspect of the internal elastic membrane may exceptionally induce foreign body granulomata.

Takayasu's arteritis (Takayasu's disease, Pulseless disease)

A progressive obliterative arteritis of the vessels arising from the arch of the aorta was first reported by Savory in 1856 [218]. Takayasu described the retinal changes in 1908 [219]. This worldwide disease [220-223] is most common in Asia [224]. There is a predilection for young women and females with this disease outnumber males by 8:1. The age at onset is 27.3 +/- 9.2 yr. [225]. Ito has recently reviewed the condition [226].

The two main pathogenic mechanisms suggested are infections or an altered immunological state. Treponema pallidum, haemolytic Streptococcus and Mycobacterium tuberculosis have all been considered responsible for Takayasu's disease via their production of antibodies [220, 227, 228]; none of these agents has been identified within the vascular lesions. The possible involvement of the immuno-reactive tissues is invoked, as frequent association of Takayasu's disease with other auto-immune disorders has been reported: disseminated lupus erythematosus, scleroderma, pyoderma gangrenosum, ankylosing spondylitis, Still's disease [229], Crohn's disease and ulcerative colitis [230-233], sarcoidosis, Behçet's disease, and immune glomerulonephritis [234]. Some data suggest that genetic factors are important in pathogenesis; there are twin sisters with Takayasu arteritis, disequilibrium of a HLA complex type (Aw24-DW52-C4A2-C4BQ0-

Dw12) in patients with the disease in Japan, and a predilection to affect young women of Mongolian ancestry in the Far East and in Latin America [235, 236].

About half of all patients develop an initial acute systemic illness with fever, night sweating, headaches, weight loss, arthralgias, and fatigue. Cutaneous lesions, such as erythema nodosa may be present [237]. Intense and spontaneous pain, occurring along the arterial paths, may be exacerbated by palpation. This episode gradually subsides and is followed by a more chronic stage characterised by ischaemic manifestations that vary depending on the vessels involved. There is weakening of the pulses with markedly low or unobtainable blood pressure in the vessels arising from the aortic arch; occular disturbances occur with various neurological deficits linked to low cerebral flow. Occlusive changes in the descending thoracic aorta sometimes lead to a form of acquired coarctation. Heart failure is common and can stem from aortic insufficiency caused by the disease, and coronary artery involvement [238, 239]. Rarely, pulmonary artery obstruction leads to pulmonary hypertension [83]. The abdominal aorta (particularly the renal arteries) may be affected, often causing serious renovascular hypertension [240, 223]. An aneurysm or a coarctation may be detected by chance or during a complication [241, 242]. In most cases, the general manifestations regress, and the diagnosis is only suggested a posteriori when symptoms of vascular insufficiency appear months or years later.

Pathology and Differential diagnosis

Although Takayasu's arteritis classically involves the aortic arch and its first order branches (most characteristically the subclavian arteries), in one-third of cases, it affects the remainder of the aorta and its branches [243] (Fig. 31).

The disease has been subdivided into four types (Table 8). Smaller arteries may also be involved.

Grossly, the arterial involvement may be segmental or multifocal [244, 223]. The external aspect of the diseased artery is considerably thickened and fused with perivascular tissue. The orifices of the major collaterals are narrowed or even obliterated. On cross

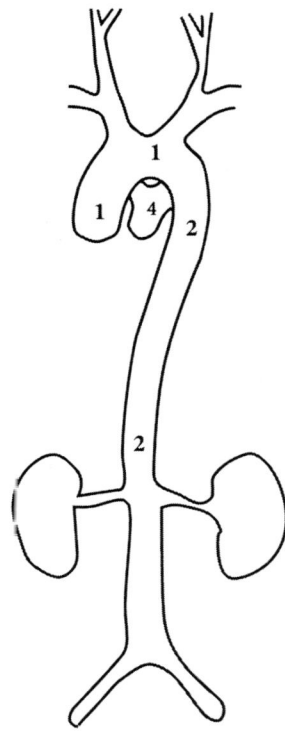

Fig. 31. Takayasu's disease. Anatomical involvement and types

section, the arterial wall appears yellow and rigid, reducing the lumen while the intima displays marked wrinkling.

Histologically, the lesion affects the junction between the adventitia and the media. Active lesions have a heavy inflammatory infiltrate made up of lymphocytes, plasma cells, histiocytes and some rare giant cells (Fig. 32-33) interspersed with newly-formed capillaries. This distorts the adventitia, and overlaps the outermost part of the media, disrupting the elastic fibres in elastic arteries, or the external elastic lamina in muscular arteries (Fig. 34). Healed lesions show fibrosis totally devoid of inflammatory cells. This pro-

Table 8. Takayasu's disease. Anatomical involvement and types

TYPES	DESCRIPTION	Fig. 31
I	Ascending aorta, aortic arch and main branches	1
II	Descending, abdominal aorta and main branches	2
III	I+II	1+2
IV	Pulmonary arteries with/without the aorta and its branches	4

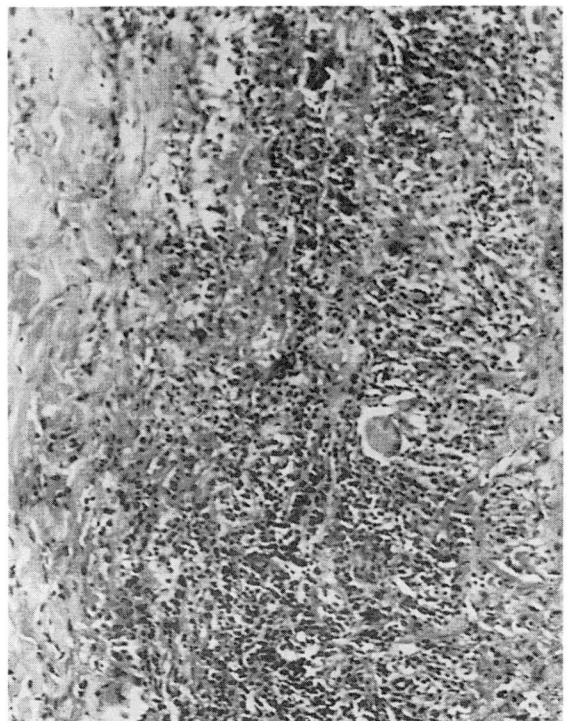

Fig. 32. Takayasu's disease of the aorta. Initial adventicitis. HES

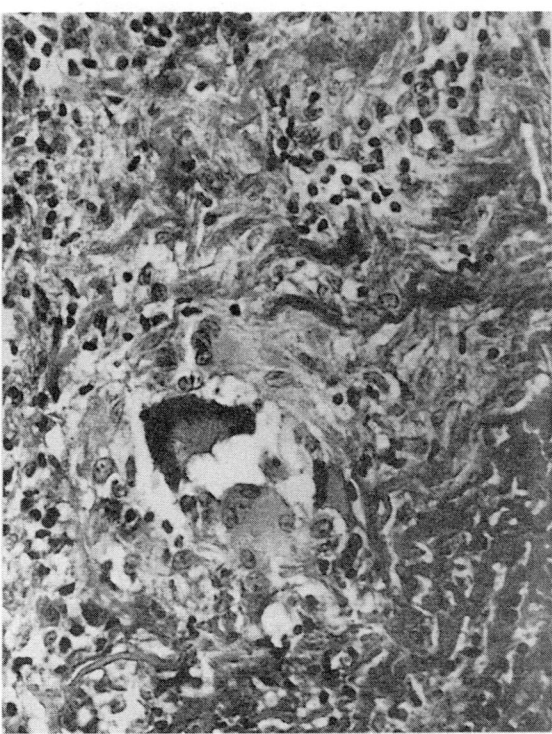

Fig. 33. Takayasu's disease of the aorta. Occasional giant cells may be seen. HES

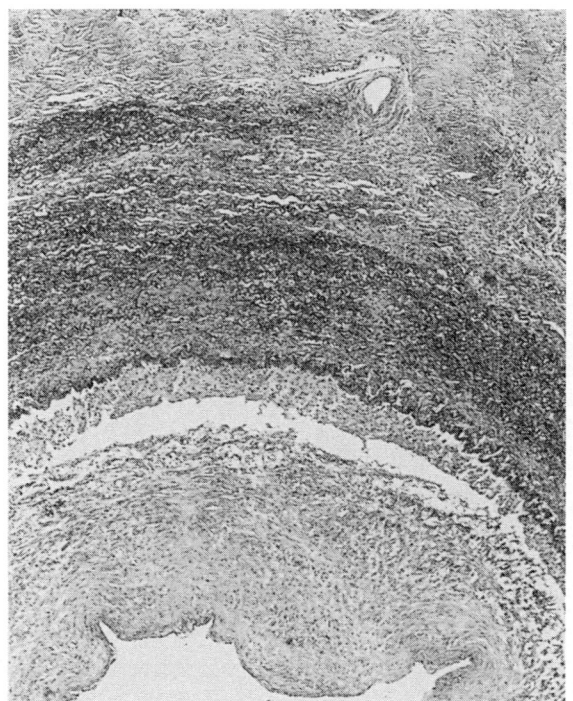

Fig. 34. Takayasu's disease of the subclavian artery. Extension of inflammatory process into the outermost part of the media. Orcein

cess encloses the vasa vasora, nerves, and lymphatics of the adventitia, and overlaps the external part of the media (Fig. 35-36). In some areas, the ingrowth of newly-formed capillaries into the media resembles an angioma. The intima shows fibroblastic thickening with oedematous changes and is usually devoid of inflammatory cells. These changes lead to marked thickening of the arterial wall.

Active and healed lesions may coexist in the same or two consecutive segments of the artery indicating that progressive development of the disease has occurred. Regional lymph nodes frequently show sinusoidal histiocytosis and sometimes epithelioid granulomata.

The differential diagnosis includes syphilitic aortitis and aortic giant cell arteritis. Syphilitic aortitis mostly involves the aortic arch and lymphocytic infiltration of the vasa vasorum and heavy infiltration of plasma cells and lymphocytes in the media is seen in active disease. Giant cell arteritis usually affects the elderly and degradation of elastic fibers with foreign body granulomata with giant cells are not seen in Takayasu's disease. Extensive fibrosis in the healed stage may simulate terminal-stage of syphilitic aortitis, and, to some extent, the post-traumatic state or the adven-

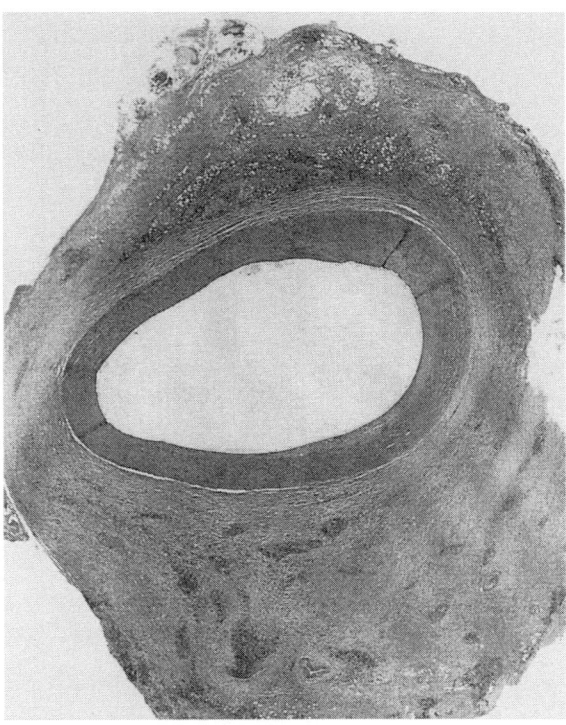

Fig. 35. Takayasu's disease of the primary carotid artery. Note marked fibrosis thickening the adventitia. HES

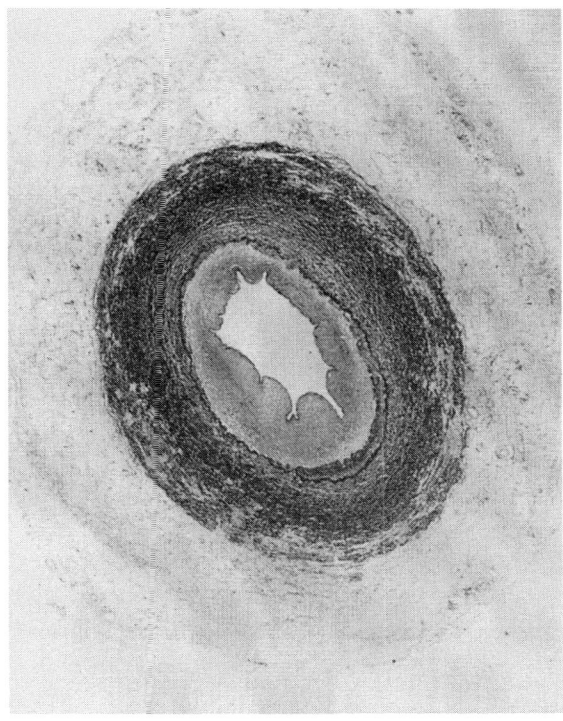

Fig. 36. Takayasu's disease of the primary carotid artery. Healed stage with tiger skin pattern in the external part of the media. Orcein

titial form of fibrodysplasia. In the latter condition, the external elastic lamina is preserved [245].

Polyarteritis nodosa (Classic polyarteritis nodosa, Kussmaul's disease)

An inflammatory process involves all three layers of the artery, with destructive medial changes leading to the formation of small aneurysms. Only medium-sized and small arteries are affected. First described by Küssmaul and Maier in 1866 [246], polyarteritis nodosa (PAN) is characterised by segmental inflammation, with infiltration by eosinophils, and necrosis of medium-sized or small arteries. Veins may also be involved.

Experimental and clinical evidence suggests that classic polyarteritis nodosa is an immune complex-mediated process [247, 248]. Experimentally, the disease has been produced by repeated injections of heterologous proteins. Many drugs have been reported to cause classic polyarteritis nodosa [249, 250].

Periarteritis nodosa is commonly associated with urticaria, hay fever and asthma, as well as with infections including hepatitis B & C infections [251-256]. About 30% of patients with PAN have hepatitis B antigen in their serum, and P-ANCA is often present in the serum and correlate with disease activity. Polyarteritis nodosa is often associated with other connective tissue diseases. There is an overlap, both clinically and histologically, with leukocytoclastic vasculitis (microscopic polyarteritis nodosa). There is a male predilection, generally in the ratio of 2:1. The disease occurs at any age but the vast majority of patients are in their fifth and sixth decades. Although PAN is said to be rare in children [257] there have been many reports [258-260].

The onset may be insidious or sudden with nonspecific manifestations of a multi-system involvement. Cardiac manifestations include pericarditis, arrhythmia and myocardial infarction caused by coronary involvement and terminal cardiac failure. Rare pulmonary involvement may manifest as Löffler's syndrome and asthma. Haemoptysis is caused by lung infarction and vascular rupture.

Pathology and differential diagnosis

The diagnosis can be established by the identification of necrotizing arteritis on tissue biopsy specimens, particularly medium-sized arteries of affected tissues. In most cases, biopsies of symptomatic sites in the active phase prior to treatment will identify lesions. "Blind" biopsies or biopsies performed late in the course of the disease are seldom informative. Specimens from muscles, nerves or viscera are preferable to those from the skin. Involvement of the skin is not necessarily indicative of systemic involvement. The most frequent sites of involvement in autopsy series are the kidneys (85%), heart (76%), liver (62%), and gastrointestinal tract (51%). Other affected organs include muscle (39%), the pancreas (35%), testes (33%), peripheral nerves (32%), central nervous system (27%) and skin (20%) [261, 262].

Grossly, the affected artery appears as a pearl-string with discrete nodules (aneurysms) 1 to 2 mm in diameter located at the branch points and bifurcations. This is particularly evident on the mesenteric border of an intestinal loop. The frequency of multiple intra-parenchymal aneurysms may be as high as 60%. Intravascular thrombosis is a frequent sequela to the acute vasculitis. Impairment of perfusion with ulceration, infarction, ischaemic atrophy, or haemorrhages in the areas supplied by these vessels may provide the first clue to the existence of the underlying disorder.

Histologically, lesions show four main stages of development, all of which may coexist. In the initial stage, focal fibrinoid necrosis, most often localised to a portion of the circumference rather than its entirety, occurs at the junction between the intima and media (Fig. 37). In small arteries this may extend to involve the full thickness of the arterial wall. This necrotic area contains nuclear debris, disintegrated fibrin, lipids, and extravasated plasma proteins, fragmented red blood cells and myocytes. The endothelial lining detaches and leukocytes begin to migrate into the arterial wall. In the skin, immunofluorescence microscopy reveals immunoglobulin and complement components in the vascular lesions, especially if these are examined within 24 hours of development. In the second stage, leukocytes, histiocytes and lymphocytes invade the necrotic area. A loose fibrinous thrombus partially occludes the lumen (Fig. 38). Weakening of the vascular wall leads to formation of aneurysms, mostly saccular (Fig. 39), which may rupture and cause haemorrhage [263]. In the third stage, granulation tissue distorts the vascular wall and considerably reduces its lumen. This tis-

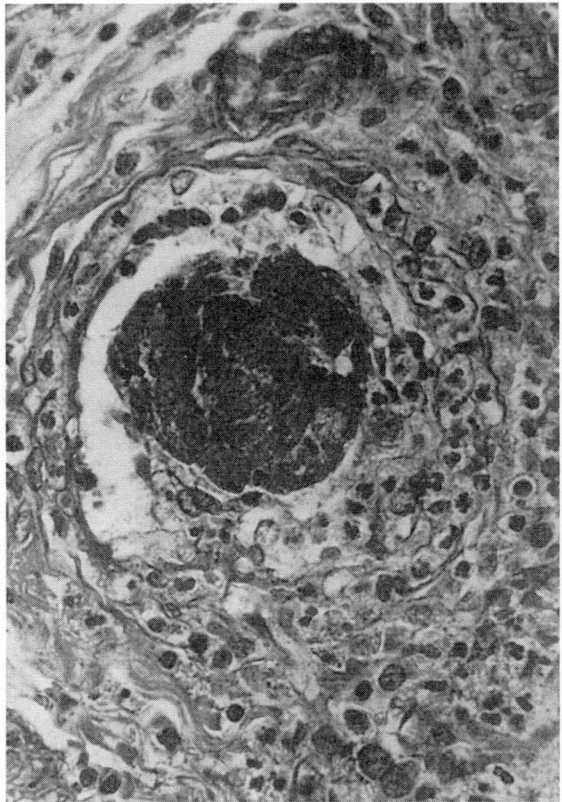

Fig. 37. Periarteritis nodosa. Initial stage with parietal infiltration of inflammatory cells and fibrinoid necrosis. HES

sue contains large number of macrophages, plasma cells and lymphocytes, intermingled with fibroblasts, and newly-formed capillaries. In the fourth stage, the lesion undergoes fibrosis and a few lymphocytes accumulate, mostly in the adventitia. Thrombosed small aneurysms shrink and become fibrotic masses. Calcium deposits may appear in the fibrotic tissue.

In the kidneys, classical lesions of periarteritis nodosa involving parenchymal medium-sized and small vessels are referred to as the macroscopic form, which leads to thrombosis, infarction and arterial hypertension. The microscopic form is characterized by segmental proliferative glomerulonephritis (Fig. 40) with deposit of IgG along the glomerular membrane (Fig. 41). In some instances the lesions of periarteritis nodosa may be indistinguishable from those of leukocytoclastic vasculitis. In muscle biopsies, vascular granulomata may involve the interstitial tissue and simulate dermatomyosis. In the heart, lesions of infantile periarteritis nodosa may mimic those of the mucocutaneous lymph node syndrome or Kawasaki's disease [163].

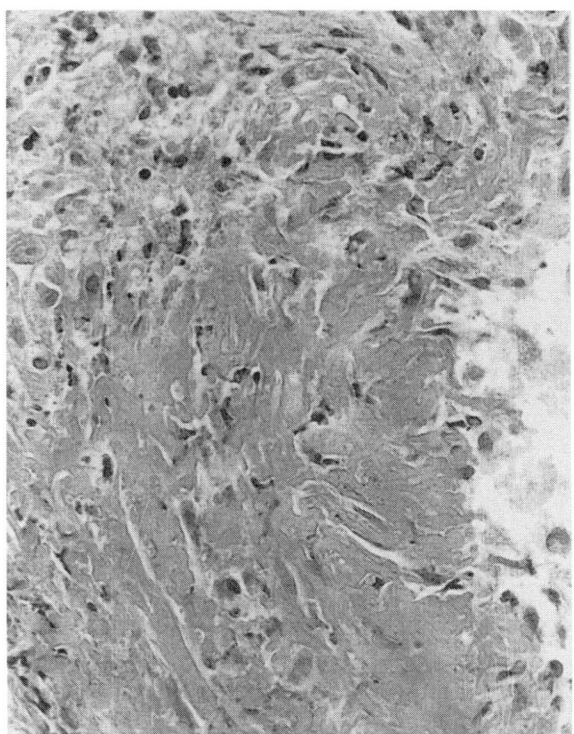

Fig. 38. Periarteritis nodosa. Vascular fibrinoid necrosis. HES

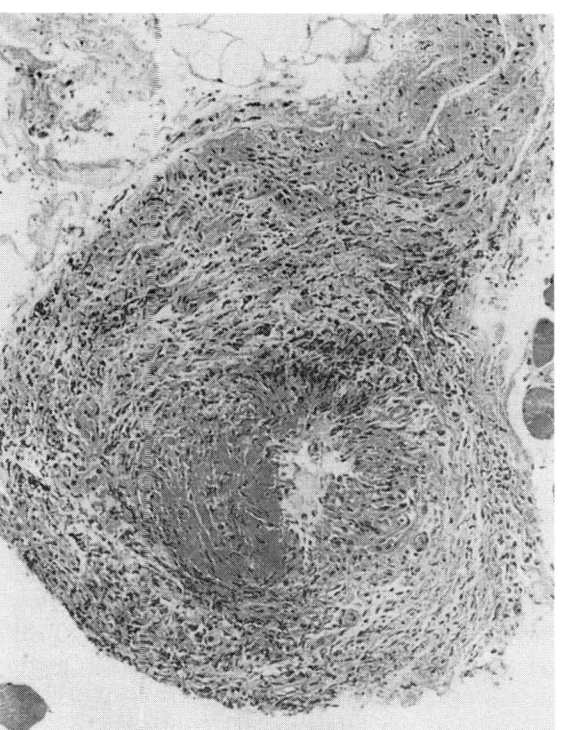

Fig. 39. Periarteritis nodosa. Saccular aneurysm. HES

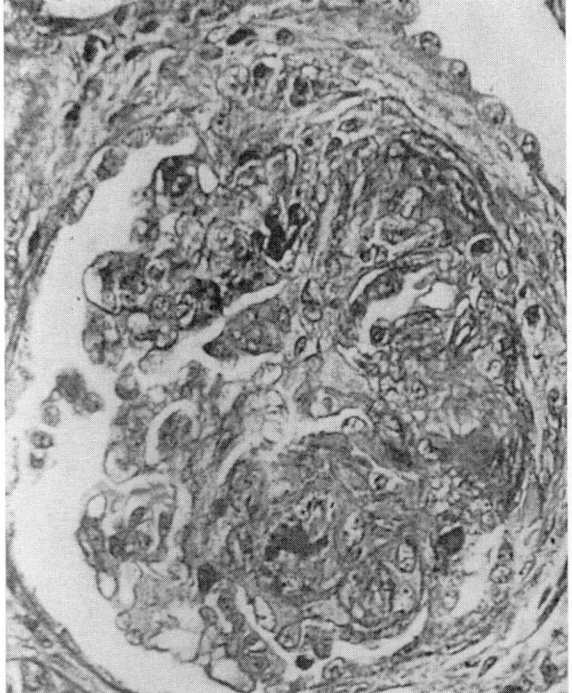

Fig. 40. Periarteritis nodosa. Renal microscopic form showing segmental proliferative glomerulonephritis. Masson's trichrome. (Courtesy Dr D. Droz)

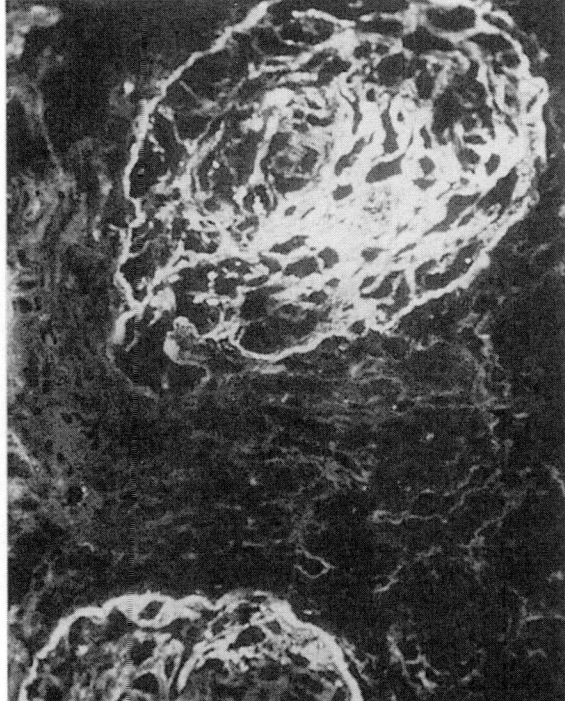

Fig. 41. Periarteritis nodosa. Renal microscopic form. Deposits of IgG along glomerular basement membrane. Immunofluorescence technique. (Courtesy Dr D. Droz)

Isolated visceral vasculitis

This uncommon clinicopathological entity is characterised by vasculitis limited to the vessels of a viscus in apparent absence of systemic vasculitis or other systemic diseases. Pathogenic mechanisms are unknown. This vasculitis often coexists with other pathological processes, including adenocarcinoma of the breast [264], cervical carcinoma after irradiation, granulomatous cholecystitis [265], acute pancreatitis [266], chronic hepatitis, rickettsial infection or in systemic disease (disseminated lupus erythematosus, coeliac disease).

There may be no symptomatology and the arteritis may be discovered in a resected specimen of appendix or gall-bladder, for example. Clinical manifestations vary but there may be associated cholecystitis [267]; appendicitis [268], digestive disorders [269], cervicitis [270], urological impairment [271], myalgia and subcutaneous nodules [272]. Any viscus may be involved, either separately (breast, uterus, testis, pancreas, gallbladder) [273-275] or together in a regional context, such as the female genital tract [276, 277]. Concomitant multifocal locations involving different arteries are rare [278]. Systemic symptoms are usually absent.

Pathology and differential diagnosis

Pathological appearances may be those of either a typical necrotizing angiitis (Fig. 42) or a giant cell vasculitis (Fig. 43-44). Associated venous involvement [279] has been reported.

Primary angiitis of the central nervous system

Although primary angiitis of the central nervous system (PACNS) is usually limited to the central nervous system, autopsies in some of the previously reported cases have demonstrated a variable degree of involvement of extracranial arteries, including the pulmonary vessels and abdominal visceral arteries. The cause of PACNS is unknown but the condition is uncommon; about 120 cases have been reported in the literature, but the incidence seems to be increasing. The average age at onset is about 45 years (range 3-75) with a male preponderance (4:3). Presenting symptoms consist in unexplained acute progressive encephalopathy without evidence of extracranial or systemic vasculitis: headache (62%), paresis (55%), decreased cognition, confusion, decreased consciousness, progressive intellectual deterioration (50,9%), or multifocal neurological defects, seizure, spinal cord problems and cerebral haemorrhage [280]. Diplopia, blurred vision, nystagmus, pupillary abnormalities

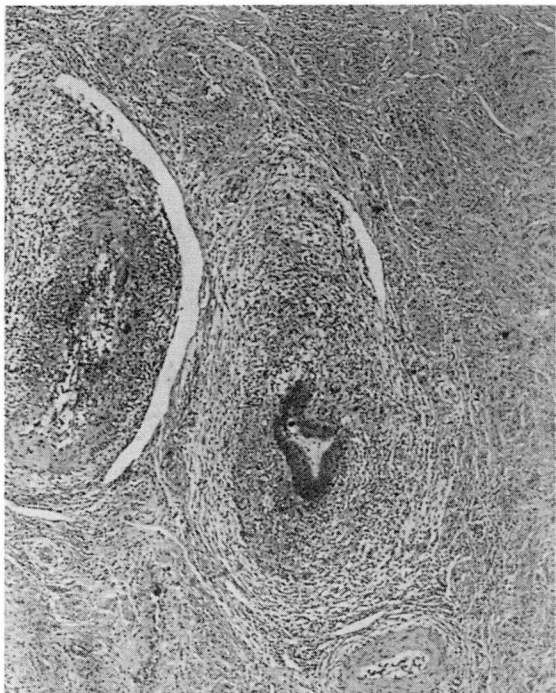

Fig. 42. Isolated visceral vasculitis. Necrotizing angiitis of the uterine cervix of a 40 year-old woman undergoing a total hysterectomy for leiomyomata. No clinical repercussion seen. HES

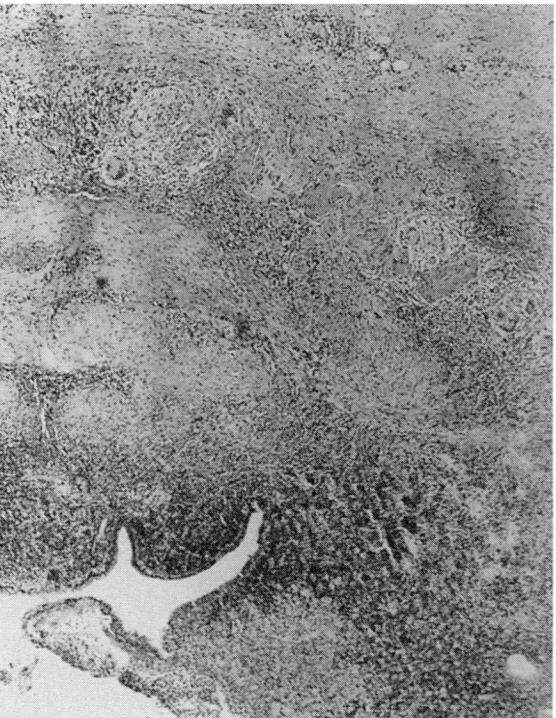

Fig. 43. Isolated visceral vasculitis. Giant cell vasculitis of the gallbladder displaying chronic cholecystitis. HES

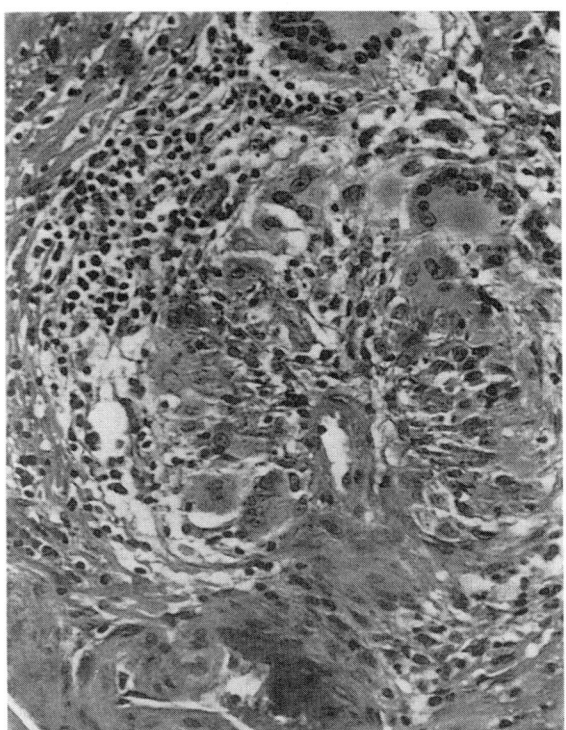

Fig. 44. Giant cell vasculitis of the gallbladder displaying chronic cholecystitis. HES

The inflammatory infiltrate is predominantly lymphocytic with a smaller number of neutrophils, eosinophils, histiocytes and plasma cells. Giant cells may be present in variable numbers. Morphologically, acute, healing and healed lesions may coexist in different segments of the same artery or adjacent arteries. In most patients, PACNS is diagnosed clinically without an histological confirmation.

Differential diagnosis should rule out non-vasculitic conditions, especially lymphomatoid granulomatosis (LMG) and the so-called "benign angiopathy of the CNS" (BACNS). LMG is a T-cell lymphoma with angioinvasive and angiodestructive features, mimicking necrotic or granulomatous vasculitis and involving capillaries and small arteries. Fifteen to twenty percent of LMG patients have central nervous system dysfunction and peripheral neuropathy. The condition is confined to the central nervous system [289]. Benign angiopathy of the CNS has an acute onset with symptoms resembling those of PACNS. The primary differences are a normal cerebrospinal fluid and a rapid and dramatic response to steroids. It is unclear how much of a role vasospasm plays in this disease since calcium channel blockers may also relieve symptoms. Vascular changes are minimal and consist mainly of intimal fibrosis.

Behçet's syndrome (Behçet's disease)

This condition is characterised by simultaneously or successively occurring recurrent attacks of genital (80-87%) and oral (98-99%) ulceration (aphthae) with uveitis or iridocyclitis (68-79%) and hypopyon [290, 291]. A seronegative arthritis is often present. A phase of a generalised disorder presents variable manifestations [292], including dermatitis (69-90%), usually in the form of erythema nodosum, cardiovascular symptoms [293], digestive, renal and cerebral involvement [14-18%) [294] and amyloidosis. Behçet's syndrome has a high incidence in the Middle East and Far East ("Silk Route disease") and in Germany and England. In the United States, this disorder is relatively rare [295]. Behçet's syndrome is most often seen in men in the third decade [296, 297].

The cause is unknown. A possible immune mechanism is suggested by diminished T suppressor cell function, the presence of a variety of autoantibodies to human oral mucosa, the presence of high levels of circulating immune complexes, and detection of immunoglobulins and complement in blood vessel walls [298]. Almost 78% of cases express HLA-B51 subtypes [299, 300] histocompatibility antigens. However, DNA-hybridisation and experimental studies favour a

and dysarthria are indications of possible cranial nerve involvement [281, 282]. A history of herpes zoster infection, Hodgkin's disease, or illicit drug use may be found. Constitutional symptoms are generally absent, except fever and weight loss [283]. The sedimentation rate is elevated in only 10% of patients. There are no consistent abnormalities in serological or autoimmune markers. Analysis of the cerebrospinal fluid is often normal but there may be an elevation of protein, often accompanied by a small number of neutrophils and/or lymphocytes. PACNS is a diagnosis of exclusion. The majority of other possibilities (infection, drugs, neoplasms, systemic vasculitis) should be excluded from the history, presentation and laboratory data. The diagnosis is made by clinical presentation together with defined angiographic changes. Biopsies of the brain parenchyma and leptomeninges, when possible, may provide additional data [284, 285]. The prognosis is poor [286].

Pathology and differential diagnosis

PANS affects the small and medium-sized arteries (rarely the veins and venules) of the leptomeninges and brain. It is characterised by a segmental, necrotizing or granulomatous vasculitis, often accompanied by thrombosis [287, 288]. Skip lesions are common.

viral aetiology involving herpes simplex virus [301, 302].

There are three groups of clinical manifestations: nervous, digestive and vascular. Thrombophlebitis with migrating phlebitis is common and may affect both superficial and deep veins, which are more frequently involved than arteries (88% versus 12%) [297]. Superior and inferior vena cava obstruction is not uncommon. Occlusion of the main hepatic vein may lead to sudden occlusion with Budd-Chiari syndrome [303]. A nephrotic syndrome occurs when renal veins are involved [304]. Arterial complications appear 3 to 8 years after the onset in 1.5 to 6% of patients [305]. There is a report of mitral valve prolapse and dilated cardiomyopathy [306]. An elevated erythrocyte sedimentation rate, elevated levels of alpha 2-globulins, and polyclonal hyperimmunoglobulinaemia have been reported in the active stage of the disease. Haematuria and proteinuria are indicative of renal involvement, either by Behçet's syndrome or associated amyloidosis. CNS manifestations and vascular involvement account for most of the mortality associated with the disease.

Pathology and differential diagnosis

Vascular involvement in Behçet's syndrome mainly involves the great vessels with venous (Fig. 45-46) and arterial thrombosis with aneurysm formation [307]. The aorta and its main branches are mostly affected [33.5% in an autopsy series in Japan [308]. Medium-sized arteries and small veins are rarely involved. Histological features include lymphocytic vasculitis (Fig. 47), leukocytoclastic vasculitis with extensive or focal fibrinoid necrosis distorting the media and adventitia (Fig. 48-49) [309]. Histiocytes and eosinophils may be present. At the periphery, fibroblasts tend to replace the smooth muscle cells while newly-formed vessels proliferate into the vascular wall. In elastic arteries, elastic fibers are fragmented and thinned. These areas become weakened and the sites of aneurysm formation [310]. Chronic lesions are characterised by dense fibrosis containing newly-formed vessels and some small collections of lymphocytes and plasma cells. Renal biopsy may demonstrate either necrotizing vasculitis or glomerulopathy. Deposits of IgM and C3 in the glomerular capillaries are seen on immunoflourescence. Behçet's syndrome should be distinguished from other vasculitides, especially Takayasu's disease. The diagnosis depends on the clinical context.

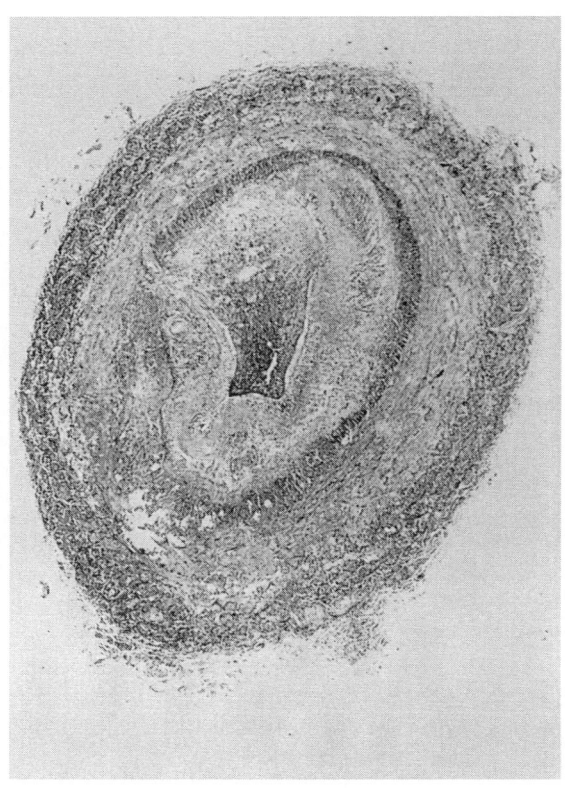

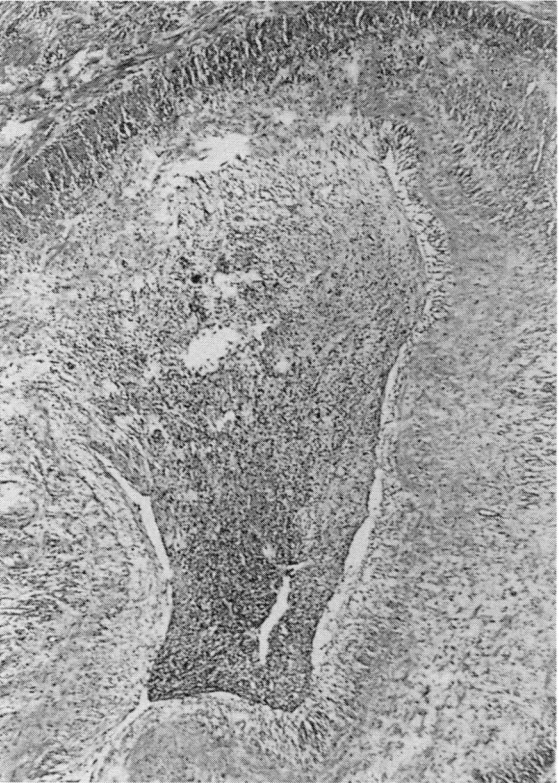

Fig. 45-46. Behçet's disease. Phlebitis with thrombosis. HES

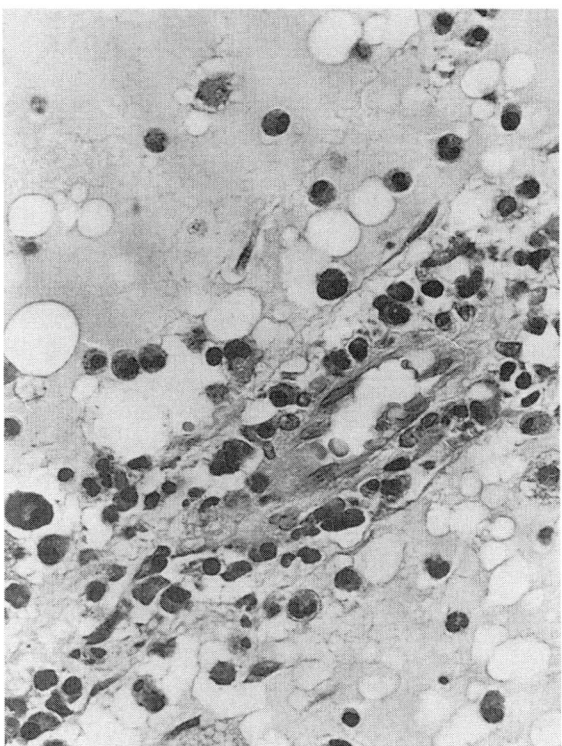

Fig. 47. Behçet's disease. Lymphocytic vasculitis. HES

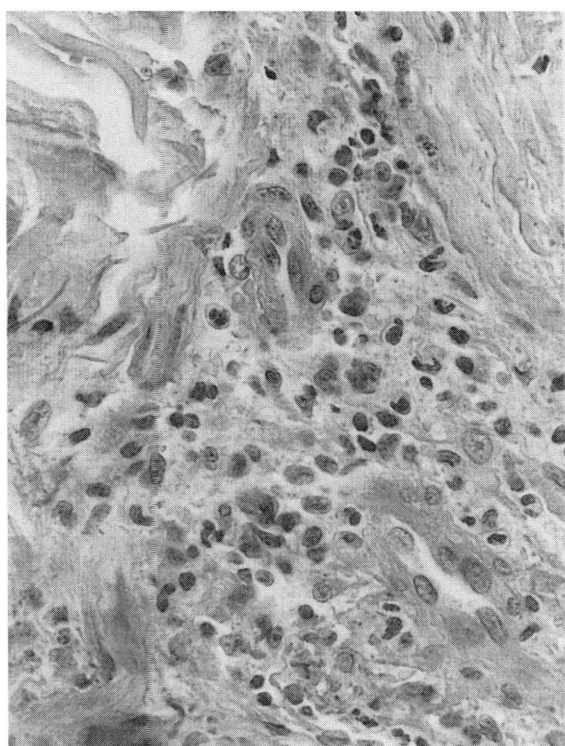

Fig. 49. Behçets disease. Leukocytoclastic vasculitis. HES

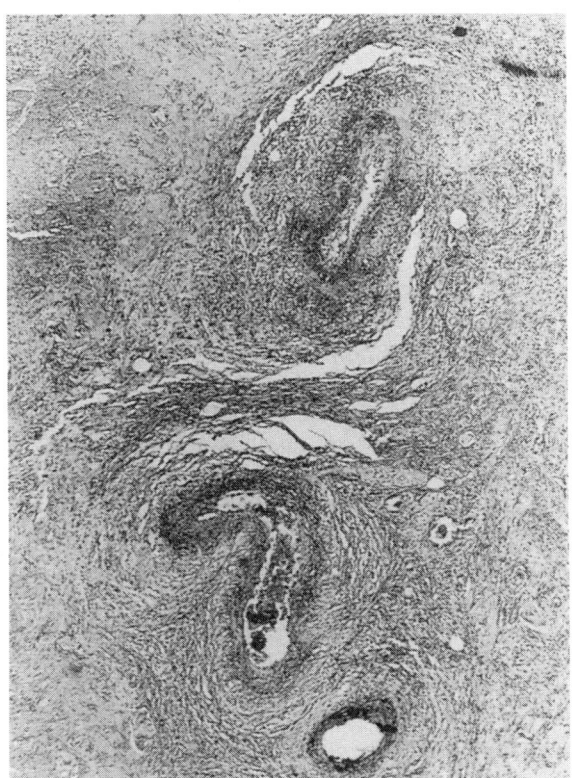

Fig. 48. Behçet's disease. Leukocytoclastic vasculitis. HES

Thromboangiitis obliterans (Buerger's disease)

This is an acute and chronic inflammation of medium-sized arteries and veins, especially of the legs of young and middle-aged men, associated with thrombotic occlusion and commonly resulting in gangrene. First reported by von Winiwarter in 1879 and by Larivière, thromboangiitis obliterans (TAO) was presented as a specific entity by Leo Buerger in 1908 [311, 312]. More recent data suggest a recent increase in the disease in women [313].

The aetiology of the disease is unknown but a relationship to cigarette smoking is a consistent aspect of this disorder. Most patients are or have been heavy smokers [314]. Thromboangiitis obliterans has occurred in non-smokers or after cessation of cigarette smoking [315] – there is one report in a child of 5 years [316] – but this is an exception. Several mechanisms have been suggested for the association, including a reaction to tobacco of persons with a specific phenotype, suggested because of the greater prevalence of HLA-A9 and HLA-B5 in patients with the disease [317]. An autoimmune disorder with lymphocytic hypersensitivity to types I and III human collagen associated with an inconsistent presence of anti-collagen and anti-elastin antibodies has been suggested

[318]. Some authors contend that the fibrotic proliferation in the wall of the vessels and the cellular organisation of the thrombi are parts of the secondary reactions in and to a thrombus. This hypothesis does not satisfactorily explain the multiple segmental localisation of the thrombi [319]. Infectious agents which have been invoked in causation include rickettsiae, but, although vasculitis can be reproduced experimentally, there is no clear evidence of a relationship between TAO and rickettsial disease [320].

Clinically, the symptoms and signs of thromboangiitis obliterans are those of arterial ischaemia and of superficial phlebitis. The onset is gradual, starting in the most distal vessels of the upper and lower extremities, and progressing proximally, culminating in distal gangrene. In many cases, it affects the arms as well as the legs. A history of migratory phlebitis, usually in the superficial veins of the foot or leg, is present in about a third of patients [321]. Early symptoms include coldness, numbness, tingling, or burning. Just over half of patients present with Raynaud's phenomenon with a long history of vasomotor impairment [322]. Amputation is required when severe tissue damage occurs. However, the amputation risk in Buerger's disease is difficult to evaluate because of the heterogeneity of the published series and the diversity of the therapy used in trials [323, 324]. Whatever the extent of the amputations, life span is similar to that of an age-matched population. This clearly contrasts the prognosis of thromboangiitis obliterans with that of an atheromatous arteriopathy.

Pathology and differential diagnosis

Thromboangiitis obliterans affects the lower extremities more commonly and more severely than the upper limbs and viscera. Occlusions of the vessels of the leg are often bilateral and asymmetrical (Fig. 50-51). Proximal stenoses, especially popliteal, are frequent. Exceptional visceral lesions in the brain, heart, kidneys and intestines may develop during exacerbations, but an exact diagnosis is always difficult to establish. In contrast to atherosclerosis, the lesions of Buerger's disease are sharply segmental and usually start in medium-sized and small vessels (posterior tibial, anterior tibial, radial, ulnar, plantar, palmar and digital arteries). The involved vascular segments appear hardened and retracted. They are clearly delineated from normal areas. Accompanying medium and small sized veins may also show a migrating phlebitis and well-demarcated occlusions without any downstream collateral compensation, but these changes remain inconsistent and non-specific [325, 326]. Larger

arteries are involved only later, as are the large venous trunks. Histological lesions are similar in arteries and veins. Acute involvement is characterised by infiltration of neutrophils in the vascular wall with mural or occlusive thrombosis of the lumen. The entirety realises a panvasculitis (Fig. 52-53). In time, the thrombus undergoes organisation and recanalization. In the chronic stage, lesions display organised luminal thrombus containing a few lymphocytic infiltrates with some giant cells and fibrosis mainly affecting the media and adventitia (Fig. 54). These coats are crisscrossed by newly-formed dilated capillaries. These nonspecific changes may result from slowing of blood flow. In advanced or old lesions, the luminal thrombus becomes less cellular and more fibrotic. Vascular thrombosis or embolism is the major differential diagnosis.

TAO is distinctive from periarteritis nodosa giant cell arteritis because of the greater extent of the lesions, the absence of medial necrosis, the absence of aneurysms and the consistent presence of an occluding mass. Other entities that should be systematically looked for include the entrapment syndrome of popliteal vessels, disseminated lupus erythematosus, Behcet's disease, haematological disorders (myeloproliferative syndromes, essential thrombocythaemia, anomalies of C, S proteins and antithrombin III) [327].

Cogan's syndrome (Oculovestibulo-auditory syndrome)

This non-syphilitic interstitial keratitis is characterised by an abrupt onset with vertigo and tinnitus followed by deafness. About 50% of patients have an associated systemic disease, most commonly polyarteritis nodosa [328]. However, urticarial vasculitis and fatal aortitis have been reported [329, 330]. The cause of Cogan's syndrome is unknown but many reports have documented an improvement in symptoms with immunosuppressive therapy [331-333]. Most patients are less than 30 years old although the age range is 4-1/2 to 63 years [334]. Systemic manifestations consist of fever, arthralgia and adenopathy. Visceral symptoms reflect ischaemia as a result of vasculitis; abdominal pain, variable neurological manifestations and aortic valvular insufficiency may be found. Leukocytosis and eosinophilia occur and the HLA phenotype BW17 is present with a greater than expected frequency [335].

Pathology and differential diagnosis

The aortitis involves the media and intima. A mixed infiltrate of neutrophils, mononuclear cells and occa-

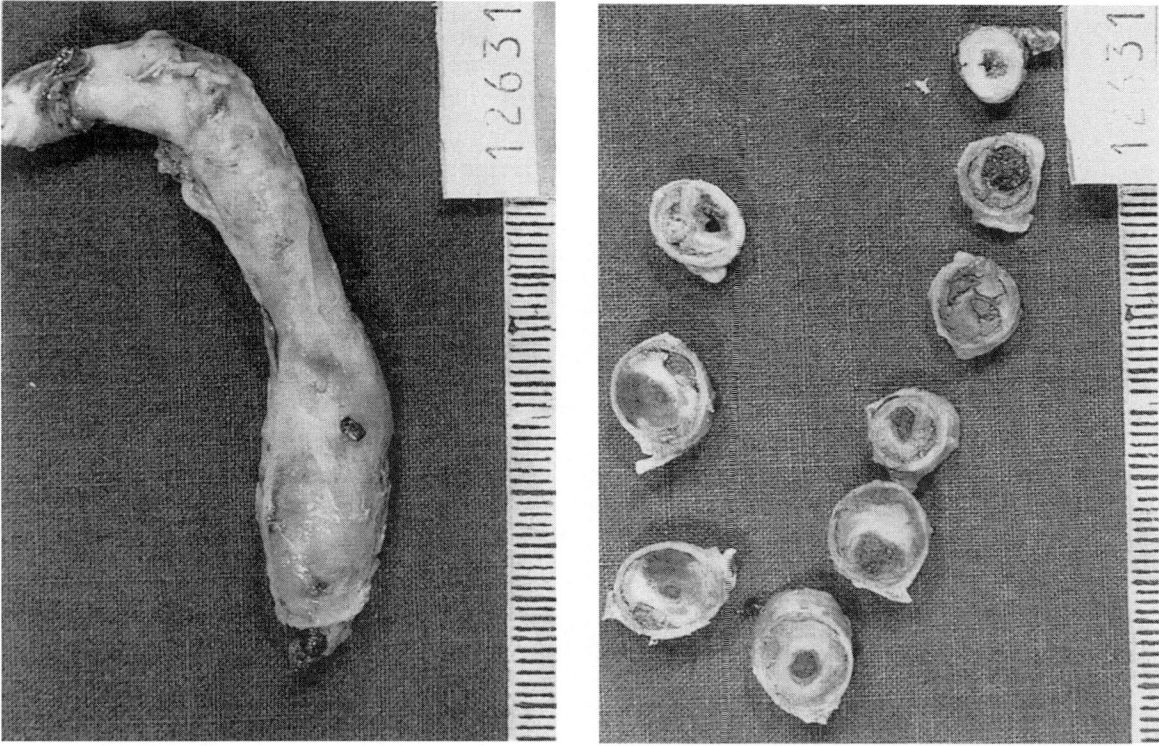

Fig. 50-51. Thromboangeitis obliterans (TAO). Occlusive thrombosis of a popliteal artery

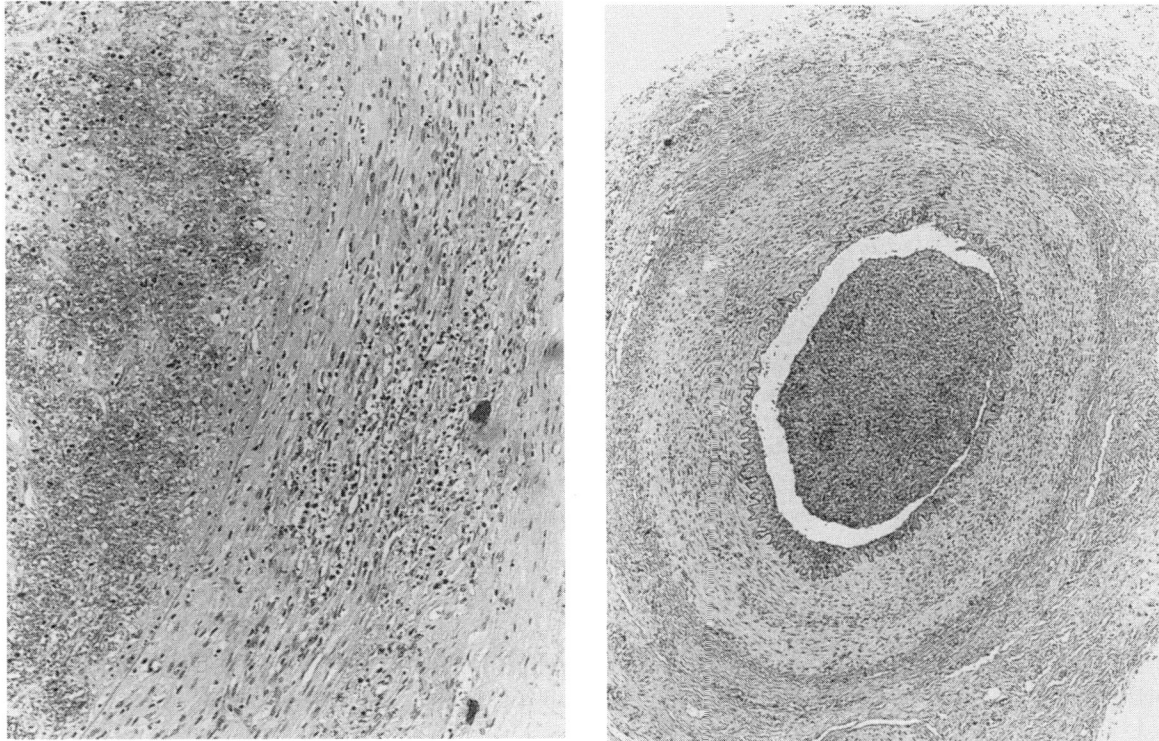

Fig. 52-53. Thromboangeitis obliterans (TAO). Panarteritis with thrombosis. Orcein

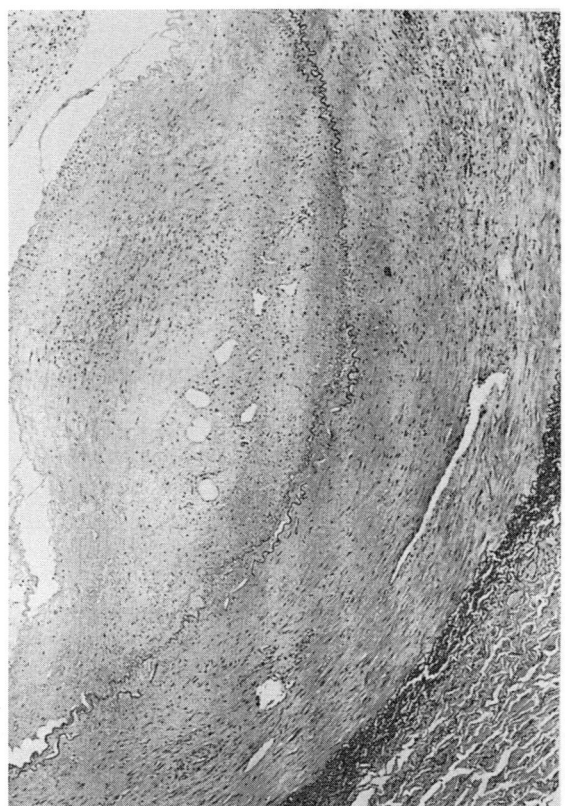

Fig. 54. Thromboangiitis obliterans. Organised occlusive thrombus with some inflammatory infiltrate in the wall. Orcein

sional giant cells is found in areas with fragmentation of the elastic framework, necrosis and fibrosis of the vessel wall.

Sarcoidosis

Vasculitis is an important component of sarcoidosis. Sarcoid vasculitis damages mostly medium-sized and small arteries but involvement of major vessels, such as the abdominal aorta, and the pulmonary, subclavian and iliac arteries, has been reported [336] (Fig. 55-56). The characteristic feature is the development of non-caseiting granulomata in the adventitia. These nodules, made up of clusters of closely packed epithelioid cells, macrophages and multinucleate giant cells surrounded by thin rims of lymphocytes, monocytes, and fibroblasts, extend to the media, weaken the vascular wall and may lead to the formation of aneurysms. Non-caseating granulomata, however, are not specific for sarcoidosis, and are seen in mycobacterial and other fungal infections, berylliosis, syphilis, and Crohn's disease. Capillaries show enlarged endothelial cells with aggregation of eosinophils, thickening of the basement membrane and thrombosis [337]. Association with leukocytoclastic vasculitis has been reported [338].

Erythema nodosum

This acute disorder is a dermatosis marked by inflammatory, nonsuppurative nodules in the skin and subcutaneous tissues of the lower extremities, with vasculitis, arthralgia and fever. The commonest cause of erythema nodosum is infection. Other causes include adverse drug reactions, sarcoidosis, Crohn's disease, non-Hodgkin lymphoma, pregnancy, discoid lupus erythematosus, Sharp's syndrome and aspartame use [339, 340] (Table 9).

The disease is more frequent in women than in men (4:1). The peak incidence occurs between the ages of 18 and 34 years. It begins with a mild fever, sore throat, malaise, and arthralgia. A modest but widespread lymphadenopathy may occur. Nodules, generally less than 1 cm in diameter, appear on the legs,

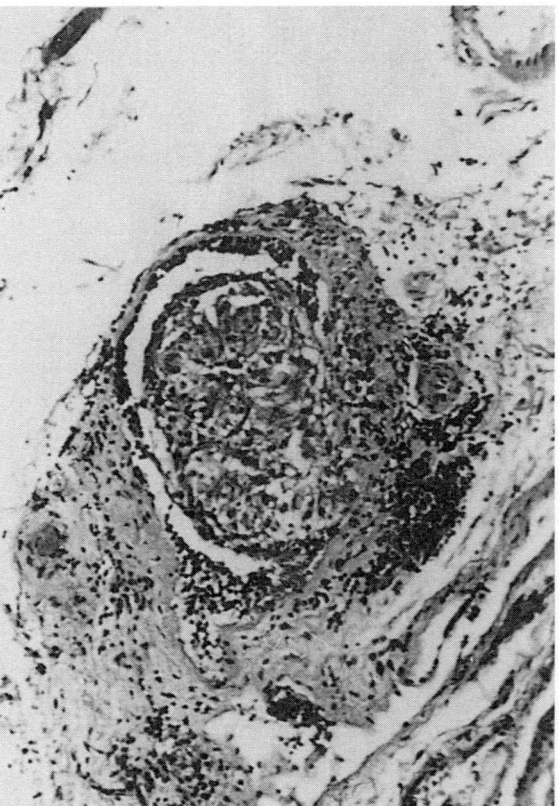

Fig. 55. Sarcoid vasculitis. Granuloma developed in the vascular wall may protrude into the lumen causing occlusion. HES

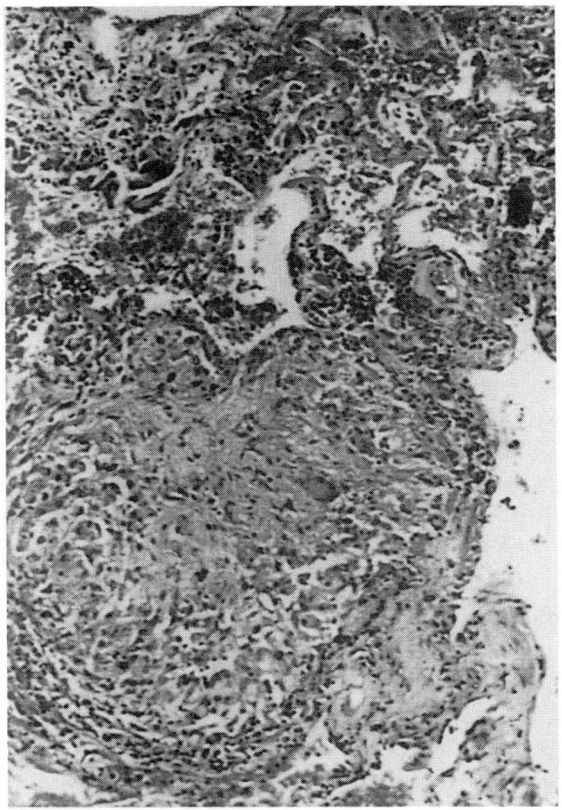

Fig. 56. Sarcoid vasculitis. Granulomatous vasculitis. HES

less commonly on the thighs, arms, and trunk, and rarely on the hands and face. They are pale or pinkish red, and painful and firm to the touch. The classic bi-

lateral distribution of the nodes on the extensor surface of the lower extremities occurs in 47% of patients. This disease is self-limited, usually lasting 2 to 6 weeks. The nodules regress in 1 to 2 weeks, but successive lesions may develop. As the lesions involute, they become brownish, mimicking haematomata. 77% of infection-induced erythema nodosum healed after 7 weeks, the longest course being 18 weeks. In contrast, 30% of idiopathic erythema nodosum lasted more than 6 months.

Pathology and Differential diagnosis

Dilated capillaries are seen in the cutis and sub-cutis. Infiltrates of neutrophils and lymphocytes accumulate around arterioles and venules in the middle and lower portion of the dermis (Fig. 57-58). The intima may show slight fibroblastic proliferation of the endothelium. Thrombus may be present. Leukocytoclastic vasculitis is seen in 30% of biopsies [340]. Generally the diagnosis presents little difficulty. Superficial thrombophlebitis, furunculosis, erythema induratum, and nodular vasculitis should be excluded.

Erythema elevatum diutinum (Bury's disease)

This is a localised variant of leukocytoclastic vasculitis with chronic symmetrical eruption of flattened nodules on the buttocks and extensor aspects of the wrists, elbows, and knees. Association with a cryoglobulin and IgA monoclonal gammopathy or human immunodeficiency virus infection has been described [341]. Any age group may be affected but 30-50 year olds are most often seen. Lesions appear as red or purplish papules and nodules (less than 1cm in dia-

Table 9. Pathological conditions associated with erythema nodosum

AETIOLOGIES	ASSOCIATED PATHOLOGICAL CONDITIONS
Viral infections	Measles, Psittacosis, Cat-scratch disease, Lymphogranuloma venereum
Bacterial infections	Syphilis, Tuberculosis, Leprosy, Diphtheria, Yersinia or Pasteurella infections, Meningococcaemia, β-haemolytic streptococcal infection, Rheumatic fever
Fungal infections	Blastomycosis, Coccidioidomycosis, Histoplasmosis
Immune diseases	Sarcoidosis, Crohn's disease, Chronic ulcerative colitis, Systemic and discoid lupus erythematosus, Behçet's disease, Sharp's syndrome
Lymphoproliferative conditions	Leukaemia, Hodgkin's disease and non-Hodgkin lymphoma
Drug sensivity	Aspartame, bromides, iodides, phenobarbital, phenolphthalein, salicylates, sulfonamides, thiouracil, oral contraceptives
Miscellaneous	Pregnancy

meter), or round, indurated elevated plaques (5 to 6 cm in diameter). Often distributed symmetrically, they involve the extensor surfaces of the joints, and itching, pain and arthralgia may be present. The course of the disease is chronic and progressive. Resolution occurs after 5 to 10 years.

Nodular vasculitis

This condition is characterised by chronic or recurrent nodular lesions of subcutaneous tissue, especially of the legs of older women (30-50 years), with lobular panniculitis, focal necrosis, and obliterative inflammation of the arteries and veins. The condition resembles erythema induratum but without evidence of associated tuberculosis [342]. The cause is unknown. Lesions are red, painful nodules varying from a few millimetres to a few centimeters in diameter. They appear in isolated instances or in waves, frequently on the lower limbs. Isolated lesions may persist for several months. Ulceration may occur.

Pathology and differential diagnosis

In the nodules, small arteries, arterioles, venules and lymphatics are surrounded by a collection of mononuclear cells, mostly lymphocytes and plasma cells. Intimal thickening and thrombosis may appear.

Nodular nonsuppurative panniculitis (Christian's disease, Weber-Christian disease)

Recurring attacks of fever and the formation of tender, red nodular, indurated skin lesions characterise this disease. The cause is unknown but there are association with acute pancreatitis, alpha 1-antitrypsin deficiency, trauma, and cold [343-346]. There is a female predominance. Patients present with chills and fever. The lesions are made up of painful plaques of varying size (from a few millimetres to a few centimeters), usually on the thighs and lower part of the abdomen. They persist for 1 to 3 weeks then regress, leaving retracted atrophic scars. Adipose tissue in other locations may also be involved (bone marrow, visceral adipose tissue, joints). Some patients develop hepatosplenomegaly. New lesions develop periodically.

Pathology and differential diagnosis

The subcutaneous fat tissue is distorted by necrosis and oedema with infiltration of neutrophils, lipophages, giant cells, and lymphocytes (Fig. 59-60). These cells also surround small arteries, arterioles, and venules [347-349] with oedema of the wall, endo-thelial proliferation, thrombosis and aneurysm [350-352]. Fibrosis occurs when the process regresses.

Granuloma faciale

Persistent, well-demarcated nodules appear on the face, consisting of a dense dermal infiltrate of eosinophils and neutrophils, with fibrinoid vasculitis and later mononuclear infiltration and fibrosis. Granuloma faciale affects mostly the middle-aged but may appear in children. Clinically, single or multiple lesions occur on the face and, to a lesser degree, the neck, chest and arms. The lesions consist of asymptomatic erythematous or brownish red, soft papules, plaques or nodules, up to several centimeters in diameter. The surface often shows fine telangiectases with dilated follicles. Itching or stinging may be present. There is no evidence of associated systemic involvement. Granuloma faciale tends to chronicity with periods of relapse and partial remissions.

Pathology and differential diagnosis

Histologically, the mid-dermis shows dilated small blood vessels (capillaries, arterioles and venules) whose walls are infiltrated by eosinophils with fibrin deposits. The surrounding connective tissue is distorted by a dense nodular infiltrate made up of large numbers of eosinophils, neutrophils displaying leucocytoclasis, and an admixture of plasma cells, mast cells and lymphocytes. Purpura is present and fibrin may be widely distributed in the dermis. Older lesions may show fibrosis and haemosiderin deposits. Immunofluorescence [353] reveals granular deposits of IgA and complement along the epidermodermal junction, and within the vascular walls. Less often, IgA and IgM may be present and there may also be abundant fibrin.

Pyoderma gangrenosum

This condition is characterised by a chronic non-infective eruption of spreading, undermined ulcers showing central healing, with diffuse dermal neutrophil infiltration, and vasculitis. Pyoderma gangrenosum affects both sexes without predilection, at any age, but most commonly patients in their fourth and fifth decades [354]. Clinically, lesions are represented by large, painful, and tender necrotic ulcers having irregular contours. These ulcers, measuring often 10 cm or more in diameter, are either solitary or multiple. They often develop after minor trauma. The lower limbs, the face, arms, trunk and buttocks may all be affected. Bullous variants may occur. Association of

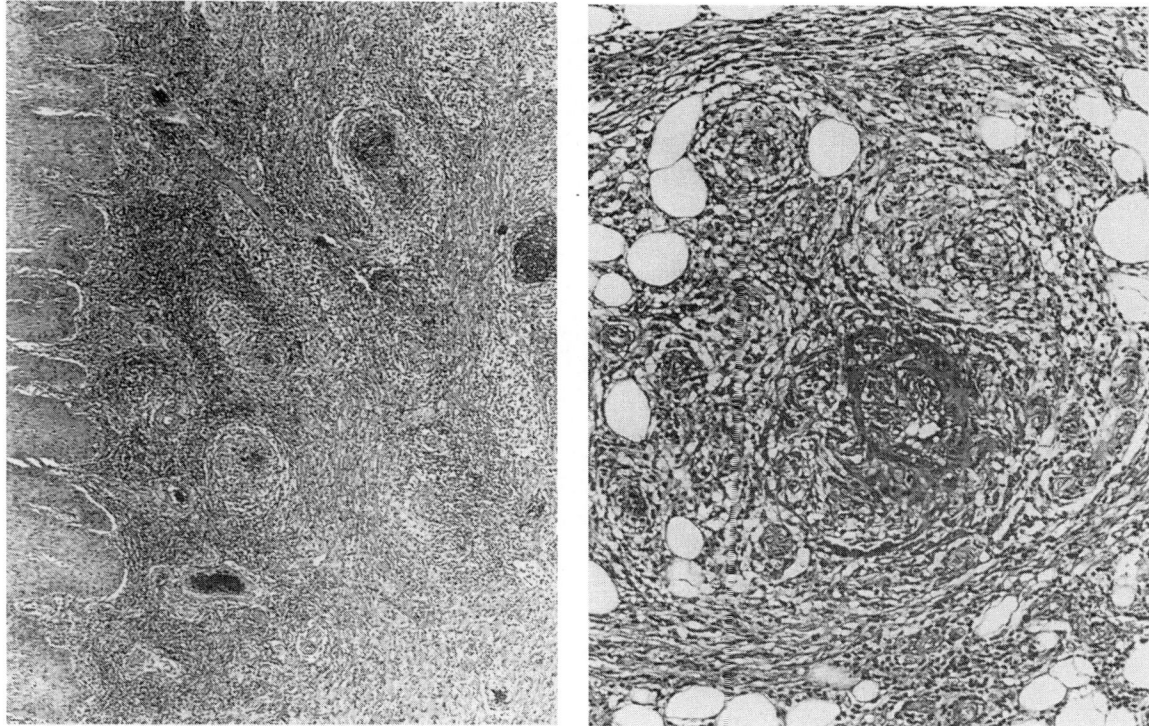

Fig. 57-58. Erythema nodosum. Leukocytoclastic vasculitis. HES

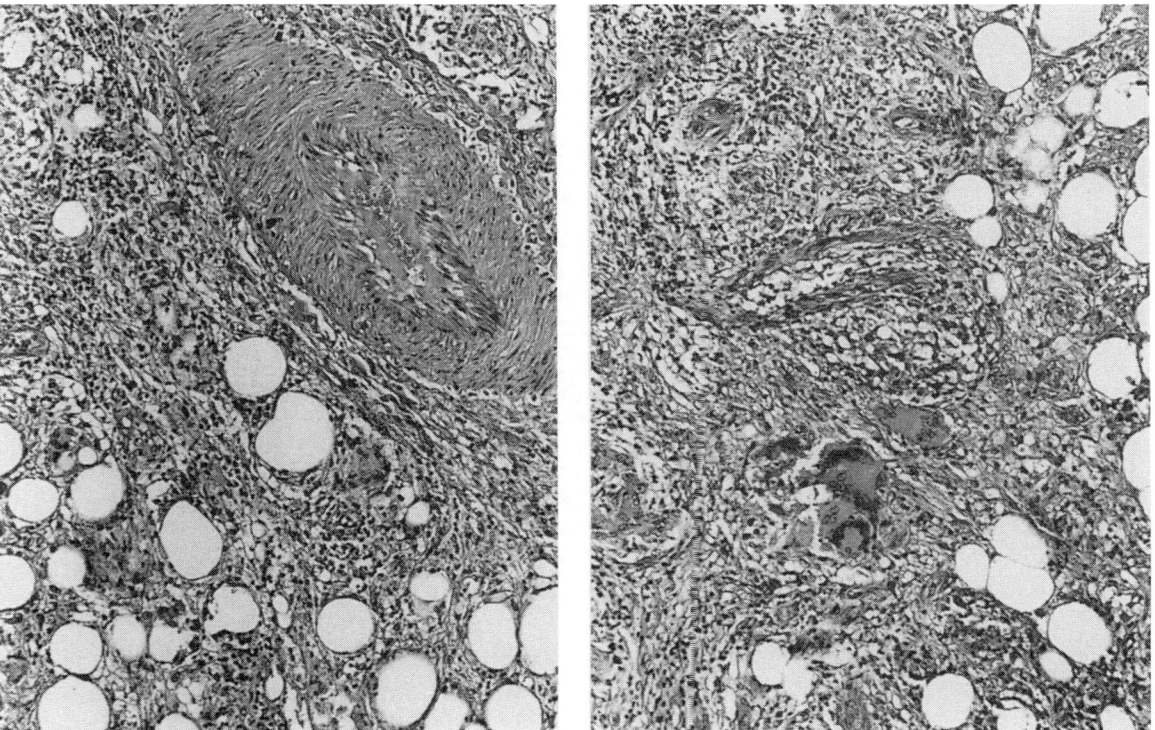

Fig. 59-60. Nodular nonsuppurative panniculitis (Christian's disease) with involvement of small calibre vessels. HES

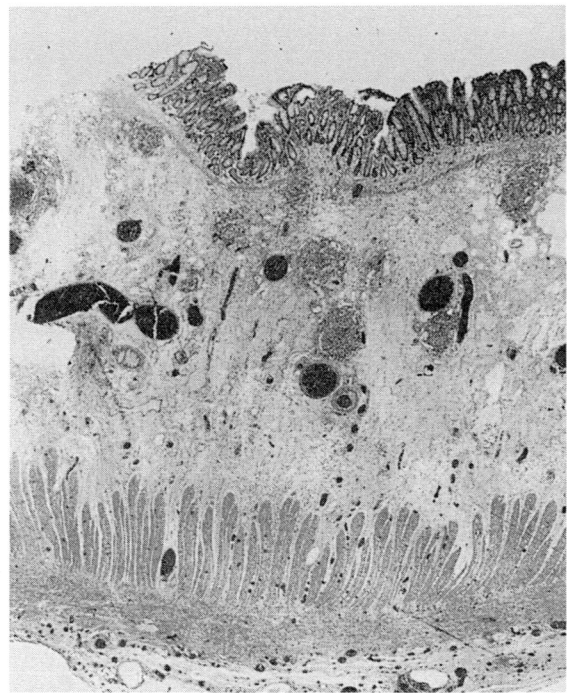

Fig. 61. Crohn's disease. Right colectomy specimen. Note multiple granulomata in the colic submucosa. HES

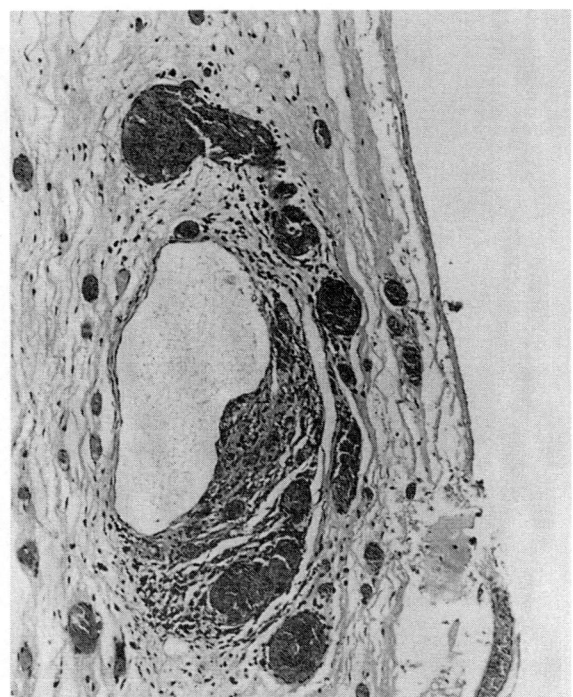

Fig. 62. Crohn's disease. Right colectomy specimen. A serosal lymphatic showing granulomatous lymphangitis. HES

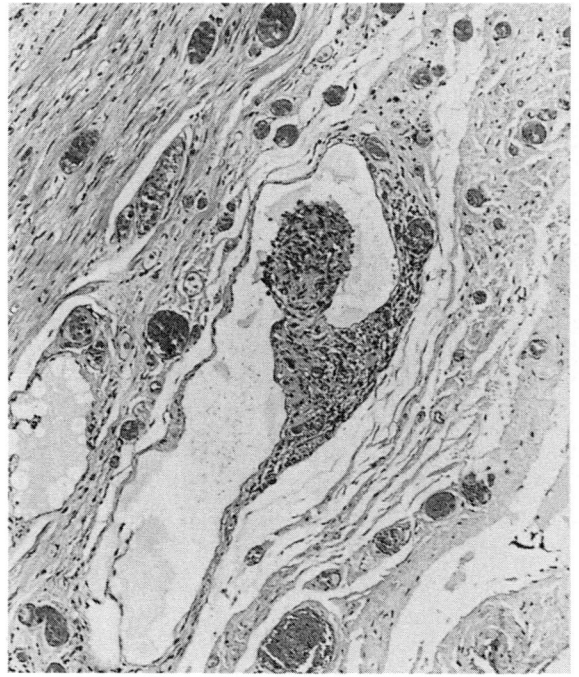

Fig. 63. Crohn's disease. Right colectomy specimen. Granulomatous lymphangitis with granuloma protruding into the lumen. HES

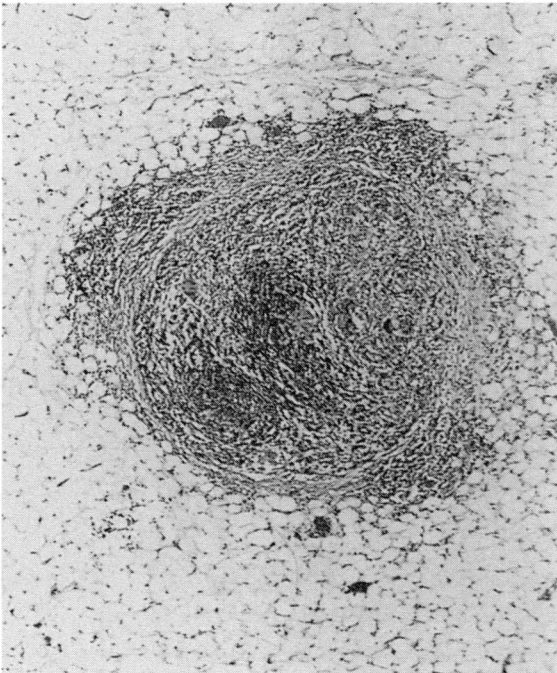

Fig. 64. Crohn's disease. Right colectomy specimen. Occlusive granulomatous lymphangitis. HES

pyoderma gangrenosum with ulcerative colitis and Crohn's disease, Behçet's syndrome, seronegative arthritis, rheumatoid arthritis, ankylosing spondylitis [355], benign monoclonal gammopathy (most often IgA), multiple myeloma, hypogammaglobulinaemia, leukaemia, and some underlying malignant tumours [356, 357] have all been reported. The histological pattern of pyoderma gangrenosum is that of non-specific cutaneous ulceration with abscess formation. Lymphocytic and/or leukocytoclastic vasculitis in 73% of the biopsy specimens obtained from the borders of the lesions [358], may be a consequence rather than a cause of the lesion.

Vasculitis associated with miscellaneous disorders

A leukocytoclastic vasculitis may be part of subacute bacterial endocarditis, ulcerative colitis, primary biliary cirrhosis, dermatomyositis, and progressive systemic sclerosis [359-361]. Granulomatous vasculitis may be associated with Crohn's disease (Fig. 61-64).

Bibliography

1. Fauci AS, Haynes BF, Katz P (1978) The spectrum of vasculitis: clinical, pathologic, immunologic, and therapeutic considerations. Ann Intern Med 89: 660-76
2. Jennette JC, Falk RJ, Andrassy K, Bacon PA, Churg J, Gross WL, Hagen EC, Hoffman GS, Hunder GG, Kallenberg CG, et al (1994) Nomenclature of systemic vasculitides. Proposal of an international consensus conference. Arthritis Rheum 37: 187-92
3. Mandell BF, Hoffman GS (1994) Differentiating the vasculitides. Rheum Dis Clin North Am 20: 409-42
4. Takeuchi K, Hirose S (1994) Vasculitis syndrome-clinical classification and diagnostic approaches. Nippon Rinsho 52: 1970-6
5. Ghersetich I, Jorizzo JL, Lotti T (1995) Working classification of vasculitis. Int Angiol 14: 101-6
6. Heller I, Isakov A, Blinder-Weiner S, Topilsky M (1995) Bayesian classification of vasculitis: a simulation study. Methods Inf Med 34: 259-65
7. Leu HJ (1995) Classification of vasculitides. A survey. Vasa 24: 319-24
8. Bruce IN, Bell AL (1997) A comparison of two nomenclature systems for primary systemic vasculitis. Br J Rheumatol 36:453-8
9. Watts RA, Scott DG (1997) Classification and epidemiology of the vasculitides. Baillieres Clin Rheumatol 11: 191-217
10. Cotran RS, Pober JS (1992) Recent insights into the mechanisms of vascular injury. Implications for the pathogenesis of vasculitis. In Simionescu N, and Simionescu M (eds) Endothelial cell dysfunctions. New York, Plenum Press p. 183
11. Jennette JC, Falk RJ, Wilkman AS (1995) Anti-neutrophil cytoplasmic autoantibodies—a serologic marker for vasculitides. Ann Acad Med Singapore 24: 248-53
12. Jennette JC (1991) Antineutrophil cytoplasmic autoantibody-associated diseases: a pathologist's perspective. Am J Kidney Dis 18: 164-70
13. Ewert BH, Jennette JC, Falk RJ (1991) The pathogenic role of antineutrophil cytoplasmic autoantibodies. Am J Kidney Dis 18: 188-95
14. Zielonka TM, Samolinski B, Tchorzewska H, Chorzelski T, Droszcz W (1991) Significance of anti-neutrophil cytoplasmic autoantibodies in the diagnosis of Wegener's granulomatosis. Pol Arch Med Wewn 86: 113-6
15. Noel LH (1994) Kidney and vasculitis. Rev Med Interne 15: 399-405
16. Cohen P, Guillevin L, Baril L, Lhote F, Noel LH, Lesavre P (1995) Persistence of antineutrophil cytoplasmic antibodies (ANCA) in asymptomatic patients with systemic polyarteritis nodosa or Churg-Strauss syndrome: follow-up of 53 patients. Clin Exp Rheumatol 13: 193-8
17. Heeringa P, Brouwer E, Cohen Tervaert JW, Weening JJ, Kallenberg CG (1998) Animal models of anti-neutrophil cytoplasmic antibody associated vasculitis. Kidney Int 53: 253-63
18. Morshuis WJ, Zeebregts CJ, Haanen HC, Elbers JR, Ernst JM, Vermeulen FE (1997) Aortitis, aortic valve incompetence, and left coronary ostium stenosis in a patient with C-ANCA-associated necrotizing vasculitis. Thorac Cardiovasc Surg 45: 97-9
19. Weir A, Taylor-Robinson SD, Poole S, Pignatelli M, Walters JF, Calam J (1997) Cytoplasmic antineutrophil cytoplasmic antibody-positive vasculitis associated with ulcerative colitis. Am J Gastroenterol 92: 506-8
20. Goeken JA (1991) Antineutrophil cytoplasmic antibody—a useful serological marker for vasculitis. J Clin Immunol 11: 161-74
21. Guillevin L, Lhote F, Brauner M, Casassus P (1995) Antineutrophil cytoplasmic antibodies (ANCA) and abnormal angiograms in polyarteritis nodosa and Churg-Strauss syndrome: indications for the diagnosis of microscopic polyangiitis. Ann Med Interne (Paris) 146: 548-50
22. Berry CL (Ed.)(1999) Transplantation pathology. A guide for practicing pathologists. Current topics in pathology. Vol 92. Springer-Verlag, Berlin Heidelberg New York Barcelona Hong Kong London Milan Paris Singapore Tokyo
23. Veraguth AJ, Hauselmann HJ, Hunziker T, Gerber NJ (1992) Vasculitic skin lesions caused by nonsteroidal anti-inflammatory agents. Schweiz Med Wochenschr 122: 923-9
24. Lowry MD, Hudson CF, Callen JP (1994) Leukocytoclastic vasculitis caused by drug additives. J Am Acad Dermatol 30: 854-5
25. Arbiser JL, Dzieczkowski JS, Harmon JV, Duncan LM (1995) Leukocytoclastic vasculitis following staphylococcal protein A column immunoadsorption therapy. Two cases and a review of the literature. Arch Dermatol 131: 707-9
26. Han BG, Choi SO, Shin SJ, Kim HY, Jung SH, Lee KH (1995) A case of Henoch-Schonlein purpura in disseminated tuberculosis. Korean J Intern Med 10: 54-9
27. Calabrese LH, Duna GF (1996) Drug-induced vasculitis. Curr Opin Rheumatol 8: 34-40
28. Wooten MD, Jasin HE (1996) Vasculitis and lymphoproliferative diseases. Semin Arthritis Rheum 26: 564-74
29. Zlatanic J, Fleisher M, Sasson M, Kim P, Korelitz BI (1996) Crohn's disease and acute leukocytoclastic vasculitis of skin. Am J Gastroenterol 91: 2410-3

30. Kao GF, Evancho CD, Ioffe O, Lowitt MH, Dumler JS (1997) Cutaneous histopathology of Rocky Mountain spotted fever. J Cutan Pathol 24: 604-10

31. Reiner MR, Brunetti VA (1997) Imipenem-cilastatin-induced leukocytoclastic vasculitis. J Am Podiatr Med Assoc 87: 245-7

32. Ekenstam EA, Callen JP (1984) Cutaneous leucocytoclastic vasculitis. Arch Dermatol 120: 484-9

33. Grunwald MH, Avinoach I, Amichai B, Halevy S (1997) Leukocytoclastic vasculitis—correlation between different histologic stages and direct immunofluorescence results. Int J Dermatol 36: 349-52

34. Aboobaker J, Greaves MW (1986) Urticarial vasculitis. Clin Exp Dermatol 11: 436-44

35. Charlesworth EN (1996) Urticaria and angioedema: a clinical spectrum. Ann Allergy Asthma Immunol 76: 484-95

36. O'Donnell B, Black AK (1995) Urticarial vasculitis. Int Angiol 14: 166-74

37. de Castro FR, Masouye I, Winkelmann RK, Saurat JH (1996) Urticarial pathology in Schnitzler's (hyper-IgM) syndrome. Dermatology 193: 94-9

38. Petruzzellis V, Florio T, Conte A, Rantuccio F (1990) Clinico-pathogenetic observations on the subject of superficial vasculitis. G Ital Dermatol Venereol 125: 7-13

39. Bonkovsky HL, Liang TJ, Hasegawa K, Banner B(1995) Chronic leukocytoclastic vasculitis complicating HBV infection. Possible role of mutant forms of HBV in pathogenesis and persistence of disease. J Clin Gastroenterol 21: 42-7

40. Johnson RJ, Gretch DR, Yamabe H, Hart J, Bacchi CE, Hartwell P, Couser WG, Corey L, Wener MH, Alpers CE, et al (1993) Membranoproliferative glomerulonephritis associated with hepatitis C virus infection. N Engl J Med 328: 465-70

41. Pawlotsky JM, Dhumeaux D, Bagot M (1995) Hepatitis C virus in dermatology. A review. Arch Dermatol 131: 1185-93

42. Schirren CA, Zachoval R, Schirren CG, Gerbes AL, Pape GR (1995) A role for chronic hepatitis C virus infection in a patient with cutaneous vasculitis, cryoglobulinaemia, and chronic liver disease. Effective therapy with interferon-alpha. Dig Dis Sci 40: 1221-5

43. Yamabe H, Johnson RJ, Gretch DR, Fukushi K, Osawa H, Miyata M, Inuma H, Sasaki T, Kaizuka M, Tamura N, et al (1995) Hepatitis C virus infection and membranoproliferative glomerulonephritis in Japan. J Am Soc Nephrol 6: 220-3

44. Kuniyuki S, Katoh H (1996) Urticarial vasculitis with papular lesions in a patient with type C hepatitis and cryoglobulinaemia. J Dermatol 23: 279-83

45. Manna R, Todaro L, Latteri M, Gambassi G, Massi G, Grillo MR, Romito A, Caputo S, Gasbarrini GB (1997) Leucocytoclastic vasculitis associated with hepatitis C virus antibodies. Br J Rheumatol 36: 124-5

46. Lind KM, Gaub J, Pedersen RS (1994) Henoch-Schonlein purpura associated with Campylobacter jejuni enteritis. Case report. Scand J Urol Nephrol 28: 179-81

47. Jessop SJ (1995) Cutaneous leucocytoclastic vasculitis: a clinical and aetiological study. Br J Rheumatol 34: 942-5

48. Maestri A, Malacarne P, Santini A (1995) Henoch-Schonlein syndrome associated with breast cancer. A case report. Angiology 46: 625-7

49. Schlehaider UK, Suckow M, Rosenthal P, Kowalzick L (1997) Cutaneous reactions in Crohn disease. Vasculitis in various skin segments. Hautarzt 48: 328-31

50. Al-Sheyyab M, El-Shanti H, Ajlouni S, Sawalha D, Daoud A (1995) The clinical spectrum of Henoch-Schonlein purpura in infants and young children. Eur J Pediatr 154: 969-72

51. Nussinovitch M, Prais D, Finkelstein Y, Varsano I (1998) Cutaneous manifestations of Henoch-Schonlein purpura in young children. Pediatr Dermatol 15: 426-8

52. Michel BA, Hunder GG, Bloch DA, Calabrese LH (1992) Hypersensitivity vasculitis and Henoch-Schonlein purpura: a comparison between the 2 disorders. J Rheumatol 19: 721-8

53. Mroczkowska-Juchkiewicz A, Pawlowska-Kamieniak A, Szczepanowska A, Papierkowski A (1997) Massive gastrointestinal hemorrhage in the course of Schoenlein-Henoch purpura in an 8-year old girl. Pol Merkuriusz Lek 3: 81-2

54. Kauffmann RH, Herrmann WA, Meyer CJ, Daha MR, Van Es LA (1980) Circulating IgA-immune complexes in Henoch-Schonlein purpura. A longitudinal study of their relationship to disease activity and vascular deposition of IgA. Am J Med 69: 859-66

55. Mills JA, Michel BA, Bloch DA, Calabrese LH, Hunder GG, Arend WP, Edworthy SM, Fauci AS, Leavitt RY, Lie JT, et al (1990) The American College of Rheumatology 1990 criteria for the classification of Henoch-Schonlein purpura. Arthritis Rheum 33: 1114-21

56. Martinez-Taboada VM, Blanco R, Garcia-Fuentes M, Rodriguez-Valverde V (1997) Clinical features and outcome of 95 patients with hypersensitivity vasculitis. Am J Med 102: 186-91

57. Calabrese LH, Michel BA, Bloch DA, Arend WP, Edworthy SM, Fauci AS, Fries JF, Hunder GG, Leavitt RY, Lie JT et al (1990) The American College of Rheumatology 1990 criteria for the classification of hypersensitivity vasculitis. Arthritis Rheum 33: 1108-13C

58. Tucker LB (1991) Systemic lupus erythematosus, dermatomyositis, scleroderma, vasculopathies, and other connective tissue disorders in children. Curr Opin Rheumatol 3: 844-53

59. Bacon PA, Carruthers DM (1995) Vasculitis associated with connective tissue disorders. Rheum Dis Clin North 2: 1077-96

60. Pelkonen P (1995) Childhood systemic lupus erythematosus, vasculitis, and rheumatic fever and neonatal lupus. Curr Opin Rheumatol 7: 430-6

61. Breedveld FC (1997) Vasculitis associated with connective tissue disease. Baillieres Clin Rheumatol 11: 315-34

62. Tan EM, Cohen AS, Fries JF, Masi AT, McShane DJ, Rothfield NF, Schaller JG, Talal N, Winchester RJ (1982) The 1982 revised criteria for the classification of systemic lupus erythematosus. Arthritis Rheum 25: 1271-7

63. Ishikawa O, Miyachi Y, Watanabe H (1997) Hypocomplementaemic urticarial vasculitis associated with Jaccoud's syndrome. Br J Dermatol 137: 804-7

64. Walts AE, Dubois EL (1977) Acute dissecting aneurysm of the aorta as the fatal event in systemic lupus erythematosus. Am Heart J 93: 378-81

65. Guard RW, Gotis-Graham I, Edmonds JP, Thomas AC (1995) Aortitis with dissection complicating systemic lupus erythematosus. Pathology 27: 224-8

66. MacLeod CB, Johnson D, Frable WJ (1992) "Tree-barking" of the ascending aorta. Syphilis or systemic lupus erythematosus? Am J Clin Pathol 97: 58-62

67. Weiner DK, Allen NB (1991) Large vessel vasculitis of the central nervous system in systemic lupus erythematosus: report and review of the literature. J Rheumatol 18: 748-51

68. Bertrand E, Kuczynska-Zardzewialy A, Palasik W, Chorzelski T (1995) Rare vascular changes in the brain in a case of subacute cutaneous lupus erythematosus. Folia Neuropathol 33: 235-40

69. D'Cruz D, Cervera R, Olcay Aydintug A, Ahmed T, Font J, Hughes GR (1993) Systemic lupus erythematosus evolving into systemic vasculitis: a report of five cases. Br J Rheumatol 32: 154-7

70. Johansson EA, Niemi KM, Mustakallio KK (1977) A peripheral vascular syndrome overlapping with systemic lupus erythematosus. Recurrent venous thrombosis and hemorrhagic capillary proliferation with circulating anticoagulants and false-positive seroreactions for syphilis. Dermatologica 155: 257-67

71. Godeau P, Piette JC, Frances C, Le Thi Huong Du, Bletry O, Wechsler B (1990) The multiple clinical aspects of lupus. Clin Exp Rheumatol 8: S27-S35

72. Hanson VG, Horowitz M, Rosenbluth D, Spiera H, Puszkin S (1992) Systemic lupus erythematosus patients with central nervous system involvement show autoantibodies to a 50-kD neuronal membrane protein. J Exp Med 176: 565-73

73. Burkholder PM (1974) Atlas of human glomerular pathology. Harper & Row, Hagerstown 433p

74. Morioka S, Makino H, Wada J, Shikata K, Yamasaki Y, Ogura T, Amano T, Asaumi A, Okada S, Ota Z (1995) A case of systemic lupus erythematosus associated with severe fibrinoid necrosis located mainly in the glomerular afferent arteriole. Nippon Jinzo Gakkai Shi 37: 69-73

75. Harris ED Jr (1990) Rheumatoid arthritis. Pathophysiology and implications for therapy. N Engl J Med 322: 1277-89

76. Arnett FC, Edworthy SM, Bloch DA, McShane DJ, Fries JF, Cooper NS, Healey LA, Kaplan SR, Liang MH, Luthra HS, et al (1988) The American Rheumatism Association 1987 revised criteria for the classification of rheumatoid arthritis. Arthritis Rheum 31: 315-24

77. Minari C, Cecconami L, Fioravanti A, Montemerani M, Scola C, Marcolongo R (1994) Lymphoedema of the limbs in rheumatoid arthritis. Clin Rheumatol 13: 464-9

78. Sant SM, Tormey VJ, Freyne P, Casey EB (1995) Lymphatic obstruction in rheumatoid arthritis. Clin Rheumatol 14: 445-50

79. Reimer KA, Rodgers RF, Oyasu R (1976) Rheumatoid arthritis with rheumatoid heart disease and granulomatous aortitis. JAMA 235: 2510-12

80. Yokoyama T, Kurosaka D, Hashimoto N (1996) An autopsy case of rheumatoid arthritis associated with proliferative endarteritis died of sudden severe melaena. Nihon Rinsho Meneki Gakkai Kaishi 19: 179-84

81. Bely M, Apathy A (1996) Vasculitis in rheumatoid arthritis. Orv Hetil 137: 1571-8

82. Sokoloff L, McCloskey RT, Bunim JJ (1953) Vascularity of the early nodule of rheumatoid arthritis. AMA Arch Pathol 55: 475-95

83. Lande A, Bard R (1976) Takayasu's arteritis: an unrecognized cause of pulmonary hypertension. Angiology 27: 114-21

84. Danning CL, Illei GG, Boumpas DT (1998) Vasculitis associated with primary rheumatologic diseases. Curr Opin Rheumatol 10: 58-65

85. Lopez-Larrea C, Gonzalez S, Martinez-Borra J (1998) The role of HLA-B27 polymorphism and molecular mimicry in spondylarthropathy. Mol Med Today 4: 540-9

86. Fujito T, Inoue T, Hoshi K, Hatano H, Kamishirado H, Takayanagi K, Hayashi T, Morooka S, Takabatake Y, Uehara Y (1995) Systemic amyloidosis following ankylosing spondylitis associated with congestive heart failure. A case report. Jpn Heart J 36: 681-8

87. Tucker CR, Fowles RE, Calin A, Popp RL (1982) Aortitis in ankylosing spondylitis: early detection of aortic root abnormalities with two dimensional echocardiography. Am J Cardiol 49: 680-6

88. De Almeida FA, Albanesi Filho FM, de Albuquerque EM, Magalhaes EC, de Menezes ME (1995) Echocardiography in the evaluation of cardiac involvement in seronegative spondylo-arthropathies. Medicina (B Aires) 55: 231-6

89. Roldan CA, Chavez J, Wiest PW, Qualls CR, Crawford MH (1998) Aortic root disease and valve disease associated with ankylosing spondylitis. J Am Coll Cardiol 32: 1397-404

90. Reveille JD (1998) HLA-B27 and the seronegative spondyloarthropathies. Am J Med Sci 316: 239-49

91. Magro CM, Crowson AN, Peeling R (1995) Vasculitis as the basis of cutaneous lesions in Reiter's disease. Hum Pathol 26: 633-8

92. Pavlica L, Mitrovic D, Mladenovic V, Popovic M, Krstic S, Andelkovic Z (1997) Reiter's syndrome—analysis of 187 patients. Vojnosanit Pregl 54: 437-46

93. Hoogland YT, Alexander EP, Patterson RH, Nashel DJ (1994) Coronary artery stenosis in Reiter's syndrome: a complication of aortitis. J Rheumatol 21: 757-9

94. Rodriguez J, Diaz F, Collazos J (1994) Thrombophlebitis and Reiter's syndrome. Postgrad Med J 70: 145-6

95. Dzhus MB, Zharinov OI, Nadashkevych ON (1995) Cardiac involvement in Reiter's disease. Lik Sprava (9-12): 168-9

96. Boehni U, Christen B, Greminger P, Michel BA (1997) Systemic vasculitis associated with seronegative spondylarthropathy (Reiter's syndrome). Clin Rheumatol 16: 610-3

97. Carrion M, Giron JA, Ventura J, Camacho A, Garcia-Diez C (1993) Airway complications in relapsing polychondritis. J Rheumatol 20: 1628-9

98. Sohi GS, Desai AM, Ward WW, Flowers NC (1981) Aortic cusp involvement causing severe aortic regurgitation in a case of relapsing polychondritis. Cathet Cardiovasc Diagn 7: 79-86

99. Bowness P, Hawley IC, Morris T, Dearden A, Walport MJ (1991) Complete heart block and severe aortic incompetence in relapsing polychondritis: clinicopathologic findings. Arthritis Rheum 34: 97-100

100. Del Rosso A, Petix NR, Pratesi M, Bini A (1997) Cardiovascular involvement in relapsing polychondritis. Semin Arthritis Rheum 26: 840-4

101. Pearson CM, Kroening R, Verity MA, Getzen JH (1967) Aortic insufficiency and aortic aneurysm in relapsing polychondritis. Trans Assoc Am Physicians 80: 71-90

102. Cipriano PR, Alonso DR, Baltaxe HA, Gay WA Jr, Smith JP (1976) Multiple aortic aneurysms in relapsing polychondritis. Am J Cardiol 37: 1097-102

103. Giordano M, Valentini G, Sodano A (1984) Relapsing polychondritis with aortic arch aneurysm and aortic arch syndrome. Rheumatol Int 4: 191-3

104. Thuaire C, Benamer H, Brochet E, Aubry P, Hayem G, Vissuzaine C, Chatel D, Assayag P (1997) Anatomoclini-

cal study of aortic insufficiency in atrophic polychondritis. Apropos of a case. Arch Mal Cœur Vaiss 90: 995-8

105. Hughes RA, Berry CL, Seifert M, Lessof MH (1972) Relapsing polychondritis. Three cases with a clinico-pathological study and literature review. Q J Med 41: 363-80

106. Sanchez-Guerrero J, Gutierrez-Urena S, Vidaller A, Reyes E, Iglesias A, Alarcon-Segovia D (1990) Vasculitis as a paraneoplastic syndrome. Report of 11 cases and review of the literature. J Rheumatol 17: 1458-62

107. Naschitz JE, Yeshurun D, Eldar S, Lev LM (1996) Diagnosis of cancer-associated vascular disorders. Cancer 77: 1759-67

108. Farcet JP, Weschsler J, Wirquin V, Divine M, Reyes F (1987) Vasculitis in hairy-cell leukaemia. Arch Intern Med 147: 660-4

109. Fain O, Guillevin L, Kaplan G, Sicard D, Lemaire V, Godeau P, Kahn MF (1991) Vasculitis and neoplasms. 14 cases. Ann Med Interne (Paris) 142: 486-504

110. Fernandez AM, Abeles M, Wong RL (1994) Recurrent leukocytoclastic vasculitis as the initial manifestation of acute myelomonocytic leukaemia. J Rheumatol 21: 1972-4

111. Farrell AM, Gooptu C, Woodrow D, Costello C, Bunker CB, Cream JJ (1996) Cutaneous lymphocytic vasculitis in acute myeloid leukaemia. Br J Dermatol 135: 471-4

112. Hasler P, Kistler H, Gerber H (1995) Vasculitides in hairy cell leukaemia. Semin Arthritis Rheum 25: 134-42

113. Jufresa J, Alegre J, Ruiz Marcellan MC, Surinach JM, Marques A, Fernandez de Sevilla T (1996) Cutaneous vasculitis during primary myelofibrosis. An Med Interna 13: 494-5

114. Pavlidis NA, Klouvas G, Tsokos M, Bai M, Moutsopoulos HM (1995) Cutaneous lymphocytic vasculopathy in lymphoproliferative disorders—a paraneoplastic lymphocytic vasculitis of the skin. Leuk Lymphoma 16: 477-482

115. Perrone A, Guida G, Leuci D, Schiraldi O (1995) Cutaneous vasculitis, mixed cryoglobulinaemia in a patient with non-secreting monolateral pheochromocytoma. A likely paraneoplastic syndrome. Recenti Prog Med 86: 499-502

116. Birchmore D, Sweeney C, Choudhury D, Konwinski MF, Carnevale K, D'Agati V (1996) IgA multiple myeloma presenting as Henoch-Schonlein purpura/polyarteritis nodosa overlap syndrome. Arthritis Rheum 39: 698-703

117. Hasegawa H, Ozawa T, Tada N, Taguchi Y, Ohno K, Chou T, Watanabe T, Kuroda T, Nakano M, Usuda H, Emura I, Arakawa M (1996) Multiple myeloma-associated systemic vasculopathy due to crystalglobulin or polyarteritis nodosa. Arthritis Rheum 39: 330-4

118. Bodokh I, Lacour JP, Perrin C, Ferrari E, Ticchioni M, Roule C, Isetta C, Jourdan J, Ortonne JP (1993) Cutaneous leukocytoclastic vasculitis with circulating anticoagulant disclosing myxoma of the left atrium. Ann Dermatol Venereol 120: 789-92

119. Kurzrock R, Cohen PR, Markowitz A (1994) Clinical manifestations of vasculitis in patients with solid tumors. A case report and review of the literature. Arch Intern Med 154: 334-40

120. Sanchez-Angulo JI, Benitez-Roldan A, Silgado-Rodriguez G, Ruiz-Campos J (1996) Leukocytoclastic vasculitis as the form of presentation of hepatocarcinoma. Gastroenterol Hepatol 19: 255-8

121. Hayem G, Gomez MJ, Grossin M, Meyer O, Kahn MF (1997) Systemic vasculitis and epithelioma. A report of three cases with a literature review. Rev Rhum Engl Ed 64: 816-24

122. Shmurun RI (1997) Allergic vasculitis in benign prostatic hyperplasia combined with a latent prostatic carcinoma. Urol Nefrol (Mosk) 5: 46-9

123. Wang H-C, Lu J-Y, Ting Y-M, Lin C-C (1996) Digital ischemia associated with lung cancer: a case report. Chin Med J (Taipei) 57: 370-4

124. Meltzer M, Franklin EC, Elias K, McCluskey RT, Cooper N (1966) Cryoglobulinaemia—a clinical and laboratory study. II. Cryoglobulins with rheumatoid factor activity. Am J Med 40: 837-56

125. McDuffie FC, Sams WM Jr, Maldonado JE, Andreini PH, Conn DL, Samayoa EA (1973) Hypocomplementemia with cutaneous vasculitis and arthritis. Possible immune complex syndrome. Mayo Clin Proc 48: 340-8

126. Goodpasture EW (1919) The significance of certain pulmonary lesions in relation to the etiology of influenza. Am J Med 158: 863-70

127. Meyers CM, Kalluri R, Neilson EG (1997) Anti-glomerular basement membrane disease In Neilson EG, Couser WG (ed) Immunologic renal diseases. Lippincott-Raven Publishers, Philadelphia.

128. Wieslander J, Heinegard D (1985) The involvement of type IV collagen in Goodpasture's syndrome. Ann N Y Acad Sci 460: 363-74

129. Butkowski RJ, Shen GQ, Wieslander J, Michael AF, Fish AJ (1990) Characterization of type IV collagen NC1 monomers and Goodpasture antigen in human renal basement membranes. J Lab Clin Med 115: 365-73

130. Morrison KE, Mariyama M, Yang-Feng TL, Reeders ST (1991) Sequence and localization of a partial cDNA encoding the human alpha 3 chain of type IV collagen. Am J Hum Genet 49: 545-54

131. Kalluri R, Gattone VHJr, Noelken ME, Hudson BG (1994) The alpha3 (IV) chain of type IV collagen induces autoimmune Goodpasture syndrome. Proc Natl Acad Sci USA 91: 6201-5

132. Sternlieb I, Bennett B, Scheinberg IH (1975) D-Penicillamine-induced Goodpasture's syndrome in Wilson's disease. Ann Intern Med 82: 673-6

133. Wilson CB (1988) Immunologic diseases of the lung and kidney (Goodpasture's syndrome) in Fisherman AP (ed.) Pulmonary diseases and disorders. 2nd ed NewYork, McGraw-Hill pp 675-82

134. Wu MJ, Rajaram R, Shelp WD, Beirne GJ, Burkholder PM (1980) Vasculitis in Goodpasture's syndrome. Arch Pathol Lab Med 104: 300-2

135. Dean SE, Saba SR, Ramirez G (1991) Systemic vasculitis in Goodpasture's syndrome. South Med J 84: 1387-90

136. Maresi E, Becchina G, Orlando E, Ottoveggio G (1995) Acute necrotizing capillaritis in an adolescent dying from a Goodpasture-like pulmonary-renal syndrome Pathologica 87: 666-71

137. Rydel JJ, Rodby RA (1998) An 18-year-old man with Goodpasture's syndrome and ANCA-negative central nervous system vasculitis. Am J Kidney Dis 31: 345-9

138. Komadina KH, Houk RW, Vicks SL, Desrosier KF, Ridley DJ, Boswell RN (1988) Goodpasture's syndrome associated with pulmonary eosinophilic vasculitis. J Rheumatol 15: 1298-301

139. Lombard CM, Colby TV, Elliot CG (1989) Surgical pathology of the lung in anti-basement membrane antibody-associated Goodpasture's syndrome. Hum Pathol 20: 445-1

140. Koffler D, Sandson J, Carr R, Kinkel HG (1969) Immunologic studies concerning the pulmonary lesions in Goodpasture's syndrome. Am J Pathol 54: 293-301.

141. Berry CL (1983) Kawasaki's disease. Pediatr Cardiol 4: 233-4
142. Dajani AS, Taubert KA, Gerber MA, Shulman ST, Ferrieri P, Freed M, Takahashi M, Bierman FZ, Karchmer AW, Wilson W, et al (1993) Diagnosis and therapy of Kawasaki disease in children. Circulation 87: 1776-80
143. Butler DF, Hough DR, Friedman SJ, Davis HE (1987) Adult Kawasaki syndrome. Arch Dermatol 123: 1356-61
144. Habon T, Toth K, Keltai M, Lengyel M, Palik I (1998) An adult case of Kawasaki disease with multiplex coronary aneurysms and myocardial infarction: the role of transesophageal echocardiography. Clin Cardiol 21: 529-32
145. Morens DM, Anderson LJ, Hurwitz ES (1980) National surveillance of Kawasaki disease. Pediatrics 65: 21-5
146. Meade RH 3d, Brandt L (1982) Manifestations of Kawasaki disease in New England outbreak of 1980. J Pediatr 100: 558-62
147. Bell DM, Brink EW, Nitzkin JL, Hall CB, Wulff H, Berkowitz ID, Feorino PM, Holman RC, Huntley CL, Meade RH 3d, Anderson LJ, Cheeseman SH, Fiumara NJ, Gilfillan RF, Keim DE, Modlin JF (1981) Kawasaki syndrome: description of two outbreaks in the United States. N Engl J Med 304: 1568-75
148. Lin FY, Bailowitz A, Koslowe P, Israel E, Kaslow RA (1985) Kawasaki syndrome. A case-control study during an outbreak in Maryland. Am J Dis Child 139: 277-9
149. Rauch AM, Glode MP, Wiggins JW Jr, Rodriguez JG, Hopkins RS, Hurwitz ES, Schonberger LB (1991) Outbreak of Kawasaki syndrome in Denver, Colorado: association with rug and carpet cleaning. Pediatrics 87: 663-9
150. Ohno S, Miyajima T, Higuchi M, Yoshida A, Matsuda H, Saheki Y, Nagamatsu I, Togashi T, Matsumoto S (1982) Ocular manifestations of Kawasaki's disease (mucocutaneous lymph node syndrome). Am J Ophthalmol 93: 713-7
151. Marchette NJ, Melish ME, Hicks R, Kihara S, Sam E, Ching D (1990) Epstein-Barr virus and other herpesvirus infections in Kawasaki syndrome. J Infectious Dis 161: 680-4
152. Rogers MF, Kochel RL, Hurwitz ES, Jillson CA, Hanrahan JP, Schonberger LB (1985) Kawasaki syndrome. Is exposure to rug shampoo important? Am J Dis Child 139: 777-9
153. Cuttica RJ (1997) Vasculitis, Kawasaki disease, and pseudovasculitis. Curr Opin Rheumatol 9: 448-57
154. Falcini F, Trapani S, Turchini S, Farsi A, Ermini M, Keser G, Khamashta MA, Hughes GR (1997) Immunological findings in Kawasaki disease: an evaluation in a cohort of Italian children. Clin Exp Rheumatol 15: 685-9
155. Leung DY, Sullivan KE, Brown-Whitehorn TF, Fehringer AP, Allen S, Finkel TH, Washington RL, Makida R, Schlievert PM (1997) Association of toxic shock syndrome toxin-secreting and exfoliative toxin-secreting Staphylococcus aureus with Kawasaki syndrome complicated by coronary artery disease. Pediatr Res 42: 268-72
156. Jason J, Montana E, Donald JF, Seidman M, Inge KL, Campbell R (1998) Kawasaki disease and the T-cell antigen receptor. Hum Immunol 59: 29-38
157. Imakita M, Sasaki Y, Misugi K, Miyazawa Y, Hyodo Y (1984) Kawasaki disease complicated with mitral insufficiency. Autopsy findings with special reference to valvular lesion. Acta Pathol Jpn 34: 605-16
158. Shapira OM, Shemin RJ (1997) Aneurysmal coronary artery disease. Atherosclerotic coronary artery ectasia or adult mucocutaneous lymph node syndrome (Kawasaki's disease)? Chest 111: 796-9
159. Bradley DJ, Glode MP (1998) Kawasaki disease. The mystery continues. West J Med 168: 23-9
160. Kim NS, Menahem S (1998) Serious sequels of Kawasaki disease. Cardiol Young 8: 386-9
161. Ohni S, Goto S, Nakamura H, Yamada T, Taira M, Sakurai I (1998) Adult multiple coronary aneurysms of Kawasaki's disease's sequelae; two autopsy cases. Rinsho Byori 46: 177-81
162. Kato H, Inoue O, Kawasaki T, Fujiwara H, Watanabe T, Toshima H (1992) Adult coronary artery disease probably due to childhood Kawasaki disease. Lancet 340: 1127-9
163. Landing BH, Larson EJ (1977) Are infantile periarteritis nodosa with coronary artery involvement and fetal mucocutaneous lymph node syndrome the same? Comparison of 20 patients from North America with patients from Hawaii and Japan. Pediatrics 59: 651-62
163. Tanaka N, Sekimoto K, Naoe S (1976) Kawasaki disease-Relationship with infantile periarteritis nodosa. Arch Pathol Lab Med 100: 81-6
165. Martelle RR (1955) Coronary thrombosis in a five-month-old infant. J Pediatr 46: 322-6
166. Leavitt RY, Fauci AS, Bloch DA, Michel BA, Hunder GG, Arend WP, Calabrese LH, Fries JF, Lie JT, Lightfoot RW Jr, et al (1990) The American College of Rheumatology 1990 criteria for the classification of Wegener's granulomatosis. Arthritis Rheum 33: 1101-7
167. Horn RG, Fauci AS, Rosenthal AS, Wolff SM (1974) Renal biopsy pathology in Wegener's granulomatosis. Am J Pathol 74: 423-40
168. Barksdale SK, Hallahan CW, Kerr GS, Fauci AS, Stern JB, Travis WD (1995) Cutaneous pathology in Wegener's granulomatosis. A clinicopathologic study of 75 biopsies in 46 patients. Am J Surg Pathol 19: 161-72
169. Carrington CB, Liebow A (1966) Limited forms of angiitis and granulomatosis of Wegener's type. Am J Med 41: 497-527
170. Cassan SM, Coles DT, Harrison EG Jr (1970) The concept of limited forms of Wegener's granulomatosis. Am J Med 49: 366-79
171. Iglesias PA, Zelman S, Guillan RA (1970) Granulomatous polyarteritis. Wegener's granulomatosis "limited form". J Kans Med Soc 71: 460-4
172. Leu HJ (1979) Pathergic granulomatoses. Pathomorphology of classical and limited form of Wegener's granulomatosis, of lymphomatoid granulomatosis and of eosinophilic granulomatous angiitis. Vasa 8: 203-12
173. DeRemee RA, McDonald TJ, Harrison EG Jr, Coles DT (1976) Wegener's granulomatosis. Anatomic correlates, a proposed classification. Mayo Clin Proc 51: 777-81
174. Krupsky M, Landau Z, Lifschitz-Mercer B, Resnitzky P (1993) Wegener's granulomatosis with peripheral eosinophilia. Atypical variant of a classic disease. Chest 104: 1290-2
175. Rosignoli M, Pezzuto RW, Galli J, D'Alatri L (1992) Midline granuloma and Wegener's granulomatosis. Acta Otorhinolaryngol Ital 12: S1-S46
176. De Gioanni PP, Bosco GF, Modica R (1993) Midline granuloma. A clinical case report. Minerva Stomatol 42: 107-12
177. Rothacher UM, Rump JA, Herbst EW, Blum U, Maier W, Peter HH (1994) Differential diagnostic aspects of lethal midline granulomas (granuloma gangraenescens). Immun Infekt 22: 158-60

178. Lee PY, Freeman NJ, Khorsand J, Weinstock MA (1997) Angiocentric T-cell lymphoma presenting as lethal midline granuloma. Int J Dermatol 36: 419-27

179. Sakata K, Hareyama M, Oouchi A, Sido M, Nagakura H, Morita K, Harabuchi Y, Kataura A, Hinoda Y (1998) Treatment of localized non-Hodgkin's lymphomas of the head and neck: focusing on cases of non-lethal midline granuloma. Radiat Oncol Investig 6: 161-9

180. Tamura S, Yamanaka N, Saito T, Takano I, Hotomi M, Yokoyama M (1996) Two cases of lethal midline granuloma thought to be of natural killer cell origin. Nippon Jibiinkoka Gakkai Kaiho 99: 46-53

181. Savage CO, Winearls CG, Evans DJ, Rees AJ, Lockwood CM (1985) Microscopic polyarteritis: presentation, pathology and prognosis. Q J Med 56: 467-83

182. Kohsokabe S, Fujita J, Tanaka M, Imai T, Fukuda J (1995) An autopsy case of microscopic polyarteritis nodosa resembling Schoenlein-Henoch purpura. Ryumachi 35: 899-903

183. Masi AT, Hunder GG, Lie JT, Michel BA, Bloch DA, Arend WP, Calabrese LH, Edworthy SM, Fauci AS, Leavitt RY, et al (1990) The American College of Rheumatology 1990 criteria for the classification of Churg-Strauss syndrome (allergic granulomatosis and angiitis). Arthritis Rheum 33: 1094-100

184. Crotty CP, Deremee RA, Wikelmann RK (1981) Cutaneous clinicopathologic correlation of allergic granulomatosis. J Am Acad Dermatol 5: 571-81

185. Trittel C, Moller J, Euler HH, Werner JA (1995) Churg-Strauss syndrome. A differential diagnosis in chronic polypoid sinusitis. Laryngorhinootologie 74: 577-80

186. Dicken CH, Wilkelmann RK (1978) The Churg-Strauss granuloma: cutaneous, necrotizing, palisading granuloma in vasculitis syndromes. Arch Pathol Lab Med 102: 576-80

187. Churg A (1991) Vasculitis and mimics of vasculitis involving the lungs. In Churg A, Churg, J. (eds.): Systemic Vasculitides. New York, Igaku-Shoin p. 121

188. Burke GW, Cirocco R, Markou M, Viciana A, Ruiz P, Allouch M, Esquenazi V, Roth D, Nery J, Miller J (1995) Acute graft loss secondary to necrotizing vasculitis. Evidence for cytokine-mediated Shwartzman reaction in clinical kidney transplantation. Transplantation 59: 1100-4

189. Aziz S, McDonald TO, Gohra H (1995) Transplant arterial vasculopathy: evidence for a dual pattern of endothelial injury and the source of smooth muscle cells in lesions of intimal hyperplasia. J Heart Lung Transplant 14: S123-36

190. Koskinen P, Lemstrom K, Bruggeman C, Lautenschlager I, Hayry P (1994) Acute cytomegalovirus infection induces a subendothelial inflammation (endothelialitis) in the allograft vascular wall. A possible linkage with enhanced allograft arteriosclerosis. Am J Pathol 144:41-50

191. Buttner T, Heye N, Przuntek H (1994) Temporal arteritis with cerebral complications: report of four cases. Eur Neurol 34: 162-7

192. Lambert M, Weber A, Boland B, De Plaen JF, Donckier J (1996) Large vessel vasculitis without temporal artery involvement: isolated form of giant cell arteritis? Clin Rheumatol 15: 174-80

193. Landrin I, Chassagne P, Bouaniche M, Dominique S, Doucet J, Nouvet G, Bercoff E (1997) Pulmonary artery thrombosis in giant cell arteritis. A new case and review of literature. Ann Med Interne (Paris) 148: 315-6

194. Thielen KR, Wijdicks EF, Nichols DA (1998) Giant cell (temporal) arteritis: involvement of the vertebral and internal carotid arteries. Mayo Clin Proc 73: 444-6

195. Vered Z, Pras M, Horowitz A, Rath S, Neufeld HN (1986) Severe aortic regurgitation: a rare presentation of giant cell arteritis. Clin Cardiol 9: 509-11

196. Cormier JM, Vuong-Ngoc P (1995) Un anévrysme inflammatoire inhabituel: maladie de Horton de l'aorte sous-rénale. Cardinale 7: 22-5

197. Bosson C, Hadrami J, Kharsa G, Lim DQ, Nitel M, Chotard Y (1996) Spontaneous rupture of the ascending aorta disclosing inflammatory arteritis. Arch Mal Cœur Vaiss 89: 1683-6

198. Manigand G, Taillandier J, Benhamou A, Barbagelatta M, Lemaigre G (1982) Aortic dissection and Horton arteritis. Mal Vasc 7: 217-20

199. Lagrand WK, Hoogendoorn M, Bakker K, te Velde J, Labrie A (1996) Aortoduodenal fistula as an unusual and fatal manifestation of giant-cell arteritis. Eur J Vasc Endovasc Surg 11: 502-3

200. Tozzi N, Kharsa G, Olivier A (1998) Giant cell arteritis and necrosis of the small intestine. Report of a case. J Mal Vasc 23: 293-6

201. Dummer W, Zillikens D, Schulz A, Brocker EB, Hamm H (1996) Scalp necrosis in temporal (giant cell) arteritis:implications for the dermatologic surgeon. Clin Exp Dermatol 21: 154-8

202. Ostberg G (1972) Morphological changes in the large arteries in polymyalgia arteritica. Acta Med Scand (Suppl) 533: 135-64

203. Klein RG, Hunder GG, Stanson AW, Sheps SG (1975) Large artery involvement in giant cell (temporal) arteritis. Ann Int Med 83: 806-12

204. Gonzalez-Gay MA, Blanco R, Abraira V, Garcia-Porrua C, Ibanez D, Garcia-Pais MJ, Rigueiro MT, Sanchez-Andrade A, Guerrero J, Casariego E (1997) Giant cell arteritis in Lugo, Spain, is associated with low longterm mortality. Rheumatol 24: 2171-6

205. Mickley V, Hutschenreiter S, Kogel H, Vogel U, Sunder-Plassmann L (1992) Giant cell arteritis of the arteries of the arm. Diagnosis, surgical indications and choice of procedure. Vasa Suppl 35: 53-4

206. Martinez-Taboada V, Brack A, Hunder GG, Goronzy JJ, Weyand CM (1996) The inflammatory infiltrate in giant cell arteritis selects against B lymphocytes. J Rheumatol 23: 1011-4

207. Martinez-Taboada V, Hunder NN, Hunder GG, Weyand CM, Goronzy JJ (1996) Recognition of tissue residing antigen by T cells in vasculitic lesions of giant cell arteritis. J Mol Med 74: 695-703

208. Brack A, Geisler A, Martinez-Taboada VM, Younge BR, Goronzy JJ, Weyand CM (1997) Giant cell vasculitis is a T cell-dependent disease. Mol Med 3: 530-43

209. Hunder GG (1998) Giant cell arteritis. Lupus 7: 266-9

210. Nordborg E, Nordborg C (1998) The inflammatory reaction in giant cell arteritis: an immunohistochemical investigation. Clinical and Experimental Rheumatology 16: 165-8

211. Knecht S, Henningsen H, Rauterberg EW (1991) Immunohistology of temporal arteritis: phenotyping of infiltrating cells and deposits of complement components. J Neurol 238: 181-2

212. Shintani S, Tsuruoka S, Tamaki M, Mihara N, Shiigai T, Kikuchi M (1995) Immunofluorescence study of immune complexes in polymyalgia rheumatica. J Neurol Sci 128: 103-6

213. Velvart M, Felder M, Fehr K, Sommermeyer G, Cancer M, Wagenhauser FJ, Boni A (1983) Temporal arteritis in polymyalgia rheumatica: immune complex deposits and the role of the leukocyte elastase in the pathogenesis. Z Rheumatol 42: 320-7

214. O'Brien JP, Regan W (1998) Actinically degenerate elastic tissue: the prime antigen in the giant cell (temporal) arteritis syndrome ? New data from the posterior ciliary arteries. Clin Exp Rheumatol 16: 39-48

215. Tomita T, Imakawa K (1998) Matrix metalloproteinases and tissue inhibitors of metalloproteinases in giant cell arteritis: an immunocytochemical study. Pathology 30: 40-50

216. Hunder GG, Bloch DA, Michel BA, Stevens MB, Arend WP, Calabrese LH, Edworthy SM, Fauci AS, Leavitt RY, Lie JT, et al (1990) The American College of Rheumatology 1990 criteria for the classification of giant cell arteritis. Arthritis Rheum 33: 1122-8

217. Rao JK, Allen NB, Pincus T (1998) Limitations of the 1990 American College of Rheumatology classification criteria in the diagnosis of vasculitis. Ann Intern Med 129: 345-52

218. Savory WS (1856) Case of a young woman in whom the main arteries of both upper extremities and of the left side of the neck were throughout completely obliterated. Med Chir Trans Lond 39: 205.

219. Numano F, Kobayashi Y, Maruyama Y, Kakuta T, Miyata T, Kishi Y (1996) Takayasu arteritis: clinical characteristics and the role of genetic factors in its pathogenesis. Vasc Med 1: 227-33

220. Luppi-Herrera L, Sanchez-Torres G, Marcushamer J, Mispireta J, Horwitz S, Vela JE (1977) Takayasu's arteritis. Clinical study of 107 cases. Am Heart J 93: 94-103

221. Fiessinger JN, Camilleri JP, Cormier JM, Housset E (1983) Takayasu's disease: diagnosis. Ann Med Interne (Paris) 134(5): 441-3

222. Hall S, Barr W, Lie JT, Stanson AW, Kazmier FJ, Hunder GG (1985) Takayasu arteritis. A study of 32 North American patients. Medicine 64: 89-99

223. Robles M, Reyes PA (1994) Takayasu's arteritis in Mexico: a clinical review of 44 consecutive cases. Clin Exp Rheumatol 12: 381-8

224. Wahab AS, Sunarto, Soebardi A, Harlistyanti R (1990) Takayasu's disease. Paediatr Indones 30: 313-8

225. Jain S, Kumari S, Ganguly NK, Sharma BK (1996) Current status of Takayasu arteritis in India. Int J Cardiol 54: S111-6

226. Ito I (1995) Aortitis syndrome (Takayasu's arteritis). A historical perspective. Jpn Heart J 36: 273-81

227. Hernandez Pando R, Espitia C, Mancilla R, Reyes PA (1994) Takayasu's arteritis. A seroimmunological test of its relationship to mycobacterial infection. Arch Inst Cardiol Mex 64: 331-7

228. Aggarwal A, Chag M, Sinha N, Naik S (1996) Takayasu's arteritis: role of Mycobacterium tuberculosis and its 65 kDa heat shock protein. Int J Cardiol 55: 49-55

229. De Bandt M, Kahn MF (1991) Takayasu's arteritis associated with Still's disease in an adult. Clin Exp Rheumatol 9: 639-40

230. Hidano A, Watanabe K (1981) Pyoderma gangrenosum and cardio-vasculopathies, particularly Takayasu arteritis. Review of the Japanese literature. Ann Dermatol Venerol 108: 13-21

231. Yoshida H, Tomokuni T, Tamura K, Watase K, Matsuwaka R, Matsuda H (1992) A surgical case of thoracic aortic aneurysm due to Takayasu's aortitis associated with ulcerative colitis. Nippon Kyobu Geka Gakkai Zasshi 40: 1135-9

232. Houman MH, Doghri A, Boubaker J, Kchir MN, Mahdhaoui A, Filali A, Miled M (1996) Takayasu disease in Crohn disease: an exceptional association. Ann Gastroenterol Hepatol (Paris) 31: 337-40

233. Aoyagi S, Akashi H, Kawara T, Ishihara K, Tanaka A, Kanaya S, Koga Y, Ishikawa R (1998) Aortic root replacement for Takayasu arteritis associated with ulcerative colitis and ankylosing spondylitis—report of a case. Jpn Circ J 62: 64-8

234. Arita M, Iwane M, Nakamura Y, Nishio I (1998) Anticoagulants in Takayasu's arteritis associated with crescentic glomerulonephritis and nephrotic syndrome: a case report. Angiology 49: 75-8

235. Numano F (1992) Hereditary factors of Takayasu arteritis. Heart Vessels Suppl 7: 68-72

236. Numano F, Kakuta T (1996) Takayasu arteritis—five doctors in the history of Takayasu arteritis. Int J Cardiol 54: S1-S10

237. Perniciaro CV, Winkelmann RK, Hunder GG (1987) Cutaneous manifestations of Takayasu's arteritis. J Amer Acad Dermatol 17: 998-1005

238. Gupta SK, Khanna MN, Lahiri TK, Goel AK (1980) Involvement of cardiac valves in Takayasu's arteritis. Report of seven cases. Indian Heart J 32: 147-55

239. Acar C, Farge A, Ramsheyi A, Julia P, Fabiani JN, Bruneval P, Fiessinger JN, Carpentier A (1993) Combined surgery of the mitral valve and the abdominal aorta in a case of Takayasu's disease. Ann Cardiol Angeiol (Paris) 42: 475-3

240. Takagi M, Ikeda T, Kimura K, Saito Y, Ishii M, Takeda T, Murao S (1984) Renal histological studies in patients with Takayasu's arteritis. Report of 3 cases. Nephron 36: 68-73

241. Lande A, Berkmen YM (1986) Radiologic aspects of aortitis In Lande A, Berkmen YM, McAllister HA Jr (ed.) Aortitis: Clinical,pathologic,and Radiographic aspects. Raven Press, NewYork 81-143

242. Lagneau P, Michel JB, Vuong PN (1987) Surgical treatment of Takayasu's disease. Ann Surg 205: 157-66

243. Ishikawa K (1988) Diagnostic approach and proposed criteria for the clinical diagnosis of Takayasu's arteriopathy. JACC 12: 964-72

244. Nasu T (1963) Pathology of pulseless disease. A systematic study and critical review of 21 autopsy cases reported in Japan. Angiology 14: 255-42

245. Camilleri JP, Bruneval P (1989) The vasculitis syndromes in aorta and large arteries. Pathological aspects. In Camilleri JP, Berry CL, Fiessinger J-N, Bariety J (eds) Diseases of the arterial wall. Springer -Verlag, London 457-82

246. Küssmaul A, Maier R (1866) Ueber eine bisher nicht beschriebene eigenthümliche Arterienerkrankung (periarteritis nodosa), die mit Morbus Brightü und rapid fortschreitender allgemeiner Muskellälmung einhergeht. Dtsch Arch Klin Med 1: 484-518

247. Diaz-Perez JL, Schroeter AL, Winkelmann RK (1980) Cutaneous periarteritis nodosa: immunofluorescence studies. Arch Dermatol 116: 56-8

248. Kelsall JT, Chalmers A, Sherlock CH, Tron VA, Kelsall AC (1997) Microscopic polyangiitis after influenza vaccination. J Rheumatol 24: 1198-202

249. Mullick FG, McAllister HA Jr, Wagner BM, Fenoglio JJ Jr (1979) Drug related vasculitis. Clinicopathologic correlations in 30 patients. Hum Pathol 10: 313-25

250. Hanton G, Le Net JL, Ruty B, Leblanc B (1995) Characterization of the arteritis induced by infusion of rats with UK-61,260, an inodilator, for 24 h. A comparison with the arteritis induced by fenoldopam mesylate. Arch Toxicol 69: 698-704

251. Sepp NT, Umlauft F, Illersperger B, Grunewald K, Schuler G, Greil R, Vogel W (1995) Necrotizing vasculitis associated with hepatitis C virus infection: successful treatment of vasculitis with interferon-alpha despite persistence of mixed cryoglobulinaemia. Dermatology 191: 43-5

252. Drueke T, Barbanel C, Jungers P, Digeon M, Poisson M, Brivet F, Trecan G, Feldmann G, Crosnier J, Bach JF (1980) Hepatitis B antigen-associated periarteritis nodosa in patients undergoing long-term hemodialysis. Am J Med 68: 86-90

253. Calabrese LH (1991) Vasculitis and infection with the human immunodeficiency virus. Rheum Dis Clin North Am 17: 131-47

254. Debat Zoguereh D, Badiaga S, Girard N (1997) Periarteritis nodosa disclosed by epilepsy in a drug addict with hepatitis B and C virus carrier state. Rev Med Interne 18: 311-5

255. Guillevin L, Lhote F (1997) Classification and management of necrotising vasculitides. Drugs 53: 805-16

256. Hartmann H (1997) Extrahepatic manifestations of HBV and HCV infection. Schweiz Rundsch Med Prax 86: 1163-6

257. Ginarte M, Pereiro M, Toribio J (1998) Cutaneous polyarteritis nodosa in a child. Pediatr Dermatol 15: 103-7

258. Kumar L, Thapa BR, Sarkar B, Walia BN (1995) Benign cutaneous polyarteritis nodosa in children below 10 years of age—a clinical experience. Ann Rheum Dis 54: 134-6

259. Gunal N, Kara N, Cakar N, Kocak H, Kahramanyol O, Cetinkaya E (1997) Cardiac involvement in childhood polyarteritis nodosa. Int J Cardiol 60: 257-62

260. Maeda M, Kobayashi M, Okamoto S, Fuse T, Matsuyama T, Watanabe N, Fujikawa S (1997) Clinical observation of 14 cases of childhood polyarteritis nodosa in Japan. Acta Paediatr Jpn 39: 277-9

261. Cupps TR, Fauci AS (1981) The vasculitides In Smith LH (ed.) Major problems in Internal Medicine, Vol XXI, WB Saunders, Philadelphia p 26-49

262. Cupps TR, Moore PM, Fauci AS (1983) Isolated angiitis of the central nervous system. Prospective diagnostic and therapeutic experience. Am J Med 74: 97-105

263. Inoue M, Akikusa B, Masuda Y, Kondo Y (1998) Demonstration of microaneurysms at the interlobular arteries of the kidneys in microscopic polyangiitis: a three-dimensional study. Hum Pathol 29: 223-7

264. Clement PB, Senges H, How AR (1987) Giant cell arteritis of the breast: case report and literature review. 18: 1186-9

265. Vuong PN, Lehir A, Nguyen H, Faucheur B (1988) Artérite à cellules géantes isolée de la vésicule biliaire. Etude anatomo-clinique d'une observation et discussion pathogénique. Arch Anat Cytol Path 36: 229-233

266. Vuong NP, Guerrieri MT, Alexandre JH, Camilleri JP (1984) Early histological changes in acute pancreatitis. A retrospective pathological study of 20 total pancreatectomy specimens. Path Res Pract 178: 273-279

267. Chen KT (1989) Gallbladder vasculitis. J Clin Gastroenterol 11: 537-40

268. Fayemi AD, Ali M, Braun EJ (1972) Necrotizing vasculitis of the gallbladder and the appendix. Am J Gastroenterol 67: 608-12

269. Desbazeille F, Soule JC (1986) Manifestations digestives des vascularites. Gastroenterol Clin Biol 10: 405-14

270. Fetissof F, Lansac J (1980) Artérite nécrosante et granulomateuse isolée du col de l'utérus. Nouv Press Med 9: 3094-5

271. Yoo B, Kim HK, Choi SW, Moon HB (1996) A case of polyarteritis nodosa with bilateral ureteral obstruction. Korean J Intern Med 11: 165-8

272. Ferreiro JE, Saldana MJ, Azevedo SJ (1986) Polyarteritis manifesting as calf myositis and fever. Am J Med 80: 312-5

273. Papaioannou CC, Hunder GG, Lie JT (1979) Vasculitis of the gallbladder in a 70 year-old man with giant cell (temporal) arteritis. J Rheumatol 6: 71-5

274. Thael JF, Saue GL (1983) Giant cell arteritis involving the breasts. J Rheumatol 10: 329-31

275. Dechelotte P, Dauplat J, Philippe P, Sauvezie B, Fonck Y (1985) Giant cell arteritis of the uterus. Apropos of a case. Ann Pathol 5: 217-9

276. Schneider V (1981) Visceral giant cell arteritis limited to the female genital tract. J Reprod Med 26: 328-31

277. Bell DA, Mondschein M, Scully RE (1986) Giant cell arteritis of the female genital tract. A report of three cases. Am J Surg Pathol 10: 696-701

278. Lie JT (1978) Disseminated visceral giant cell arteritis. Am J Clin Pathol 69: 299-305

279. Zerbino DD (1981) Giant cell vasculitis (arteries and phlebitis). Arkhiv Pathologit 43: 42-7

280. Calabrese LH, Furlan AJ, Gragg LA, Ropos TJ (1992) Primary angiitis of the central nervous system: diagnostic criteria and clinical approach. Cleve Clin J Med 59: 293-306

281. Moore PM, Fauci AS (1981) Neurologic manifestations of systemic vasculitis. A retrospective and prospective study of the clinico-pathologic features and response to therapy in 25 patients. Am J Med 71: 517-24

282. Rothenberg R (1985) Isolated angiitis of the brain. Case in a renal transplant recipient. Am J Med 79: 629-32

283. Wenzel RP, Hayden FG, Groschel DH, Salata RA, Young WS, Greenlee JE, Newman S, Miller PJ, Hechemy KE, Burgdorfer W, et al (1986) Acute febrile cerebrovasculitis: a syndrome of unknown, perhaps rickettsial, cause. Ann Intern Med 104: 606-15

284.-Rush PJ, Inman R, Berstein M (1986) Isolated vasculitis of the central nervous system in a patient with celiac disease. Am J Med 81: 1092-4

285. Parisi J, Moore P (1994) The role of biopsy in vasculitis of the central nervous system. Seminars in Neurology. 14: 341-8

286. Chu CT, Gray L, Goldstein LB, Hulette CM (1998) Diagnosis of intracranial vasculitis: a multi-disciplinary approach. J Neuropathol Exp Neurol 57: 30-8

287. Girard PL, Dumas M, Escourolle R, Ciudad MA, Gray MF, Ndiaye IP (1976) Giant cell granulomatous angiitis of the central nervous system. Rev Neurol (Paris) 132: 369-82

288. Calvani M (1989) Cerebral vasculitis in children. Pediatr Med Chir 11: S57-S61

289. Kokmen E, Bilman JrK, Abell MR (1977) Lymphomatoid granulomatosis clinically confined to the CNS. Arch Neurol 34: 782-4

290. James DG, Spiteri MA (1982) Behçet's disease. Ophthalmology 89: 1279-84

291. Michaelson JB, Friedlander MH (1990) Behçet's disease. Int Ophthalmol Clin 30: 271-8

292. Wechsler B, Le Thi Huong Du, De Gennes, Bletry O, Piette JC, Mathieu A et al (1989) Manifestations arté-

rielles de la maladie de Behçet. Douze observations. Rev Méd Interne 10: 303-11

293. Hamza M (1987) Large artery involvement in Behcet's disease. J Rheumatol 14: 554-9

294. O'Duffy JD, Goldstein NP (1976) Neurologic involvement in seven patients with Behcet's disease. Am J Med 61: 170-8

295. Mangelsdorf HC, White WL, Jorizzo JL (1996) Behcet's disease. Report of twenty-five patients from the United States with prominent mucocutaneous involvement. J Am Acad Dermatol 34: 745-50

296. Lie JT (1992) Vascular involvement in Behçet's disease arterial and venous and vessels of all sizes. J Rheumatol 19: 341-3

297. Koc Y, Gullu I,Akpek G, Akpolat T, Kans VE, Kiraz et al (1992) Vascular involvement in Behçet's disease. J Rheumatol 19: 402-10

298.-Sakane T, Suzuki N, Nagafuchi H (1997) Etiopathology of Behcet's disease: immunological aspects. Yonsei Med J 38: 350-8

299. Benezra D (1998) Primary association of HLA-B51 with Behcet's disease in Ireland (letter) Br J Ophthalmol 82: 715

300. Gonzalez-Escribano MF, Rodriguez MR, Walter K, Sanchez-Roman J, Garcia-Lozano JR, Nunez-Roldan A (1998) Association of HLA-B51 subtypes and Behcet's disease in Spain. Tissue Antigens 52: 78-80

301. Lee S, Bang D, Cho YH, Lee ES, Sohn S (1996) Polymerase chain reaction reveals herpes simplex virus DNA in saliva of patients with Behcet's disease. Arch Dermatol Res 288: 179-83

302. Sohn S, Lee ES, Bang D, Lee S (1998) Behcet's disease-like symptoms induced by the herpes simplex virus in ICR mice. Eur J Dermatol 8: 21-3

303. Chajek T, Fainara J (1975) Behcet's disease: Report of 41 cases and a review of the literature. Medicine (Baltimore) 54: 179-96

304. Piers A (1977) Behcet's disease with arterial and renal manifestations. Proc R Soc Med 70: 540-4

305. Hamza M, Horchani H, Elleuch M, Hamza K, Chaker C, Fourati M, Hamza R, Zribi A, Ennabli E (1988) Arterial involvement in Behcet's disease. J Mal Vasc 13: 245-9

306. Giordano N, Senesi M, Mondillo S, Palumbo F, Battisti E, D'Aprile N, Faglia S, Mangiacotti L, Palazzuoli V, Nami R, Gennari C (1996) Heart involvement in Behcet's disease: a personal caseload en review of the literature. G Ital Cardiol 26: 519-25

307. Matsumoto T, Uekusa T, Fukuda Y (1991) Vasculo-Behcet's disease: a pathologic study of eight cases. Hum Pathol 22: 45-51

308. Honma M, Hamauzu N, Honma M, Takeuchi A, Hashimoto T, Imamura T, Inaba G (1991) Histopathological examination of a case of Behcet's disease with aortic regurgitation. Ryumachi 31: 62-7

309. Chen KR, Kawahara Y, Miyakawa S, Nishikawa T (1997) Cutaneous vasculitis in Behcet's disease: a clinical and histopathologic study of 20 patients. J Am Acad Dermatol 36: 689-96

310. Gotor MA, Medrano J, Ruiz C, Alfonso ER, Guerrero J, de Gregorio MA (1997) Pulmonary artery aneurysm and thrombosis caused by vasculitis in Behcet's disease. Arch Bronconeumol 33: 591-3

311. Buerger L (1908) Thrombo-angiitis obliterans: a study of the vascular lesions leading to the presenile spontaneous gangrene. Am J Med Sci 136: 567-80

312. Lie JT, Mann RJ, Ludwig J (1979) The brothers von Winiwarter, Alexander (1848-1917) and Felix (1852-1931),

313. Lie JT (1987) Thromboangiitis obliterans (Buerger's disease) in women. Medicine (Baltimore) 66: 65-72

314. Lie JT (1989) The rise and fall and resurgence of thromboangiitis obliterans (Buerger's disease). Acta Pathol Jpn 39: 153-8

315. Lie JT (1987) Thromboangiitis obliterans (Buerger's disease) in an elderly man after cessation of cigarette smoking—a case report. Angiology 38: 864-7

316. Marandian MH, Saboury-Deilami M, Rakchan M, Lessani M, Behvad A, Grouhi M (1985) Thromboangiitis obliterans and distal gangrene in a 5-year-old child. Pediatrie 40: 553-7

317. McLoughlin GA, Helsby CR, Evans CC, Chapman DM (1976) Association of HLA-A9 and HLA-B5 with Buerger's disease. Br Med J 2: 1165-6

318. Adar R, Papa MZ, Halpern Z, Mozes M, Shoshan S, Sofer B, Zinger H, Dayan M, Mozes E (1983) Cellular sensitivity to collagen in thromboangiitis obliterans. N Engl J Med 308 1113-6

319. Juergens JL (1980) Thromboangiitis obliterans (Buerger's disease, TAO) In Juergens JL, Spittell JA, Fairbairn II JF (ed) Peripheral vascular diseases. Saunders, Philadelphia, London, Toronto 469-91

320. Feng HM, Wen J, Walker DH (1993) Rickettsia australis infection: a murine model of a highly invasive vasculopathic rickettsiosis. Am J Pathol 142: 1471-82

321. Belcaro G Nicolaides AN, Veller M (1995) Venous disorders. A manual of diagnosis and treatment. Saunders, London, Philadelphia, Toronto, Sidney, Tokyo

322. Goodmar RM, Elian B, Mozes M, Deutsch V (1965) Buerger's disease in Israel. Am J Med 39: 601-15

323. Ohta T, Shionoya S (1988) Fate of the ischemic limb in Buerger's disease. Br J Surg 75: 259-62

324. Dehaine-Bamberger N, Amar R, Touboul C, Emmrich J, Fiessinger J-N (1993) Aspects cliniques et prognostic de la maladie de Buerger. 83 observations. Presse Méd (Paris) 22: 945-8

325. Hagen B, Lohse S (1984) Clinical and radiologic aspects of Buerger's disease. Cardiovasc Intervent Radiol 7: 283-93

326. Kurata A, Franke FE, Machinami R, Schulz A (2000) Thromboangiitis obliterans: classic and new morphological features.Virchows Arch 436: 59-67

327. Davis RB (1985) Acute thrombotic complications of myeloproliferative disorders in young adults. Am J Clin Pathol 84: 180-5

328. Cheson BD, Bluming AZ, Alroy J (1976) Cogan's syndrome: a systemic vasculitis. Am J Med 60: 549-55

329. Vollertsen RS (1990) Vasculitis and Cogan's syndrome. Rheum Dis Clin North Am 16: 433-9

330. Ochonisky S, Chosidow O, Kuentz M, Man N, Fraitag S, Pelisse JM, Revuz J (1991) Cogan's syndrome. An unusual etiology of urticarial vasculitis. Dermatologica 183: 218-20

331. Hughes GB, Kinney SE, Barna BP, Tomsak RL, Calabrese LH (1983) Autoimmune reactivity in Cogan's syndrome: a preliminary report. Otolaryngol Head Neck Surg 91: 24-32

332. Majoor MH, Albers FW, van der Gaag R, Gmelig-Meyling F, Huizing EH (1992) Corneal autoimmunity in Cogan's syndrome? Report of two cases. Ann Otol Rhinol Laryngol 101: 679-84

333. Oldenski R (1993) Cogan syndrome: autoimmune-mediated audiovestibular symptoms and ocular inflammation. J Am Board Fam Pract 6: 577-81

334. Hulse M, Partsch CJ (1975) The Cogan syndrome. Laryngol Rhinol Otol (Stuttg) 54: 977-85

335. Kaiser-Kupfer MI, Mittal KK, Del Valle LA, Haynes BF (1978) The HLA antigens in Cogan's syndrome. Am J Ophthalmol 86: 314-6

336. Takemura T, Matsui Y, Saiki S, Mikami R (1992) Pulmonary vascular involvement in sarcoidosis: a report of 40 autopsy cases. Hum Pathol 23: 1216-23

337. Mochizuki I, Kobayashi T, Wada R, Kawaguchi T, Ozawa K, Fukushima M, Hirose Y, Kono H, Takeda J, Kusama S, et al (1990) Vascular lesions in the biopsied bronchus of patients with sarcoidosis changes of the endothelial cells in aggregation of eosinophils. Sarcoidosis 7: 35-41

338. Garcia-Porrua C, Gonzalez-Gay MA, Garcia-Pais MJ, Blanco R (1998) Cutaneous vasculitis: an unusual presentation of sarcoidosis in adulthood. Scand J Rheumatol 27: 80-2

339. Blomgren SE (1974) Erythema nodosum. Semin Arthritis Rheum 4: 1-24

340. Bohn S, Buchner S, Itin P (1997) Erythema nodosum: 112 cases. Epidemiology, clinical aspects and histopathology. Schweiz Med Wochenschr 127: 1168-76

341. Dronda F, Gonzalez-Lopez A, Lecona M, Barros C (1996) Erythema elevatum diutinum in human immunodeficiency virus-infected patients—report of a case and review of the literature. Clin Exp Dermatol 21: 222-5

342. Montgomery H, O'Leary PA, Barker NW (1945) Nodular vascular diseases of the legs: erythema induratum and allied conditions. JAMA 128: 335-40

343. Beacham BE, Cooper PH, Buchanan CS, Weary PE (1980) Equestrian cold panniculitis in women. Arch Dermatol 116: 1025-7

344. Gombergh R, Blanchet-Bardon C, Delmas PF, Sohier J, Laval-Jeantet M, Puissant A (1981) Weber-Christian syndrome and chronic pancreatitis. Ann Radiol (Paris) 24: 651-5

345. Lonchampt F, Blanc D, Terrasse F, Humbert P, Kienzler JL, Agache P (1985) Weber-Christian disease associated with familial alpha-1-antitrypsin deficiency. Apropos of a case. Ann Dermatol Venereol 112: 35-9

346. Smith KC, Pittelkow MR, Su WP (1987) Panniculitis associated with severe alpha 1-antitrypsin deficiency. Treatment and review of the literature. Arch Dermatol 123: 1655-61

347. Panush RS, Yonker RA, Dlesk A, Longley S, Caldwell JR (1985) Weber-Christian disease. Analysis of 15 cases and review of the literature. Medicine (Baltimore) 64: 181-91

348. Kiguchi H, Kasahara K, Mochizuki M, Yasuda Y, Ishibashi T, Konishi F, Kanazawa K, Saitoh K, Waza K, Kawa-

mura H (1989) Weber-Christian disease associated with multiple perforations of the ileum and colon. Am J Gastroenterol 84: 808-10

349. White JW Jr, Winkelmann RK (1998) Weber-Christian panniculitis: a review of 30 cases with this diagnosis. J Am Acad Dermatol 39: 56-62

350. Förström L, Winkelmann RK (1977) Acute panniculitis: a clinical and histologic study of 34 cases. Arch Dermatol 113: 909-17

351. Ricevuti G, Balduini CL, Marabelli S, Ricevuti GP, Rizzo SC (1981) Non-suppurative recurrent febrile nodular panniculitis (Weber-Christian disease). Description of a case with disseminated intravascular coagulopathy. Recenti Prog Med 71: 30-40

352. Oyama H, Ueda M, Kida Y, Tanaka T, Iwakoshi T, Niwa M, Kitamura R, Taira M, Kobayashi T(1995) Subarachnoid hemorrhage of unknown origin associated with Weber-Christian disease – case report. Neurol Med Chir (Tokyo) 35: 454-7

353. Nieboer C, Kalsbeek GL (1978) Immunofluorescence studies in granuloma eosinophilicum faciale. J Cutan Pathol 5: 68-75

354. Powell FC, Schroeter AL, Su WPD, Perry HO (1985) Pyoderma gangrenosum: a review of 86 patients. Q J Med (NS) 55: 173-86

355. Holt PJA, Davies MG, Saunders KC, Nuki G (1980) Pyoderma gangrenosum: clinical and laboratory findings in 15 patients with special reference to polyarthritis. Medicine (Baltimore) 59: 114-33

356. Hickman JG, Lazarus GS (1980) Pyoderma gangrenosum: a reappraisal of associated systemic diseases. Br J Dermatol 102: 235-7

357. Hay CRM, Messenger AG, Cotton DWK, Bleehen SS, Winfield DA (1987) Atypical bullous pyoderma gangrenosum associated with myeloid malignancies. J Clin Pathol 40: 387-92

358. von den Driesch P (1997) Pyoderma gangrenosum: a report of 44 cases with follow-up. Br J Dermatol 137: 1000-5

359. Gilliam JN, Smiley JD (1976) Cutaneous necrotizing vasculitis and related disorders. Ann Allergy 37: 328-39

360. Oddis CV, Eisenbeis CH Jr, Reidbord HE, Steen VD, Medsger TA Jr (1987) Vasculitis in systemic sclerosis: association with Sjogren's syndrome and the CREST syndrome variant. J Rheumatol 14: 942-8

361. Abu-Shakra M, Koh ET, Treger T, Lee P (1995) Pericardial effusion and vasculitis in a patient with systemic sclerosis. J Rheumatol 22: 1386-1388

XII
Operative pathology

We use the term "operative pathology" here to describe lesions related to vascular surgical techniques, the implantation of a foreign body within the vascular wall, or changes which occur at the blood-arterial wall interface as a result of operative interference.

1 – Surgical procedures

Surgery is a form of controlled trauma with the potential to produce complications. Pre-operative assessment of the patient must take into account both the risks of the natural outcome of the untreated disease, and of the complications induced by the surgical repair of a vessel [1-4].

Vascular puncture and catheter procedures

Localised injury of the vascular wall is produced by puncture or catheterisation and endothelial denudation often leads to the formation of a thrombus [5]. The complication rate depends on a number of variables including the width, length, and composition of the catheter, the number of times catheters are exchanged, and the duration of the procedure. Arterial spasm may lead to thrombosis, particularly in children and young women [6]. Long-term central venous catheters may develop a thin, white adherent covering of tissue that has been referred to as a fibrin sheath. This tissue starts as thrombus and organises within 60 days postimplantation. This sheath is not dissolved by fibrinolytic agents such as urokinase, streptokinase, or tissue plasminogen activator and may interfere with catheter function [5, 7]. Superimposed *Candida* endomycoses may result in fatal systemic candidiasis [8]. Accidental catheter embolism is exceptional [9,10].

Vascular exposure and mobilisation

Exposure requires the separation of the peri-adventitia from the vessel with a temporarily disconnection of the affected segment from its nutrient vessels and nerves. This appears to be a practical problem only for diseased vessels with inflammation of the peri-adventitia. The problem is greater in re-operation, when fibrosis thickens the peri-adventitia and causes the vessel to stick to adjacent structures. Operative complications include extensive bleeding in the peri-adventitia, wounding of the exposed vessel, and inadvertent sectioning of a collateral vessel. Acute intraoperative arterial elongation leads to minor and patchy endothelial sloughing that heals in 72 hours; the inherent contractility of the vessel wall remains unchanged [11].

Vascular clamping

The arrest of blood flow may be partial, in lateral clamping, or total, when transverse clamping is used (whether by digital compression, loop compression, a metal clamp, or balloon catheter). Complications may be secondary either to cessation of flow or to the traumatic injury caused by the procedure itself. Cessation of flow induces acute thrombosis of a stenosed vessel, or ischaemia in its distribution if the collateral circulation is insufficient. Traumatic clamping injuries include crushing and necrosis of the vessel wall, detachment of a calcified atheromatous plaque, and plaque dissection. Forceps-type clamps with fine points on each blade impress multiple pricks or puncture injuries in the wall. Over-inflation of a balloon catheter used to clamp a vessel from inside the lumen causes abrasion of the endothelium with "compression" of intimal lesions into the media (a mechanism used in transluminal angioplasty). Excessive tightening of a loop tourniquet may produce a partial rupture, affecting the intima and media. When a loop is applied twice, the vessel is both strangled and pivoted on its axis, and the line of rupture is thus spiral in shape.

Vascular incision

In a diseased vessel a vascular incision shakes loose parts of the structure, for example necrotic or calcified atheromatous plaques. Complications depend on the site of the incision; there may be parietal dissection, mural thrombosis and distal embolism.

Vascular occlusion or ligation

During surgery, haemostasis of small vessels by means of a clip or by electric cauterization causes coagulative necrosis of the vascular wall. This process causes the vascular wall to retract, resulting in a thrombosis that leads to complete occlusion of the lumen.

Ligation exerts concentric compression on the arterial wall with reduction of the lumen and formation of a thrombus. This extends on both sides of the ligated area. Once organised, the thrombus occludes the ligated area permanently. Complications include haemorrhage and extensive thrombosis. Haemorrhage often results from loosening of the band of an unsecured ligature, or when the vascular segment to be ligated is incompletely exposed. An extensive thrombosis usually occurs in a vascular fork when one of the ligated collaterals has a long dead-end stump, leading to progressive and complete occlusion of the vascular lumen.

Vascular suture

During suturing, the needle must necessarily penetrate the vascular wall with each stitch causing a microscopic parietal wound. Histologically, each hole caused by the needle corresponds to a very limited detachment of the vascular endothelium, exposing the connective tissue below the intima. When suturing is complete, this area of detachment facilitates the adhesion of a layer of fibrin and platelets for 24 to 48 hrs. The process may be disturbed in a number of ways which include overtightening – when sutures are too tight, the thread may shear the edges of the vascular incision, resulting in haemorrhage with secondary loosening of the suture and delayed haematoma. The placement of stitches in continuous sutures with "bites" too far apart may cause leakage with haemorrhage or formation of a false aneurysm. Other faults occur with an overcast-type suture, composed of either simple stitches or mattress stitches, which may cause a defect in lining up the faces of the wound. An overcast stitch which is too tight may create a stenosis and stitches which are too close together increase fibrosis, making the wall of the artery rigid and giving rise to progressive stenosis [12, 13]. Healing of the sutured areas depends on the type of suture used and determines the haemodynamic profile of the injured area.

Arterial anastomosis

The aim of an anastomosis is not only to restore the continuity of the vessel but to preserve its anatomical configuration. Anastomoses may be side-to-side, end-to-end or end-to-side. Complications may follow inadequate geometrical configuration and will depend on the type of anastomosis for their rheological effects.

Side-to-side anastomosis

Anatomical complications affecting flow are rare.

End-to-side anastomosis

This is the most commonly used technique for connecting a long bypass or to implant one vessel in another while preserving collaterals in the excised segment. However, haemodynamic complications depend on the outline of the section of the vessel to be implanted. Stenosis may occur when the vascular end is perpendicular (Fig. 1). A bevelled cut permits an angular configuration and, in general, it is fair to say that the greater the angle of connection, the greater the turbulence in the blood flow. Turbulence predisposes to thrombosis, dilatation and aneurysm formation with decreased blood flow below the anastomosis. A 45° connecting angle produces blood flow close to normal. When the bevel is too long, the end may fold just in front of the anastomosis after suturing. Too great a tension at this end both flattens and causes a "Y" deformity of the recipient side branch.

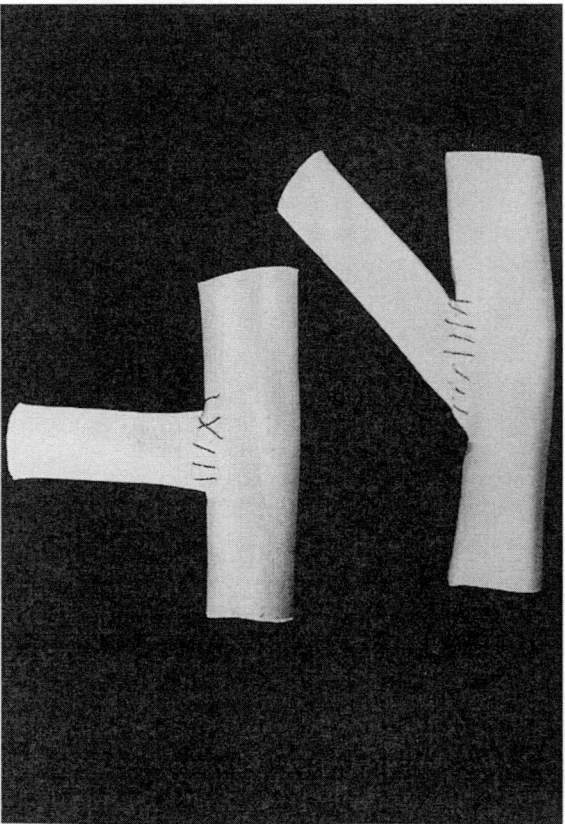

Fig. 1. Side-to-end anastomosis. (Courtesy Dr P. Desoutter)

Insufficient tension causes redundancy or a "dolicho-collateral". All of these defects in vascular geometry cause turbulent blood flow.

End-to-end anastomosis

The pattern of organization of an end-to-end anastomosis of two blood vessels having the same diameter is similar to that of a vascular suture. When the vessels have different diameters (Fig. 2), the anastomosis must lead to a functional stenosis with compliance mismatch. When the bypass has a smaller diameter, the larger recipient vessel behaves as a post-stenotic dilatation with consequent turbulent blood flow with a potential for thrombosis. This complication can be avoided in two ways: the end of the smaller vessel can be enlarged by two slits, thus allowing it to line up adequately with the larger vessel; it is also possible to make an oblique incision or a wide cut at both ends of both vessels. A single slit in one vessel can cause an angulation just before the anastomosis, after it is sutured. This defect in the configuration of the artery

causes the later development of fibroblastic endarteritis in arterial anastomosis.

Late complications

Intimal hyperplasia

This process is permanent, whatever type of anastomosis is performed, and contributes to changes in vascular compliance, frequently producing stenosis, thrombosis and favoring the development of atherosclerosis [14]. It occurs near the distal or lower end of bypasses, and, in the femoro-popliteal segment, usually becomes manifest at 3 to 12 months. Proximally, intimal hyperplasia is likely to be severe when the angle of incidence of the two segments is greater than 55 [15]. Grossly, there is whitish bulging of the intima, including the suture line. This bump is circumferential in an end-to-end, but more limited in an end-to-side anastomosis. Histologically, the intima of the recipient vessel shows fibrotic thickening, producing an intimal flap that overlaps the anastomotic line.

False aneurysm

Overtight suturing of the anastomotic line, and inappropriate suture material and angle of incidence of sutured vessels will cause necrosis in the wall and damage to the ends of prostheses. This disruption produces haemorrhage or fluid leakage with surrounding haematomas, and the process of organisation may lead to a false aneurysm [16]. The incidence of para-anastomotic false aneurysms increases with time (0.8, 6.2, and 35.8%, at 5, 10, and 15 years respectively) [17].

2 – Pathology related to surgical techniques

Thrombo-endarterectomy

This procedure excises the internal occluding atheromatous deposits in order to restore the patency of the vascular lumen. The remaining wall is composed of the external portion of the media, the external elastic lamina and the adventitia.

Techniques

There are three commonly used techniques: direct excision, eversion and gas endarterectomy. The

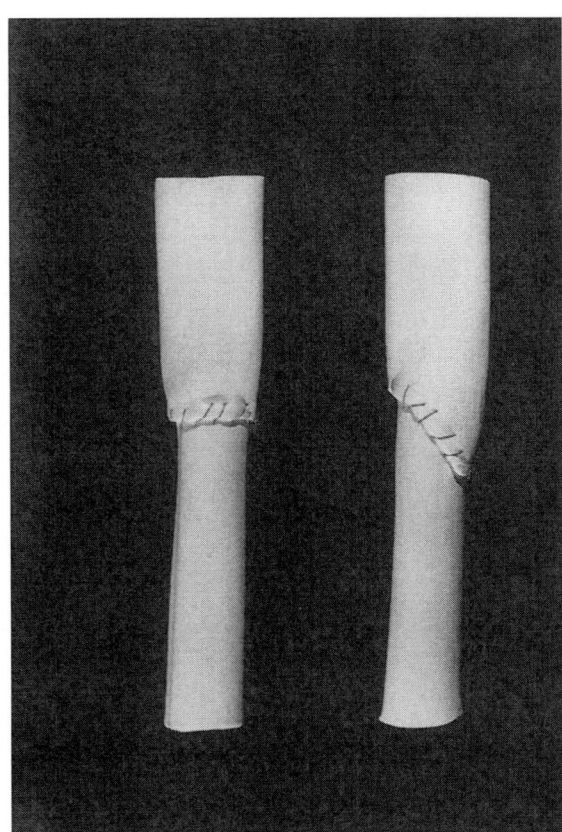

Fig. 2. End-to-end anastomosis. (Courtesy Dr P. Desoutter)

conventional or direct endarterectomy encompasses two variants : semi-closed and open.

Semi-closed endarterectomy

After exposure and mobilization of the diseased vessel, a longitudinal arteriotomy is performed at each end of the involved segment through the subadventitial cleavage plane (Fig. 3A). A ring dissector is introduced through the distal end, passing over the occluding core into the cleavage plane upwards (Fig. 3B). After a sharp transection at both ends, the occluding core is extruded through either the lower or upper incision by traction and slight torsion. Proximal and distal intimal edges are then fixed to the arterial wall with interrupted stitches (Fig. 3C).

Open endarterectomy

The artery is exposed along its entire length. The arteriotomy may be longitudinal (Fig. 4A), oblique or transverse (an eversion or "turn over" procedure). Initial separation of the cleavage plane is carried out with a dissector or spatula. Whenever possible an extraluminal dissection of the occluding core is desirable (Fig. 4B). The "atheromatous" core is removed either by direct visualization (Fig. 4C), by a stripping instrument, or by injection of pressurised water or gas. Whatever the technique used, the limits of the unblocked area must be clear and gently sloped at the distal extremity to avoid detachment of the intima secondary to the blood flow. It is not mandatory to reattach

the proximal and distal ends of the intimal flap, although in some instances it may be necessary to do so.

Pathology and complications

The core of the thrombo-endarterectomy (TEA) is a cylinder; its luminal face is irregularly lined with atheromatous plaques, some of which are ulcerated with a thrombus on the surface. The external face corresponds to the plane of cleavage (Fig. 5). In the part of the artery that remains, the endarterectomised area is smooth. The newly-formed artery often has a larger external diameter than it did before surgery (Fig. 6-7). An experimental study in dogs undergoing carotid endarterectomy shows a fibrin-platelet carpet on the endarterectomised surface immediately after flow is established. This phenomenon is maximal 1 hr after surgery and appears to stabilise towards 24 hr. By 48 hr there is little evidence of active thrombus formation, or re-endothelialisation from existing endothelial cells. However in non-heparinised animals, a typical thrombus may develop. One week later, most of the mural thrombus has disappeared and regeneration of the endothelial monolayer occurs by migration from the endarterectomy end points and suture lines. Rapid smoothing over of the "steps" along the side of the recanalised segment results from proliferation of smooth muscle cells from the remaining media. The thinner the residual media, the thicker the neointima grows. Occasionally elastic lamellae reminiscent of an internal elastic lamina develop close to the arterial lumen [18-21].

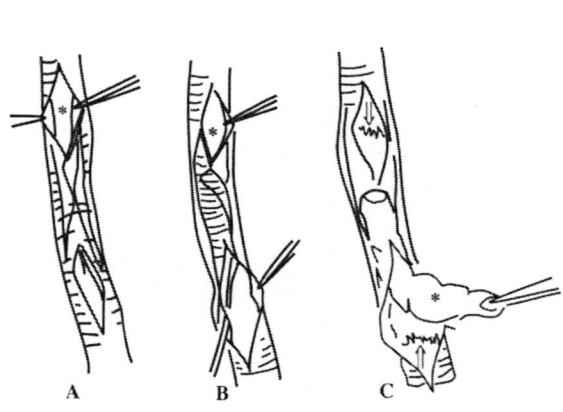

Fig. 3. Semi-closed endarterectomy. (*): occluding core; (=>): proximal and distal intimal edges

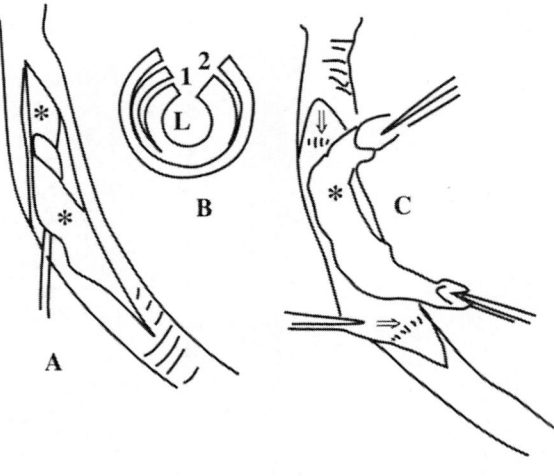

Fig. 4. Open endarterectomy. (*): occluding core; (=>): proximal and distal intimal edges (1): luminal endarterectomy; (2): extraluminal endarterectomy; (L): vascular lumen

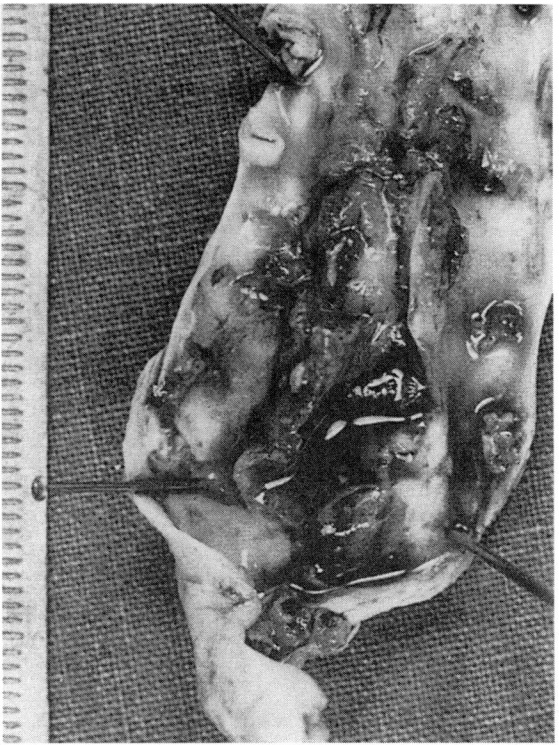

Fig. 5. Endarterectomy core

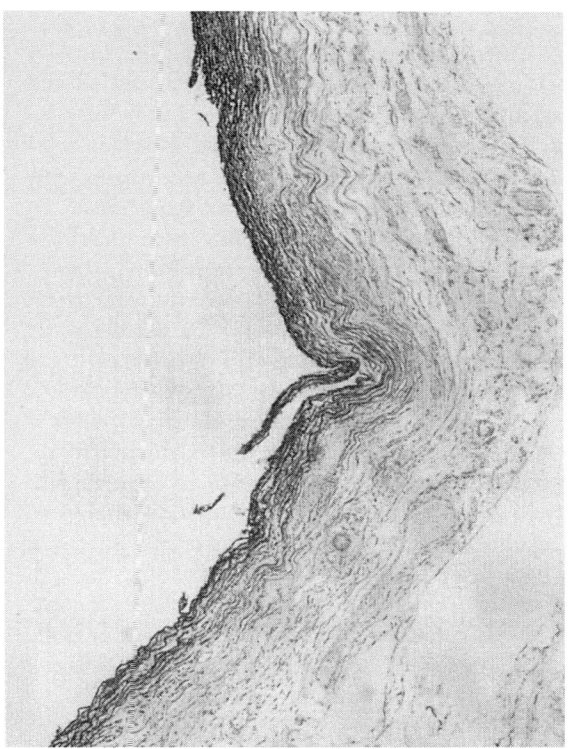

Fig. 6. Endarterectomy. Remaining arterial wall consisting of the outermost part of the media and the adventitia. Orcein elastic stain. (Orcein)

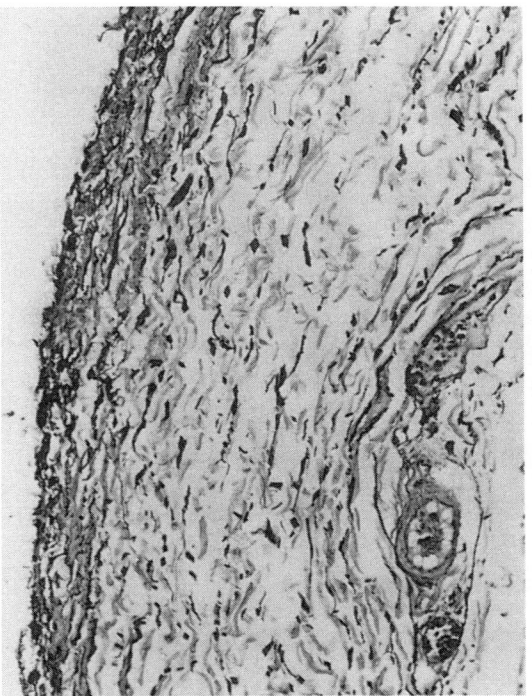

Fig. 7. Endarterectomy. Well preserved external lamella in the remaining arterial wall. Orcein

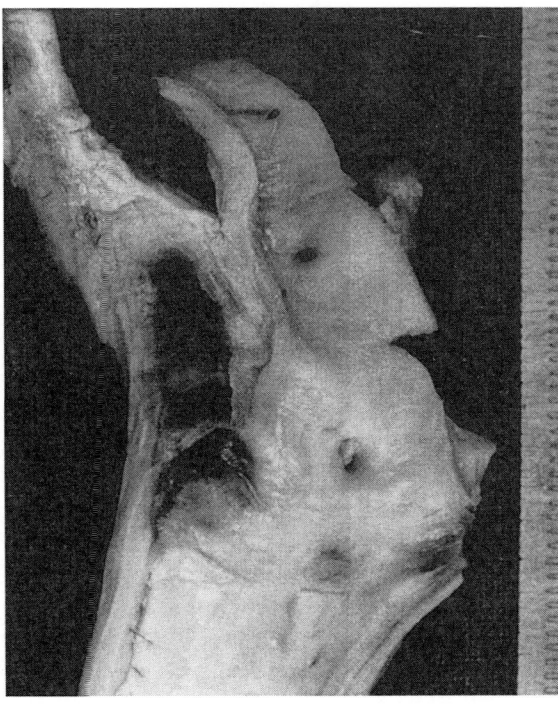

Fig. 8. Endarterectomy. Thrombosis developed on the surface of the endarterectomised area

Early complications include thrombosis (Fig. 8) and embolism. Surface thrombosis on the endarterectomised area may give rise to distal emboli and detachment of the distal edge of the intima may induce an acute occlusive thrombosis. Destruction of the lymphatic vessels may produce a seroma or lymphocele, which requires either drainage or re-exploration of the wound. So-called pseudoaneurysms and recurrent atherosclerosis represent the two most frequent late complications. After TEA, the artery no longer possesses the architecture of a normal vessel and large arteries may dilate, often as much as 10 to 12 years after surgery. The use of patches increases the risk of false aneurysm approximately four fold [22]. Medium-sized arteries, however, are more likely to develop a gradual stenosis, which becomes evident 5 or 6 years postoperatively. This is a dynamic process probably influenced by surgical technique as well as by anatomic, hemodynamic, and patient factors. Early restenosis (between 3 and 18 months), and late restenosis (between 18 and 60 months) should be distinguished from residual disease (which tends to present within 3 months of operation).

In the internal carotid artery, stenosis has been studied extensively and results either from intimal hyperplasia (24% of patients) (Fig. 9), kinking and coiling (3.3% of patients) or recurrent atherosclerosis (72,7% of patients) [23-26]. Recurrent atherosclerosis, involving 10% to 15% of patients, is evident as early as 6 months and worsens for 12 to 18 months. Fortunately it becomes symptomatic in only 3% to 5% of patients [27, 28].

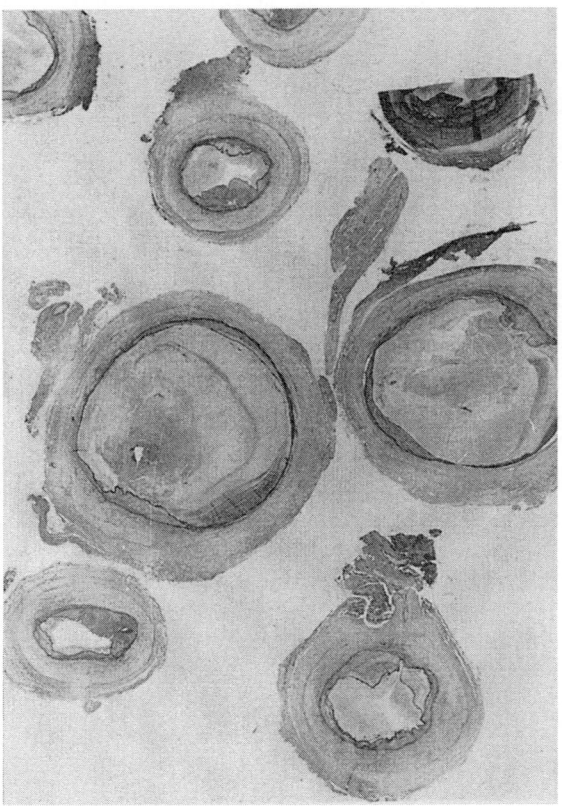

Fig. 9. Endarterectomy. Occluding intimal hyperplasia. Orcein

Direct re-establishment of vascular patency

The vessel is opened to remove an embolus or a thrombus and closed under direct vision. A less invasive method is a retrograde technique using clamping forceps or a Fogarty catheter having an inflatable balloon near its tip (Fig. 10). These approaches are more likely to be successful when the clot is recent, but are difficult when the clot adheres closely to the intima or produces extensive thrombosis in the distal vascular segment. Insertion of a Fogarty catheter may cause abrasion of the endothelial lining, a source of recurrent thromboses in small vessels. In atheromatous arteries, the catheter may detach or dissect a calcified plaque [29]. Faulty technique gives rise to complications; excessive "sweeping" causes intimal (Fig. 11) or intimal and medial rupture with dissection (Fig. 12-13) and thrombosis; perforation with arteriovenous fistula is rare. Rupture of the Fogarty

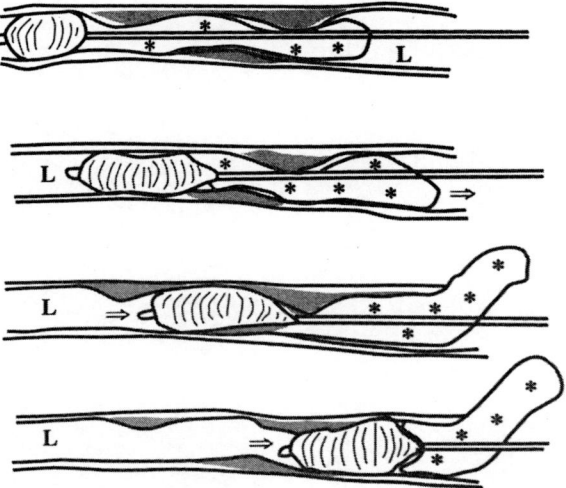

Fig. 10. Vascular unblocking with an inflatable balloon catheter (Fogarty). (asterisk): occluding clot; L: vascular lumen

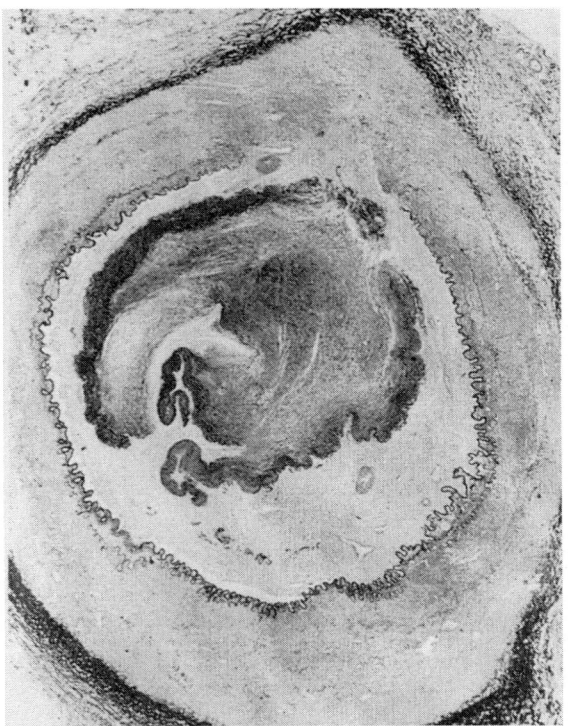

Fig. 11. Vascular unblocking with an inflatable balloon catheter (Fogarty). Intimal detachment with total occlusion of the lumen. Orcein

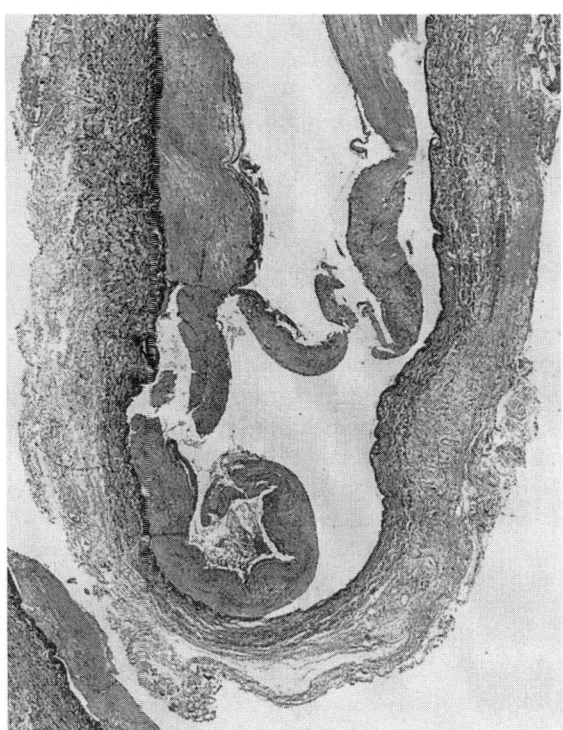

Fig. 12. Vascular unblocking with an inflatable balloon catheter (Fogarty). Rupture of the intima and media after balloon catheter angioplasty. Orcein

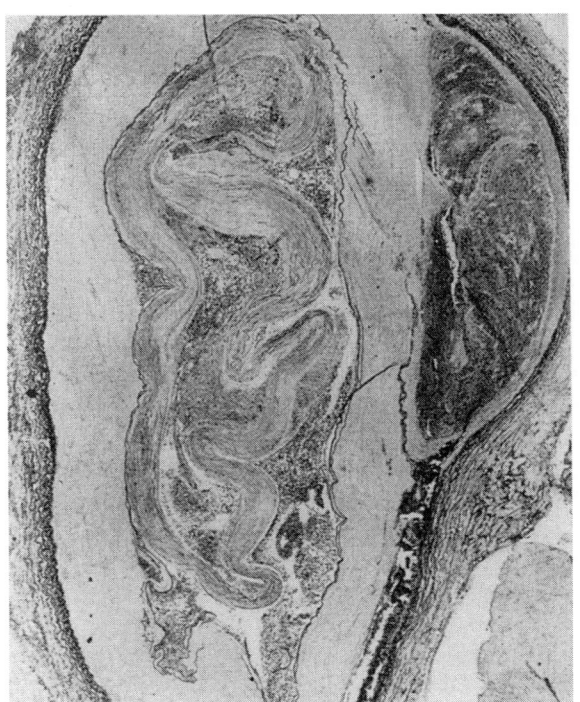

Fig. 13. Vascular unblocking with an inflatable balloon catheter (Fogarty). Detachment of the intima with subadventitial haematoma. Orcein

balloon catheter with distant and fatal migration is an exceptional event [30, 31].

Percutaneous angioscopy

This type of procedure has become a reality thanks to major advances in catheter technology and miniaturisation of fiber optics. It provides direct visualisation of the endoluminal surface of coronary vessels, evaluation of atherosclerotic plaques, and traumatic intimal defects [32-34]. Complications are similar to those with the Fogarty catheter when a rigid or overlarge apparatus is used.

Angioplasty

There are many methods of reconstructing a blood vessel; those which give rise to particular pathological problems are considered here.

Percutaneous transluminal angioplasty

Balloon dilatation of narrowed segments as an alternative to bypass surgery was first described by Dotter and Judkins in 1964 to "revascularize" the lower limbs

[35]. The application field of this procedure is wide; iliac, femoro-popliteal, renal and coronary arteries are all dealt with as a routine. The initial technique consisted of introducing rigid coaxial teflon dilators sequentially over a guide wire, but this was applicable only to relatively straight arteries. It was originally assumed that angioplasty worked by compression and remodelling of the atheromatous material, but, in reality, angioplasty works by controlled trauma. In atherosclerotic arteries, the calcified plaque is compressed, fragmented longitudinally and circumferentially, with the cracks also tearing into the intima and the media. Atheromatous plaques are disrupted, impacted into the vascular wall, calcified lesions show longitudinal cracks, and intra-plaque dissections may occur [36]. In ostial stenosis angioplasty is less efficient; the balloon acts on the plaque longitudinally. Soon after deflation, the atherosclerotic plaque recoils and stenosis reappears.

The myocytes of the media are stretched (Fig. 14), the adventitia is dilated and the atheromatous material is redistributed radially and laterally into the over-dilated adventitia, thus leaving a large patent central lumen that is kept open by the increased flow. In intimal fibrodysplasia, the initial technique is disappointing despite repeated inflations at high pressures : inflation dilates the vessel wall, but spasm and the large tissue mass produces residual stenosis. In medial fibromuscular dysplasia, overdilation of stenotic segments leads to dilation with luminal patency. Most vessels show the best effect from low pressure inflation of the balloon. The media becomes thinner while smooth muscle cells are crushed and lengthened.

Complications of transluminal angioplasty occur in 5 to 10% of patients. Arterial spasm may increase the risks of thrombosis, dissection or perforation. A thrombus may form on the catheter and guide wire. Dislodging of weakened atherosclerotic plaques may cause cholesterol crystal embolism. In arteries harbouring fibrodysplasia, the intima may detach, giving rise to a flap floating into the vascular lumen, thus inducing thrombosis. Intramedial haemorrhage, parietal dissection, intimal and/or medial breaks are common. Organisation of parietal breaks or dissection leads to development of a false aneurysm. Aggressive dilation may lead to complete vessel rupture.

Around 30-40% of patients undergoing PTA experience restenosis of the widened segment within six months of the procedure [37, 38]. Restenosis results from a complex process, including intimal hyperplasia (Fig. 15) [39-44]. This response to injury may only develop after repeated PTA or bypass surgery [45-47]. Intravascular irradiation has been proposed as a me-

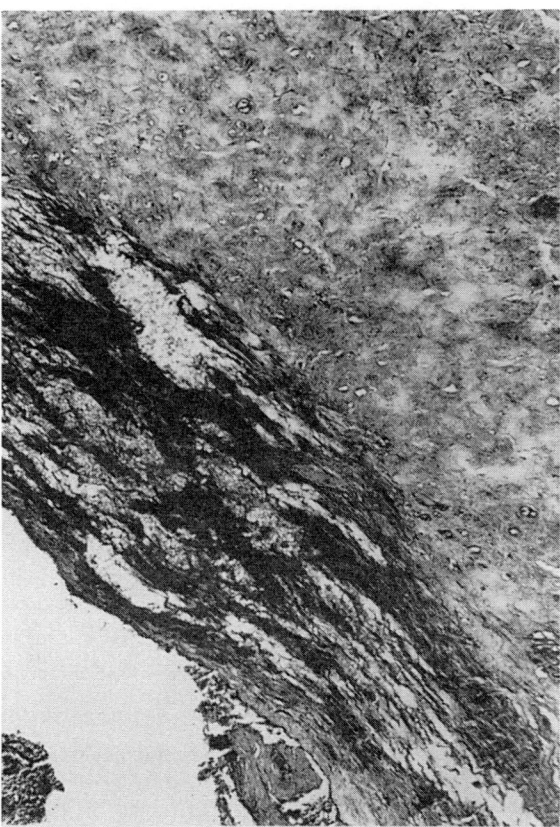

Fig. 14. Percutaneous transluminal angioplasty. Dilaceration of the media with interstitial haemorrhage. Masson's trichrome stain

thod for the prevention of re-stenosis by inhibition of VSMC proliferation [48-51].

Endoluminal vascular stenting

Stenting is the use of a wire mesh tube to prop open a vessel, often recently cleared using angioplasty. The stent is collapsed, placed over an angioplasty balloon catheter, and manœuvred into the constricted area. When the balloon is inflated, it locks into place and forms a rigid support to hold the vessel open. Stenting has also been used to treat true or false aneurysms, arterio-venous fistulae and dissection [52, 53]. The use of stents to release drugs that interfere with cell proliferation in the vessel or which minimise thrombotic risk may improve the long-term success of this procedure. Vascular stenting is usually reserved for near ostial lesions that do not respond to percutaneous transluminal angioplasty. In the aorta, the stent should be placed so that it extends slightly into the lumen (approximately 1-2mm) to ensure that it covers the ostium adequately; this may be evident at autopsy, even after an interval.

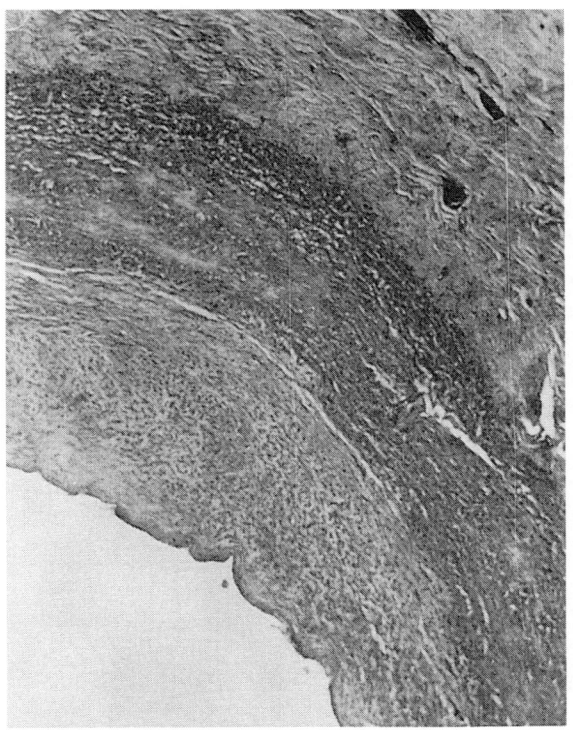

Fig. 15. Percutaneous transluminal angioplasty. Intimal hyperplasia. Masson's trichrome

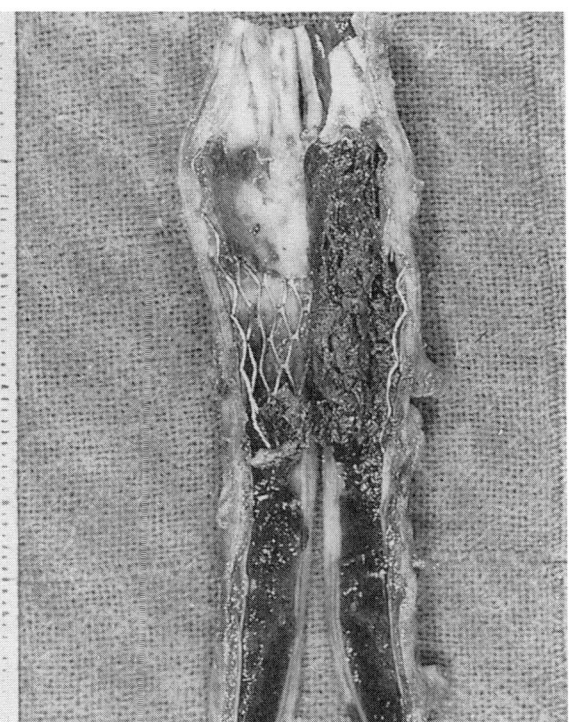

Fig. 16. Endoluminal vascular stenting. Intimal hyperplasia engulfing the stent mesh with superimposed thrombosis. (Courtesy Dr P. Desoutter)

Pathological examination of the specimens of carotid endarterectomy performed after progressive stenosis following endoluminal stenting show incorporation of the stent into the atheromatous plaque (Fig.16-17-18) [54]. Complications include infection, soft-tissue oedema, rupture, perforation,arterio-venous fistula especially when the artery is of small calibre and flanked by a satellite vein, thrombosis and embolism [55-57].

Frank rupture requires surgical repair; perforation by a guide wire is almost always self-sealing. Embolization of plaque, thrombus, and cholesterol may occur. Restenosis complicates long-term clinical outcomes in one third of the patients [58]. The strongest predictors of restenosis are diabetes mellitus, multiple lesions and persistence of a small diameter lumen after stenting [59, 60].

Laser angioplasty

This procedure has been used alone and in conjunction with balloon angioplasty. Conventional thermal lasers remove plaque by applying heat, and may cause parietal coagulative necrosis and perforation. This complication can be avoided by using a "cool" laser

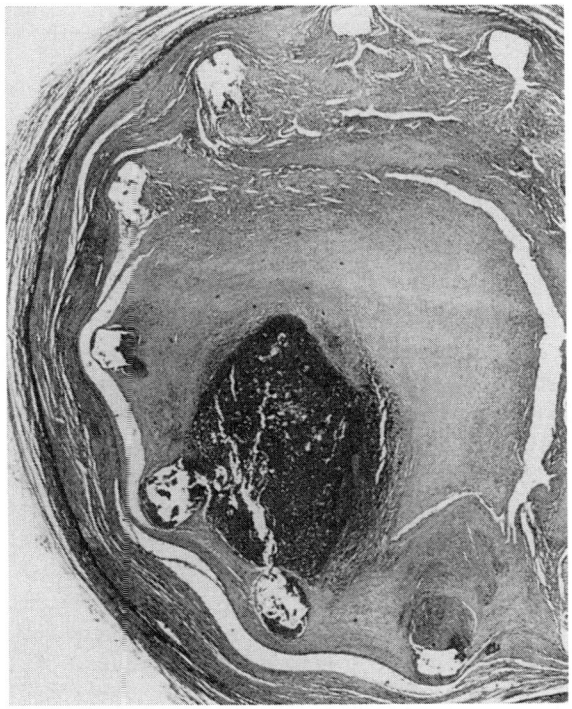

Fig. 17. Endoluminal vascular stenting. Intimal hyperplasia enclosing stenting mesh. Masson's trichrome

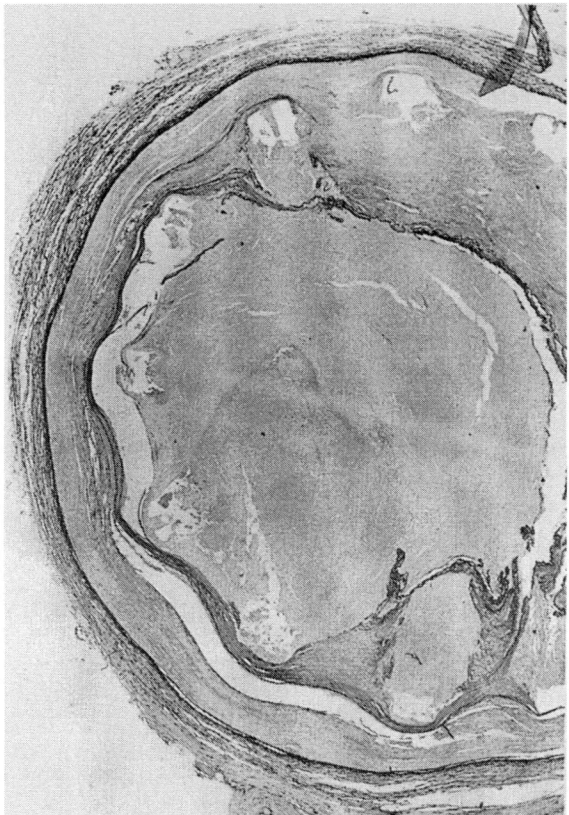

Fig. 18. Endoluminal vascular stenting. Incorporation of the stent in the atheromatous plaque. Note disruption of the internal elastic lamella and penetration of the media. Orcein

capable of generating laser energy and delivering it precisely to the target. The vascular changes caused by lasers are discussed in chapter VII.

Rotating shaver angioplasty

This procedure may precede a balloon angioplasty. The catheter is threaded through the blood vessels into the blocked area. The tip of the catheter has a high-speed rotating shaver which is a disk or "burr" device, grinding the plaque up into minute particles. One such device, called the Rotablator, rotates at close to 200 000 rpm, and grinds away atherosclerotic plaques [61, 62]. Balloon angioplasty may then be used on the artery.

It has been suggested that the rotating burr "shaved" the fibrous cap of the plaque, thus exposing the underlying crater. This structure is then compressed by balloon dilatation that expands the true lumen [63]. The primary success rate for high frequency rotational atherectomy alone is 50-60% [64], with complications similar to those of balloon catheter angioplasty.

Dislocation of the rotating blade due to pressure from hard plaque tissue is a severe technical pitfall [65]. The rate of long-term restenosis is between 40-50% with or without adjunctive balloon angioplasty [64].

Patch-graft angioplasty

This technique is used to close a longitudinal arteriotomy in a small or medium-calibre vessel by covering the vascular opening with a piece of tissue (arterial autograft, venous autograft, or synthetic prosthesis) to prevent stenosis (Fig. 19).

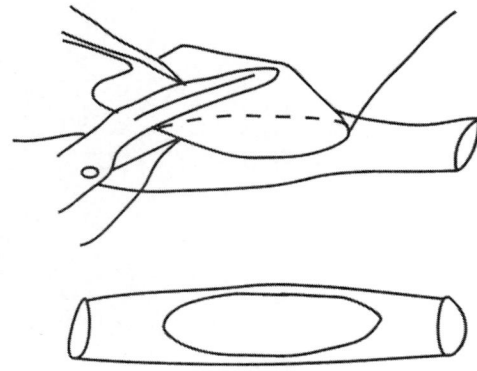

Fig. 19. Patch-graft angioplasty

In an operative specimen, the contour of the patch-graft is delineated by sutures (Fig. 20). Complications may result from faulty surgical technique or from the disintegration of the graft material itself (Fig. 21-22). Too large a patch can cause turbulence, leading to thrombosis and the formation of an aneurysm (Fig. 23-24) [22, 66]. Complications related to the changes in the patch are those that occur with any graft or prosthesis [67].

Vascular bypass

Bypasses are performed with grafts or prostheses. Grafts may be autografts or xenografts and arteries or veins. An ideal graft or prosthesis should be easy to obtain, handle and suture, mechanically resistant, biocompatible, resistant to infection, and free of toxic or oncogenic effects

The clinical course of a bypass.

Healing of sutures and lines of anastomosis

No continuity is developed between the recipient artery and the bypass at the line of anastomosis. Non-

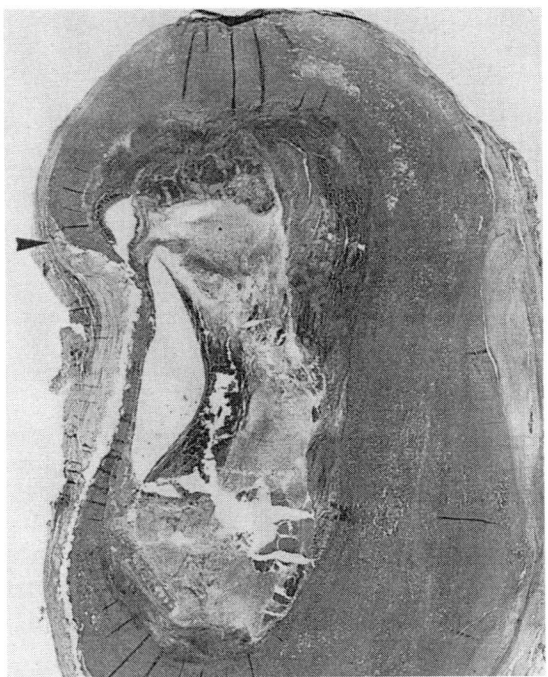

Fig. 20. Dacron patch-graft angioplasty. Patch-graft (arrow heads) in a thrombosed endarectomised artery. Note artefactual detachment of the patch from the remaining arterial wall. Masson's trichrome

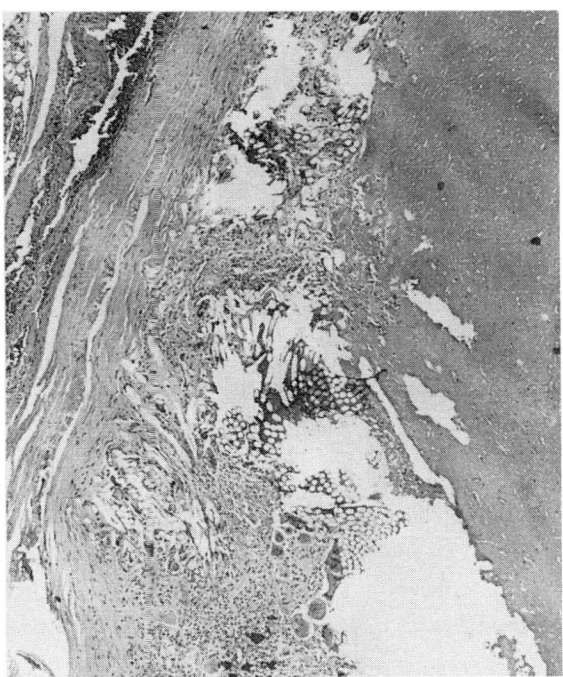

Fig. 21. Dacron patch-graft angioplasty. Desintegration of a long-term patch-graft with separation of prosthetic mesh. HES

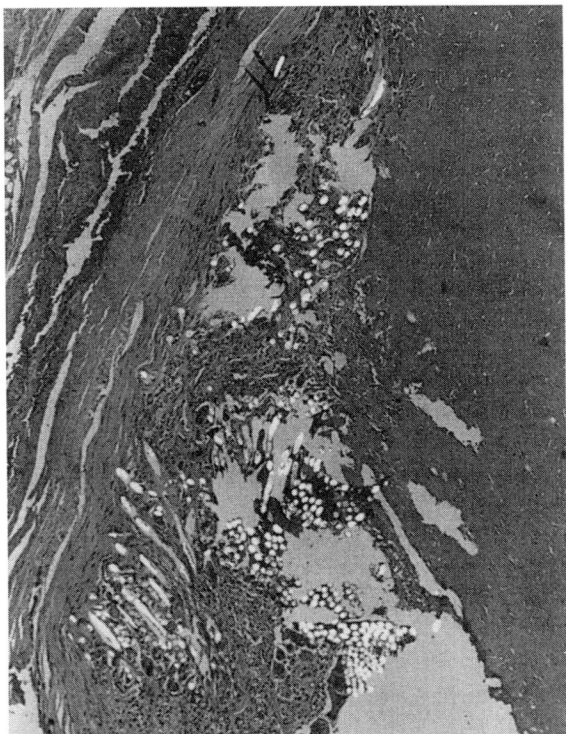

Fig. 22. Dacron patch-graft angioplasty. Polarized light helps identify remnants of prosthetic mesh

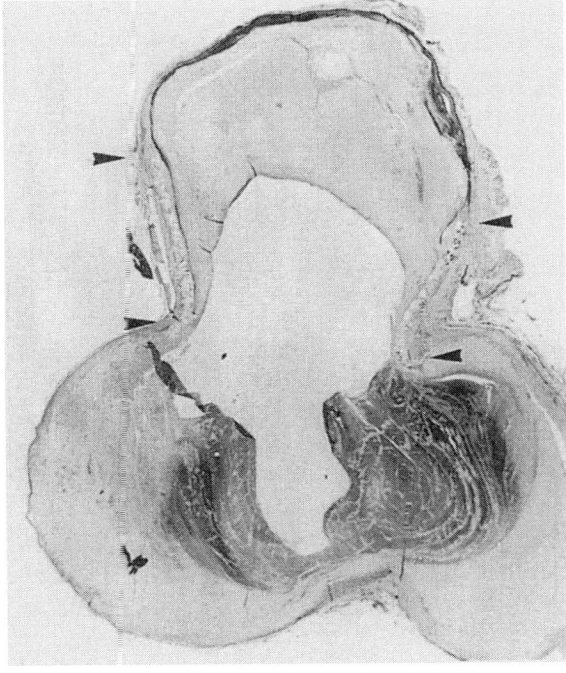

Fig. 23. Dacron patch-graft angioplasty. Partially thrombosed aneurysm developed in a ruptured patch-graft (arrow heads). Prosthetic material is present at the neck of the aneurysm. Black line corresponds to the external elastic membrane of the recipient artery. Orcein

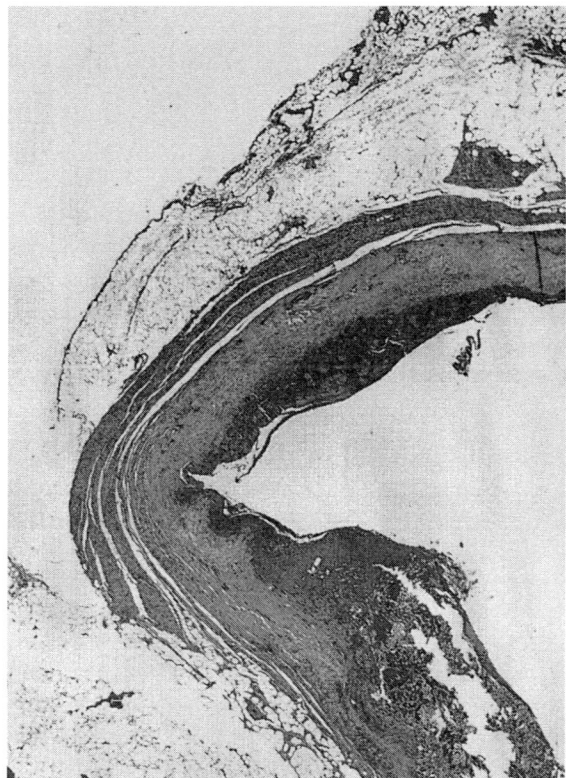

Fig. 24. Dacron patch-graft angioplasty. Fibrotic aneurysmal wall containing prosthetic debris. Masson's trichrome

absorbable sutures produce a foreign body granuloma in the recipient artery and behave as a wick, allowing plasma to ooze and inflammatory cells to penetrate. This phenomenon results in an inflammatory granuloma that is replaced by fibrosis.

Adaptation of the bypass to the neighbouring tissue and the recipient artery

Perigraft connective tissue forms an external capsule, often with foreign body granulomata, depending on the nature of the material. At the blood interface, different changes occur in different parts of the vessel. Immediately after implantation, the luminal aspect of the middle portion is covered with a thin layer of fibrin containing some platelets, monocytes, and polymorphonuclear leukocytes. Organisation of this layer from the 1st to 3rd weeks gives rise to an internal capsule or pseudo-intima. However, its organization remains very slow and is almost never completed [68]. At the line of anastomosis, endothelial cells coming from the endothelium of the recipient artery slide over the bypass, a partial re-endothelialisation which extends for a few millimetres [4, 69, 70].

Protein kinase C (PKC) may play a role in this process [71].

General complications of bypasses

In general, complications are commoner in bypasses which do not mimic normal anatomy. It is generally true to say that the longer the bypass the higher the risk of complications.

Thrombosis

This usually occurs at the line of anastomosis and may extend to the arterial side. There are many potentially contributory factors, including surgery which results in poor junctional configurations, poor alignment of bypasses or any defect affecting flow, intimal hyperplasia, defective anastomotic compliance and progression of the atherosclerotic process. Certain types of material may favour the onset of extensive thrombosis in the bypass [72-74].

Rupture of anastomosis

The probability of rupture is increased by a number of factors, including shearing of the arterial edge by the suture thread with anastomotic dehiscence, breakage of sutures, sepsis, dilatation or post-operative peri-bypass oedema with seroma and lymphocele [75-79].

Changes in shape or size of the prosthesis

Lack of tolerance for the graft material and mechanical fatigue occurring following the haemodynamic constraints created by the new anatomical site will cause alterations, especially in regions (crural area, popliteal fossa) that undergo extensive tension and frequent flexion and extension. The bypass may undergo bending or kinking, flattening or twisting and become aneurysmal [16, 17, 80]. An excessive inflammatory reaction triggered by the prosthetic material produces excessive fibrosis of the external capsule. Regular follow-ups of patients with aged vascular grafts and the precise documentation of implanted materials are necessary to estimate graft degradation [81-83].

Infection

Infection may occur either immediately or long after surgery, with a median time of 10 months [84]. Rupture of the bypass, haemorrhage and septic shock or embolism may follow, requiring graft excision [85-88].

Fistula

Fistulae develop as a result of erosion of an organ by the often pulsating bypass, or by rupture of an aneurysm into the viscus [89, 90].

Further development of atheroseleromatosis

Lipid deposits and calcification may affect the new vessel wall.

Pathology of biological grafts

Xenografts

The commonly used form is from bovine carotid arteries, taken from adult cattle, immersed in a proteolytic enzyme solution (1% ficin) and treated with dialdehyde or glutaraldehyde solution [91, 92]. The grafts are thereby transformed into a tubular segment of connective tissue, devoid of any antigenic action. Other techniques (such as the No-react aldehyde detoxification processes) have been tested to avoid the cytotoxicity of the xenograft and to inhibit calcium deposition [93]. Storage is possible for up to 3 years. Bovine arterial xenografts are used to fashion arteriovenous fistulas for renal dialysis, to perform coronary revascularisation, to administer chemotherapeutic agents, and for repeated blood transfusions [94, 95, 96, 97, 98]. After implantation, the xenograft is rapidly surrounded by dense connective tissue. In man, it is still recognizable for some years. Good tolerance is reported in iliac artery bypasses over a 13 year period [99]. However, calcific degeneration of the graft is the major problem [100]. The long-term course is peppered with possible complications: recurrence of atheroma, anastomotic stenosis and true aneurysm (3-6% of implanted xenografts) [101]. An external Dacron tulle support is helpful in strengthening the graft and preventing its dilation. In practice it has proved necessary to temper the early enthusiasm reported from various centers [96].

Allografts

Allografts or homografts should be collected less than 12 hours after death. The homograft is then treated by absolute alcohol or a 4% solution of formaldehyde; alternatively freezing and lyophylization may be used [102-104]. Glycerol preservation has been experimentally tried [105]. A history of septicaemia, neoplasia, and relevant viral infections in the donor history contraindicates the use of vessels. Generally, fresh allografts undergo rapid rejection. However, preserved allografts have a longer, but still limited, clinical life [106].

1. Arterial allografts. Once implanted, the allograft behaves in exactly the same way regardless of the preservation technique used. The endothelium and the intima disappear before implantation. Myocytes and fibroblasts in the media disappear after a few days. In the first weeks thereafter, the media continues to be denuded of its component cells (Fig. 25). Elastic lamellae fragment. One month later, fibrosis surrounds the adventitia [107, 108]. Eighteen months post-operatively, the homograft appears as a fibrohyaline tube whose softness and elasticity are reduced. Calcification may appear in the wall (Fig. 26) [109].

2. Venous allografts. Saphenous homografts retain all the vessel characteristics necessary for the creation of an arterio-venous fistula or for revascularization procedures [110]. Human umbilical veins treated with glutaraldehyde and secondarily reinforced with a surrounding polyester mesh are increasingly being used Once implanted, umbilical vein grafts appear to be well tolerated. The gross appearance after implantation is similar to that of the preimplant graft except for thinning of the wall leading to dilatation with aneurysm formation (17% of grafts) [111]. The jugular vein has been used for mesocaval graft interposition in the management of portal cavernoma in children [112].

Histologically, the venous architecture remains recognisable; it is hyalinised in some places and cracked in others (Fig. 27-28). In older specimens, the internal elastic membrane shows discontinuity or fragmentation; the medial smooth muscle cells undergo degeneration and hyalinization. A foreign body reaction develops with fibrosis at the periphery of the polyester mesh in sheathed grafts. Long term complications include infection (Fig. 29), thromboses, development of atheromatous lesions and transverse cracks in the wall, the latter probably secondary to elongation of the wall of the vein compared with the Dacron coat. All these complications limit the indication for venous homografts [113, 114].

Autografts

The ability to use a healthy artery segment exists only in patients with arteries free from atherosclerosis or where it is possible to re-use a thrombo-endarterectomised segment. Arterial autografts exhibit all of the disadvantages observed with an endarterectomised artery, especially stenosis and aneurysmal dilatation. There are three ways to use an autograft; as a non-inverted in-situ venous graft, where the vein remains in its tissue bed and can substitute for the companion

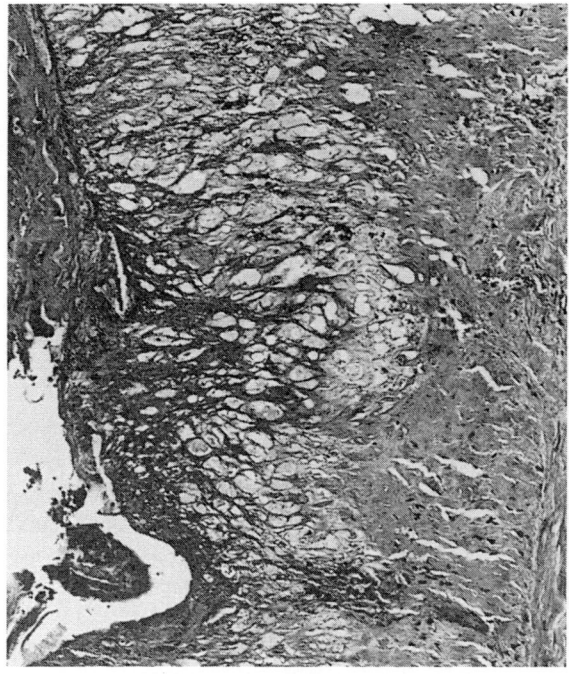

Fig. 25. Arterial allograft showing denuded media. Masson's trichrome

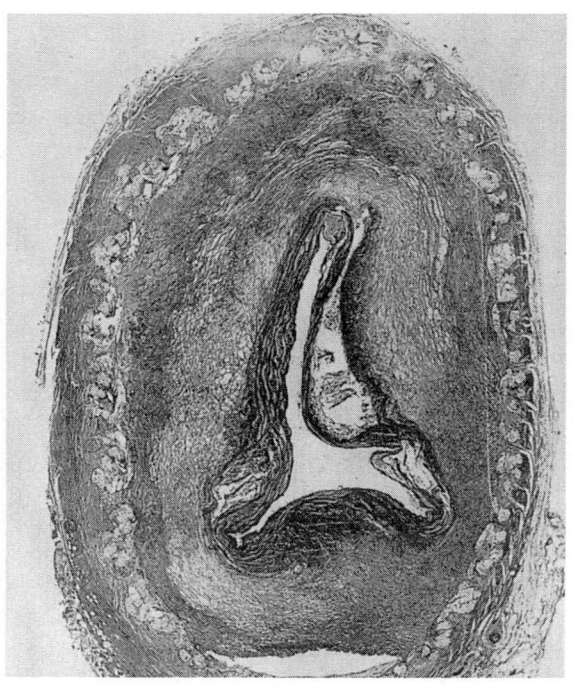

Fig. 27. Venous allograft. Partially thrombosed umbilical vein graft reinforced by Dacron coat. Masson's trichrome

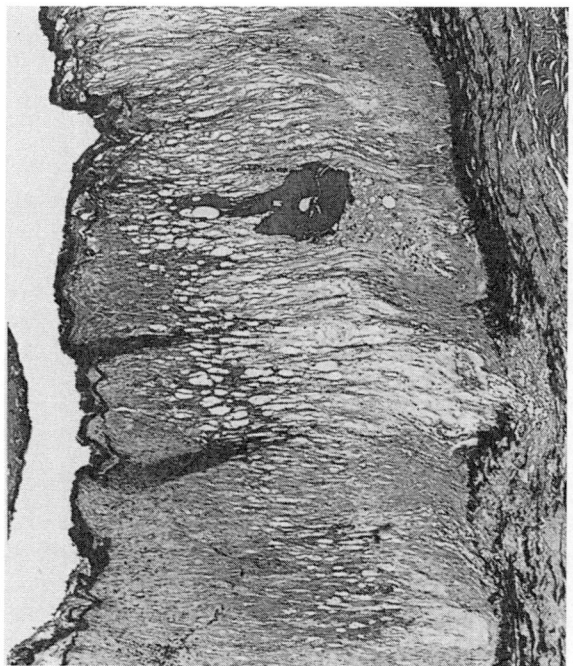

Fig. 26. Arterial allograft. Fibrohyaline transformation and calcification of an arterial homograft. Orcein

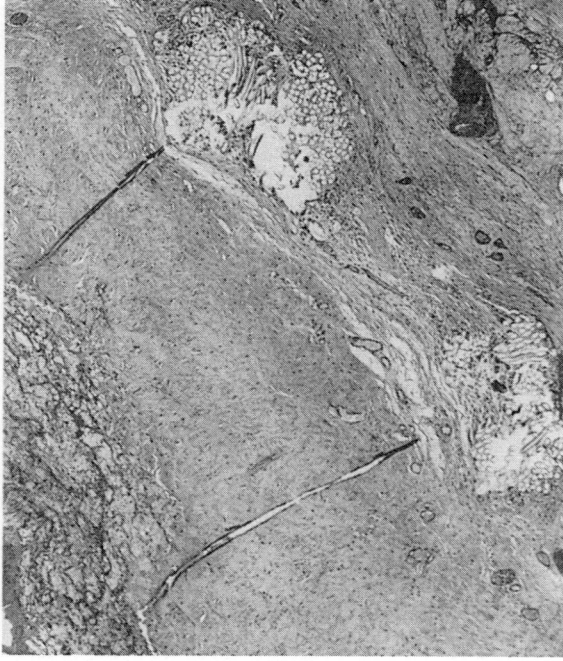

Fig. 28. Venous allograft. Dacron-reinforced umbilical vein graft showing degeneration with hyalinization. Note transverse cracks in the media. Haematoxylin, eosin and saffron stain. (HES)

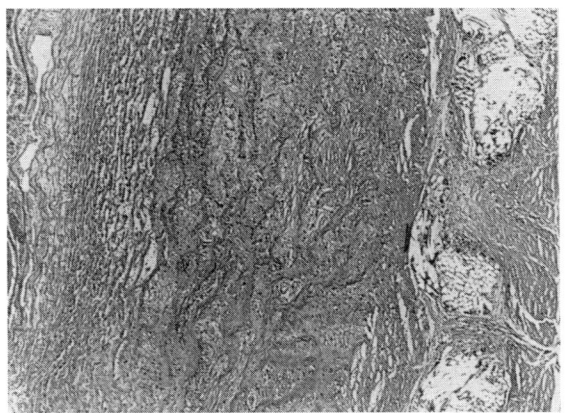

Fig. 29. Venous allograft. Dacron-reinforced umbilical vein graft. Sepsis with heavy infiltration of leukocytes. HES

artery, but destruction of the valves may produce operative or post-operative complications. Venous autographs may also be non-inverted ex-situ grafts, which may be placed at a distant site, or may be used as inverted grafts where there is no valvular destruction (Fig. 30).

For a non-inverted *in situ* venous autograft, the cusps of the first valve can be excised under direct vision as they are visible on opening. At the other valves, the cusps can be broken by use of a smooth-nosed metal or plastic internal stripper. As the vein tapers, correctly sized strippers are necessary to evert the valves and ensure destruction of valvular competence. For *ex situ* bypasses, the vein must be of sufficient size. The specimen is collected by spread incisions after ligation of all collateral vessels and gentle dilatation with the heparinized patient's blood or with Collin's solution, the medium in which the vein is immersed before being surgically implanted. Intravascular administration of nitroglycerin may help preserve the vaso-

dilatory capacity of the transposed, denervated, and devascularised venous graft [115]. Immediately after implantation, the endothelial lining is detached from the endovein [116]. The denuded sub-endothelial layer and the inner portion of the media are infiltrated by inflammatory elements. The whole area is covered by a fibrinous coating (Fig. 31). From 4 weeks after surgery, the venous intima becomes thicker with proliferation of smooth muscle cells, which are often arranged parallel to the blood flow. Maximum thickening of the intima occurs after 12 months and is combined with a newly-formed internal elastic lamella, which is often interrupted in places. Anastomotic intimal hyperplasia is evident 14 to 31 days after implantation and gradually increases, particularly at the distal portion of the anastomosis. This change is greater after end-to-side anastomosis than after end-to-end anastomosis [117, 118]. However, the graft will remain patent if the surgical technique is good. The possible mechanisms of intimal hyperplasia include interruption of vasa vasorum, surgical trauma, exposure to arterial pressure, turbulence flow caused by poor size match, or abnormal hydraulic force created by the anastomotic angle [119, 120]. In the media, relative ischaemia of the autograft when it

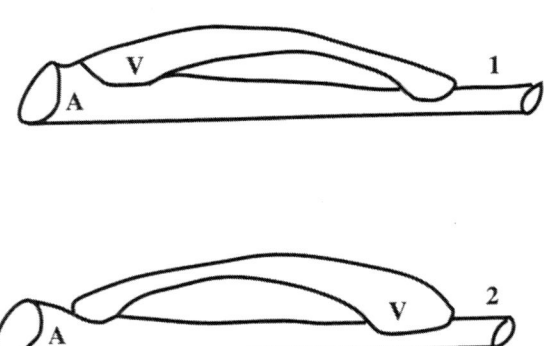

Fig. 30. *In situ* non-inverted venous autograft (1) and *ex situ* inverted autograft (2) bypass (A. artery; V. venous autograft)

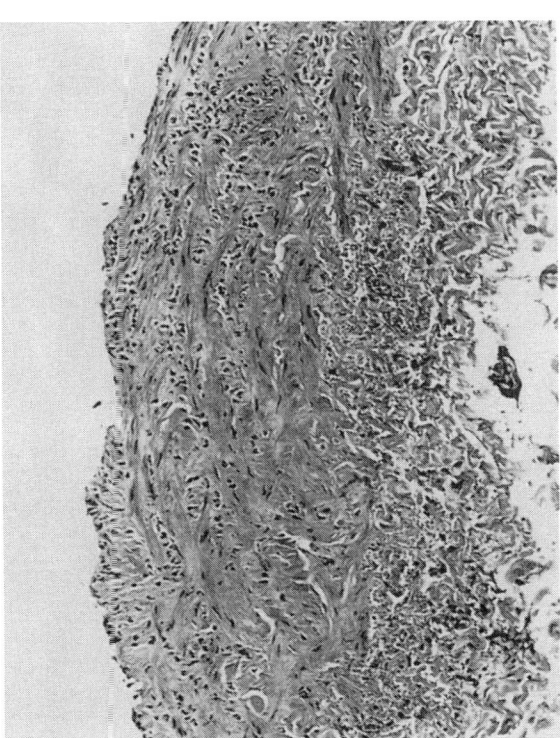

Fig. 31. Venous autograft. Early changes with infiltration of inflammatory cells. HES

is collected causes a loss of cellular elements, which are replaced by sclerotic tissue, but the configuration of the autograft remains unchanged. The entirety results in vein graft disease. New techniques such as covering the grafts with microporous, compliant biodegradable polyurethane prosthesis, and external stenting are under investigation to prevent overdistension, fibrosis and intimal hyperplasia [121, 122].

Complications of autografting include thrombosis, which may occur as a result of stenosis due to faulty surgery (Fig. 32), intimal hyperplasia (Fig. 33), or deterioration of the distal vascular bed through progressive vascular disease. Aneurysmal dilation or local stenosis may develop when collaterals are inadequately ligated; a long collateral stump favours formation of an aneurysm, a too tight stump reduces the main graft diameter and leads to graft wall fibrosis. Progressive intimal proliferation with superimposed thrombosis also occurs in an overlong "dead end" of a venous collateral. Localised ischaemia of the venous wall, secondary to a fault in autograft preparation, may be the starting point for tubular stenosis to develop at a distance from the anastomotic lines. Thus careful surgical preparation of the graft is of upmost importance in avoiding these complications. In long-

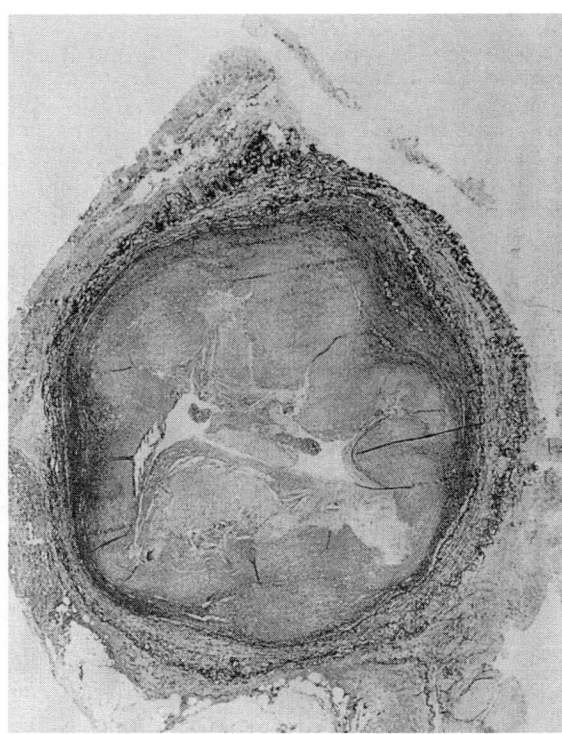

Fig. 33. Venous autograft. Occlusive intimal hyperplasia. Orcein

term venous grafts, degenerative changes may result in multi-aneurysmal dilation (Fig. 34) [123]. Accelerated atherosclerosis (Fig. 35) may appear [124] and contribute to the development of stenotic lesions, requiring reoperation from 7 months to 12 years postoperatively [125]. Composition of recurrent newly-formed plaques in vein grafts is similar to that in the native arteries of the same patients [34, 126].

Pathology of vascular prostheses

The ideal prosthesis must be capable of being sterilised without alteration, be chemically inert, should not induce inflammatory or foreign body reactions, should not produce a state of allergy or hypersensitivity, should not be modified by tissue fluids, must be capable of supporting mechanical loads, be non-carcinogenic and be easy and cheap to make [127]

Construction and material base of the major types of prosthesis

Prostheses made of Vinyon N (acrilonitril, vinyl chloride), Nylon (polyunethame), Orlon (polyacrylonitride), Ivalon, Silastic, Dacron (polyethylene terephthalate) (Fig. 36-37) and Teflon (polytetrafluoroethylene) are in current use but Dacron and Teflon are the most favoured [128]. Experimentally, polyurethane

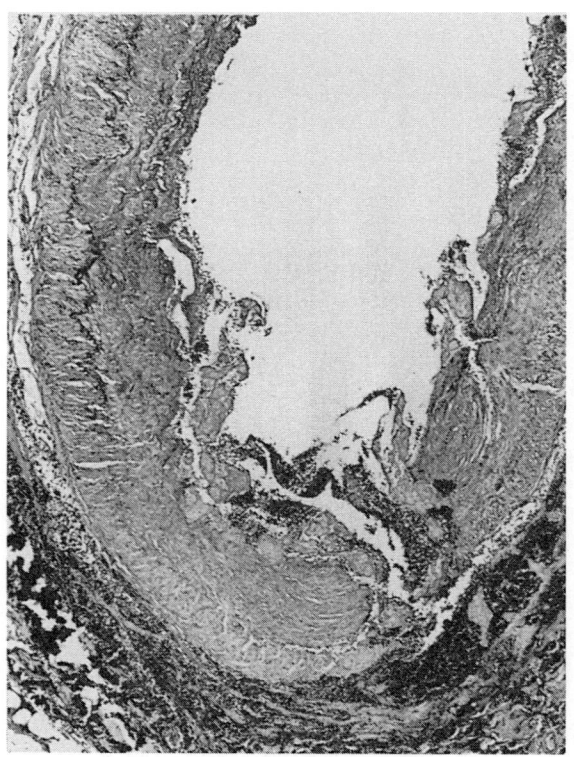

Fig. 32. Venous autograft. Intimo-medial rupture with adventitial haemorrhage caused by faulty surgery. Masson's trichrome

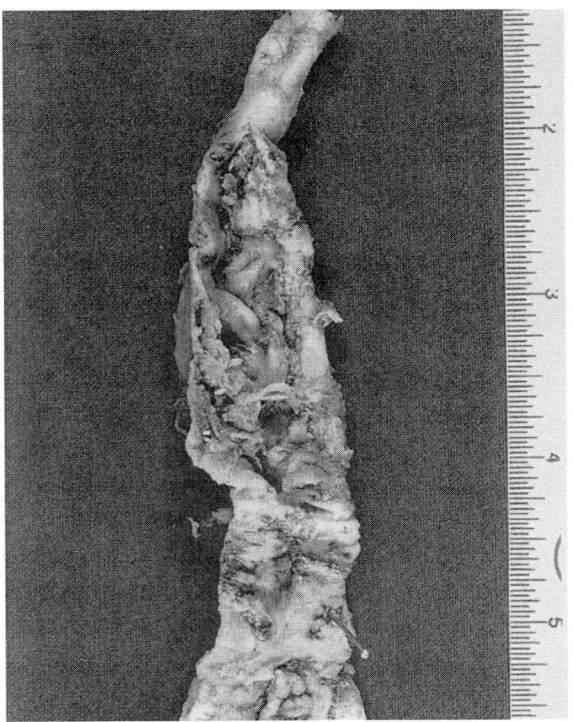

Fig. 34. Venous autograft. Accelerated atherosclerosis with aneurysmal dilation

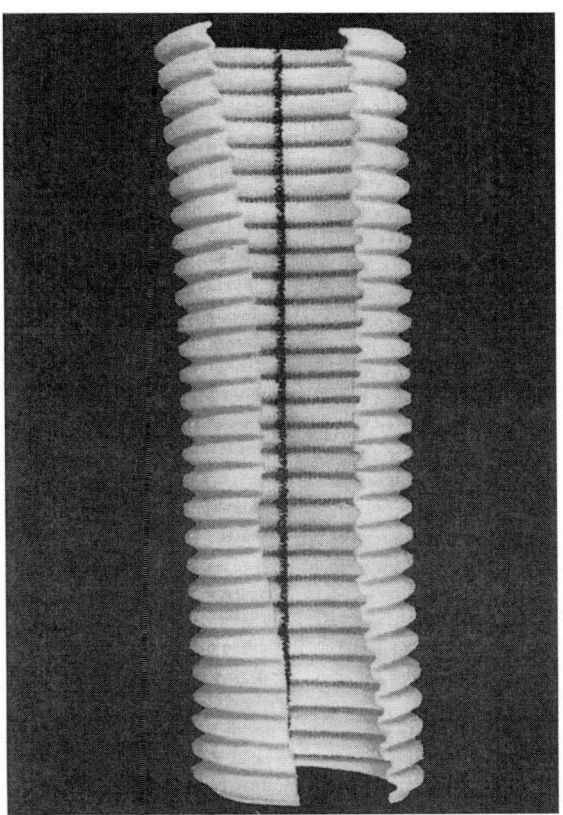

Fig. 36. Dacron vascular prosthesis with black landmark fibres

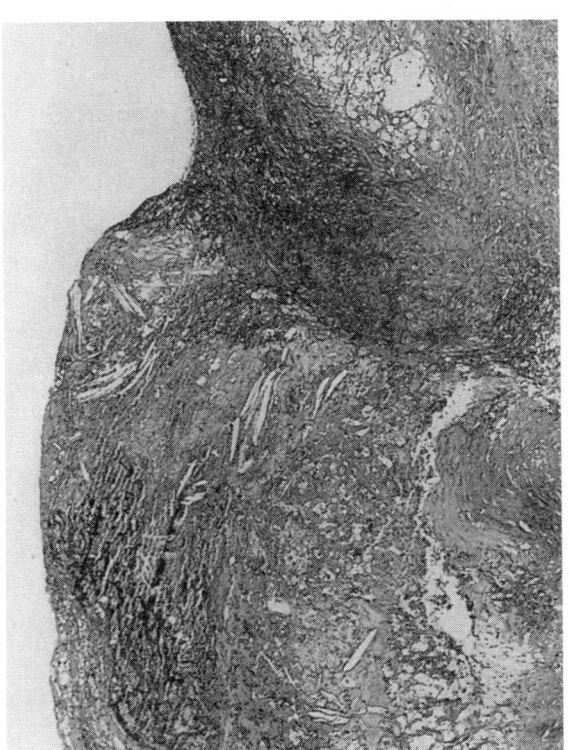

Fig. 35. Venous autograft. Newly-formed atherosclerotic plaque. HES

grafts and graft materials containing carbon fibres providing a negative charge to the luminal aspect or impregnated with basic fibroblast growth factor and heparin have been used in smaller vessels [129, 130]. Combined synthetic and biological grafts might have real advantages when used as bypasses. They consist of a pretreated venous allograft (human umbilical vein), rendered inert with glutaraldehyde and rein-forced by a Dacron polyester mesh [131, 132]. Grafts made by implanting a synthetic framework into the recipient to ensure in situ fibrous infiltration (5 to 6 weeks) are also promising. The Spark-mandril device is an example [133, 134], but has not proved success-ful in clinical use. Endothelial seeding technology is under investigation to prevent prostheses from deve-loping thrombosis,and from the effects of prolonged pulsatile shear stress [135-137]. This method [138, 139] is also used in vitro to engineer bioprothetic heart valves [140]. Other trials, such as prostheses bonded with heparin, and pretreated with fibroblast growth factor, are under way [141-143].

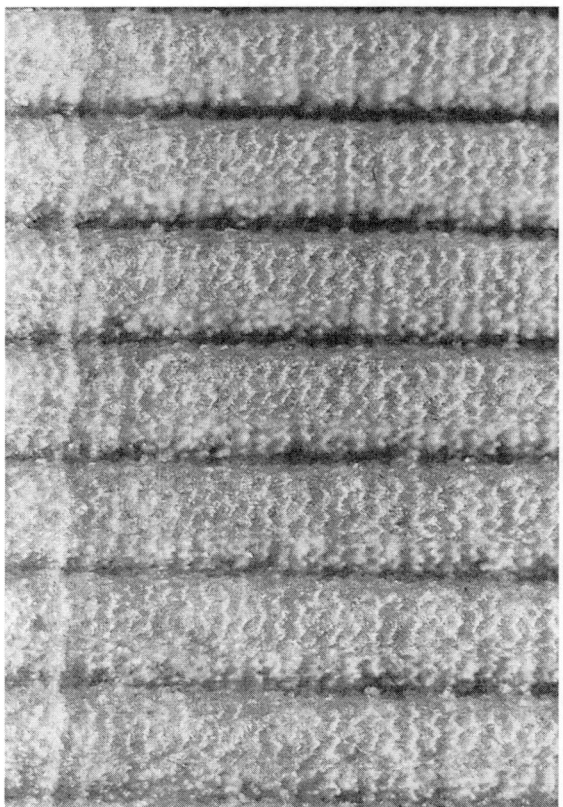

Fig. 37. Dacron vascular prosthesis. Note good porosity between meshes

Types of synthetic prostheses

1. Crepe-type prostheses (Wesolowki's prostheses) are soft and possess good porosity but permit fibroblast ingrowth through the interstices of the graft. With time, fibrosis and foreign body reaction lead to cracking and leaking with detachment from the prosthetic bed. Peri-prosthetic haematomata are common. For these reasons their use has been abandoned but they may be found at autopsy.
2. Knitted prostheses (DeBakey's ultra-light prostheses) allow good cell permeability but need careful pre-coagulation, a disadvantage if anti-coagulant drugs are to be administered.
3. Woven prostheses are stiffer, waterproof and have a low cellular permeability. They are used when patients are receiving anti-coagulant drugs or if they have disorders of haemostasis.
4. Velvet prostheses are covered by a velvet dacron material that resists thrombosis and cellular penetration.

5. Expanded reinforced porous prostheses (PET or polyethylene terepthalate and PTFE or polytetrafluoroethylene.) This porous expanded form of polymer Teflon material is composed of 15% pure tetrafluoroethylene and 85% air by volume. The expansion of a standard ePTFE leads to a maze-like microtexture consisting of solid nodes linked by thin fibrils. This highly electronegative and hydrophobic material confers chemical inertness and stability on the polymer. In the first series of femoro-popliteal bypasses using these grafts half of these bypasses exhibited fusiform dilation in the following months, resulting from a defect in circumferential tensile strength [144, 145]. The ePTFE was then reinforced with a bandage composed of layers of expanded PTFE film (Fig. 38). The resultant bilayer pattern provides superior circumferential and longitudinal strength and decreases radial dilation. Recent study has demonstrated that under static pressure between 0 and 300 mmHg the in-vitro tranverse dilatation of PTFE grafts is 8.4% [83]. A reinforced ePTFE prosthesis does not require previous clotting before its implantation. Other subtypes of ePTFE prostheses harbour carbon fibres providing a ne-

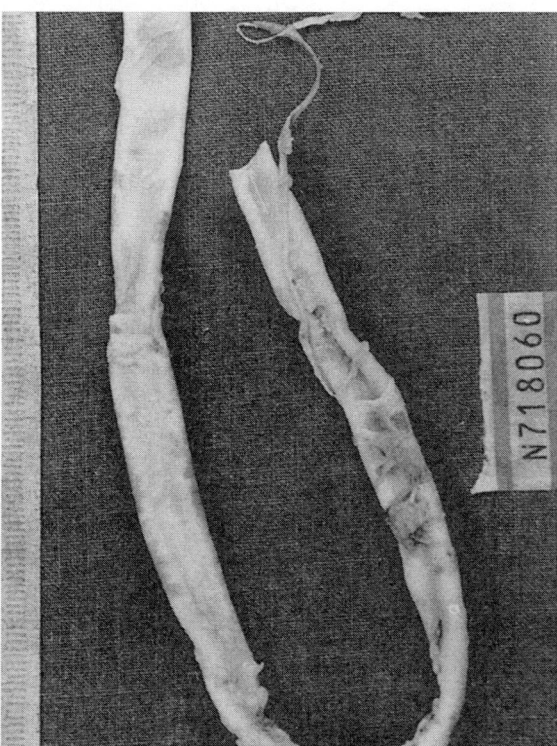

Fig. 38. ePTFE vascular prosthesis. Removed PTFE prosthesis displaying detachment of the reinforcement bandage. (Courtesy Dr J.-M. Fichelle)

gative charge to the luminal side (Fig. 39) with additional reinforcement (Fig. 40). A new ePTFE proshesis (Goretex Stretch, W.L. Gore & Associates Inc.,USA) was introduced for clinical use in 1991 [146]. This novel graft is constructed in the same double layer technique. Longitudinal extensibility is the result of microcrimping of the inner tube. This Stretch ePTFE facilitates sizing and anastomotic accuracy during implantation and has been used for aortic reconstruction, lower extremity revascularization and arteriovenous shunting.

Behaviour of the implanted prosthesis according to its type

1. Dacron. The Dacron prosthesis is made of texturised multifilamentous yarn with extended porosity. The "knitted" type offers superior handling characteristics and has less tendency to fray, but needs preclotting prior to implantation. The "woven" type is less porous and does not require preclotting. Porosity permits fibroblast ingrowth through the interstices of the graft with development of foreign body granulomata and fibrosis, leading to firm incorporation of the graft (Fig. 41). Under static pressure between 0 and 300 mmHg [83], the *in vitro* transverse dilatation of a dacron prosthesis

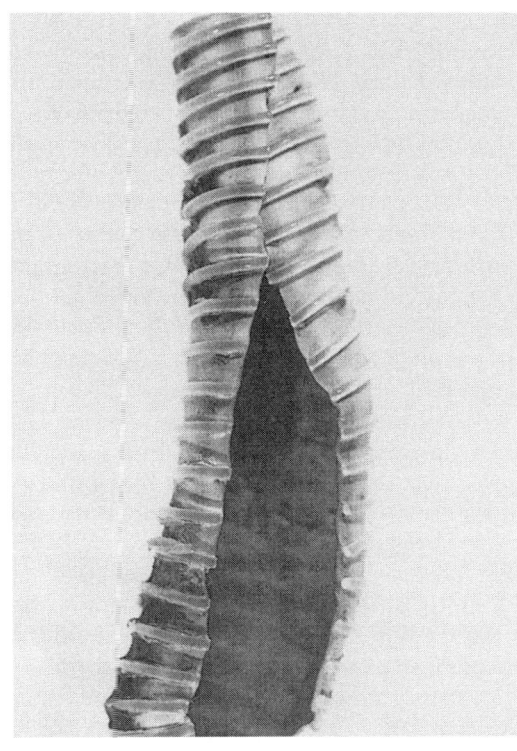

Fig. 40. ePTFE vascular prosthesis harbouring carbon fibres in the luminal side with additional external reinforcement bandage

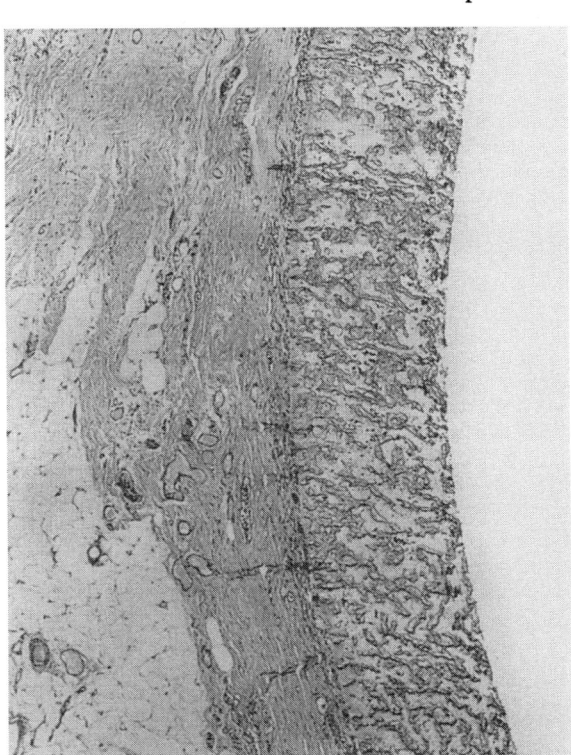

Fig. 39. ePTFE vascular prosthesis containing carbon fibres in the luminal aspect. HES

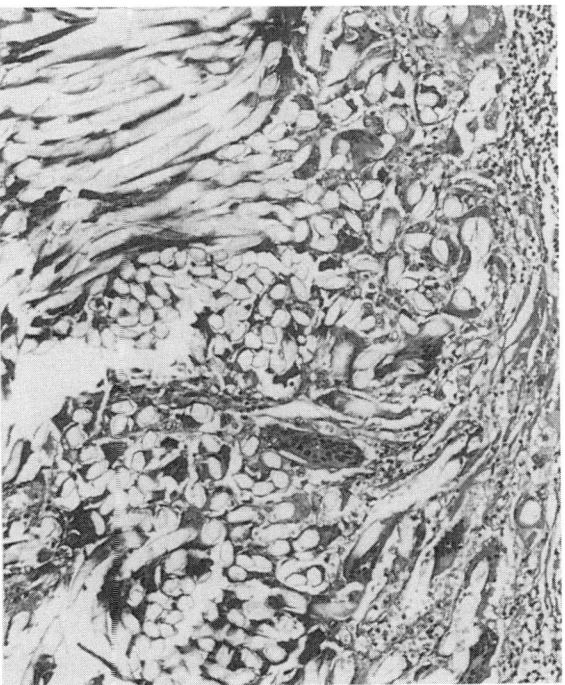

Fig. 41. Dacron vascular prosthesis. Fibrosis with foreign body granulomata developed in the interstices of the graft. HES

is 6.9%. On a long-term basis, the prosthesis undergoes gradual disintegration (Fig. 42) with separation of fibers leading to prosthetic fatigue, and
possible rupture (Fig. 43) with aneurysmal dilation (Fig. 44). So its functional durability depends
on the haemodynamic flow and the size of the
graft. Dacron grafts are less compliant (five to ten
times) when compared with native arteries, thus
producing a compliance mismatch. Dacron grafts
to small and medium-sised arteries, such as tibioperoneal arteries, give significantly poorer results
when compared with the outcome in large arteries
[147, 148].

2. Teflon prostheses. These grafts have a tensile wall
   strength that remains unchanged for years. Once
   implanted, these prosthesis dilate by 15-20% over
   the pulse pressure range and are thus often useful
   in small calibre vessels.

3. Expanded tetrafluoroethylene prostheses (ePTFE).
   The main difference between ePTFE and synthetic
   prostheses is that in the external capsule, the
   connective tissue penetration stops at the reinforcing sheath, which seems to limit the foreign body
   reaction (Fig. 45-46-47). The organization of the
   internal capsule or neo-intima has been a matter
   of controversy. Campbell demonstrated penetration of connective tissue containing newly-formed
   vessels giving rise to a true neo-intima in dogs and
   later in man [149]. A study of biopsies of permeable TFEP implanted for a period longer than
   60 months in man seemed to refute these results
   [150] and demonstrated a lack of connective tissue
   penetration and neovascularization. Endothelial
   proliferation was limited to the anastomotic lines
   (Fig. 48). The neo-intima is basically made of fibrin, platelets, blood cells and cell debris (Fig. 49).
   Collagen and elastin fibers are never seen, even in
   a long-standing prosthesis. In the prosthetic matrix, plasma with a few blood cells oozes inside the
   interstitial space. With time this material becomes
   hyalinised. Some areas of calcification may be seen
   (Fig. 50). Detachment of the reinforcing bandage
   may lead to distortion of the matrix by foreign
   body granulomata, fibrosis (Fig. 51-52) and rupture (Fig. 53).

The provision of repeated vascular access

Temporary access

If access is required for a few hours or days, a semi-rigid catheter of Teflon or a similar material is passed
over a guide wire by the Sedinger technique into the
appropriate vessel. In this way measurements of the

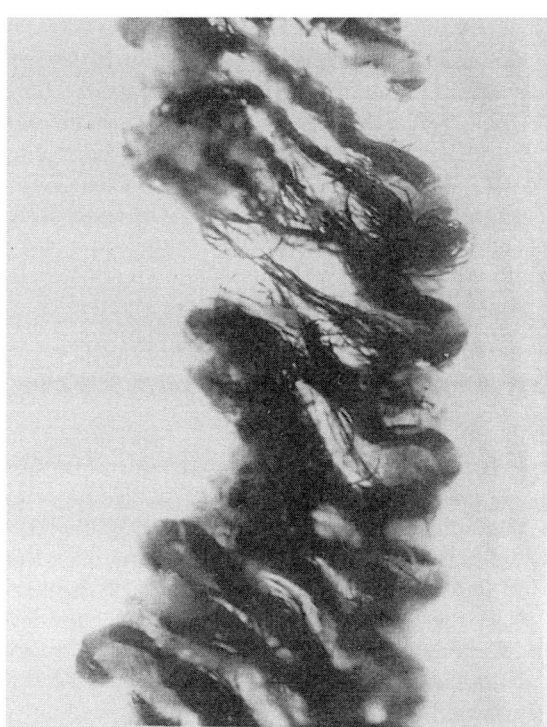

Fig. 42. Dacron vascular prosthesis. Uneven separation of the
black landmark fibres caused by prosthetic fatigue

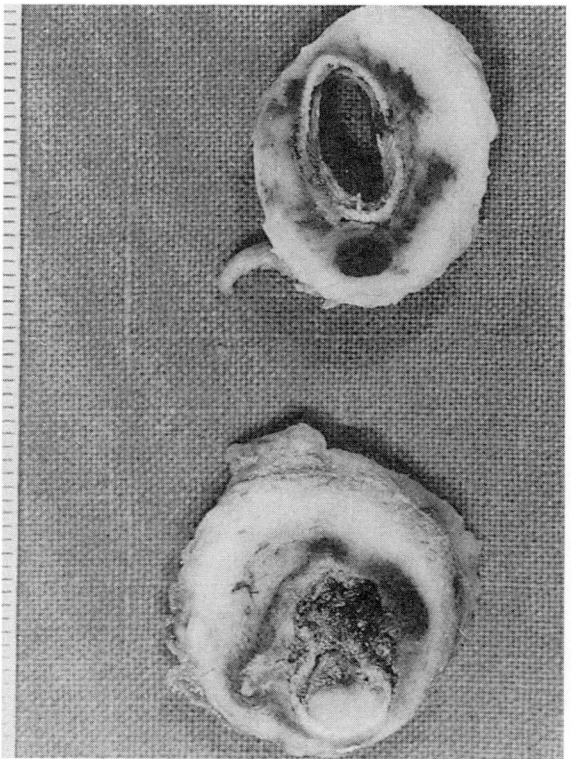

Fig. 43. Dacron vascular prosthesis. Prosthetic rupture with
dissecting haematoma uplifting the external capsule

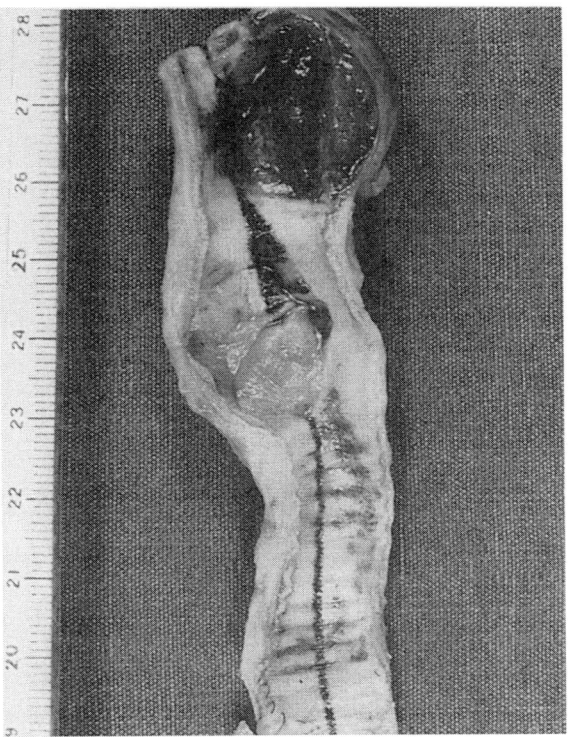

Fig. 44. Dacron vascular prosthesis. Rupture with aneurysm formation

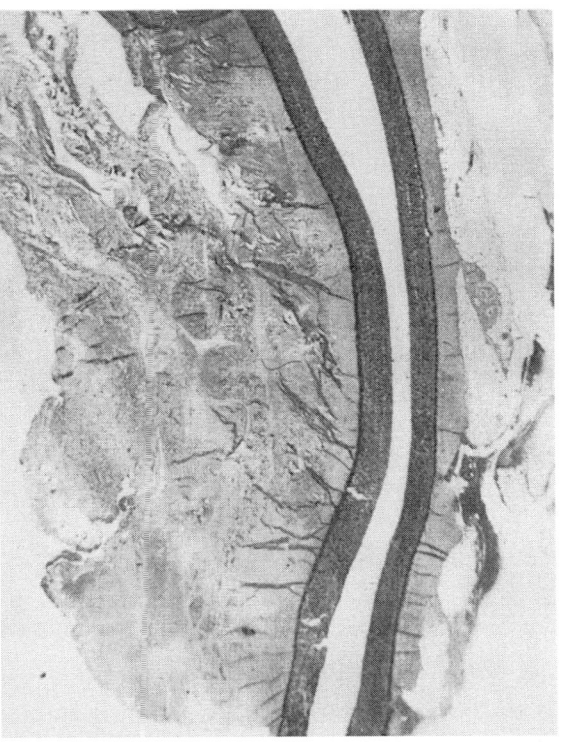

Fig. 45. ePTFE prosthesis. External capsule with fibrotic engulfment of the reinforcement bandage. HES

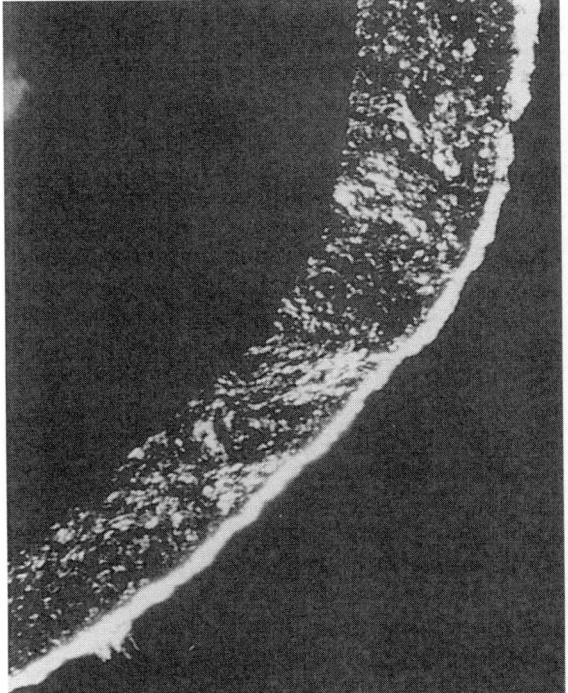

Fig. 46. ePTFE prosthesis. Strongly refringent reinforcement bandage surrounding the prosthetic matrix made up of juxtaposed knots under polarized light

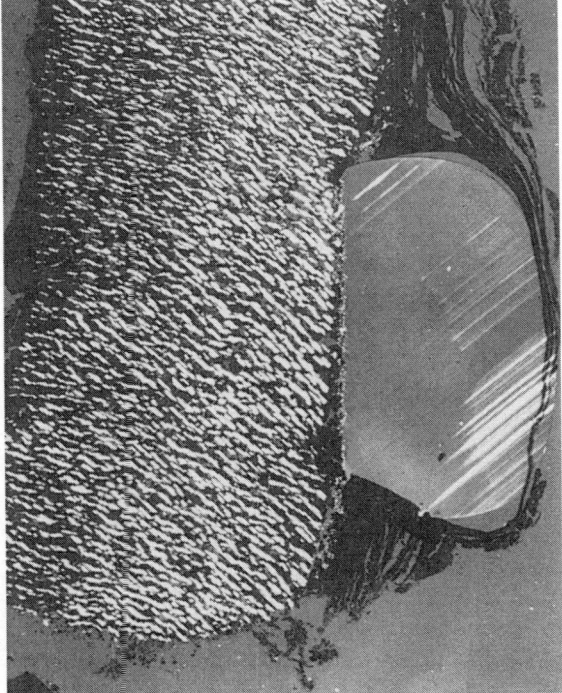

Fig. 47. ePTFE prosthesis with additional reinforcement bandage (see Fig. 40). Polarized light

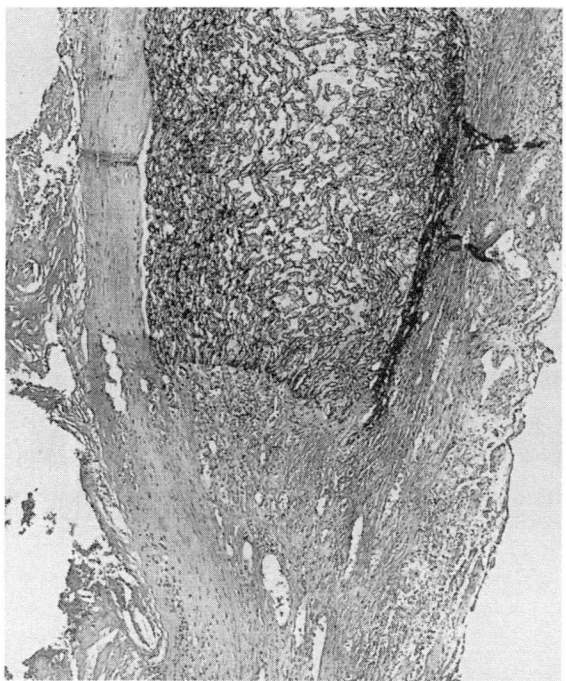

Fig. 48. ePTFE prosthesis. Internal capsule or neo-intima at the anastomotic line. HES

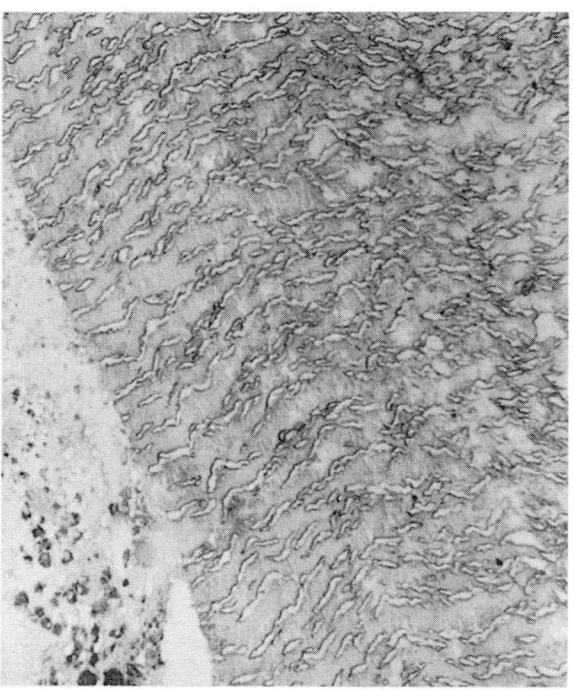

Fig. 49. ePTFE prosthesis. Internal capsule far away from the anastomotic line. Note presence of fibrin, blood cells and cell debris. No immunohistochemically confirmed endothelial cells seen. Per-oxidase antiperoxidase immunohistochemical technique (PAP)

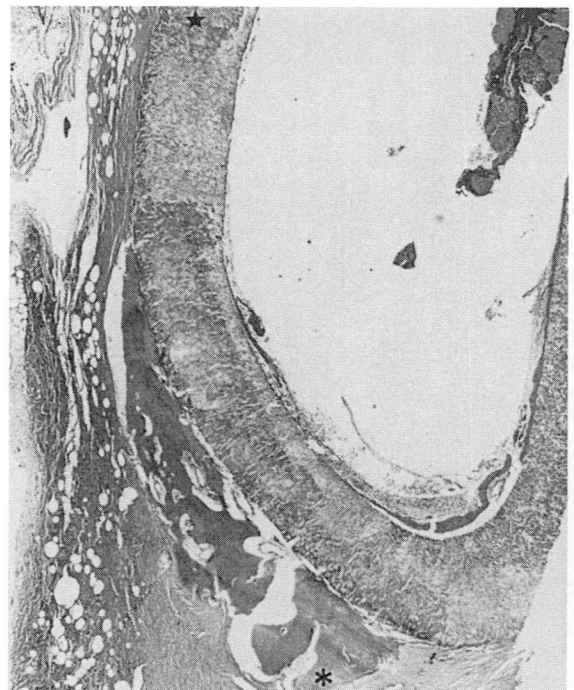

Fig. 50. ePTFE prosthesis. Calcifications of the matrix with osseous metaplasia in the external capsule. HES

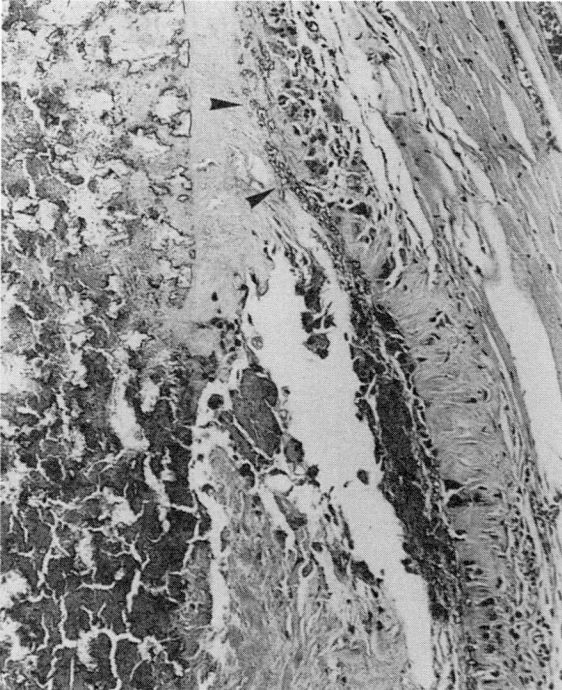

Fig. 51. ePTFE prosthesis. Detachment of the reinforcement bandage (arrow heads) with foreign body granulomata separating the matrix from the external capsule. HES

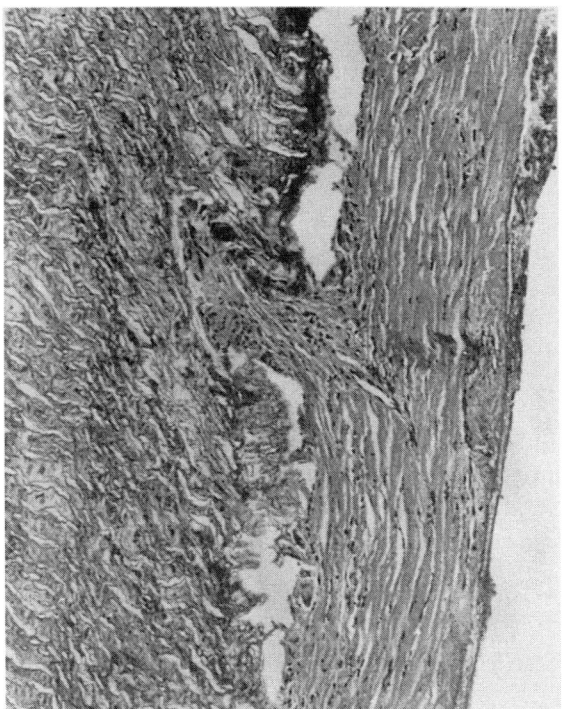

Fig. 52. ePTFE prosthesis. Small area of matrix rupture sealed by fibrotic strands. HES

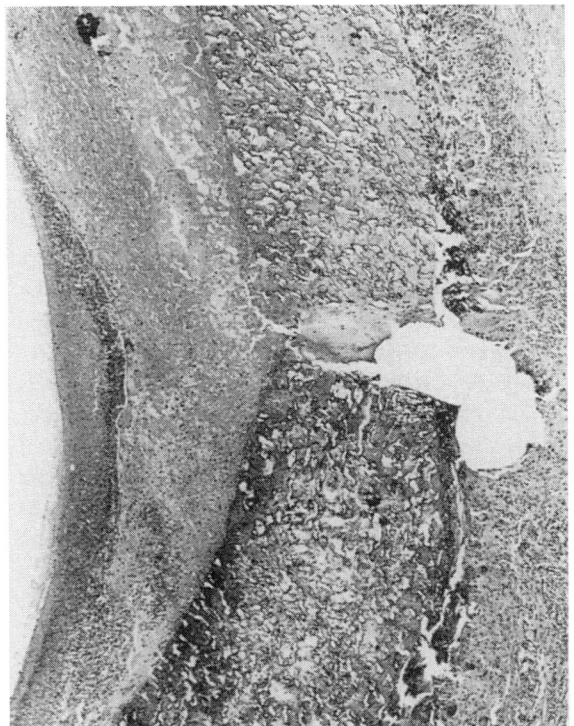

Fig. 53. ePTFE prosthesis. Complete rupture of the matrix caused by a misplaced suture stitch

central venous pulmonary artery pressure, intermittent femoral vein cannulation for maintenance haemodialysis and chemotherapy can be carried out. However, semi-rigid catheters are prone to infection and thrombosis [8, 151, 152].

Permanent access

Many techniques have been used, each with advantages and disadvantages. Direct cannulation for renal dialysis damaged vessels repeatedly until exhaustion of potential puncture sites led to the death of the patient. Teflon-Silastic external arteriovenous shunts or prolonged peritoneal dialysis [153] were a practical but not permanent solution. Internal side-to-side arteriovenous fistula – AVF provides a lifetime of access in patients with normal blood vessels. An arteriovenous bridge using an autogenous vein [154], a bovine heterograft or a prosthetic graft (GoreTex polytetrafluoroethylene PTFE, polyurethane) for older and sicker patients permits direct puncture [101, 129, 128]. There is no ideal material for permanent vascular access and selection of the best method depends on the patient as well as the indication.

The simple side-to-side AVF remains the ideal. The aim is to cannulate two veins easily and rapidly, obtaining a flow of 200ml or more per minute, three times weekly for a lifetime. AVF can be carried out at the wrist and midforearm; at the wrist, the radial artery should always be used because in the event of occlusion, the ulnar artery can almost always supply blood flow to the hand [155]. The brachial artery is rarely used for an antecubital AVF. It is rarely practical to use femoro-popliteal vessels. When an AVF is not feasible, a gap between a suitable artery and vein must be bridged by a graft, usually in the upper extremity. Bovine arterial xenografts can be used; however, PTFE is generally agreed to be the most suitable material for this purpose. Complications include:

1. Occlusion. In a long functioning fistula, occlusion may result from repeated use of the same vein, thrombosis, intimal hyperplasia (Fig. 54-55) and dyslipidemia [156-158]. Unblocking is carried out by introducing Fogarty catheters, dilators and heparinised solution into both artery and vein. Thrombectomy can be performed after vascular incision. This procedure can be repeated in PTFE grafts.

2. Ischaemia. After functioning for a period, an AVF may cause ischemia of the hand by diversion of blood from the palmar arch into the low resistance of the venous system and ischaemic neuropathy may result from an arterial steal syndrome. Digital compression of the AVF produces perceptible im-

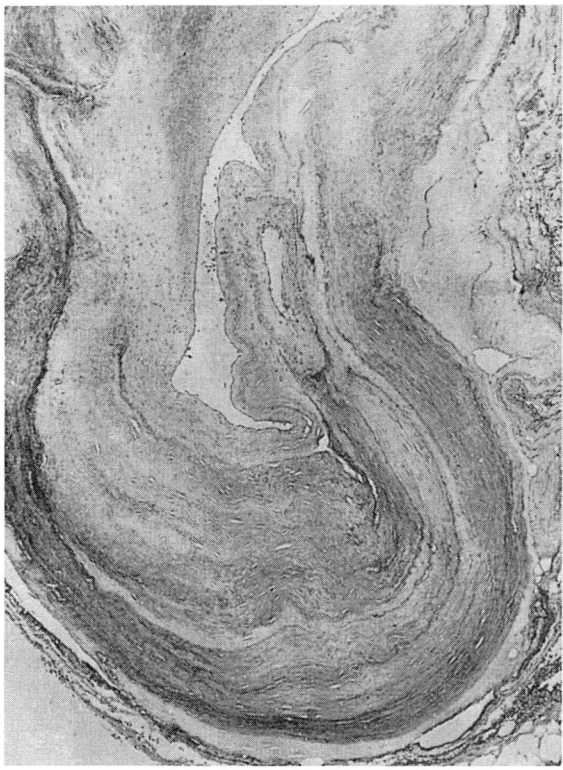

Fig. 54. Permanent vascular access. Surgical arterio-venous fistula for haemodialysis. Marked intimal hyperplasia occluding in the venous loop. ...Orcein...

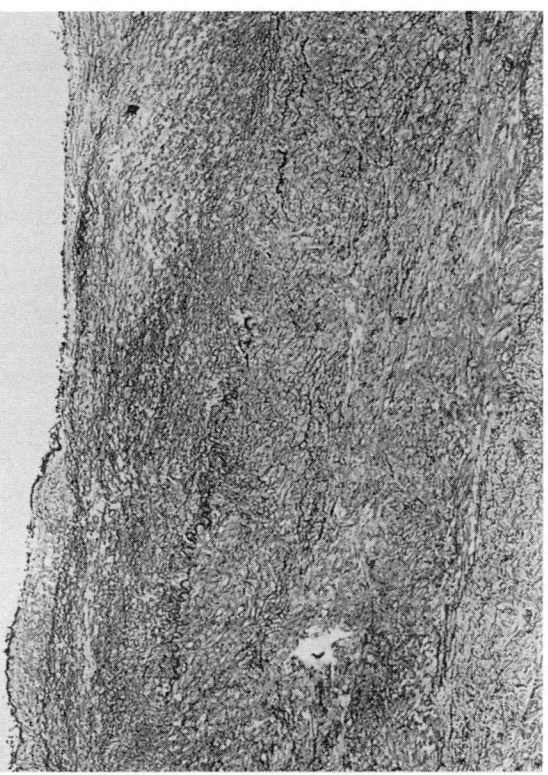

Fig. 55. Permanent vascular access. Surgically-confected arterio-venous fistula for haemodialysis. Newly-formed internal elastic membrane developed in the arterialized venous loop. ...Orcein...

provement of the digital pulses. Ligation of the radial artery distal to the fistula often resolves the problem and preserves access.

3. Venous hypertension. This occurs when the limb proximal to a functioning fistula or graft is occluded and the arterialised blood is pumped into a hand with inadequate venous drainage, resulting in long-term cutaneous dystrophic changes [159-161] Ligation of the distal vein relieves the hypertension. If venous hypertension results from brachial artery inflow into the axillary vein of an extremity that has had considerable venous compromise, the only treatment alternatives may be banding of the graft or closure of the access.

4. Venous atherosclerosis. In long term haemodialysis, the venous loops fashioned into arteriovenous anastomoses may develop irregularity and narrowing of the lumen by atherosclerosis (Fig. 56-57) [158, 162].

5. Neural compression. Neural compression is rare. Local oedema may produce a carpal tunnel syndrome.

6. Aneurysm formation. An aneurysm must be distinguished from a perigraft hematoma or false aneurysm with its extraluminal turbulent blood flow. Aneurysms may develop at the site of repeated punctures, on the graft material, or at the arterial or venous site of the anastomosis (Fig. 58). Infection, distal outflow obstruction and the type of graft material may all play a role in their development [161]. The incidence of false aneurysms and puncture site complications differs markedly between the material used, for example 0.96% and 1.92% per patient year with Omniflow vascular grafts, and 2.38% per patient with PTFE grafts [128]. True venous aneurysms have been reported proximal to PTFE bridge grafts. In most cases, frank or occult infection is the main cause [163]. Other causes include suture failure, graft degeneration, arterial or venous wall degeneration, multiple previous operations at the anastomotic area, and mechanical tension.

7. Congestive heart failure. This may occur with large shunts and occurs more commonly if the

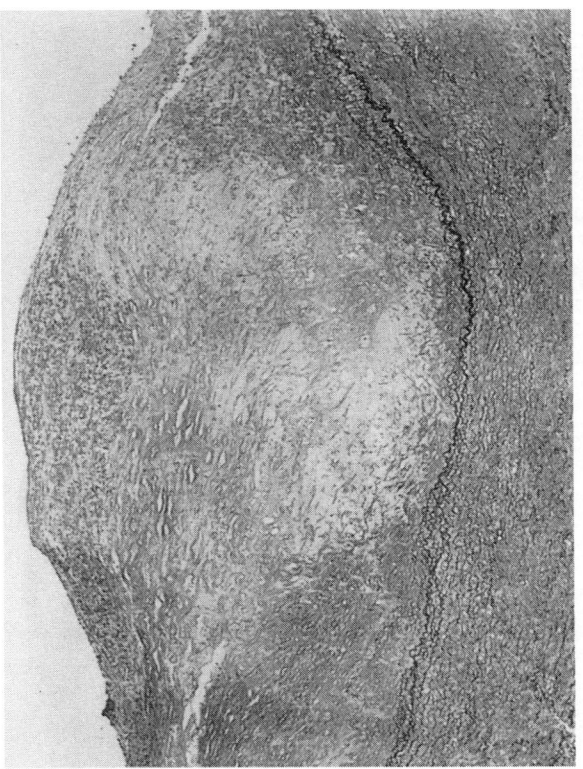

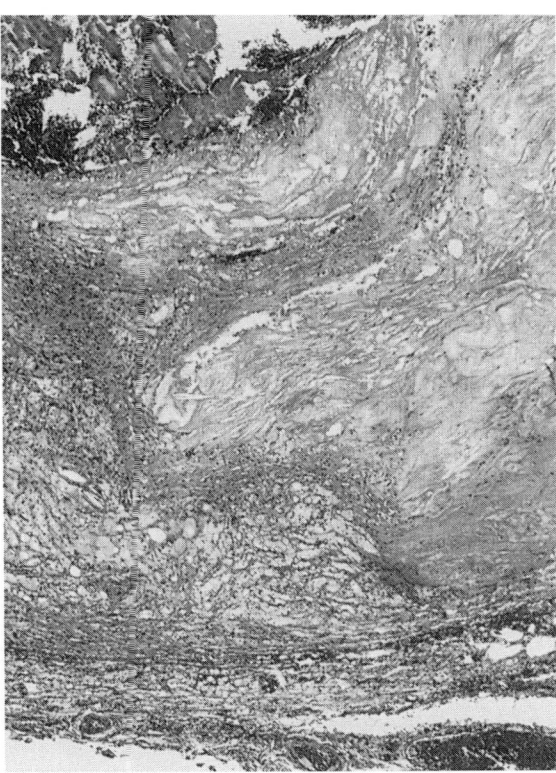

Fig. 56. Permanent vascular access. Surgically-confected arterio-venous fistula for haemodialysis. Fibroatheroma developed in the venous loop. ...Orcein...

Fig. 57. Permanent vascular access. Surgically-confected arterio-venous fistula for haemodialysis. Complicated atherosclerotic plaque with thrombosis in the venous loop. Masson's trichrome

brachial or femoral artery is used. Treatment of an excessively large flow involves banding of the graft.

8. Skin erosion and infection. Skin erosions with graft or vessel exposure can occur at repeated puncture sites when the bypass is placed too superficially, giving the potential for bleeding, infection, and false aneurysm formation. The graft should be removed in any postoperative graft infection [161, 164]

9. Bluefarb-Stewart syndrome (Kaposiform angiodermatitis or pseudo-Kaposi's sarcoma). This rare syndrome is characterised by proliferation of fibroblasts and of blood vessels, leading to tortuosity and elongation of cutaneous capillaries. The cause is an altered oxygen saturation. Some lesions arise after local trauma, amputation [165] or at the site of a surgical arteriovenous shunt [166, 167]. Others are congenital and may present in the first and second decades of life [168-170]. Clinically, the lesions appear as violaceous ma-

cules or patches that lead to soft, smooth, non-tender, reddish or purplish nodules on a limb with an underlying arteriovenous fistula. Thrills or bruits are rarely found. Varicose veins may be present. Pain may occur after repeated ulceration with secondary infection. Bluefarb-Stewart syndrome is punctuated by intermittent infections and haemorrhage. When infection, haemorrhage, pain, deformity and cardiovascular decompensation become severe, amputation of the limb may be the only course.

Histologically, the skin lesions are characterised by a markedly increased number of thick-walled blood vessels in the dermis (Fig. 59). These vessels, lined with plump endothelial cells, are interspersed with extravasated red blood cells, haemosiderin-loaded macrophages and fibroblasts (Fig. 60-61). The blood vessels may gather in discrete lobules separated by fibrous septa. The overlying epidermis may be hyperplastic. The major diffe-

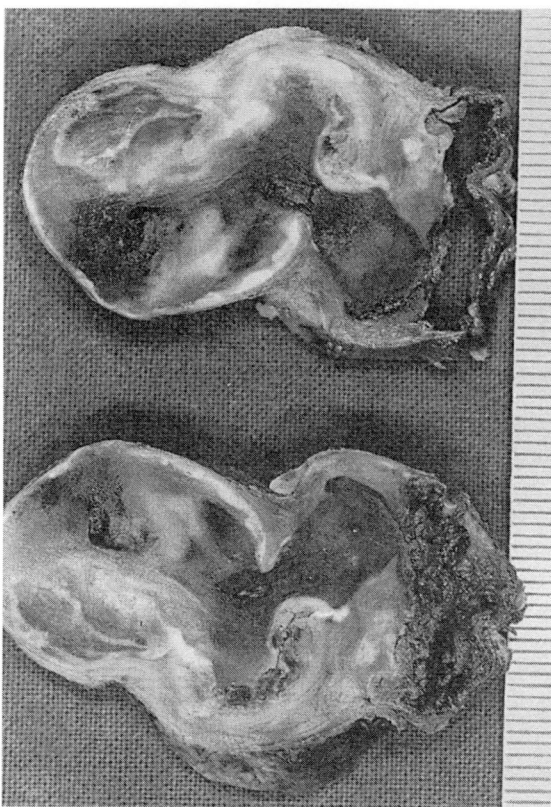

Fig. 58. Permanent vascular access. Surgically-confected arterio-venous fistula for haemodialysis. Thrombosed aneurysm. Note whitish calcified atherosclerotic plaques lining the venous loop. (Courtesy Dr M. Cogan)

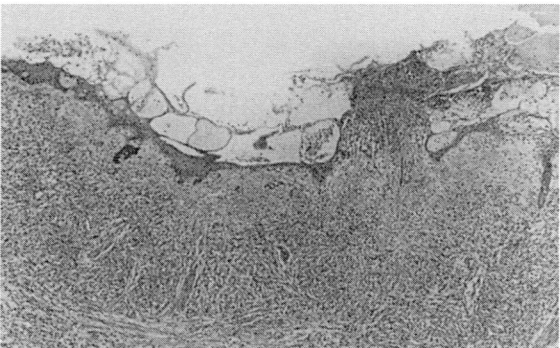

Fig. 59. Permanent vascular access. Surgically-confected arterio-venous fistula for haemodialysis. Bluefarb-Stewart syndrome. Dense proliferation of capillaries, distorting the dermis, eroding and uplifting the epidermis

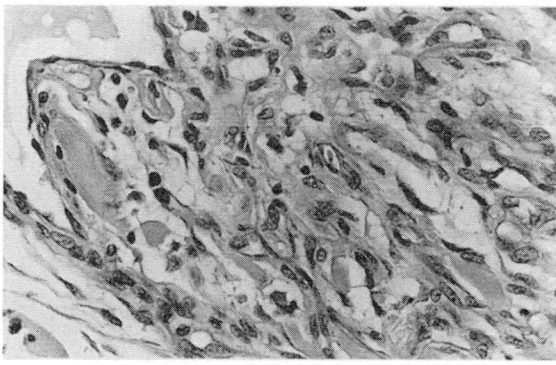

Fig. 60. Permanent vascular access. Surgically-confected arterio-venous fistula for haemodialysis. Bluefarb-Stewart syndrome. Newly formed capillaries lined with plump endothelial cells. HES

rential diagnosis is Kaposi's sarcoma but the characteristic features of Kaposi's sarcoma such as protrusion of preexisting normal venules into bizarre-shaped, thin-walled neoplastic vessels, fascicles of oval and spindle tumour cells separated by slit-like spaces that contain red blood cells, are lacking.

Operative procedures for veins

Sclerotherapy

This procedure is reserved for venous stars or small veins that are not amenable to surgical stripping, for occlusion of venous segments, either distal or proximal to the point of ligation of the major trunk, and for veins that may reappear in the years following an adequate vein removal. Sclerotherapy produces permanent fibrosis and deposits of haemosiderin pigment may stain the injection site for some months.

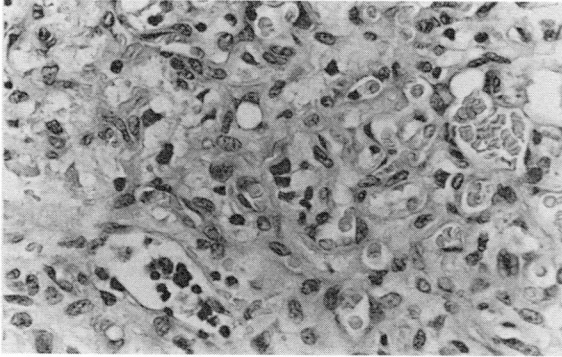

Fig. 61. Permanent vascular access. Surgically-confected arterio-venous fistula for haemodialysis. Bluefarb-Stewart syndrome. Immature capillaries mimicking Kaposi's sarcoma. HES

Stripping of varicose veins

Stripping is indicated when varicosities are large or produce significant symptoms (varicose eczema, skin pigmentation, and ulceration) (Fig. 62). Minor complications, such as haematomas and wound infection, usually reflect errors in surgical technique, but these are now rare. Trauma to the neighbouring saphenous or sural nerves is possible and excessive trauma or exposure of the common femoral vein may cause deep venous thrombosis. Cryosurgery allows complete invaginated stripping and represents an important technical improvement [171]. Recurrent varicose veins occur in over 20% of patients undergoing vein surgery [172]. This frequency appears higher [65.7%) in some multicenter studies. Causes of recurrency include incomplete surgical removal of varicosities (78.7%), diagnostic error (9.2%) [173], and pronounced inherent weakness of the veins, which appear normal at the time of surgery. Saphenous vein saving surgery, consisting of occlusion of incompetent perforators, may be an alternative to stripping [174].

Vena cava surgery

Balloon catheter dilation, stent placement, thrombolytic therapy [175], and vena cava interruption may all be performed. The first two procedures are not as successful in veins as in arteries because of the lower flow in venous beds.

Lytic therapy for pulmonary embolism is very effective [176-178]. In this site, it is easy for the lytic agent to bathe the emboli continuously. In other venous beds, the lytic agent may bypass the thrombosed area via collaterals and the procedure is thus less effective.

Vena cava interruption for thromboembolic disease permits the trapping of emboli at the inferior vena cava (less commonly at the superior vena cava) in more than 95% of cases. A large number of conditions may be treated in this way, including recurrent pulmonary embolism in patients receiving adequate anticoagulation therapy, and chronic pulmonary embolism with associated pulmonary hypertension and cor pulmonale. Recent pulmonary embolectomy with residual thrombi in distal veins [179-181], suppurative pelvic thrombophlebitis with possible showers of infected pulmonary emboli, and documented thromboembolism in a patient who has a contraindication to anticoagulation or complications of therapy, may also be treated by interruption [182]. Ligation or partial interruption using sutures or clips or filters may be extraluminal and require direct exposure of the

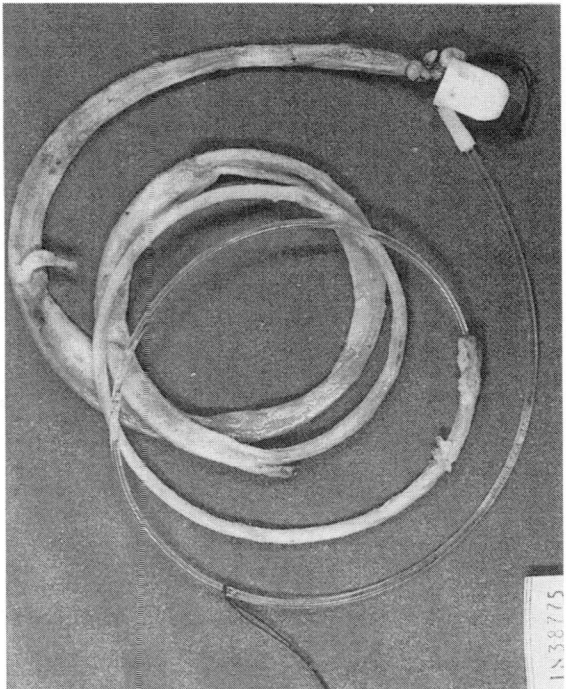

Fig. 62. Stripped varicose saphenous vein. (Courtesy Dr C. Lebard)

vein. In general, methods using plastic clips are superior to suture techniques. They do not damage the luminal surface, and are more reliable in compressing or dividing the vein into channels of appropriate size [183, 184]. External clips also prevent progressive dilation of the vein with subsequent enlargement of compartments.

In patients having preexisting cardiac disease with low-output myocardial failure, the complications of ligation include the sudden pooling of blood in the lower extremities with a sudden decrease in the venous return to the heart. This condition, like a pulmonary embolism, results in fatal shock with oedema and pain in the lower extremities [185]. The sequelae in the lower limbs resulting from this acute venous hypertension may be aggravated by the presence of prexisting thrombosis, and may lead to phlegmasia cerulea dolens and the postphlebitic syndrome [186]. Recurrent pulmonary embolism occurs in 5-15% of patients undergoing interruption of the inferior vena cava, and in 10-25% of patients having a femoral vein interruption [187, 188]. Clip unfastening is an exceptional event [189].

Intraluminal interruption is generally made by placing filters in the lumen of the vena cava from a venous catherization entry point (Fig. 63-64). They can be delivered to a precise location and several designs of filters are available [190-193]. Complications of intraluminal filters include difficulties with placement, perforation of an anchoring leg with retroperitoneal bleeding and haematoma, poor fixation leading to detachment and migration of the filter with fatal embolization [194], thrombotic occlusion of the vena cava – this may be caused by efficient clot trapping rather than by local mechanical influences – or recurrent pulmonary embolism (less than 10% of insertions with a 1% incidence of fatal embolism)[195-198]. Major disadvantages of the umbrella filter (Mobin-Uddin) are laceration of the vena cava wall and a tendency to become occluded rapidly, if a high load of emboli is presented. For these reasons the incidence of late morbidity following insertion of the umbrella filter is high, approaching that of inferior vena cava ligation.

In patients with malignancy or suprainguinal venous thrombus, insertion of an IVC filter gives little or no survival benefit these patients [199]. At least two thirds of patients with the Mobin-Uddin umbrella filter ultimately develop complete caval occlusion, compared with an approximate 10 occlusion rate for patients with the Kimray-Greenfield cone filter [191, 200].

Venous valve reconstruction

This is indicated when chronic venous insufficiency is caused by redundant valves. The surgical techniques include internal intravenous direct valve repair and extravenous tightening of the vein wall around the valve cusp [201-203]. Complications include technical stenosis, thrombosis, haematoma and infection [204].

Operative procedures for lymphoedema

In patients with lymphoedema, the goal of medical management (gravitational drainage, elastic support) is to manipulate or alter the pathological state so that the oedema is stabilised or reduced. Percutaneous

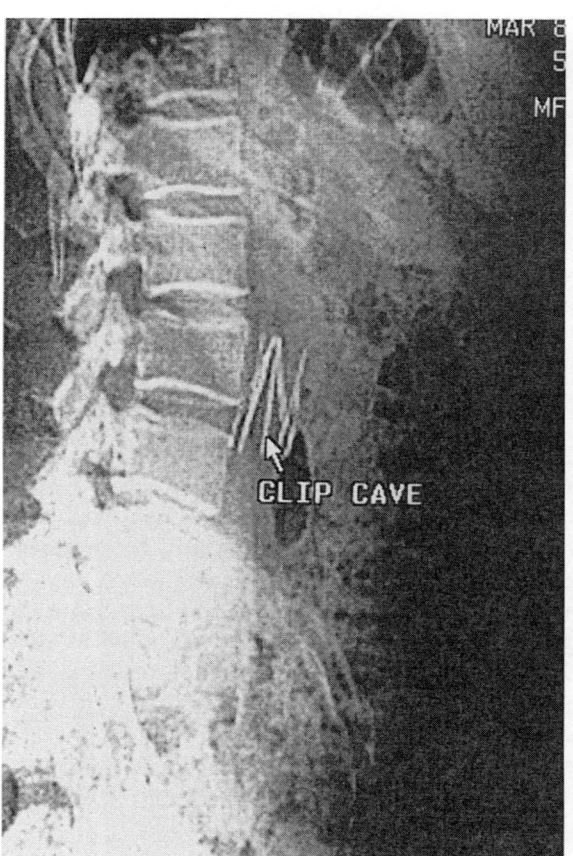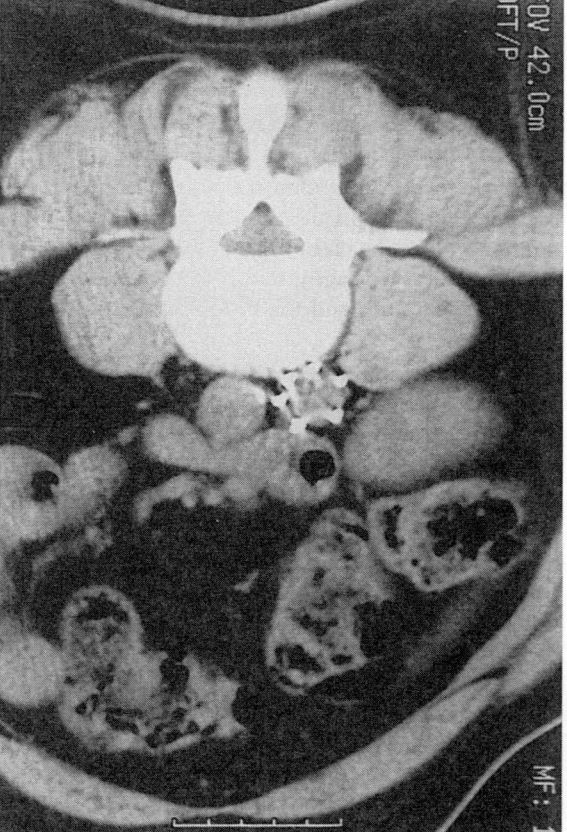

Fig. 63-64. Partial interruption of the vena cava by means of a cone filter. (Courtesy Dr B. Augustin)

sclerotherapy to the regional lymph nodes may improve lymphoedema [205]. Surgery becomes necessary when the change is progressive. The surgical procedures are of two kinds: excisional techniques and bridging drainage techniques. Radical or partial excision removes the entire diseased area including the skin, fat and usually the deep fascia (Fig. 65-66). The denuded limb is then resurfaced by either free thick-split grafts, full-thickness grafts or flaps (Charles operation), often taken from the excised specimen [206-209]. Thompson's technique and variants [210] consist of transposing the superficial lymphatics or the adipo-lymphatico-venous tissues from an unaffected limb into the deep compartment of the oedematous limb by burying the skin flap from which the epidermis has been shaved. Microsurgical lymphatic anastomosis to vein (nodo-venous then lymphovenous), and to lymphatic themselves are now performed. To date, none of the procedures described can be considered curative.

Possible complications of the surgery of lymphoedema include skin loss, especially in dermal-flap procedure, occlusion of lymphovenous anastomoses after microsurgery, reaccumulation of lymph from failure to remove affected tissue completely, secondary cellulitis, hypertrophic scarring with keloid formation and verrucal hyperkeratosis, caused by superimposed fungus infection at the site of surgery [207].

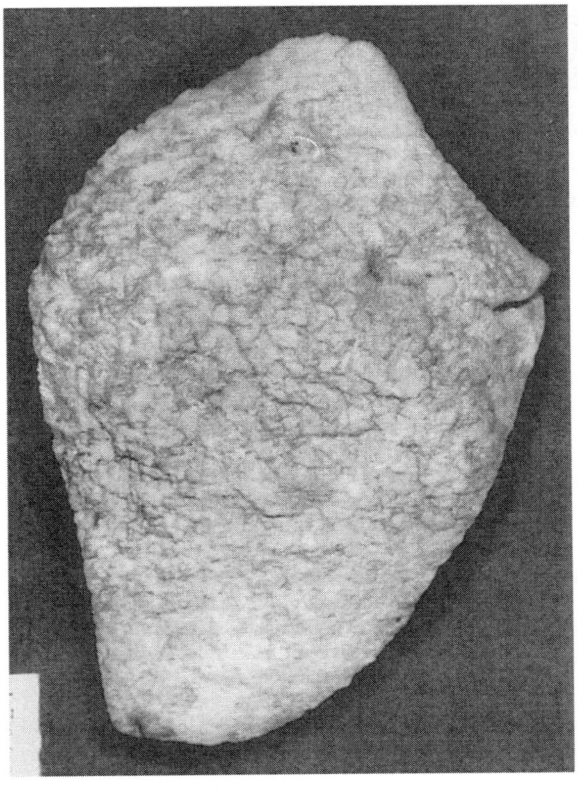

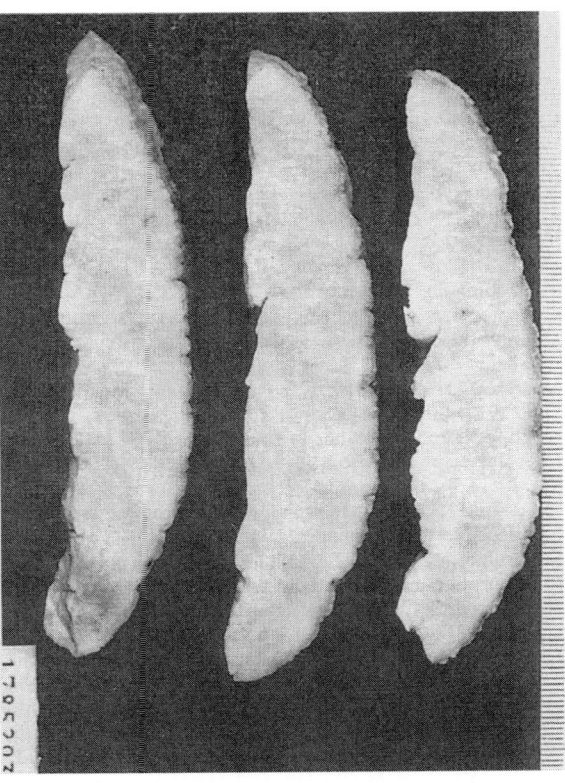

Fig. 66. Lymphoedema excisional specimen. Cut section showing marked oedema and fibrosis thickening the sub-cutaneous tissue

Fig. 65. Lymphoedema excisional specimen. Peau-d'orange pattern of the skin. (Courtesy Dr P. Trévidic)

Bibliography

1. M, Sautot J, Frileux C (1977) Artères-Veines-Lymphatiques *In* Patel J, Leger L, Patel JC (eds.) Nouveau traité de techniques chirurgicales -Tome 4, Masson, Paris, 691p
2. Haimovici H (1984) Vascular surgery: Principle and Techniques. Appleton-Century-Crofts, Northwalk, 1187p
3. Bernhard VM, Towne JB (1985) Complications in vascular surgery. Grune Stratton, Orlando, 793p
4. Vuong PN, Cormier JM (1987) Pathologie de l'artère opérée *In* Camilleri JP, Berry CL, Fiessinger JN, Bariety J: Les maladies de la paroi artérielle, Flammarion, Paris, pp 591-611
5. Lajvardi A, Trerotola SO, Strandberg JD, Samphilipo MA, Magee C (1995) Evaluation of venous injury caused by a percutaneous mechanical thrombolytic device. Cardiovasc Intervent Radiol 18: 172-78

6. Sprayregren S (1984) Principles of arteriography. In Haimovici H (Ed) Vascular surgery. Appleton-Century-Crofts, Northwalk pp 65-91

7. O'Farrell L, Griffith JW, Lang CM (1996) Histologic development of the sheath that forms around long-term implanted central venous catheters. JPEN J Parenter Enteral Nutr 20: 156-8

8. Hantschke D (1989) The significance of central venous catheters in the genesis of Candida endomycoses. Mycoses 32: 235-8

9. Bloom AI, Woolf YG, Cuenca A (1996) Accidental embolization of an intravenous cannula in the upper limb: retrieval following computed tomography localization. Eur J Emerg Med 3: 106-7

10. Ranchere JY, Thiesse P, Gordiani B, Perol M (1997) Peripheral venous catheter embolism. Ann Fr Anesth Reanim 16: 196-8

11. Ruiz-Razura A, Williams JL Jr, Reilly CL, Cohen BE, Schini VB, Vanhoutte PM, Thomsen S (1994) Acute intraoperative arterial elongation: histologic, morphologic, and vascular reactivity studies. J Reconstr Microsurg 10: 367-73

12. Starr DS, Weatherford SC, Lawrie GM, Morris GC Jr (1979) Suture material as a factor in the occurrence of anastomotic false aneurysms. An analysis of 26 cases. Arch Surg 114: 412-5

13. Klein SR, Goldberg L, Miranda RM, Bosco P, Nelson RJ, White RA (1982) Effect of suture technique on arterial anastomotic compliance. Arch Surg 117: 45-7

14. Butany JW, David TE, Ojha M (1998) Histological and morphometric analyses of early and late aortocoronary vein grafts and distal anastomoses. Can J Cardiol 14: 671-7

15. Bond MG, Hostetler JR, Karayannacos PE, Geer JC, Vasko JS (1976) Intimal changes in arteriovenous bypass grafts. Effects of varying the angle of implantation at the proximal anastomosis and of producing stenosis in the distal runoff artery. J Thorac Cardiovasc Surg 71: 907-16

16. Chen FZ, Xu X, Fu WG, Wu ZG (1994) Anastomotic false aneurysm following abdominal aortic aneurysmectomy and prosthetic grafting. Chin Med J 107: 832-5

17. Mii S, Mori A, Sakata H, Kawazoe N (1998) Para-anastomotic aneurysms: incidence, risk factors, treatment and prognosis. J Cardiovasc Surg (Torino) 39: 259-66

18. Lusby RJ, Ferrell LD, Englestad BL, Price DC, Lipton MJ, Stoney RJ (1983) Vessel wall and indium-111-labelled platelet response to carotid endarterectomy. Surgery 93: 424-32

19. Dirrenberger RA, Sundt TM Jr (1987) Carotid endarterectomy. Temporal profile of the healing process and effects of anticoagulation therapy. J Neurosurg 48: 201-19

20. Stewart GW, Bandyk DF, Kaebnick HW, Storey JD, Towne JB (1987) Influence of vein-patch angioplasty on carotid endarterectomy healing. Arch Surg 122: 364-71

21. Burrig KF, Schrix T (1995) Arterial wall texture after uncomplicated endarterectomy. Pathologe 16: 336-41

22. Zanetti PP, Sorisio V, Rosa G, Accordino R, Amerio GM, Cavanenghi D, Zappa A, Dutto C, Novellone GL, Duc E (1995) Pseudoaneurysms after carotid endarterectomy. Minerva Chir 50: 889-93

23. Collins PS, Orecchia P, Gomez E (1991) A technique for correction of carotid kinks and coils following endarterectomy. Ann Vasc Surg 5: 116-20

24. Valentine RJ, Myers SI, Hagino RT, Clagett GP (1996) Late outcome of patients with premature carotid atherosclerosis after carotid endarterectomy. Stroke 27: 1502-6

25. Marek JM, Koehler C, Aguirre ML, Westerband A, Gentile AT, Mills JL, Hunter GC (1998) The histologic characteristics of primary and restenotic carotid plaque. J Surg Res 74: 27-33

26. Moore WS, Kempczinski RF, Nelson JJ, Toole JF (1998) Recurrent carotid stenosis: results of the asymptomatic carotid atherosclerosis study. Stroke 29: 2018-25

27. Edwards WH Jr, Edwards WH Sr, Mulherin JL Jr, Martin RS 3d (1989) Recurrent carotid artery stenosis. Resection with autogenous vein replacement. Ann Surg 209: 662-8

28. Johnson BL, Gupta AK, Bandyk DF, Shulman C, Jackson M (1996) Anatomic patterns of carotid endarterectomy healing. Am J Surg 172: 188-90

29. Mitusch R, Stierle U, Sheikhzadeh A (1998) Atherosclerosis of the aorta as a source of arterial embolisms. Z Kardiol 87: 789-96

30. Mahler F, Triller J, Weidmann P, Nachbur B (1986) Complications in percutaneous transluminal dilatation of renal arteries. Nephron 44: S60-S63

31. Volk EE, Prayson RA, Perl J 2nd (1997) Autopsy findings of fatal complication of posterior cerebral circulation angioplasty. Arch Pathol Lab Med 121: 738-40

32. Serra A, Pereira H, Betriu A (1993) Percutaneous coronary angioscopy. Rev Port Cardiol 12: 1005-12

33. Alfonso F, Almeria C, Fernandez-Ortiz A, Segovia J, Ferreiros J, Goicolea J, Hernandez R, Banuelos C, Gil-Aguado M, Macaya C (1997) Aortic dissection occurring during coronary angioplasty: angiographic and transesophageal echocardiographic findings. Cathet Cardiovasc Diagn 42: 412-5

34. Silva JA, White CJ, Collins TJ, Ramee SR (1998) Morphologic comparison of atherosclerotic lesions in native coronary arteries and saphenous vein graphs with intracoronary angioscopy in patients with unstable angina. Am Heart J 136: 156-63

35. Dotter CT, Judkins MP (1964) Transluminal treatment of arteriosclerotic obstruction. Circulation 30: 654-70

36. Bauters C, Lablanche JM, Renaud N, McFadden EP, Hamon M, Bertrand ME (1996) Morphological changes after percutaneous transluminal coronary angioplasty of unstable plaques. Insights from serial angioscopic follow-up. Eur Heart J 17: 1554-9

37. Simonetti G, Bonomo L, Cornalba GP, De Caro G, Falappa P, Feltrin G, Gandini G, Grosso M, Iaccarino V, Lupattelli L, et al (1993) Percutaneous transluminal renal angioplasty. Italian experience at 13 centers. Radiol Med (Torino) 86: 503-8

38. Abe S, Handa S (1994) Percutaneous transluminal coronary angioplasty and directional coronary atherectomy: a short review of recent progress. Rinsho Kyobu Geka 14: 115-20

39. Capron L, Bruneval P (1989) Influence of applied stress on mitotic response of arteries to injury with a balloon catheter: quantitative study in rat thoracic aorta. Cardiovasc Res 23: 941-8

40. MacLeod DC, Strauss BH, de Jong M, Escaned J, Umans VA, van Suylen RJ, Verkerk A, de Feyter PJ, Serruys PW (1994) Proliferation and extracellular matrix synthesis of smooth muscle cells cultured from human coronary atherosclerotic and restenotic lesions. J Am Coll Cardiol 23: 59-65

41. Schwartz SM, Majesky MW, Murry CE (1995) The intima: development and monoclonal responses to injury. Atherosclerosis 118 S125-S140

42. Caramori PR, Eggers EE, Silva Filho AP, Uchoa DM, Jung F, Zago AC, Cerski CT, Schwartsmann G, Zago AJ (1997)

Postangioplasty restenosis: a practical model in the porcine carotid artery. Braz J Med Biol Res 30: 1087-91

43. Tschopl M, Tsakiris DA, Marbet GA, Labs KH, Jager K (1997) Role of hemostatic risk factors for restenosis in peripheral arterial occlusive disease after transluminal angioplasty. Arterioscler Thromb Vasc Biol 17: 3208-14

44. Inoue T, Sakai Y, Fujito T, Hoshi K, Hayashi T, Takayanagi K, Morooka S (1998) Clinical significance of neutrophil adhesion molecules expression after coronary angioplasty on the development of restenosis. Thromb Haemost 79: 54-8

45. Essed CE, Brand MVD, Becker AE (1983) Transluminal coronary angioplasty and early restenosis. Br Heart J 49: 393-6

46. Austin GE, Ratliff NB, Hollman J, Tabei S, Phillips DF (1985) Intimal proliferation of smooth muscle cells as an explanation for recurrent coronary artery stenosis after percutaneous transluminal coronary angioplasty. J Am Coll Cardiol 6: 369-75

47. Bruneval P, Guermonprez JL, Perrier P, Carpentier A, Camilleri JP (1986) Coronary artery restenosis following transluminal coronary angioplasty. Arch Pathol Lab Med 110: 1186-7

48. Hirai T, Korogi Y, Harada M, Takahashi M (1996) Prevention of intimal hyperplasia by irradiation. An experimental study in rabbits. Acta Radiol 37: 229-33

49. Wilcox JN, Waksman R, King SB, Scott NA (1996) The role of the adventitia in the arterial response to angioplasty: the effect of intravascular radiation. Int J Radiat Oncol Biol Phys 36: 789-96

50. Weinberger J, Simon AD (1997) Intracoronary irradiation for the prevention of restenosis. Curr Opin Cardiol 12: 468-74

51. Fortunato JE, Glagov S, Bassiouny HS (1998) Irradiation for the treatment of intimal hyperplasia. Ann Vasc Surg 12: 495-503

52. Hashimoto M, Sawada S, Morioka N, Kotani K, Iwamiya T, Senda T, Tanigawa N, Kobayashi M, Okuda Y, Ohta Y, et al (1995) Percutaneous placement of intraluminal stent-graft for aortic dissection: experimental study. Nippon Igaku Hoshasen Gakkai Zasshi 55: 939-45

53. Blum U, Langer M (1996) Vascular stents and development of endoluminal therapy of aortic aneurysm. Zentralbl Chir 121: 714-20

54. Vale FL, Fisher WS 3rd, Jordan WD Jr, Palmer CA, Vitek J (1997) Carotid endarterectomy performed after progressive carotid stenosis following angioplasty and stent placement. Case report. J Neurosurg 87: 940-3

55. Link J, Muller-Hulsbeck S, Brossmann J, Steffens JC, Heller M (1996) Perivascular inflammatory reaction after percutaneous placement of covered stents. Cardiovasc Intervent Radiol 19: 345-7

56. Bouchart F, Dubar A, Bessou JP, Redonnet M, Berland J, Mouton-Schleifer D, Haas-Hubscher C, Soyer R (1997) Pseudomonas aeruginosa coronary stent infection. Ann Thorac Surg 64: 1810-3

57. Desoutter P, Houissa-Vuong S, Van T, Vuong PN (2000) Faux-anévrysme avec fistule artério-veineuse compliquant une endoprothèse. Angéiologie 52: 45-6

58. Anzuini A, Rosanio S, Legrand V, Tocchi M, Coppi R, Marazzi G, Vicedomini G, Pagnotta P, Montorfano M, Bonnier H, Sheiban I, Kulbertus HE, Chierchia SL (1997) Immediate and long-term clinical and angiographic re-

sults of the Wiktor stent in the treatment of chronic coronary occlusions. G Ital Cardiol 27: 881-91

59. Elezi S, Kastrati A, Neumann FJ, Hadamitzky M, Dirschinger J, Schomig A (1998) Vessel size and long-term outcome after coronary stent placement. Circulation 98: 1875-80

60. Kastrati A, Schomig A, Elezi S, Schuhlen H, Dirschinger J, Hadamitzky M, Wehinger A, Hausleiter J, Walter H, Neumann FJ (1997) Predictive factors of restenosis after coronary stent placement. J Am Coll Cardiol 30: 1428-36

61. Brown DL, George CJ, Steenkiste AR, Cowley MJ, Leon MB, Cleman MW, Moses JW, King SB 3rd, Carrozza JP, Holmes DR, Burkhard-Meier C, Popma JJ, Brinker JA, Buchbinder M (1997) High-speed rotational atherectomy of human coronary stenoses: acute and one-year outcomes from the New Approaches to Coronary Intervention (NACI) registry. Am J Cardiol 80: 60K-7K

62. Waksman R, Popma JJ, Kennard ED, George CJ, Douglas JS Jr, Cowley M, Leon MB, Holmes DR, Hinohara T, Safian RD, Hornung CA, Brinker JA, Roubin GS, Bonan R, Kereiakes D, Matthews RV, Baim DS (1997) Directional coronary atherectomy (DCA): a report from the New Approaches to Coronary Intervention (NACI) registry. Am J Cardiol 80: 50K-59K

63. Bucay M, Zacca NM, Trakhtenbroit AD, Asimacopoulos PJ, Master H, Raizner AE (1992) Rotablator induced "shave" of intraluminal cap exposing intramural plaque crater. Cathet Cardiovasc Diagn 25: 209-12

64. Haude M, Eick B, Baumgart D, Caspari G, Ge J, Liu F, Gorge G, Erbel R (1996) High frequency rotational angioplasty. Z Kardiol 85: S17-S23

65. Bauriedel G, Schluckebier S, Welsch U, Werdan K, Hofling B (1995) Dislocation of the rotating cutter during directional coronary atherectomy: a note of caution. Cathet Cardiovasc Diagn 35: 244-9

66. Okita Y, Takamoto S, Ando M, Morota T, Yamaki F, Matsukawa R, Kawashima Y, Nakajima N (1997) Long-term results of patch repair for saccular aneurysms of the transverse aortic arch. Eur J Cardiothorac Surg 11: 953-6

67. Sottiurai VS, Jones R, Nakamura YA, Boustany C, Sue SL, Batson RC (1994) The role of vein patch in distal anastomotic intimal hyperplasia: an histologic characterization. Int Angiol 13: 96-102

68. Rahlf G, Urban P, Bohle RM (1986) Morphology of healing in vascular prostheses. Thorac Cardiovasc Surg 34: 43-8

69. Pasquinelli G, Freyrie A, Preda P, Curti T, D'Addato M, Laschi R (1990) Healing of prosthetic arterial grafts. Scanning Microsc 4: 351-62

70. Wu MF, Shi Q, Ahmad A, Fujita Y, Ishida A, Sauvage LR (1998) Dynamic and comparative vascular graft healing studies using multiple sequential biopsies. J Invest Surg 11: 275-80

71. Yamamura S, Nelson PR, Kent KC (1996) Role of protein kinase C in attachment, spreading, and migration of human endothelial cells. J Surg Res 63: 349-54

72. Usui Y, Goff SG, Sauvage LR, Wu HD, Robel SB, Walker M (1988) Effect of healing on compliance of porous Dacron grafts. Ann Vasc Surg 2: 120-6

73. Marois Y, Guidoin R, Roy R, Vidovsky T, Jakubiec B, Sigot-Luizard MF, Braybrook J, Mehri Y, Laroche G, King M (1996) Selecting valid in vitro biocompatibility tests that predict the in vivo healing response of synthetic vascular prostheses. Biomaterials 17: 1835-42

74. Chinn JA, Sauter JA, Phillips RE Jr, Kao WJ, Anderson JM, Hanson SR, Ashton TR (1998) Blood and tissue

compatibility of modified polyester: thrombosis, inflammation, and healing. J Biomed Mater Res 39: 130-40

75. Carson RJ, Edwards A, Szycher M (1996) Resistance to biodegradative stress cracking in microporous vascular access grafts. J Biomater Appl 11: 121-34

76. Haaverstad R, Urnes O, Dahl T, Myhre HO (1996) Lymphatic complications after lower limb vascular surgery. Tidsskr Nor Laegeforen 116: 1886-8

77. Qiu Y, Tarbell JM (1996) Computational simulation of flow in the end-to-end anastomosis of a rigid graft and a compliant artery. ASAIO J 42: M702-M709

78. Fink AM, Ditchfield MR (1997) Wall enhancement of leaking polytetrafluoroethylene grafts: a new CT sign. Pediatr Radiol 27: 327-9

79. Soong CV, B'Sa AA (1998) Lower limb oedema following distal arterial bypass grafting. Eur J Vasc Endovasc Surg 16: 465-71

80. Chakfe N, Jahn C, Nicolini P, Kretz JG, Edah-Tally S, Beaufigeau M, Lebras Y, Beaujeux R, Durand B, Eisenmann B (1997) The impact of knee joint flexion on infrainguinal vascular grafts: an angiographic study. Eur J Vasc Endovasc Surg 13: 23-30

81. Reichert V, Addili F, Schmitz-Rixen T (1997) Changes in biomechanical properties of biological and synthetic prostheses. Khirurgiia (Mosk) 4: 29-35

82. Riepe G, Loos J, Imig H, Schroder A, Schneider E, Petermann J, Rogge A, Ludwig M, Schenke A, Nassutt R, Chakfe N, Morlock M (1997) Long-term in vivo alterations of polyester vascular grafts in humans. Eur J Vasc Endovasc Surg 13: 540-8

83. Shekarriz H, Wenk H, Muller G, Bruch HP (1997) In vitro evaluation of blood vessel prosthesis dilatation – Dacron and PTFE – a new measuring technique. Zentralbl Chir 122: 805-8

84. Jones L, Braithwaite BD, Davies B, Heather BP, Earnshaw JJ (1997) Mechanism of late prosthetic vascular graft infection. Cardiovasc Surg 5: 486-9

85. Mertens RA, O'Hara PJ, Hertzer NR, Krajewski LP, Beven EG (1995) Surgical management of infrainguinal arterial prosthetic graft infections: review of a thirty-five-year experience. J Vasc Surg 21: 782-90

86. Bergamini TM, McCurry TM, Bernard JD, Hoeg KL, Corpus RA, James BE, Peyton JC, Brittian KR, Cheadle WG (1996) Antibiotic efficacy against *Staphylococcus epidermidis* adherent to vascular grafts. J Surg Res 60: 3-6

87. Mingoli A, Sapienza P, di Marzo L, Sgarzini G, Burchi C, Modini C, Cavallaro A (1997) Management of abdominal aortic prosthetic graft infection requiring emergent treatment. Angiology 48: 491-5

88. Gutowski P (1998) Aortoiliac graft infection as a diagnostic and treatment problem. Ann Acad Med Stetin 41: S1-S72

89. Fiorani P, Speziale F, Rizzo L, Sbarigia E, Massucci M, Rached HA (1996) Treatment of prostheto-digestive fistulas using in situ prosthetic bypass. J Mal Vasc 21: S162-S6

90. van Baalen JM, Kluit AB, Maas J, Terpstra JL, van Bockel JH (1996) Diagnosis and therapy of aortic prosthetic fistulas: trends over a 30-year experience. Br J Surg 83: 1729-34

91. Keshishian JM (1978) Experiences with the use of bovine heterografts in the arterial position. Vascular grafts 24: 271-2

92. Oakes DD, Spees EK Jr, Light JA, Flye MW (1978) A three year experience using modified bovine arterial hetero-

grafts for vascular access in patients requiring hemodialysis. Ann Surg 187: 423-9

93. Abolhoda A, Yu S, Oyarzun JR, Allen KR, McCormick JR, Han S, Kemp FW, Bogden JD, Lu Q, Gabbay S (1996) No-react detoxification process: a superior anticalcification method for bioprostheses. Ann Thorac Surg 62: 1724-30

94. Teijeira FJ, Marois Y, Aguiar L, Guidoin R, Bauset R, Lamoureux G, Downs A, Marois M, Boyer D (1989) Comparison of processed bovine internal mammary arteries and autologous veins as arterial femoral substitutes in dogs: blood compatibility and pathological characteristics. Can J Surg 32: 180-7

95. Welz A, Triefenbach R, Murrmann G, Grenzner S, Hammer C (1992) Experimental evaluation of the dialdehyde starch preserved bovine internal mammary artery as a small diameter arterial substitute. J Card Surg 7: 163-9

96. Mitchell IM, Essop AR, Scott PJ, Martin PG, Gupta NK, Saunders NR, Nair RU, Williams GJ (1993) Bovine internal mammary artery as a conduit for coronary revascularization: long-term results. Ann Thorac Surg 55: 120-2

97. Esposito F, Vitale N, Crescenzi B, Scardone M, de Luca L, Cotrufo M (1994) Short-term results of bovine internal mammary artery use in cardiovascular surgery. Tex Heart Inst J 21: 193-7

98. Tomizawa Y, Moon MR, DeAnda A, Castro LJ, Kosek J, Miller DC (1994) Coronary bypass grafting with biological grafts in a canine model. Circulation 90: II160-II166

99. Rosenberg N (1983) The modified bovine arterial graft *In* Wright CB, Hobson II RW, Hiratzka LF et al (eds.) Vascular grafting. Clinical applications and techniques. John Wright -PSG, Boston, p. 148

100. Liao K, Frater RW, La Pietra A, Ciuffo G, Ilardi CF, Seifter E (1995) Time-dependent effect of glutaraldehyde on the tendency to calcify of both autografts and xenografts. Ann Thorac Surg 60: S343-S347

101. Guidoin R, Marois D, Zelter J, Bonnaud P, Marois M, Leblond P, Sheiner N, Gosselin C, Roy P (1984) Progressive complications associated with the use of a bovine heterograft for vascular access. Can J Surg 27: 72-7

102. Lupinetti FM, Tsai TT, Kneebone JM, Bove EL (1993) Effect of cryopreservation on the presence of endothelial cells on human valve allografts. J Thorac Cardiovasc Surg 106: 912-7

103. Crowe D, O'Loughlin K, Knox L, Mitchell G, Hurley J, Romeo R, Morrison W (1995) Morphologic change in rabbit femoral arteries induced by storage at four degrees Celsius and by subsequent reperfusion. J Vasc Surg 22: 769-79

104. Vogt PR, Brunner-La Rocca HP, Carrel T, von Segesser LK, Ruef C, Debatin J, Seifert B, Kiowski W, Turina MI (1998) Cryopreserved arterial allografts in the treatment of major vascular infection: a comparison with conventional surgical techniques. J Thorac Cardiovasc Surg 116: 965-72

105. Wolff KD, Dienemann D (1990) Vessel preservation with glycerol: an experimental study in rats. J Oral Maxillofac Surg 48: 914-8

106. Callow AD (1996) Arterial homografts. Eur J Vasc Endovasc Surg 12: 272-81

107. Muller-Schweinitzer E, Mihatsch MJ, Schilling M, Haefeli WE (1997) Functional recovery of human mesenteric and coronary arteries after cryopreservation at -196 degrees C in a serum-free medium. J Vasc Surg 25: 743-50

108. van Son JA, Falk V, Walther T, Smedts FM, Mohr FW (1997) Low-grade intimal hyperplasia in internal mammary and right gastroepiploic arteries as bypass grafts. Ann Thorac Surg 63: 706-8

109. Yankah AC, Wottge HU (1997) Allograft conduit wall calcification in a model of chronic arterial graft rejection. J Card Surg 12: 86-92

110. Ruddle AC, George S, Armitage WJ, MacGowan A, McCulloch S, Brookes ST, Mitchell DC (1998) Venous allografts prepared from stripped long saphenous vein. Is there a need for antibiotic sterilisation? Eur J Vasc Endovasc Surg 15: 444-8

111. Strobel R, Boontje AH, Van Den Dungen JJ (1996) Aneurysm formation in modified human umbilical vein grafts. Eur J Vasc Endovasc Surg 11: 417-20

112. Broto J, Infante D, Tormo R, Marhuenda C, Gil Vernet JM, Boix-Ochoa J (1995) Our experience in the management of portal cavernoma in children. Cir Pediatr. 8: 99-101

113. Guidoin R, Gagnon Y, Roy PE, Marois M, Johnston KW, Batt M (1986) Pathologic features of surgically excised human umbilical vein grafts. J Vasc Surg 3: 146-54

114. Miyata T, Tada Y, Takagi A, Sato O, Oshima A, Idezuki Y, Shiga J (1989) A clinico-pathologic study of aneurysm formation of glutaraldehyde-tanned human umbilical vein grafts. J Vasc Surg 10: 605-11

115. Berglund H, Luo H, Nishioka T, Eigler NL, Kim CJ, Tabak SW, Siegel RJ (1996) Preserved vasodilatory response to nitroglycerin in saphenous vein bypass grafts. Circulation 94: 2871-6

116. Mordick TG 2nd, Romanowski L, Eaton C, Siemionow M (1995) Microvascular application of the nonreversed vein graft. Plast Reconstr Surg 95: 731-6

117. Dobrin PB, Littooy FN, Golan J, Blakeman B, Fareed J (1988) Mechanical and histologic changes in canine vein grafts. J Surg Res 44: 259-65

118. Shiroma H, Kusaba A (1996) Ultrastructural features of progressive intimal hyperplasia at the distal end-to-side anastomosis of vein grafts. Cardiovasc Surg 4: 393-8

119. Lie JT (1980) The structure of the normal vascular system and its reactive changes. *In* Juergens JL, Spittell JA, Fairbairn II JF (ed) Peripheral vascular diseases. Saunders, Philadelphia, London, Toronto 51-81

120. Davies MG, Barber L, Dalen H, Svendsen E, Hagen PO (1994) Control of the structural and functional consequences of vein graft intimal hyperplasia with a 21-aminosteroid—U74389G. Eur J Vasc Surg 8: 448-56

121. Sato S, Niu S, Kanda K, Oka T, Wildevuur CR (1992) Development of a method to prevent degenerative changes of the vein graft for arterial reconstruction. Nippon Geka Gakkai Zasshi 93: 419-28

122. Mehta D, George SJ, Jeremy JY, Izzat MB, Southgate KM, Bryan AJ, Newby AC, Angelini GD (1998) External stenting reduces long-term medial and neointimal thickening and platelet derived growth factor expression in a pig model of arteriovenous bypass grafting. Nat Med 4: 235-39

123. Bastounis E, Balas P, Hadjinikolaou L, Papalambros E (1994) Multi-aneurysmatic degeneration of an autogenous venous graft inserted as femoro-popliteal by-pass. Int Angiol 13: 164-7

124. Bulkley BH, Hutchins GM (1977) Accelerated "atherosclerosis". A morphologic study of 97 saphenous vein coronary artery bypass grafts. Circulation 55: 163-9

125. Kobayashi T, Fuse K, Naruse Y, Watanabe Y, Konishi H (1993) Histological study of saphenous vein graft disease after coronary artery bypass grafting. Nippon Kyobu Geka Gakkai Zasshi 41: 592-7

127. Vuong NP, Cheilan F, Houissa-Vuong S (1999) Pathology of vascular prostheses. Ann Pathol 19: 195-202

126. Mautner SL, Mautner GC, Hunsberger SA, Roberts WC (1992) Comparison of composition of atherosclerotic plaques in saphenous veins used as aortocoronary bypass conduits with plaques in native coronary arteries in the same men. Am J Cardiol 70: 1380-7

128. Wang SS, Chu SH (1996) Clinical use of omniflow vascular graft as arteriovenous bridging graft for hemodialysis. Artif Organs 20: 1278-81

129. Nakagawa Y, Ota K, Sato Y, Teraoka S, Agishi T (1995) Clinical trial of new polyurethane vascular grafts for hemodialysis: compared with expanded polytetrafluoroethylene grafts. Artif Organs 19: 1227-32

130. Doi K, Matsuda T (1997) Enhanced vascularization in a microporous polyurethane graft impregnated with basic fibroblast growth factor and heparin. J Biomed Mater Res 34: 361-70

131. Dardik H, Miller N, Dardik A, Ibrahim I, Sussman B, Berry SM, Wolodiger F, Kahn M, Dardik I (1988) A decade of experience with the glutaraldehyde-tanned human umbilical cord vein graft for revascularization of the lower limb. J Vasc Surg 7: 336-46

132. -Dardik H (1995) The second decade of experience with the umbilical vein graft for lower – limb revascularization. Cardiovasc Surg 3: 265-9

133. Sparks CH (1973) Silicone mandril method for growing reinforced autogenous femoro-popliteal artery grafts in situ. Ann Surg 177: 293-300

134. Pietri P, Alagni G, Domeniconi (1976) Sparks-mandril prosthesis and a new alternative in obstructions of the femoro-popliteal axis. Minerva Chir 31: 473-87

135. Leseche G, Ohan J, Bouttier S, Bertrand P, Andreassian B (1995) Above-knee femoropopliteal bypass grafting using endothelial cell seeded PTFE grafts: five-year clinical experience. Ann Vasc Surg 9: S15-S23

136. Sipehia R, Martucci G, Lipscombe J (1996) Transplantation of human endothelial cell monolayer on artificial vascular prosthesis: the effect of growth-support surface chemistry, cell seeding density, ECM protein coating, and growth factors. Artif Cells Blood Substit Immobil Biotechnol 24: 51-63

137. Giudiceandrea A, Seifalian AM, Krijgsman B, Hamilton G (1998) Effect of prolonged pulsatile shear stress in vitro on endothelial cell seeded PTFE and compliant polyurethane vascular grafts. Eur J Vasc Endovasc Surg 15: 147-54

138. Flugelman MY (1995) Inhibition of intravascular thrombosis and vascular smooth muscle cell proliferation by gene therapy. Thromb Haemost 74: 406-10

139. Flugelman MY (1995) Vascular gene therapy. Adv Exp Med Bio 382: 269-77

140. Zund G, Breuer CK, Shinoka T, Ma PX, Langer R, Mayer JE, Vacanti JP (1997) The in vitro construction of a tissue engineered bioprosthetic heart valve. Eur J Cardiothorac Surg 11: 493-7

141. Lanzetta M, Crowe DM, Hickey MJ (1996) Fibroblast growth factor pretreatment of 1-mm PTFE grafts. Microsurgery 17: 606-11

142. Becquemin JP, Riff Y, Kovarsky S, Ardaillou N, Benhaien-Sigaux N (1997) Evaluation of a polyester collagen-coated heparin bonded vascular graft. J Cardiovasc Surg (Torino) 38: 7-14

143. Laemmel E, Penhoat J, Warocquier-Clerout R, Sigot-Luizard MF (1998) Heparin immobilised on proteins usable for arterial prosthesis coating: growth inhibition of smooth-muscle cells. J Biomed Mater Res 39: 446-52

144. Veith FJ, Moss CM, Fell SC, Rhodes BA, Somberg E, Weiss P, Boley SJ, Haimovici H (1978) Expanded polytetrafluoroethylene grafts in reconstructive arterial surgery. Preliminary report of the first 110 consecutive cases for limb salvage. JAMA 240: 1867-9

145. Mohr L, Smith L (1980) Polytetrafluoroethylene graft aneurysm. Arch Surg 115: 1467-70

146. Chiesa R, Melissano G, Castellano R, Astore D, Castrucci M, Del Maschio A, Grossi A (1995) A new ePTFE stretch graft for aorto-iliac reconstructions. Surgical evaluation and one year follow-up with Magnetic Resonance Imaging. J Cardiovasc Surg 36: 135-41

147. Descotes J, Brudon JR, Zabot JM, Vinard E, Eloy R, Chignier E, Guidollet J, Louisot P (1989) The neoartery, myth or reality? Study of 79 explanted arterial prostheses. Chirurgie 115: 58-65

148. Esato K, Kubo Y, Yasuda K, Shigematsu H, Iwai T, Ishimaru S, Uchida H, Ishii K (1998) Satigrel, a new anti-platelet agent, inhibits platelet accumulation in prosthetic arterial grafts. Am J Surg 175: 56-60

149. Campbell CD, Brooks DH, Webster MW, Diamond DL, Peel RL, Bahnson HT (1979) Expanded microporous polytetrafluoroethylene as a vascular substitute: a two year follow-up. Surgery 85: 177-83

150. Camilleri JP, Vuong NP, Bruneval P, Tricotet V, Balaton A, Fiessinger JN, Cormier JM (1985) Surface healing and histologic maturation of patent polytetrafluoroethylene grafts implanted in patients for up to 60 months. Arch Pathol Lab Med 109: 833-7

151. Simmons JR, Buzdar AU, Ota DM, Marts K, Hortobagyi GN (1992) Complications associated with indwelling catheters. Med Pediatr Oncol 20: 22-5

152. Gould JR, Carloss HW, Skinner WL (1993) Groshong catheter-associated subclavian venous thrombosis. Am J Med 95: 419-23

153. Palmer RA, Newell JE, Gray EJ, Quinton WE (1966) Treatment of chronic renal failure by prolonged peritoneal dialysis. N Engl J Med 274: 248-54

154. Bonnaud P, Lebkiri B, Boudier L, Man NK (1994) Preserved saphenous grafts in hemodialysis. 20 years' experience. Nephrologie 15: 177-80

155. Deshmukh N, Reppert M (1993) Venous ulceration of the hand secondary to a cimino fistula. Mil Med 158: 752-3

156. Mashiah A, Liebergall M, Pasik S, David A, Bar-Khayim Y (1986) Axillary vein thrombosis: a rare complication following creation of arteriovenous fistula for hemodialysis. J Cardiovasc Surg (Torino) 27: 291-3

157. Windus DW (1993) Permanent vascular access: a nephrologist's view. Am J Kidney Dis 21: 457-71

158. Cheung AK, Wu LL, Kablitz C, Leypoldt JK (1993) Atherogenic lipids and lipoproteins in hemodialysis patients. Am J Kidney Dis 22: 271-6

159. Swayne LC, Manstein C, Somers R, Cope C (1983) Selective digital venous hypertension: a rare complication of hemodialysis arteriovenous fistula. Cardiovasc Intervent Radiol 6: 61-2

160. Roca-Tey R, Ramirez de Arellano M, Codina S, Olmos A, Piera L, Gonzalez U (1992) Cutaneous trophic disorders secondary to arteriovenous fistula for hemodialysis. Med Clin (Barc) 98: 58-60

161. Nakagawa Y, Ota K, Sato Y, Fuchinoue S, Teraoka S, Agishi T (1994) Complications in blood access for hemodialysis. Artif Organs 18: 283-8

162. Stehbens WE, Karmody AM (1975) Venous atherosclerosis associated with arteriovenous fistulas for hemodialysis. Arch Surg 110: 176-80

163. Patel KR, Chan FA, Batista RJ, Clauss RH (1992) True venous aneurysms and arterial "steal" secondary to arteriovenous fistulae for dialysis. J Cardiovasc Surg (Torino) 33: 185-8

164. McMullen K, Hayes D, Hussey JL, Boudreaux JP (1991) Salvage of hemodialysis access in infected arteriovenous fistulas. Arch Surg 126: 1303-5

165. Kolde G, Worheide J, Baumgartner R, Brocker EB (1989) Kaposi-like acroangiodermatitis in an above-knee amputation stump. Br J Dermatol 120: 575-80

166. Lemarchand-Venencie F, Boisnic S, Riche MC, Merland JJ (1991) Pseudo-Kaposi syndromes of vascular origin. J Mal Vasc 16: 153-7

167. Kim TH, Kim KH, Kang JS, Kim JH, Hwang IY (1997) Pseudo-Kaposi's sarcoma associated with acquired arteriovenous fistula. J Dermatol 24: 28-33

168. Ueki H, Inagaki Y, Kohda M, Takei Y (1986) Stewart-Bluefarb syndrome. Hautarzt 37: 673-5

169. Calzavara Pinton P, Carlino A, Manganoni AM, Donzelli C, Facchetti F (1990) Epidermal nevus syndrome with multiple vascular hamartomas and malformations. G Ital Dermatol Venereol 125: 251-4

170. Koppel RA, Marrogi AJ, Fishman SJ (1994) Unilateral pseudo-Kaposi's sarcoma (Bluefarb-Stewart type). Cutis 54: 257-60

171. Constantin JM, Etienne G, Hevia M (1997) Technique and results of cryo-stripping in the treatment of varicose veins of the lower limbs. Ann Chir 51: 745-8

172. Lofgren EP (1984) Varicose veins In Haimovici H: Vascular surgery, Principles and techniques. Appleton-Century-Crofts, Norwalk, Connecticut 979-1006

173. Berni A, Tromba L, Mosti G, Mele R, Tombesi T, Bedoni P, Avruscio GP, Neroni G, Ofria F, Lantone G, Selvaggio M, Amicucci G, Iabichella ML (1998) Recurrence of varicose veins after treatment. Multicenter study by the Italian Doppler Club, Clinical and Technological Society. Minerva Cardioangiol 46: 87-90

174. Hammarsten J (1997) Saphenous vein-saving surgery—an alternative to stripping. Nord Med 112: 361-4

175. Castaneda-Zuniga WR, Tadavarthy SM (1992) Interventional radiology, 2nd edn, Williams and Wilkins, Baltimore

176. de Bono DP, Pringle S (1991) Local inhibition of thrombosis using urokinase linked to a monoclonal antibody which recognises damaged endothelium. Thromb Res 61: 537-45

177. Comerota AJ, Aldridge SC, Cohen G, Ball DS, Pliskin M, White JV (1994) A strategy of aggressive regional therapy for acute iliofemoral venous thrombosis with contemporary venous thrombectomy or catheter-directed thrombolysis. J Vasc Surg 20: 244-54

178. Tarry WC, Makhoul RG, Tisnado J, Posner MP, Sobel M, Lee HM (1994) Catheter-directed thrombolysis following vena cava filtration for severe deep venous thrombosis. Ann Vasc Surg 8: 583-90

179. Adams JT, Deweese JA (1984) Venous interruptions In Haimovici H: Vascular surgery, Principles and techniques. Appleton-Century-Crofts, Norwalk, Connecticut 991-1006

180. Lurquin P, Mendes da Costa P (1993) Surgical interruption of the inferior vena cava. Rev Med Brux 14: 23-7

181. Cotroneo AR, Di Stasi C, Cina A, Di Gregorio F (1996) Venous interruption as prophylaxis of pulmonary embolism: vena cava filters. Rays 21: 461-80

182. Braverman SJ, Battey PM, Smith RB 3d (1992) Vena caval interruption. Am Surg 58: 188-92

183. Perhoniemi V, Salmenkivi K, Kivisaari A, Hastbacka J (1986) Caval ligation versus clipping to counteract pulmonary embolism. Ann Chir Gynaecol 75: 325-7

184. Heaps JM, Lagasse LD (1990) Use of the inferior vena cava clip in patients at high risk for pulmonary embolism. Gynecol Oncol 39: 277-83

185. Abu Rahma AF, Boland J, Lawton WE Jr, Kusminsky R (1981) Long term follow-up of prophylactic caval clipping. J Cardiovasc Surg (Torino) 22: 550-4

186. Feinman LJ, Meltzer AJ (1989) Phlegmasia cerulea dolens as a complication of percutaneous insertion of a vena caval filter. J Am Osteopath Assoc 89: 63-8

187. Adams JT, DeWeese JA (1970) Comparative evaluation of ligation and partial interruption of the femoral vein in the treatment of thromboembolic disease. Ann Surg 172: 795-803

188. Donaldson MC, Wirthlin LS, Donaldson GA (1980) Thirty-year experience with surgical interruption of the inferior vena cava for prevention of pulmonary embolism. Ann Surg 191: 367-72

189. Rudondy P, Jausseran JM, Bergeron P, Courbier R (1988) Unfastening of an Adams-de Weese clip: an uncommon cause of recurrent pulmonary embolism after interruption of the inferior vena cava. Ann Vasc Surg 2: 235-6

190. Cimochowski GE, Evans RH, Zarins CK, Lu CT, DeMeester TR (1980) Greenfield filter versus Mobin-Uddin umbrella: the continuing quest for the ideal method of vena caval interruption. J Thorac Cardiovasc Surg 79: 358-65

191. Milleret R, Amat G, Curnier JM (1983) Comparative results of the use of Greenfields' filter, an umbrella filter, and a caval clip for vena cava interruption. J Mal Vasc 8: 211-3

192. Darcy MD, Cardella JF, Hunter DW, Smith TP, Castaneda-Zuniga WR, Lund G, Amplatz K (1986) Experience with the Amplatz retrievable vena caval filter. Work in progress. Radiology 161: 611-4

193. Greenfield LJ, Proctor MC (1997) Endovascular methods for caval interruption. Semin Vasc Surg 10: 310-4

194. Nevin WS, Beddingfield GW (1972) Migration of vena cava filter. JAMA 222: 88

195. Gomez GA, Cutler BS, Wheeler HB (1983) Transvenous interruption of the inferior vena cava. Surgery 93: 612-9

196. Rudondy P, Ferdani M, Reggi M, Jausseran JM (1994) Interruption of the inferior vena cava using the Vascor filter: preliminary series of 51 cases. Cardiovasc Surg 2: 344-9

197. Matchett WJ, Jones MP, McFarland DR, Ferris EJ (1998) Suprarenal vena caval filter placement: follow-up of four filter types in 22 patients. J Vasc Interv Radiol 9: 588-93

198. Zwaan M, Lorch H, Kulke C, Kagel C, Schweider G, Siemens HJ, Muller G, Eberhardt I, Wagner T, Weiss HD (1998) Clinical experience with temporary vena caval filters. J Vasc Interv Radiol 9: 594-601

199. Rosen MP, Porter DH, Kim D (1994) Reassessment of vena caval filter use in patients with cancer. J Vasc Interv Radiol 5: 501-6

200. Belcaro G, Nicolaides AN, Veller M (1995) Venous disorders. A manual of diagnosis and treatment. Saunders, London, Philadelphia, Toronto, Sydney, Tokyo, 194 p

201. Rai DB, Lerrer R (1991) Chronic venous insufficiency disease. Its etiology. A new technique for vein valve transplantation. Int Surg 76: 174-8

202. Kistner RL, Eklof B, Masuda EM (1995) Deep venous valve reconstruction. Cardiovasc Surg 3: 129-40

203. Jamieson WG, Chinnick B (1997) Clinical results of deep venous valvular repair for chronic venous insufficiency. Can J Surg 40: 294-9

204. Raju S, Hardy JD (1997) Technical options in venous valve reconstruction. Am J Surg 173: 301-7

205. Maeda Y, Arima K, Matsuura H, Hayashi N, Yanagawa M, Kawamura J (1998) Percutaneous sclerotherapy for chyluria with leg oedema: a case report. Hinyokika Kiyo 44: 25-7

206. Miller TA (1980) Charles procedure for lymphoedema: a warning. Am J Surg 139: 290-2

207. Miller TA, Wyatt LE, Rudkin GH (1998) Staged skin and subcutaneous excision for lymphoedema: a favorable report of long-term results. Plast Reconstr Surg 102: 1486-98

208. Mavili ME, Naldoken S, Safak T (1994) Modified Charles operation for primary fibrosclerotic lymphoedema. Lymphology 27: 14-20

209. Dandapat MC, Mukherjee LM, Patra SK (1991) Evaluation of different surgical procedures in filarial of lower extremity. J Indian Med Assoc 89: 127-9

210. Tanaka Y, Tajima S, Imai K, Tsujiguchi K, Ueda K, Yabu K (1996) Experience of a new surgical procedure for the treatment of unilateral obstructive lymphoedema of the lower extremity: adipo-lymphatico venous transfer. Microsurgery 17: 209-16

XIII
The pathology of veins, lymphatics, arteriovenous anastomoses and the erectile vascular tissue

1 – Pathology of the venous system

Phlebitis

Bacterial infections in veins may be a complication of local or systemic infections. Infected wounds, superimposed infections in eczema or mycosis or septicaemia may all have a venous component (Fig. 1). Iatrogenic infections are most frequently caused by a venous catheter or systems for long term vascular access [1]. A purulent and necrotic phlebitis with secondary thrombosis may develop (Fig. 2-3-4). Tuberculosis (Fig. 5) and syphilis can also affect veins and viral and rickettsial phlebitis can give rise to microabscesses (particularly frequent in cat-scratch disease) [2]. Migrating phlebitis may result from hypersensivity. Mondor's disease is a variant of migrating phlebitis with marked fibrosis transforming the affected vein into a fibrous cord. The commonest site of this condition is the lateral thoracic area [3]. No cause is evident in most cases but some are part of a systemic disease, including Buerger's disease, Behçet's syndrome and connective tissue diseases, including the granulomatoses and polymyalgia (See chapter XI). The lesions are multinodular and segmental. Affected veins displayed granuloma-

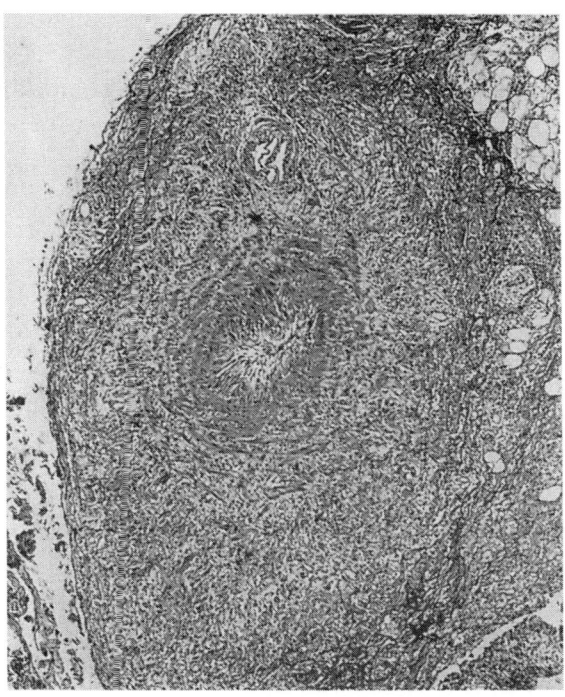

Fig. 1. Phlebitis. Haematoxylin, eosin and saffron stain. (HES)

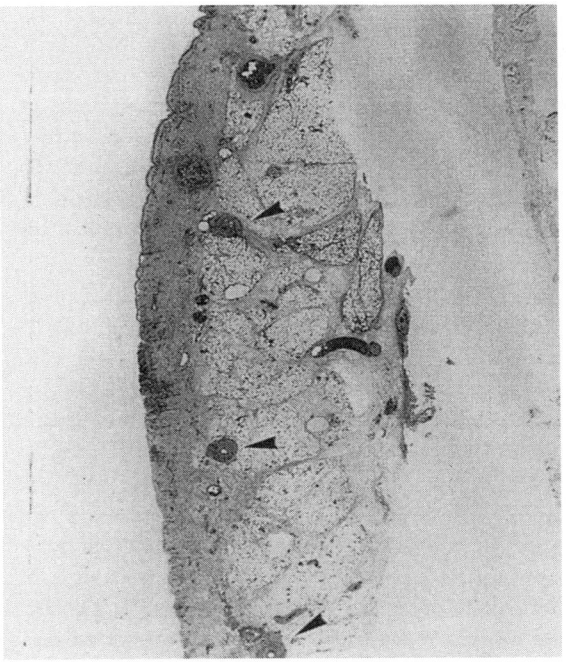

Fig. 2. Diffuse purulent phlebitis in an AIDS patient dying of Gram-negative septicemia. Note multiple abscesses (arrow heads) in the skin and subcutaneous tissue. HES

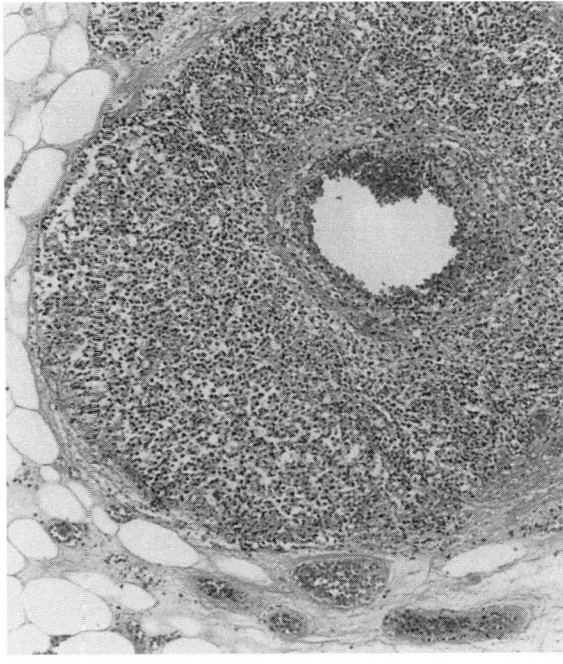

Fig. 3. Purulent phlebitis. Note dense infiltration of leukocytes thickening the venous wall. HES

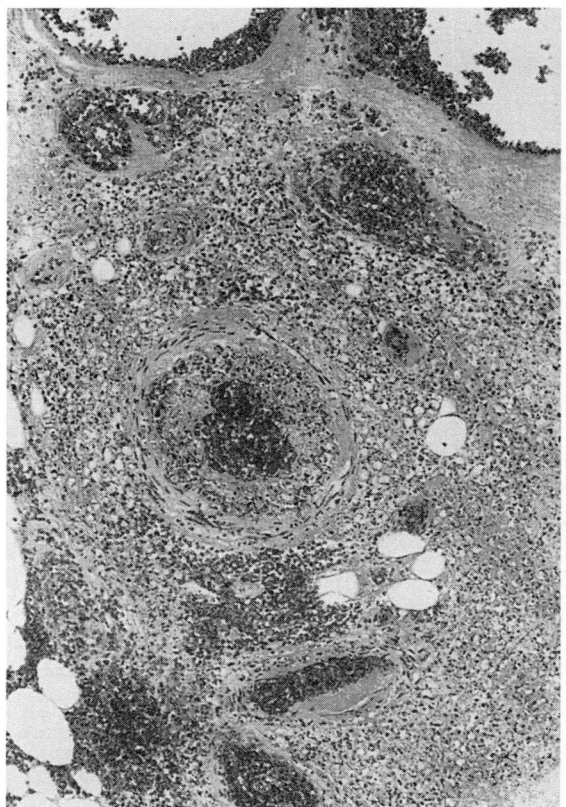

Fig. 4. Purulent phlebitis with superimposed thrombosis. HES

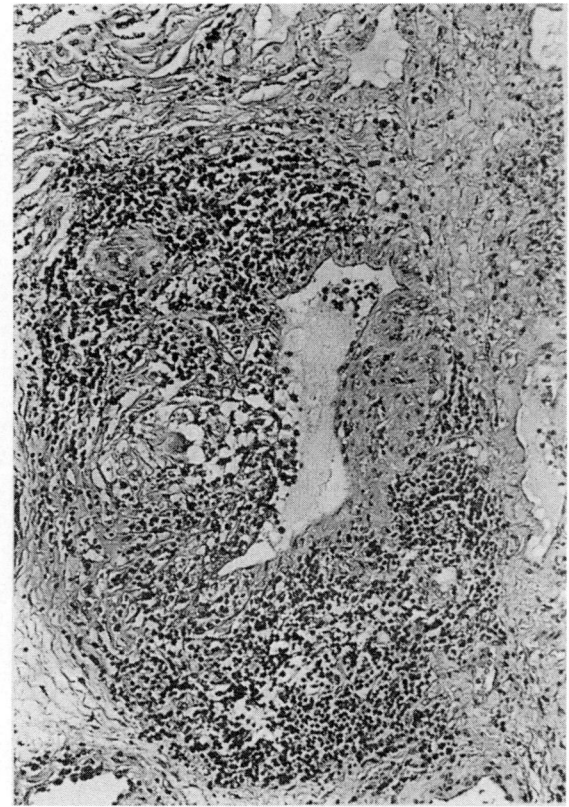

Fig. 5. Granulomatous phlebitis. HES

tous phlebitis with or without giant cells and localised fibrinoid necrosis [4]. The intima is frequently thickened.

Varicose veins

Varicose veins are characterised by dilatation, elongation and tortuosity without associated inflammation (Fig. 6). They reflect a chronic venous insufficiency (CVI) [5] but do not specify its site. Some 10-20% of the world population may have varicose veins in the legs [6]. Vulvar varicosities appear in some 2% of pregnant women and most disappear completely within 4-6 weeks of delivery [7]. Age is the main risk factor: 20% of the subjects around 20 years and 80% of those around 60 years are affected by varicose veins. Other factors include gender, hereditary factors, obesity, number of pregnancies, age at menarche, and hormonal contraceptives [8]. Varicose veins are more susceptible to injury and acute complications include

haemorrhage and thrombosis. Long-standing varicosities may be associated with microvascular changes, chronic oedema, skin hyperpigmentation, induration and malleolar ulceration with local infection [9]. Varicophlebitis can be regarded as a typical late complication of varicosities in the superficial venous system [1].

Varicose veins develop after obstruction, damage or both. An acquired or congenital arteriovenous fistula may be causative, especially when varicose veins are unilateral, present in an unusual location, or when they are associated with ulceration and elongation of the limb.

The causes of primary varicose veins are unknown. Two partially satisfactory hypotheses have been proposed; there may be progressive incompetence of the venous valves resulting from high venous pressure in the main superficial trunks and in the communicating veins [10] or there may be a primary weakness of the venous wall caused by a connective tissue failure of some kind [11]. Venous wall weakness may result from changes in smooth muscle cells, which are transformed from a contractile to a secretory mode leading to collagen deposition with reduced elasticity. Retinoblastoma protein (pRb) may play a role as a possible subcellular regulator [12]. All of these mechanisms lead to an increase in the venous pressure, and further destruction of the valve cusps connecting the deep and superficial systems, giving rise to valvular incompetence, dilatation of the collateral channels, and, in some circumstances, reversal of the venous flow.

Pathology and differential diagnosis

Whatever the age or sex of the patient, the histological appearance of the veins is identical. Dilatation, tortuosity, muscular atrophy and hypertrophy occur together in the early stages. The media and adventitia remain unchanged. The intima may be thickened, with cushions, bumps or "rugs" made up of a thin layer of connective tissue with scattered elastic fibers (Fig. 7-8). Fibers containing elastin decrease in quantity and show dystrophic changes. With time, fibrosis develops in both media and adventitia. The early signs of this process include the appearance of a thin mantle of glycosamonoglycans around smooth muscle cells. In the next step, this mantle will transform into collagen, giving rise to a collagen network that progressively replaces the muscular layers. The content of collagen I and III decreases ; conversely, the quantity of collagen IV, V and VI increases [13]. This process may sometimes involve either the intima, media and adventitia or all three layers simultaneously (Fig. 9). Intimal fibrosis is not more frequent or more severe than in non-varicose veins. Fibrosis of the media is more marked in varicose veins than in normal veins, especially in the advanced stage when the vein becomes a rigid irregular tube. In some areas the wall develops muscular hypertrophy, but in areas of low pressure muscular atrophy occurs, a change particularly prominent on the internal border of the venous meander. Venous valves may remain thin and non retracted even when the vein presents advanced degeneration. Fibrous thickening of the intima should be differentiated from post-thrombotic or inflammatory fibrosis ; this usually contains newly-formed vessels. The architecture of varicose veins is totally different from that of aged veins.

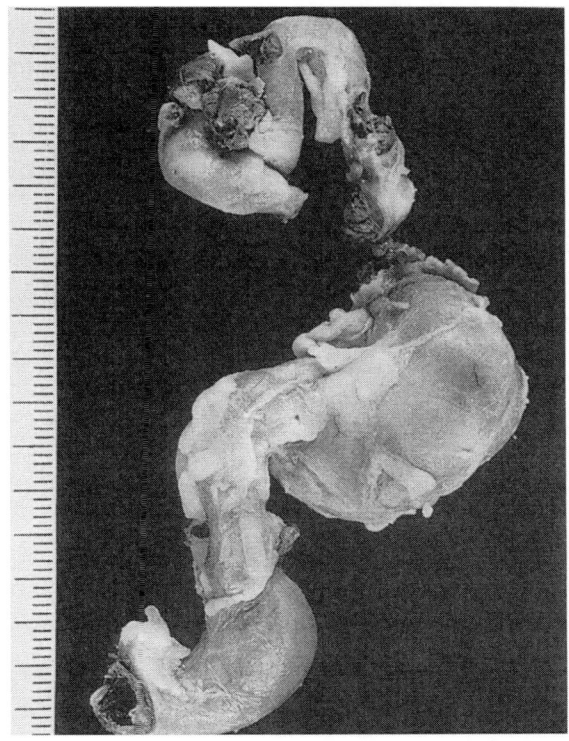

Fig. 6. Stripped varicose vein. Note uneven venous calibre and luminal thrombosis. (Courtesy Dr P. Desoutter)

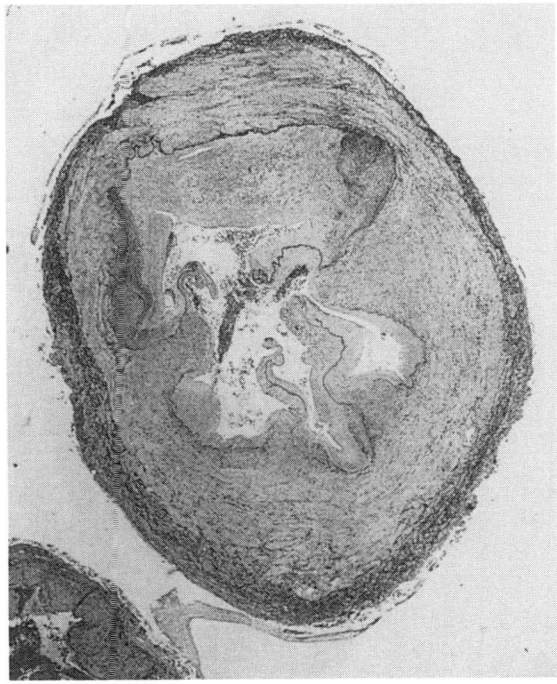

Fig. 7. Varicose vein. Cushion-like thickening of the intima in early stage of varicosis. Orcein elastic stain (Orcein)

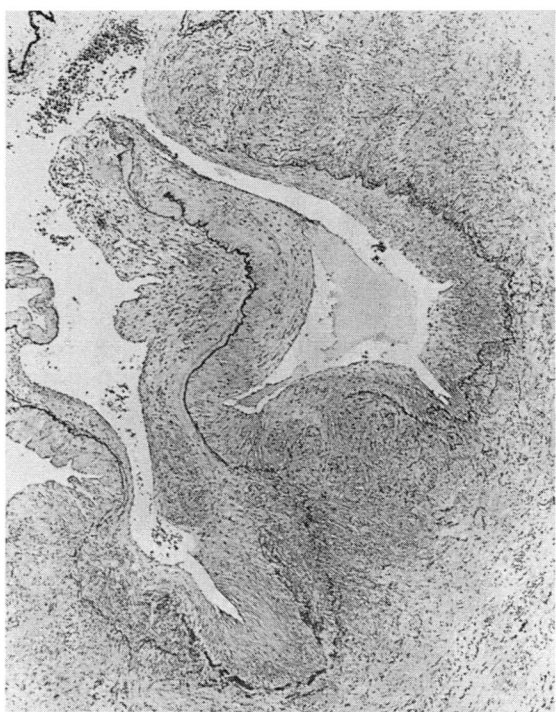

Fig. 8. Varicose vein. Marked thickening of the valvular rugs. ...Orcein...

Phlebosclerosis (Venofibrosis, fibrous endophlebitis, hyperplastic phlebitis, venous hypertrophy, endophlebosclerosis)

This condition is part of the venous ageing process but it may be observed in very young subjects, even in infants, and may predispose to thrombosis. Prolonged increase in intravenous pressure (congestive heart failure, portal or pulmonary hypertension, arteriovenous fistula) or incorporation of thromboses into the intima are thought to lead to the thickening of the venous wall. Pathologically, there is fibrotic thickening of one, two or often all three coats of the vein. Initially the thickened intima contains myocytes; later this layer becomes acellular (Fig. 10).

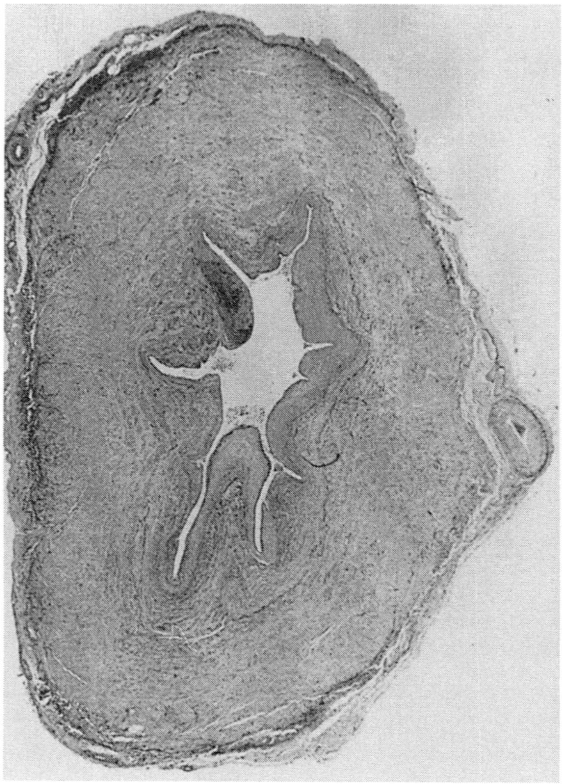

Fig. 9. Varicose vein. Fibrotic thickening of the media. ...Orcein...

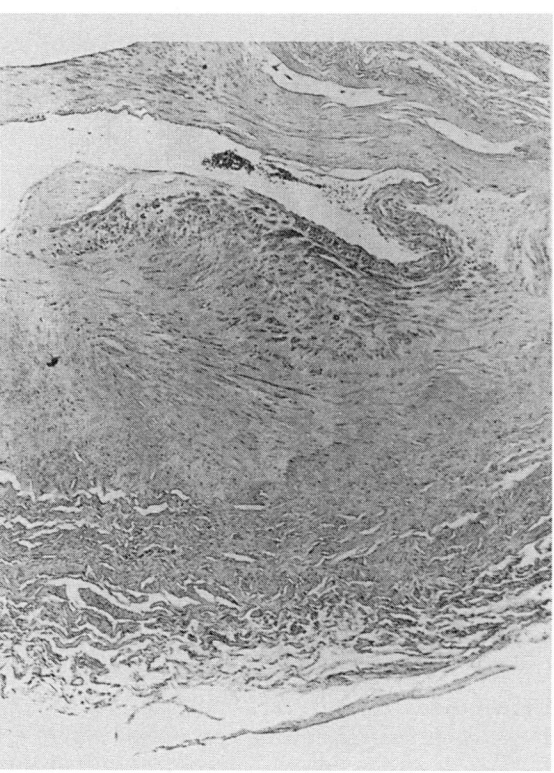

Fig. 10. Phlebosclerosis. Diffuse fibrosis involving the venous intima and media. HES

Chronic venous insufficiency and postphlebitic syndrome

This descriptive term embraces all the changes resulting from an increase in venous pressure in both deep and superficial veins. Eighty-six percent of patients suffering from an episode of deep vein thrombosis are expected to develop chronic venous insufficiency and postphlebitic syndrome with a venous ulcer within 10 years. The lapse of time between the two events may be as long as 15 years. Ten percent of patients are hospitalized at least once because of recurrent thrombosis, cellulitis, lipodermatosclerosis and venous ulcer. Female patients are twice as common as males, with a mean age of 55 [6]. Clinical features include nocturnal swelling progressing to irreversible chronic oedema, muscular pain after prolonged standing, severe bursting pain on walking (venous claudication), skin hyperpigmentation and hardening, dermatitis, and itching lipodermosclerosis of the extremities and ankle. Secondary varicoses may be present. The outcome includes venous obstruction and reflux leading to venous ulcer. The sequelae of deep venous thrombosis are uncertain. In the months that follow deep vein thrombosis, recanalization restores patency but valvular competence is lost forever. An incompetent venous segment transmits an abnormally high pressure to the next distal one, which dilates, loses its valvular competence and may produce reflux of venous flow with changes in posture [14]. These changes, more frequent in perforating veins (60%) than in deep (27%) [6, 15] ones, lead to impairment of the microcirculation [9]. These changes almost always develop in the lower limb. Most cases are the aftermath of deep venous thrombosis, hence the term "postphlebitic syndrome". Exceptional cases are caused by congenital absence or incompetence of valves [16].

Diagnostic entities

Primary pulmonary veno-occlusive disease

This poorly understood condition is characterised by occlusion of pulmonary veins and venules in the absence of left-sided cardiac failure [17, 18]. Suggested aetiologies include viral infection [19, 20], immune complex disease, and drugs [21]. The disease is rare and usually diagnosed at autopsy. This condition occurs in both sexes and all ages and a febrile illness often precedes the condition. Patients present with chemosis, facial swelling, dyspnea, radiological signs of congestion, pleural effusions and pericardial tamponade [22].

Pathology and differential diagnosis

Many or most medium and small veins show occlusive intimal hyperplasia, but the condition also involves large pulmonary and bronchial veins. The media may be normal, thickened, or arterialized with formation of internal and external elastic lamellae. Adventitial fibrosis extends from the veins into interlobular or interalveolar septa. The pulmonary arteries develop intimal and medial hypertrophy. Haemorrhage and haemosiderin deposition occur. An interstitial lymphocytic and histiocytic infiltrate is found in the majority of cases. A histological diagnosis should be made with caution in the elderly as pulmonary veins may undergo progressive mural thickening with age. The combination of diffuse interstitial fibrosis and haemosiderin pigment deposits may mimic idiopathic pulmonary haemosiderosis. Inflammatory infiltrates simulate interstitial pneumonitis.

Obstructive membranes in the inferior vena cava

This change is defined as the presence of a localised fibrotic thickening of the intima of the vena cava. There is no plausible explanation regarding this intracaval location for membrane formation. Two hypotheses have been suggested to explain the development of this condition [23]. It may represent a congenital fusion defect of the five distinctive embryonal segments of the retrohepatic portion of the inferior vena cava [24] but many features discredit this theory; there is only an exceptional association with other malformations of this region, such as agenesis of the left hepatic lobe [25]. Children are rarely affected and the mean age at presentation is 36 yrs [26, 27].

Traumatic causes include contusion [28], Cockett's syndrome [29], and repeated compression caused by respiration (via the diaphragm), leading to turbulence of the blood flow at the level of the hepatic veins [24] and thrombus formation in the predisposed vena cava. An intra-abdominal infection may induce a thrombus in the vena cava, resulting in membrane formation; in some countries, membranous obstruction of the vena cava is frequent in people living in poor conditions, walking bare foot and developing frequent cutaneous infections [30]. Retroperitoneal fibrosis and Behçet's disease may play a role in the pathogenesis. Membranes result from organization of a thrombus. Since IVC thrombosis occurs in many diseases, an association with membranes is frequently reported in a wide variety of conditions [31-36].

Clinical manifestations may be latent and include hepatomegaly, jaundice, ascites, oesophageal varices, and abdominal pains. Liver enlargement (71-86%), ascites (31-69%), abdominal pain (26-62%), varicoses and collateral circulation are the most prominent symptoms and signs [33]. When the membrane is suprahepatic the Budd-Chiari syndrome results. Jaundice and proteinuria are exceptional events [23, 28].

The mean survival with a membrane is about 5 years although this may be less when severe systemic disease has existed for some time (for example, in systemic lupus erythematosis). Acute liver insufficiency and fatal digestive haemorrhage dominate the outcome [23]. Treatment is mostly surgical. In complete obstruction, the membrane is first perforated with a metallic guide then secondarily dilated [37, 38]. Other techniques, such as laser angioplasty with Nd-YAG, have been tried, but the limited number of patients undergoing this procedure and the insufficient passage of time do not allow us to judge their efficiency. Surgical procedure consists of either transcardiac membranotomy [39] or direct membranectomy with thrombus removal [40, 41]. An alternative procedure is a cavo-atrial bypass using a PTFE prosthesis [42].

Pathology and differential diagnosis

Externally, the vena cava appears normal or may present a minor surface indentation. The obliteration may be partial or complete. All the supra-hepatic veins are occluded in 40% of cases. There are two main classifications. The first is based on the macroscopic appearance of the membrane [43] (Table 1). The second [44] takes into account the membrane site with regard to the hepatic veins, which may be patent or obliterated (Table 2). Hirooka's classification is more frequently used than Dubost's; type 1b is the most frequent.

Histologically, the intima shows fibrotic thickening with a plaque that often contains incorporated thrombotic material and shows calcification [44]. The media and adventitia almost always remain unchanged but there are reports of fibrosis extending to the underlying media and adventitia, leading to stenosis [28]. Dilatation of sinusoids, haemorrhage and pericentrolobular necrosis typify a supra-hepatic block. In the advanced stage, centrolobular fibrosis or cirrhosis is seen.

Differential diagnosis includes clotting disorders and the use of indwelling catheters, external compression or extension of malignant disease. In the latter circumstance, the site of a "pseudo-thrombotic" tumour may be below the liver, retrohepatic or below or/at the entrance to the right atrium [23].

Table 1. Dubost's classification of membranous obstruction of the inferior vena cava

Type	Membrane	Inferior vena cava stenosis
a	thin, complete or incomplete	None
b	thin, complete	Loose
c	thick, complete	Tight
d	thick, complete	Tight with additional thrombus

Table 2. Hirooka's classification of membranous obstruction of the inferior vena cava (RHV: right hepatic vein, LHV: left hepatic vein)

Type	Subtype	Description
1	a	above patent RHV, above patent LHV
	b	below obliterated RHV, above patent LHV
	c	below patent RHV, below patent LHV
2	a	above obliterated RHV, above obliterated LHV
	b	below obliterated RHV, below obliterated LHV

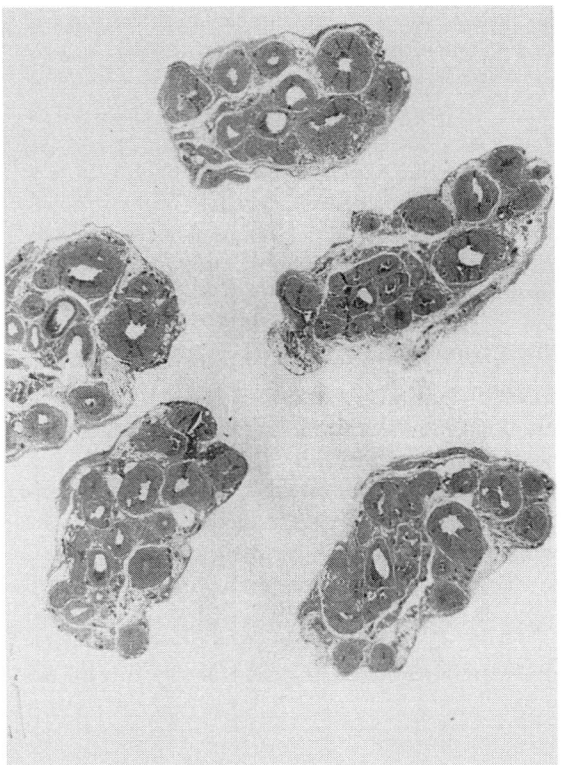
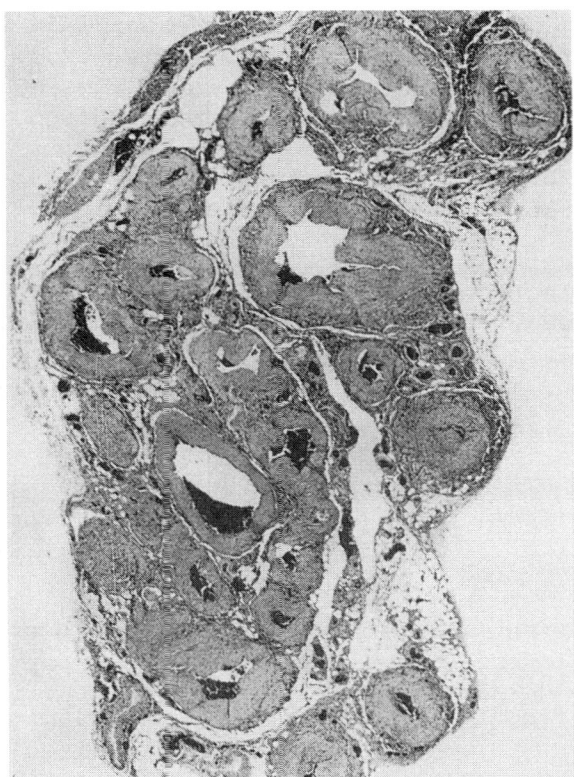

Fig. 11-12. Varicocele. Note dilatation and tortuosity of the pampiniform plexus. HES

Varicocele

This condition is caused by the incompetence of valves in the spermatic and testicular veins, with an increase in venous pressure in the pampiniform plexus leading to dilatation and tortuosity (Fig. 11). Ninety percent of varicoceles are on the left side where the spermatic vein ends in the left renal vein [6, 45]. This connection allows transmission of more retrograde pressure to the contents of the scrotum. Overt varicoceles cause enlargement of the left hemiscrotum and testis. The pampiniform plexus is tortuous, dilated, clearly visible and palpable in a standing position. The venous wall present dystrophic changes with fibrosis similar to those developed in varicose vein (Fig. 12-13). In infants and adolescents, varicocele is often associated with a smaller and hypotrophic testis, with impaired fertility [46-48].

Pelvic congestion syndrome

The patients often present with vulvar varicosities and pelvic pain of variable intensity, worsening during premenstrual episodes, extended menstrual periods, and intercourse [49, 50]. A similar syndrome

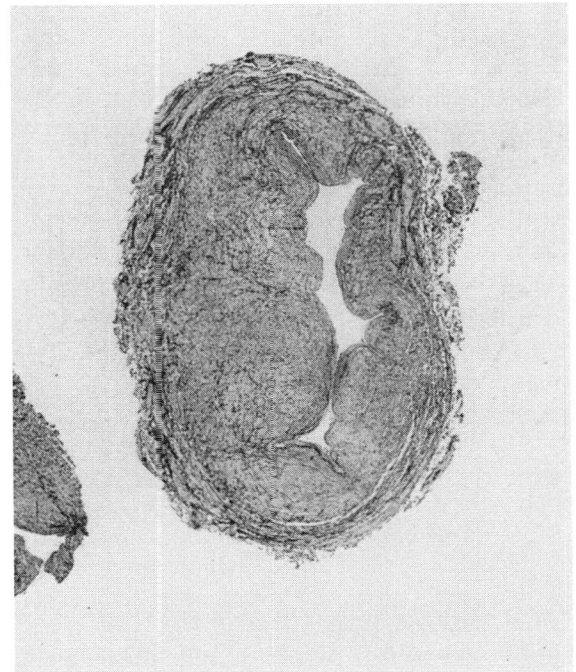

Fig. 13. Varicocele. Marked dystrophic changes of the venous wall with disappearance of the valvular apparatus. Orcein.

also affects women working under conditions where activity is limited [51, 52]. This syndrome may occur during pregnancy and disappears after delivery but reappearance of the symptoms is possible in later pregnancies. Some multiparous women also develop varicoceles in the broad ligament and others in the ovary [53]. Untreated, the syndrome tends to regress after the menopause. The morphological appearances are similar to those of varicose veins.

Venous atherosclerotic-like lesions (See chapter IV)

2 – Pathology of the lymphatic system

Lymphangitis

Lymphangitis is part of the inflammatory process. It is difficult to distinguish true infiltration of the lymph vessels and inflammatory congestion of the lumen and filling of lymph vessels by an inflammatory cell population. In lymphangitis, the surrounding connective tissue will contain more inflammatory cells than the lymph vessel wall itself. This process may be an important component of the vasculitides (see chapter XI).

Lymphangiosis

Colonisation of the lymphatic vessels by **tumour** cells **or** parasites is sometimes referred to by this term. It differs from lymphangitis even if associated with an inflammatory reaction in the lymph vessels and the formation of granulomata. Lymphangiosis carcinomatosum describes the filling of long lymphovascular segments by aggregates or complexes of tumour cells, the serous membranes in particular showing fine moniliform gray-white networks.

Lymphoedema

Lymphoedema results from the accumulation of lymph in the tissues [54, 55]. Clinically, lymphoedema may be preceded by recurrent lymphangitis and cellulitis. Commonly unilateral and beginning in the lower leg, it progresses proximally, overflows onto the genitals and involves the entire limb in 1 to 2 years, leading to permanent enlargement and disfiguration. There are four stages : latent, reversible, irreversible and elephantiasis [56]. Association with chronic ve-

nous insufficiency is frequent, leading to varicosities, skin pigmentation, recurrent dermatitis and ulceration. Associated deep venous thrombosis may occur [57-59] and much more rarely, angiosarcoma or Kaposi's sarcoma may develop [60]. There are two types of lymphoedema. Primary lymphoedema is a congenital developmental abnomality of the lymphatics. Secondary or obstructive lymphoedema results from mechanical blockage of previously normal proximal lymphatics.

Primary lymphoedema

Primary lymphoedema may be present at birth but more often begins at puberty (Fig. 14), and becomes obvious in the second and third decades [61-63]. It occurs predominantly in young women. Milroy's disease should be diagnosed only in cases where the lymphoedema is both congenital and familial in origin [62, 64]. Primary lymphoedema results from congenital obstruction of lymphatic vessels and can occur from agenesis, hypoplasia, and varicose dilatation where valves are incompetent, aggravating the ac-

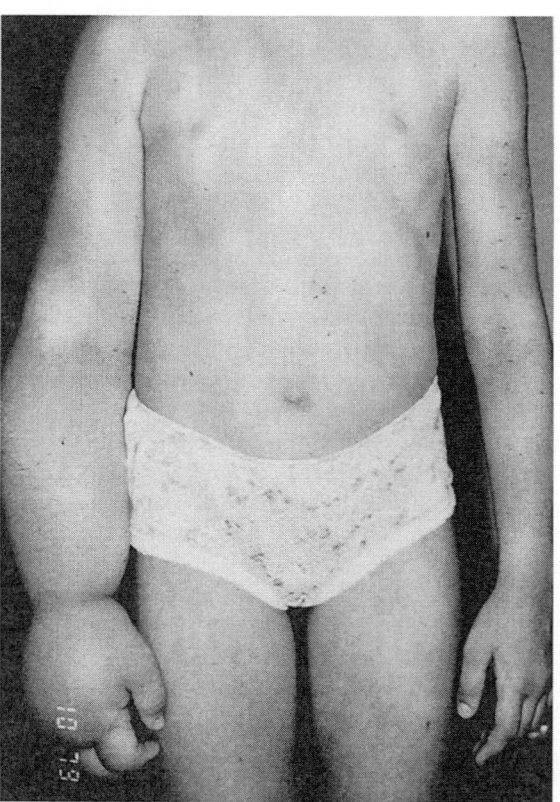

Fig. 14. Primary lymphoedema of a right superior limb in a child. (Courtesy Ms F. Alliot)

cumulation of interstitial fluid [56, 57, 59]. Total agenesis of lymphatic vessels is vanishingly rare and what is found is extreme rarity of lymphatic vessels. Malformations of the lymphovascular system are more frequent than is generally reported [63] in syndromes of limb malformation.

Acquired lymphoedema

This condition is caused by an acquired mechanical blockage of normal lymphatics, [65, 66]. Tumours and inflammatory conditions (filariasis, erysipelas) [67, 68] may block nodal filtration, producing lymphatic occlusion and stasis. Irradiation of node-bearing areas may impede lymphatic flow as will surgical or traumatic removal of nodes (Fig. 15). Very obese subjects may show some degree of reversible lymphoedema, if a significant loss of weight or an increase in exercise is achieved. This type of oedema is characterized by mild bilateral and symmetrical swelling in the pretibial areas without involvement of the feet [69]. Obstruction of veins and lymphatics combined with reduced muscle pumping and lowered cabin pressure may all contribute to triggering, or worsening, of lymphoedema during aircraft flights [70].

Pathology and differential diagnosis

The subcutaneous tissue is thickened and oedematous (Fig. 16). Fibrosis surrounds numerous dilated lymphatic vessels, blood capillaries, nerve fibers and the adnexa, giving rise to whitish strands (Fig. 17) reflecting the honeycoomb pattern revealed by CT scan (Fig. 18,19). Lymphatics are dilated and tortuous ; valves are incompetent and backflow occurs. The wall of the vessels show fibrosis with hypertrophy of muscle cells. Surrounding tissue is distorted by mononuclear cell infiltration and lymphoid follicles (Fig. 20-22). In some areas, lymphatic vessels undergo marked dilatation and fibrosis (Fig. 23). Some small muscular arteries display hypertrophy of the media (Fig. 24) as do arrectores pilora. In the chronic stage, a verrucous pattern may appear with hyperkeratosis and papillomatosis of the covering epidermis [66] (Fig. 25-26). These changes lead to elephantiasis (Fig. 27). In regional lymph nodes, fibrosis develops in both cortical and medullary parenchyma [71].

Particular entities

In blood vessels, arteritis or phlebitis is often associated with inflammatory infiltration of the adventitial lymph vessels. In the lungs, a rapid distension of peribronchial lymphatics is observed in pulmonary oedema of any cause, following inhalation of hot or toxic gases or in pneumonia or tuberculosis. In the

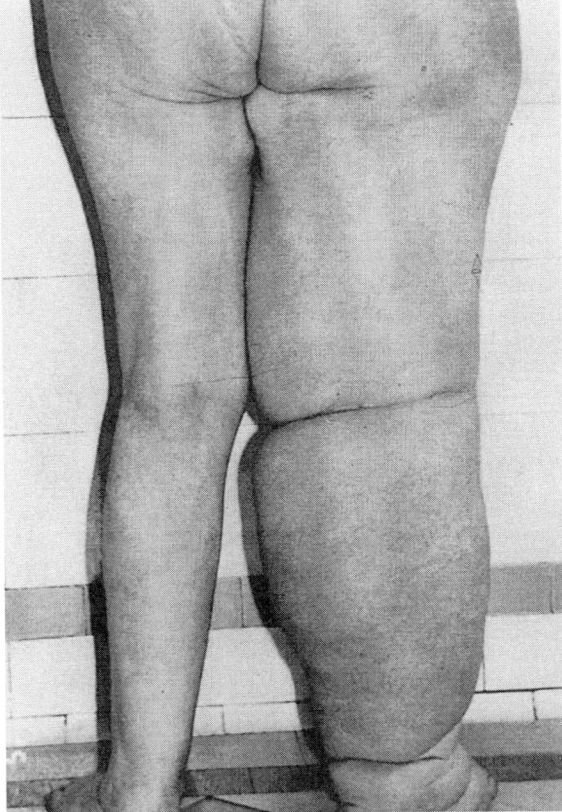

Fig. 15. Acquired lymphoedema. Female patient suffering from invasive carcinoma of the cervix. Lymphoedema of the right inferior limb occuring after a Wertheim's hysterectomy procedure with bilateral iliac lymph node curage. (Courtesy Dr R. Cluzan)

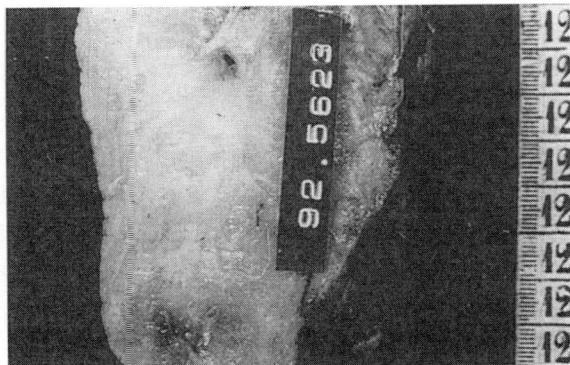

Fig. 16. Lymphoedema. Cut section of a lymphoedema resection specimen. Marked oedematous and fibrotic thickening of the skin and subcutaneous tissues

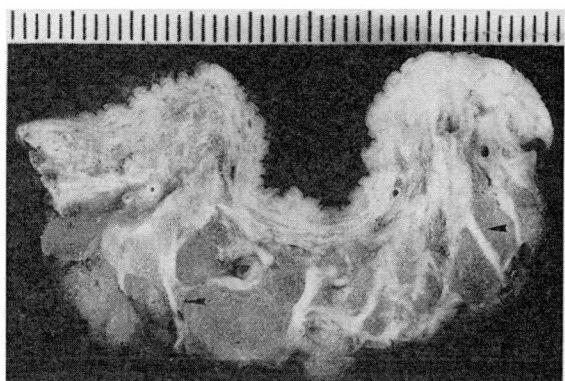

Fig. 17. Lymphoedema. Fibrotic strands enclosing numerous ectatic lymphatic vessels

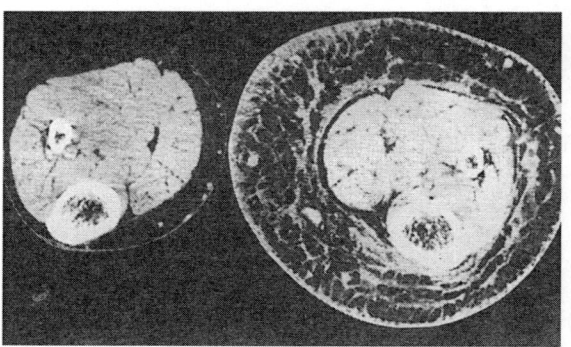

Fig. 18. Lymphoedema. Honeycomb pattern evidenced by CT scan (Courtesy Dr M. Marotel)

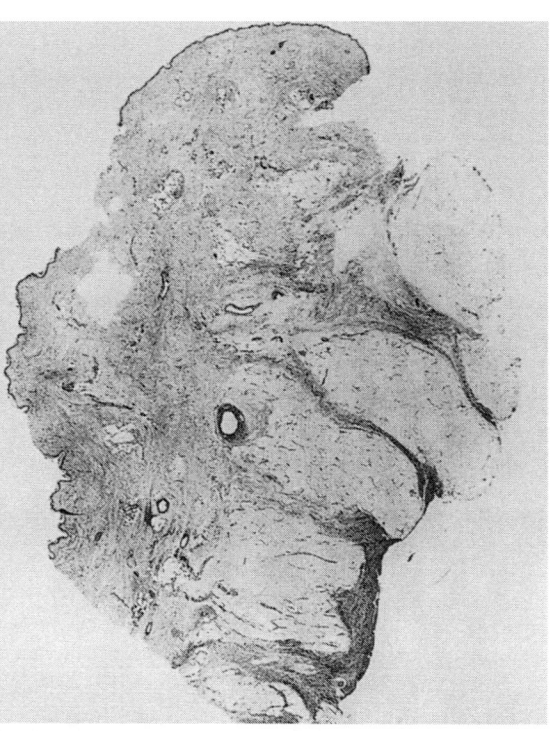

Fig. 19. Lymphoedema. Fibrotic strands enclosing dilated vessels, nerve fibres, cutaneous adnexa and extending to the subcutaneous tissue. HES

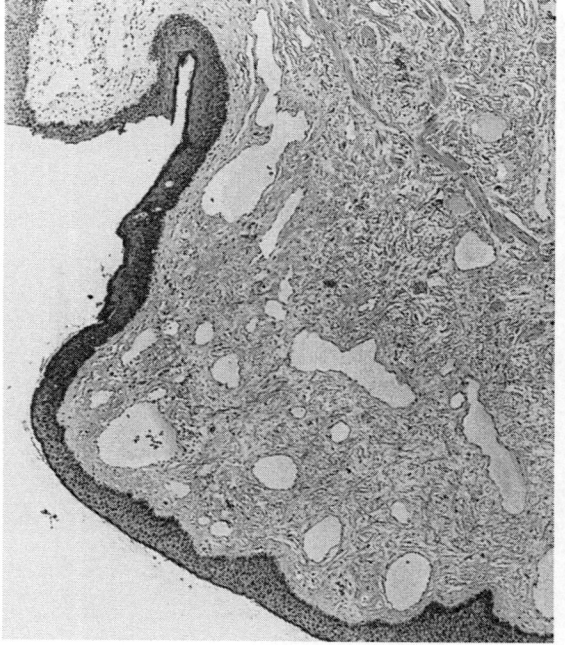

Fig. 20. Lymphoedema. Dilatation of superficial lymphatic capilaries. Note hypertrophy of arrectores pilora. HES

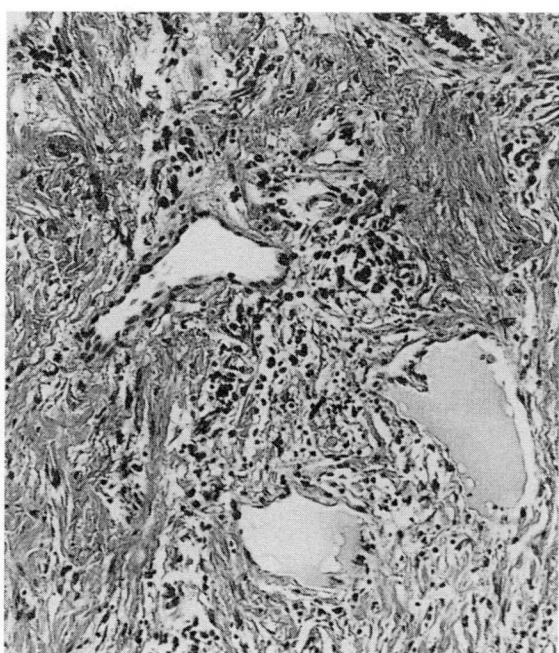

Fig. 21. Lymphoedema. Chronic inflammation surrounding dilated lymphatic vessels. HES

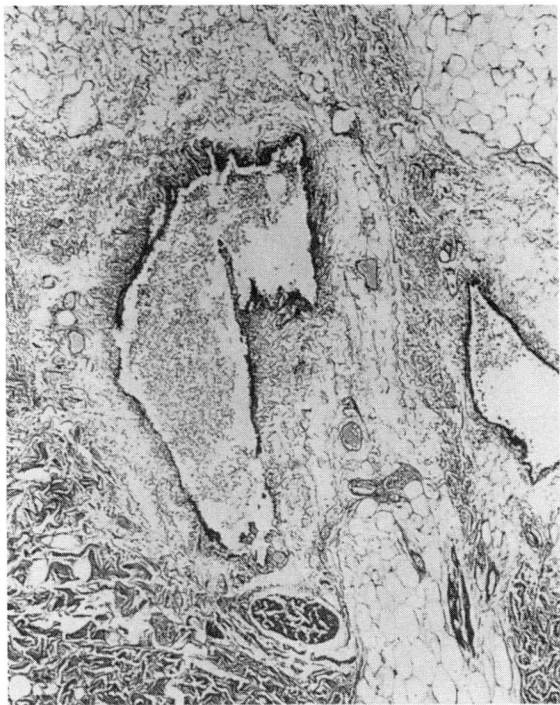

Fig. 22. Lymphoedema. Dilated lymphatic vessels with incompetent valves. HES

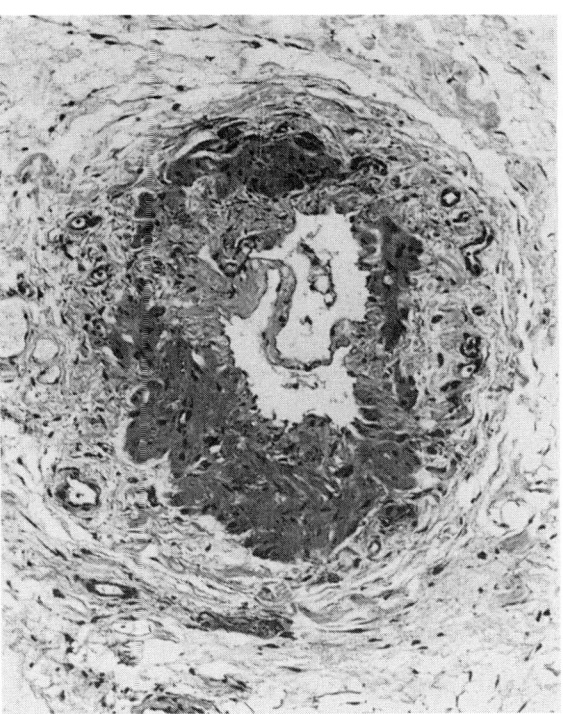

Fig. 23. Lymphoedema. Collecting lymph vessel displaying parietal fibrosis. Note thickening of the valvular apparatus. Masson's trichrome stain

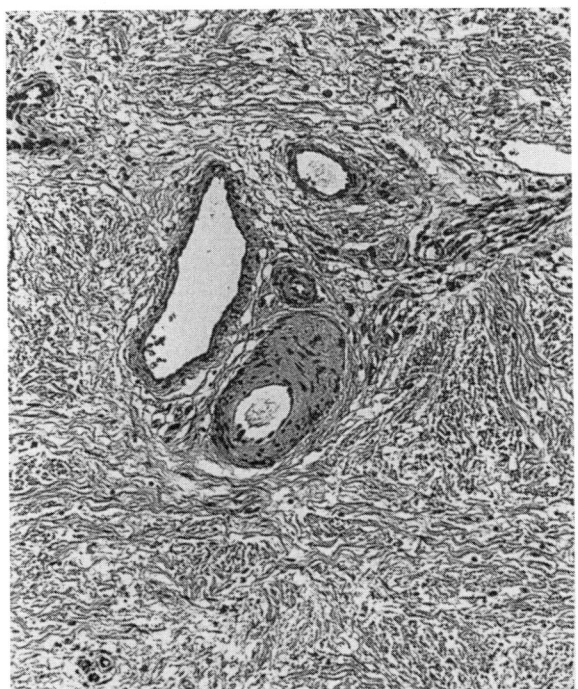

Fig. 24. Lymphoedema. Small dermic muscular artery showing hypertrophy of the media. HES

kidneys, changes in the renal lymph vessel system occur whenever the interstitium is overloaded by preceding tubular damage, or interstitial nephritis with increased high-protein and high-lipid oedema. The anatomical ramification of the lymphatic branches within the connective tissue septa of the liver is particularly dense and experimental blockage of the biliary tract leads to a compensatory outflow of bile via the hepatic lymph vessels. A comparable compensation mechanism has been demonstrated after disturbances to the venous outflow from the liver.

Vascular proliferation in lymph nodes (vascular transformation of lymphatic node sinuses, nodal angiomatosis)

First reported by Haferkamp et al [72], vascular proliferation in lymph nodes (VPLN) is characterized by a proliferation of capillaries within the dilated sinuses of lymph nodes, usually axillary or iliac, removed at the time of radical mastectomy or prostatectomy. The vascular transformation of the lymphonodular sinuses has been attributed to extensive obstruction of collecting nodal veins with opening of communicating channels between the blood vessels and lympha-

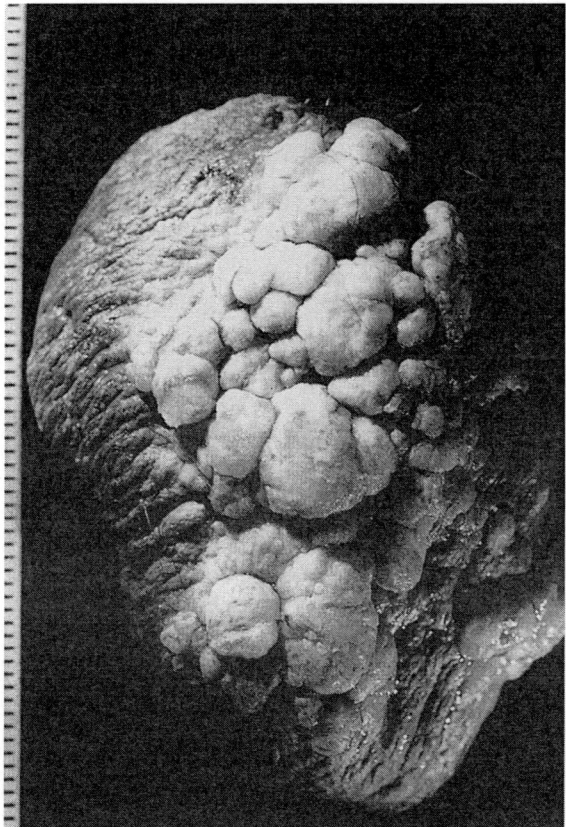

Fig. 25. Verrucous lymphoedema. (Courtesy Dr P. Trévidic)

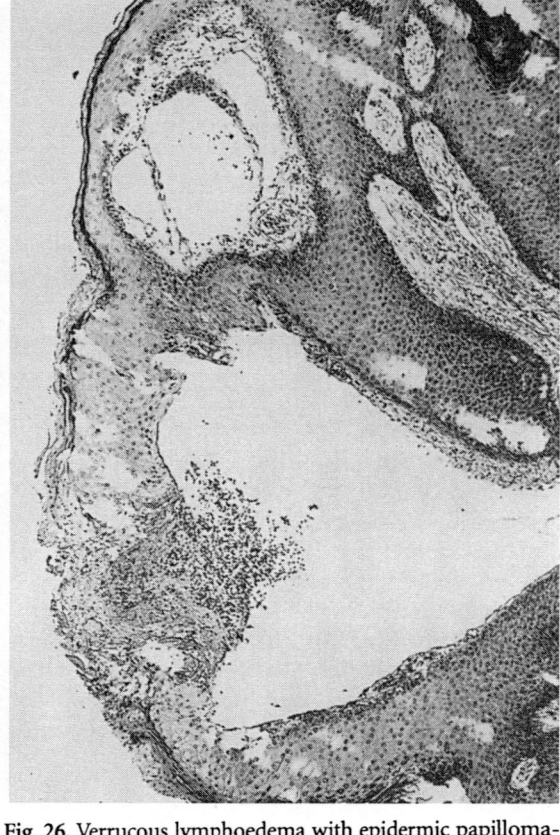

Fig. 26. Verrucous lymphoedema with epidermic papillomatosis and hyperkeratosis. HES

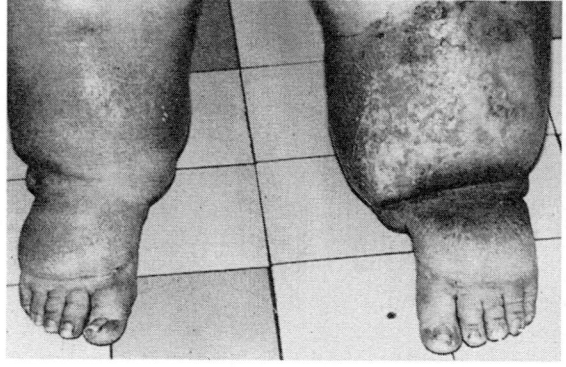

Fig. 27. Elephantiasis of both inferior limbs with dermatitis. (Courtesy Dr R.V. Cluzan)

tics. This gives rise to a shunt causing nodal sinuses to be filled with red cells [72], but this can also occur after a blockade of the efferent lymph vessels of the nodes. Concomitant severe venous and lymphatic stasis may play a role [73, 74]. In rabbits, experimental VPLN appears at day 7 postoperatively after partial ligation of the nodal veins together with all efferent lymphatics. Isolated ligation of nodal veins is not sufficient to produce VPLN, while complete ligation of all efferent veins and lymphatics leads to necrosis [75].

Pathology and differential diagnosis

Grossly, the lymph node is large but its consistency remains normal. Some degree of congestion is seen on cross section. Histologically, the change involves the subcapsular spaces and sinuses and consists of a proliferation of capillaries (Fig. 28-29). These vessels form an anastomotic network lined with plump endothelial cells which show some mitoses (Fig. 30-31).Some endothelial cells are spindle shaped [76-79]. The entire area is surrounded by an intra-sinusoidal fibrotic reaction. The transformed sinuses crush the nearby lymphoid tissue leading to parenchymal atrophy and thrombosis of the collecting veins. The lymph node capsule may be thickened by fibrosis. This uncommon lesion should not be misinterpreted as an hamartoma [80] or a vascular tumour, although it may, superficially, resemble Kaposi's sarcoma (KS), malignant haemangioendothelioma (MH), or metastatic haemangiopericytoma. Primary KS commonly develops in the medullary part of the node then extends to the remaining parenchyma. Sarcomatous spindle cells are surrounded by a fine reticulin network. Infiltration of lymphocytes and plasma cells may be diffuse or located around the tumour. Nearby lymphoid tissue shows follicular hyperplasia. VPLN and MH both present anastomotic vascular slits lined with an endothelium (angiomatoid MH) and compact areas of epithelioid cells (undifferentiated MH). MH not only involves the lymphatic sinuses, but also displays cellular atypia and nuclear hyperchromatism together with an inflammatory stroma. Metastatic haemangiopericytomata may form compact tumours

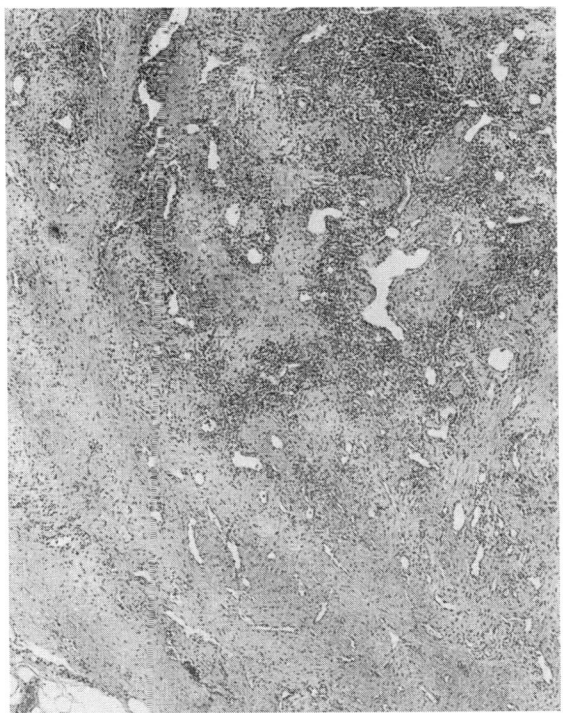

Fig. 29. Vascular proliferation in a lymph node. Atrophy of the lymph node parenchyma. HES

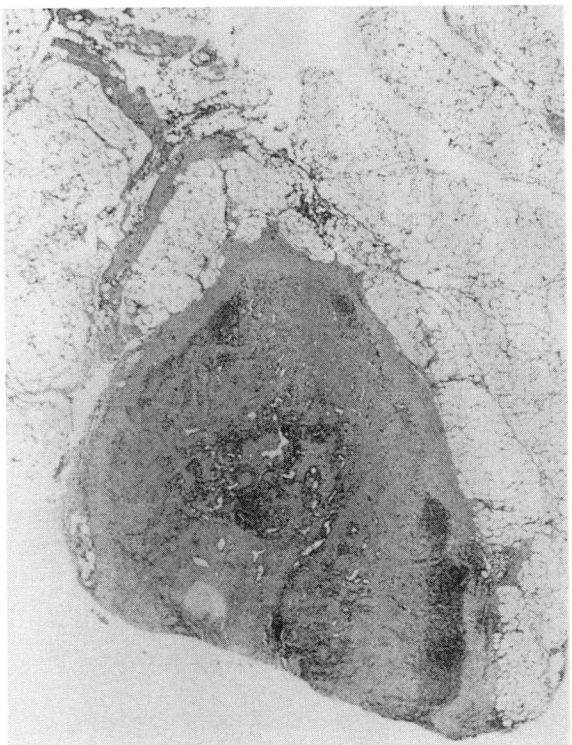

Fig. 28. Vascular proliferation in a lymph node. Note involvement of the subcapsular spaces and sinuses. HES

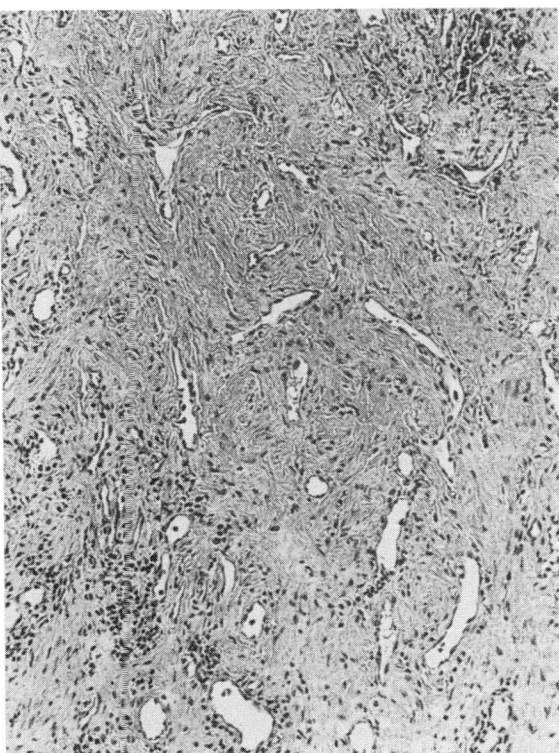

Fig. 30. Vascular proliferation in a lymph node. Anastomotic vessels surrounded by fibrosis. HES

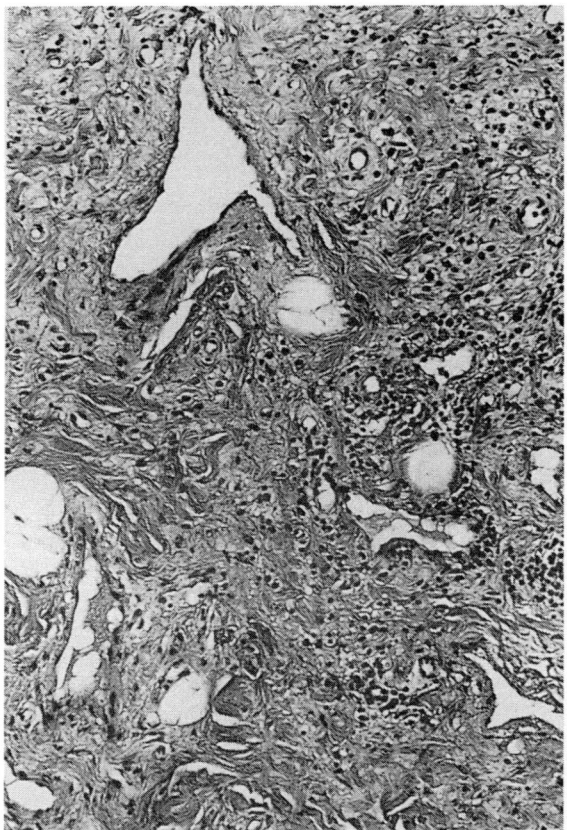

Fig. 31. Vascular proliferation in a lymph node. Most vessels are lined with plump endothelial cells. HES

with pericytes enclosed individually by reticulin fibers and arranged around variable-sized vascular cavities. The endothelial lining is well-differentiated and non-proliferating.

Acquired lymphangiectasia, lymphatic cysts and lymphocoeles

Acquired lymphangiectasia

This condition is caused by neoplastic obstruction of lymph vessels, lymph node metastases, parasitic infestation of the lacteals, non-specific inflammation, Behcet's disease, adhesions after surgery, or lymphatic fistulae [81]. Lymphangiectasia may be isolated or diffuse. The extremities, the retroperitoneal spaces, the mediastinum and the neck are most frequently involved. In the skin and mucosa, acquired lymphangiectasia gives rise to lymphoedema. In the digestive tract, lymphangiectases often occur in the small intestine, rarely in the wall of the colon, and may cause a protein-losing enteropathy.

Lymph cysts and lymphoceles

Differentiation between lymphangiectases, lymph cysts and lymphoceles may be difficult. Lymph cysts and lymphoceles may vary between a few millimetres to up to 20 cm in diameter. The clinical presentation varies with their location. Histologically, lymph cysts are surrounded by smooth muscle cells. True lymphocele should be differentiated from a collection of lymph or seroma formed after surgery. They may be a particular problem following renal transplantation [82] where lymphoceles develop within from 1 week to 5 years after transplantation. Although uncommon and benign, this lesion may compress the ureter and vein, thus reducing the renal function and mimicking either rejection or deep venous thrombosis.

3 – Pathology of the arteriovenous anastomoses

Raynaud's phenomenon and Raynaud's disease

Raynaud's phenomenon is a change produced by episodic constriction of small arteries and arterioles of the extremities. There are intermittent attacks of blanching or cyanosis of the digits, precipitated by exposure to cold or by emotional upsets [83, 84]. The major sign is colour change on exposure to cold. Colour changes do not occur above the metacarpophalangeal joints and rarely involve the thumb. They may be triphasic (pallor, cyanosis, redness or reactive hyperemia) or biphasic (cyanosis, then reactive hyperemia). Pain, paraesthesia (numbness, feeling of tightness or sticking in the fingers) may be present. Ultimately, gangrenous ulceration may occur. Rewarming the hands restores normal colour and sensation.

Raynaud's disease should be differentiated from Raynaud's phenomenon. Raynaud's phenomenon often accompanies or precedes an underlying disease that usually becomes manifest within 2 yrs, and is equally prevalent in men (18.6%) and women (19.7%) [85]. Primary Raynaud's disease occurs in those with no evidence of an underlying cause, with bilateral involvement and a history of symptoms for more than or equal to 2 yrs without progression. Its prevalence is somewhat higher in women (9.6%) than in men (8.1%). A small percentage of patients suffering from Raynaud's disease develop a connective-tissue disease (CTD) or systemic sclerosis over a period of around 10 years from the onset [86]. Nailfold capillary microscopy (NCM) helps predict this situation [87].

The pathogenesis of Raynaud's disease remains an enigma [88] and even the mechanism of Raynaud's phenomenon is not understood, although a growing number of neurovascular abnormalities have been identified [89]. Table 3 lists the established causes and clinical entities of Raynaud's phenomenon [84,90-104].

Pathology and differential diagnosis

There are no established early lesions and, in mild forms, the arteries remain normal. In warm-handed adults, the digital arteries usually show slight thickening of the intima and, after 60, pronounced thickening may be found. In patients with severe Raynaud's phenomenon, intimal thickening is greater than in warm-handed adults (Fig. 32). Arteriovenous anastomosis may show hyperplasia of epithelioid glomic cells (Fig. 33). Trophic lesions are more frequent with gangrenous ulceration. In patients with scleroderma and lupus erythematosus who have Raynaud's phenomenon, ultrastructural study reveals loss of capillaries, endothelial swelling, endothelial inclusions in residual capillaries and reduplication of the basement membrane in the microvascular bed of muscle, skin and renal capillaries. Raynaud's phenomenon should be distinguished from thromboangiitis oblitearns, arteriosclerosis obliterans, acrocyanosis and scleroderma. Thromboangiitis obliterans usually involves the lower limbs with a history of recurrent superficial thrombophlebitis. Arteriosclerosis obliterans rarely starts before the age of 50. The lower extremities are

Table 3. Major causes and clinical entities of Raynaud's phenomenon

Causes	Clinical entities
Occupational vascular diseases	Vibration syndrome (hand-transmitted vibration tools)
Occlusive vascular disease and neurogenic associated lesions	Arteriosclerosis, Buerger's disease or thromboangiitis obliterans, Carpal tunnel syndrome, Thrombotic or post-embolic arterial occlusion, Thoracic outlet syndrome.
Connective tissue diseases	Dermatomyositis, Disseminated lupus erythematous, Goujerot-Sjögren syndrome, Rheumatoid arthritis, Scleroderma, Sharp's syndrome.
Vasculitides	Cold agglutinins disease, Cryoglobulinaemia, Horton's disease, Periarteritis nodosa, Wegener's disease.
Chemical agents	Amantadine hydrochloride (1-Adamantanamine), Arsenic (As), Ergotamine and its derivatives (C33H35N5O5), Nitroglycerin, Silica and Silicone gel, Toxic oil syndrome, Vinyl chloride (chloroethylene).
Drugs	Amphetamine sulfate, Amphoterin B, Beta-blocker agents, Bleomycin sulfate, Bromocriptine, Cisplatin, Clonidine hydrochloride, Cyclosporine, Ergot derivatives, Estrogen, Imipramine hydrochloride, Interferon-alpha, Progesterone, Vincristine sulfate.
Haemopathies and coagulation disorders	Antiphospholipid syndromes, Disseminated intravascular coagulation (DIC), Hypergammaglobulinaemia (IgM), Polycythaemia, Thrombocythaemia
Miscellaneous conditions	Arteriovenous fistula for haemodialysis, Fabry's disease, Helicobacter pylori infection, Myxoedema, Neoplasias (Ovarian adenocarcinoma), Oxalosis, Primary pulmonary hypertension

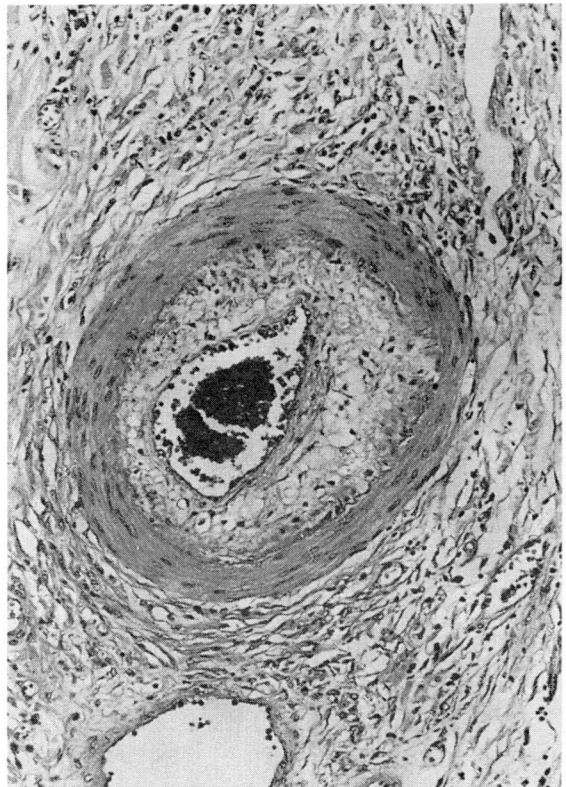

Fig. 32. Raynaud's phenomenon. Intimal thickening of digital arteries. HES

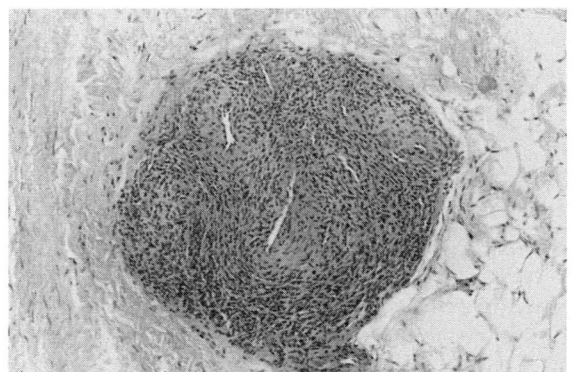

Fig. 33. Raynaud's phenomenon. Hyperplasia of epithelioid glomic cells surrounding an arteriovenous anastomosis. HES

first and more extensively involved. Acrocyanosis usually affects women, as does Raynaud's phenomenon, but the change in colour of the skin is a diffuse and more permanent cyanosis than is that of Raynaud's phenomenon. Scleroderma may be associated with Raynaud's phenomenon and it is important to determine whether Raynaud's phenomenon precedes or follows the onset of scleroderma. A story of telangiectasia preceding fibrosis of the skin lends support to the diagnosis of scleroderma.

Haemorrhoids

Normally, closure of the anal canal is ensured by cushions of tissue containing sac-like or serpiginous venous plexuses. Haemorrhoids result from permanent dilatation of these venous plexuses with significant development of the arteriovenous anorectal cavernous bodies leading to anal cushion enlargement and symptoms. When the dilatation is persistent, arterial blood passes from the peripheral branches of the superior rectal artery directly to the vein lumen, resulting in the ultimate development of varicose angioma-like phlebectasia [105-107].

In the early stages, little may be found other than an increased size of the cushions at the anal verge. As the condition develops, the anal verge may protrude and the mucosa becomes visible (Fig. 34) first on straining, and later in the resting state [108] Uncomplicated haemorrhoids cannot be palpated. When patients present with troublesome bleeding with early prolapse, sclerotherapy may be added to medical treatment. The sclerosing agent (5% phenol in vegetable oil) is injected submucosally into the loose areolar tissue above the haemorrhoids. Rubber band ligation is indicated for much enlarged and prolapsing haemorrhoids causing ischaemic necrosis followed by fibrosis and fixation of the tissues. Cryosurgery destroys haemorrhoids by cold necrosis using a cryoprobe (CO_2 or N_2O). Complications of surgery include ulceration, thrombosis and prolapse. An ulcerative cryptitis may develop between two haemorrhoids and give rise to abscess formation.

Pathology and differential diagnosis

Haemorrhoids consist of large blood-filled cavities measuring from 2 to 15 mm in diameter. Some are veins limited by a dystrophic varicose thick wall made up of collagen and elastic fibers ; others are dilated thin-walled capillaries lined with a single endothelial layer with some collagen fibers beneath it (Fig. 35). Some veins present prominent intraluminal fibrous cushions (Fig. 36). Inflammatory infiltration, edema, and red blood cell diapedesis are not uncommon (Fig. 37), nor are recent and old thromboses (Fig. 38). The covering ano-rectal mucosa presents significant crypt distortion. These changes are remarkably similar to those seen in mucosal prolapse syndrome [109].

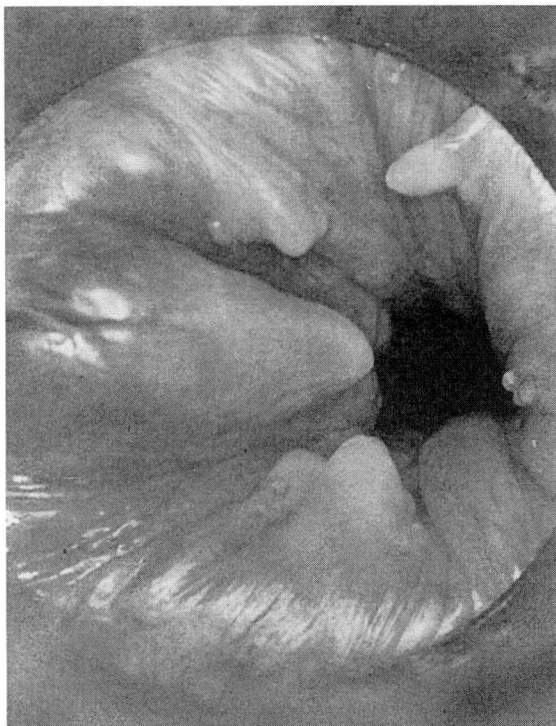

Fig. 34. Prolapsed haemorrhoids. (Courtesy Pr J. Denis)

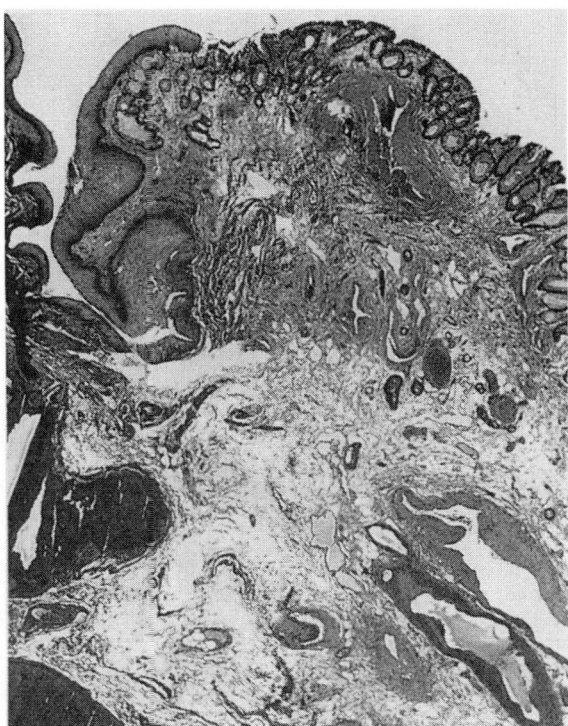

Fig. 35. Haemorrhoid. Dystrophic ectatic veins interspersed with dilated thin-walled capillaries. HES

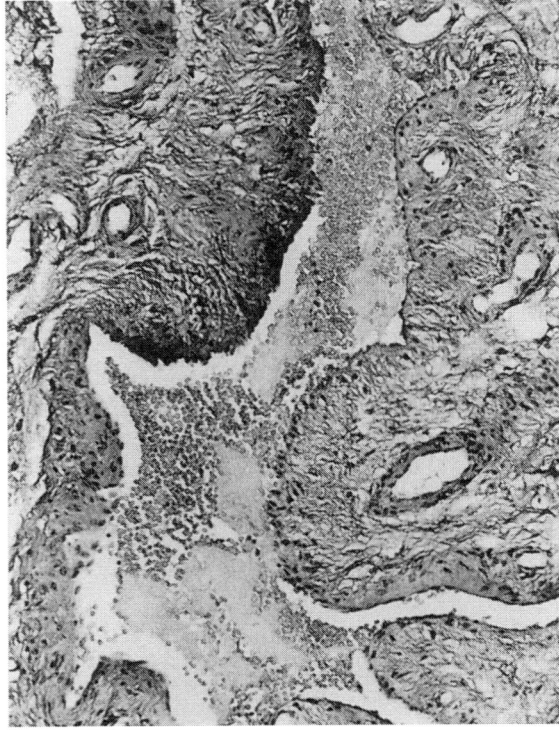

Fig. 36. Haemorrhoid. Prominent fibrous cushions reducing the lumen of haemorrhoidal vessels. HES

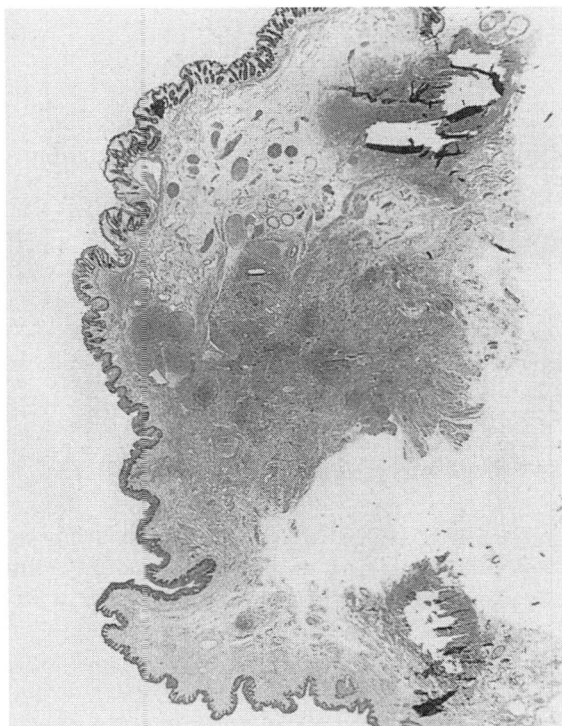

Fig. 37. Prolapsed haemorrhoid with diffuse haemorrhage and thrombosis HES

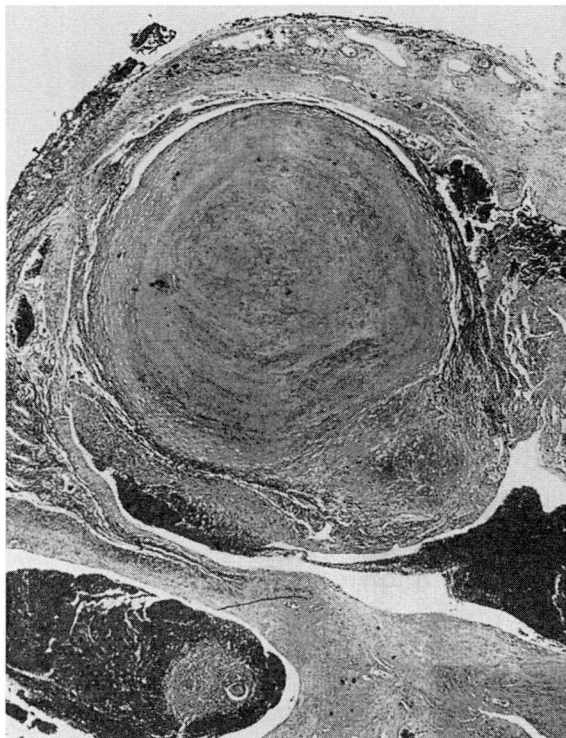

Fig. 38. Haemorrhoid with fresh and organised thrombi or phleboliths. HES

4 – Pathology of the erectile vascular tissue

This section is concerned with the morphological aspects of male erectile dysfunction which encompasses vasculogenic dysfunction and priapism.

Vasculogenic impotence

This condition is defined as a persistent inability to attain and maintain an erection adequate to permit satisfactory sexual performance. This condition affects 10% of the male population and about 52% of men between 40 70 [110, 111]. Vascular impairment is the major cause : alterations in the inflow (cavernosal artery insufficiency, arteriogenic impotence) and outflow (corporal veno-occlusive dysfunction, venous leak, failure to store) [112].

Inflow disorder (Cavernosal-artery insufficiency, arteriogenic impotence, failure to fill)

Atherosclerotic disease may involve the hypogastric cavernous arterial bed diffusely leading to cavernosal-artery insufficiency [113]. Thirty five % of male patients (20-59 years) suffering from severe diabetic microangiopathy have erectile impotence [114]. Trauma to the pelvis [115, 116], and ionising radiation (X-Ray) are other potential causes (Fig. 39-40).

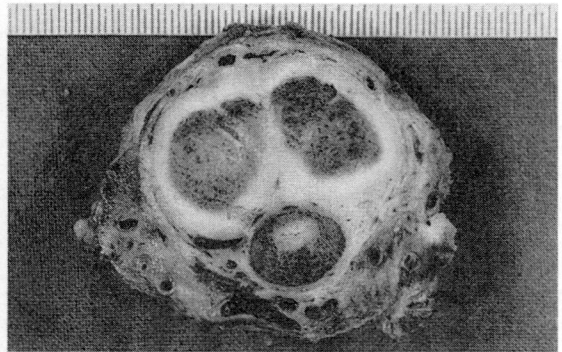

Fig. 39. Vasculogenic impotence. Male patient undergoing resection and post-operative radiation for an epidermoid carcinoma of penis. Note fibrosis of the corpus cavernosum and corpus spongiosum

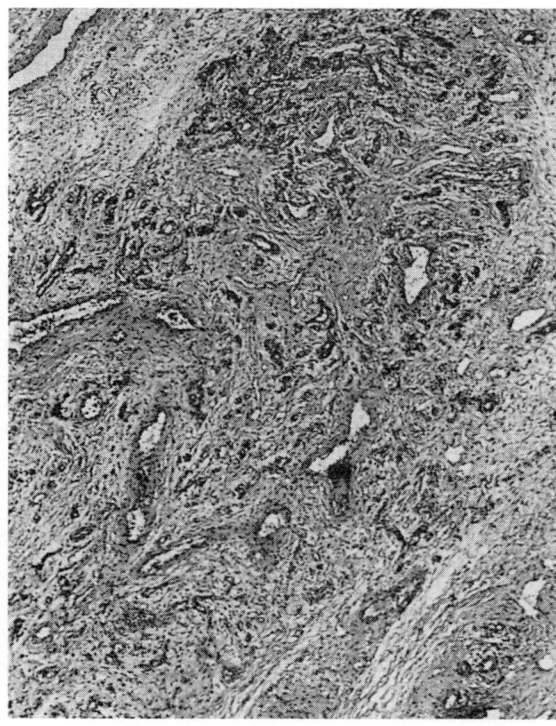

Fig. 40. Vasculogenic impotence. Penis. Diffuse fibrosis of the cavernous arterial bed. HES

Outflow disorder

Cavernosal veno-occlusive dysfunction, venous leak, and failure to store, result from impairment of trabecular smooth muscle relaxation [117, 118]. Alteration in the physiological mechanisms regulating the autonomic dilator nerves or the endothelium and release of the endothelium derived relaxing factor (EDRF) may be important causes. Structural changes in the fibers of collagen and elastin may also occur, secondary to nonenzymatic glycosylation of proteins associated with ageing, diabetes mellitus, and collagen vascular diseases, such as systemic sclerosis [117, 119, 120].

Histologically, the corpus cavernosum and tunica albuginea testis show severe fibrosis while the deep and superficial veins do not show significant differences from normal.

Priapism

Persistent erection of the penis, often accompanied by pain and tenderness, defines priapism. There are two types [121, 122].

Low flow veno-occlusive priapism (Type I)

This type is characterised by severe blood stasis within the corpora cavernosa and reduction of arterial perfusion through compression of the deep arteries of the penis. The mean age of the patients is 36 years and consultation is often delayed for some days. Pripism has been associated with alcoholism, abuse of amphetamines, cocaine, opioids, sedatives and psychotropic drugs, radiotherapy, thrombosis, sickle-cell anaemia, and chronic myeloid leukaemia. In one-third of cases, no cause has been identified [123-126].

High flow arterial priapism (Type II)

This is typified by arterial hyperperfusion. Outflow obstruction is absent. The penis is erect but of an elastic consistence, pain and ischaemia are lacking. Causes of high flow arterial priapism include trauma, accidental arterial-lacunar fistula after intracavernosal self-injection with papaverine and phentolamine, hypervascularization following deep dorsal vein arterialization to treat arteriogenic or mixed arteriogenic and venogenic impotence [127] and drug abuse including marijuana, ethanol, and cocaine [126, 128]. Even with a delay of treatment of up to 6 months the corpora cavernosa remain intact, and normal erectile function is preserved.

Bibliography

1. Rudofsky G (1989) Pathogenesis, diagnosis and therapy of thrombophlebitis and varicophlebitis. Herz 14: 283-6
2. Jordaan HF (1986) Widespread superficial thrombophlebitis as a manifestation of secondary syphilis—a new sign. A report of 2 cases. S Afr Med J 70: 493-4
3. Pugh CM, DeWitty RL (1996) Mondor's disease. J Natl Med Assoc 88: 359-63
4. Sharma MC, Deshpande V, Sharma R, Pal S, Sahni P (1998) Giant cell phlebitis as a cause of large intestinal stricture. J Clin Gastroenterol 27: 79-81
5. Berni A, Cavaiola S, Tombesi T, Mele R, Tromba L, Fiorellino A, Corbellini L (1997) A new classification of varicose veins to compare various surgical strategies. Eur Rev Med Pharmacol Sci 1: 157-9
6. Belcaro G, Nicolaides AN, Veller M (1995) Venous disorders. A manual of diagnosis and treatment. Saunders, London, Philadelphia, Toronto, Sydney, Tokyo
7. Davy A (1994) Chapitre 8 In Barthelemy P, Lefebvre D (eds.) Insuffisance veineuse des membres inférieurs. Masson, Paris 75-85
8. Krasinski Z, Kotwicka M, Oszkinis G, Dzieciuchowicz L, Borkiewicz P, Wasko R, Gabriel M (1997) Investigations on the pathogenesis of primary varicose veins. Wiad Lek 50: 275-80
9. Bollinger A, Leu AJ, Hoffmann U, Franzeck UK (1997) Microvascular changes in venous disease: an update. Angiology 48: 27-32
10. Haimovici H (1987) Role of precapillary arteriovenous shunting in the pathogenesis of varicose veins and its therapeutic implications. Surgery 101: 515-22
11. Clarke H, Smith SR, Vasdekis SN, Hobbs JT, Nicolaides AN (1989) Role of venous elasticity in the development of varicose veins. Br J Surg 76: 577-80
12. Pappas PJ, Gwertzman GA, DeFouw DO, Padberg FT Jr, Silva MB Jr, Duran WN, Hobson RW 2nd (1998) Retinoblastoma protein: a molecular regulator of chronic venous insufficiency. J Surg Res 76: 149-53
13. Bouissou H, Pieraggi MT, Julian M, Maurel E, Thiers J-C (1994) Anatomo-pathologie de la veine variqueuse. In Barthelemy P, Lefebvre D (eds.) Insuffisance veineuse des membres inférieurs. Masson, Paris 17-25
14. Labropoulos N, Giannoukas AD, Delis K, Mansour MA, Kang SS, Nicolaides AN, Lumley J, Baker WH (1997) Where does venous reflux start? J Vasc Surg 26: 736-42
15. Kistner RL (1986) Diagnosis of chronic venous insufficiency. J Vasc Surg 3: 185-8
16. Kistner RL, Eklof B, Masuda EM (1996) Diagnosis of chronic venous disease of the lower extremities: the "CEAP" classification. Mayo Clin Proc 71: 338-45
17. Mark EJ (1984) Lung biopsy interpretation. Williams and Wilkins, Baltimore London, p 284
18. Justo RN, Dare AJ, Whight CM, Radford DJ (1993) Pulmonary veno-occlusive disease: diagnosis during life in four patients. Arch Dis Child 68: 97-100
19. Ruchelli ED, Nojadera G, Rutstein RM, Rudy B (1994) Pulmonary veno-occlusive disease. Another vascular disorder associated with human immunodeficiency virus infection? Arch Pathol Lab Med 118: 664-6
20. Escamilla R, Hermant C, Berjaud J, Mazerolles C, Daussy X (1995) Pulmonary veno-occlusive disease in a HIV-infected intravenous drug abuser. Eur Respir J 8: 1982-4
21. Palmer SM, Robinson LJ, Wang A, Gossage JR, Bashore T, Tapson VF (1998) Massive pulmonary edema and death after prostacyclin infusion in a patient with pulmonary veno-occlusive disease. Chest 113: 237-40

22. Liang MH, Stern S, Fortin PR, Louie DC, Marsh JD, Mudge GH Jr, Murphy G (1991) Fatal pulmonary venoocclusive disease secondary to a generalized venulopathy: a new syndrome presenting with facial swelling and pericardial tamponade. Arthritis Rheum 34: 228-33

23. Kieffer E, Ruotolo C, Richard T, Lesaget F, Moro N (1985) Membranes et hypopasies de la veine cave inférieure terminale In Kieffer E (Ed) Chirurgie de la veine cave inférieure et de ses branches. Expansion Scientifique Française, Paris p 117-31

24. Hirooka M (1969) Membranous obstruction of the inferior vena cava on the hepatic portion. Hypothetical etiology based on developmental abnormality. Acta Hepatol Jpn 10: 566-77

25. Lu CL, Chou YH, Hwang SJ, Chan CY, Lee SD (1995) Membranous obstruction of the inferior vena cava in Taiwan. J Gastroenterol Hepatol 10: 287-94

26. Okuda H, Yamagata H, Obata H, Iwata H, Sasaki R, Imai F, Okudaira M, Ohbu M, Okuda K (1995) Epidemiological and clinical features of Budd-Chiari syndrome in Japan. J Hepatol 22: 1-9

27. Rector WG, Xu Y, Goldstein L, Peters RL, Reynolds TB (1985) Membranous obstruction of the inferior vena cava in the United States. Medicine 64: 134-43

28. Coue O, Fornes P, Paraf F, Couetil JP, Bruneval P (1996) Budd-Chiari syndrome secondary to post-traumatic stenosis of the inferior vena cava. Gastroenterol Clin Biol 20: 196-9

29. Pinsolle J, Videau J (1982) Anomalies du carrefour iliocave: interprétation du syndrome de Cockett d'après 180 dissections. Chirurgie 108: 451-8

30. Shrestha SM, Okuda K, Uchida T, Maharjan KG, Shrestha S, Joshi BL, Larsson S, Vaidya Y (1996) Endemicity and clinical picture of liver disease due to obstruction of the hepatic portion of the inferior vena cava in Nepal. J Gastroenterol Hepatol 11: 170-9

31. Simpson IW (1982) Membranous obstruction of the inferior vena cava and hepatocellular carcinoma in South Africa. Gastroenterology 82: 171-8

32. Dhiman RK, Saraswat VA, Radhakrishnan S, Parashar A, Agarwal DK, Naik SR (1992) Multiple venous thromboses and membranous obstruction of inferior vena cava in association with hereditary protein C deficiency: a case report. J Gastroenterol Hepatol 7: 434-8

33. Balian A, Naveau S, Chaput J-C (1997) Obstruction membraneuse de la veine cave inférieure. Gastroenterol Clin Biol 21: 265-73

34. Okuda K, Kage M, Shrestha SM (1998) Proposal of a new nomenclature for Budd-Chiari syndrome: hepatic vein thrombosis versus thrombosis of the inferior vena cava at its hepatic portion. Hepatology 28: 1191-8

35. Wechsler B, Fassin D, Godeau P (1985) Thromboses de la veine cave inférieure. Bilan étiologique In Kieffer E (Ed.) Chirurgie de la veine cave inférieure et de ses branches. Expansion Scientifique Française, Paris p 193-8

36. Kraut J, Berman JH, Gunasekaran TS, Allen R, McFadden J, Messersmith R, Pellettiere E (1997) Hepatic vein thrombosis (Budd-Chiari syndrome) in an adolescent with ulcerative colitis. J Pediatr Gastroenterol Nutr 25: 417-20

37. Hunter JA, Sessions R, Buenger R (1970) Experimental balloon obstruction of the inferior vena cava. Ann Surg 171: 315-20

38. Yamada R, Sato M, Kawabata M, Nakatsuka H, Nakamura K, Kobayashi N (1983) Segmental obstruction of the hepatic inferior vena cava treated by transluminal angioplasty. Radiology 149: 91-6

39. Kimura C, Shirotami H, Kuma T (1962) Transcardiac membranotomy for obliteration of the inferior vena cava in the hepatic portion. J Cardiovasc Surg 3: 393-404

40. Dumanian AV, Giragos HG, Sanders A, Frahm HJ, Hadidian HA (1971) The Budd-Chiari syndrome. A new method in the surgical treatment of the disease. Ann Thorac Surg 7: 79-84

41. Michot F, Tubiana JM, Chermet J, Lévy VG, Huguet C (1980) Oblitération membraneuse de la veine cave inférieure inter-hépato-diaphragmatique. La membranectomie est-elle la meilleure opération ? Ann Chir 34: 299-304

42. Maillard JN, Elman A, Erlinger S, Sanguinetti J (1982) Syndrome de Budd-Chiari par obstruction membraneuse de la veine cave inférieure. Traitement par anastomose mésentérico-cave et prothèse cavo-auriculaire. Gastroenterol Clin Biol 6: 748-51

43. Dubost C, Piwnica A, Carpentier A, Kieffer E (1969) Traitement chirurgical des oblitérations membraneuses du segment terminal des veines caves. A propos de deux observations. Ann Chir Thorac Cardio Vasc 8: 433-43

44. Hirooka M, Kimura C (1970) Membranous obstruction of the hepatic portion of the inferior vena cava. Arch Surg 100: 656-63

45. Agger P, Johnsen SG (1978) Quantitative evaluation of testicular biopsies in varicocele. Fertil Steril 29: 52-7

46. Preite M, Rotta L, Meneghelli R, Veronese E, Ferrari G, Pazzaglia M (1987) The varicocele today. Chir Ital 39: 415-22

47. Kass EJ, Reitelman C (1995) Adolescent varicocele. Urol Clin North Am 22: 151-9

48. D'Agostino S, Musi L, Belloli G (1996) Primary varicocele: a substimated pathology in pediatrico-adolescent age. Pediatr Med Chir 18: S21-S26

49. Charles G (1995) Congestive pelvic syndromes. Rev Fr Gynecol Obstet 90: 84-90

50. Mathis BV, Miller JS, Lukens ML, Paluzzi MW (1995) Pelvic congestion syndrome: a new approach to an unusual problem. Am Surg 61: 1016-8

51. Pilawski Z, Kosmider M, Lazar W (1987) Evaluation of work systems in the textile industry in relation to the development of pathological changes in the genital organs of seamstresses. Med Pr 38: 66-71

52. Menkiszak J (1989) Pain in the lumbosacral region in pelvic congestion syndrome in women working under conditions of limited motor activity. Ann Acad Med Stetin 35: 167-78

53. Fernandez-Samos R, Zorita A, Ortega JM, Moran C, Moran O, Vazquez J, Vaquero F (1993) Female gonadal venous insufficiency. Angiologia 45: 203-9

54. Merli GJ (1984) Lymphoedema. Clin Podiatry 1: 363-72

55. Browse NL, Stewart G (1985) Lymphooedema: pathophysiology and classification. J Cardiovasc Surg (Torino) 26: 91-106

56. Dustmann HO (1982) Diagnosis, differential diagnosis and therapy of lymphoedema. Z Orthop 120: 76-82

57. Wright NB, Carty HM (1994) The swollen leg and primary lymphooedema. Arch Dis Child 71: 44-9

58. Cox NH, Paterson WD, Popple AW (1996) A reticulate vascular abnormality in patients with lymphooedema: observations in eight patients. Br J Dermatol 135: 92-7

59. Mehta SD, Robinson RJ, Bern SA (1996) Pedal manifestations of Milroy's disease. J Am Podiatr Med Assoc 86: 400-2

60. Brostrom LA, Nilsonne U, Kronberg M, Soderberg G (1989) Lymphangiosarcoma in chronic hereditary ooedema (Milroy's disease). Ann Chir Gynaecol 78: 320-3

61. Ijaiya K, Modder U, Heinisch HM (1976) Primary lymphoedema of the lower limbs in childhood. Klin Padiatr 188: 203-8

62. Gregl A, von Heyden D, Jentsch F, Yu D (1983) Primary lymphoedema. Z Lymphol 7: 21-8

63. Hanssler L, Metz KA, Roll C, Hennecke KH (1990) Primary lymphatic dysplasia in a newborn infant. Monatsschr Kinderheilkd 138: 772-4

64. Blagowidow N, Page DC, Huff D, Mennuti MT (1989) Ullrich-Turner syndrome in an XY female fetus with deletion of the sex-determining portion of the Y chromosome. Am J Med Genet 34: 159-62

65. Esato K, Ohara M, Seyama A, Akimoto F, Kuga T, Takenaka H, Zempo N (1991) 99mTc-HSA lymphoscintigraphy and leg oedema following arterial reconstruction. J Cardiovasc Surg (Torino) 32: 741-6

66. Schissel DJ, Hivnor C, Elston DM (1998) Elephantiasis nostras verrucosa. Cutis 62: 77-80

67. Vuong PN, Cluzan RV, Trévidic P (1997) Récidive d'un cancer gastrique révélée par un lymphoedème après une plongée sous-marine: une observation. J Mal Vasc 22 (Suppl A): .68-69

68. Kasseroller R (1998) Sodium selenite as prophylaxis against erysipelas in secondary lymphoedema. Anticancer Res 18: 2227-30

69. Rudkin GH, Miller TA (1994) Lipoedema: a clinical entity distinct from lymphoedema. Plast Reconstr Surg 94: 841-7

70. Casley-Smith JR, Casley-Smith JR (1996) Lymphoedema initiated by aircraft flights. Aviat Space Environ Med 67: 52-6

71. Maiborodin IV, Shevela AI, Titova LV (1998) Variants and stages of regional lymph nodes sclerosis in lymphoedema. Arkh Patol 60: 47-51

72. Haferkamp O, Rosenau W, Lennert K (1971) Vascular transformation of lymph node sinuses due to venous obstruction. Arch Pathol 92: 81-3

73. Scherrer C, Maurer R (1985) La transformation vasculaire sinusienne du ganglion lymphatique. Analyse morphologique et immuno-histochimique de six cas. Ann Pathol 5: 231-8

74. Di Blasi A, Ferbo U (1989) Ischemic stenosis of the ileum with reactive parietal and lymph-nodal angioendotheliomatous hyperplasia. Pathologica 81: 63-9

75. Steinmann G, Földi E, Földi M, Racz, Lennert K (1982) Morphologic findings in lymph nodes after occlusion of their efferent lymphatic vessels and veins. Lab Invest 47: 43-50

76. Michael M, Koza V (1989) Vascular transformation of lymph node sinuses – a diagnostic pitfall. Histopathologic and immunohistochemical study. Pathol Res Pract 185: 441-4

77. Ostrowski ML, Siddiqui T, Barnes RE, Howton MJ (1990) Vascular transformation of lymph node sinuses. A process displaying a spectrum of histologic features. Arch Pathol Lab Med 114: 656-60

78. Chan JK, Warnke RA, Dorfman R (1991) Vascular transformation of sinuses in lymph nodes. A study of its morphological spectrum and distinction from Kaposi's sarcoma. Am J Surg Pathol 15: 732-43

79. Cook PD, Czerniak B, Chan JK, Mackay B, Ordonez NG, Ayala AG, Rosai J (1995) Nodular spindle-cell vascular transformation of lymph nodes. A benign process occurring predominantly in retroperitoneal lymph nodes draining carcinomas that can simulate Kaposi's sarcoma or metastatic tumour. Am J Surg Pathol 19: 1010-20

80. Magro G, Grasso S (1997) Angiomyomatous hamartoma of the lymph node: case report with adipose tissue component. Gen Diagn Pathol 143: 247-9

81. Brun JL (1995) Postoperative lymphoceles and lymphatic fistula in gynecologic and breast neoplasms. Bull Cancer 82: 711-6

82. Ward K, Klingensmith WC 3d, Sterioff S, Wagner HN Jr (1978) The origin of lymphoceles following renal transplantation. Transplantation 25: 346-7

83. Raynaud M (1888) On local asphyxia and symmetrical gangrene of the extremities and new researches on the nature and treatment of local asphyxia of the extremities. Selected Monographs. London, New Sydenham Soc Publ, Vol 121, pp 1-199

84. Lekakis J, Mavrikakis M, Emmanuel M, Prassopoulos V, Papazoglou S, Papamichael C, Moulopoulou D, Kostamis P, Stamatelopoulos S, Moulopoulos S (1998) Cold-induced coronary Raynaud's phenomenon in patients with systemic sclerosis. Clin Exp Rheumatol 16: 135-40

85. Brand FN, Larson MG, Kannel WB, McGuirk JM (1997) The occurrence of Raynaud's phenomenon in a general population: the Framingham Study. Vasc Med 2: 296-301

86. Spencer-Green G (1998) Outcomes in primary Raynaud phenomenon: a meta-analysis of the frequency, rates, and predictors of transition to secondary diseases. Arch Intern Med 158: 595-600

87. Luggen M Belhorn L, Evans T, Fitzgerald O, Spencer-Green G (1995) The evolution of Raynaud's phenomenon: a longterm prospective study. J Rheumatol 22: 2226-32

88. Marcolongo R, Cora F, Laveder F, Cavallo M, Busato A, Rigoli AM (1997) Raynaud's phenomenon. Practical considerations on the forms secondary to immunomediated systemic diseases. Minerva Med 88: 307-10

89. Walmsley D, Goodfield MJD (1990) Evidence for an abnormal peripherally mediated vascular response to temperature in Raynaud's phenomenon. Br J Rheumatol 29: 181-4

90. Nielsen SL, Parving HH, Hansen JE (1982) Myxoedema and Raynaud's phenomenon. Acta Endocrinol (Copenh) 101: 32-4

91. Alonso-Ruiz A, Calabozo M, Perez-Ruiz F, Mancebo L (1993) Toxic oil syndrome. A long-term follow-up of a cohort of 332 patients. Medicine (Baltimore) 72: 285-95

92. Blann AD, Illingworth K, Jayson MI (1993) Mechanisms of endothelial cell damage in systemic sclerosis and Raynaud's phenomenon. J Rheumatol 20: 1325-30

93. Berger CC Bokemeyer C, Schneider M, Kuczyk MA, Schmoll HJ (1995) Secondary Raynaud's phenomenon and other late vascular complications following chemotherapy for testicular cancer. Eur J Cancer 31A: 2229-38

94. Kohli M, Bennett RM (1995) Raynaud's phenomenon as a presenting sign of ovarian adenocarcinoma. J Rheumatol 22: 1393-4

95. Lavras Costallat LT, Valente Coimbra AM (1995) Raynaud's phenomenon in systemic lupus erythematosus. Rev Rhum Engl Ed 62: 349-53

96. Anderson DR, Schwartz J, Cottrill CM, McClain SA, Ross JS, Magidson JG, Klainer A, Bisaccia E (1996) Silicone granuloma in acral skin in a patient with silicone-gel breast implants and systemic sclerosis. Int J Dermatol 35: 36-8

97. Bachmeyer C, Farge D, Gluckman E, Miclea JM, Aractingi S (1996) Raynaud's phenomenon and digital

necrosis induced by interferon-alpha. Br J Dermatol 135: 481-3

98. Field T, Bridges AJ (1996) Clinical and laboratory features of patients with scleroderma and silicone implants. Curr Top Microbiol Immunol 210: 283-90

99. Harazin B, Langauer-Lewowicka H (1996) Raynaud's phenomenon in different groups of workers using hand-held vibrating tools. Cent Eur J Public Health 4: 130-2

100. Haustein UF (1996) Raynaud phenomenon and scleroderma. Hautarzt 47: 336-40

101. Hladunewich M, Sawka C, Fam A, Franssen E (1997) Raynaud's phenomenon and digital gangrene as a consequence of treatment for Kaposi's sarcoma. J Rheumatol 24: 2371-5

102. Sibilia J, Rey D, Beck-Wirth G, Fraisse P, Chakfe N, Grunebaum L, Wiesel ML, Partisani ML, Lang JM (1997) Acrosyndromes induced by bleomycin in HIV 1 related Kaposi's disease. 5 cases. Presse Med 26: 1564-7

103. Zernikow B, Fleischhack G, Hasan C, Bode U (1997) Cyanotic Raynaud's phenomenon with conventional but not with liposomal amphotericin B: three case reports. Mycoses 40: 359-61

104. Gasbarrini A, Franceschi F, Cammarota G, Pola P, Gasbarrini G (1998) Vascular and immunological disorders associated with Helicobacter pylori infection. Ital J Gastroenterol Hepatol 30: 115-8

105. Datsun IG, Mel'man EP (1992) Role of glomus shunts of the anorectal cavernous bodies in the mechanism of hemorrhoid development. Arkh Patol 54: 28-31

106. Loder PB, Kamm MA, Nicholls RJ, Phillips RK (1994) Haemorrhoids: pathology, pathophysiology and aetiology. Br J Surg 81: 946-54

107. Delco F, Sonnenberg A (1998) Associations between hemorrhoids and other diagnoses. Dis Colon Rectum 41: 1534-41

108. Shafik A (1988) A new concept of the anatomy of the anal sphincter mechanism and the physiology of defecation. XXXI. "Strainodynia": an etiopathologic study. J Clin Gastroenterol 10: 179-84

109. Kaftan SM, Haboubi NY (1995) Histopathological changes in haemorrhoid associated mucosa and submucosa. Int J Colorectal Dis 10: 15-8

110. Feldman HA, Goldstein I, Hatzichristou DG, Krane RJ, McKinlay JB (1994) Impotence and its medical and psychosocial correlates: results of the Massachusetts Male Aging Study. J Urol 151: 54-61

111. Ludwig G (1998) Diagnosis and therapy of erectile dysfunction. Z Arztl Fortbild Qualitatssich 92: 335-42

112. Goldstein I (1996) Vasculogenic impotence In Loscalzo J, Creager MA, Dzau VJ (ed) Vascular medicine. A textbook of vascular biology and diseases. Little, Brown and Cie, Boston, pp 885-900

113. Azadzoi KM, Siroky MB, Goldstein I (1996) Study of etiologic relationship of arterial atherosclerosis to corporal veno-occlusive dysfunction in the rabbit. J Urol 155(5): 1795-800

114. McCulloch DK, Campbell IW, Wu FC, Prescott RJ, Clarke BF (1980) The prevalence of diabetic impotence. Diabetologia 18: 279-83

115. Godec CJ, Reiser R, Logush AZ (1988) The erect penis – injury prone organ. J Trauma 28: 124-6

116. Penson DF, Seftel AD, Krane RJ, Frohrib D, Goldstein I (1992) The hemodynamic pathophysiology of impotence following blunt trauma to the erect penis. J Urol 148: 1171-80

117. Azadzoi KM, Goldstein I (1992) Erectile dysfunction due to atherosclerotic vascular disease: the development of an animal model. J Urol 147(6): 1675-81

118. Azadzoi KM, Kim N, Brown ML, Goldstein I, Cohen RA, Saenz de Tejada I (1992) Endothelium-derived nitric oxide and cyclooxygenase products modulate corpus cavernosum smooth muscle tone. J Urol 147(1): 220-5

119. Krane RJ, Goldstein I, Saenz de Tejada I (1989) Impotence. N Engl J Med 321: 1648-59

120. Nehra A, Hall SJ, Basile G, Bertero EB, Moreland R, Toselli P, de las Morenas A, Goldstein I (1995) Systemic sclerosis and impotence: a clinicopathological correlation. J Urol 153: 1140-6

121. Bruhlmann W, Zollikofer C, Hauri D (1987) Angiographic, cavernosonographic and clinical differentiation of two forms of priapism with different prognoses. ROFO Fortschr Geb Rontgenstr Nuklearmed 147: 165-8

122. Magoha GA (1995) Priapism: a historical and update review. East Afr Med J 72: 399-401

123. Levine JF, Saenz de Tejada I, Payton TR, Goldstein I (1991) Recurrent prolonged erections and priapism as a sequela of priapism: pathophysiology and management. J Urol 145: 764-7

124. Dunn EK, Miller ST, Macchia RJ, Glassberg KI, Gillette PN, Sarkar SD, Strashun AM (1995) Penile scintigraphy for priapism in sickle cell disease. J Nucl Med 36: 1404-7

125. Benchekroun A, Lachkar A, Soumana A, Farih MH, Belahnech Z, Marzouk M, Faik M (1998) Priapism in adults. 16 cases. Ann Urol (Paris) 32: 103-6

126. Altman AL, Seftel AD, Brown SL, Hampel N (1999) Cocaine associated priapism. J Urol 161: 1817-8

127. Wolf JS Jr, Lue TF (1992) High-flow priapism and glans hypervascularization following deep dorsal vein arterialization for vasculogenic impotence. Urol Int 49: 227-9

128. Myrick H, Markowitz JS, Henderson S (1998) Priapism following trazodone overdose with cocaine use. Ann Clin Psychiatry 10: 81-3

XIV
Developmental anomalies and hereditary diseases of vessels

Congenital vascular anomalies can be divided into three groups : those developing during intra-uterine life, those associated with karyotype aberrations, and those arising from the effects of single genes or complex polygenic mutations. There are no good data on the incidence of these lesions; a recent Finnish study on 4346 new-borns showed a 3.8% rate of vascular lesions excluding salmon patches on the head and neck, in general agreement with other studies [1]. Seventy to 80% of lesions are said to regress spontaneously by the age of seven years. In most instances of this type of lesion both blood and lymphatic vessels may be affected.

1 – Developmental vascular anomalies

Most of these, including aberrations of the usual anatomical branching and anastomosing pattern, are of surgical interest and their significance is often related to the danger which attends on their presence in an operative field. Rarely, some anomalies may be an advantage for the patient; for example, a supernumerary vascular supply may prevent infarction when the primary vessel is occluded.

Telangiectases

Naevus flammeus (Flame nevus, naevus telangiectaticus)

This term embraces both the salmon patch (starry or deep naevus, nevus simplex, stork bite, birthmark, angel's kiss) and port-wine stains (planar naevus or naevus vinosus). These lesions belong to a wide scope of congenital macular stains that represent marked capillary ectasia. Clinically, these lesions are common on the head and neck. A salmon patch is a faint intradermal lesion of a light pink to rust colour. It is ordinarily flat and blanches on pressure. A port-wine stain is much darker than a salmon patch and the overlying skin often undergoes thickening with hyperkeratosis. When present in the distribution of the trigeminal nerve, a port-wine stain may be associated with Sturge-Weber syndrome and other extensive un-

derlying vascular malformations such as Klippel-Trenaunay, Shapiro-Shulman, Bonnet-Dechaume-Blanc, Cobb, Fegeler, Robert and Parkes-Weber syndromes [2]. The vast majority of salmon patches remain stable, persisting throughout life, or ultimately regressing and need no treatment. A port-wine stain grows allometrically and has no tendency to fade. Inoperable lesions which have been irradiated may become malignant [3]; currently laser treatment is used where cosmetic improvement is necessary [4].

Pathology and differential diagnosis

The salmon patch and port-wine stain are made up of widely dilated venules of variable size in the mid and deep dermis, with a decrease in the number of perivascular nerves. These vessels may develop to resemble those in a true haemangioma. The differential diagnosis includes cutis marmorata telangiectatic congenita and senile ectasia (senile vascular naevus, cherry angioma). The abnormal venules in nevus flammeus are much more dilated than those in cutis marmorata telangiectatic congenita, which mostly affects children. In "senile" ectasia, elastic fibres are seen in the reticular dermis.

Lymphangiectasia (lymphangiectasis, lymphectasia, telangiectasia lymphatica)

Abnormal dilatation of pre-existing lymph channels is seen, giving rise to multiple cystic spaces. The change may be isolated or diffuse. The lesion may be a congenital dysplasia of the lymphatics, with hypoplasia or aplasia of the larger lymph collectors, lymph trunks and cisterna chyli, or may result from the functional consequences of these malformations or stasis [5]. Lymphangiectasia may be associated with chromosomal aberrations (Turner's, Ullrich-Turner and Noonan's syndromes [6, 7] or be part of complex syndromes, such as osseous lymphangiomatosis with osteolysis (Gordham-Stout's disease or disappearing bone disease) [8] (Fig. 1). Lymphangiectasia often presents as a diffuse swelling of part or all of an extremity with considerable deformation. It also involves viscera, including the lungs, pericardium, digestive tract, urinary tract, uterus and brain with subsequent chylothorax, chylopericardium, intestinal chylorrhoea, chyluria, chylometrorrhea and lymphostatic encephalopathy. Congenital pulmonary lymphangiec-

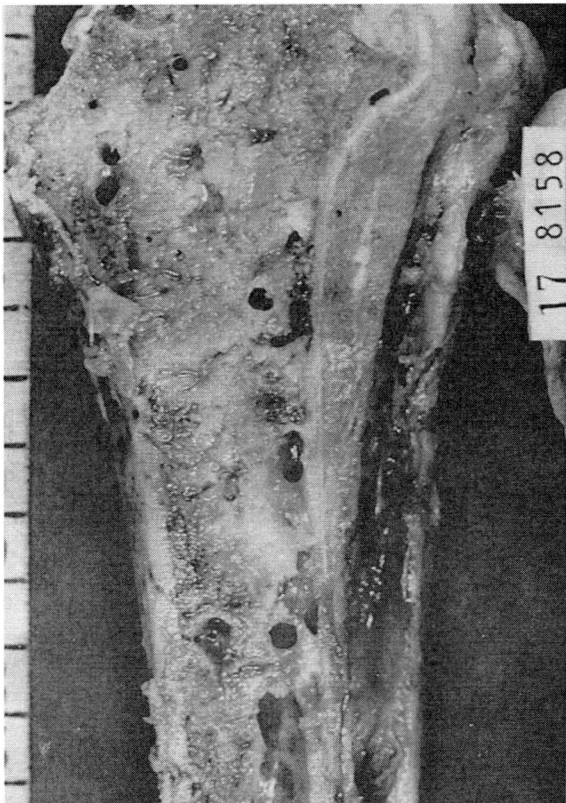

Fig. 1. Lymphangiomatosis of the tibia. Note marked osteolysis around dilated lymphatic vessels

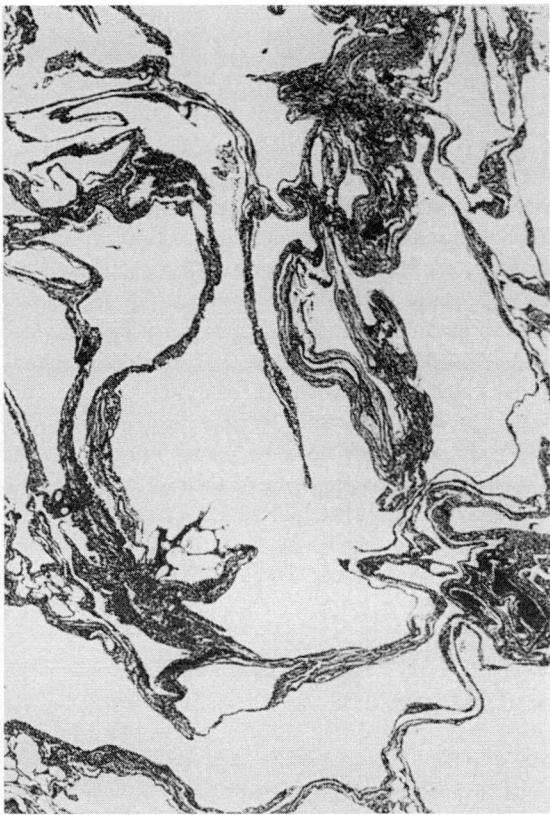

Fig. 2. Congenital pulmonary lymphangiectasia. Haematoxylin, eosin and saffron stain (HES). (Courtesy Pr P. Hofman)

tasia occurs in the newborn, presenting as severe respiratory distress. Most patients die within a few days of birth [9-12]. Primary intestinal lymphangiectasia causes a protein-losing enteropathy [13]. In the skin and mucosa, secondary lymphangiectasia causes local lymph oedema and may lead to difficult corrective cosmetic management. Chylometrorrhea may be a manifestation of chylous reflux caused by megalymphatics and lymphatic hypoplasia [14].

Pathology and differential diagnosis

The dilated lymphatic vessels are separated by strands of fibrous tissue and lined with a flattened normal endothelium. In the lungs, congenital lymphangiectasia (Fig. 2-3) may involve either a single lobe or the entire lung.

Haemangiomatous syndromes

These syndromes are rare. A characteristic feature is the extension of angiomatous lesions into multiple organ systems, often associated with non-vascular hamartomatous components and visceral abnormalities. In neurocutaneous syndromes, skin vascular lesions permit early diagnosis, which may help to prevent complications [2]. There is a well-marked tendency to infiltrative changes at the margins of the lesions, making surgical excision difficult.

Klippel-Trenaunay-Weber syndrome (Angio-osteo-hypertrophy syndrome, congenital dysplastic angiectasia, haemangiectatic hypertrophy)

Klippel-Trenaunay-Weber syndrome is characterised by a triad of capillary malformations, atypical varicosities of veins, and bony or soft tissue abnormalities usually involving one extremity with localised gigantism (Fig. 4-5) [15, 16]. The port-wine stains occur in almost all patients, and limb hypertrophy in about two-thirds. Varicosities and abnormal veins may require surgery [17]. The disease may cause heart failure in neonates due to venous shunting [18] and pul-

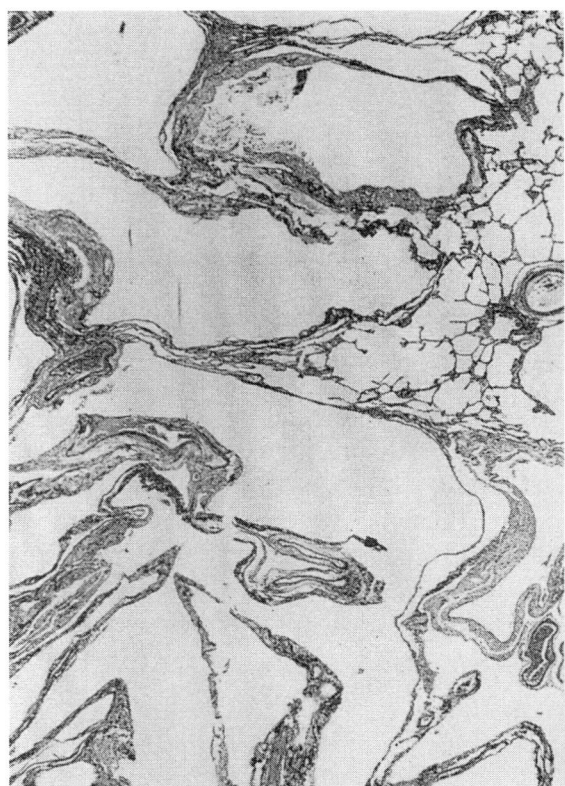

Fig. 3. Congenital pulmonary lymphangiectasia with honeycomb pattern. HES (Courtesy Pr P. Hofman)

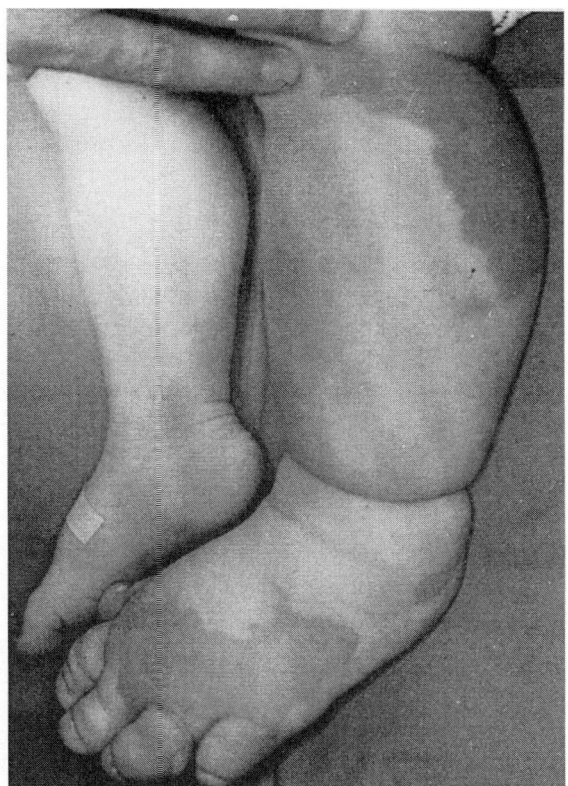

Fig. 4. Klippel-Trenaunay-Weber syndrome leading to hypertrophy of the right leg. (Courtesy Dr R. Malek)

monary involvement has been described. The Parke-Weber syndrome is a variant of angio-osteohypertrophy where the arteriovenous fistulae involve large vessels. There have been reports of autosomal dominant inheritance [19, 20] and familial cases have been described [21]. One report of a possible defect at 5q or 11p has been made on the basis of a reciprocal translocation [22]. In most instances, the lower limb is affected and the lesions may extend into the lower trunk. The skin surface reveals fine telangiectases or deeply coloured port-wine stains, which may be of metameric distribution. An arteriovenous fistula should be suspected when the skin temperature is greatly increased. The occurrence of small and raised papules oozing lymph reflects participation of lymphatic structures. A radiograph usually reveals lengthening of the underlying skeletal parts. Computed tomography and angiography help outline the extent of visceral involvement (kidneys, bladder, vagina, liver, peritoneum and pleura), which may be much greater than expected from clinical evaluation alone.

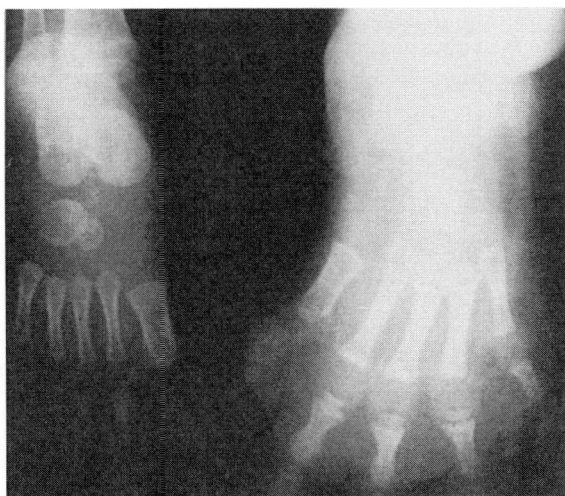

Fig. 5. Klippel-Trenaunay-Weber syndrome with asymetrical osteo-hypertrophy evidenced by X-ray (Courtesy Dr R.Malek)

Syndactyly is frequent. The lesions usually continue to enlarge allometrically and remain stable after the age of 20. Severe bleeding may occur even after minor trauma [23], and infection is common when a large lymphatic component is present. The major problem is cosmetic, except when the lesions are extensive enough to cause mechanical complications or congestive cardiac failure. Definitive surgery is rarely possible. Protection and support of the involved area are the best therapeutic measures. A limb amputation may be required to relieve any physical incapacity or congestive cardiac failure. In Parke-Weber syndrome, the major therapeutic priority is to reduce or eliminate the arteriovenous fistulas in order to prevent congestive heart failure.

Pathology and differential diagnosis

Cutaneous tissue displays a widespread increased vascularity. Numerous angiomatous thick-walled vessels of the cavernous, capillary or venous type are seen in the subcutis (Fig. 6-7). It is usually difficult or impossible to localize the arterio-venous anastomoses. Abnormalities of veins include agenesis or hypoplasia, persistence of embryonic veins, defects of venous valves, and varicosities. The Proteus syndrome [24] is a very variable syndrome of hemihypertrophy, macrodactyly and exostoses with pigmented naevi and subcutaneous tumours, which should be distinguished from true Klipple-Trenaunay-Weber.

Sturge-Weber syndrome (Sturge-Weber disease, encephalotrigeminal angiomatosis, Sturge-Kalischer-Weber syndrome, encephalo-facial angiomatosis)

This is a triad of congenital cutaneous angioma in the distribution of the trigeminal or fifth cranial nerve (usually unilateral), homolateral meningeal angioma with intracranial calcification and neurological signs and an angioma of choroid, often with secondary glaucoma. Incomplete forms of the syndrome may exhibit any two of the major features in variable degrees, occasionally with angiomas elsewhere. Sturge-Weber syndrome is considered to belong to the same group as the Klippel-Trenaunay syndrome [25]. A few familial cases, reported in the literature, favour an hereditary basis for the disease. The true prevalence is unknown but is clearly very low. The syndrome is characterised by a port-wine stain present at birth in one or more territories supplied by the divisions of the trigeminal nerves associated with ipsilateral venous angiomatous masses in the leptomeninges. The underlying cerebral cor-

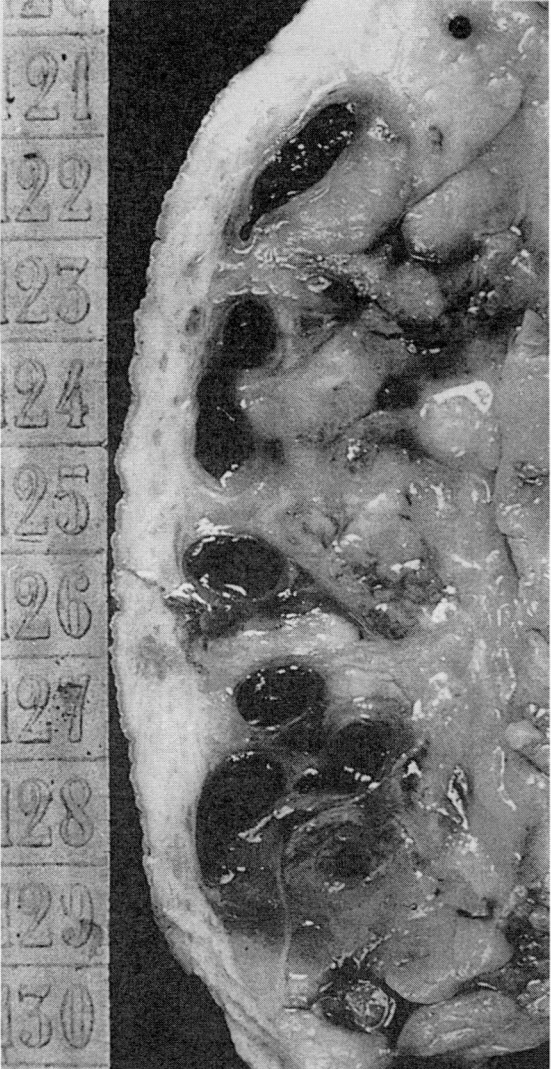

Fig. 6. Klippel-Trenaunay-Weber syndrome. Numerous angiomatous cavities distorting the subcutis

tex undergoes progressive calcification. The resulting cerebral atrophy is responsible for seizures, hemiplegia, mental retardation and radio-opacities in the skull. Haemangiomas may occur elsewhere in the skin or in the viscera [25]. Sujansky and Conradi [26] found that 45% of their 171 cases had non-trigeminal haemangiomas and 80% of cases had experienced regular seizures beginning at times between birth and 23 years. Glaucoma was common. Pheochromocytomas occur at a high frequency in these patients. The prognosis is poor [27].

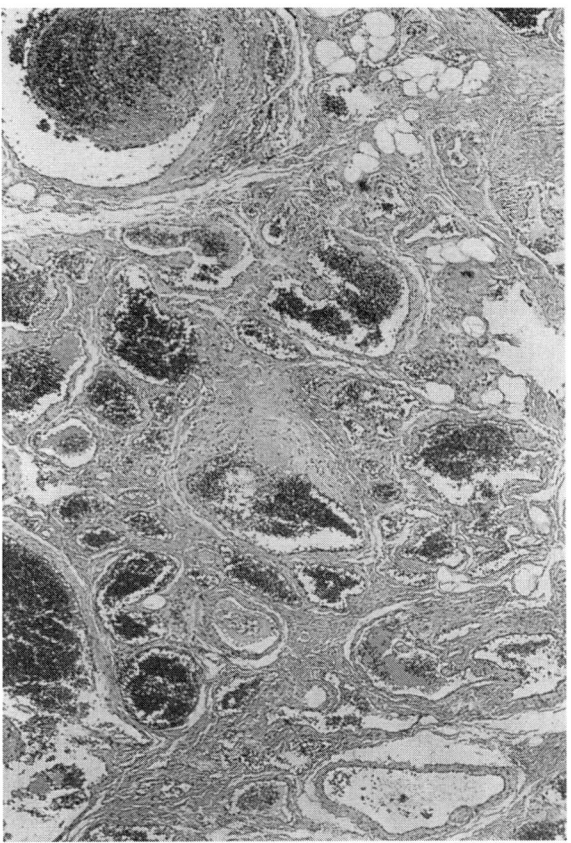

Fig. 7. Klippel-Trenaunay-Weber syndrome. Angiomatous vessels are of the cavernous, venous, capillary types. HES

Pathology and differential diagnosis

The skin lesions consist of venous haemangiomas. In the nervous system, the thickened leptomeninges harbour numerous thin-walled veins and capillaries. Haemangiomatous vessels rarely penetrate the cortex, although there is some increase in vascularity, and the affected brain undergoes atrophy. The adjacent parenchyma undergoes atrophy with reactive gliosis and patchy loss of nerve cells. Progressive calcification may appear in large vessel walls. Small cortical vessels may be occluded by thromboses. These changes explain the typical radiological findings: asymmetry of the skull, and cortical calcifications arranged in a sinuous double-contoured "tramline" or "railroad track" pattern.

Cobb's syndrome (Cutaneomeningospinal angiomatosis)

This rare syndrome is characterized by vascular cutaneous nevi distributed in dermatomes, associated with an angioma of the spinal cord and resulting neurological symptoms [28]. Association with visceral angiomatosis (broncho-pulmonary, digestive, genitourinary) and extradural lymphatic anomalies such as lymphangioma [29-31] has been reported.

Pathology and differential diagnosis

Vascular anomalies of the spinal cord consist of intramedullary, and peridural arteriovenous fistula associated with vertebral angioma. Cutaneous angiomas are either verrucous, acanthoma-like or flat.

Maffucci's syndrome (Dyschondroplasia with haemangiomas, Dyschondroplasia with vascular hamartomas)

In this syndrome there are multiple cavernous haemangiomas with enchondromatosis. About 100 cases have been reported. Haemangiomas are usually present at birth or prior to puberty, with no sex predilection. The cartilaginous tumours develop after the occurrence of vascular lesions, in the metaphyseal region of tubular bones, especially of the hands and feet. The deformities of cartilage and bone result in warping, bending and predisposition to pathological fracture. Other skeletal anomalies include fibrous dysplasia, aneurysmal bone cyst, and ossifying fibroma. Chondrosarcoma may appear in 15-20% of patients [32-34]. Malignancy arising from the vascular component, however, has only been reported in two cases [33]. Patients with Maffucci's syndrome also have a tendency to develop other types of neoplasms, including gliomas and ovarian adenocarcinomas.

Pathology and differential diagnosis

The haemangiomas are often found in the bones and the soft tissues of the limbs. They are of the cavernous type. Spindle cell haemangioendothelioma (SCH) has also been reported and Fanburg et al [35] have suggested that many of the haemangiomas reported in this syndrome may, in fact, have been SCH. Enchondromas usually measure less than 3 cm and are well circumscribed, translucent and grayish blue. Histologically, these nodules present a hyaline matrix, containing chondrocytes that reside in lacunae. As in Ollier's disease, the enchondromas in Maffucci's syndrome may demonstrate a greater degree of cellularity and cytological atypia than is typical for these lesions and can be difficult to distinguish from chondrosarcoma.

Lymphangiomatous syndromes

Benign lymphangioendothelioma (Progressive lymphangioma)

Compact, irregular groups or small masses of endothelial cells, and collections of irregular, delicate vessels resembling lymphatics form these lesions. It is not clear whether benign lymphangioendothelioma is a hamartoma or a true benign neoplasm and the prevalence is unknown. Lymphangioendotheliomata usually affect the limbs and trunk of infants and young adults. The lesion consists of well-defined, pink to reddish-brown macules or plaques, which tend to increase in size. Their average diameter is about 3 cm and they do not recur after complete excision [36, 37].

Pathology and differential diagnosis

Vascular spaces are found, distorting the upper dermis and filled with proteinaceous material without red blood cells. Endothelial cell proliferation may lead to intraluminal papillary projections or compact cellular masses. The differential diagnosis includes low-grade Stewart-Treves angiosarcoma; however, cellular atypia is absent and cutaneous angiosarcomas usually develop on the face and scalp of elderly patients. Absence of red blood cells, haemosiderin pigment deposits and a paucity of plasma cells favors the diagnosis of benign lymphangioendothelioma over Kaposi's sarcoma.

Lymphangiomatosis

This disorder is the result of a multifocal and diffuse proliferation of lymphatic vessels [34, 38]. Lymphangiomatosis affects children and young adults with a slight predominance in males (1.7: 1). The prevalence is unknown but the bone and lungs are most frequently involved. Diffuse systemic cases have been reported [39-41]. In the bone, lymphangiomatosis causes extensive decalcification with osteolysis, limb deformities and spontaneous fractures – Gorham's disease (phantom bone disease, disappearing bone disease, massive osteolysis). There are fewer than 150 reported cases in the literature [8]. Most patients are under 35, but all ages [5 to 65] may be affected. Changes are usually limited to one bone, but several bones may be affected [42-44]. Involvement of the lung results in shortness of breath, cyanosis and chylothorax [45]. The clinical course is unpredictable and spontaneous regression has been reported. Depending on the extent of the disease death may occur from 1 to 12 years after diagnosis [46]. In Gorham's disease, extension to the entire limb wi-

thout malignant transformation may occur [47]. In lymphangiomatosis of the lung the prognosis is poor when serosal surfaces are involved. Surgical excision is the only treatment. In Gorham's disease, bone grafts undergo lysis. Radiotherapy may be useful in extensive lymphangiomatosis of the lung [48]. Partial splenic embolization may help to treat associated disseminated intravascular coagulation when medical therapy fails [49].

Pathology and differential diagnosis

In skin, lymphangiomatosis produces cystic lymphatic cavities lined with flattened endothelium raising the epidermis (Fig. 8). In most cases of visceral lymphangiomatosis, the diagnosis is made at autopsy. Histologically the bone is replaced by fibrotic areas containing lymphatics. The pulmonary parenchyma is distorted by numerous anastomotic lymphatic channels of variable size. These diffusely-distributed vessels are surrounded by smooth muscle cells and bordered by a flat endothelium. The vascular lumen contains lymph and lymphocytes. Immuno-histochemically, the endothelial cells react strongly with

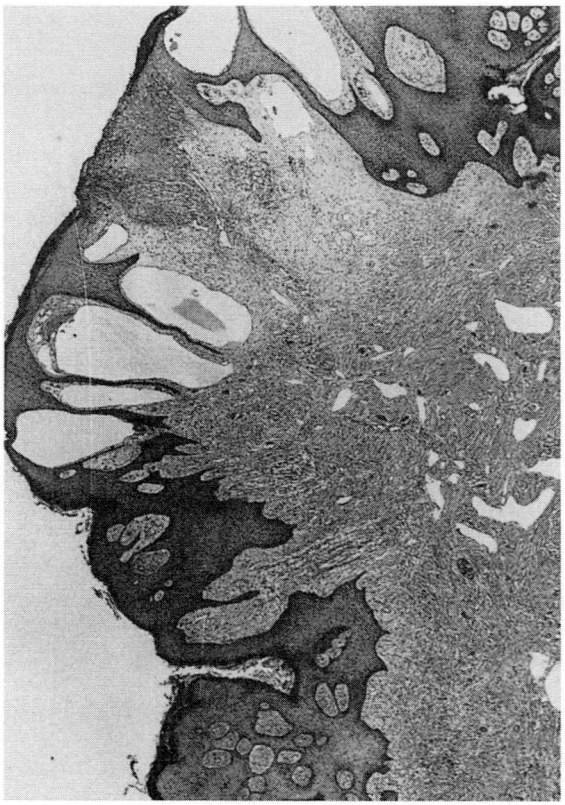

Fig. 8. Lymphangiomatosis. Skin involment. HES

FVIII-RAg and CD 31. Reactivity with CD34 and UEA-1 is unexpected, although the latter marker is considered more reliable than FVIII-RAg [50, 51]. Differential diagnoses include diffuse haemangiomatosis and other lymphatic disorders (lymphangiectasia, lymphangiomyomatosis). In the lungs, persistent interstitial emphysema in ventilated neonates produces a similar appearance of "cysts" around broncho-vascular pedicles, but often lined with multinucleated giant cells rather than endothelial cells. Pulmonary lymphangiectasia is characterized by a marked dilatation of normal lymphatics.

Lymphangioleiomyomatosis (Lymphangiopericytoma, lymphangiomyoma)

Proliferation of smooth muscle cells in the wall of lymphatic vessels gives rise to multiple parietal leiomyomatous nodules, beginning in the pelvic or retroperitoneal lymphatics with slow extension into the thoracic duct and pulmonary lymphatics [10, 41, 52-55]. The prevalence is unknown. Lymphan giomyomatosis mostly affects women in their reproductive years [56]. Clinical manifestations depend on the location of the lesion. Pulmonary involvement is manifest by progressive dyspnea and cyanosis, chylothorax, or chylopericardium. A chest roentgenogram first displays predominant fine, linear or nodular opacities in the bases. These opacities become diffuse and interspersed with bullous areas. Chylous ascites, protein losing enteropathy, intestinal bleeding, acute and chronic pericholangiolitis or chronic pancreatitis reveal intra-abdominal involvement [57-60]. Ultrasonography, computed tomography, and magnetic resonance imaging help locate these cystic tumours. Associated pathology includes trisomy 21, renal angiomyolipoma and Bourneville's tuberous sclerosis [7, 61-63]. The clinical course of pulmonary lymphangiomyomatosis consists of successive episodes leading to right heart failure from pulmonary hypertension. The prognosis depends on the extent of the lesion and survival varies from 6 months to 10 years in the context of rapidlyprogressive dyspnea [49].

Pathology and differential diagnosis

Lymphatic vessels at any site may be affected but superficial or lymph nodal involvement is rare. Lesions consist of variable-sized cysts randomly distributed in the affected tissue. Histologically, these cysts are lymphatic vessels surrounded by hyperplastic smooth muscle cells, forming leiomyomatous nodules (Fig. 9-10-11). The smooth muscle cells may have enlarged and pleomorphic nuclei, but there are no atypical mitoses. The surrounding stroma shows lymphocytic in-

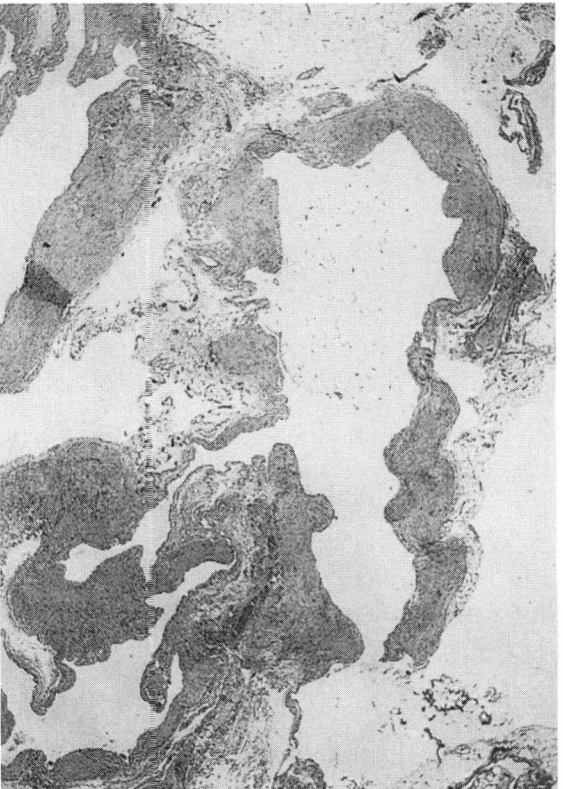

Fig. 9. Lymphangiomyomatosis. Note hyperplasia of the smooth muscle cells in the lymphatic vascular wall. HES

filtration with germinal center formation. In the lungs, concomitant hyperplasia of smooth muscle cells may be seen in the bronchiolar and venous walls. The overall appearance is one of progressive stenosis of bronchioles, bullous emphysema, pneumothorax, haemorrhage, congestive vasculopathy associated with hypertrophic cardiomyopathy and multiple venous thromboses [64]. The differential diagnosis includes lymphangiomatosis, but there is no leiomyomatous hyperplasia in the walls of vessels in this entity. In the mesentery, lymphangiomyomatosis may mimic intestinal duplication as the leiomyomatous component may simulate the muscular layer of the digestive wall. The presence of lymphocytic infiltrates and the absence of other intestinal structures (mucosa, myenteric plexuses) confirm the diagnosis. Immunohistochemically there is expression of estrogen, of progesterone receptors and of HMB-45 in the smooth muscle cells [56]. Factor VIII-related antigen and CD31 highlight the endothelial cells [50].

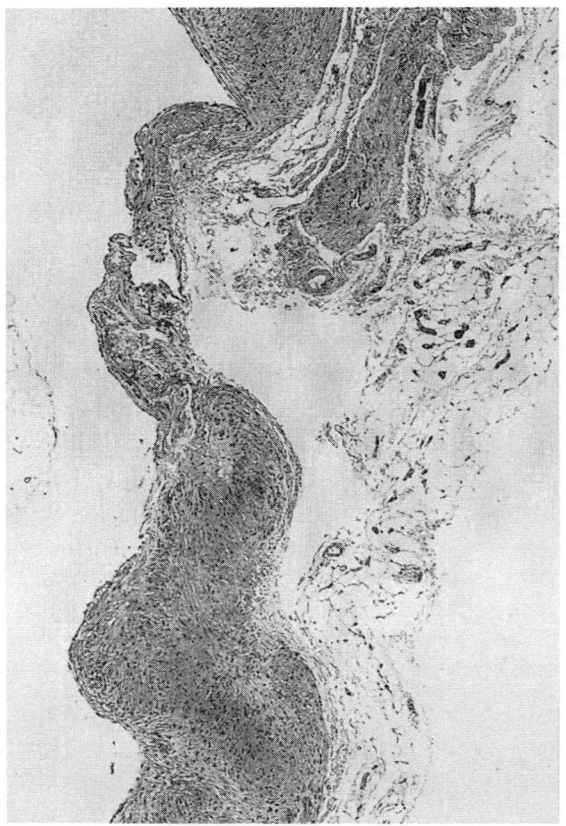

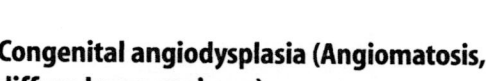

Fig. 10. Lymphangiomyomatosis. In some areas, smooth muscle cell hyperplasia leads to genuine leiomyoma thickening the vascular wall. HES

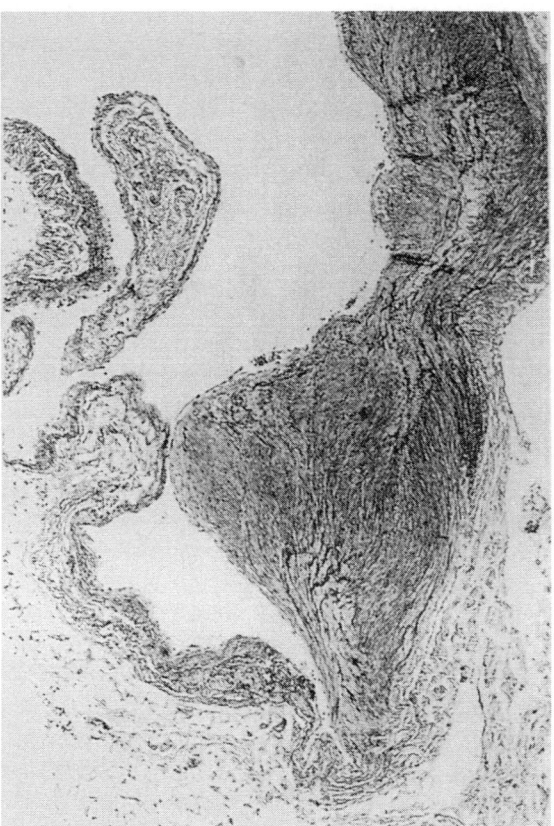

Fig. 11. Lymphangiomyomatosis. Some parietal leiomyomas protrude into the vascular lumen. Orcein elastic stain (Orcein)

Congenital angiodysplasia (Angiomatosis, diffuse haemangioma)

This is a poorly defined entity in which vascular lesions appear as large masses of dysplastic vessels of variable size and shape in any part of the body [65]. In some areas, anastomoses or fistulae produce racemose haemangiomas or cirsoid aneurysms. Recently a more extensive clinical variant has been reported, characterized by multiple angiomas developed contiguously in large segments of the body, involving multiple tissue planes, or spreading extensively in tissues of the same type [66]. The vast majority of cases occur during childhood or infancy and hypertrophy of an extremity may be noted. Persistent swelling, pain and tenderness are common symptoms. Skin involvement gives rise to proliferative plaque-like lesions [67]. Angiomatosis is rare in the viscera. Malignant transformation has not been reported. Iatrogenic embolism is one therapeutic option; however, adequate

surgical excision is the best treatment. In cases presenting in the neonatal period there is a high mortality both from the lesion and frequently from a superimposed consumption coagulopathy and the Kasabach-Merritt syndrome of disseminated intravascular coagulopathy, microangiopathic anaemia and thrombocytopaenia may develop [68].

Pathology and differential diagnosis

The lesion consists of an interwoven mixture of all kinds of vessel (Fig. 12). Some are true arteries, veins, capillaries and lymphatics, others the intermediate states between arteries and veins (Fig. 13). A glomus-like component may be present (Fig. 14). One component, frequently venous, may predominate. Capillaries often gather in bunches (Fig. 15), and may develop within a vascular wall; capillary-sized vessels may proliferate close to or within the walls of the disorganised venous segments. Angiodysplastic arteries or veins are delineated by irregularly thickened and cellular walls with variable degrees of intimal and me-

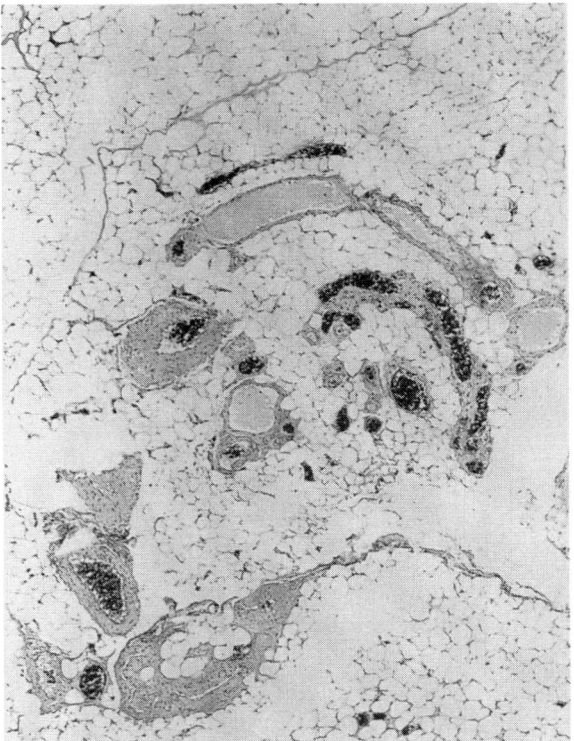

Fig. 12. Congenital angiodysplasia showing an interwoven mixture of all kinds of vessels: arteries, veins, capillaries. (Courtesy Dr S. Houissa-Vuong)

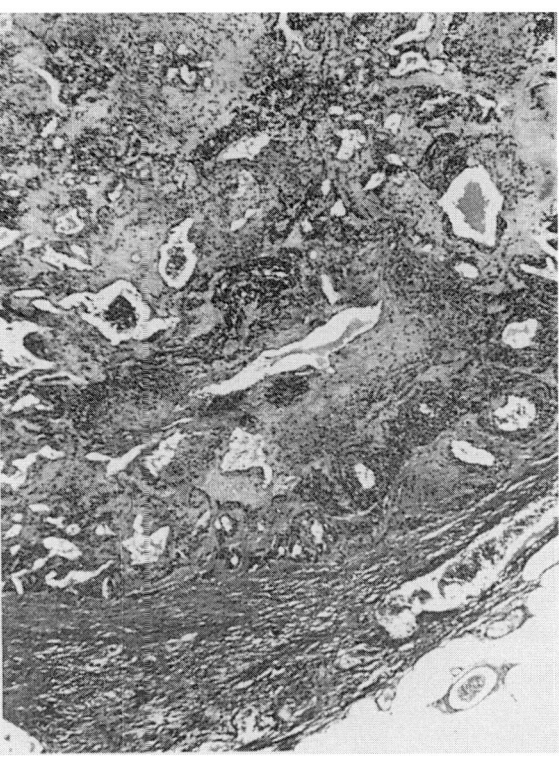

Fig. 13. Congenital angiodysplasia. Some vessels are of the intermediate states between arteries and veins. Masson's trichrome stain

dial fibrosis. The muscle within the vascular wall is less well organised than that of a normal vessel and elastic lamellae may be lacking or rudimentary. Fresh, or organised and calcified thrombi may be present (Fig. 16). The component vessels of these lesions are distinctive; unlike classical haemangiomas their walls are thick. Extravasated red blood cells, haemosiderin pigment and inflammatory infiltrates are present in the mass and thus this variant may mimic Kaposiform infantile haemangioendothelioma [67, 69, 70].

Major developmental anomalies of great vessels

These anomalies are frequently associated with heart defects.

Patent Ductus Arteriosus

The ductus arteriosus may be persistently patent in the premature infant and in infants with hypoxaemia or respiratory distress syndrome. As an abnormality it is common in Down's syndrome, and as a consequence of rubella. Females are affected more than males (4:1). Ten to fifteen percent of PDAs are associated with ventricular septal defect (VSD), pulmonary or aortic valvular stenosis or atresia and aortic coarctation. Aneurysm dilatation is rare [71].

Pathology and differential diagnosis

The length of the ductus arteriosus varies widely from 0.4cm to 1cm, and the diameter may vary from a few millimetres to 1 cm. On opening, the intimal surface presents a corrugated appearance. Histologically, the ductus arteriosus has a pattern resembling a musculoelastic artery. The relatively thick intima is underlined by a partly disrupted internal elastic lamina. The media, made up of bundles of smooth muscle cells (SMCs) is distorted by clear spaces containing a metachromatic ground substance interspersed with scattered elastic fibers. Pathologists should be aware that prostaglandin E1 (PGE1) administration has a profound weakening effect on the structure of the wall of

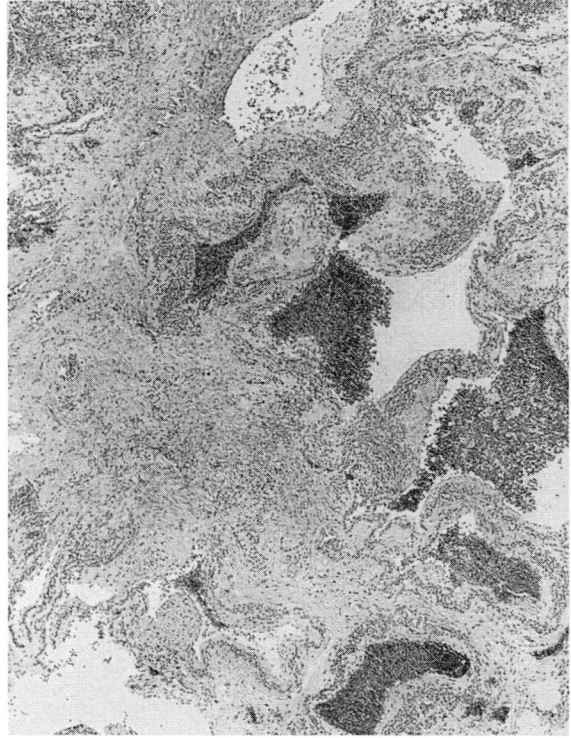

Fig. 14. Congenital angiodysplasia. Note an associated glomic component. HES

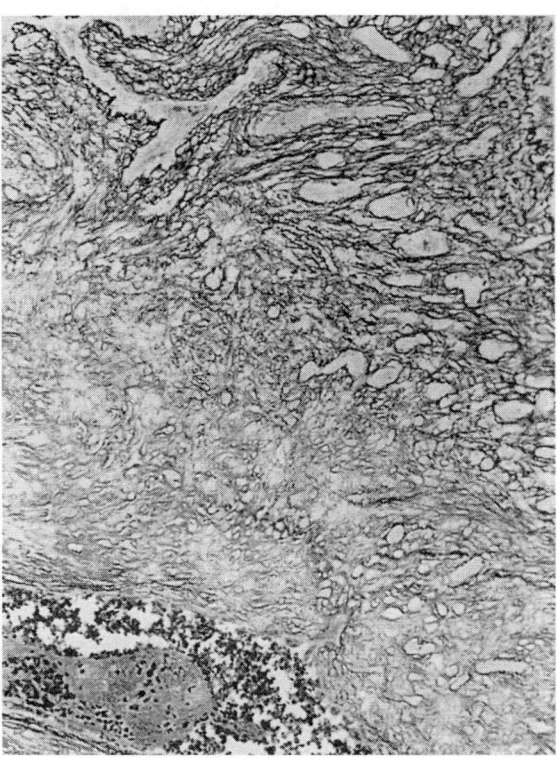

Fig. 15. Congenital angiodysplasia. Bunches of blood capillaries inside an angiodysplastic vessel. Orcein

the ductus arteriosus, rendering the vessel prone to laceration. The changes consist of oedema of the media with separation of medial components by clear spaces, pathological interruptions of the internal elastic lamina, and intimal lacerations, some of which extend into the media. In congenital rubella, the ductus is very immature with extensive subendothelial elastic lamina [72-74].

Pulmonary-aortic window

This results from failure of complete separation of the common truncus leading to a persistent communication between the ascending aorta and the pulmonary artery above the aortic and pulmonary valve level. The anomaly may be associated with a ventricular septal defect.

Aortic coarctation

A focal constriction or stricture or narrowing of the aorta at or near the site of the insertion of the ductus occurs in the classical form.

Coarctation of the thoracic aorta

Coarctation may be proximal or distal to the ductus arteriosus or its remains, the ligamentum arteriosum. The anomaly is usually classified as pre-ductal (infantile) and post-ductal (adult type) (Fig. 17). The prevalence is 1 in 2,000 births. There is a male predilection (1.9M/1F), although females with Turner's syndrome frequently have coarctation. The age at presentation varies enormously (1 month to 63 years) [75] and is mainly determined by the associated defects. The clinical features depend almost entirely on the severity of the narrowing and the patency of the ductus arteriosus.

The preductal "infantile" type (20.7% of the total in one series) [75] presents by 2 to 3 weeks after birth with caudal cyanosis. The post-ductal type more frequently affects older children and adults [76]. The preductal type is more often associated with other cardiovascular anomalies including Marfan's syndrome, hypoplastic left heart syndrome, atrial and ventricular septal defects and a bicuspid aortic valve [77-79]. Congenital intracranial aneurysms, usually involving the circle of Willis, and facial cavernous haemangioma are well established associations [80].

In the preductal type, blood flows from a patent ductus into the distal aorta. When the coarctation is juxtaductal or postductal, blood flows to the lower extremities by way of the subclavian arteries and collaterals. The raised intravascular pressure in the upper part of the body may induce pulmonary hypertension and hyperplasia of sustentacular (type II) cells of the carotid bodies [81, 82, 83]. A case of necrotizing enterocolitis caused by spontaneous closure of the ductus arteriosus in the 1st week of life, has been reported in a term infant [84]. Untreated, 60-70% of patients with coarctation of the aorta die before the age of 40 years from congestive heart failure, thrombosis [85], intracranial haemorrhage caused by rupture of aneurysms [86], infective aortitis at the point of narrowing, and rupture or dissection of the precoarcted aorta related to hypertension and degenerative structural changes in the aortic wall [87, 88].

Pathology and differential diagnosis

Encroachment on the aortic lumen is of variable severity, sometimes leaving only a small channel or, at other times, producing only minimal narrowing. The coarcted segment is a shelf-like obstruction in the lumen (Fig. 18). Rarely, it consists of a diaphragm with a central pinpoint lumen measuring less than 1mm in diameter. The diameter of the upstream aorta tapers progressively as the coarctation is approached. In the part of the aorta lying distal to the coarctation, the intima presents a localised corrugated jet-lesion and post-stenotic dilatation may be seen. Histologically, the ridge consists mainly of thickening plus some infolding of the aortic wall that protrudes into the lumen, making it narrow and eccentric (Fig. 19-20). Ductal tissue forms the inner part of the ridge for more than half of its total circumference. Secondary fibroblastic proliferation of the intima may develop and accentuates the stenosis (Fig. 21). In longitudinal sections, the coarcted segment has a triangular shape, its base being attached to the thickened media and its apex directed toward the opposite wall. In the downstream aorta, the jet-lesion is characterised by localised fibrous intimal thickening [89, 90].

Primary aortic coarctation at unusual sites

Unusual sites include the ascending aorta, the aortic arch between the innominate artery (truncus brachiocephalicus), the left common carotid artery, and the left subclavian artery, and the lower part of the thora-

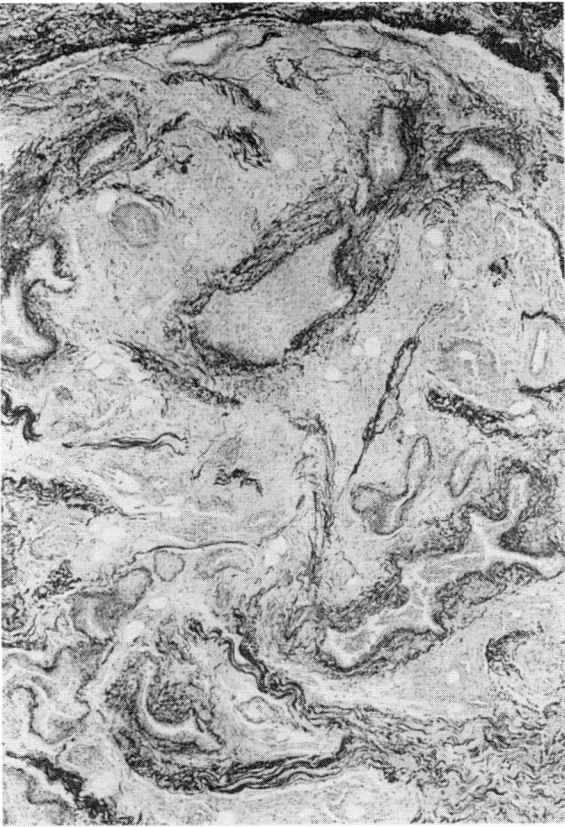

Fig. 16. Congenital angiodysplasia. Some dysplastic vessels are occluded by fresh and old thrombi. Orcein

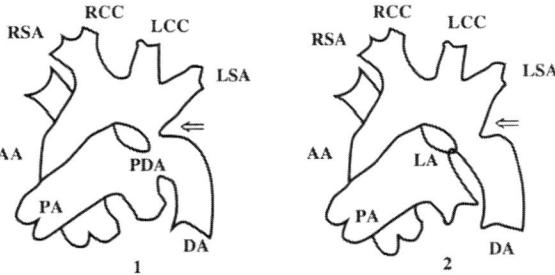

Fig. 17. Pre-ductal (1) and post-ductal (2) types of aortic coarctation. (AA: ascending aorta; CA: carotid artery; DA: descending aorta; LA: ligamentum arteriosum; LCC: left common carotid artery; LSA: left subclavian artery; PA: pulmonary artery; PDA: patent ductus arteriosus; RCC: right common carotid artery; RSA: right subclavian artery; => coarctation)

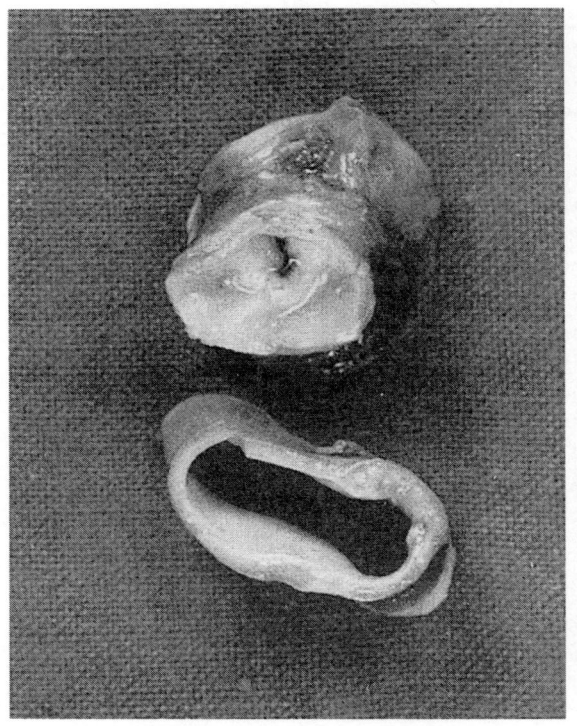

Fig. 18. Aortic coarctation. Shelf-like coarctation of the aortic arch centered by a slit-like lumen. Note post-stenotic dilatation in the distal portion

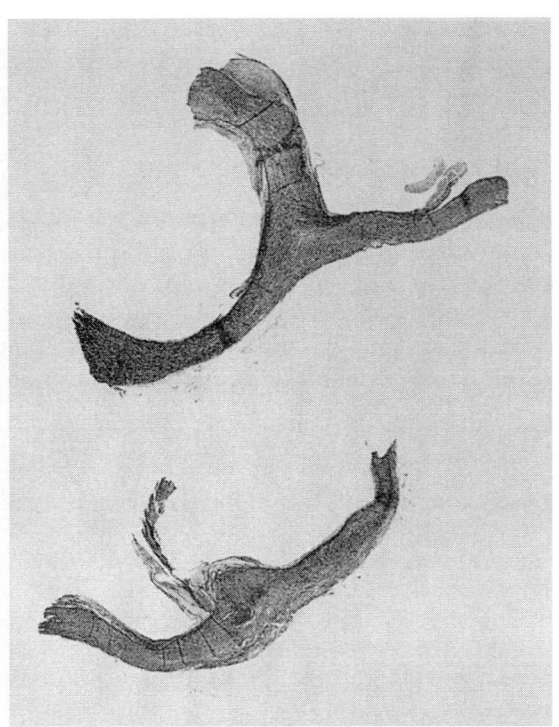

Fig. 19. Aortic coarctation. Coarctation ridge. Orcein

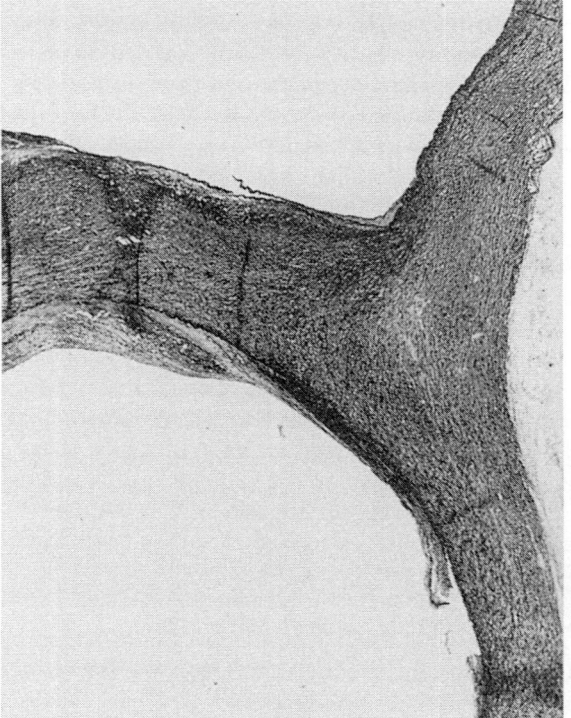

Fig. 20. Aortic coarctation. Infolding of the aortic wall. Orcein

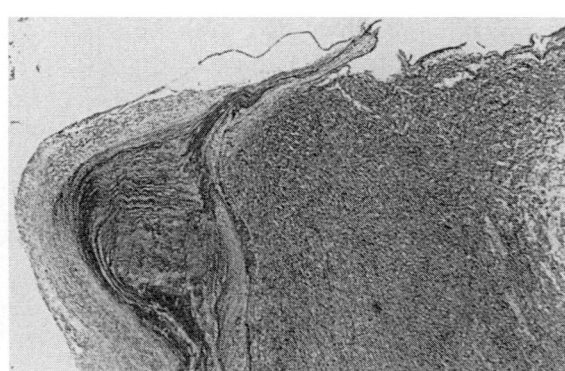

Fig. 21. Intimal fibroblastic thickening. Orcein

cic aorta or the abdominal aorta (Fig. 22). Association of suprarenal coarctation of the abdominal aorta with other anomalies (Williams syndrome, bilateral renal artery stenoses and poststenotic aneurysm) has been reported [91, 92]. Renovascular hypertension occurs when the suprarenal and/or inter-renal segment is involved.

Pathology and differential diagnosis

When the constricted area measures more than 1 cm in length, the anomaly is probably better described as tubular hypoplasia rather than coarctation. The histological pattern appears similar to that observed in classical coarctation.

Interrupted aortic arch (atresia of aortic arch)

This anomaly is characterised by a congenital absence of the aortic arch. There are three types [93], classified by the origin of major collaterals of the proximal aorta (Fig. 23). Clinically, the condition resembles preductal coarctation. The descending thoracic aorta is fed through the ductus arteriosus. Its prevalence, associated anomalies, clinical course and treatment are summarised in table 1.

Pathology and differential diagnosis

The aortic arch is reduced to a fibrotic strand connecting the proximal and distal segments of the aorta.

Anomalous innominate artery or truncus brachiocephalicus

The right innominate artery in a patient with a left aortic arch arises more distally than usual – typically to the left of the trachea. As the vessel courses to the right, it may produce an anterior tracheal indentation and occasionally these patients may be symptomatic. This anomaly is noted somewhat more frequently in children with underlying congenital heart disease. Treatment consists of surgical reposition of the vessel for symptomatic patients.

Vascular rings

Anomalies of the origin or position of the aortic arch or its branches may give rise to vascular rings that encircle the trachea and/or oesophagus, and at times produce pressure symptoms. An anomalous aberrant right subclavian artery originating from the descending aortic arch may cause symptoms in childhood. A double aortic arch becomes symptomatic in the first 6 months of life, a right aortic arch and left ligamentum

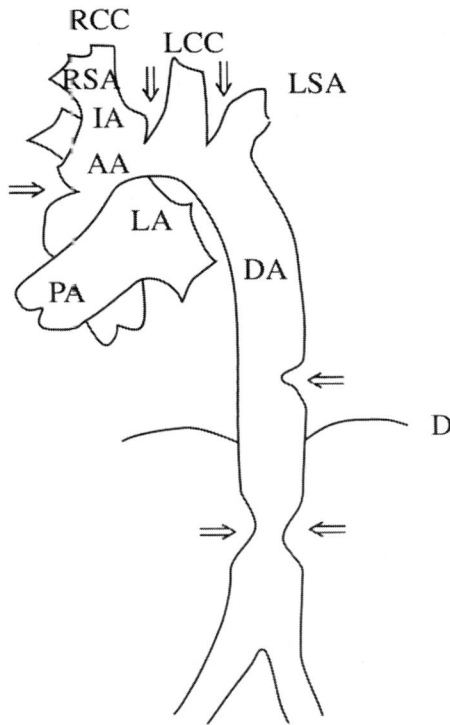

Fig. 22. Primary aortic coarctation at unusual sites (AA: ascending aorta; D: diaphragm; DA: descending aorta; IA: innominate artery or truncus brachiocephalicus; LCC: left common carotid artery; LA: Ligamentum arteriosum; LSA: left subclavian artery; PA: pulmonary artery; RCC: right common carotid artery; RSA: right subclavian artery, =>: aortic coarctation)

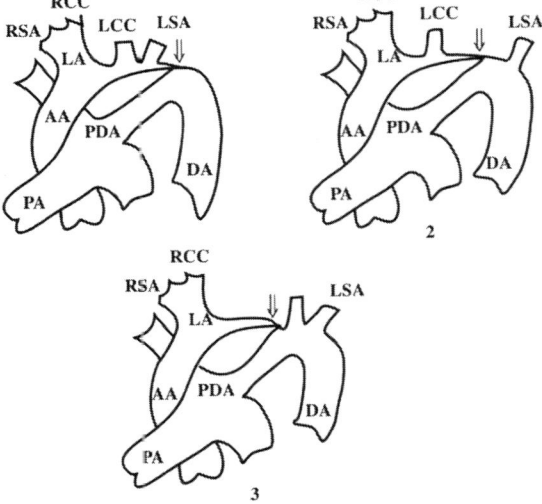

Fig. 23. Types (1, 2, 3) of interrupted aortic arch (AA: ascending aorta; DA: descending aorta; IA: innominate artery or truncus brachiocephalicus; LCC: left common carotid artery; LSA: left subclavian artery; PA: pulmonary artery; PDA: patent ductus arteriosus; RCC: right common carotid artery; RSA: right subclavian artery; =>: Interrupted area)

Table 1. Types of infantile interrupted aortic arch

TYPES	1	2	3
Frequency	Common	Common	Rare
Interruption	Distal to the left subclavian artery	Between the left subclavian and the left carotid artery.	Distal to the innominate artery
Continuation	The descending aorta is a continuation of the ductus	The left subclavian originates from the descending aorta.	Both the left carotid artery and left sub-clavian artery are connected to the descending aorta.
Associated disorders	Ventricular and atrial septal defect; bicuspid aortic valve; muscular subaortic stenosis; ductus arteriosus; anomalous origin of brachiocephalic vessels (95%).	Congenital absence of the thymus and parathyroid glands, without agammaglobulinaemia but with selective T-cell deficiency, frequent infections and delayed development, tetany (DiGeorge syndrome in 10% of cases)	Ventricular and atrial septal defect; bicuspid aortic valve; muscular subaortic stenosis; ductus arteriosus; anomalous origin of brachio-cephalic vessels (95%).
Treatment	Prosthetic bypass	Prosthetic bypass	Prosthetic bypass

(or ductus) arteriosum usually causes symptoms after 1 year of age. Oesophageal compression may produce a cough when eating and difficulty in swallowing. Tracheal compression may result in stridor and recurrent respiratory infections. Angiography is necessary for diagnosis and surgical treatment is indicated when oesophageal or tracheal compression is apparent.

Pathology and differential diagnosis

There are three types of vascular rings (Table 2, Fig. 24): aberrant right subclavian artery, double aortic arch, right aortic arch and left ligamentum (or ductus) arteriosum. None of these interferes with cardiac function. The histological pattern of the vessels in the vascular rings is unremarkable.

Anomalies of the pulmonary artery

These include aberrant origins of the pulmonary artery from the descending aorta, the ductus arteriosus and vascular sling.

Pulmonary artery arising from ascending aorta

A pulmonary artery arising from the ascending aorta is generally large. There are two types; the anterior involves the left pulmonary artery, and the posterior the right (Fig. 25). The diagnosis can be established by angiocardiography.

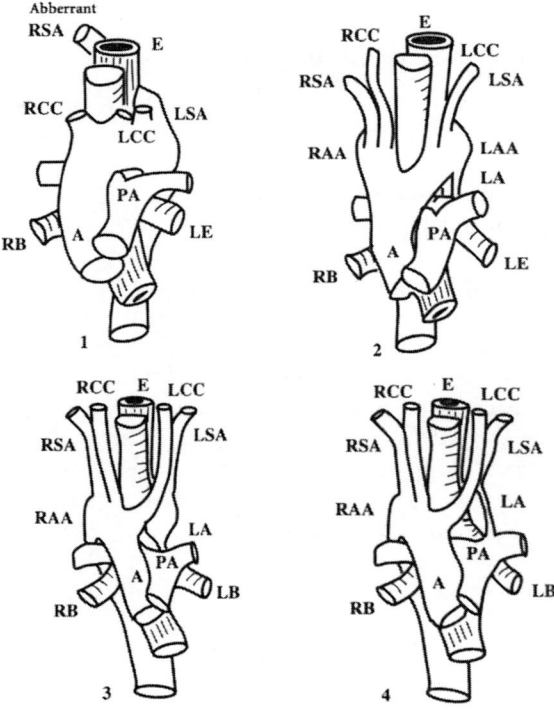

Fig. 24. Types of vascular rings (AA: ascending aorta; E: oesophagus; LA: Ligamentum arteriosum; LAA: left aortic arch; LB: left bronchus; LCC: left common carotid artery; LSA: left subclavian artery; PA: pulmonary artery; RAA: right aortic arch; RCC: right common carotid artery; RSA: right subclavian artery; RB: right bronchus; T: trachea)

Table 2. Types of vascular rings.

TYPES OF VASCULAR RINGS	ABERRANT RIGHT SUBCLAVIAN ARTERY	DOUBLE AORTIC ARCH	RIGHT AORTIC ARCH AND LEFT-SIDE CONTRO-LATERAL DUCTUS ARTERIOSUS
Description	The anomalous artery originates from the descending aortic arch, and encircles the trachea and oesophagus.	The right-side arch is usually dominant, and, at times, the left arch is atretic. Rarely is the ductus arteriosusbilateral. Left and right common carotid and subclavian arteries arise from their corresponding arches	The ductus arteriosus originates posteriorly from the descending aorta. A ring is formed by the right arch, left ductus arteriosus and pulmonary artery. Conversely, when the ductus arteriosus originates from the bifurcation of the left brachiocephalic trunk or innominate artery, no ring is formed.

Pulmonary artery arising from ductus arteriosus

The artery arises from the ductus arteriosus originating from the aortic arch if the arch is on the same side (left aortic arch) or from the innominate artery if the aortic arch is on the opposite side (right aortic arch) (Fig. 26). There is a tendency for the ductus arteriosus to close and a large left-to-right shunt is not usually present. In many cases, the ductus arteriosus is completely obliterated and the involved lung is then supplied by collaterals of the bronchial artery.

Pulmonary vascular sling

This malformation is characterized by an anomalous left pulmonary artery arising from the posterior aspect of the right pulmonary artery. The overall appearance resembles a sling at the level of the right main

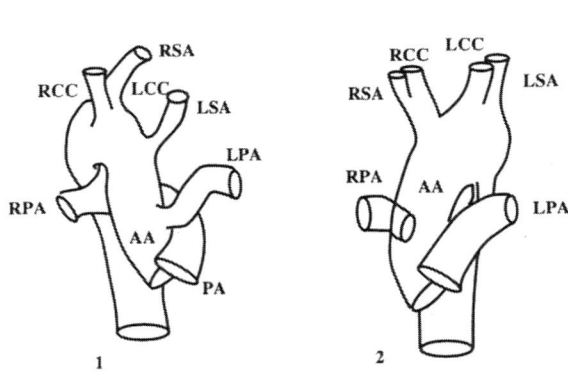

Fig. 25. Pulmonary artery arising from ascending aorta (1: anterior type; 2: posterior type; AA: ascending aorta; LCC: left common carotid artery; LPA: left pulmonary artery; LSA: left subclavian artery; PA: pulmonary artery; RCC: right common carotid artery; RPA: right pulmonary artery; RSA: right subclavian artery)

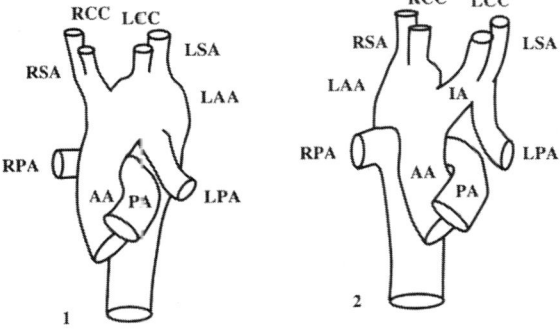

Fig. 26. Pulmonary artery arising from ductus arteriosus (AA: ascending aorta; IA: inominate artery; LAA: left aortic arch; LCC: left common carotid artery; LPA: left pulmonary artery; LSA: left subclavian artery; PA: pulmonary artery; RAA: right aortic arch RCC: right common carotid artery; RPA: right pulmonary artery; RSA: right subclavian artery; 1: type 1. Left pulmonary artery from L ductus arteriosus originating from the left aortic arch; 2: type 2. left pulmonary artery from innominate artery with right aortic arch.)

bronchus and carina (Fig. 27). The aberrant left pulmonary artery runs between the trachea and the oesophagus to the left lung. Other associated cardiovascular and tracheo-bronchial anomalies, such as a complete tracheal ring, and a right upper bronchus arising independently from the trachea, have been reported. Clinically, severe respiratory difficulty is manifest at a very early age with stridor, emphysema, atelectasis, and pneumonitis of the right upper lobe or even of the entire right lung.

Anomalies of great systemic veins

These are uncommon. They rarely cause functional changes and are usually discovered by chance at postmortem examination or in the course of cardiovascular check-up or surgical procedures. They may be isolated or associated with other cardiovascular anomalies.

Left superior vena cava (Left SVC)

A persistent left superior vena cava is the most clinically significant venous anomaly. The left jugular and left subclavian vein join to form the left superior vena cava, which descends into the chest parallel to the right superior vena cava, anterior to the left lung hilus and always enters a markedly dilated coronary sinus. The accessory hemiazygos vein may resemble the normal right-side azygos vein. The right superior vena cava is usually present. A bridging vein often connects the two cavae across the anterior mediastinum. Patients with this anomaly present moderate central cyanosis. There is no murmur and left ventricular hypertrophy may be present.

Azygos drainage of the inferior vena cava

Normally, the azygos vein arises from the right ascending lumbar vein or the inferior vena cava, ascends through the aortic orifice of the diaphragm, lies in the posterior mediastinum, and terminates in the superior vena cava (Fig. 28/1). Azygos drainage of the inferior vena cava occurs when the hepatic segment of the inferior vena cava is absent. The prehepatic portion of the inferior vena cava drains into the right atrium by means of an enlarged azygos vein. The hepatic veins empty into the right atrium by way of a short common trunk that forms the most proximal part of the inferior vena cava. This condition is rarely isolated; other cardiac anomalies may be present, such as the asplenia or polysplenia syndromes.

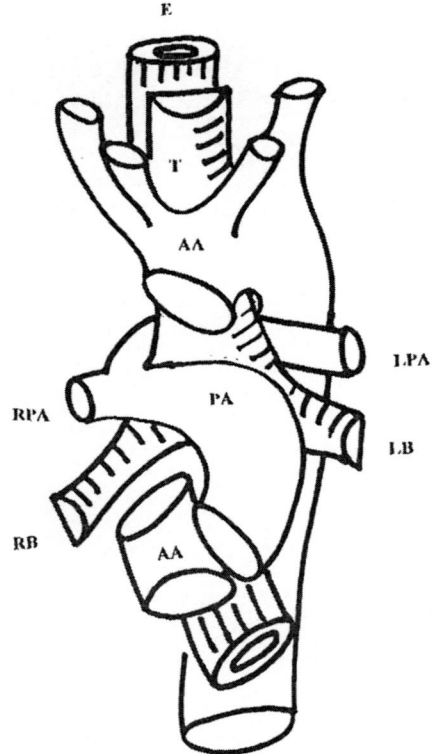

Fig. 27. Pulmonary vascular sling (AA: ascending aorta; E: oesophagus; LB: left bronchus; LPA: left pulmonary artery; PA: pulmonary artery; RB: right bronchus; RPA: right pulmonary artery; T: trachea)

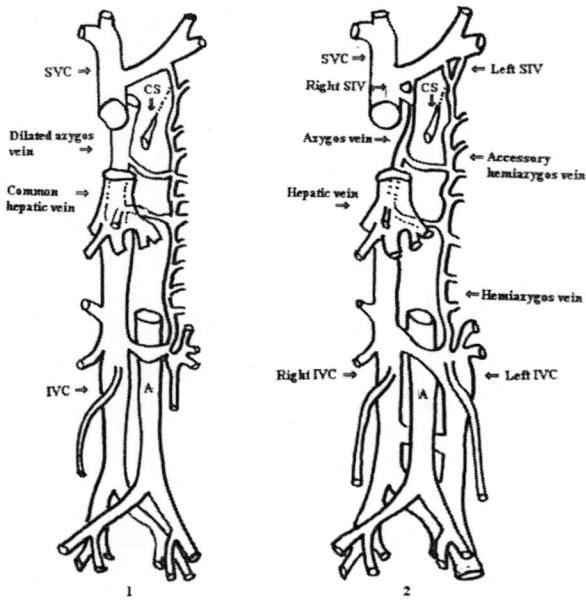

Fig. 28. Azygos drainage of the inferior vena cava (1) and double inferior vena cava (2) (A: abdominal aorta; CS: coronary sinus; IVC: inferior vena cava; SVC: superior vena cava; SIV: superior intercostal vein)

Double inferior vena cava

Patients with cardiac anomalies associated with the various types of situs inversus may have this anomaly, which causes difficulty at surgery (Fig. 28/2). Its presence should be established by angiocardiography during diagnostic work-up.

2 – Pathological entities

Vascular anomalies associated with cytogenetic disorders

Autosomal disorders

Vascular anomalies are frequently associated with cardiac abnormalities, including patent ductus arteriosus, ventricular septal defect, atrio-ventricular canal, transposition of the great vessels, and endocardial cushion defects. In trisomy 21 (Down's syndrome), 18 (Edward's syndrome), 13 (Patau's syndrome), or deletion of the short arm of chromosome 5 (5p-) (cri-du-chat, Lejeune syndrome) vascular anomalies are common.

Cri-du-chat syndrome (Lejeune syndrome)

There is deletion of the short arm of chromosome 5 (5p-). Characteristic features consist of microcephaly, round facies with antimongoloid palpebral fissures, epicanthal folds, micrognathia, strabismus, mental and physical retardation, and a characteristic high-pitched catlike whine. In general, these children thrive better than those with the trisomies, and some survive into adult life. As the infant grows older, the kitten cry and high vocal register improve, rendering clinical diagnosis more difficult. Cardiovascular anomalies consist of patent ductus arteriosus and ventricular septal defect (50%). The prevalence is about 1/50,000 births, with a female preponderance.

Patau's syndrome (13 trisomy, D1 trisomy, D trisomy, 13-15 trisomy)

This is a variable syndrome of malformation in infants with 47 chromosomes, the extra chromosome being of group D, no. 13. Most cases result from meiotic non-disjunction. Severe and wide-ranging malformations consist of microcephaly, arhinencephaly with mental and motor retardation, cyclops, anophthalmia, microphthalmia or coloboma; low-set ear; polydactyly with dermatoglyphic anomalies, single palmar flexion crease; polycystic kidneys and hydronephrosis, cryptorchism, bicornuate uterus, umbilical hernia, and malrotation of intestines. Cardiovascular anomalies include patent ductus arteriosus and ventricular septal defect. Rarely do these infants survive beyond the first year of life; most die within a few weeks to months. The prevalence is about 1/7000. There is no sex predominance.

Edwards' syndrome (18 trisomy, E trisomy, 17 trisomy, 16-18 trisomy)

Most cases result from meiotic non-disjunction and therefore carry a complete extra copy of a chromosome of group E, no. 18. This variable syndrome of malformations includes mental retardation, abnormal skull shape, prominent occiput, epicanthic folds, low-set and malformed ears, micrognathia, narrow palate, Meckel's diverticulum, inguinal hernia, small pelvis, renal anomalies, cryptorchism, abnormal flexion of fingers, and dermatoglyphic anomalies. The major vascular malformation is patent ductus arteriosus associated with ventricular septal defect in almost all patients (99%). These infants rarely survive beyond the first year of life.

Down's syndrome (trisomy 21 syndrome)

This well known syndrome is one of mental retardation associated with a variable constellation of malformations. The region of chromosome 21 that is required for the expression of the facial, neurologial, and cardiovascular changes is limited to the 21q 22.2 and 21q 22.3 region [94]. The prevalence is about 1/800 newborns [95]. There is a strong influence of maternal age on the incidence of Down's syndrome with an incidence of 1 in 1550 live births in women under 20 years rising to 1 in 25 live births for mothers over 45. Forty percent of patients present defects of the endocardial cushions with ostium primum, atrial septal defect, atrioventricular valve malformations and prolapse, but classical ventricular septal defects, transposition of the great vessels and patent ductus arteriosus are also common [96]. Rarely trisomy 21 gives rise to a Noonan syndrome phenotype with nuchal and thoracic lymphangiomatosis, oedema of the dorsum of hands and feet, and bicuspid pulmonary valve [7]. Most deaths in infancy and early childhood are caused by cardiac anomalies.

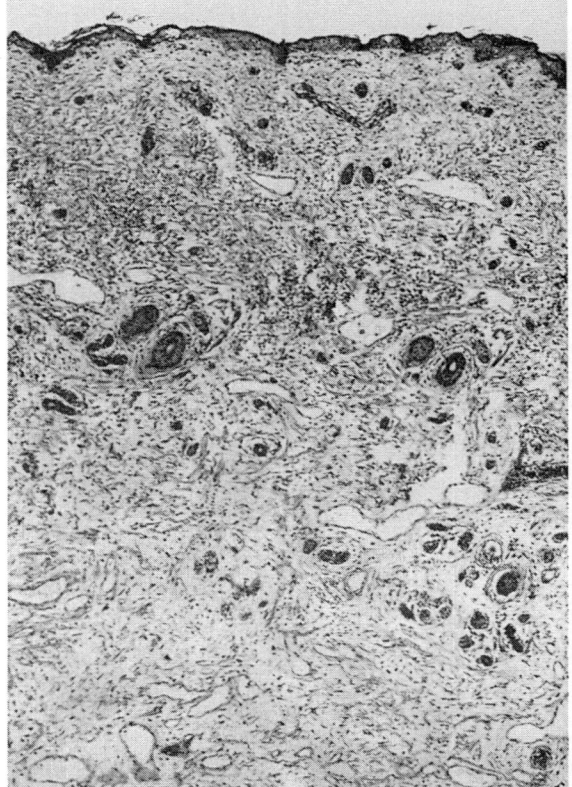 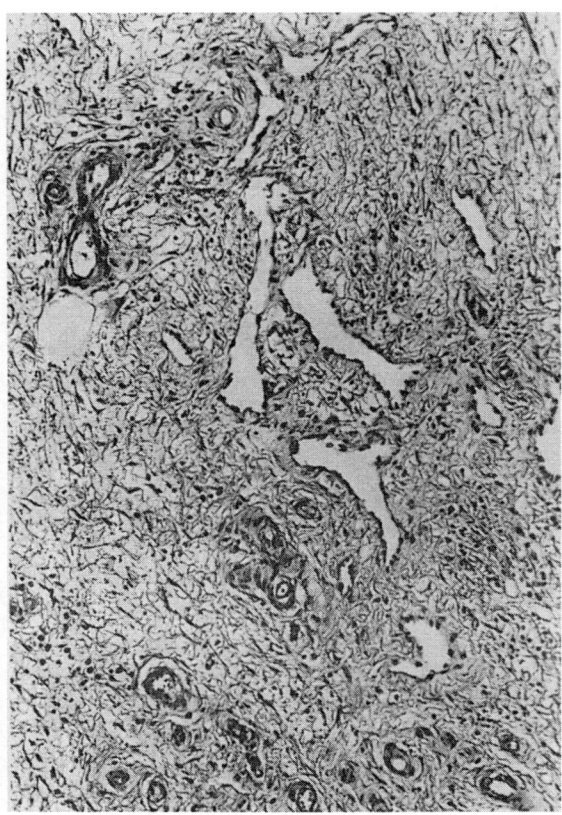

Fig. 29. Turner syndrome.Cystic hygroma of the neck. HES

Fig. 30. Turner syndrome. Cystic hygroma of the neck. Markedly dilated lymphatic vessels. HES

Sex chromosome disorders

Turner's syndrome (XO)

The prevalence of this syndrome is around 1/5,000 births but many affected embryos are known to be eliminated spontaneously. Echocardiographic fetal studies find the commonest cardiovascular abnormalities to be hypoplastic aortic arch in combination with hypoplastic left ventricle and outflow tract [97]. Between 50 and 60% of living patients with Turner's syndrome have a vascular system abnormality which may be a patent ductus arteriosus, coarctation, anomalous pulmonary venous connections, lympho-oedema of the extremities or cystic lymphangioma (Fig. 29-30-31) [98, 99]. Associated cardiac anomalies include pulmonary stenosis, and aortic and pulmonary valve dysplasia [100, 101].

Penta X syndrome

These patients are severely retarded and have mongoloid facies, prominent epicanthic folds, hypertelorism, colobomata and simian palmar lines. Patent ductus arteriosus is the major vascular anomaly [102-104].

XXXXY syndrome

Common vascular anomalies include patent ductus arteriosus, abnormal pulmonary venous connections, aortic coarctation and cystic lymphangioma [102, 105, 106].

Fragile X syndrome (Martin-Bell syndrome)

This relatively common syndrome is characterized by an inheritable, unstable DNA in a portion of the X chromosome with methylation of the cytosine bases and inactivation of the FMR-1 gene, the fragile site

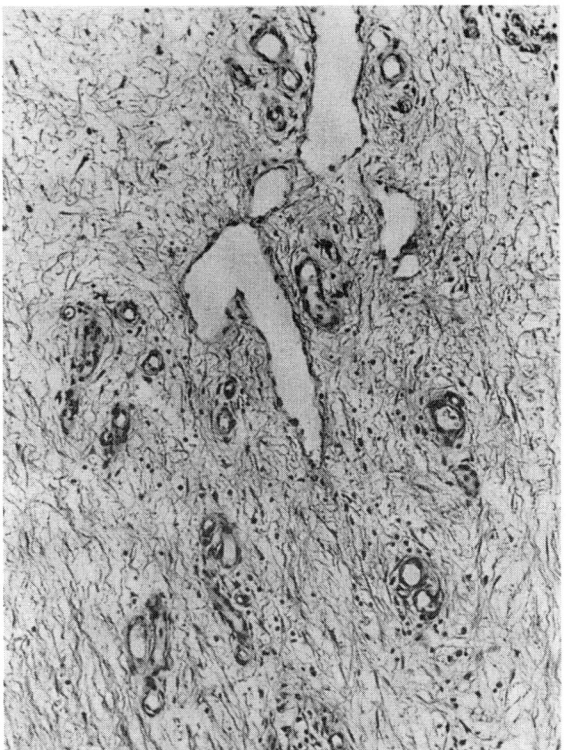

Fig. 31. Turner syndrome. Cystic hygroma of the neck. Note lymphocyte infiltrates around dilated lymphatic vessels. HES

being located on the long arm of the X chromosome. The fragile X chromosome may affect both sexes. Clinical manifestations encompass mental retardation [107], long face with prognathism, and prominent ears, and macro-orchidism in males. Impaired left ventricular filling, mitral valve prolapse, dilatation of the aortic root [108-112], diffuse tubular hypoplasia and mild coarctation of the aorta [113] have been reported. Histologically, marked alterations in elastin structure and distribution are seen in the base of the mitral and tricuspid valves.

Vascular anomalies associated with single-gene mutations

X-linked anomalies

Fabry's disease (Anderson-Fabry's disease, Angiokeratoma corporis diffusum, Glycolipid lipidosis)

This X-linked recessive disorder is caused by deficiency of alpha-galactosidase A, an enzyme that breaks down ceramide trihexose. Mutations are found in the alpha-galactosidase gene at Xq22.1 [114]. There is an accumulation of neutral glycolipids in histiocytes in the blood vessel walls, lymphatics, heart, lungs, renal glomeruli, peripheral nerves, skin, smooth muscle, and small intestine [115, 116]. Clinical features include angiokeratomas on the thighs, buttocks, and genitalia, hypohidrosis, paresthesia in extremities, cornea verticillata, and spoke-like posterior subcapsular cataracts. Death results from renal, cardiac, or cerebrovascular complications. Cardiomyopathy has been reported in carriers [117].

Hunter's syndrome

Mucopolysaccharidosis type I is a lysosomal storage disease caused by iduronate-2-sulphatase deficiency [118]. Acid mucopolysaccharides (heparan and dermatan sulfates) accumulate in the central nervous system and peripheral tissues. Cardiovascular manifestations (valvular dysfunction, myocardial thickening, coronary artery narrowing, myocardial infarction) leading to congestive heart failure are parts of the more severe clinical variants and occur as a result of glycosaminoglycan accumulation.

Ehlers-Danlos syndrome

Types V and IX are X-linked recessive diseases (see below).

Autosomal dominant diseases

Cerebral autosomal dominant arteriopathy with subcortical infarcts and leukoencephalopathy (CADASIL)

This newly described inherited arterial disease has an autosomal dominant transmission with the gene mapped to chromosome 19. It affects the small vessels of the brain and more than two hundred cases have now been reported, belonging to at least 30 unrelated pedigrees in Europe, America and Asia [119]. The age at onset of symptoms is in the forties, mean 45 years, with attacks of migraine occurring earlier in life (38.1 years) than ischaemic events (49.3 years). The penetrance of the disease appears complete between 30 and 40 years of age [120, 121]. The patients are free of classical vascular risk factors [122]. The clinical features include four major neurological presentations associated in variable degrees during the course of the disease; migraine with or without aura, epileptic seizures, mood disorders with severe depressive episodes, and strokes or stroke-like episodes with major psychiatric symptoms and dementia. The disease has a progressive course and a mean duration of 13.6

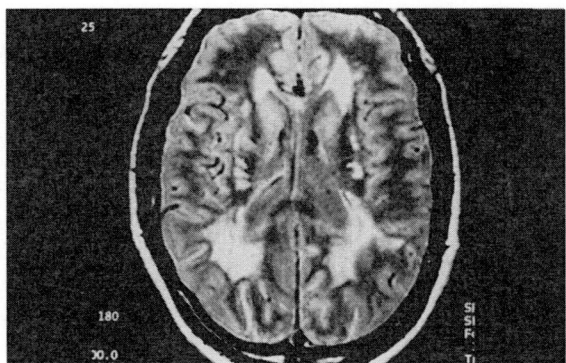

Fig 32. CADASIL. Axial image (3200/17-Rho) in a 54 year-old woman affected by CADASIL with pseudo-bulbar syndrome. Symmetrical hyperintense perventricular lesions associated with punctuated lesions in the basal ganglia and both external capsules. (Courtesy Dr P. Davous)

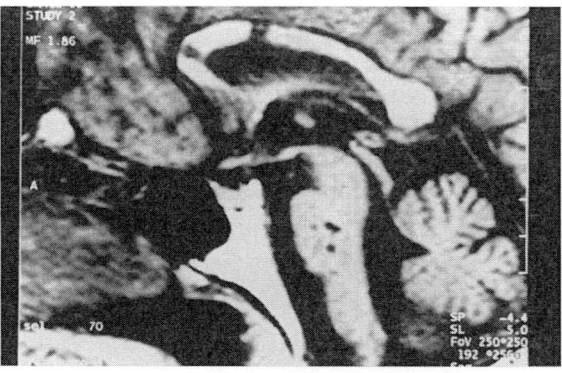

Fig 33. CADASIL. Same patient as Fig 1. T1 weighted sagittal image (500/12) showing multiple small infarcts in the corpus callosum and pons as low signal lesions. (Courtesy Dr P. Davous)

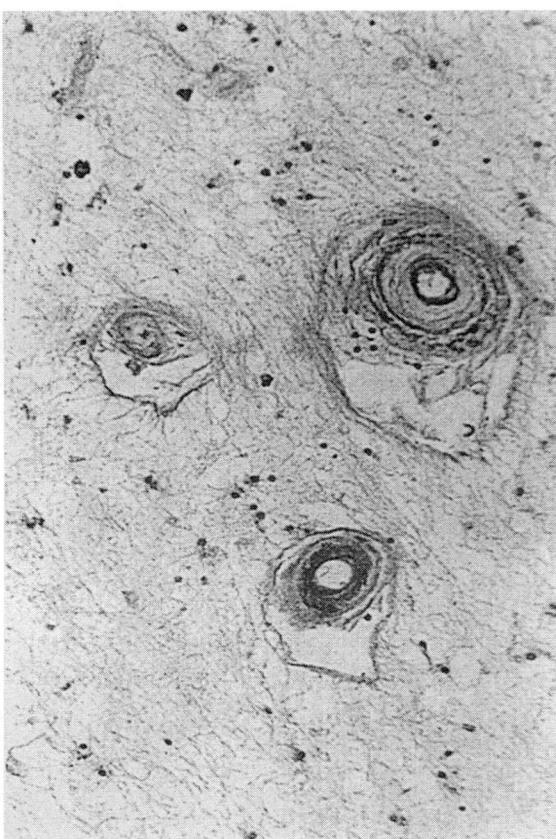

Fig 34. CADASIL. The white matter is extremely rarefied (little myelin and few axons), and the vessel structure is clearly abnormal. Periodic Acid Schiff staining technique. (PAS)

years. Death occurs in the fifties with a pseudo-bulbar syndrome and subcortical dementia. Cerebral magnetic resonance imaging shows a diffuse leukoencephalopathy with subcortical infarcts in the basal ganglia and white matter (Fig. 32-33). The disease is genetically homogeneous and caused by missense point mutations in the Notch3 gene, which encodes a transmembrane receptor protein. Each defect leads to either a gain or loss of a cysteine residue in the extracellular, N-terminal domain of the molecule, which most probably results in conformational alteration. The function of Notch3 in adults and the pathogenesis of CADASIL are uncertain, but in development the products of the gene have a role in cell/cell communication [123]. Presently, no specific therapy is available.

Pathology and differential diagnosis

Macroscopic lesions are similar to Binswanger's encephalopathy [122]. The cerebral white matter shows oedema with secondary demyelination and multiple lacunar infarcts develop, mainly in the basal ganglia and frontal white matter (Fig. 34). These lead to a cognitive decline and finally to dementia. These infarcts result from a thickening and fibrosis of the walls of the small and medium-sized penetrating arteries with consequent obliteration and/or thrombosis. Basophilic, periodic acid-Schiff-positive material accumulates between degenerating smooth muscle cells. (Fig. 35). Ultrastrucurally, this granular, electron dense and osmiophilic material is also seen in the basal layer of both arterioles and capillaries (Fig. 36-37) [124, 125]. Vascular endothelial cells are swollen with destruction of tight junctions. These findings suggest that impaired permeability of vascular endothelium may play a role in the destruction of vascular smooth muscle cells [126]. Although the symptoms are almost

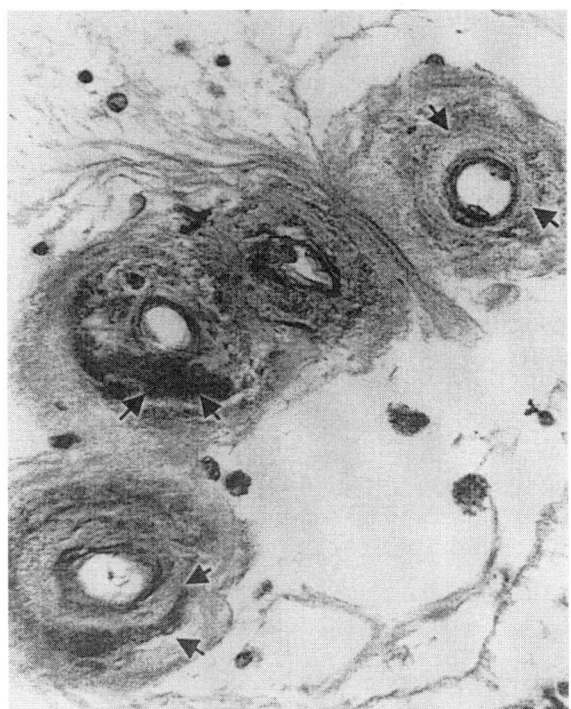

Fig 35. CADASIL. High power view of more vessels, showing the fragmented wall. The arrows point to the rather smudgy granular typical deposits. PAS

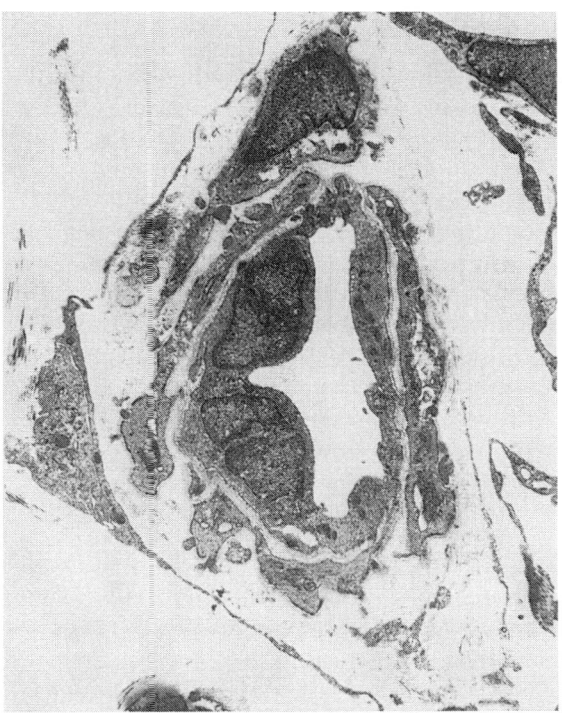

Fig 36. CADASIL. Electron micrograph of a small arteriole from the skin biopsy showing degenerative changes of smooth muscle cells. (Courtesy Dr M. Ruchoux and Dr H. Chabriat)

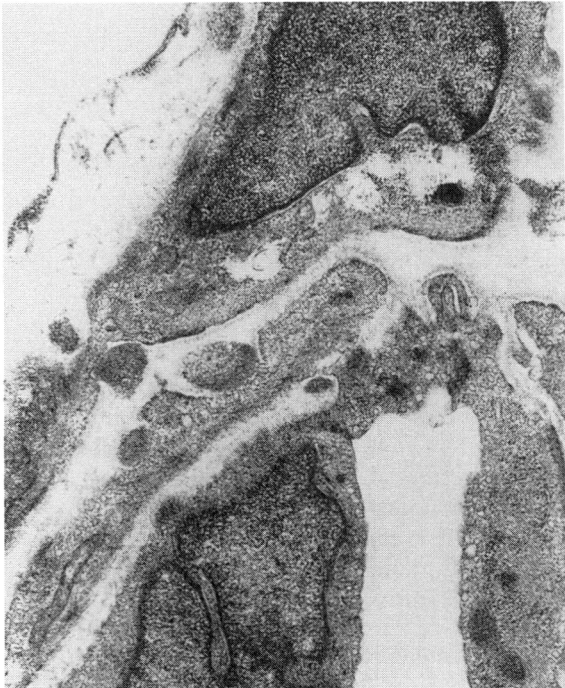

Fig 37. CADASIL. Electron micrograph of a small arteriole from the skin. Note characteristic deposits of granular osmiophilic material beyond the basement membrane. (Courtesy Dr M.Ruchoux and Dr H. Chabriat)

exclusively neurological, the arteriopathy is generalized and dermal and muscular arteries and small vessels are involved in the early phase of the disease with or without clinical manifestations. Thus skin and muscle are useful targets for diagnostic biopsy [119, 123].

Crouzon's syndrome (Craniofacial dysostosis)

A mutation in the fibroblast growth factor gene *FGFR2* is found in the Crouzon's syndrome, where the skull is affected but the limbs are normal. Cardiovascular malformations include coarctation of the aorta and aortic stenosis. The Crouzon's syndrome is related to Alpers syndrome; the closest mutation is only 14 amino acids away from the mutations causing the Alpers syndrome (C to G transversions). Studies of allele specific amplifications have shown that these occur in spermatogenesis (fathers, but not mothers of Alpers babies, tend to be older than average). The characteristic features include premature synostosis of cranial sutures, beaked nose, exophthalmos, hypertelorism with progressive visual impairment, hypoplasia of the maxilla, and a high-arched short palate.

Ehlers-Danlos syndrome (Cutis hyperelastica)

This is a group of generalised connective tissue diseases characterised by overelasticity and friability of the skin, excessive extensibility of the joints, and fragility of the small blood vessels and sometimes large arteries, due to a deficient quality or quantity of collagen. At present at least 11 forms are recognised on the basis of their clinical characteristics, methods of transmission and biochemical defect.The first four types of the Ehlers-Danlos syndrome (EDS) account for approximately 95% of cases. Almost all forms are transmitted with a dominant autosomal pattern [127]; however, Ehlers-Danlos type VI, VII and X syndromes are autosomal recessive, and Ehlers-Danlos type V and IX syndromes X-linked recessive [128, 129]. Ehlers-Danlos type 1 syndrome is the most frequent and most severe form [127]. The cardiovascular system is mostly affected in Type IV. Mutations in the COL3A1 gene [130, 131] are central to this type in which rupture of large vessels caused by abnormalities of type III collagen is a common cause of death [132-135]. In reality, this is a heterogeneous group genetically encompassing at least three distinct mutations: deletions, RNA splice mutations, and point mutations all occur. Some affect the synthesis rate of pro A1 (III) chains, others the type III pro-collagen secretion, and others lead to the synthesis of structurally abnormal type III collagen. Other cardiovascular anomalies include mitral valve prolapse, atrial and/or ventricular septal defect, patent ductus arteriosus, diffuse aneurysmal formation with spontaneous arteriovenous fistulae, and microangiopathy [136-140]. Spontaneous rupture of the colon and small intestine may occur [141]. Types I and III also present an apparent high prevalence of cardiovascular abnormalities: dilatation of the aortic root and the pulmonary artery, ectasia of the sinuses of Valsalva and various valvular and septal malformations are found [142].

Pathology and Differential diagnosis

In the cardiovascular system, the lesions are similar to those of Marfan's syndrome. Histologically, elastic arteries present coarse fragmented elastic fibers in the media, which displays severe degeneration with large deposists of acid mucopolysaccharides. These changes result in aneurysmal dilatation [143]. Spontaneous rupture is the most frequent and severe complication.

von Hippel-Lindau disease (Retinocerebral angiomatosis)

This condition is a phacomatosis, with haemangiomas of the retina, often multiple and bilateral, associated with haemangioblastomas, primarily of the cerebellum and walls of the fourth ventricle, occasionally involving the spinal cord. There are associated cysts or hamartomas of the kidneys, adrenal glands, pancreas and other organs. This disorder is transmitted in an autosomal dominant pattern. The tumour suppressor gene for VHL is on the short arm of chromosome 3 (3p 25-26) and encodes a protein involved in signal transduction or cell adhesion [144, 145]. About two-thirds of patients develop bilateral, often multiple, renal cell carcinomas. Polycythaemia is present in about 10% of cases and the haemangioblastomas may be the source of erythropoietin, although the cell origin of the growth factor is not known. Treatment includes resection of the cerebellar hemangioblastomas, laser therapy for retinal lesions, and partial nephrectomies for bilateral renal carcinomas. The prognosis is poor.

Pathology and differential diagnosis

Capillary haemangioblastomas commonly present as a cystic lesion with a mural nodule. Histologically, there is a mixture of variable proportions of delicate capillaries with "stromal" cells between them. These cells, with abundant vacuolated cytoplasm, are of uncertain histogenesis.

Hypercholesterolemic xanthomatosis

The familial hyper-cholesterolaemias are a complex group. This autosomal dominant disease features plasma cholesterol levels of around 300-500 mg/dl. Clinical features include xanthelasma and xanthomas. Xanthelasmas mostly develop in the eyelids and are associated with arcus senilis surrounding the cornea. Xanthomas are painless nodules that are found in either the subcutaneous tissues (elbows, knees, buttocks) or tendons (fingers, knees and heels) and, sometimes, mucosa. In arteries, massive lipid deposition may obstruct the coronary arteries causing angina and myocardial infarction at an early age. Deficiency of Low Density Lipoprotein (LDL) receptors leads to deficient hepatic clearance of VLDL (Very Low Density Lipoprotein). Non-receptor-mediated LDL uptake then becomes chaotic, and results in lipid-bloated cells forming xanthomas and severe atherosclerosis-like lesions.

Pathology and differential diagnosis

Xanthomata are characterized by infiltration of xanthomatous and Touton multinucleated giant cells. In arteries, these cells may accumulate in the intima, thickening this layer and causing stenosis.

Marfan's syndrome

This is a heterogeneous group of genetic disorders with a defect of the mesodermal connective tissues resulting in skeletal and articular, ocular, cardiovascular and, to some extent, cerebral disorders. The syndrome occurs in all races and ethnic groups with no sex predominance. About 70 to 85% of the cases are familial and transmitted as an autosomal dominant trait. The remainder are sporadic. This syndrome results from mutations in the fibrillin gene [146], mapped to chromosome 15q15-q21. Point mutations in the fibrillin gene were found in some patients with the sporadic form [147, 148]. Fibrillin is a large connective tissue glycoprotein which is a major component of elastic microfibrils, produced by fibroblasts that aggregate either alone or in combination with other proteins to give rise to a microfibrillar network in the extracellular matrix. The microfibrillary fibers act as scaffolding for elastin deposits. These widely distributed microfibrillar fibers are particularly abundant in ligaments, in the ocular ciliary zonules and in the aorta. In Marfan's syndrome, fibrillin is either abnormal or deficient because of defective secretion from fibroblasts, easy degradation by matrix metalloproteinases (MMPs) and/or poor incorporation into the extracellular matrix [149, 150]. The abundance of abnormal microfibrillar fibers in the tissues of patients with Marfan's syndrome may explain the degenerative, generalized nature of this disease. The fibers cannot resist normal tissue stress and they progressively elongate over time, which causes them to overstretch or break. DNA polymorphism in the fibrillin gene clone was shown to be tightly linked to the Marfan phenotype by family linkage studies. The Marfan locus is mapped to chromosome 15q15-21.3 [148, 149, 151]. A number of authors have identified new point mutations in fibrillin genes 1 and 2. Fibrillin 1 (FBN1) codes for the main constitutive protein of the elastic tissue that resists load and stress (aortic adventitia, suspending ligament of the lens, skin), fibrillin 2 (FBN2) for the orientation of the elastin present in cartilage, the aortic media and the bronchi [152]. The most significant of the defects is enlargement of the aortic root with dilatation of the aortic ring. Mitral valves become floppy, and redundant with attenuated chordae. Severe heart failure results. Dilatation of the ascending aorta results from mucoid degeneration of the media. Life expectancy is reduced by one-third. Cardiovascular lesions are life-threatening in about 1/3 of patients. Most deaths are caused by rupture of aortic dissections, bacterial endocarditis, heart failure or sudden death [153]. The risk of aortic valvae insufficiency [154], acute aortic dissections and arterial rupture is increased in women of childbearing age with Marfan's syndrome, as it is in Ehlers-Danlos disease [155-157]. The outlook for Marfans disease appears good when the patients undergo elective aortic root replacement [158]. From the cardiovascular standpoint, prophylactic ascending aortic resections are recommended when the aortic root grows to 60 mm diameter or more, because postoperative mortality rates are less than 2% and five-year survival rates are more than 85%, if the surgery is performed at this stage [159, 160]. Extracardiovascular complications include intestinal perforation and/or rupture; cervical incompetence and placenta praevia have been reported [161, 162].

Pathology and differential diagnosis

The two most common lesions are dilatation of the ascending aorta owing to cystic medial degeneration and mitral valve prolapse. In the aorta, the histological changes in the media are identical to those found in non-Marfan cystic degeneration. These degenerative changes range from mild fragmentation of elastic tissue to overt cystic change with focal separation of the elastic and fibromuscular elements of the media. Formation of small cleft-like or cystic spaces haphazardly distributed throughout the thickness of the media, filled with amorphous material resembling the ground substance of connective tissue; ultimately, loss of elastic laminae occurs. Weakening of the media favours progressive dilatation of the aortic valve ring and the root of the aorta, and predisposes to intimal tears with fatal intramural dissection and aneurysms. The mitral valve leaflets appear floppy, while the chordae tendineae undergo myxomatous degeneration and become elongated and thinned. The collagenous structure of the chordae tendineae is also attenuated; they lengthen and may rupture. Similar changes may involve the tricuspid valve and, rarely, the aortic or pulmonic valves (or both) may be affected. Secondary induced injuries caused by the prolapsing leaflets include fibrosis of the valve leaflets, ventricular endocardial surface and endocardium, mural thrombosis and focal calcification at the base of the leaflet. About 3% of patients with floppy valves develop serious complications, such as infective endocarditis, valvular insufficiency, embolism of leaflet thrombi resulting in a stroke or other systemic infarcts, and arrhythmias.

Neurofibromatosis

This phacomatosis occurs in two main types: neurofibromatosis 1 and 2 [163]. Half of the cases present with an autosomal dominant transmission, the remainder result from new mutations. Neurofibromatosis-1 is related to tumour suppressor genes mapped to chromosome 17q11 [164]. These genes encode a protein called neurofibromin, which down-regulates the function of the p21 ras oncoprotein. The tumour suppressor gene of neurofibromatosis-2 is mapped to chromosome 22 [165] and encodes a protein that links integral membrane proteins with the cytoskeleton. Vascular manifestations of neurofibromatosis include coarctation of the aorta and obstructive aortic arch syndrome, arterial fibromuscular dysplasia, and arterial or venous aneurysm [166-169]. Renovascular hypertension may be related to extrinsic compression of the renal artery by a neurofibroma, or primary medial fibrodysplasia [170] or to associated pheochromocytoma.

Pathology and differential diagnosis

Vascular lesions of von Recklinghausen's disease include fibromuscular dysplasia and proliferative nodules of smooth muscle cells in vessel walls. Fibromuscular dysplasia may involve any point of the arterial tree, including the coronary vessels. Histologically, the lesions may be intimal or medial with occasional aneurysm formation (Fig. 38-39-40). Proliferative nodules of smooth muscle cells usually develop at the junction of the intima and media and protrude into the lumen of arteries and arterioles. In some areas, they may involve the intima and the media in a concentric fashion.

Noonan's syndrome

Most features of this syndrome mimic those of Turner's syndrome. Vascular anomalies found include patent ductus arteriosus, abnormal pulmonary venous connections, aortic coarctation, cystic lymphangioma or hygroma and lymphoedema [171, 172]. Fifty to sixty percent of patients have outlet valve anomalies with pulmonary stenosis and aortic and pulmonary valve dysplasia.

Osler-Weber-Rendu disease (Osler's disease, Hereditary haemorrhagic telangiectasia)

Multiple small aneurysmal telangiectases are distributed over the skin and mucous membranes with many (often small) arterio-venous fistulae.This rare disorder is transmitted as a dominant Mendelian trait and affects both sexes equally. In about 20% of cases, however, a family history is missing. The disease usually becomes manifest after puberty. Clinically the lesions may develop anywhere in the body, but particularly occur in the nasal mucosa and the mouth. They

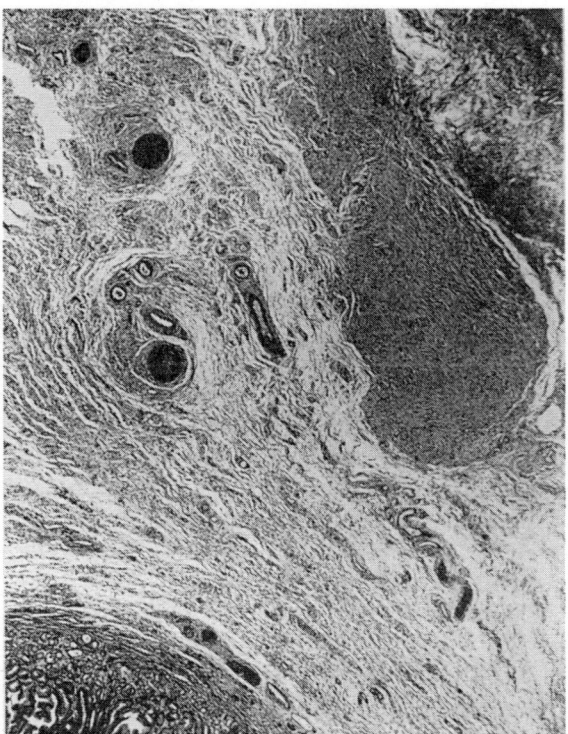

Fig. 38. Neurofibromatosis. Female patient, 78 yo, having a long course von Recklinghausen's disease, suffering from suspect gastric ulcer. Gastrectomy specimen, free of malignancy, showing thickening of the submucosa with neurofibromas and occluded small arteries. HES

consist of flat or slightly raised, irregularly shaped red spots measuring from 1 to less than 5 mm in diameter, located directly beneath the skin or mucosal surfaces of the oral cavity, and lips. They blanch upon application of pressure and bleed very readily, epistaxis being the most common symptom. Similar lesions may be found in the alimentary, respiratory, and urinary tracts as well as in the brain, liver and spleen [173]. Other associated lesions include aneurysms, vascular malformations and arteriovenous fistulas in the lungs, brain and liver. Complex arteriovenous fistulae occur in the spinal cord [174]. Laboratory data include marked hypochromic anaemia, and normal coagulation tests, although von Willebrand's disease has been reported in some cases [175]. Symptoms appear more pronounced with increasing age, but life expectancy is normal.

Pathology and differential diagnosis

In the skin and mucosa, the lesions consist of dilated capillaries with thin walls, made up of a single layer of

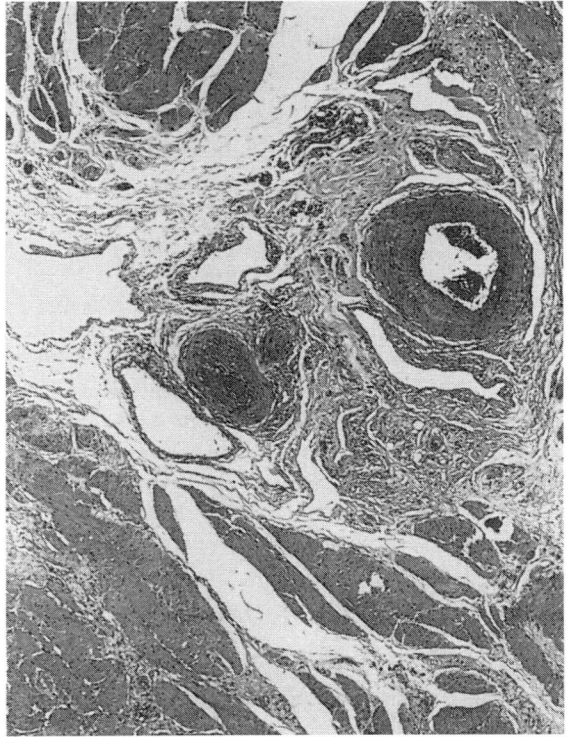

Fig. 39. Neurofibromatosis. Same patient. Submucosal small arteries showing either total occlusion or intimal thickening. HES

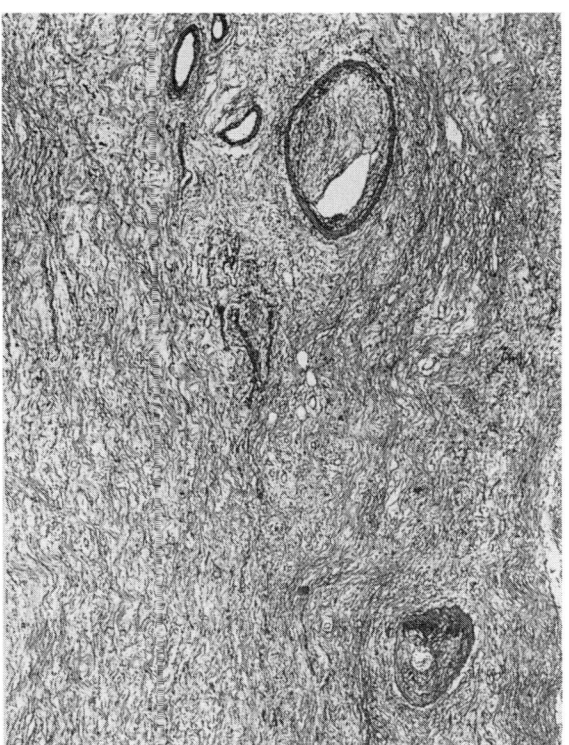

Fig. 40. Neurofibromatosis. Same patient. Vascular changes corresponding to typical intimal fibromuscular dysplasia. ...Orcein...

endothelial cells. These capillaries lie immediately beneath a greatly thinned epithelium. The lesions can be distinguished from petechiae by their peculiar distribution, and by their tendency to blanch on pressure from a glass slide.

Progeria (Hutchinson-Gilford disease)

Gilford [176] first gave the name "progeria" to this disease. This condition is characterised by normal development in the first year followed by gross retardation of growth, with a senile appearance mimicking sclereodema in early infancy [177]. Premature arteriosclerosis leads to coronary artery disease with angina pectoris and fatal myocardial infarction, senile aortic calcific stenosis leading to aortic regurgitation and congestive heart failure [178-180]. The age at death ranges from 7 to 27.5 years, with a median age of 13.4 years. Some patients need coronary artery bypass surgery and percutaneous transluminal angioplasty [81]. The syndrome is probably autosomal dominant with

rare instances of affected sibs due to germinal mosaicism [182, 183].

Pathology and differential diagnosis

Vascular changes in progeria and related syndromes (Werners' syndrome) are simply severe atherosclerosis causing occlusion of coronary, cerebral and renal arteries with fatal consequences [184].

Tuberous sclerosis (Bourneville's disease, Epiloia)

Multisystem hamartomas produce the typical triad of seizures, mental retardation, and skin nodules (angiofibromas) of the face. Cerebral and retinal lesions consist of glial nodules. Vascular involvement is uncommon. Some reports have described renal angiomyolipomas, aortic aneurysm and fibromuscular dysplasia of renal arteries to be responsible for renovascular hypertension [185].

Autosomal recessive anomalies

Alkaptonuria (Ochronosis, Homogentisuria)

A congenital lack of the enzyme homogentisate 1,2-dioxygenase, which mediates an essential step in the metabolism of phenylalanine-tyrosine, allows homogentisic acid to accumulate in the body. This is excreted, imparting a black colour to the urine after oxidation [186] The remaining homogentisic acid selectively binds to collagen in connective tissues, tendons, and cartilage, giving to these structures a blueblack pigmentation (ochronosis) most evident in the ears, nose, and cheeks. Interstitial tissue of viscera (pancreas, prostate, and kidneys), and membranes (sclera, cornea, tympanic membrane) are also affected; so are the heart valves and large arteries [187].

Pathology and differential diagnosis

The gross appearance of pigment deposits is striking. The surface of the cardiac valves and the arterial intima remains intact, while a deeper black layer is visible through it.

Ataxia-telangiectasia (Louis-Bar syndrome)

This entity is part of a group of degenerative diseases affecting the cerebellar cortex, spinal cord, peripheral nerves, and other regions of the neuraxis. Progressive cerebellar ataxia, oculocutaneous telangiectases and immune deficiency with proneness to pulmonary infections are the main characteristics [188]. T cell leukaemia and lymphomas may develop [189] There is a mutation of the so-called ATM gene, a "checkpoint" gene in cell cycling, on chromosome 11. Neurological signs of cerebellar disease usually predate the appearance of the numerous oculocutaneous telangiectases.

Pathology and differential diagnosis

The vascular lesions are characterised by groupings of dilated capillaries with thin walls, lined with a single endothelial layer.

Homocystinuria

This disease is an inborn error of methionine metabolism. Normally cystathionine beta-synthetase (21q22.3) catalyses the conversion of homocysteine and serine to cystathionine. The incidence of the homozygous disease of cystathionine beta-synthetase is estimated to be 1:200,000, that of the heterozygous form 1: 300. There are, however, numerous other causes of a mild to moderate homocysteinemia, for example, a deficiency of the cofactors vitamin B6, B12 and folic acid. [190]. Deficiency of cystathionine (bêta-synthetase activity induces accumulation of homocysteine and methionine in the blood and tissues resulting in ocular, musculo-skeletal, central nervous system, and vascular manifestations.

Pathology and differential diagnosis

Data on arterial histology in homocystinuria and mild hyperhomocysteinaemia are limited. Experimentally, hyperhomocysteinaemia promotes intimal injury, induces dysfunction of the vascular endothelium, oxidation of cholesterol and unsaturated lipids, platelet aggregation, thrombogenic factors, myointimal hyperplasia, deposition of sulfated glycosaminoglycans, fibrosis and calcification. It is thought that in Man these changes lead to early atherosclerotic vascular changes, occlusive complications, venous thrombosis and aneurysm [191-195].

Mucopolysaccharidoses

These syndromes result from deficiencies of specific lysosomal enzymes involved in the degradation of mucopolysaccharides or glycosaminoglycans (dermatan sulfate, heparan sulfate, keratan sulfate, and chondroitin sulfate) [196]. The enzymes involved in the degradation of these molecules cleave terminal sugars from the polysaccharide chains disposed along a polypeptide or "core protein". When there is a block in the removal of a terminal sugar, the remainder of the polysaccharide chain is not further degraded, and thus these chains accumulate within lysosomes in various cells throughout the body, including endothelial cells and smooth muscle cells and viscera, including the blood vessels and heart. Severe neurologic, vascular and somatic changes result. The mucopolysaccharidoses occur in around 0.04-0.3% of newborns and represents 1.5% of all congenital disorders [197]. Around 13 types of MPS have been identified and numerically classified from MPS-I to MPS-VIII, based upon symptoms [197, 198] and specific enzyme deficiencies. Seven out of the remaining types present involvement of heart and blood vessels (Table 3). There is one case report of repair of an aortic aneurysm following aortic valve replacement in an 8 year old child with mucopolysaccharidosis. The value of this report lies in the illustration of the infiltration of the aortic wall by stored glycosaminoglycan [143] although the precise enzyme defect was not identified.

Within a given type, the clinical pattern varies widely in severity resulting from different mutant alleles at the same genetic locus.

Table 3. Biochemical characteristics and mode of inheritance of mucopolysaccharidoses with cardiovascular involvement (AR: autosomal recessive inheritance, I: inheritance, X-R: X-linked recessive inheritance)

SYNDROMES	DEFICIENT ENZYME	I	GENE MAP LOCUS	NON-ENZYMATIC BREAKDOWN PRODUCTS
MPS I-H (Hurler)	alpha-L-iduronidase	AR	4p16.3	dermatan and heparan sulfates
MPS I-S (Scheie)	alpha-L-iduronidase	AR	4p16.3	dermatan and heparan sulfates
MPS I-H-S (Hurler-Scheie)	alpha-L-iduronidase	AR	4p16.3	dermatan and heparan sulfates
MPS II (Hunter)	iduronate 2-sulfatase	X-R	Xq27.3-q28	dermatan and heparan sulfates
MPS IV A (Morquio A)	N-acetyl galacto-samine-6 sulfatase	AR	?	keratan sulfate
MPS IV B (Morquio B)	beta-galactosidase A	AR	3p21.33	keratan sulfate
MPS VI (Maroteaux-Lamy) (1963)	arylsulfatase B(ARSB)	AR	5p11-q13	dermatan sulfate

MPSI (Hurler and Scheie's syndrome)

MPSI results from deficiency of (alpha-L-iduronidase. Dermatan and heparan sulfates (DS, HS) accumulate in the central nervous system and peripheral tissues. Cardiovascular manifestations include coronary artery narrowing, myocardial fibrosis, and cardiac valve and endocardial thickening, which lead to congestive heart failure. Life expectancy is about 10 years.

MPS IV (Morquio A and Morquio B syndromes)

MPS IV A (Morquio A) is caused by a deficiency in N-acetyl-galactosamine-6-sulfatase, and MPS IV B (Morquio B) by a deficiency in (beta-galactosidase A. In the two variants, keratan sulfate accumulates in the cells of the musculoskeletal system. Coronary artery intimal sclerosis has been described [199]. Cardiac valvular lesions are evident with aortic regurgitation and are an important cause of premature death.

MPS VI (Maroteaux-Lamy syndrome)

This syndrome is caused by arylsulfatase B (ARSB) (5p11-q13) deficiency with accumulation of acid mucopolysaccharide (dermatan sulfate), primarily in the cells of the musculoskeletal system, causing severe musculoskeletal changes. Cardiovascular changes consist of aortic and mitral valvular dysfunction and are an important cause of death, as in other disorders of this type.

Pathology and differential diagnosis

The affected cells are distended and have apparent clearing of the cytoplasm. The clear cytoplasm can sometimes be resolved into numerous minute vacuoles, which correspond to swollen lysosomes filled with a finely granular, water soluble, PAS-positive material (Fig. 41). In fresh tissue, this material can be identified biochemically as glycosaminoglycan. Hepatosplenomegaly, skeletal deformities, cerebral damage, valvular lesions (Fig. 42-43) and subendothelial arte-

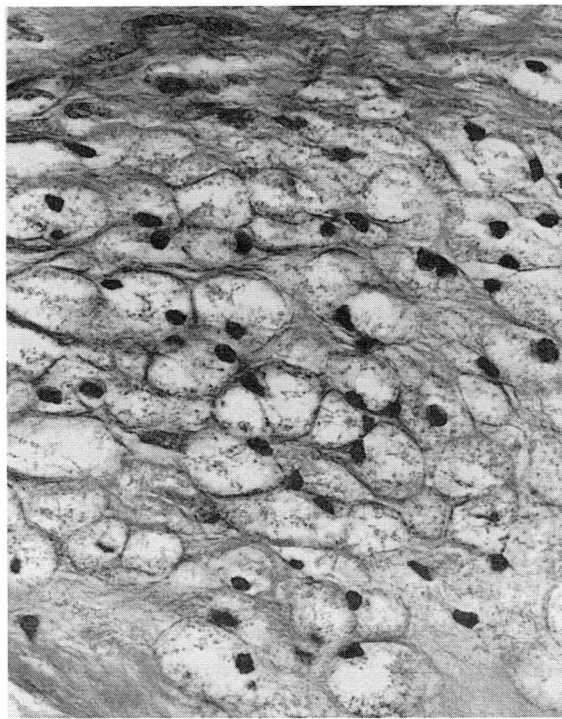

Fig. 41. Mucopolysaccharidoses. Affected cells with clear cytoplasm filled with granular, PAS-positive material. PAS

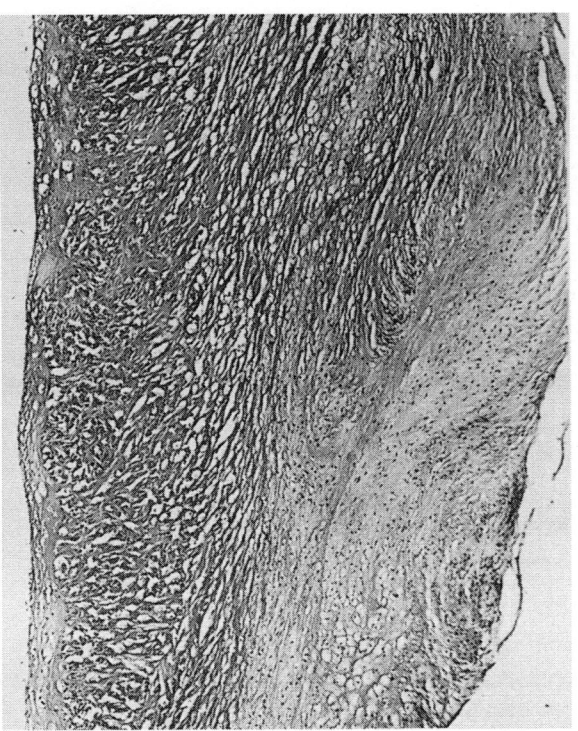

Fig. 42. Mucopolysaccharidoses. Valvular envolvement. PAS

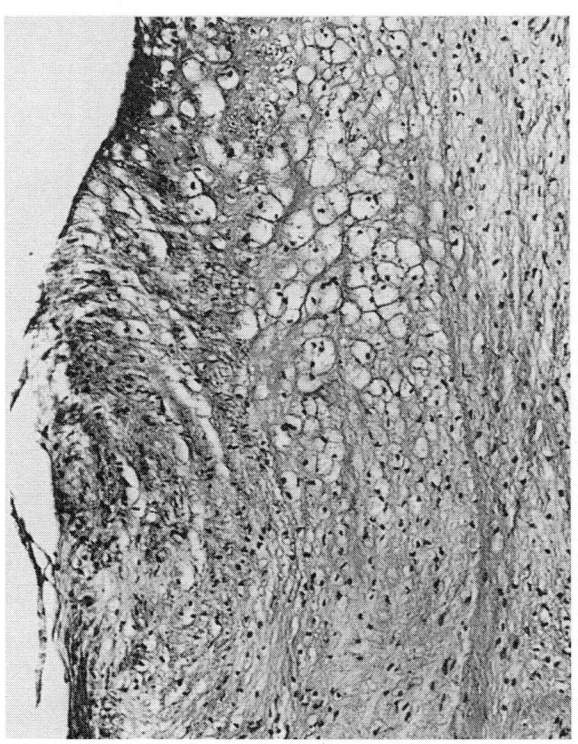

Fig. 43. Mucopolysaccharidoses. Valvular envolvement. PAS

rial deposits (Fig. 44-45), particularly in the coronary arteries, are common complications of all the MPS.

Primary hyperoxaluria and oxalosis

This disorder is characterised by calcium oxalate nephrocalcinosis and nephrolithiasis, extrarenal oxalosis, and increased urinary output of oxalic and glycolic acids; it is usually evident clinically in the first decade of life, with progressive renal failure and uraemia. There are two autosomal recessive forms: Primary Hyperoxaluria Type I and Type II. Primary Hyperoxaluria Type I (PHI) is caused by a defect in alanine glyoxalate (AGT) which is normally found in the peroxisome of liver cells. Primary Hyperoxaluria Type II (PHII), also caused by a defective gene in liver cells and other cells, is a milder disease and does not usually present the long-term kidney impairment that is seen with PHI. Extrarenal deposition of calcium oxalate involves several tissues, including the heart. Cardio-vascular complications include conduction disorders, embolic stroke, pulmonary hypertension, peripheral vasospasm with acrocyanosis and Raynaud's phenomenon, distal pulse loss, and peripheral gangrene. A fulminating vascular syndrome may develop some days after bilateral nephrectomy

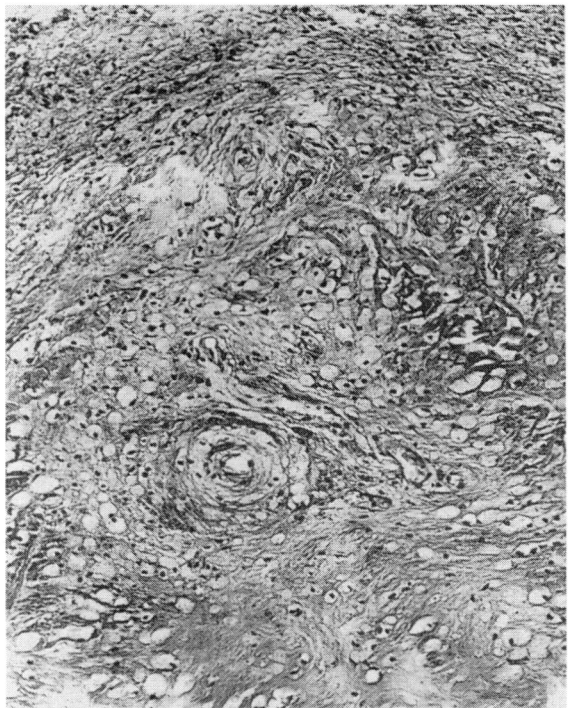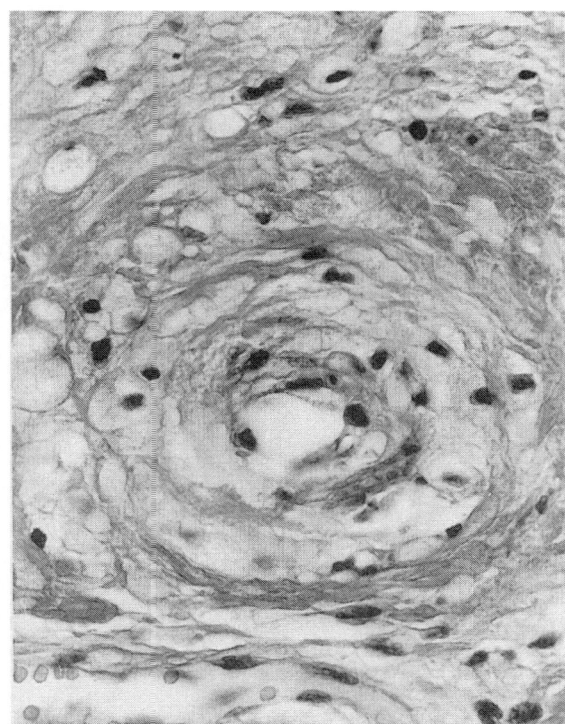

Fig. 44-45. Mucopolysaccharidoses. Subendothelial deposits of PAS-positive material in coronary artery. PAS

[200-207]. Treatment of vascular oxalosis is directed towards relief of occlusive lesions and includes vasodilators, steroids, heparin, phenylbenzoamine, epidural block, surgical sympathectomy and hyperbaric oxygen.

Pathology and differential diagnosis

Arteries are more commonly involved than veins and the myocardium. Oxalate crystals pile up in all arteries (Fig. 46), whatever their size. Crystal deposits producing, foreign body granulomas (Fig. 47-48), subintimal fibrosis and occlusion with occasional thrombosis are seen in the media.

Sickle cell disease

Homozygotes develop "crises" characterised by episodes of severe pain caused by capillary stasis and microvascular occlusions with thrombosis [208, 209]. Bone infarcts, leg ulcers, and autoinfarction of the spleen are all associated with increased susceptibility to bacterial infections.

Werner's syndrome

There are scleroderma-like skin changes, general microsplanchnia, extreme hypogonadism, bilateral juvenile cataracts, diabetes mellitus and progeria [210, 211]. This syndrome has an autosomal recessive inheritance. Vascular anomalies and calcified aortic atherosclerosis occur, as in progeria. Many factors are implicated in the pathogenesis of these changes: the hypercoagulable state [212], high concentrations of blood plasminogen activator inhibitor-1(PAI-1) and intercellular adhesion molecule-1 (ICAM-1) [213], and abnormal lipoprotein metabolism [214].

Vascular anomalies associated with complex or polygenic inheritance

Blue rubber-bleb nevi syndrome

First reported by Gascoyen in 1860, this syndrome, so named by Bean in 1958, is characterized by bluish, erectile, easily compressible, nipple-like or dome-shaped thin-walled haemangiomatous nodules, widely distributed in the skin (Fig. 49-50), mucous membranes (Fig. 51) and other parts of the body, especially in the alimentary tract [215]. There is some evidence that this syndrome has an autosomal dominant mode

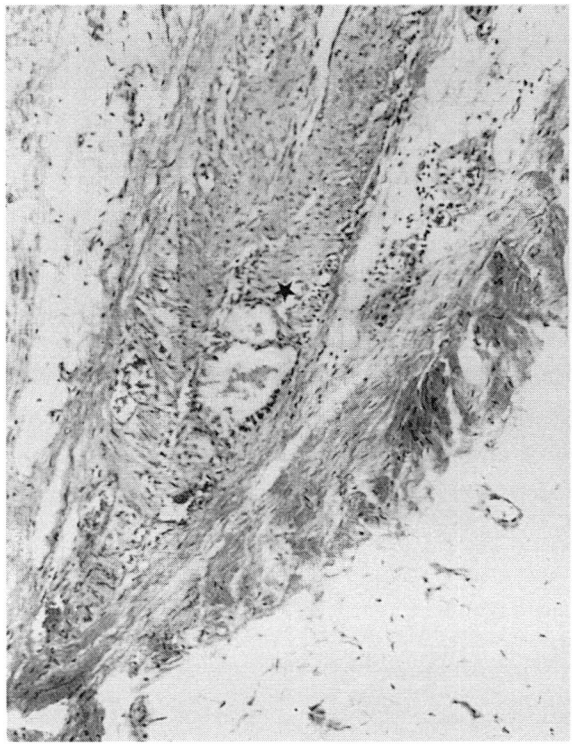

Fig. 46. Oxalosis. Oxalate crystals accumulate in an arterial wall. HES

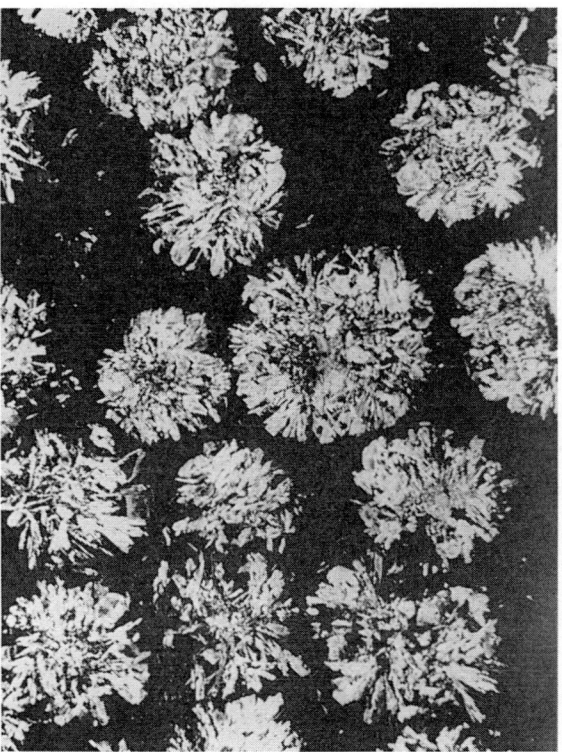

Fig. 47. Refringent firework-like oxalate crystals under polarized light

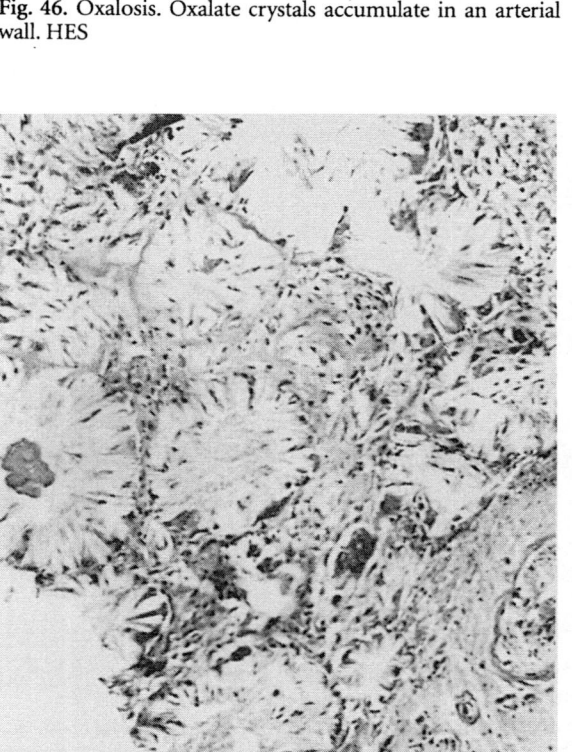

Fig. 48. Oxalate crystals surrounded by foreign body granulomas. HES

of inheritance [216] and Gallione et al [217] have suggested it is part of a group of venous malformations linked to chromosome 9 in a region encompassing a tumour suppressor gene and the interferon gene cluster. It is often detected at birth or in early infancy. Lesions may be few or numerous, sometimes numbering hundreds, and involve large cutaneous areas on both trunk and limbs. Other sites involved include the lips, oral cavity, glans penis, and nasopharynx. Some lesions may be painful, especially at puberty, and may be associated with hyperhidrosis. In about 90% of patients, similar lesions develop in the viscera, especially in the digestive tract, and cause gastrointestinal bleeding and intussusception [216]. Digestive blue rubber-bleb nevi commonly bleed, causing severe iron-deficiency anemia and even death. Fatal haemorrhage may result from rupture of angiomas in other viscera. In the brain, thrombosis is frequent; focal irreversible neurologic deficits may result from patchy areas of infarction. In the digestive tract, haemorrhage may be controlled by cauterization applied via an endoscope or by resection of the bleeding lesion. In the skin, the carbon dioxide laser has been used to remove the vascular nevi with excel-

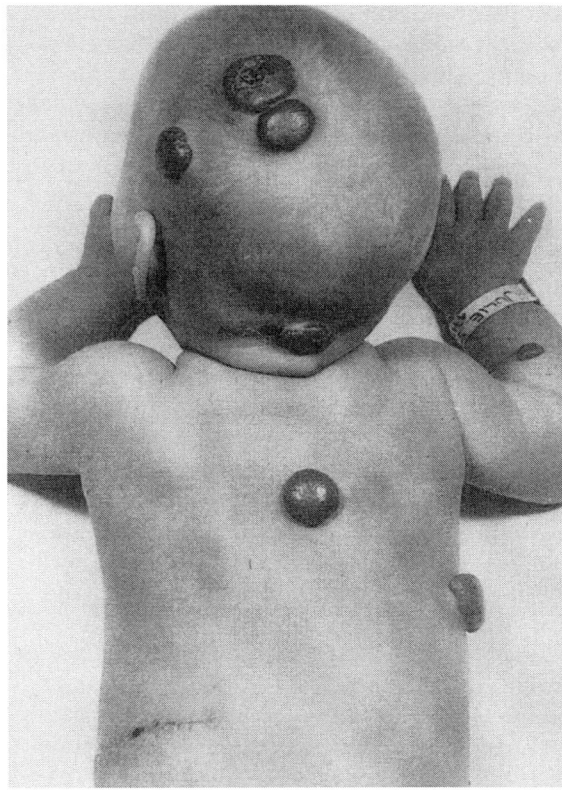

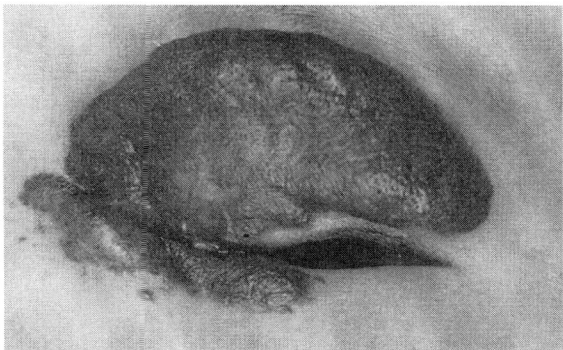

Fig. 50. Blue rubber-bleb nevi syndrome. Same infant. Confluent blue rubber-bleb nevi cordoning the right eyelids

Fig. 49. Blue rubber-bleb nevi syndrome with widely distributed haemangiomatous nodules in the scalp, neck, thorax and back of an infant, already operated on for a splenic haemangioma

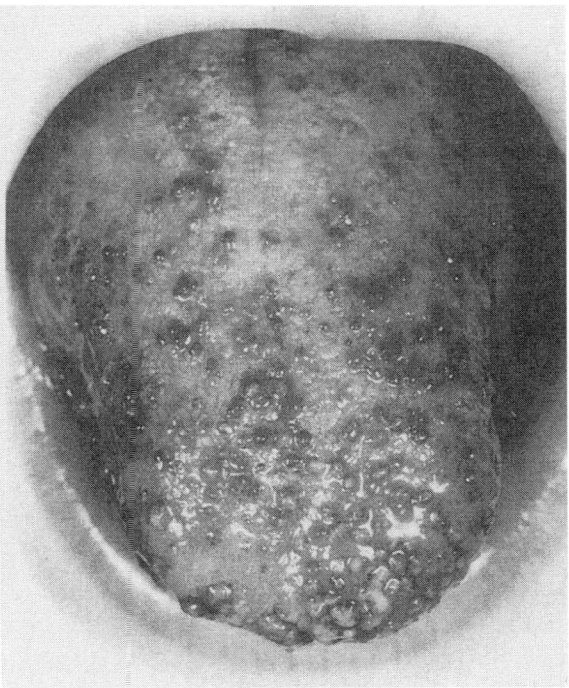

Fig. 51. Blue rubber-bleb nevi syndrome. Same infant. Diffuse blue rubber-bleb nevi distorting the tongue

lent results. Protection and support are indicated for lesions involving extremities, but marked disfigurement, pain or bleeding may impose amputation.

Pathology and differential diagnosis

Blue rubber-bleb nevi are a variant of cavernous haemangioma. In the skin, the lesions involve the dermis and subcutis; in the gastro-intestinal tract, they distort the lamina propria and submucosa. The nevi consist of very large, endothelium-lined cavities separated from one another by fibrous septa. Smooth muscle may be prominent within the wall of some cavern-like vessels. Some vein-like cavities may contain phleboliths. Theoretically, vascular malformations from other causes could mimic blue rubber-bleb nevi, but the clinical pattern and morphologic findings are sufficiently distinctive to establish the diagnosis. Other differential diagnoses include glomangiomas, angiokeratomas, and familial hemorrhagic telangiectasia (Osler-Weber-Rendu disease).

Cutis laxa (Dermatochalasis)

This is characterized by degeneration of elastic fibers with patients appearing to have an excessive amount of skin. Patients have an aged appearance with drooping jowls, blood-hound facies, a deep voice, unwrinkled and sagging folds of skin on the trunk and extremities, hip dislocation, pulmonary emphysema, inguinal, umbilical and diaphragmatic hernias, gastrointestinal and urinary diverticula, and diverticula of the alimentary tract or bladder. Vascular anomalies include stenoses of pulmonary artery branches with hypertension, dilatation and elongation with tortuosity of the aorta and its major branches, sudden fatal occlusive coronary arterial disease [218, 219, 220].

Osteogenesis imperfecta

The inheritance is autosomal dominant in most families, but a rare autosomal recessive type also exists. There is premature arteriosclerosis, stenosis of the aortic isthmus, mucoid changes in cardiac valves leading to aortic regurgitation, and aneurysm of the sinus of Valsalva [221, 222].

Pulmonary capillary haemangiomatosis

There are multiple thin-walled capillaries, grouped in nodules, distorting the lung parenchyma and causing pulmonary hypertension. Sporadic cases are regarded as congenital hamartomas [223-226] but an hereditary form with probable autosomal recessive inheritance seems to exist [227]. Progressive shortness of breath, recurrent haemoptysis, and occasional digital clubbing are the most frequent symptoms and generally occur between 20-40 years. A diffuse micronodular pattern can be viewed on a chest X-ray, while a perfusion scan displays segmental defects caused by chronic micro-thromboembolism. According to Tron et al [228], pulmonary capillary haemangiomatosis is a low-grade malignant vascular neoplasm with an aggressive growth pattern of the proliferating vessels. Most patients die within one to five years from the onset of the clinical symptoms [51, 224].

Pathology and differential diagnosis

The lung parenchyma is firm, congested and scattered with multiple, small, yellowish-gray nodules associated with haemorrhagic areas. These nodules surround the bronchi and vessels, while the peripheral parenchyma remains normal. Histologically, the nodules consist of a proliferation of small capillary-sized vessels. In some areas, these vessels form glomerular-like tufts jutting into the alveolar spaces containing fresh haemorrhages and haemosiderin-laden macrophages. These capillaries develop from the adventitia of nearby arterioles and venules. In some areas, they disrupt the vascular wall. The capillary proliferation also infiltrates the interstitium and the outermost parts of the bronchi and bronchioles. The vessels are lined with regular endothelial cells. The differential diagnosis includes pulmonary veno-occlusive disease where the lung parenchyma presents segmental areas of congestion and haemorrhage. Histological changes consist of a thickening of the intima of most medium

and small veins and venules by a myxoid fibrosis, which may extend to the interlobular septa. Large pulmonary and bronchial veins may be involved. The intimal hyperplasia reduces the venous lumen, which may be totally occluded by a thrombus. Orcein stain may unveil arterialization with elastic fibers seen in the intima and around the media. Venous infarcts may occur with haemorrhage, haemosiderin deposits and calcification. Secondary diffuse interstitial fibrosis with haemosiderin deposits, can mimic idiopathic pulmonary haemosiderosis. Interstitial fibrosis is usually more nodular than diffuse. The presence of an interstitial inflammatory infiltrate made up of lymphocytes and histiocytes can simulate an interstitial pneumonitis, but the veins present a normal intima. Lymphangiectasis, diffuse pulmonary lymphangiomatosis, lymphangiomas and lymphangio leiomyomatosis may theoretically cause confusion but in these conditions, the vascular cavities are filled with lymph. The distinction from a well-differentiated angiosarcoma may be difficult. In a well-differentiated angiosarcoma, vascular cavities present a heterogeneous distribution, being closely spaced in some areas and widely separated in others. In contrast, angiomatosis corresponds to a diffuse proliferation of blood vessels that are distributed uniformly throughout the tumour. In Kaposi's sarcoma, most patients are young adult males. Lung parenchyma shows red-blue discoloration. Histologically there is a mitotically active spindle cell proliferation around cleft-like vascular spaces. Some tumour cells have PAS-positive hyaline globules. Haemosiderin pigment is present.

Supravalvular aortic stenosis

This anomaly may occur as an isolated finding in an autosomal dominant form without other evidence of dysmorphology [229, 230]. It may represent an autosomal dominant inherited variant of aortic dysplasia caused by mutations in the elastin gene [231] but is more commonly part of a developmental disorder, Williams syndrome, affecting multiple organ systems, including the vascular system and with hypercalcemia [232, 233]. Affected individuals present with moderate mental and growth retardation, "elfin" facies (prominent cheeks, pouting lower lip, hypertelorism, retroussé nose, small mandible, prominent ears and stellate irides) [234]. Hypertension, nephrocalcinosis and coeliac disease complicate severe cases [235, 236]. Patients with Williams syndrome show a hemizygous submicroscopic deletion of the elastin locus on chromosome 7 (7q11.23) detectable by FISH (fluorescent *in situ* hybridation). Deletion occurs in the elastin gene where abnormalities are also found in the isolated form [237-243]. Cardiovascular anomalies include supravalvular aortic stenosis, stenosis of multiple peripheral pulmonary artery branches and, occasionally, supravalvular pulmonic stenosis. Total anomalous pulmonary venous connection has been also reported [91, 244-246]. The ascending aorta and other arteries display marked wall thickening or dysplasia with distortion of elastic lamellae and smooth muscle cells (Fig. 52-53). Calcification is seen in the media (Fig. 54). These changes cause vascular narrowing and rigidity [247, 248].

Vascular anomalies related to environmental influences

Viral infections, exposure to drugs, and irradiation may induce vascular malformations in the fetus and infant. Experimentally, teratogenic effects in the cardiovascular system may be found in animals exposed to ionizing radiation, hypoxaemia, and drugs, including folate antagonists, androgenic hormones, alcohol, anticonvulsants, warfarin and 13-cis-retinoic acid.

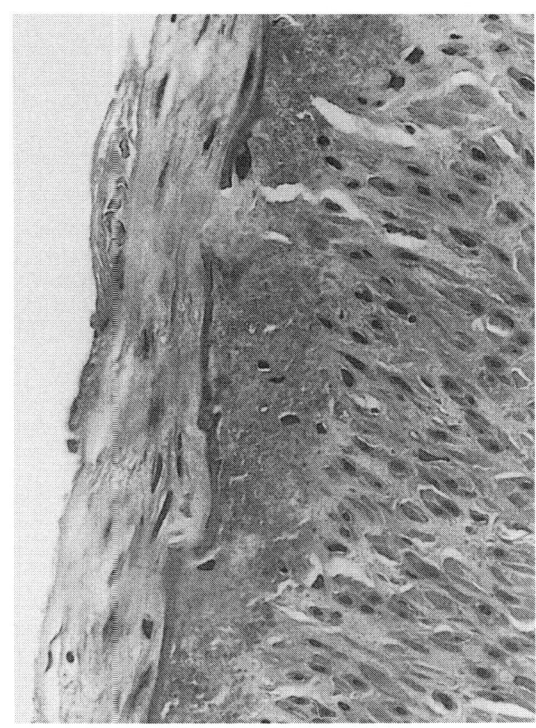

Fig. 53. Supravalvular aortic stenosis. Fragmentation of the internal elastic membrane. HES

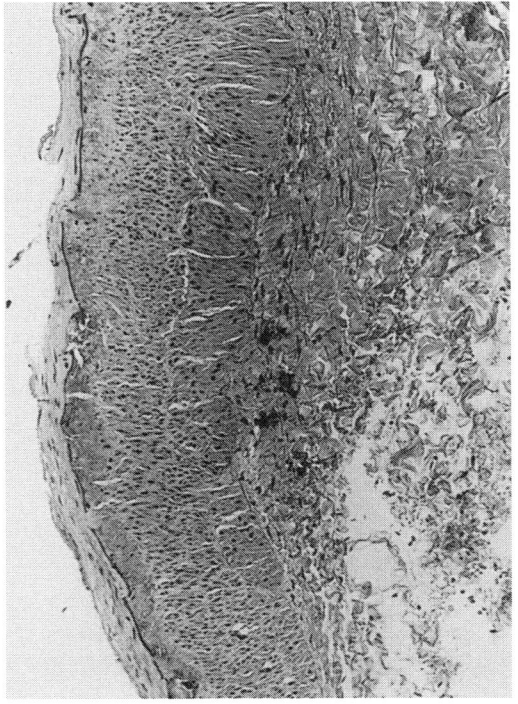

Fig. 52. Supravalvular aortic stenosis. Muscular artery displaying distortion of the internal elastic membrane and smooth muscle cells in the media. Orcein

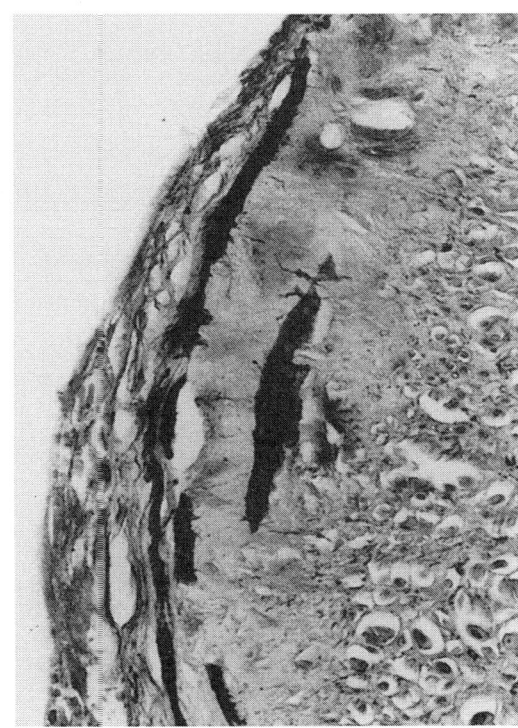

Fig. 54. Supravalvular aortic stenosis. Calcification in the inner part of the media. HES

Bibliography

1. Karvonen SL, Vaajalahti P, Marenk M, Janas M, Kuokkanen K (1992) Birthmarks in 4336 Finish newborns. Acta Derm Venereol 72: 55-7

2. de Felipe I, Quintanilla E (1997) Neurocutaneous syndromes with vascular alterations. Rev Neurol 25: S250-S258

3. Handfield-Jones SE, Kennedy CT, Bradfied JB (1988) Angiosarcoma arising in an angiomatous naevus following irradiation in childhood. Br J Dermatol 118: 109-12

4. Landthaler M, Hohenleutner U, el-Raheem TA (1995) Laser therapy of childhood haemangiomas. Br J Dermatol 133: 275-81

5. Distefano G, Rodono A, Betta P, Di Bella D, Gelardi S, Di Fede GF, Romeo MG (1996) Congenital pulmonary lymphangiectasia with chylothorax. Different evolution of 2 cases with severe neonatal respiratory distress. Pediatr Med Chir 18: 519-23

6. Blagowidow N, Page DC, Huff D, Mennuti MT (1989) Ullrich-Turner syndrome in an XY female fetus with deletion of the sex-determining portion of the Y chromosome. Am J Med Genet 34: 159-62

7. Fryns JP, Moerman P (1998) Trisomy 21 in a second trimester male hydropic fetus with "Noonan-syndrome-phenotype": nuchal and thoracic lymphangiomatosis, oedema of the dorsum of hands and feet, and bicuspid pulmonary valve. Genet Couns 9: 59-60

8. Green HD, Mollica AJ, Karuza AS (1995) Gorham's disease: a literature review and case reports. J Foot Ankle Surg 34: 435-41

9. Askin FB (1991) Respiratory tract disorders In Wigglesworth JM, Singer DB (eds.) Textbook of fetal and perinatal pathology. Blackwell Scientific Publications, Boston, p.659

10. Gilewski MK, Statler CC, Kohut G, Toriello HV (1996) Congenital pulmonary lymphangiectasia and other anomalies in a child: provisionally unique syndrome? Am J Med Genet 66: 438-40

11. Kerhoas Nicolas CK, Le Bidaut M, Dosquet C, Enjolras O, Stalder JF (1997) Kasabach-Merritt syndrome of the leg associated with osteolysis or Gorham sign. Ann Dermatol Venereol 124: 852-4

12. Njolstad PR, Reigstad H, Westby J, Espeland A (1998) Familial non-immune hydrops fetalis and congenital pulmonary lymphangiectasia. Eur J Pediatr 157: 498-501

13. Misery L, Lachaux A, Chambon M, Faure M, Claudy A (1996) Waldman's disease. Primary intestinal lymphangiectasis. Ann Dermatol Venereol 123: 567-8

14. Dellamonica P, Lapeyre L, Martin J (1975) Chylometrorrhea. Clinical manifestation of primary chyle reflux. Nouv Presse Med 4: 3129-31

15. Klippel M, Trénaunay P (1900) Du naevus variqueux ostéo-hypertrophique. Arch Gen Med (Paris) 185: 641-72

16. Weber FP (1907) Angioma-formation in connection with hypertrophy of limbs and hemi-hypertrophy. Br J Dermatol 19: 231-5

17. Jacob AG, Driscoll DJ, Shaughnessy WJ, Stanton AW, Clay RP, Gloviczki P (1998) Klippel-Trenaunay syndrome: spectrum and management. Mayo Clin Proc 73: 28-36

18. Christenson L, Yankowitz J, Robinson R (1997) Prenatal diagnosis of Klippel-Trenaunay syndrome as a cause for in utero heart failure and severe postnatal sequelae. Prenat Diagn 17: 1176-80

19. Ceballos-Quintal JM, Pinto-Escalante D, Castillo-Zapata I (1996) A new case of Klippel-Trenaunay-Weber (KTW) syndrome: evidence of autosomal dominant inheritance. Am J Med Genet 63: 426-7

20. Lorda-Sanchez I, Prieto L, Rodriguez-Pinilla E, Martinez-Frias ML (1998) Increased parental age and number of pregnancies in Klippel-Trenaunay-Weber syndrome. Ann Hum Genet 62: 235-9

21. Craven N, Wright AL (1995) Familial Klippel-Trenaunay syndrome: a case report. Clin Exp Dermatol 20: 76-9

22. Whelan AJ, Watson MS, Porter FD, Steiner RD (1995) Klippel-Trenaunay-Weber syndrome associated with a 5: 11 balance translocation. Am J Med Genet 59: 492-4

23. Aronoff DM, Roshon M (1998) Severe hemorrhage complicating the Klippel-Trenaunay-Weber syndrome. South Med J 91: 1073-5

24. Reize P, Schonthaler M, Sell S (1997) Proteus syndrome: a case report. Z Orthop Ihre Grenzgeb 135: 174-8

25. Furukawa T, Igata A, Toyokura Y (1970) Ikeda S: Sturge-Weber and Klippel-Trenaunay syndrome with nevus of Ota and Ito. Arch Dermatol 102: 640-5

26. Sujansky E, Conradi S (1995) Outcome of Sturge-Weber syndrome in 52 adults. Am J Med Genet 57: 35-45

27. Sujansky E, Conradi S (1995) Sturge-Weber syndrome: age of onset of seizures and glaucoma and the prognosis for affected children. J Child Neurol 10: 49-58

28. Jessen RT, Thompson S, Smith EB (1977) Cobb syndrome. Arch Dermatol 113: 1587-90

29. Kraus GE, Bucholz RD, Weber TR (1990) Spinal cord arteriovenous malformation with an associated lymphatic anomaly. Case report. J Neurosurg 73: 768-73

30. Stein J, Myers SJ (1992) Spinal cord arteriovenous malformation in a person with congenital lymphatic abnormalities. Am J Phys Med Rehabil 71: 349-51

31. Shim JH, Lee DW, Cho BK (1996) A case of Cobb syndrome associated with lymphangioma circumscriptum. Dermatology 193: 45-7

32. Lewis RJ, Ketcham A (1973) Maffucci's syndrome: functional and neoplastic significance. J Bone Joint Surg 55A: 1465-79

33. Davidson TI, Kissin MW, Bradish CF, Westbury G (1985) Angiosarcoma arising in a patient with Maffucci syndrome. Eur J Surg Oncol 11: 381-4

34. Mazabraud A (1994) Anatomie pathologique osseuse tumorale. Springer-Verlag, Paris Berlin Heidelberg NewYork Londres Tokyo HongKong Barcelone Budapest

35. Fanburg JC, Meis-Kindblom JM, Rosenberg AE (1995) Multiple endochondromas associated with spindle-cell hemangioendotheliomas. An overlooked variant of Maffuci's syndrome. Am J Surg Pathol 19: 1029-38

36. Tadaki T, Aiba S, Masu S, Tagami H (1988) Acquired progressive lymphangioma as a flat erythematous patch on the abdominal wall of a child. Arch Dermatol 124: 699-701

37. Wilson Jones E, Winkelmann RK, Zachary CB, Reda AM (1990) Benign lymphangio-endothelioma. J Am Acad Dermatol 23: 229-35

38. Needleman RL (1996) Gorham's disease: a literature review and case reports (letter). J Foot Ankle Surg 35: 369

39. Panich V (1994) Splenic cystic lymphangiomatosis: an unusual cause of massive splenomegaly: report of a case. J Med Assoc Thai 77: 165-8

40. de Souza LM, Bentlin MR, de Abreu ES, Bacchi CE (1996) Systemic congenital lymphangiomatosis. Rev Paul Med 114: 1278-81

41. Dutheil P, Leraillez J, Guillemette J, Wallach D (1998) Generalized lymphangiomatosis with chylothorax and skin lymphangiomas in a neonate. Pediatr Dermatol 15: 296-8

42. Van den Houten BR, Kate T, Gerding JC (1985) The Hajdu-Cheney syndrome. A review of the literature and report of three cases. Int J Oral Surg 14: 113-25

43. Takeda Y, Kuroda M, Suzuki A, Fujioka F, Takayama K (1987) Massive osteolysis of the mandible. Acta Pathol Jpn 37: 677-84

44. Damron TA, Brodke DS, Heiner JP, Swan JS, De Souky S (1993) Gorham's disease (Gorham-Stout syndrome) of scapula. Case report. Skeletal Radiol 22: 464-7

45. Swensen SJ, Hartman TE, Mayo JR, Colby TV, Tazelaar HD, Muller NL (1995) Diffuse pulmonary lymphangiomatosis: CT findings. J Comput Assist Tomogr 19: 348-52

46. Gutierrez RM, Spjut HJ (1972) Skelettal angiomatosis: report of three cases and review of the literature. Clin Orthop Rel Res 85: 82-97

47. Najman E, Fabeici-Sabadi V, Temmer B (1967) Lymphangioma in the inguinal region with cystic lymphangiomatosis of bone. J Pediatr 71: 561-6

48. Kandil A, Rostom AY, Mourad WA, Khafaga Y, Gershuny AR, el-Hosseiny G (1997) Successful control of extensive thoracic lymphangiomatosis by irradiation. Clin Oncol (R Coll Radiol) 9: 407-11

49. Patton DF, Kaye R, Dickman P, Blatt J (1998) Partial splenic embolization for treatment of disseminated intravascular coagulation in lymphangiomatosis. J Pediatr 132: 1057-60

50. Ramani P, Shah A (1993) Lymphangiomatosis. Histologic and immunohistochemical analysis of four cases. Am J Surg Pathol 17: 329-35

51. Tazelaar HD, Kerr D, Yousem SA, Saldana MJ, Langston C, Colby TV (1993) Diffuse pulmonary lymphangiomatosis. Hum Pathol 24: 1313-22

52. Carlson KC, Parnassus WN, Klatt EC (1987) Thoracic lymphangiomatosis. Arch Pathol Lab Med 111: 475-7

53. Bloch P, Meshaka G, Takeara E, Hamdan M (1989) Diffuse retroperitoneal lymphangioleiomatosis. Presse Med 18: 2011-3

54. Younathan CM, Kaude JV (1992) Renal peripelvic lymphatic cysts (lymphangiomas) associated with generalized lymphangiomatosis. Urol Radiol 14: 161-4

55. Brown RR, Pathria MN, Ruggieri PM, Jacobson JA, Craig JG, Resnick D (1997) Extensive intraosseous gas associated with lymphangiomatosis of bone: report of three cases. Radiology 205: 260-2

56. Ohori NP, Yousem SA, Sonmez-Alpan E, Colby TV (1991) Estrogen and progesterone receptors in lymphangioleiomyomatosis, epithelioid hemangioendothelioma, and sclerosing hemangioma of the lung. Am J Clin Pathol 96: 529-35

57. Sathyavagiswaran L, Sherwin RP (1989) Acute and chronic pericholangiolitis in association with multifocal hepatic lymphangiomatosis. Hum Pathol 20: 601-3

58. Houissa H, Jouini M, Kacem M, Safta ZB, Belaid S (1994) Cystic lymphangioma of the spleen. An exceptional site. Ann Gastroenterol Hepatol (Paris) 30: 215-7

59. Takami A, Nakao S, Sugimori N, Ishida F, Yamazaki M, Nakatsumi Y, Saito M, Otake S, Nakamura S, Matsuda T (1995) Management of disseminated intra-abdominal lymphangiomatosis with protein-losing enteropathy and intestinal bleeding. South Med J 88: 1156-8

60. Iwabuchi A, Otaka M, Okuyama A, Jin M, Otani S, Itoh S, Sasahara H, Odashima M, Kotanagi H, Satoh M, Masuda H, Masamune O (1997) Disseminated intra-abdominal cystic lymphangiomatosis with severe intestinal bleeding. A case report. J Clin Gastroenterol 25: 383-6

61. Barrière H, Stalder JF, Chailleux E, De Kersaint-Gily A, Bolz JL (1981) Sclérose tubéreuse de Bourneville et lymphangiomyomatose. Sem Hôp Paris 57: 321-6

62. Capron F, Ameille J, Leclerc P, Mornet P, Barbagellata M, Reynès M, Rochemaure J (1983) Pulmonary lymphangioleiomyomatosis and Bourneville's tuberous sclerosis with pulmonary involvement: the same disease ? Cancer 52: 851-5

63. About I, Capdeville J, Voigt JJ, Bernard P, Michetti C, Faizon R (1994) Renal angiomyolipoma and pulmonary lymphangiomyomatosis: a non-fortuitous association. Rev Med Interne 15: 279-81

64. Bradley SL, Dines DE, Soule EH, Muhm JR (1980) Pulmonary lymphangiomatosis. Lung 158: 69-80

65. Malan E, Fuglionisi A (1964) Congenital angiodysplasias of the extremities (note I: generalities and classification; venous dysplasia). J Cardiovasc Surg (Torino) 5: 87-130

66. Rao VK, Weiss SW (1992) Angiomatosis of soft tissue: an analysis of the histologic features and clinical outcome in 51 cases. Am J Surg Pathol 16: 764-71

67. Allen PW (1994) Three new vascular tumors– Tufted angioma, Kaposiform infantile hemangioendothelioma and Proliferative cutaneous angiomatosis. Int J Pathol 2: 63-72

68. Szlachetka DM (1998) Kasabach-Merritt syndrome: a case review. Neonatal Netw 17: 7-15

69. Brooks J, Elenitsas R, Hicks D, Elder D (1993) Proliferative cutaneous angiomatosis: A cellular tumor mimicking angiosarcoma and Kaposi's sarcoma (abstract). Mod Pathol 6: 5A

70. Vin-Christian K, McCalmont TH, Frieden IJ (1997) Kaposiform hemangioendothelioma. An aggressive, locally invasive vascular tumor that can mimic hemangioma of infancy. Arch Dermatol 133: 1573-8

71. d'Udekem Y, Rubay JE, Sluysmans T (1997) A case of neonatal ductus arteriosus aneurysm. Cardiovasc Surg 5: 338-9

72. Gittenberger-de Groot AC (1977) Persistent ductus arteriosus: most probably a primary congenital malformation. Br Heart J 39: 610-8

73. Gittenberger-de Groot AC, Moulaert AJ, Harinck E, Becker AE (1978) Histopathology of the ductus arteriosus after prostaglandin E1 administration in ductus dependent cardiac anomalies. Br Heart J 40: 215-20

74. Gittenberger-de Groot AC, Moulaert AJ, Hitchcock JF (1980) Histology of the persistent ductus arteriosus in cases of congenital rubella. Circulation 62: 183-6

75. Valenzuela Garcia LF, Vazquez Garcia R, Pastor Morales L, Calvo Jambrina R, Rodriguez Hernandez MJ, Font Cabrera I Cubero Garcia J, Pastor Torres L, Cruz Fernandez JM, Infantes Alcon C (1998) Aortic coarctation: different anatomo-clinical forms depending on the age of presentation. Rev Esp Cardiol 51: 572-81

76. Elzenga NJ, Gittenberger-de Groot AC (1983) Localised coarctation of the aorta. An age dependent spectrum. Br Heart J 49: 317-23

77. Machii M, Becker AE (1995) Nature of coarctation in hypoplastic left heart syndrome. Ann Thorac Surg 59: 1491-4

78. Sarigul A, Yurdakul Y, Isbir S, Mercan S, Celiker A (1997) Bicuspid aortic valve and coarctation of aorta. Turk J Pediatr 39: 429-32

79. Yamaguchi A, Adachi H, Kamio H, Murata S, Okada M, Adachi K, Ino T, Ichikawa T, Nagai J, Yamada S (1998) A combination of preductal aortic coarctation and type B dissection: report of a case. Surg Today 28: 435-7

80. Goh WH, Lo R (1993) A new 3C syndrome: cerebellar hypoplasia, cavernous haemangioma and coarctation of the aorta. Dev Med Child Neurol 35: 637-41

81. Heath D, Smith P, Hurst G (1986) The carotid bodies in coarctation of the aorta. Br J Dis Chest 80: 122-30

82. Deluca SA (1990) Coarctation of the aorta. Am Fam Physician 42: 1285-8

83. Aota M, Nomoto S, Yamaki S, Ban T (1997) Pulmonary hypertension caused by medial hypertrophy associated with aortic stenosis and preductal coarctation. Ann Thorac Surg 64: 244-7

84. Hasegawa T, Yoshioka Y, Sasaki T, Iwasaki Y, Miki Y, Sumimura J, Koyama H, Dezawa T (1997) Necrotizing enterocolitis in a term infant with coarctation of the aorta complex. Pediatr Surg Int 12: 57-8

85. Bonhoeffer P, Bonnet D, Sidi D, Kachaner J (1997) Thrombus in coarctation of the aorta masquerading as an interrupted aortic arch. Heart 77: 183-4

86. Mitchell IM, Pollock JC (1990) Coarctation of the aorta and post-stenotic aneurysm formation. Br Heart J 64: 332-3

87. Kido M, Ueda T, Mitsumaru A, Nakamichi T, Yasudo M, Kawada S (1997) A case report of postcoarctation mycotic aneurysm after surgical treatment for cerebral arterial aneurysms. Nippon Kyobu Geka Gakkai Zasshi 45: 1006-10

88. Kurien A, John PR, Milford DV (1997) Hypertension secondary to progressive vascular neurofibromatosis. Arch Dis Child 76: 454-55

89. Elzenga NJ, Gittenberger-de Groot AC (1985) Coarctation and related aortic arch anomalies in hypoplastic left heart syndrome. Int J Cardiol 8: 379-93

90. Elzenga NJ, Gittenberger-de Groot AC, Oppenheimer-Dekker A (1986) Coarctation and other obstructive aortic arch anomalies: their relationship to the ductus arteriosus. Int J Cardiol 13: 289-308

91. Bergamini TM, Bernard JD, Mavroudis C, Backer CL, Muster AJ, Richardson JD (1995) Coarctation of the abdominal aorta. Ann Vasc Surg 9: 352-6

92. Mickley V, Lang G, Fleiter T, Sunder-Plassmann L (1997) Atypical aortic coarctations in type I neurofibromatosis. Zentralbl Chir 122: 735-42

93. Edwards JE, Titus Jl (1995) Congenital anomalies of blood vessels and their complications In Stehbens WE, Lie JT (Eds.) Vascular Pathology, Chapman&Hall, London pp21-61

94. Korenberg JR, Kawashima H, Pulst SM, Allen L, Magenis E, Epstein CJ (1990) Down syndrome: toward a molecular definition of the phenotype. Am J Med Genet Suppl 7: 91-7

95. Cooley WC, Graham JM Jr (1991) Down syndrome—an update and review for the primary pediatrician. Clin Pediatr (Phila) 30: 233-53

96. Geggel RL, O'Brien JE, Feingold M (1993) Development of valve dysfunction in adolescents and young adults with Down syndrome and no known congenital heart disease. J Pediatr 122: 821-3

97. Gembruch U, Baschat AA, Knopfle G, Hansmann M (1997) Results of chromosomal analysis in fetuses with cardiac anomalies as diagnosed by first– and early second-trimester echocardiography. Ultrasound Obstet Gynecol 10: 391-6

98. Chervenak FA, Isaacson G, Blackemore KJ, Breg WR, Hobbins JC, Berkowitz RL, Tottora M, Mayden K, Mahonay M (1983) Fetal cystic hygroma. N Engl J Med 309: 822-5

99. Descamps P, Jourdain O, Paillet C, Toutain A, Guichet A, Pourcelot D, Gold F, Castiel M, Body G (1997) Etiology, prognosis and management of nuchal cystic hygroma: 25 new cases and literature review. Eur J Obstet Gynecol Reprod Biol 71: 3-10

100. Couceiro Gianzo JA, Perez Cobeta R, Fuster Siebert M, Barreiro Conde J, Pombo Arias M (1996) The Turner syndrome and cardiovascular changes. An Esp Pediatr 44: 242-4

101. Ruibal Francisco JL, Sanchez Buron P, Pinero Martinez E, Bueno Lozano G, Reverte Blanc F (1997) Turner's syndrome. Relationship between the karyotypes and malformations and associated diseases in 23 patients. An Esp Pediatr 47: 167-71

102. Nora JJ, Clarke Fraser F (1974) Medical genetics: Principles and practice. Lea & Febiger, Philadelphia, 399 p

103. Gomez-Valencia L, Najera-Martinez P, Morales-Hernandez A, Martinez-Diaz De Leon A (1989) Penta-X syndrome. Report of a case with 47, XXX/48, XXXX/49, XXXXX mosaicism. Bol Med Hosp Infant Mex 46: 417-21

104. Kassai R, Hamada I, Furuta H, Cho K, Abe K, Deng HX, Niikawa N (1991) Penta X syndrome: a case report with review of the literature. Am J Med Genet 40: 51-6

105. Karsh RB (1975) Congenital heart disease in 49, XXXXY syndrome. Pediatrics 56: 462-4

106. Muis N, Cats BP, Ippel PF, Beemer FA (1982) A newborn infant with the XXXXY-syndrome. Tijdschr Kindergeneeskd 50: 112-6

107. Sutherland GR, Mulley JL, Richards RI (1993) Fragile X syndrome. The most common cause of familial intellectual handicap. Med J Aust 158: 482-5

108. Hagerman RJ, Synhorst DP (1984) Mitral valve prolapse and aortic dilatation in the fragile X syndrome. Am J Med Genet 17: 123-31

109. Loehr JP, Synhorst DP, Wolfe RR, Hagerman RJ (1986) Aortic root dilations and mitral valve prolapse in the fragile X syndrome. Am J Med Genet 23: 189-94

110. Sreeram N, Wren C, Bhate M, Robertson P, Hunter S (1989) Cardiac abnormalities in the fragile X syndrome. Br Heart J 61: 289-91

111. Nadazdin A, Shahi M, Foale RA (1991) Impaired left ventricular filling during ST-segment depression provoked by dipyridamole infusion in patients with syndrome X. Clin Cardiol 14: 821-6

112. Crabbe LS, Bensky AS, Hornstein L, Schwartz DC (1993) Cardiovascular abnormalities in children with fragile X syndrome. Pediatrics 91: 714-5

113. Waldstein G, Hagerman R (1988) Aortic hypoplasia and cardiac valvular abnormalities in a boy with fragile X syndrome. Am J Med Genet 30: 83-98

114. Eng CM, Ashley GA, Burgert TS, Enriquez AL, D'Souza M, Desnick RJ (1997) Fabry disease: thirty five mutations in the alpha-galactosidase A gene in patients with classic and variant phenotypes. Mol Med 3: 174-82

115. Le Bodic MF, Le Bodic L, Buzelin F, Bureau B, Mussini-Montpellier J (1978) Vascular lesions of Fabry's disease. Optical, histochemical and ultrastructural studies. Ann Anat Pathol (Paris) 23: 23-39

116. Smith P, Heath D, Rodgers B, Helliwell T (1991) Pulmonary vasculature in Fabry's disease. Histopathology 19: 567-9

117. Kanda A, Nakao S, Tsuyama S, Murata F, Kanzaki T (2000) Fabry disease: ultrastructural lectin histochemical analyses of lysosomal deposits. Virchows Arch 436: 36-42

118. Li P, Thompson JN, Hug G, Huffman P, Chuck G (1996) Biochemical and molecular analysis in a patient with the severe form of Hunter syndrome after bone marrow transplantation. Am J Med Genet 64: 531-5

119. Davous P (1998) CADASIL: a review with proposed diagnostic criteria. Eur J Neurol 5: 219-33

120. Chabriat H, Vahedi K, Iba-Zizen MT, Joutel A, Nibbio A, Nagy TG, Krebs MO, Julien J, Dubois B, Ducrocq X, et al (1995) Clinical spectrum of CADASIL: a study of 7 families. Cerebral autosomal dominant arteriopathy with subcortical infarcts and leukoencephalopathy. Lancet 346(8980): 934-9

121. Dichgans M, Mayer M, Uttner I, Bruning R, Muller-Hocker J, Rungger G, Ebke M, Klockgether T, Gasser T (1998) The phenotypic spectrum of CADASIL: clinical findings in 102 cases. Ann Neurol 44: 731-9

122. Desmond DW, Moroney JT, Lynch T, Chan S, Chin SS, Mohr JP (1999) The natural history of CADASIL: a pooled analysis of previously published cases. Stroke 30: 1230-3

123. Kalimo H, Viitanen M, Amberla K, Juvonen V, Marttila R, Poyhonen M, Rinne JO, Savontaus M, Tuisku S, Winblad B (1999) CADASIL: hereditary disease of arteries causing brain infarcts and dementia. Neuropathol Appl Neurobiol 25: 257-65

124. Ebke M, Dichgans M, Bergmann M, Voelter HU, Rieger P, Gasser T, Schwendemann G (1997) CADASIL: skin biopsy allows diagnosis in early stages. Acta Neurol Scand 95: 351-7

125. Mayer M, Straube A, Bruening R, Uttner I, Pongratz D, Gasser T, Dichgans M, Muller-Hocker J (1999) Muscle and skin biopsies are a sensitive diagnostic tool in the diagnosis of CADASIL. J Neurol 246: 526-32

126. Ruchoux MM, Maurage CA (1998) Endothelial changes in muscle and skin biopsies in patients with CADASIL. Neuropathol Appl Neurobiol 24: 60-5

127. Paradisi M, Giubilei L, Canzona F, Angelo C, Onetti Muda A, Puddu P (1997) Ehlers-Danlos syndrome type I. Ultrastructural study. Minerva Pediatr 49: 215-9

128. Beighton P, Curtis D (1985) X-linked Ehlers-Danlos syndrome type V; the next generation. Clin Genet 27: 472-8

129. Byers PH, Holbrook KA (1990) Ehlers-Danlos syndrome In Emery AE, Rimoin DL (eds.): Principles and Practice of Medical Genetics, 2nd ed. New York, Churchill Livingstone, p. 1065

130. Germain D (1995) Ehlers-Danlos syndromes. Clinical, genetic and molecular aspects. Ann Dermatol Venereol 122: 187-204

131. Smith LT, Schwarze U, Goldstein J, Byers PH (1997) Mutations in the COL3A1 gene result in the Ehlers-Danlos syndrome type IV and alterations in the size and distribution of the major collagen fibrils of the dermis. J Invest Dermatol 108: 241-7

132. Albat B, Boismenu L, Thevenet A (1993) Aortic rupture in a patient with Ehlers-Danlos type IV syndrome. Presse Med 22: 1975-6

133. de Wazières B, Coppère B, Durieu I, Fest T, Ninet J, Levrat R, Vuitton DA, Dupond JL (1995) Vascular and/or cardiac manifestations of type IV Ehlers-Danlos syndrome. 9 cases. Presse Med 24: 1381-5

134. Wimmer PJ, Howes DS, Rumoro DP, Carbone M (1996) Fatal vascular catastrophe in Ehlers-Danlos syndrome: a case report and review.J Emerg Med 14: 25-31

135. Brandt T, Hausser I, Orberk E, Grau A, Hartschuh W, Anton-Lamprecht I, Hacke W (1998) Ultrastructural connective tissue abnormalities in patients with spontaneous cervicocerebral artery dissections. Ann Neurol 44: 281-5

136. Lach B, Nair SG, Russel NA, Benoit BG (1987) Spontaneous carotid-cavernous fistula and multiple arterial dissections in type IV Ehlers-Danlos syndrome. J Neurosurg 66: 462-7

137. Superti-Furga A, Saesseli B, Steinmann B, Bollinger A (1992) Microangiopathy in Ehlers-Danlos syndrome type IV. Int J Microcirc Clin Exp 11: 241-7

138. Olgunturk FR, Tunaoglu FS, Gumus H, Beyazova U, Turkyilmaz C (1993) Diffuse arterial aneurysms in a case of Ehlers-Danlos syndrome—a case report. Angiology 44: 909-13

139. Minola E, Maculotti L (1994) Multiple vascular lesions in a patient with Ehlers-Danlos type IV. Pathologica 86: 61-5

140. Maeda T, Suzuki Y, Haeno S, Asada M, Hiramatsu R, Tanaka F, Okada M, Suzuki T (1996) Ehlers-Danlos syndrome and congenital heart anomalies. Intern Med 35: 200 -2

141. Henry C, Geiss S, Wodey E, Pennerath A, Zabot MT, Peyrol S, Plauchu H (1995) Spontaneous colonic perforations revealing Ehlers-Danlos syndrome type IV. Arch Pediatr 2: 1067-72

142. Tiller GE, Cassidy SB, Wensel C, Wenstrup RJ (1998) Aortic root dilatation in Ehlers-Danlos syndrome types I, II and III. A report of five cases. Clin Genet 53: 460-5

143. Engle J, Safi HJ, Abassi O, Iliopoulos DC, Dorsay D, Cartwright J Jr, Weilbaecher D (1997) Muco-polysaccharidosis presenting as paediatric multiple aortic aneurysm: first reported case. J Vasc Surg 26: 704-10

144. Latif F, Tory K, Gnarra J, Yao M, Duh FM, Orcutt ML, Stackhouse T, Kuzmin I, Modi W, Geil L et al (1993) Identification of the von Hippel-Lindau disease tumor suppressor gene. Science 260(5112): 1317-20

145. Szymanski SC, Hummerich H, Latif F, Lerman MI, Rohrborn G, Schroder E (1993) Long range restriction map of the von Hippel-Lindau gene region on human chromosome 3p. Hum Genet 92: 282-8

146. McKusick VA (1991) The defect in Marfan syndrome. Nature 352(6333): 279-81

147. Pyeritz, RE (1990) Marfan's syndrome In Emery AE, Rimoin DL (eds.) Principles and Practice of Medical Genetics, 2nd ed. New York, Churchill Livingstone, p 1047

148. Dietz HC, Pyeritz RE, Hall BD, Cadle RG, Hamosh A, Schwartz J Meyers DA, Francomano CA (1991) The Marfan syndrome locus: confirmation of assignment to chromosome 15 and identification of tightly linked markers at 15q15-q21.3. Genomics 9: 355-61

149. Milewicz DM, Pyeritz RE, Crawford ES, Byers PH (1992) Marfan syndrome: defective synthesis, secretion, and extracellular matrix formation of fibrillin by cultured dermal fibroblasts. J Clin Invest 89: 79-86

150. Segura AM, Luna RE, Horiba K, Stetler-Stevenson WG, McAllister HA Jr, Willerson JT, Ferrans VJ (1998) Immunohistochemistry of matrix metalloproteinases and their inhibitors in thoracic aortic aneurysms and aortic valves of patients with Marfan's syndrome. Circulation 98: SII331-SII337

151. Raghunath M, Superti-Furga A, Godfrey M, Steinmann B (1993) Decreased extracellular deposition of fibrillin and decorin in neonatal Marfan syndrome fibroblasts.Hum Genet 90: 511-5

152. Boileau C, Collod G, Bonnet D (1997) Contribution of genetics to pathogenicity and diagnosis of Marfan syndrome. Arch Mal Cœur Vaiss 90: S1707-S1712

153. Prahlow JA, Barnard JJ, Milewicz DM (1998) Familial thoracic aortic aneurysms and dissections. J Forensic Sci 43: 1244-9

154. Kudlicki J, Drozd J, Oleszczuk J (1997) Pregnancy in women with Marfan's syndrome. Ginekol Pol 68: 94-101

155. Brees CK, GRll SA (1995) Rupture of the external iliac artery during pregnancy: a case of type IV Ehlers-Danlos syndrome. J Ky Med Assoc 93: 553-5

156. Babatasi G, Massetti M, Saloux E, Grollier G, Agostini D, Potier JC, Khayat A (1998) Ehlers-Danlos disease revealed during pregnancy through the diagnosis of aortic dissection. Arch Mal Cœur Vaiss 91: 83-6

157. Rasmussen LA, Lund JT, Pettersson G (1998) Marfan syndrome and pregnancy. Ugeskr Laeger 160: 6219-20

158. Gott VL (1998) Antoine Marfan and his syndrome: one hundred years later. Md Med J 47: 247-52

159. Antman EM (1994) Current diagnosis and prescription for Marfan's syndrome: When to operate? Journal of Cardiac Surgery 9: S174-S176

160. Gott VL, Cameron DE, Pyeritz RE, Gillinov AM, Greene PS, Stone CD, Alejo DE, McKusick VA (1994) Composite graft repair of Marfan aneurysm of the ascending aorta: results in 150 patients. J Card Surg 9: 482-9

161. Eliashar R, Sichel JY, Biron A, Dano I (1998) Multiple gastrointestinal complications in Marfan syndrome. Postgrad Med J 74: 495-7

162. Paternoster DM, Santarossa C, Vettore N, Dalla Pria S, Grella P (1998) Obstetric complications in Marfan's syndrome pregnancy. Minerva Ginecol 50: 441-3

163. Mulvihill JJ, Parry DM, Sherman JL, Pikus A, Kaiser-Kupfer MI, Eldridge R (1990) NIH conference. Neurofibromatosis 1 (Recklinghausen disease) and neurofibromatosis 2 (bilateral acoustic neurofibromatosis). An update. Ann Intern Med 113: 39-52

164. Gutmann DH, Collins FS (1993) The neurofibromatosis type 1 gene and its protein product, neurofibromin. Neuron 10: 335-43

165. Rouleau GA, Merel P, Lutchman M, Sanson M, Zucman J, Marineau C, Hoang-Xuan K, Demczuk S, Desmaze C, Plougastel B, et al (1993) Alteration in a new gene encoding a putative membrane-organizing protein causes neuro-fibromatosis type 2. Nature 363(6429): 515-21

166. Vuong PN, Le Bourgeois P, Houissa-Vuong S, Martin P, Berrod J-L (2001) Intimal muscular fibrodysplasia responsible for an ischemic gastric ulcer in a patient with a von Recklinghausen's disease: a case report. J Mas Vas (Paris) 26: 65-68

167. Planche C, Camilleri JP, El Abdel Hafez A, Zannier D, Mercier JN, Artru B (1983) Lesions of the aortic arch in Recklinghausen's disease. Arch Mal Cœur Vaiss 76: 607-13

168. Debure C, Fiessinger JN, Bruneval P, Vuong NP, Cormier JM, Housset E (1984) Multiple arterial lesions in von Recklinghausen's disease. A case. Presse Med 13: 1776-8

169. Nopajaroonsri C, Lurie AA (1996) Venous aneurysm, arterial dysplasia, and near-fatal hemorrhages in neurofibromatosis type 1. Hum Pathol 27: 982-5

170. Finley JL, Dabbs DJ (1988) Renal vascular smooth muscle proliferation in neurofibromatosis. Hum Pathol 19: 107-10

171. Edwards MJ, Graham JM Jr (1990) Posterior nuchal cystic hygroma. Clin Perinatol 17: 611-40

172. Langer JC, Fitzgerald PG, Desa D, Filly RA, Golbus MS, Adzick NS, Harrison MR (1990) Cervical cystic hygroma in the fetus: clinical spectrum and outcome. J Pediatr Surg 25: 58-61

173. Roth A (1984) Lymphangiectasies disséminées cutanées congénitales, pleurales et intestinales. Arch Anat Cytol Pathol 32: 349-52

174. Pruvo JP, Rufenacht D, Leclerc X, Merland JJ (1996) Malformations vasculaires de la moelle. Feuillets de Radiologie 36: 471-84

175. Ahr DJ, Rickles FR, Hoyer LW, O'Leary DS, Conrad ME (1977) von Willebrand's disease and hemorrhagic telangiectasia: association of two complex disorders of hemostasis resulting in life-threatening hemorrhage. Am J Med 62: 452-8

176. Gilford H (1904) Ateleiosis and progeria: continuous youth and premature old age. Brit Med J 2: 914-8

177. Erdem N, Gunes AT, Avci O, Osma E (1994) A case of Hutchinson-Gilford progeria syndrome mimicking scleredema in early infancy. Dermatology 188: 318-21

178. Baker PB, Baba N, Boesel CP (1981) Cardiovascular abnormalities in progeria. Case report and review of the literature. Arch Pathol Lab Med 105: 384-6

179. Ha JW, Shim WH, Chung NS (1993) Cardiovascular findings of Hutchinson-Gilford syndrome – a Doppler and two-dimensional echocardiographic study. Yonsei Med J 34: 352-5

180. Matsuo S, Takeuchi Y, Hayashi S, Kinugasa A, Sawada T (1994) Patient with unusual Hutchinson-Gilford syndrome (progeria). Pediatr Neurol 10: 237-40

181. Dyck, J D, David TE, Burke B, Webb GD, Henderson MA, Fowler RS (1987) Management of coronary artery disease in Hutchinson-Gilford syndrome. J. Pediat. 111: 407-10

182. Monu JU, Benka-Coker LB, Fatunde Y (1990) Hutchinson-Gilford progeria syndrome in siblings. Report of three new cases. Skeletal Radiol 19: 585-90

183. Parkash H, Sidhu SS, Raghavan R, Deshmukh RN (1990) Hutchinson-Gilford progeria: familial occurrence. Am J Med Genet 36: 431-3

184. Riedel H (1980) Morphologic contribution to a progeria syndrome (Hutchinson-Gilford). Zentralbl Allg Pathol 124: 410-5

185. Paraf F, Bruneval P (1996) Arterial fibromuscular dysplasia and Bourneville's tuberous sclerosis. Ann Pathol 16: 203-6

186. Gaines Jr JJ (1989) The pathology of alkaptonuric ochronosis. Hum Pathol 20: 40-6

187. Kenny D, Ptacin MJ, Bamrah VS, Almagro U (1990) Cardiovascular ochronosis: a case report and review of the medical literature. Cardiology 77: 477-83

188. Moghadam BK, Zadeh JY, Gier RE (1993) Ataxia-telangiectasia. Review of the literature and a case report. Oral Surg Oral Med Oral Pathol 75: 791-7

189. Amromin GD, Boder E, Teplitz R (1979) Ataxia-telangiectasia with a 32 year survival. A clinico-pathological report. J Neuropathol Exp Neurol 38: 621-43

190. Donner MG, Schwandt P, Richter WO (1997) Homocysteine and coronary heart disease. Is slight or moderate homocysteinemia related to increased risk of coronary heart disease? Fortschr Med 115: 24-30

191. Almgren B, Eriksson I, Hemmingsson A, Hillerdal G, Larsson E, Aberg H (1978) Abdominal aortic aneurysm in homocystinuria. Acta Chir Scand 144: 545-8

192. McCully KS (1993) Chemical pathology of homocysteine. I. Atherogenesis. Ann Clin Lab Sci 23: 477-93

193. D'Angelo A, Mazzola G, Crippa L, Fermo I, Vigano D'Angelo S (1997) Hyperhomocysteinemia and venous thromboembolic disease. Haematologica 82: 211-9

194. Bakker RC, Brandjes DP (1997) Hyperhomo-cysteinae-mia and associated disease. Pharm World Sci 19: 126-32

195. de Jong SC, van den Berg M, Rauwerda JA, Stehouwer CD (1998) Hyperhomocysteinemia and atherothrombotic disease. Semin Thromb Hemost 24: 381-5

196. Muenzer J (1986) Mucopolysaccharidoses. Adv Pediatr 33: 269-302

197. Pagni L, Bartolozzi L, Giacchetti D (1992) Mucopoly-saccharidosis. A case report of Morquio's type-A disease (MPS IV-A). Minerva Stomatol 41: 527-33

198. Balcavage WX, King MM (1995) Biochemistry: Examination and Board Review. Appleton and Lange, Norwalk

199. Factor SM, Biempica L, Goldfischer S (1978) Coronary intimal sclerosis in Morquio's syndrome. Virchows Arch A Pathol Pathol Anat 379: 1-10

200. Blackburn WE, McRoberts JW, Bhathena D, Vasquez M, Luke RG (1975) Severe vascular complications in oxalosis after bilateral nephrectomy. Ann Intern Med 82: 44-6

201. Baethge BA, Sanusi ID, Landreneau MD, Rohr MS, McDonald JC (1988) Livedo reticularis and peripheral gangrene associated with primary hyperoxaluria. Arthritis Rheum 31: 1199-203

202. Di Pasquale G, Ribani M, Andreoli A, Zampa GA, Pinelli G (1989) Cardioembolic stroke in primary oxalosis with cardiac involvement. Stroke 20: 1403-6

203. Brett F, Kealy WF, Murnaghan D, Hogan JM (1990) Primary hyperoxaluria—a case report. Ir J Med Sci 159: 78-9

204. Spiers EM, Sanders DY, Omura EF (1990) Clinical and histologic features of primary oxalosis. J Am Acad Dermatol 22: 952-6

205. Winship IM, Saxe NP, Hugel H (1991) Primary oxalosis – an unusual cause of livedo reticularis. Clin Exp Dermatol 16: 367-70

206. Magnani G, Fatone F, Martella D, Binetti G, Magnani B (1992) A case of oxalosis with heart and lung involvement. Cardiologia 37: 507-11

207. Farreli J, Shoemaker JD, Otti T, Jordan W, Schoch L, Neu LT, Bastani B (1997) Primary hyperoxaluria in an adult with renal failure, livedo reticularis, retinopathy, and peripheral neuropathy. Am J Kidney Dis 29: 947-52

208. Chopdar A (1975) Multiple major retinal vascular occlusions in sickle cell haemoglobin C disease. Br J Opthalmol 59: 493-6

209. Gerry Jr JL, Bulkley BH, Hutchins GM (1978) Clinicopathologic analysis of cardiac dysfunction in 52 patients with sickle cell anemia. Am J Cardiol 42: 211-6

210. Ishii T, Hosoda Y (1975) Werner's syndrome: autopsy report of one case, with a review of pathologic findings reported in the literature. J Am Geriatr Soc 23: 145-54

211. Tokunaga M, Mori S, Sato K, Nakamura K, Wakamatsu E (1976) Postmortem study of a case of Werner's syndrome. J Am Geriatr Soc 24: 407-11

212. Goto M, Kato Y (1995) Hypercoagulable state indicates an additional risk factor for atherosclerosis in Werner's syndrome. Thromb Haemost 73: 576-8

213. Murano S, Nakazawa A, Saito I, Masuda M, Morisaki N, Akikusa B, Tsuboyama T, Saito Y (1997) Increased blood plasminogen activator inhibitor-1 and intercellular adhesion molecule-1 as possible risk factors of atherosclerosis in Werner syndrome. Gerontology 43 S43-S52

214. Saito Y (1991) Receptor function of low-density lipoproteins in Werner's syndrome. Gerontology 37: S48-S55

215. Fine RM, Derbes VJ, Clark WH (1961) Blue rubber bleb nevus. Arch Dermatol 84: 144-7

216. Kisu T, Yamaoka K, Uchida Y, Mori H, Nakama T, Hisatsugu T, Miyaji H, Motooka M (1986) A case of blue rubber bleb nevus syndrome with familial onset. Gastroenterol Jpn 21: 262-6

217. Gallione CJ, Pasyk KA, Boon LM, Lennon F, Johnson DW, Helmbold EA, Markel DS, Vikkula M, Mulliken JB, Warman ML et al (1995) A gene for familial venous malformations maps to chromosome 9p in a second large kindred. J Med Genet 32: 197-9

218. Sayers CL, Goltz RW, Mottiaz J (1975) Pulmonary elastic tissue in generalized elastolysis (cutis laxa) and Marfan's syndrome: a light and electron microscopic study. J Invest Dermatol 65: 451-7

219. Mehregan AH, Lee SC, Nabai H (1978) Cutis laxa (generalized elastolysis). A report of four cases with autopsy findings. J Cutan Pathol 5: 116-26

220. Muster AJ, Bharati S, Herman JJ, Esterly NB, Gonzales-Crussi F, Holbrook KA (1983) Fatal cardiovascular disease and cutis laxa following acute febrile neutrophilic dermatosis. J Pediatr 102: 243-8

221. Heppner RL, Babbit HI, Bianchine JW, Warbasse JR (1973) Aortic regurgitation and aneurysm of sinus of Valsalva associated with osteogenesis imperfecta. Am J Cardiol 31 654-7

222. Sigmund J, Sperl W, Fink FM, Stos H (1986) Aorteisthmus-stenosen und osteogenesis imperfecta. Pediatr Pathol 21: 343-9

223. Vevaina JR, Mark J (1988) Thoracic hemangiomatosis masquerading as interstitial lung disease. Chest 93: 657-9

224. Faber CN, Yousem SA, Dauber JH, Griffith BP, Hardesty RL, Paradis IL (1989) Pulmonary capillary hemangiomatosis. A report of three cases and a review of the literature. Am J Resp Dis 140: 808-13

225. Domingo C, Encabo B, Roig J, Lopez D, Morena J (1992) Pulmonary capillary hemangiomatosis: report of a case and review of the literature. Respiration 59: 178-80

226. Mazur Y, Remberger K (1996) Pulmonary capillary hemangiomatosis as a rare cause of pulmonary hypertension. Path Res Pract 192: 290-5

227. Langleben D, Heneghan JM, Batten AP, Wang NS, Fitch N, Schlesinger RD, Guerraty A, Rouleau JL (1988) Familial pulmonary capillary hemangiomatosis resulting in primary pulmonary hypertension. Ann Intern Med 109: 106-9

228. Tron V, Magee F, Wright JL, Colby T, Churg A (1986) Pulmonary capillary hemangiomatosis. Hum Pathol 17: 1144-50

229. Burnel P, Marcon F, Lucron H, Bosser G, Gilgenkrantz S, Jonveaux P, Chery M, Worms AM (1997) Familial supravalvular aortic stenosis. Investigation in a family and review of the literature. Arch Mal Cœur Vaiss 90: 719-24

230. Ozergin U, Sunam GS, Yeniterzi M, Yuksek T, Solak T, Solak H (1996) Supravalvular aortic stenosis without Williams syndrome. Thorac Cardiovasc Surg 44: 219-21

231. Curran ME, Atkinson DL, Ewart AK, Morris CA, Leppert MF, Keating MT (1993) The elastin gene is disrupted by a translocation associated with supravalvular aortic stenosis. Cell 73: 159-68

232. Kruse K, Pankau R, Gosch A, Wohlfahrt K (1992) Calcium metabolism in Williams-Beuren syndrome. J Pediatr 121: 902-7

233. Folger JrGM (1977) Further observations on the syndrome of idiopathic infantile hypercalcemia associated with supravalvular aortic stenosis. Am Heart J 93: 455-62

234. Karmiloff-Smith A, Tyler LK, Voice K, Sims K, Udwin O, Howlin P, Davies M (1998) Linguistic dissociations in

Williams syndrome: evaluating receptive syntax in on-line and off-line tasks. Neuropsychologia 36: 343-51

235. Chiaravalloti G, Rossomando V, Quinti S, Assanta N, Ughi C, Ceccarelli M (1995) Williams-Beuren syndrome and celiac disease. Minerva Pediatr 47: 43-6

236. Wessel A, Motz R, Pankau R, Bursch JH (1997) Arterial hypertension and blood pressure profile in patients with Williams-Beuren syndrome. Z Kardiol 86: 251-7

237. Joyce CA, Zorich B, Pike SJ, Barber JC, Dennis NR (1996) Williams-Beuren syndrome: phenotypic variability and deletions of chromosomes 7, 11, and 22 in a series of 52 patients. J Med Genet 33: 986-92

238. Brondum-Nielsen K, Beck B, Gyftodimou J, Horlyk H, Liljenberg U, Petersen MB, Pedersen W, Petersen MB, Sand A, Skovby F, Stafanger G, Zetterqvist P, Tommerup N (1997) Investigation of deletions at 7q11.23 in 44 patients referred for Williams-Beuren syndrome, using FISH and four DNA polymorphisms. Hum Genet 99: 56-61

239. Teo SH, Chan DK, Yong MH, Ng IS, Wong KY, Knight L, Ho LY (1997) Williams syndrome – the Singapore General Hospital experience. Ann Acad Med Singapore 26: 360-4

240. Elcioglu N, Mackie-Ogilvie C, Daker M, Berry AC (1998) FISH analysis in patients with clinical diagnosis of Williams syndrome. Acta Paediatr 87: 48-53

241. Hou JW, Wang JK, Wang TR (1998) FISH analysis in both classical and atypical cases of Williams-Beuren syndrome. Chung Hua Min Kuo Hsiao Erh Ko I Hsueh Hui Tsa Chih 39: 398-403

242. Morris CA (1998) Genetic aspects of supravalvular aortic stenosis. Curr Opin Cardiol 13: 214-9

243. Tassabehji M, Metcalfe K, Karmiloff-Smith A, Carette MJ, Grant J, Dennis N, Reardon W, Splitt M, Read AP, Donnai D (1999) Williams syndrome: use of chromosomal microdeletions as a tool to dissect cognitive and physical phenotypes. Am J Hum Genet 64: 118-25

244. Lopez-Rangel E, Maurice M, McGillivray B, Friedman JM (1992) Williams syndrome in adults. Am J Med Genet 44: 720-9

245. Shimamoto T, Ikeda T, Koshiji T, Nishimura K, Nomoto S, Matsuda K, Ban T (1997) A successful surgical repair of total anomalous pulmonary venous connection associated with Williams syndrome. Kyobu Geka 50: 405-8

246. Uchita S, Fujiwara T, Matsuo K, Suetsugu F, Aotsuka H, Okajima Y (1998) A surgical case of supravalvular aortic stenosis with severe hypoplastic ascending aorta (diffuse type) in Williams-Beuren syndrome. Jpn J Thorac Cardiovasc Surg 46: 928-32

247. van Son JA, Edwards WD, Danielson GK (1994) Pathology of coronary arteries, myocardium, and great arteries in supravalvular aortic stenosis. Report of five cases with implications for surgical treatment. J Thorac Cardiovasc Surg 108: 21-8

248. Sadler LS, Gingell R, Martin DJ (1998) Carotid ultrasound examination in Williams syndrome. J Pediatr 132: 354-6

XV
Vascular changes in metabolic and endocrine disorders

1 – Metabolic disorders

In a number of metabolic diseases, involvement of the heart and blood vessels is a central part of the disease process ; in some the disease is manifest by virtue of a cardiovascular change or complication [1] It is these conditions which will be considered here.

Diseases of carbohydrate metabolism

Five categories are considered: the glycogen storage diseases, the mucopolysaccharidoses, the mucolipidoses, the hyperoxalurias, and diabetes mellitus.

Glycogen storage diseases

Of the 12 types of glycogen storage diseases, only type II or Pompe's disease, caused by a deficit of lysosomal enzyme acid maltase (alpha-1-glucosidase) produces vascular lesions. Smooth muscle cells and the pericytes of cerebral arteries, containing dilated lysosomes filled with glycogen, undergo degeneration and necrosis. Extensive involvement of the vascular smooth muscle cells may lead to development of fusiform aneurysms of the cerebral basilar artery [2-4].

Mucolipidoses

All of the mucolipidoses are inherited as autosomal recessive traits and four clinical types are recognized. The enzyme defects in types II and III are similar. Table 1 lists the different types ; mucolipidoses II, III, IV and fucosidosis have cardiovascular involvement [5, 6].

Mucolipidosis II (I-cell disease)

Clinical manifestations include coarsened facies, severe psychomotor retardation and striking dysostosis multiplex. The atrioventricular valves and the aortic intima show marked thickening with foam cell infiltration. A variety of cells (fibroblasts, cardiac myocytes) contain large pleomorphic inclusions. Deposits are also seen in perivascular connective tissue [5].

Mucolipidosis III (Pseudo-Hurler dystrophy)

Corneal clouding, coarse facies, mild mental retardation, skeletal dysplasia, joint contractures and valvular heart disease are found [6]

Mucolipidosis IV

Clinical features include corneal opacities, strabismus, psychomotor retardation, and hypotonia. A variety of cells (skeletal muscle cells, fibroblasts, neurons, endothelial cells, hepatocytes, epithelial cells including conjunctival cells and goblet cells) contain cytoplasmic inclusions, made up of membranous bodies, vesicles and concentric lamellae with a periodicity of 4.2 nm similar to those found in Fabry's disease. Numerous small, dense granules are also observed in the smooth muscle cells of blood vessels in the skin [6-8].

Table 1. Biochemical characteristics and mode of inheritance of mucolipidoses

SYNDROMES	ENZYME DEFECT
Mucolipidosis I (lipomucopolysaccharidosis or sialidosis)	Glycoprotein sialidase
Mucolipidosis II (I-cell disease)	N-acetylglucosamine-1-phosphatase transferase
Mucolipidosis III (pseudo-Hurler dystrophy)	
Mucolipidosis IV	mucolipidin gene mutations
Fucosidosis	alpha-L-fucosidase
alpha-Mannosidosis	alpha-mannosidase
beta-Mannosidosis	beta-mannosidase

Fucosidosis

Clinical features resemble those of Hurler's syndrome. Some patients have angiokeratomas similar to those seen in Fabry's disease. Endothelial cells in skin capillaries show cytoplasmic vacuoles with lucent amorphous contents [9, 10].

Diseases of lipid metabolism

Deficiencies of lysosomal enzymes of lipid metabolism

Gaucher's disease (Glucosyl ceramide lipidosis)

The accumulation of glucosyl ceramide in cells in the cardiovascular system in the adult form of this disease involves vessels (Fig. 1-2), rather than the myocardium. Patients with Gaucher's disease develop atherosclerosis, specific changes with intimal and perivascular fibrosis relating to deposits and involving the cardiac valves [11, 12], resulting in mitral and aortic stenosis and secondary cardiac hypertrophy and dilatation. In the lungs, alveolar capillaries may be occluded by Gaucher's cells, with pulmonary hypertension and cor pulmonale [13].

Farber's disease (Disseminated lipogranulomatosis)

This autosomal recessive inherited lipidosis is caused by a defect in acid ceramidase, a lysosomal enzyme that hydrolyses ceramide to sphingosine and a free fatty acid in viscera, leukocytes and cultured fibroblasts [14-16]. This defect leads to accumulation of ceramide in cells with formation of granulomata containing lipid-filled histiocytes. Many viscera may be affected: the larynx, lungs, liver, joints, skeletal tissues and peripheral nerves [17]. In the cardiovascular system, accumulation of ceramide leads to yellow plaques thickening the pericardium, cardiac valves, and the intima of arteries [18, 19], leading to severe luminal narrowing. Arterial tortuosity and dilatation have been also reported [20, 21].

Pathology

Cardiac valves and arteries are distorted by lipogranulomata with yellow plaques visible on the luminal aspect. Ultrastructural study demonstrates inclusions containing either parallel lamellae or curvilinear tubules [22]. In addition to granulomatous changes, extracellular deposits considered to contain glycolipids are also seen extracellularly in the three vascular coats in vessels and in the perivascular connective tissue.

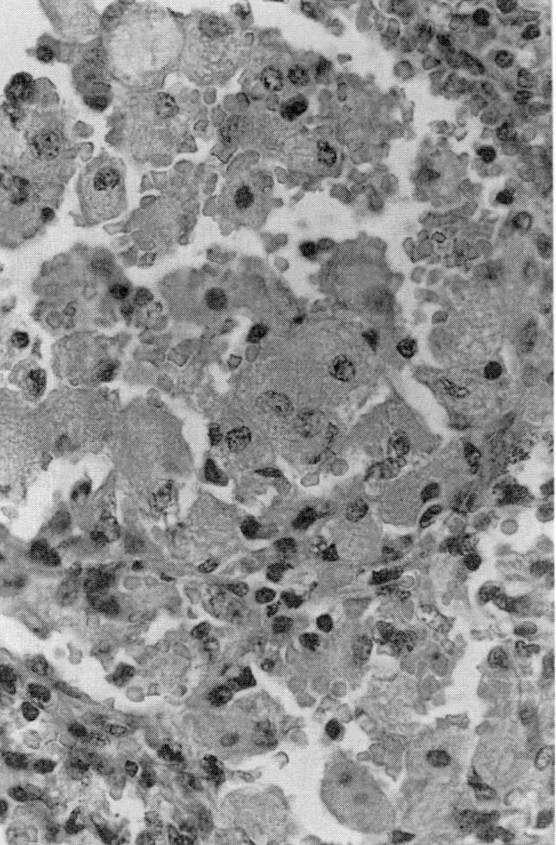

Fig. 1. Gaucher's cells lining a splenic sinusoid. Haematoxylin, eosin and saffron stain. ...HES...

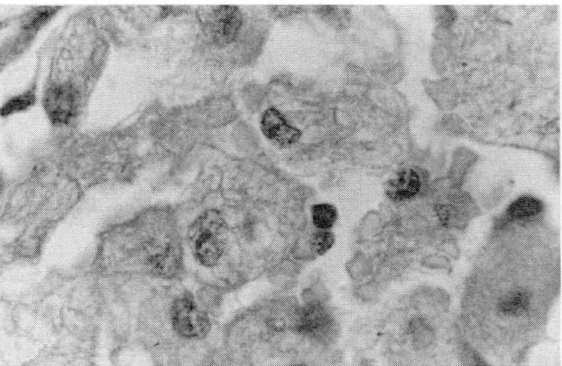

Fig. 2. Gaucher's cells. HES

Acid lipase deficiency

This condition, transmitted as a recessive autosomal trait, results from a defect of an acid lipase that hydrolyses cholesteryl ester. There are two forms; the first, Wolman's disease, leads to death in infancy; the second, cholesteryl ester storage disease, is relatively benign. The arterial intima displays marked infiltration by foamy histiocytes. Endothelial cells contain cytoplasmic round or spindle-shaped inclusions, surrounded by a double membrane [23]. Patients with cholesteryl ester storage disease also develop accelerated atherosclerosis; however, this complication is a consequence of of type IIb hyperlipoproteinaemia [24].

Neuronal ceroid lipofuscinosis

In the various forms of Batten's disease granular deposits of material mimicking lipofuscin (yellow-brown colour, yellow-orange autofluorescene, positive reaction with lipid stains, PAS -positivity) but with an ultrastructural appearance of curvilinear and rectilinear bodies [25] occur in endothelial cells. These contain abnormal lysosomes with pigment deposits.

Hyperlipoproteinaemias

Lipoproteins and apolipoproteins

Table 2 shows some essential data on these compounds [26]

There are eleven major types of apoproteins (Table 3). They have three functions: dissolution of cholesterol and triglycerides by interaction with phospholipids, regulation of enzymatic reactions (lecithine cholesterol acyl-transferase or LCAT and lipoprotein

lipase), and interactions between lipids and receptors [27].

The hyperlipoproteinaemias are a group of syndromes characterized by abnormally high concentrations of various lipoproteins. The majority of these are familial and are classified into 5 types according to the nature of the liporotein particles and their levels in plasma (Table 4).

Primary hyperlipoproteinaemias include familial lipoprotein lipase deficiency, familial apoprotein CII deficiency, familial hypercholesterolaemia, dys-beta-lipoproteinaemia, familial hypertriglyceridaemia, and familial combined hyperlipidaemia. Primary ...hyperlipoproteinaemias... without a clearly defined genetic aetiology include polygenic hypercholesterolaemia, sporadic hypertriglyceridaemia and familial hyper-alpha-lipoproteinaemia [28]. Acquired secondary hyperlipoproteinaemia results from diabetes mellitus, consumption of alcohol and ingestion of oral contraceptives [29].

Familial lipoprotein lipase deficiency (Type I)

An autosomal recessive disorder resulting from the absence of or marked reduction in the activity of lipoprotein lipase, an enzyme that hydrolyzes chylomicrons and is located in the plasma membrane of the endothelial cells. Chylomicrons accumulate massively in the plasma. Patients with familial lipoprotein lipase deficiency present with recurrent episodes of abdominal pain caused by pancreatitis, eruptive xanthomas, and small painless, yellowish papules on pressure-sensitive areas (elbows, knees and buttocks) or in tendons (fingers, knees and heels) in childhood. They do not develop accelerated atherosclerosis.

Table 2. Types of plasma lipoproteins according to molecular weight and mass composition (C: cholesterol; CE: cholesteryl ester; HDL: high density lipoproteins; IDL: intermediate density lipoproteins; LDL: low density lipoproteins; Lp(a): minor lipoprotein; MW: molecular weight; PL: phospholipid; PROT: apoproteins; TG: triglyceride; VLDL: very low density lipoproteins)

PLASMA LIPOPROTEINS	MW (kDA)	TG	CE	PL	C	PROT
Chylomicrons	400 000	86	3	7	2	2
VLDL	10 000-80 000	55	12	18	7	8
IDL	5 000-10 000	23	29	19	9	19
LDL	2 300	6	42	22	8	22
Lp(a)	3 000-5 000	3	35	22	10	30
HDL2	360	5	17	33	5	40
HDL3	175	3	13	25	4	55

Table 3. Type of apoproteins (APO) (HDL: high density lipoproteins; IDL: intermediate density lipoproteins; LDL: low density lipoproteins; MW: Molecular weight; VLDL: very low density lipoproteins)

APO	MW (kDa)	LIPID COMPONENT	ROLE
A-I	28 000	HDL, chylomicrons	Activation of lecithin-cholesterol acyltransferase
A-II	17 000	HDL, chylomicrons	Unknown
A-IV	46 000	HDL, chylomicrons	Unknown
B-48	264 000	Chylomicrons and remnants	Structural role in intestine-derived lipoproteins
B-100	550 000	LDL, IDL, VLDL, chylomicrons	Ligand for LDL receptor binding
C-I	5 800	HDL, IDL, VLDL, chylomicrons	Activation of lecithin-cholesterol acyltransferase
C-II	9 100	VLDL, IDL, HDL, chylomicrons	Activation of lipoprotein lipase
C-III	8 750	VLDL, IDL, HDL, chylomicrons	Inhibits hepatic uptake of lipoproteins
D	22 000	HDL	Unknown, may participate in cholesteryl ester transfer
E	34 000	IDL, VLDL, chylomicrons, HDL,	Ligand for binding to chylomicron remnant receptor and to LDL receptor
(a)	500 000	Lp(a), chylomicrons	Unknown

Familial apoprotein CII deficiency (Type I)

This autosomal recessive condition results in the absence of apoprotein CII, an essential cofactor for lipoprotein lipase. Clinical features and pathologic changes are similar to those of familial lipoprotein lipase deficiency.

Table 4. Types of hyperlipoproteinaemia by lipoprotein particle type and plasma level (HDL: high density lipoproteins, I: increased; IDL: intermediate density lipoproteins, LDL: low density lipoproteins, N: normal; VLDL: very low density lipoproteins)

TYPES	PRIMARY HYPERLIPO-PROTEINAEMIAS	CHYLO-MICRONS	LDL	IDL	VLDL	HDL
I	Familial lipoprotein lipase deficency Familial apoprotein CII deficiency	Increased	N	N	N	N
II	Familial hypercholesterolaemia	N	I	N	N	N
III	Dys-beta-lipoproteinaemia	N	N	I	N	N
IV	Familial hypertriglyceridaemia	N	N	N	I	N
V	Familial combined hyperlipidaemia	Increased	N	N	N	N

Familial hypercholesterolaemia (Type II)

This is an autosomal dominant disorder resulting from a mutation in the gene for the LDL receptor. LDL receptors control intracellular entry of LDL, an initial step in degradation and cholesterol synthesis. Associated deficiency of apoprotein B-100 (LDL or Low Density Lipoprotein) receptors also leads to deficient hepatic clearance of VLDL (Very Low density lipoprotein) remnants leaving them in the plasma to form LDL's. Non-receptor-mediated LDL uptake is chaotic, and lipid-bloated cells form, causing xanthomas and atherosclerosis. Classic familial hypercholesterolaemia shows a 50% reduction in B-100 apoprotein receptor effectiveness and plasma cholesterol levels of around 300-500 mg/dl. Homozygotes and heterozygotes differ in the age at onset of clinical manifestations and in their severity. The total plasma cholesterol is increased six to eightfold in the first form, and two to threefold in the second. Homozygotes die in their teens of severe accelerated atherosclerosis, usually from myocardial infarction. Other clinical symptoms include xanthelasma and xanthomas.

Pathology and differential diagnosis

Ascending aortic atherosclerosis predominates in these patients [30]. There is ostial narrowing of aortic branches including the coronary carotid arteries and cerebral arteries are heavily involved [31-33]. Florid atherosclerotic plaques also develop in the pulmonary trunk and its branches. In the heart, foam cells infiltrate the endocardium, and thicken mitral and pulmonary valves, causing both valvular stenosis and regurgitation.

Familial dys-beta-lipoproteinaemia (Type III)

The gene encoding apoprotein E, which mediates the rapid uptake of IDL and chylomicron remnants in the liver, is mutated. Clinically, this condition is associated with premature coronary, aortic and peripheral vascular disease, a marked increase in plasma cholesterol and triglyceride [34, 35], and characteristic tuberous and palmar xanthomas. However, clinical expression of the defect requires some environmental change [29, 36, 37]. Obesity and glucose intolerance are common, the two perhaps being interrelated [38]. Hypothyroidism can produce type III hyperlipoproteinaemia, and thyroid function should always be assessed in these patients [39].

Familial hypertriglyceridaemia (Type IV)

This autosomal dominant trait produces obesity, hypertension and atherosclerosis [29, 40]. Laboratory findings include high plasma concentration of VLDL, hyperglycaemia, hyperinsulinaemia, and hyperuricaemia.

Familial combined hyperlipidaemia (Type V) or Multiple lipoprotein-type hyperlipidaemia

This autosomal dominant disorder has three different lipoprotein patterns: type II, IV and V. The age onset is at puberty. Clinical symptoms manifest by premature atherosclerosis [41].

Lipoprotein deficiencies

Hypo-alpha-lipoproteinaemia

Relevant syndromes are shown in the table 5.

The major constituents of mobile lipoproteins (HDL) are apolipoproteins AI and AII; minor apolipoproteins are B, Lp(a), CI, CII, CIII, D, E, F, and G. Lecithin-cholesterol acyltransferase (LCAT) plays a major role in the transfer of cholesterol from cells to plasma, and its esterification and incorporation into HDL.

Familial apo-AI and CIII deficiency and HDL deficiency with xanthomas favor development of accelerated atherosclerosis with severe coronary artery disease.

1. **Tangier disease.** Low plasma levels of HDL, LDL and total cholesterol are seen. The decrease in plasma levels of HDL cholesterol and apo-AI results from rapid catabolism rather than decreased synthesis of HDL. There is accumulation of cholesteryl esters in various tissues, including the tonsils, lymph nodes, thymus, bone marrow, intestinal mucosa, liver, spleen, skin and cornea. In vessels, endothelial cells and smooth muscle cells show lipid vacuoles and inclusions in the cytoplasm. These changes were noted in the normal-appearing aorta of a 5-year old boy with Tangier disease [42]. Patients have a high risk for premature atherosclerosis before the age of 40.

2. **Fish-eye disease.** This condition results from mutations in the LCAT gene or on the gene for its cofactor apo-AI [43]. with deficient LCAT. LCAT activity is absent in HDL- or apo-AI-containing proteoliposomes (alpha-LCAT activity) but is normal in VLDL and LDL (beta-LCAT activity). Thus

Table 5. Biochemical characteristics and mode of inheritance of lipoprotein deficiencies (AD: autosomal dominant; AR: autosomal recessive inheritance, I: inheritance)

SYNDROMES	DEFICIENT ENZYME	I	BREAKDOWN PRODUCTS
Familial apo-AI and CIII deficiency			
HDL deficiency with xanthomas			
Tangier disease		AD	Cholesteryl esters
Fish-eye disease	Deficient LCAT		
Familial lecithin-cholesterol acyltransferase (LCAT) deficiency and familial hypo-alpha-lipoproteinaemia	Mutations in the LCAT gene or on the gene for its cofactor apo-AI	AR	Disturbance of esterification of cholesterol in all lipoprotein classes, leading to an increase in the non-esterified/esterified ratio.

the in vivo ratios of nonesterified/esterified cholesterol is near the normal limits. Clinical features include marked corneal opacity, but the risk for atherosclerosis is normal or only moderately increased.

3. **Familial lecithin-cholesterol acyltransferase (LCAT) deficiency and familial hypo-alpha-lipoproteinaemia.** This autosomal recessive condtion results from mutations in the LCAT gene or on the gene for its cofactor apo-AI [44]. Esterification of cholesterol is disturbed in all lipoprotein classes, resulting in an increase in the non-esterified/esterified ratio. An anaemia with target cells, corneal opacity with arcus formation, proteinuria and progressive renal disease, lipid deposits in bone marrow, renal glomeruli and other viscera are the main clinical symptoms. The large arteries show increased lipid deposits, hyalinization of the vessel wall and proliferation of intimal smooth muscle cells.

Familial disorders associated with low levels of low-density lipoproteins (hypo- and a-beta-lipoproteinaemia)

There are two types of apo-B: large apo-B100 and apo-B48. Apo-B100, produced in the liver, is the major component of serum VLDL and LDL and contains a binding domain for LDL receptors. Apo-B48, derived from the intestine, is devoid of LDL-receptor binding sequence [45].

1. **Hypo-beta-proteinaemia** is associated with prolonged longevity and the rarity of coronary artery disease [46].

2. **A-beta-lipoproteinaemia (Bassen-Kornweig syndrome).** This recessive inherited syndrome is characterized by the metabolic assembly or secretion defect of all lipoproteins containing apo-B. Clinical manifestations include acanthocytosis, fat malabsorption, retinitis pigmentosa, external opthalmoplegia, and a degenerative disease of the cerebellum mimicking Fiedreich's ataxia. Cardiovascular changes consist of cardiomagely with marked fibrosis involving the endo-myocardium, and the intima of arteries. There is marked hyalinization of the vascular walls of retinal blood vessels [47].

Diseases involving storage of cholesterol, other sterols, phytanic acid and related metabolic products

Cerebrotendinous xanthomatosis

This is an autosomal recessive inherited defect in the hepatic mitochondrial steroid 26-hydroxylase. The disease is manifested by subnormal intelligence, progressive cerebellar ataxia, spinal cord paresis, cataracts, and xanthomas developed in the brain, tendons and lungs. Cholesterol levels are normal or low; cholestanol and biliary alcohols in the serum and urine are abnormally elevated. Large amounts of cholestanol accumulate in various tissues leading to premature atherosclerosis [48].

Pseudoxanthoma elasticum (elastoma)

Common cardiovascular complications of pseudoxanthoma elasticum (PXE) include premature coronary artery disease with aneurysms, renovascular hypertension, and calcification of peripheral arteries frequently leading to intermittent claudication. Fibrous thickening of the endocardium and atrioventricular valves, resulting in restrictive cardiomyopathy, aneurysmal dilatation of the aortic annulus and/or mitral valve prolapse have been also described [49, 50]. Capillary microscopy reveals distorted capillaries, most of them with a normal lumen.

Refsum's disease

To our knowledge, no cardiovascular disorder has been reported to present in infantile Refsum's disease. In the adult form, clinical manifestations include peripheral neuropathy, ataxia, retinitis pigmentosa, and changes in the skin and bones. Premature degeneration of the aortic media has been described but the relationship of these lesions to the metabolic defect remains undetermined [51, 52].

Diseases of amino-acid and protein metabolism

Larsen's syndrome

This syndrome, which occurs in autosomal dominant or recessive forms is a generalized mesenchymal disorder affecting connective tissue and synthesis of collagen [53]. Patients present with skeletal dysplasia, multiple joint dislocations and a characteristic facies. A skin biopsy evidences marked fragmentation of the elastic fibres (Fig. 3-4-5). Cardiovascular anomalies consist of cardiac septal defects, prolapse of tricuspid and mitral valves (Fig. 6), dilatation of the aorta with regurgitation, ectasia and tortuosity of carotid and cerebral arteries, and aneurysm of the ductus arteriosus [20, 21]. Histologically, lesions of the aortic wall are similar to those of Marfan's syndrome: paucity and disruption of the elastic fibers, myxoid change (Fig. 7) with cyst formation.

Diseases of extracellular accumulation of fibrillar proteins

Amyloidosis

Amyloid infiltration may be systemic or localized, involving various viscera, including the cardiovascular system (Table 6), giving rise to various anatomo-clinical entities [54].

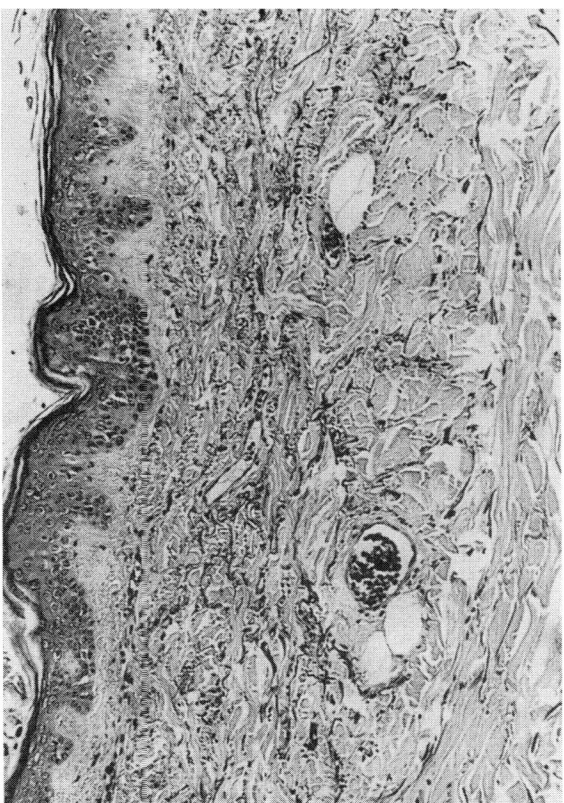

Fig. 3. Larsen's syndrome. Skin biopsy shows frgamented elastic fibres. HES

Cardiovascular amyloidosis includes senile aortic amyloidosis, isolated deposits and isolated atrial amyloidosis. Senile aortic amyloidosis is a form of ATTR amyloidosis and may not be functionally significant. In isolated atrial amyloidosis, the amyloid deposits are derived from atrial natriuretic factor [55] or a variant of apolipoprotein A1 [56-58].

Pathology and differential diagnosis

In vessels, amyloid infiltration is subtle at first but will ultimately result in occlusion of vessels with ischaemic manifestations. All types of vessel may be involved (Fig. 8-9-10-11). Aortic involvement is common in senile amyloidosis and cardiac amyloid deposits can result in significant cardiac dysfunction. Aortic amyloid deposits are predominantly in the inner third of the media, appearing in lumps or lines oriented parallel to the smooth muscle cells [56]. Cardiac amyloid deposits occur in myocardial interstitium, conduction tissue, valves, the endocardium, pericardium and in small intramural coronary arteries, veins

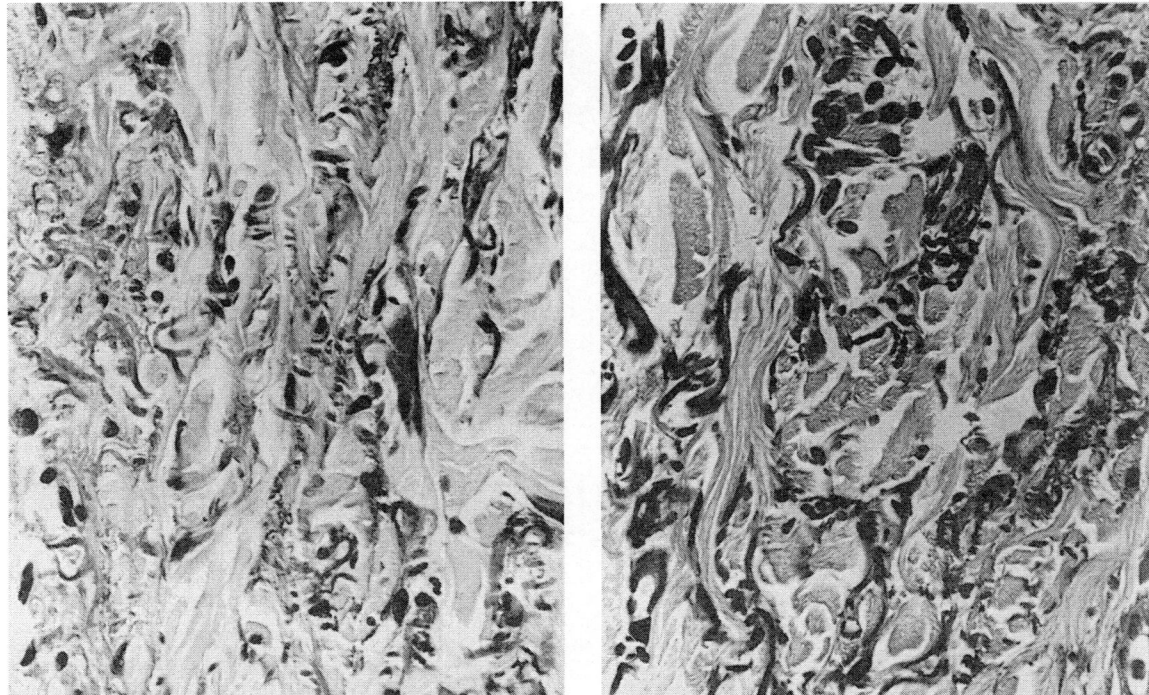

Fig. 4-5. Larsen's syndrome. Fragmented elastic fibres are gathered in clumps. Orcein elastic stain. (Orcein)

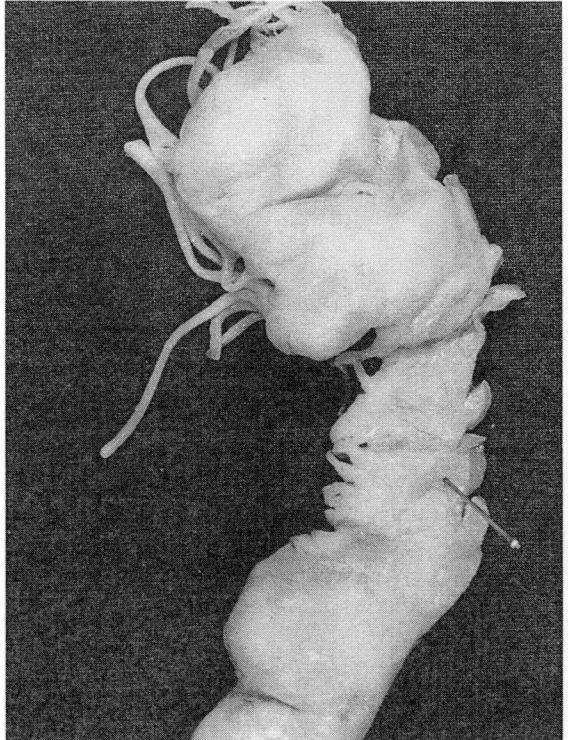

Fig. 6. Larsen's syndrome. Ballooned mitral valves

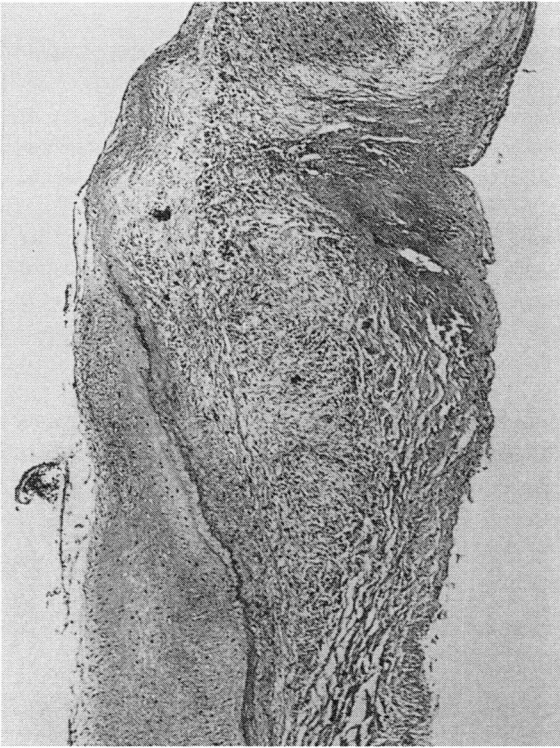

Fig. 7. Larsen's syndrome. Myxoid changes thickens the valvular leaflet. HES

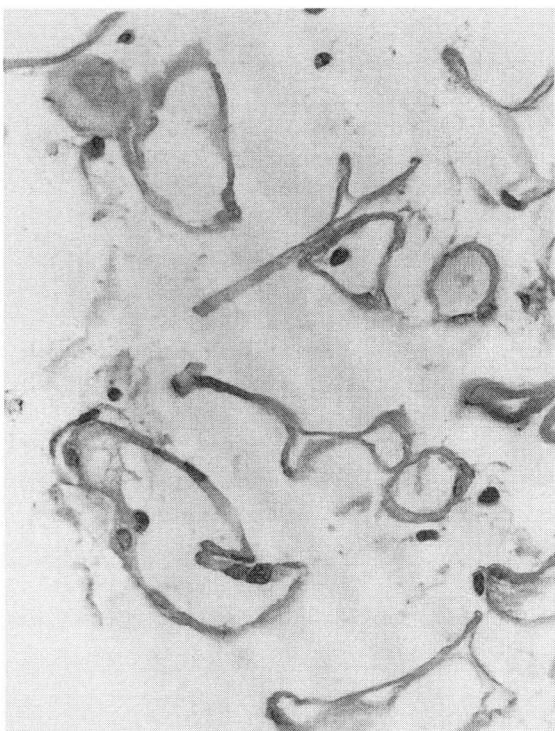

Fig. 8. Amyloidosis. Amyloid deposits along capillary basement membrane with wire-loop contour. HES

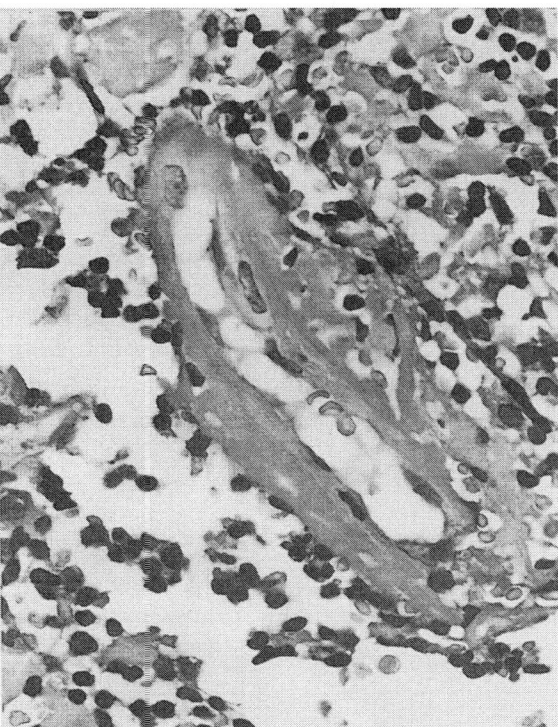

Fig. 9. Amyloidosis. Amyloid accumulation of amyloid in the three layers of a muscular artery. HES

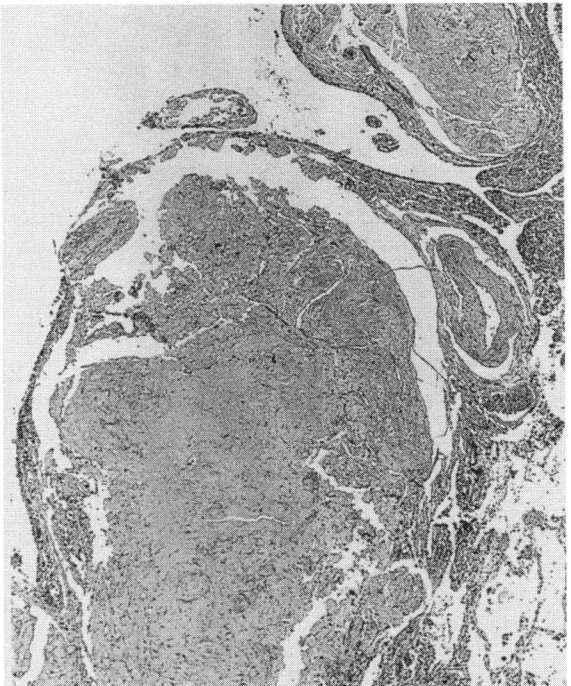

Fig. 10. Amyloidosis. Pseudo-tumoural amyloidosis of the lung with vascular amyloid accumulation mimicking thrombosis. HES

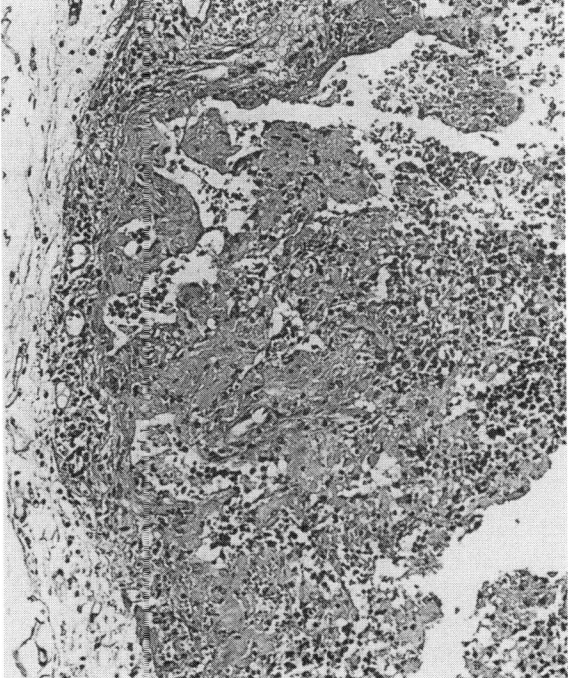

Fig. 11. Amyloidosis. Amyloid infiltration of a lymph node. Note thickening of subcapsular sinus wall. Congo Red stain

Table 6. Cardiovascular involvement in amyloidosis

TYPES	ENTITIES	TARGETS	AETIOLOGY	PRECURSORS
Systemic	Primary (AL)	Various viscera (heart, vessels, muscles, and digestive mucosa), skin	AL with/without dysglobulinaemia (multiple myeloma, Waldelström)	Immunoglobulin κ, λ, light chains
	Secondary or acquired (A)	Various viscera (liver, spleen, kidney, digestive tract) and endocrine glands...	Chronic infection, Inflammation, Haemodialysis	Serum amyloid associated protein (SA) bêta2-macro-globulins
	Hereditary	Peripheral and visceral nerves	Mediterranean fever Familial polyneuro-pathy	Serum amyloid associated protein (SA) Mutant forms of transthyretin (ATTR)
	Senile	Various viscera, including the cardiovascular system		ATTR derivative amyloid
Localized		Heart	Isolated atrial amyloidosis	Natriuretic factor Apolipoprotein A1 variant
		Heart and aorta	Senile aortic amyloidosis	ATTR derivative amyloid
		Brain	Senile cerebral amyloidosis (Alzheimer's disease)	bêta2-amyloid protein (A4)
		Tumour stroma	APUD tumours	Hormone polypep-tides (AMCT)
		Skin	Amyloid lichen, Adnexial tumours	Cytokeratins (Ad)

and capillaries. Deposits often form rings around the cardiac muscle cells and capillaries. Deposits in coronary vessels involve layers of the wall and can lead to luminal obliteration [59, 60]. In the familial neuropathic syndromes, amyloid deposits in blood vessels are prominent in the Portugese type but the myocardial interstitium is involved to a lesser extent. In familial Mediterranean fever, arterioles throughout the body are the site of amyloid deposition but cardiac interstitial involvement is extremely rare. Atypical presentation of cerebral amyloid angiopathy has been reported [61].

Light chain deposition disease

Involvement of the kidneys in this disease includes involvement of arterioles and interlobular arteries [62, 63].

Hypertrophic cardiomyopathy

This condition is an important cause of sudden death, especially in children and young adults [64, 65]. Genetic alterations are found in more than 60% of the cases, with an autosomal dominant mode of inheritance. More than 50 different mutations involving six genes have so far been associated with the development of hypertrophic cardiomyopathy. These mutations are located to genes coding for several of the proteins in the cardiac sarcomere and protein changes compromise contractility as well as sarcomere assembly, resulting in compensatory hypertrophy [66, 67]. The major vascular change is narrowing of the intramural coronary arteries [68, 69]. The arterial wall is thickened by fibrosis with hypertrophy of the smooth muscle cells in the media. These lesions may worsen the prognosis in the late stages of the disease.

Diseases of mineral and vitamin metabolism

Secondary hyperoxaluria or oxalosis

Oxalate deposition, similar to that seen in primary oxalosis, may be seen in the cardiovascular system (Fig. 12-13) [70, 71]. In the lungs, deposition of calcium oxalate in the arteries causes secondary chronic pulmonary hypertension [72] and interstitial deposition of calcium oxalate induces foreign body granulomata.

Causes include chronic renal insufficiency [73], ingestion of ethylene glycol, oxalic acid, and dietary oxalates. Intravenous feeding with xylitol and use or abuse of the anesthetic methoxyflurane, may produce the change of oxalosis and enteric hyperoxaluria occurs in patients with extensive disease of the small intestine or resection of the small intestine [74]. Pyridoxine deficiency [75], Aspergillus niger infection [76] may also cause secondary oxalosis.

Calcification

Idiopathic infantile hypercalcaemia (see chapter XIV)

Idiopathic arterial calcification of infancy

This rare cardiovascular disease is characterized by calcification of the internal elastic membrane and intimal proliferation in smaller and bigger arteries. This disease is inherited in an autosomal recessive pattern [77]. First described by Bryant and White in 1901 [78], the condition occurs mostly in neonates or infants younger than 6 months, with no sex predilection but may be seen in utero. The mean age at onset in symptomatic cases is 2 months. Respiratory dis-

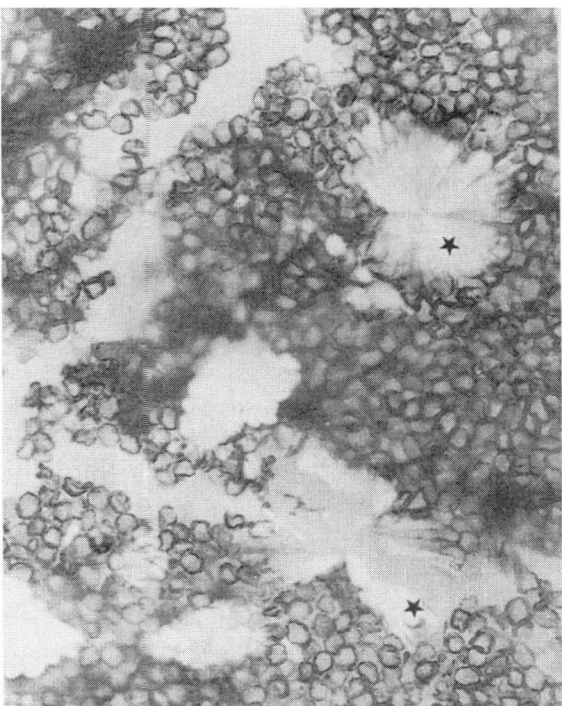

Fig. 12. Secondary oxalosis. Fatal oxalosis caused by accidental ingestion of ethylene glycol. Oxalate cristals (stars) in vascular lumen. HES

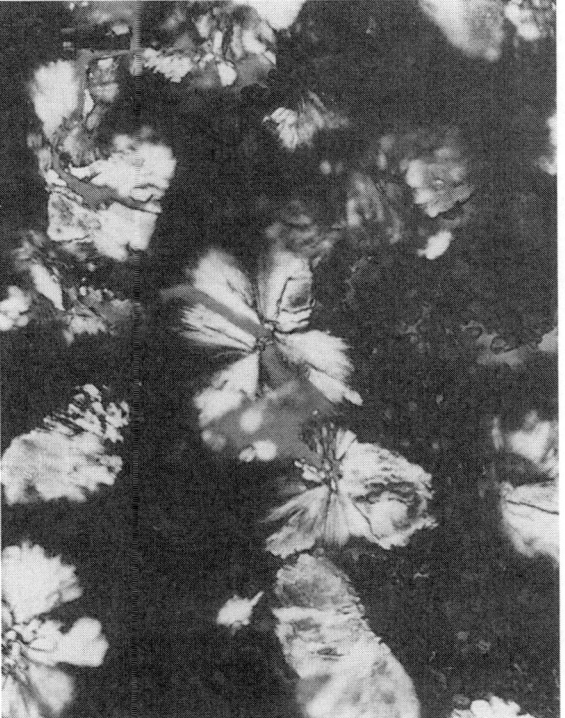

Fig. 13. Secondary oxalosis. Refringent oxalate crystals under polarized light

tress is the most common presenting symptom, followed by arterial hypertension and heart failure.
Transient renal insufficiency by nephrocalcinosis, and
skeletal abnormalities are also observed [79, 80].
Eighty five percent of patients die within the first 6
months of life with a mean survival time of 4.2
months [81-84].

Pathology and differential diagnosis

The coronary arteries are calcified in 85% of cases
with morphological changes in the aorta and aortic
valves, the arteries of the lungs, kidneys, extremities
mesentery, spleen, brain and the aorta. Extravascular
calcification (kidney, soft tissue) is evident in 37% of
the patients [82, 85-87]. There are massive calcium
deposits along the internal elastic lamella or in the
media of the coronary and systemic arteries throughout the body, with the exception of the brain and
spinal cord. There is intimal proliferation but no superimposed inflammation (Fig. 14-15). All these
changes cause arterial rigidity, loss of contractility,
and thrombosis leading to ischaemia and sometimes
fatal pulmonary thromboembolism [88].

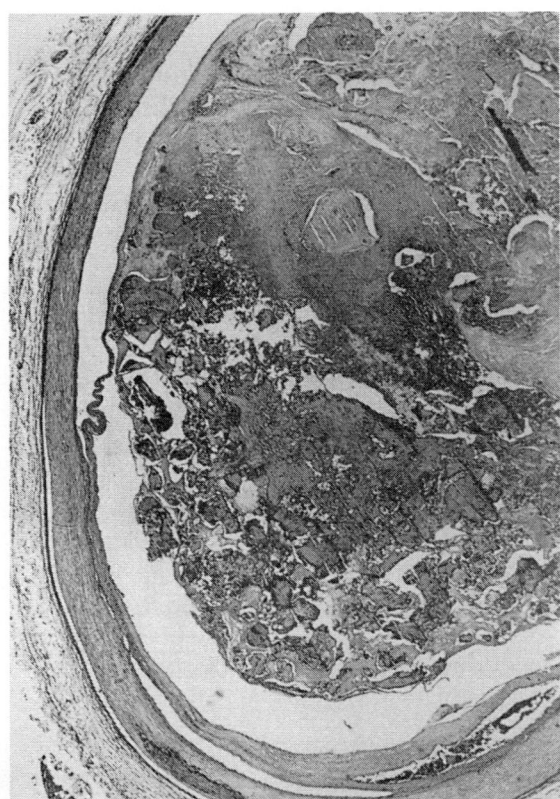

Fig. 15. Idiopathic arterial calcification of infancy. Massive
calcification deposits occluding the arterial lumen. Note intimal thickening and underlying mediacalcosis. ...Orcein...

Disorders of copper metabolism

Menke's syndrome

This condition is an X-linked disorder characterized
by abnormal transportion and sequestration of copper. The basic defect involves a deficiency in the activity of a copper-transporting ATPase leading to impaired incorporation of copper into lysyl oxidase. Low
levels of lysyl oxidase activity result in defective cross-
linking of collagen and elastin. Clinical manifestations
include growth retardation, progressive cerebral degeneration, distinctive facial features, hypopigmentation
of skin and hair, kinky hair [89] and recurrent episodes of hypothermia. Vessels display patchy degenerative changes. Superficial vessels often appear tortuous or dilated. Aneurysms may develop in major
arteries and veins. Histologically, the vessels show subintimal oedma and marked collagenous thickening
with extensive loss of elastin and smooth muscle cells
from the media. In the aorta, the elastic lamellae are
poorly formed and are composed of clumps of elastin
surrounded by large numbers of microfibrils [90].

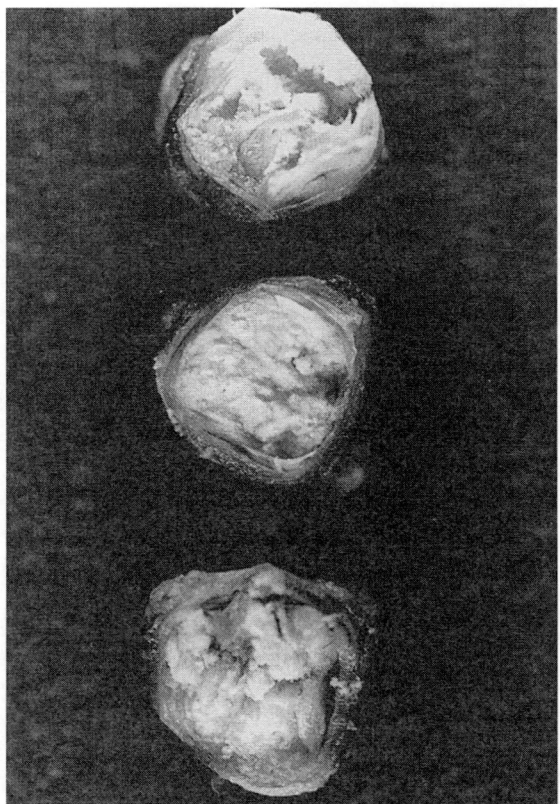

Fig. 14. Idiopathic arterial calcification of infancy. Massive
occluding calcification of the superficial femoral artery.
(Courtesy Pr D. Guilmet)

Vitamin disorders

Vitamin B12 related metabolic defects with methyl-malonic acidaemia and homocystinuria (Cbl-C type)

Cbl-C mutation results in a deficiency of both me-thylfolate-H(4) methyltrans-ferase and methylmalo-nyl CoA isomerase. These enzymes are necessary for the activation of vitamin B12, which plays a role in the methylation of homocysteine [91]. Clinical mani-festations are similar to those of homocystinuria with lethargy, feeding difficulties, mental retardation with seizures, retinal changes, cor pulmonale and right ventricular dilatation [92]. Laboratory findings in-clude megaloblastic anaemia, methylmalonic acidae-mia and homocystinuria, hypomethioninaemia. Vascular lesions include multiple pulmonary throm-boemboli and renal changes resembling those noted in thrombotic thrombocytic purpura. The mecha-nism of thromboembolism is similar to that of homo-cystinuria.

Vitamin C deficiency

Vascular changes noted in experimental scurvy in ani-mals show disruption of capillary basement mem-branes, depletion of pericapillary collagen and separa-tion of endothelial cell junctions leading to haemorrhage [93]. Acute scurvy is characterized by microvascular complications with widespread capil-lary haemorrhage [94].

Vitamin D overdosage or deficiency

Experimental administration of this vitamin to rab-bits produces extensive arterial calcification and gross irregularity of the arterial wall. The calcification has a predilection for the arterial forks and at sites initially spared in dietary-induced lipid deposition. In experi-mental arteriovenous shunts, the artery is the most frequently involved [95]. In humans, the possibility that excess vitamin D intake from vitamin D-fortified milk may induce vascular calcification is questio-nable. Vitamin D deficiency and osteoporosis are also implicated in the development of arterial calcifica-tion. Experimentally, essential fatty acid deficient ani-mals develop severe osteoporosis coupled with increa-sed renal and arterial calcification [96]. Large epidemiological studies have demonstrated a relation-ship between bone mineral density and mortality cau-sed by cerebral vascular events. Several hypotheses have been proposed to explain this relationship inclu-ding lower endogenous estrogen levels, and arterios-clerosis of the renal vessels leading to perturbed vita-min D metabolism via hyperparathyroidism and ischaemia [97, 98].

Deficiency of selenium and Vitamin E

Experimetal deficiency of selenium and vitamin E in swine results in necrosis of the myocardium, skeletal muscle, liver, pancreas and the central nervous system [99, 100]. In man, selenium deficiency leads to myo-cardial necrosis with extensive myocytolysis and fibrosis resulting in congestive heart failure, dilated cardiomyopathy, sudden death, cardiac mural throm-boses and embolic strokes [101, 102]. This condition (Keshan disease) occurs mostly in China in a zone in which the selenium content of the soil is particulary low [103].

2 – Endocrine diseases

Diabetes mellitus

Seventy percent of all deaths in the diabetic popula-tion are caused by vascular disease. This figure is about two and a half times the death rate from the same causes among non diabetic patients of all ages. In diabetics, vascular lesions occur at much a younger age in both sexes, with a faster rate of progression [104]. Although a number of cardiovascular risk fac-tors are more common in diabetics than non diabe-tics, these do not entirely account for the increased frequency of cardiovascular disease [105]. Several fac-tors have been implicated in the genesis of diabetic angiopathies: the relationship between hyperglycae-mia and vascular lesions in diabetics is difficult to de-termine in epidemiological studies.

Diabetic macroangiopathy

This condition is mainly characterized by atheroscle-rosis and medial calcification or Monckeberg's sclero-sis (arteriosclerosis) (Fig. 16) [106].

Pathology and differential diagnosis

Great vessels and coronary arteries are widely invol-ved by atherosclerotic lesions, conversely to cerebral vessels. These lesions are more extensive in the small peripheral arteries, especially in the lower limbs (Fig. 17) [107]. This location limits the development of an effective compensating collateral circulation in case of proximal stenoses or thromboses. Histologically, athe-rosclerotic lesions of diabetic macroangiopathy are si-milar to those of non-diabetic patients.

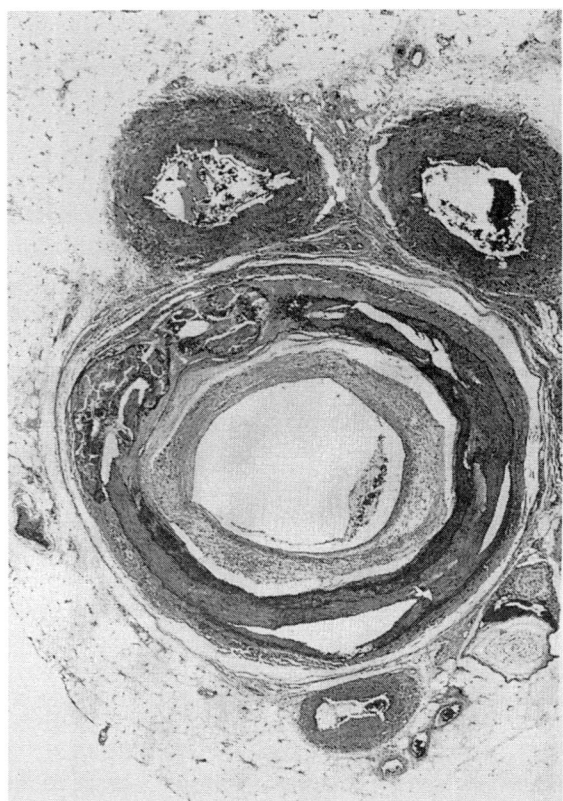

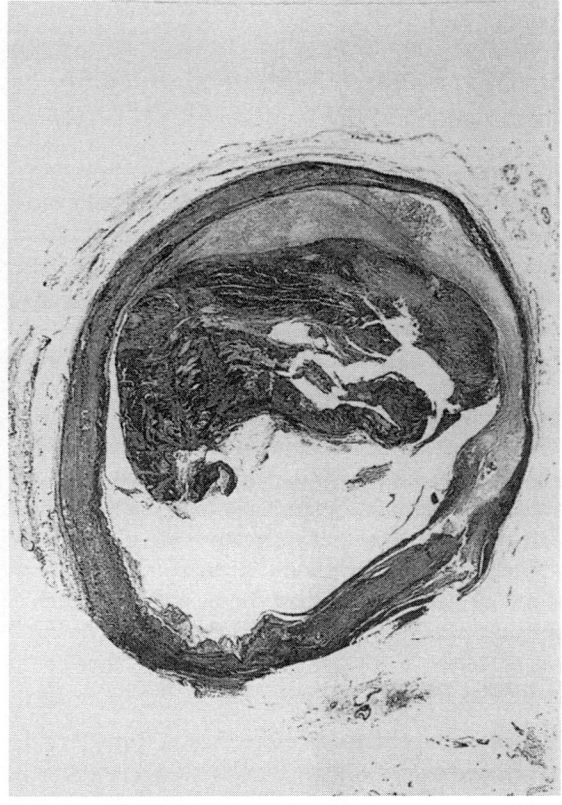

Fig. 16. Diabetes mellitus. Monckeberg's sclerosis of the tibial artery in an amputation specimen for extensive diabetic gangrene. HES

Fig. 17. Diabetes mellitus. Diabetic macroangiopathy involving the femoral artery with mediacalcosis, florid atheromatous plaques and superimposed luminal thrombosis. HES

Diabetic microangiopathy

The mechanisms by which diabetic microangiopathy develop are not known, but the HLA-DR4 gene is more frequent in diabetic patients with background or proliferative retinopathy [108]. Strict control of hyperglycaemia is crucial in the prevention of vascular complications [109-111]. A potentially atherogenic mix of elevated low-density lipoprotein cholesterol and low high-density lipoprotein cholesterol levels is found in uncontrolled diabetes mellitus. Lowering of HDL (high density lipoproteins) also occurs in sedentary and obese diabetics [112, 113]. At least one of the dyslipoproteinaemias – hypertriglyceridaemia – is associated with insulin resistance and aggravated glucose intolerance [114]. Endothelium-derived nitric oxide (NO) mediated vasodilatation is impaired in animal models of diabetes and in patients with insulin-dependent and non-insulin-dependent diabetes mellitus. It is likely that hyperglycaemia may initiate this abnormality with decreased production of NO,

inactivation of NO by oxygen-derived free radicals, and/or increased production of endothelium-derived contracting factors. These factors inhibit the protective activity of NO [115] leading to a decrease in fibrinolytic activity (plaminogen activator activity), and an increase in plasma concentrations of Willebrand factor (blood clotting factor VIII). Some investigators also reported that platelets synthetize more thromboxane A2, which is a vasoconstrictor and platelet aggregant [112].

Pathological mechanisms of microangiopathy

The stratified arrangement of hyaline material in the microvascular system suggests an accelerated loss of endothelial cells with successive elaboration of a newly-formed basement membrane [116, 117]. Pericytes are also involved and show eosinophilic degeneration [118]. These changes confirm a relationship between diabete mellitus and an increase in carbohydrate and protein complex deposits in the ground substance and connective tissue [119]. Endothelial hyperplasia leads to focal capillary deformation. Formation of microaneurysms depends on several factors: changes in the basement membrane, degenerative alterations of pericytes, and increased intraluminal pressure. There is an increase in extracellular matrix associated with a proliferation of myofibroblast-like cells, first in the subendothelial space and the adventitia while the size of the medial smooth muscle cells is reduced. These changes, superimposed on ageing changes, lead to loss of arterial compliance (See chapter II) [120, 121]. Other characteristic lesions include medial calcification and marked atherosclerosis [122-124]. Atherosclerosis is more extensive in the smaller peripheral arteries, especially in the lower limbs [110, 125-127], which limits the development of an effective compensating collateral circulation when proximal stenoses or thromboses occur.

Microangiopathy involves capillaries, arterioles, venules and lymphatic capillaries [128]. Hyalinosis, eosinophilic degeneration of pericytes, formation of loops and twisted cord-shaped capillaries, and development of microaneurysms occur (Fig. 18). Homogenous hyaline material thickens the vascular wall and immunohistochemistry reveals intense labelling with fibronectin, laminin, type IV collagen and proteoglycan containing heparan-sulfate [129]. This material piles up in the sub-endothelial space of capillaries, and thickens the basement membrane. These changes are found in the retina, skin, muscle, heart and glomeruli. In arterioles and venules, hyaline material accumulates in the subendothelial space and sometimes between smooth muscle cells of the media, a change particularly marked in the preglomerular arterioles. The basement membrane of lymphatic vessels is thickened. Deposits of hyaline material are also noted in basement membranes in the glomerular mesangium, Bowman's capsule, renal tubules, seminiferous tubules, breast ducts, sweat glands and in the ciliary process of the eye.

Morphological changes occur in capillaries, which are often looped and twisted. Microaneurysms occur at the margins of unperfused capillary areas and usually predominate in the venous side of the capillary bed [130]. In the retina, microaneurysms generally persist for several months and then disappear, while new aneurysms develop in other areas [108]. They may rupture into the vitreous. Microvasculitis and inflammatory reactions may contribute to some forms of diabetic neuropathy [131].

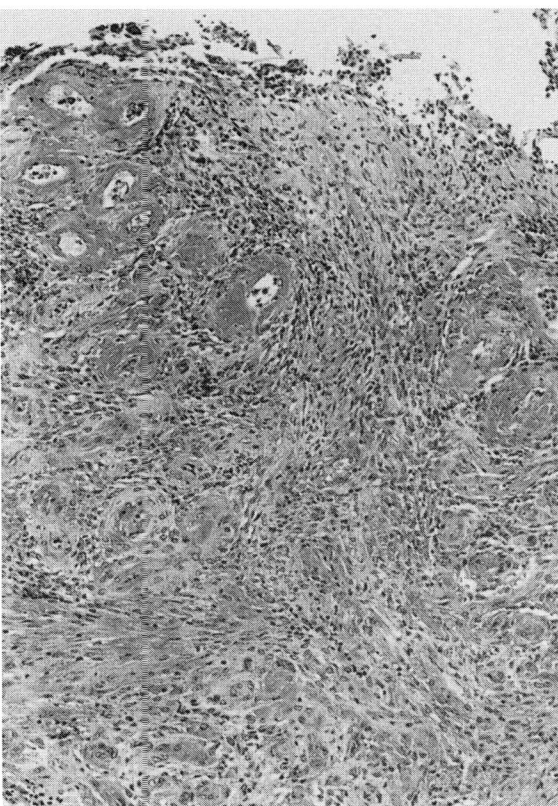

Fig. 18. Diabetes mellitus. Diabetic microangiopathy. Hyalinosis of arterioles and capillaries. HES

Specific changes

Diabetic nephropathy is probably related to angiotensin II-induced vascular endothelial growth factor expression [132].It typically gives rise to a nephrotic state with oedma, albuminuria, urinary casts and hypertension [130]. A combination of vascular obstruction and ascending infection may lead to necrosis of the renal papillae. Alterations in the microcirculatory bed give rise to a "diabetic foot" (Fig. 19) [133-135] with neuropathic and ischaemic injury. In the corpora cavernosa, associated impeded inflow disorder leads to vasculogenic impotence (Fig. 20) [134, 136, 137].

Myxoedema

Tri-iodothyronine (T3)-induced changes in cardiac function can result from direct or indirect routes. T3 increases the heart transcription of the myosin heavy chain (MHC) alpha-gene and decreases the transcription of MHC beta-gene leading to an increase of myosin V1 and a decrease in myosin V3 isoenzymes. The

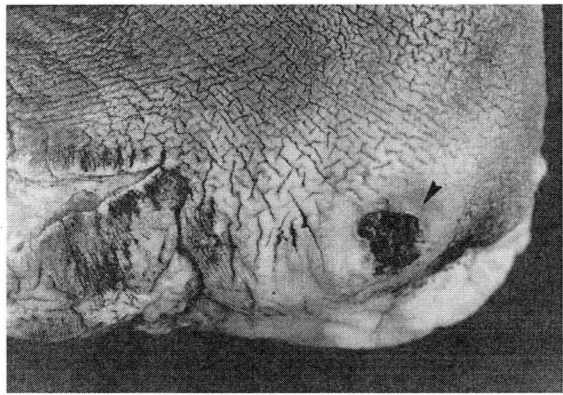

Fig. 19. Diabetes mellitus. Diabetic foot with "mal perforant" chronic heel ulcer (arrow head). (Courtesy Dr P. Desoutter)

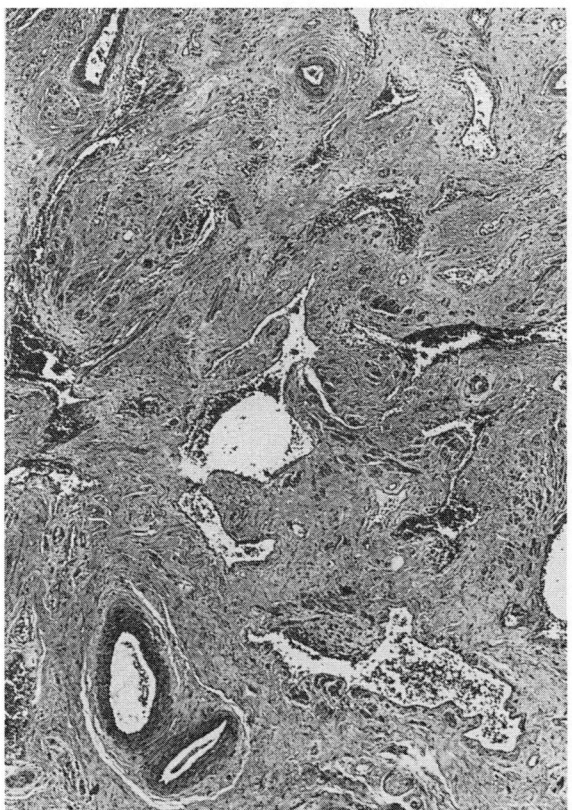

Fig. 20. Diabetes mellitus. Vasculogenic impotence caused by diffuse fibrosis of the cavernous arterial bed. HES

the sarcoplasmic reticulum (SR) [138]. The hypothyroid heart shows myofibrillar swelling with loss of striation and interstitial fibrosis. Accumulation of glycosaminoglycans is seen. On ultrastructural examination, mitochondria show disruption and lipid inclusion. Hypercholesterolaemia and impairment of fatty acid mobilization, together with decreases in peripheral oxygen consumption and changes in haemodynamic variables, favour the occurence of atherosclerosis [113, 139-142].

Hyperparathyroidism

The cells of the cardiovascular sysyem are targets for parathyroid hormone (PTH) and the structurally related peptide parathyroid hormone-related peptide (PTH-rP). PTH activates protein kinase C (PKC) of cardiomyocytes via a PKC activating domain previously identified on chondrocytes. Activation of PKC leads to hypertrophic growth and re-expression of fetal type proteins in cardiomyocytes. This hypertrophic effect of PTH is thought to contribute to the left ventricular hypertrophy seen in haemodialysis patients with secondary hyperparathyroidism [143]. The formation of calcium phosphate and calcium oxalate stones in the urinary tract with nephrocalcinosis may cause renal damage and hypertension.

Cushing's syndrome

Arteriosclerosis is common in this syndrome with hypertension and myocardial ischaemia [144-146].

Acromegaly

Goldberg et al (147) reported a case of extensive coronary collateral formation in a patient with untreated acromegaly. It is not clear if this is related to growth hormone production.

Pregnancy

Circumstantial data provide evidence of the influence of pregnancy on the cardiovascular system. Varicosities, spider naevi and enlargement of arteriovenous malformations are common [148]. Steroids may impair reparative growth of connective tissues or alter the tensile strength of vascular connective tissue. During pregnancy, decidual changes involve the smooth muscle cells of the media of the uterine spiral arteries (Fig. 21-22). These cells become enlarged, thicken the arterial wall and reduce the arterial lumen. In the aorta, straightening and fragmentation of the elastic fibers may be seen and may explain an increased incidence of dissection [149-151].

globular head of myosin V1, with its higher ATPase activity, leads to a more rapid movement of the globular head of myosin along the thin filament, resulting in an increased velocity of contraction. T3 also induces an increase in the speed of diastolic relaxation, which results from pumping by the calcium ATPase of

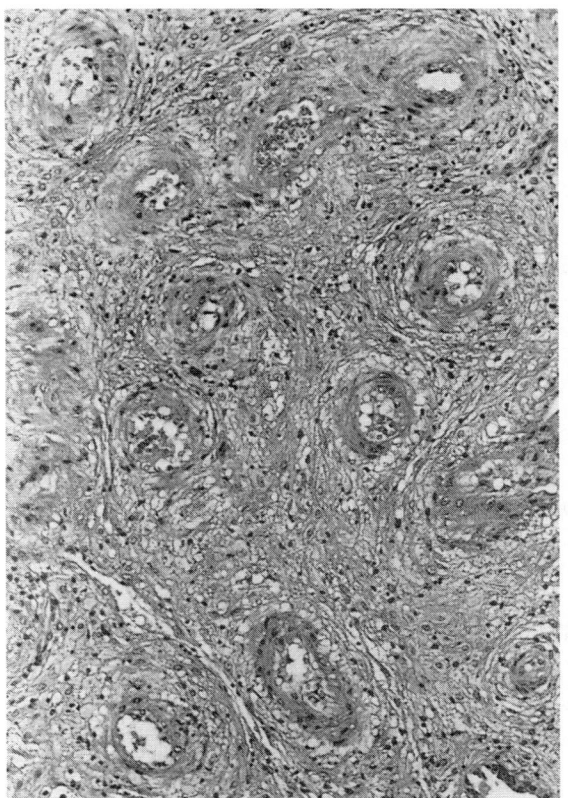

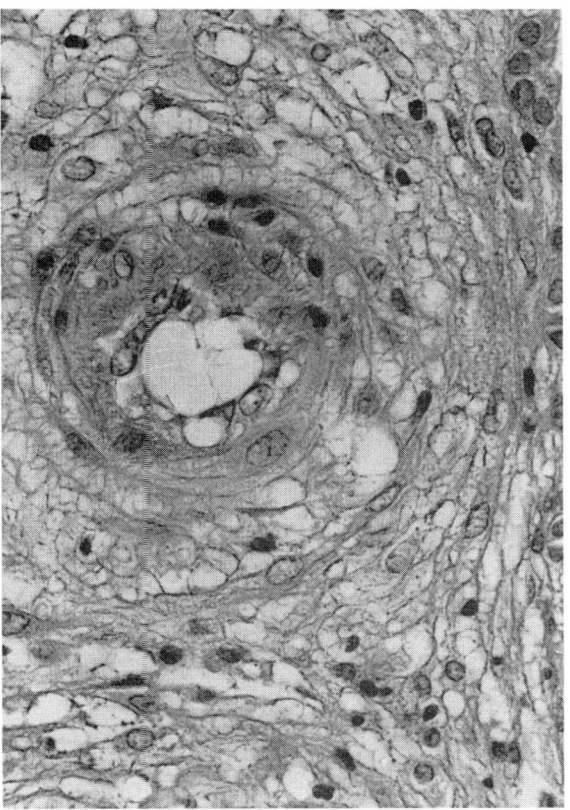

Fig. 21. Pregnancy. Hysterectomy specimen for post-partum metrorrhagia. Decidual changes of smooth muscle cells in uterine spiral arteries. HES

Fig. 22. Pregnancy. Decidual-like changes of smooth muscle cells of a spiral artery. HES

Bibliography

1. Gilbert EF (1987) The effects of metabolic diseases on the cardiovascular system. Am J Cardiovasc Pathol 1: 189-213
2. Makos MM, McComb RD, Hart MN, Bennett DR (1985) Alpha-glucosidase deficiency and basilar artery aneurysm: report of a sibship. Ann Neurol 22: 629-33
3. Matsuoka Y, Senda Y, Hirayama M, Matsui T, Takahashi A (1988) Late-onset acid maltase deficiency associated with intracranial aneurysm. J Neurol 235: 371-3
4. Iwamasa T, Chinen K, Hirayasu T (1993) Pompe's disease – acid alpha-glucosidase deficiency – a review. Nippon Rinsho 51: 2324-9
5. Okada S, Owada M, Sakiyama T, Yutaka T, Ogawa M (1985) I-cell disease: clinical studies of 21 Japanese cases. Clin genet 28: 207-15
6. Wenger D (1987) Defects in metabolism of lipids In Behrman R, Vaughan V (eds.) Nelson textbook of Pediatrics. WB Saunders Co, Philadelphia pp 329-38
7. Weitz R, Kramer I, Nissenkorn I, Shapira Y, Ben-David E, Kohn G (1990) Muscle involvement in mucolipidosis IV. Brain Dev 12: 524-8
8. Chitayat D, Meunier CM, Hodgkinson KA, Silver K, Flanders M, Anderson IJ, Little JM, Whiteman DA, Carpenter S (1991) Mucolipidosis type IV: clinical manifestations and natural history. Am J Med Genet 41: 313-8
9. Honjoh M, Yamaguchi S, Kohda N, Mori Y, Nishimura H (1985) Fucosidosis type 3 with angiokeratoma corporis diffusum. J Dermatol 12: 174-82
10. Carpenter S, Karpati G (1986) Lysosomal storage in human skeletal muscle. Hum Pathol 17: 683-703
11. Wilson ER, Barton NW, Barranger JA (1985) Valvular involvement in type 3 neuronopathic Gaucher's disease. Arch Pathol Lab Med 109: 82-4
12. Uyama E, Takahashi K, Owada M, Okamura R, Naito M, Tsuji S, Kawasaki S, Araki S (1992) Hydrocephalus, corneal opacities, deafness, valvular heart disease, deformed toes and leptomeningeal fibrous thickening in adult siblings: a new syndrome associated with -glucocerebrosidase deficiency and a mosaic population of storage cells. Acta Neurol Scand 86: 407-20
13. Roberts WC, Fredrickson DS (1967) Gaucher's disease of the lung causing severe pulmonary hypertension with associated acute recurrent pericarditis. Circulation 35: 783-9
14. Toppet M, Vamos-Hurwitz E, Jonniaux G, Cremer N, Tondeur M, Pelc S (1978) Farber's disease as a ceramidosis: clinical, radiological and biochemical aspects. Acta Paediatr Scand 67: 113-9
15. Jameson RA, Holt PJ, Keen JH (1987) Farber's disease (lysosomal acid ceramidase deficiency). Ann Rheum Dis 46: 559-61

16. Zappatini-Tommasi L, Dumontel C, Guibaud P, Girod C (1992) Farber disease: an ultrastructural study. Virchows Arch A Pathol Anat Histopathol 420: 281-90

17. Vital C, Battin J, Rivel J, Hehunstre JP (1976) Ultra-structural aspects of peripheral nerve lesions in one case of Farber's disease. Rev Neurol (Paris) 132: 419-23

18. Farber S, Cohen J, Uzman LL (1957) Lipogranu-lomatosis: a new lipoglycoprotein "storage" disease. Mt Sinai J Med 24: 816-37

19. Tanaka T, Takahashi K, Hakozaki H, Kimoto H, Suzuki Y (1979) Farber's disease (disseminated lipogranulomato-sis) – a pathological, histochemical and ultrastructural study. Acta Pathol Jpn 29: 135-55

20. Rassoly R, Gomori JM, BenEzra D (1988) Arterial tor-tuosity and dilatation in Larsen syndrome. Neuro-radiology 30: 258-60

21. Sathy N, Krishnamoorthy KM (1992) Larsen syndrome with cardiac anomaly. Indian Pediatr 29: 783-5

22. Dustin P, Tondeur M, Jonniaux G, Vamos-Hurwitz E, Pelc S (1973) Farber's disease. Anatomoclinical and ultra-structural study. Bull Acad R Med Belg 13: 733-62

23. Roytta M, Fagerlund AS, Toikkanen S, Salmi TT, Jorde LB, Forsius HR, Eriksson AW (1992) Wolman disease: morphological, clinical and genetic studies on the first Scandinavian cases. Clin Genet 42: 1-7

24. Elleder M, Ledvinova J, Cieslar P, Kuhn R (1990) Subclinical coure of cholesterol ester storage disease (CESD) diagnosed in adulthood. Virchows Arch A Pathol Anat Histopathol 416: 357-65

25. Dolman CL, Chang E (1972) Visceral lesions in amauro-tic familial idiocy with curvilinear bodies. Arch Path 94: 425-30

26. Via DP, Guyton JR, Gotto AM (1996) Pathogenesis of atherosclerosis: lipid metabolism In Loscalzo J, Creager MA, Dzau VJ (eds) Vascular Medicine. A textbook of vas-cular biology and diseases. Little Brown Company. Boston, Newyork, Totronto, London pp 307-32

27. Puchois P, Alaupovic P, Fruchart JC (1985) Mise au point sur les classifications des lipoprotéines plasmatiques. Ann Biol Clin 43: 831-40

28. Matsushima T (1994) Genotyping of hyperlipoprotei-naemia. Nippon Rinsho 52: 3203-9

29. Brown MS, Goldstein JL (1991) The hyperlipoproteinae-mias and other disorders of lipid metablism In Wilson JD, Braunwald E, Isselbacher KJ et al (eds.): Harrison's principles of internal medicine, McGraw-Hill, NewYork, pp 1814-25

30. Stehbens WE, Martin M (1991) The vascular pathology of familial hypercholesterolaemia. Pathology 23: 54-61

31. Postiglione A, Nappi A, Brunetti A, Soricelli A, Rubba P, Gnasso A, Cammisa M, Frusciante V, Cortese C, Salvatore M, et al (1991) Relative protection from cerebral atheros-clerosis of young patients with homozygous familial hy-percholesterolaemia. Atherosclerosis 90: 23-30

32. Virkola K, Pesonen E, Akerblom HK, Siimes MA (1997) Cholesterol and carotid artery wall in children and ado-lescents with familial hypercholesterolaemia: a controlled study by ultrasound. Acta Paediatr 86: 1203-7

33. Windhagen-Mahnert B, Paul T, Offner G, Mugge A, Amende I (1997) Severe stenosis of the right coronary ar-tery in a 15-year-old girl with type IIa hypercholestero-laemia: successful treatment with stent implantation. Z Kardiol 86: 727-31

34. Feussner G, Wagner A, Kohl B, Ziegler R (1993) Clinical features of type III hyperlipoproteinaemia: analysis of 64 patients. Clin Investig 71: 362-6

35. Feussner G (1996) Severe xanthomatosis associated with familial apolipoprotein E deficiency. J Clin Pathol 49: 985-9

36. Brewer HB Jr, Zech LA, Gregg RE, Schwartz D, Schaefer EJ (1983) NIH conference. Type III hyperlipoproteinae-mia: diagnosis, molecular defects, pathology, and treat-ment. Ann Intern Med 98: 623-40

37. Feussner G, Piesch S, Dobmeyer J, Fischer C (1997) Genetics of type III hyperlipoproteinaemia. Genet Epidemiol 14: 283-97

38. Sniderman AD, Cianflone K (1996) The atherogenic dys-lipoproteinaemias In Loscalzo J, Creager MA, Dzau VJ (eds) Vascular Medicine. A textbook of vascular biology and diseases. Little Brown Company. Boston, Newyork, Totronto, London p 587-607

39. Hazzard WR, Bierman EL (1972) Aggravation of broad-beta disease (type 3 hyperlipoproteinaemia) by hypothy-roidism. Arch Intern Med 130: 822-8

40. Foger B, Patsch JR (1994) Hypertriglyceridaemia. Wien Med Wochenschr 144: 308-11

41. Nagai T, Tomizawa T, Saito T, Nakano T, Nakajima K, Mori M (1996) Familial type V hyperlipoproteinaemia with hyper-remnant-like particle-cholesterol accompa-nied with apolipoprotein E3/E4 phenotype. Intern Med 35: 388-91

42. Haust MD (1992) Aortic features in Tangier disease and pathogenetic considerations– Part I. Fatty dots and streaks. Eur J Epidemiol 8: S36-S47

43. Plump AS, Azrolan N, Odaka H, Wu L, Jiang X, Tall A, Eisenberg S, Breslow JL (1997) ApoA-I knockout mice: characterization of HDL metabolism in homozygotes and identification of a post-RNA mechanism of apoA-I up-regulation in heterozygotes. J Lipid Res 38: 1033-47

44. Kuivenhoven JA, Pritchard H, Hill J, Frohlich J, Assmann G, Kastelein J (1997) The molecular pathology of leci-thin: cholesterol acyltransferase (LCAT) deficiency syn-dromes. J Lipid Res 38: 191-205

45. Qiu S, Bergeron N, Kotite L, Krauss RM, Bensadoun A, Havel RJ (1998) Metabolism of lipoproteins containing apolipoprotein B in hepatic lipase-deficient mice. J Lipid Res 39: 1661-8

46. Kwiterovich Jr PO, Sniderman AS (1983) Atherosclerosis and apoproteins B and A-I. Prev Med 12: 815-34

47. Dische MR, Porro RS (1970) The cardiac lesions in Bassen-Kornweig syndrome. Report of a cse, with au-topsy findings. Am J Med 49: 568-71

48. Baumgartner RW, Hauser V, Grob P, Waespe W (1991) Cerebrotendinous xanthomatosis. Schweiz Med Wschr 121: 858-64

49. Bertulezzi G, Paris R, Moroni M, Porta C, Nastasi G, Amadeo A (1998) Atrial septal aneurysm in a patient with pseudoxanthoma elasticum. Acta Cardiol 53: 223-5

50. Heno P, Fourcade L, Duc HN, Bonello R, Roux O, Van de Walle JP, Mafart B, Touze JE (1998) Aorto-coronary dys-plasia and pseudoxanthoma elastica. Arch Mal Cœur Vaiss 91: 415-8

51. Refsum S (1975) Heredopathia atactica polyneuritifor-mis. Phytanic acid storage disease (Refsum's disease) In Vinken PJ, Bruyn GW (eds) Handbook of clinical neuro-logy, Vol 21 System disorders and atrophies, American Elsevier, NewYork p181

52. Allen IV, Swallow M, Nevin NC, Mc Cormick D (1978) Clinicopathological study of Refsum's disease with parti-cular reference to fatal complications. J Neurol. Neurosurg. Psychiatry 41: 323-32

53. McKusick VA (1990) Larsen syndrome In Mendelian in-heritance in man. Catalogs of autosomal dominant, auto-

somal recessive and X-linked phenotypes, 9th edn, Johns Hopkins University Press, Baltimore pp 560, 1291,1292

54. Cohen AS (1991) Amyloidosis. Bulletin on the rheumatic diseases. 40: 1-12

55. Johansson B, Westermark P (1990) The relation of atrial natriuretic factor to isolated atrial amyloid. Exp Mol Pathol 52: 266-78

56. Cornwell GG III, Westermark P, Murdoch W, Pitkanen P (1982) Senile aortic amyloid. A third distinctive type of age-related cardiovascular amyloid. Am J Pathol 108: 135-9

57. Asl LH, Liepnieks JJ, Asl KH, Uemichi T, Moulin G, Desjoyaux E, Loire R, Delpech M, Grateau G, Benson MD (1999) Hereditary amyloid cardiomyopathy caused by a variant apolipoprotein A1. Am J Pathol 154: 221-7

58. Santarone M, Corrado G, Tagliagambe LM (1999) Images in cardiology: Biatrial thrombosis in cardiac amyloidosis. Heart 81: 302

59. Smith RR, Hutchins GM, Sack Jr GH, Ridolfi RL (1979) Ischemic heart disease secondary to amyloidosis of intramyocardial arteries. Am J Cardiol 44: 413-7

60. Olson LJ, Gertz MA, Edwards WD, Li CY, Pellikka PA, Holmes DR Jr, Tajik AJ, Kyle RA (1987) Senile cardiac amyloidosis with myocardial dysfunction. Diagnosis by endomyocardial biopsy and immunohistochemistry. N Engl J Med 317: 738-42

61. Bonaventura I, Munoz E, Aguilar M, Tarroch J (1998) Cerebral amyloid angiopathy. Atypical presentation. Neurologia 13: 436

62. Randall RB, Williamson WC, Mullinax F, Tung MY, Still WJS (1976) Manifestations of light chain deposition. Am J Med 60: 293-9

63. Ganeval D, Noel LH, Preud'homme JL, Droz D, Grunfeld JP (1984) Light-chain deposition disease: its relation with AL-type amyloidosis. Kidney Int 26: 1-9

64. Fujiwara H, Tanaka M, Onodera T, Kawai C (1987) Hypertrophic cardiomyopathy: mode of death and pathological findings. J Cardiol 16: S3-S8

65. Futterman LG, Myerburg R (1998) Sudden death in athletes: an update. Sports Med 26: 335-50

66. Bundgard H, Havndrup O, Host U, Kelbaek H (1998) Hypertrophic cardiomyopathy. Ugeskr Laeger 160: 5478-83

67. Kai H, Muraishi A, Sugiu Y, Nishi H, Seki Y, Kuwahara F, Kimura A, Kato H, Imaizumi T (1998) Expression of proto-oncogenes and gene mutation of sarcomeric proteins in patients with hypertrophic cardiomyopathy. Circ Res 83: 594-601

68. Tanaka M, Fujiwara H, Onodera T, Wu DJ, Matsuda M, Hamashima Y, Kawai C (1987) Quantitative analysis of narrowings of intramyocardial small arteries in normal hearts, hypertensive hearts, and hearts with hypertrophic cardiomyopathy. Circulation 75: 1130-9

69. Takemura G, Takatsu Y, Fujiwara H (1998) Luminal narrowing of coronary capillaries in human hypertrophic hearts: an ultrastructural morphometrical study using endomyocardial biopsy specimens. Heart 79: 78-85

70. Salyer WR, Hutchins GM (1974) Cardiac lesions in secondary oxalosis. Arch Intern Med 134: 250-2

71. Fayemi AO, Ali M, Braun EV (1979) Oxalosis in hemodialysis patients: a pthologic study of 80 cases. Arch Pathol Lab Med 103: 58-62

72. Magnani G, Fatone F, Martella D, Binetti G, Magnani B (1992) A case of oxalosis with heart and lung involvement. Cardiologia 37: 507-11

73. Blackburn WE, McRoberts JW, Bhathena D, Vasquez M, Luke RG (1975) Severe vascular complications in oxalosis after bilateral nephrectomy. Ann Intern Med 82: 44-6

74. Kiss D, Meier R, Gyr K, Wegmann W (1992) Secondary oxalosis following small bowel resection with kidney insufficiency and oxalate vasculopathy. Schweiz Med Wochenschr 122: 854-7

75. Chaplin A (1977) Histopathological occurrence and characterization of calcium oxalte: a review. J Clin Pathol 30: 800-11

76. Severo LC, Londero AT, Geyer GR, Picon PD (1981) Oxalosis associated with an aspergillus niger fungus ball. Report of a case. Mycopathologia 73: 29-31

77. Hajdu J, Marton T, Papp C, Hruby E, Papp Z (1998) Calcification of the fetal heart—four case reports and a literature review. Prenat Diagn 18: 1186-90

78. Moran JJ (1975) Idiopathic arterial calcification of infancy: a clinicopathologic study. Pathol Annu 10: 393-417

79. Van Reempts PJ, Boven KJ, Spitaels SE, Roodhooft AM, Vercruyssen EL, Van Acker KJ (1991) Idiopathic arterial calcification of infancy. Calcif Tissue Int 48: 1-6

80. Hodson EM, Antico VF, O'Neill P (1992) Hypertension associated with diffuse small artery calcification: a casereport. Pediatr Nephrol 6: 556-8

81. Carles D, Serville F, Dubecq JP, Alberti EM, Horovitz J, Weichhold W (1992) Idiopathic arterial calcification in a stillborn complicated by pleural hemorrhage and hydrops fetalis. Arch Pathol Lab Med 116: 293-5

82. Schiffmann JH, Wessel A, Bruck W, Speer CP (1992) Idiopathic infantile arterial calcinosis. A rare cardiovascular disease of uncertain etiology—case report and review of the literature. Monatsschr Kinderheilkd 140: 27-33

83. Saetung P, Punyathunya R (1995) Idiopathic arterial calcification of infancy: a case report. J Med Assoc Thai 78: 369-73

84. Pao DG, DeAngelis GA, Lovell MA, McIlhenny J, Hagspiel KD (1998) Idiopathic arterial calcification of infancy: sonographic and magnetic resonance findings with pathologic correlation. Pediatr Radiol 28: 256-9

85. Stuart G, Wren C, Bain H (1990) Idiopathic infantile arterial calcification in two siblings: failure of treatment with diphosphonate. Br Heart J 64: 156-9

86. Thiaville A, Smets A, Clercx A, Perlmutter N (1994) Idiopathic infantile arterial calcification: a surviving patient with renal artery stenosis. Pediatr Radiol 24: 506-8

87. Samon LM, Ash KM, Murdison KA (1995) Aorto-pulmonary calcification: an unusual manifestation of idiopathic calcification of infancy evident antenatally. Obstet Gynecol 85: 863-5

88. Champ C, Byard RW (1994) Pulmonary thromboembolism and unexpected death in infancy. J Paediatr Child Health 30: 550-1

89. Martin JJ, Flament-Durand J, Farriaux JP, Buyssens N, Ketelbant-Balasse P, Jansen C (1978) Menkes kinky-hair disease. A report on its pathology. Acta Neuropathol (Berl) 42: 25-32

90. Oakes BW, Danks DM, Campbell PE (1976) Human copper deficiency: ultrastructural studies of the aorta and skin in a child with Menke's syndrome. Exp Mol Pathol 25: 82-98

91. Cooper BA, Rosenblatt DS (1987) Inherited vitamin B12 defects. Ann Rev Nutr 7: 308-12

92. Brandstetter Y, Weinhouse E, Splaingard ML, Tang TT (1990) Cor pulmonale as a complication of methylmalonic acidaemia and homocystinuria (Cbl-C type). Am J Med Genet 36: 167-171

93. Gore I, Wada M, Goodman ML (1968) Capillary hemorrhage in ascorbic-acid-deficient guinea pigs. Ultrastructural basis. Arch Pathol 85: 493-502

94. Gazave JM, Pfister A, Degeorges M, Mousseron S (1980) Part of ascorbic acid in the maintenance of the blood capillary wall. New data. J Mal Vasc 5: 67-71

95. Stehbens WE (1988) Localization of experimental calcification in rabbit blood vessels with particular references to haemodynamics. Angiology 39: 597-608

96. Kruger MC, Horrobin DF (1997) Calcium metabolism, osteoporosis and essential fatty acids: a review. Prog Lipid Res 36: 131-51

97. Laroche M, Puech JL, Pouilles JM, Arlet J, Boccalon H, Puel P, Mazieres B, Arlet P, Ribot C (1992) Lower limb arteriopathy and male osteoporosis. Rev Rhum Mal Osteoartic 59: 95-101

98. Laroche M (1996) Arteriosclerosis and osteoporosis. Presse Med 25: 52-4

99. Van Vleet JF, Ferrans VJ, Ruth GR (1977) Ultrastructural alterations in nutritional cardiomyopathy of selenium-vitamine E deficient swine. I. Fiber lesions. Lab Invest 37: 188-200

100. Van Vleet JF, Ferrans VJ, Ruth GR (1977) Ultrastructural alterations in nutritional cardiomyopathy of selenium-vitamine E deficient swine. II. Vascular lesions. Lab Invest 37: 201-11

101. Baker SS, Lerman RH, Krey SH, Crocker KS, Hirsh EF, Cohen H (1983) Selenium deficiency with total parenteral nutrition: reversal of biochemical and functional abnormalities by selenium supplementation: a case report. Am J Clin Nutr 38: 769-74

102. Ferrans VJ, Van Vleet JF (1988) Cardiac lesions of selenium-vitamine E deficinecy in animals In Sekiguchi M, Olsen EGJ, Goodwin JF: Myocarditis and related disorders. Springer Verlag, Tokyo pp 294-7

103. Keshan Disease Research Group of the Chinese Academy of Medical Sciences, Beijing (1979) Epidemiologic studies on the etiologic relationship of selenium and Keshan disease. Chinese Med J 92: 477-82

104. Legg MA, Harawi SJ (1985) The pathology of diabetes mellitus In Marble A, Krall LP, Bradley RF et al (eds.) Joslin's Diabetes Mellitus, 4th ed, Lea & Febiger, Philadelphia pp 298-331

105. Stout RW (1993) Diabetes and atherosclerosis. Biomed Pharmacother 47: 1-2

106. Edmonds ME, Morrison N, Laws JW, Watkins PJ (1982) Medial arterial calcification and diabetic neuropathy. Br Med J (Clin Res Ed) 284: 928-30

107. Mossaz A, Assal JP (1987) Aspects physiopathologiques et cliniques de l'angiopathie diabétique. In Camilleri JP, Berry CL, Fiessinger J-N, Bariety J (eds): Les maladies de la paroi artérielle. Flammarion, Paris, 313-321

108. Dornan TL, Ting A, McPherson CK, Peckar CO, Mann JI, Turner RC, Morris PJ (1982) Genetic susceptibility to the development of retinopathy in insulin-dependent diabetics. Diabetes 31: 226-31

109. Chait A, Bierman EL, Brunzell JD (1985) Diabetic macroangiopathy In Alberti KG, Krall L(eds.) The diabetes annual. Elsevier Science Publishers, Amsterdam, pp 323-49

110. Sowers JR, Standley PR, Ram JL, Jacober S, Simpson L, Rose K (1993) Hyperinsulinaemia, insulin resistance, and hyperglycaemia: contributing factors in the pathogenesis of hypertension and atherosclerosis. Am J Hypertens 6: S260-S270

111. Capron L (1996) Atherosclerosis and cardio-vascular complications of diabetes. Ann Endocrinol (Paris) 57: 161-5

112. Colwell JA, Winocour PD, Lopes-Virella M, Halushka PV (1983) New concepts about the pathogenesis of atherosclerosis in diabetes mellitus. Am J Med 75: 67-80

113. Stehbens WE, Wierzbicki E (1988) The relationship of hypercholesterolaemia to atherosclerosis with particular emphasis on familial hypercholesterolaemia, diabetes mellitus, obstructive jaundice, myxedema, and the nephrotic syndrome. Prog Cardiovasc Dis 30: 289-306

114. Steiner G (1994) The dyslipoproteinaemias of diabetes. Atherosclerosis 110: S27-S33

115. Cosentino F, Luscher TF (1998) Endothelial dysfunction in diabetes mellitus. J Cardiovasc Pharmacol 32:S54-S61

116. Tominaga M (1995) Risk factor: diabetes mellitus. Rinsho Byori 43: 111-6

117. Dahl-Jorgensen K (1998) Diabetic microangiopathy. Acta Paediatr 425: S31-S34

118. Addison DJ, Garner A, Ashton N (1970) Degeneration of intramural pericytes in diabetic retinopathy. Br Med J 1: 246-66

119. Masmiquel L, Burgos R, Simo R (1997) Basal membrane and diabetes mellitus. Med Clin (Barc) 109: 302-10

120. Capron L (1994) Mechanisms of macrovascular involvement in diabetic subjects. Diabete Metab 20: 357-61

121. Vranes D, Cooper ME, Dilley RJ (1999) Cellular mechanisms of diabetic vascular hypertrophy. Microvasc Res 57: 8-18

122. Fuchs U, Caffier P, Schulz HG, Wieniecki P (1985) Arterial calcification in diabetics. Virchows Arch A Pathol Anat Histopathol 407: 431-9

123. Gentile S, Bizzarro A, Marmo R, de Bellis A, Orlando C (1990) Medial arterial calcification and diabetic neuropathy. Acta Diabetol Lat 27: 243-53

124. Cronin CC, O'Sullivan DJ, Mitchell TH (1996) Medial arterial calcification, calcific aortic stenosis and mitral annular calcification in a diabetic patient with severe autonomic neuropathy. Diabet Med 13: 768-70

125. Marin R, Fernandez-Vega F, Escalada P, Estevan JM, Barreiro A, Alvarez J (1993) Cardiovascular risk factors in peripheral arterial disease. A study of 403cases. Rev Clin Esp 193: 357-62

126. Simon A (1997) Diabetic macroangiopathy in humans. Therapie 52: 423-8

127. Verhaeghe R (1998) Epidemiology and prognosis of peripheral obliterative arteriopathy. Drugs 56: S1-S10

128. Orcel L (1978) Pathologie non tumorale des vaisseaux sanguins In Delarue J, Laumonier R (eds.) Anatomie pathologique. Pathologie spéciale. Flammarion, Paris p.155

129. Hiscott PS, Gierson I, Trombetta CJ (1984) Retinal and epiretinal glia; an immunohistochemical study. Br J Ophthalmol 68: 698-707

130. Nakamoto Y, Takazakura E, Hayakawa H, Kawai K, Dohi K, Fujioka M, Kida H, Hattori N, Takeuchi J (1980) Intrarenal microaneurysms in diabetic nephropathy. Lab Invest 42: 433-9

131. Llewelyn JG, Thomas PK, King RH (1998) Epineurial microvasculitis in proximal diabetic neuropathy. J Neurol 245: 159-65

132. Williams B (1998) A potential role for angiotensin II-induced vascular endothelial growth factor expression in the pathogenesis of diabetic nephropathy? Miner Electrolyte Metab 24: 400-5

133. Levin ME (1980) The diabetic foot. Angiology 31:375-85

134. Logerfo FW, Coffman JD (1984) Vascular and microvascular disease of the foot in diabetes. Implication for foot care. NEJM 311: 1615-9

135. Briza J, Krska Z (1996) Diabetic gangrene and amputation. Sb Lek 97: 493-7

136. McCulloch DK, Campbell IW, Wu FC, Prescott RJ, Clarke BF (1980) The prevalence of diabetic impotence. Diabetologia 18: 279-83

137. Azadzoi KM, Saenz de Tejada I (1992) Diabetes mellitus impairs neurogenic and endothelium-dependent relaxation of rabbit corpus cavernosum smooth muscle. J Urol 148: 1587-91

138. Mohr-Kahaly S, Kahaly G, Meyer J (1996) Cardiovascular effects of thyroid hormones. Z Kardiol 85: S219-S231

139. Kirk SJ, O'Kane HO, Morton P (1987) Coronary artery surgery and myxoedema. Br Heart J 58: 674-5

140. Toft J, Toft H (1989) Hypothyroidism and coronary artery bypass surgery. Ugeskr Laeger 151: 3406-7

141. Nyrop M, Bjornholm KI, Nielsen FE, Haedersdal C (1991) Cardiovascular manifestations of hypothyroidism. Ugeskr Laeger 153: 1849-51

142. Shigeta O, Makuuchi H, Kaneko Y, Takuma S, Konishi T, Omura M (1994) A case of acute aortic dissection associated with myxedema. Nippon Kyobu Geka Gakkai Zasshi 42: 1096-100

143. Schluter KD, Piper HM (1998) Cardiovascular actions of parathyroid hormone and parathyroid hormone-related peptide. Cardiovasc Res 37: 34-41

144. Mantero F, Boscaro M (1992) Glucocorticoid-dependent hypertension. J Steroid Biochem Mol Biol 43: 409-13

145. Takeda R (1993) Endocrine hypertension. Nippon Ronen Igakkai Zasshi 30: 182-7

146. Mizokami T, Okamura K, Sato K, Kuroda T, Sadoshima S, Fujishima M (1996) Risk factors for brain infarction in patients with Cushing's disease. Case reports. Angiology 47: 1011-7

147. Goldberg E, Berger M, Garber M (1983) Extensive coronary collateral formation in a patient with untreated acromegaly. Angiology 34: 306-10

148. Robinson JL, Hall CS, Sedzimir CB (1974) Arteriovenous malformations, aneurysms and pregnancy. J Neurosurg 41: 63-70

149. Vuong PN, Janneau D, Jousse-Hua D, Bensaïd P (1996) Anévrysme disséquant de l'aorte sous-rénale de découverte fortuite: un cas (lettre).Sem Hôp Paris 72: 628

150. Bercau G, Castaigne V, Mihaileanu S, Couetil JP, Freund M, Sauvanet E (1997) Dissection of the ascending aorta in pregnancy. Apropos of a case and review of the literature. J Gynecol Obstet Biol Reprod (Paris) 26: 540-2

151. Cheng TO (1998) Aortic dissection during pregnancy. Ann Thorac Surg 65: 1511-2

XVI
Hypertension and vessels

1 – Systemic arterial hypertension

Arterial hypertension is commonly classified as primary (essential) or secondary. Two clinical forms occur; by far the most common is a chronic or slowly developing elevation of the blood pressure leading to structural and functional changes in vessels, mediated primarily by vascular smooth muscle [1]. The aetiology is complex and depends on the interaction of a number of genetic factors and events during development, with environmental factors playing a part in some populations [2]. Information on genetic factors (genes coding for renin, angiotensin converting enzyme, angiotensinogen and the AT1 receptor) is well reviewed by Peters [3] and Morgan et al [4] have investigated the significance of polymorphism in the angiotensinogen gene.

So-called malignant hypertension is now rare in countries with effective health care; it is usually manifest by superimposed acute changes on chronically altered vessels, with insudation of plasma components and necrosis. Scarpelli et al [5] found that just under half of their cases of malignant hypertension were in patients with long established hypertension and Bohle et al [6] found secondary malignant nephrosclerosis in 151 of 1177 renal biopsies made in the evaluation of patients with essential hypertension. When this type of hypertension occurs ab initio, it is often associated with tumours (notably pheochromocytoma and renin secreting tumours). Renal failure and cerebrovascular injury are common consequences of accelerated hypertension.

The effects of hypertension on arteries resemble those of ageing, with exaggerated thickening of the intima and changes in the media. The process of arteriosclerosis is accelerated [7, 8] and increase in endothelial permeability facilitates the development of atherosclerosis [9]. As a generalisation atherosclerotic changes predominate in conduit arteries, while an increased medial thickness is seen in resistance arteries [10].

Vascular smooth muscle cell (SMC) hypertrophy, a process triggered by angiotensin II and transforming growth factor [11-13], is a major factor in the pathogenesis of vascular change and also results in an increased synthesis of extracellular matrix. In experimental models, a decrease in blood pressure and especially its long-term normalization, is followed by regression of aortic medial hypertrophy and a reduc-

tion of collagen synthesis by myofibroblasts. The same phenomenon is noted in small arteries [14].

Vascular changes in systemic hypertension

Hypertension increases the permeability of the intima to plasma proteins, blood-borne mononuclear cells and other materials. The infiltrating cells and plasma material accumulate in the intima immediately adjacent to defects of the internal elastic lamella and in the intimal musculoelastic cushions [15]. In longstanding hypertension, the intima [8] and media [16, 17] undergo marked thickening. In the media of elastic arteries the number of medial lamellar units remains unchanged, but the extracellular matrix, medial elastin and collagen increase in mass in a manner directly proportional to the mural stress [18].

Intimal thickening

In the aorta, changes are most pronounced after the third decade in both sexes. In slowly developing hypertension, the subendothelial layer shows proliferation of poorly differentiated connective cells with accumulation of elastin and collagen. The internal elastic lamella is usually disrupted and duplicated. In malignant hypertension, the intimal thickening often appears oedematous, cellular, and is basophilic.

Medial changes

The medial myocyte mass increases either by hypertrophy (large elastic arteries) or by proliferation of fibromyoblasts (small arteries and arterioles). The overall picture is of a concentric thickening of the arterial wall (in a layered or onion pattern). These changes decrease the compliance of arteries.

Necrotizing changes

These may occur in arteries, arterioles and the transitional segment in malignant hypertension. A rapid increase in eosinophilic granular material having a staining reaction akin to that of fibrin is seen with the disrupted arteriolar wall infiltrated by red cells. An inflammatory reaction develops around the vessel and the change is described as fibrinoid necrosis or necrotizing vasculitis [19]. Fibrinoid necrosis is followed by fibrosis.

Changes in specific parts of the vascular tree

Kidney

Hypertension is associated with contraction of the glomerular afferent arterioles, which protect the glomerular capillaries against excessive intravascular pressure. There is a reduction in the capillary luminal diameter with secondary thickening of the walls. Progressive deposition of matrix and collagen in the mesangial areas causes collapse of the capillary tuft and loss of glomerular function. These changes, called ischaemic glomerulosclerosis, are often accompanied by a thickening of Bowman's capsule (Fig. 1). Tubular atrophy and interstitial fibrosis follow arteriolar and glomerular changes. Renal changes in malignant hypertension display more severe arteriolar and glomerular lesions: segmental necrosis and thrombosis, mild cellular proliferation in the mesangial areas, adhesions to the Bowman capsule and sometimes crescent formation. Marked arteriolar narrowing en-

hances the ischaemic change produced by glomerular capillary collapse (Fig. 2). Hyperplasia and hypergranularity of the juxtaglomerular apparatus (Fig. 3) are found in association with high levels of renin and angiotensin in the blood [20]. Overlapping of vascular lesions (ischemic glomerulosclerosis and malignant nephrosclerosis) may occur in the same patient and even in different segments of the same artery when malignant hypertension is superimposed upon a long-standing preexistent benign hypertension (Fig. 4-5).

Heart

Hypertensive cardiomegaly is directly related to the degree of hypertension, but not necessarily to its duration [20]. Concentric left ventricular hypertrophy results in a small chamber with a thick wall (greater than 18 mm in the outflow tract). The weight of the enlarged heart is usually over 500 g but rarely exceeds 700 g. Histologically, individual myocardial fibres are enlarged; many undergo degeneration and are replaced by fibrous tissue. Myocardial hypertrophy is often

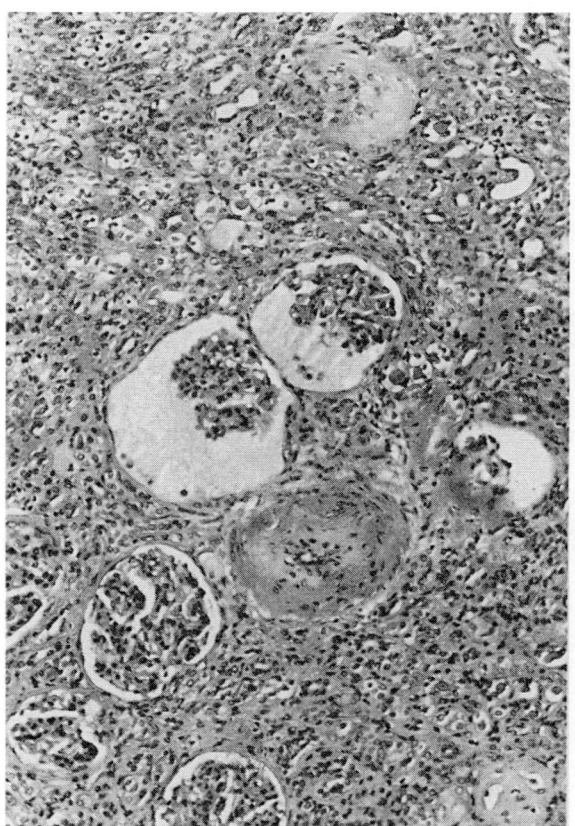

Fig. 1. Arterial hypertension. Ischaemic glomerulosclerosis. Haematoxylin, eosin and saffron stain. (HES)

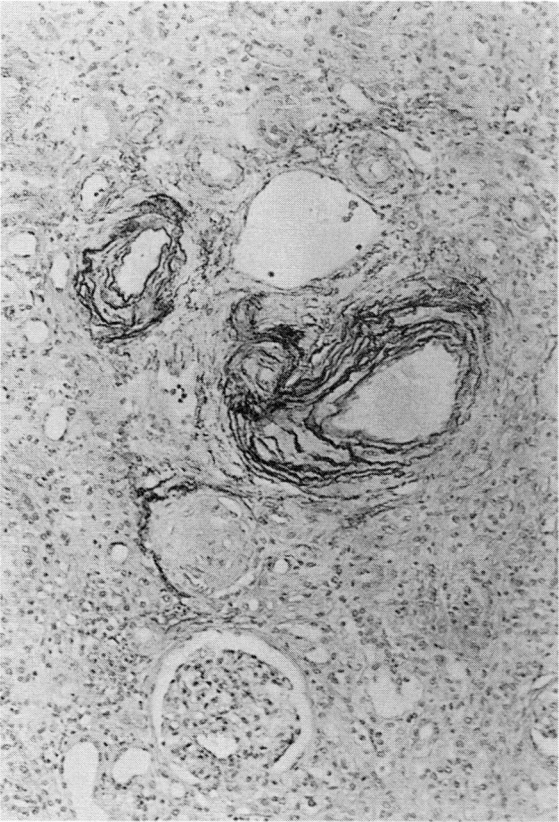

Fig. 2. Arterial hypertension. Intrarenal arteriolar stenosis. Orcein elastic stain. (Orcein)

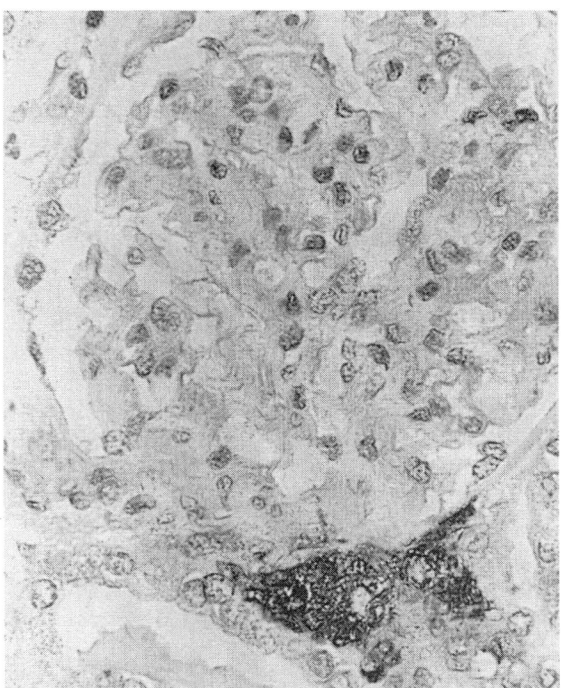

Fig. 3. Arterial hypertension. Hyperplasia of the juxtaglomerular apparatus evidenced by anti-renin antibody labelling. Peroxidase antiperoxidase immunohistochemical technique. (PAP)

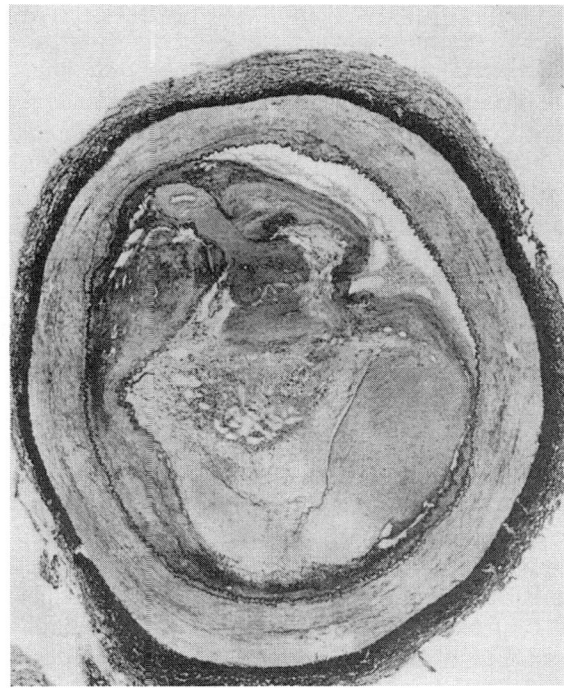

Fig. 4. Renal hypertension caused by occlusive atherosclerotic lesions. ...Orcein...

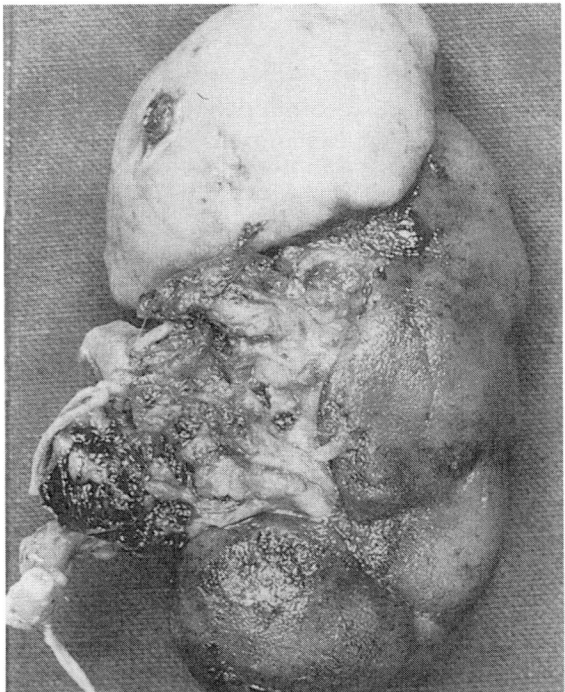

Fig. 5. Renal hypertension. Large polar infarction. Note marked retraction of the remaining renal cortex. (Courtesy Dr P. Lagneau)

accompanied by sub-endocardial fibrosis. Aggravation of coronary atherosclerosis by hypertension further enhances myocardial ischemia and fibrosis.

Brain

The principle effect of hypertension is an acceleration of atherosclerosis and the secondary effect is ischaemia, both result from the vascular narrowing produced by this disease and the effects of treatment– related fluctuations in pressure. Hypertensive encephalopathy may occur in conditions with only moderately elevated blood pressure (notably in eclampsia). Hypertension may contribute to development of intracranial aneurysms.

Post-coarctation surgery

Ten percent of patients undergoing surgical repair of aortic coarctation develop a hypertension syndrome with arterial and arteriolar fibrinoid necrosis [20]. The symptoms usually appear on the third postoperative day with elevation of the blood pressure above the preoperative level. Affected vessels include the arteries of the mesentery, abdominal viscera and gastrointestinal tract, as well as the intercostal, diaphragmatic arteries and the main branches of the abdominal aorta. Fibrinoid necrosis, leukocyte infiltration, thrombosis and aneurysm formation are common histological features. Abdominal pain, vomiting and gastrointestinal bleeding, fever, and leukocytosis occur and intestinal gangrene, perforation and peritonitis may follow. This syndrome is caused by sudden exposure of the previously protected arteries below the coarctation to a high systolic pressure.

2 – Pulmonary hypertension

In general, vascular morphology is not a good indicator of pulmonary pressure or resistance; however, the effects of hypertension may be quantified in small muscular arteries [21-24]. Pulmonary hypertension can be demonstrated in a number of chronic pulmonary diseases and in congenital heart disease where left to right shunting is significant.

Major pulmonary arteries

At birth, the pulmonary trunk and the aorta have a similar morphology. During the first weeks of life, the media of the pulmonary trunk becomes thinner, and the elastic lamellae fragment and decrease in number. The histological pattern of the pulmonary trunk in infants indicates whether pulmonary hypertension was present at birth or has occurred more recently. Intimal atherosclerosis with foam cell plaques also occurs in adults with chronic lung disease and cor pulmonale.

Small artery and arteriolar pulmonary changes in pulmonary hypertension

The effects of pulmonary hypertension were classified into 4 grades by Heath et al in 1959 [25], a classification still used today in modified form (Table 1).

Medial hypertrophy (Grade 1)

This is the earliest and most common sign of hypertension (Fig. 6). This change includes thickening of the media and extension of medial myocytes into distal vessels; myocytes can be observed down to an external diameter of 20 μ. The media increases in thickness and measures from 15 to 35% of its diameter. Medial myocytes increase both in size and number. The nuclei are oriented both parallel to and tangential to the long axis of the artery. At this level, they are best appreciated in cross-section as circular nuclei surrounded by clear rims of cytoplasm beneath the endothelium.

Intimal hyperplasia (Grade 2)

This change mostly involves arteries with an external diameter of 100 to 300 μ. The intima thickens. Intimal cells increase in size and number and tend to be oriented radially rather than concentrically (Fig. 7-8). They are separated by an abundant, clear ground substance that stains positively with Alcian blue. Over time, this myxoid character disappears and the intima becomes hyalinized. Concentrically intimal hyperplasia is distinctive from eccentric intimal cushions at bifurcation points, which are common in open lung biopsies from elderly patients and which are part of the vascular ageing process. Intimal hyperplasia follows medial hypertrophy if pulmonary hypertension develops slowly but may occur as an isolated change when pulmonary hypertension occurs rapidly in infants suffering from some types of congenital heart

Table 1. Grading of pulmonary hypertension in small arteries and arterioles

GRADE	TERMINOLOGY	DESCRIPTION
1	Medial hypertrophy	Medial thickening with extension of medial smooth muscle cells into distal vessels
2	Intimal hyperplasia	Concentric intimal thickening
3	Intimal fibroelastosis	Appearance of collagen and elastic fibers in the hypertrophied intima
4	Plexiform arteriopathy and segmental vascular ectasias	Congeries of channels developed within the arterial wall, directly next to venules and veins

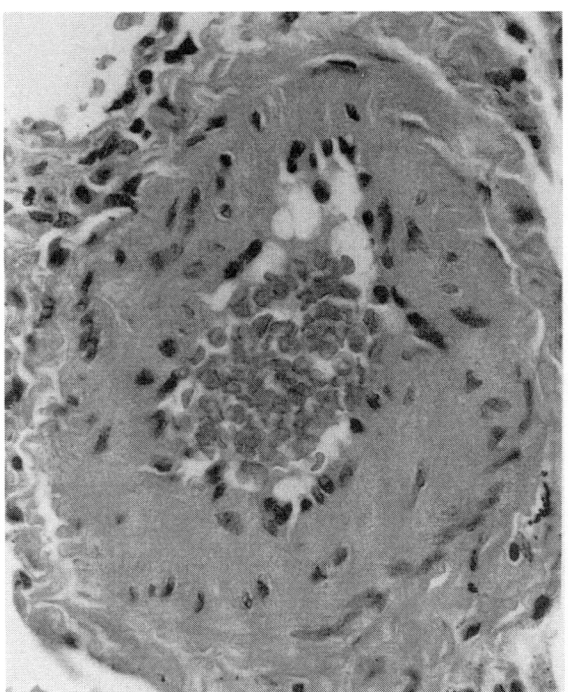

Fig. 6. Pulmonary hypertension (Grade 1). Medial hypertrophy. HES

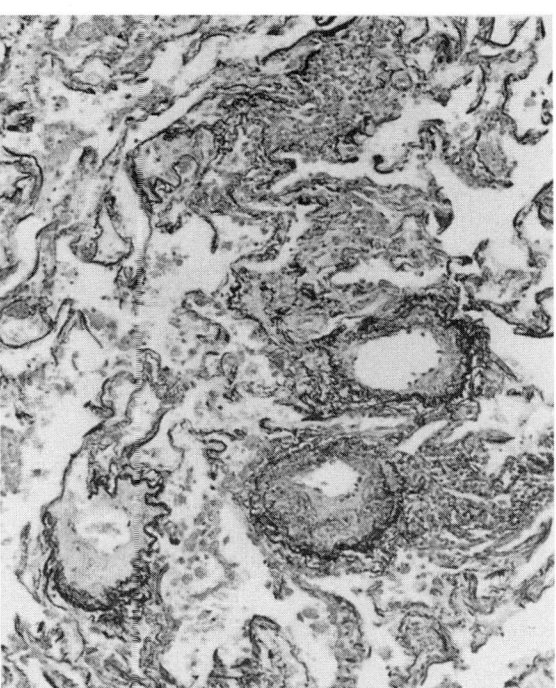

Fig. 7. Pulmonary hypertension (Grade 2). Intimal hyperplasia. ...Orcein...

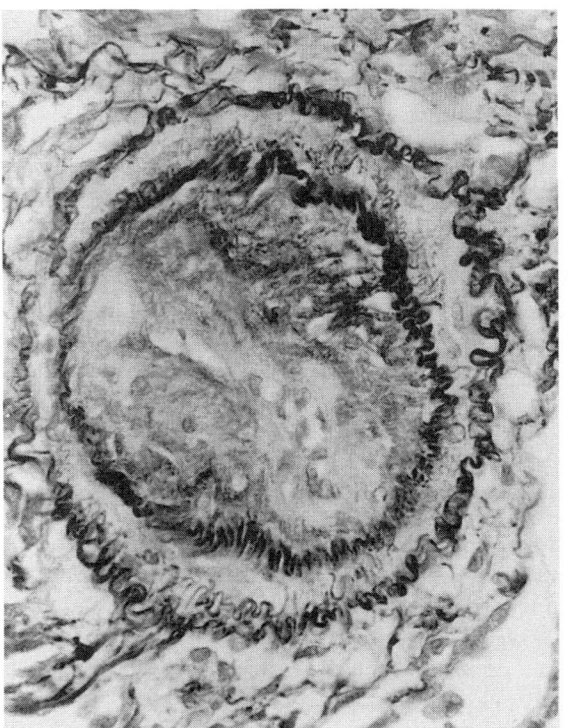

Fig. 8. Pulmonary hypertension (Grade 2). Occlusive intimal hyperplasia. ...Orcein...

disease and in adults suffering from diffuse alveolar damage or scarring fibrosis [26]. In these cases the lesion is most severe in the midst of the scarring.

Intimal fibroelastosis (Grade 3)

Larger arteries up to 500 μ in diameter are frequently involved. There are collagen and elastic fibers in the hypertrophied intima. Both the fibers and intimal cells form concentric lamellae (Fig. 9-10). With time, collagen increases in quantity and the intima becomes hyalinized. Intimal fibroelastosis indicates irreversible vascular changes and suggests a poor prognosis in congenital heart disease. However, it can also be seen in patients with scleroderma, lupus erythematosus and rheumatoid disease. Occlusive intimal fibroelastosis should be distinguished from organizing pulmonary emboli.

Advanced lesions (Grade 4)

Changes caused by severe pulmonary hypertension include plexiform arteriopathy, fibrinoid necrosis and segmental vascular ectasias. Plexiform arteriopathy is seldom seen in pulmonary hypertension, unless this is part of the change seen in high flow from congenital heart disease, which can be an important feature

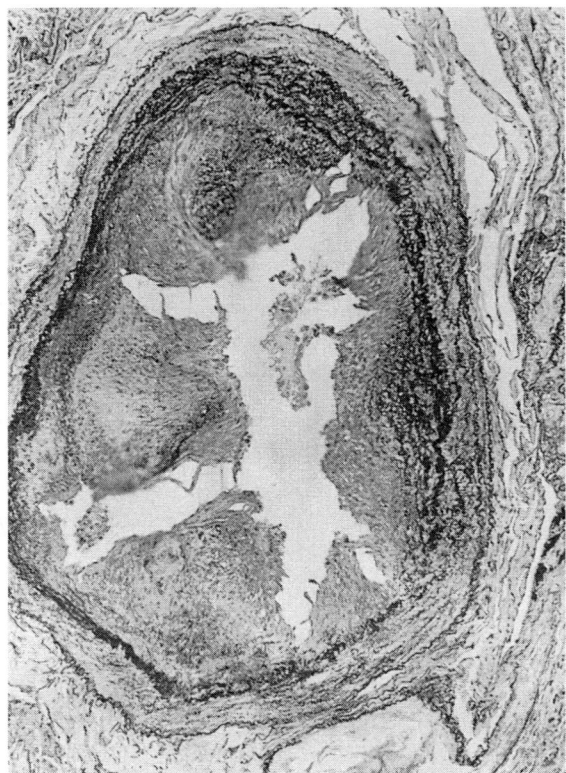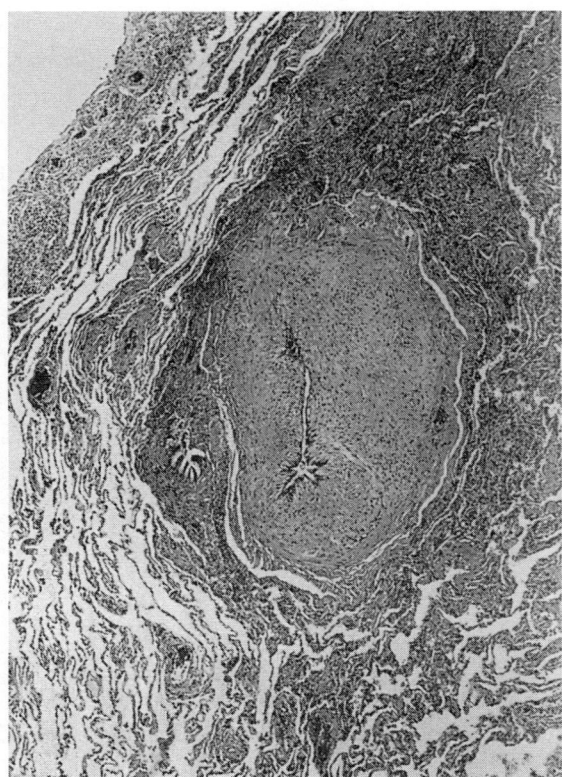

Fig. 9-10. Pulmonary hypertension (Grade 3). Intimal fibroelastosis. ...Orcein...

in differential diagnosis. However, the change is not specific and may be observed in cirrhosis, pulmonary schistosomiasis, and in pulmonary hypertension from the appetite-suppressing drug aminorex [21, 27].

Plexiform arteriopathy

Congeries of channels develop within the arterial wall, directly next to venules and veins [28, 29]. These vascular slits are lined with endothelial cells (Fig. 11-12). Plexiform lesions are scattered and only one or two may be present per slide; at least ten blocks of tissue should be examined before concluding that no plexiform lesions exist. They can measure up to 1mm in diameter, causing a "lump" on the main artery. When a plexiform lesion is small, slit-like vessels vaguely resembling Kaposi's sarcoma appear (Fig. 13). Plump endothelial cells of newly-formed vessels may mimic a glomus tumour adjacent to the artery. At other times, the newly-formed vessels may be widely patent; the lesion then resembles an arteriovenous fistula. When these vessels are obstructed, the lesion should be distinguished from an organising thrombus.

Fibrinoid necrosis

In severe pulmonary hypertension fibrinoid necrosis may involve muscular arteries or arterioles. The necrosis is often segmental, and leads to vascular rupture with aneurysm formation, followed by haemorrhage into the interstitium or alveoli and later by haemosiderosis. Organization of the fibrin clot with ingrowth of fibroblasts and newly-formed capillaries gives rise to a plexiform lesion that re-establishes the continuity of the blood flow. Fibrinoid necrosis and plexiform lesions are usually not seen under 2 years of age.

Segmental vascular ectasias

These are often associated with plexiform lesions. Occasionally, they occur in lesser degrees of pulmonary hypertension in the absence of plexiform lesions. The segment of dilated vessel may be straight, fusiform, or coiled. It may realize a localized, bulbous, thin-walled swelling mimicking an aneurysm. In the artery, the media becomes thinner and seems to have vanished. Vascular ectasias may result from proximal luminal narrowing by intimal fibrosis with post-ste-

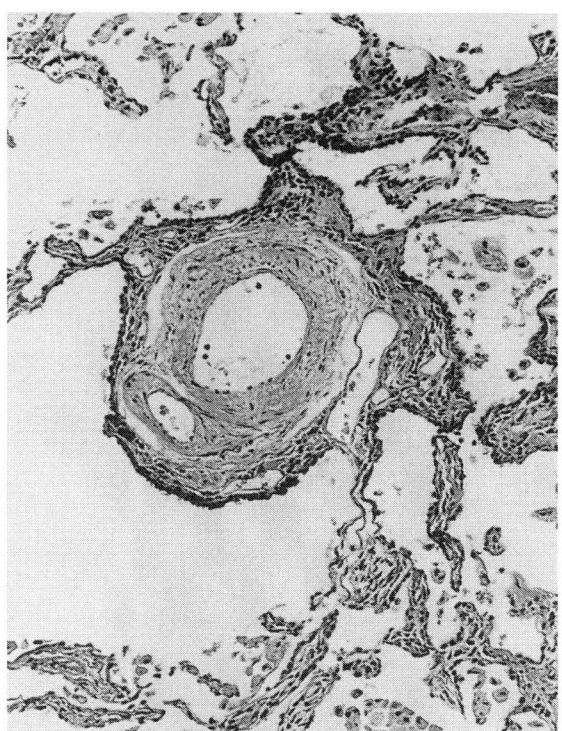

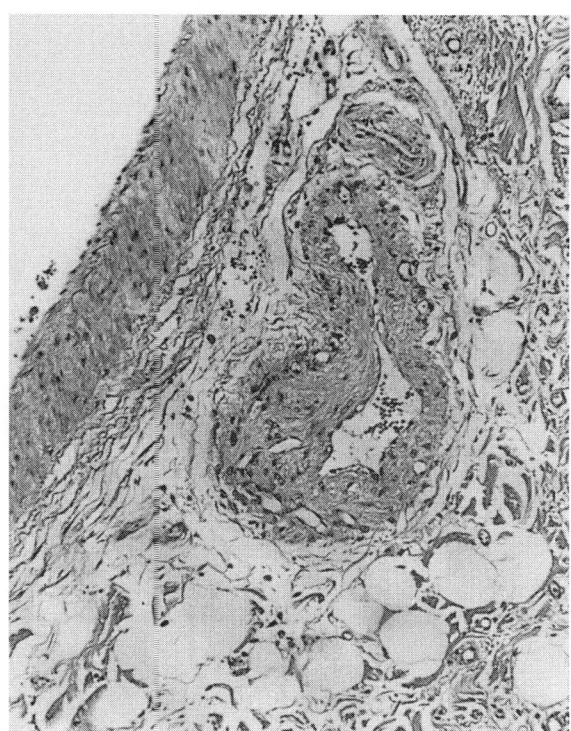

Fig. 11-12. Pulmonary hypertension (Grade 4). Plexiform arteriopathy. HES

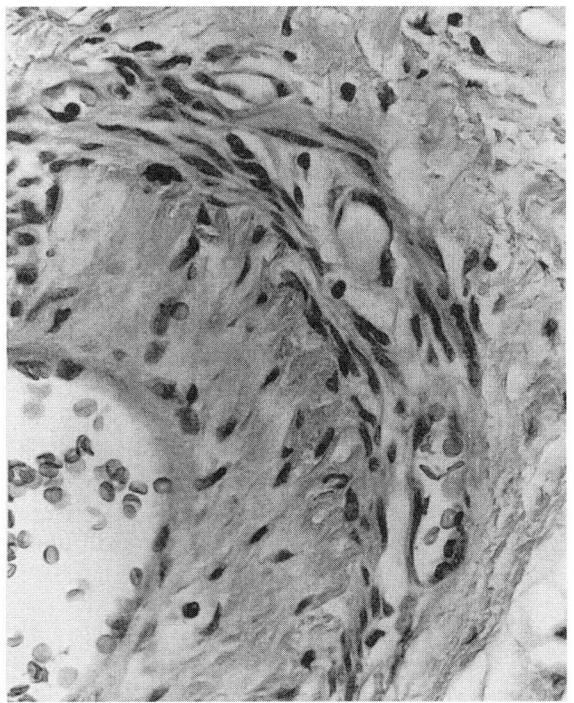

Fig. 13. Pulmonary hypertension (Grade 4). Plexiform arteriopathy. HES

notic dilatation. It is our view that these lesions are not a direct result of necrotizing arteritis.

Arterial pulmonary hypertension in congenital heart diseases

Patients with congenital heart defects are at risk of developing pulmonary artery hypertension. In the presence of pulmonary hypertension, the pulmonary vasculature fails to remodel after birth. Secondary changes then develop, and do so more rapidly than in the adult lung because the cells are exposed to the insult whilst still relatively undifferentiated [30]. Histological morphometry of arterial pulmonary hypertension is critical in choosing the optimal time for surgery and in predicting the prognosis. This approach allows the detection of arterial lesions that qualitative analysis would not identify. Three degrees of severity (A, B and C) of early pulmonary vascular changes are identified and correlated with hemodynamic evidence of progressive functional impairment (Table 2) [31, 32].

Table 2. Degrees of severity of pulmonary hypertension in small arteries and arterioles in congenital heart diseases with haemodynamic and standard grading corespondences

DEGREE OF SEVERITY (Rabinovitch 1980)	DESCRIPTION	HAEMODYNAMIC CORESPONDENCES	STANDARD GRADING (Heath 1959)
A	Abnormal extension of muscle into peripheral arteries	Increased pulmonary blood flow but pulmonary artery pressure normal	
B	Degree A changes with increased medial wall thickness of the normally muscular arteries	Increased pulmonary blood flow with increased pulmonary artery pressure	Grade 1
C	Degree B changes with a reduction in the number of small peripheral arteries	Increased pulmonary vascular resistance	

Degree A

Myocytes extend into smaller and more peripheral arteries than would normally be expected, a change which may remain isolated as a finding. Quantification of myocyte extension must take the age of the patient into account. Pulmonary blood flow is increased. Degree A change is potentially reversible and is not associated with an increase in pulmonary artery pressure.

Degree B

The media of peripheral arteries increases in thickness with myocyte hypertrophy and hyperplasia. This degree corresponds to grade 1 of the standard classification [25]. In its mild form this change is not associated with pulmonary artery hypertension, in contrast to marked degree B change, which has both increased pulmonary blood flow and pulmonary artery pressure. According to Yamaki et al [33], when a patient has less than 7% of small pulmonary arteries involved, operative repair is likely to be effective. When the value is higher than 10%, neither operative repair nor pulmonary artery banding can be recommended; both will be ineffectual and dangerous.

Degree C

Small arteries and arterioles decrease in number, probably resulting from progressive medial hypertrophy leading to luminal obliteration, atrophy and resorption of blood vessels. Pulmonary vascular resistance is increased. The changes are irreversible and the prognosis after surgery is poor.

Venous pulmonary hypertension

In adults, this condition is caused by left-sided cardiac failure, especially mitral stenosis, and pulmonary veno-occlusive disease (PVOD) of various aetiologies [34-38]. In most instances, arteriolar hypertension develops along with venous hypertension. The earliest change is hypertrophy of the media with an increase in the number of myocytes, leading to medial thickening. This is followed by intimal hyperplasia and adventitial fibrosis. Elastic fibers in veins, normally distributed throughout the media, become condensed into internal and external elastic lamellae. The "arterialized" vein is thus histologically indistinguishable from an artery, except with regard to the anatomic location. In severe venous hypertension, poorly cellular intimal fibrosis deforms and occludes the lumen. Intraparenchymal varices rarely develop. In addition to the venous changes, the parenchyma is distorted by oedema and fibrosis and this, together with the haemosiderin pigment deposited within interstitium and alveoli, gives rise to brown induration of the lung.

3 – Portal hypertension and Budd-Chiari syndrome

Portal hypertension

This condition is present when the portal pressure is over 12 mmHg, leading to a pressure gradient between the portal and the caval territories equal to or greater than 5 mmHg [39]. Splenomegaly and oesophageal varices are usually present and may cause upper gastrointestinal bleeding [40]. Portal hypertension is subdivided into supra-, intra- or infra-hepatic when occlusion develops in the portal vein, in the liver, or at a downstream hepatic level respectively.

Pathology and differential diagnosis

In supra-hepatic hypertension, partial occlusion results in downstream, liver segments becoming congested. Very soon, compensative anastomoses develop in non-occluded segments with reactive hypertrophy while obstructed segments become atrophic. Once the collaterals have developed, stasis decreases in intensity and the clinical symptoms regress

Budd-Chiari syndrome

This rare condition is characterized by venous outflow obstruction of the liver, usually occurring as a consequence of thrombosis of the hepatic veins and, sometimes, of the inferior vena cava [41]. It leads to portal hypertension [42].

There is no sex predilection and any age may be affected [42, 43]. The mean age of male patients is 36.4, that of female patients 46.5. The clinical course may be acute or chronic; however, the average period from the likely onset to the first medical consultation is 6.6 years [44]. The onset may be insidious with anaemia, thrombocytopaenia, pleural effusion, leg oedema, and venous dilatation over the trunk but presentation with right upper quadrant abdominal pain, hepatomegaly, and ascites may occur. The diagnosis is confirmed by inferior vena caval and hepatic venous catheterization. Involvement of the inferior vena cava may be of two types, primary hepatic vein thrombosis (classical Budd-Chiari) and obliterative disease predominantly affecting the hepatic portion of the IVC [45]. Okuda et al [45] suggested the term "obliterative hepato-cavopathy" (OHC) to designate the second category, which constitutes the vast majority of cases of outflow block in developing countries. OHC is frequently complicated by hepatocellular carcinoma and primary hepatic vein thrombosis (classical Budd-Chiari) is not.

Usually no cause is found, but many diseases are implicated: Behçet's disease [46, 47], hepatic and digestive amyloidosis [48], conditions associated with a thrombotic tendency, such as polycythemia vera, paroxysmal nocturnal haemoglobinuria, myeloproliferative disease [45, 49, 50], systemic lupus erythematosus [51] and Sjogren's syndrome [52], the use of oral contraceptive agents [53] or after pregnancy [54]. Closure of an atrial septal defect [55], or the presence of a vena cava membrane [56] may predispose to this condition [57, 58]. Blunt trauma with formation of haematoma, echinococcosis [59, 60] may lead to compression block of the suprahepatic vessels [61, 62, 63]. Rarely tumours such as primary leiomyosarcoma or secondary extension of a renal clear cell adenocarcinoma induce this syndrome [64, 65, 66].

Pathology and differential diagnosis

In these occlusive lesions, the basic structure of the venous wall is maintained. The intima is transformed into a fibrous laminar structure with a superimposed mixture of fresh thrombi and organized thrombi of varying ages. Recanalisation with calcifications may occur [42, 67]. The liver parenchyma presents chronic congestion, haemorrhage, and cell necrosis with a scant inflammatory reaction. Cirrhosis may be a long-term complication.

Bibliography

1. Husken BC, van der Wal AC, Teeling P, Mathy MJ, Mertens MJ, Pul AJ, Pfaffendorf M, van Zwieten PA (1997) Heterogeneity in morphological characteristics of coronary arteries and aortae in various models of hypertension. Blood Press 6: 242-9
2. Belkic K, Emdad R, Theorell T (1998) Occupational profile and cardiac risk: possible mechanisms and implications for professional drivers. Int J Occup Med Environ Health 11: 37-57
3. Peters J (1995) Molecular basis of human hypertension: the role of angiotensin. Baillieres Clin Endocrinol Metab 9: 657-78
4. Morgan L, Broughton Pipkin F, Kalsheker N (1996) DNA polymorphisms and linkage disequilibrium in
5. Scarpelli PT, Livi R, Caselli GM, Di Maria L, Teghini L, Montemurro V, Toti G, Becucci A (1997) Accelerated (malignant) hypertension: a study of 121 cases between 1974 and 1996. J Nephrol 10: 207-15
6. Bohle A, Wehrmann M, Greschniok A, Junghans R (1998) Renal morphology in essential hypertension: analysis of 1177 unselected cases. Kidney Int Suppl 67: S205-6
7. Cliff WJ (1970) The aortic tunica media in aging rats. Exp Mol Pathol 13: 172-89
8. Haudenschild CC, Prescott MF, Chobanian AV (1980) Effects of hypertension and its reversal on aortic intima lesions of the rat. Hypertension 2: 23-44

9. Folkow B (1992) Hypertension and endothelial function – aspects of atheroma protection. Blood Press 1: S11-S12

10. Luscher TF (1995) Hypertension and vascular diseases: molecular and cellular mechanisms. Schweiz Med Wochenschr 125: 270-82

11. Barrett TB, Sampson P, Owens GK, Schwartz SM, Benditt EP (1983) Polyploid nuclei in human artery wall smooth muscle cells. Proc Natl Acad Sci USA 80: 882-85

12. Geisterfer AAT, Peach MJ, Owens GK (1988) Angiotensin II induces hypertrophy, not hyperplasia, of cultured rat aortic smooth muscle cells. Hypertension 13: 305-4

13. Owens GK, Geisterfer AAT, Wei-Hwa Yang Y, Komoriya A (1988) Transforming growth factor-beta-induced growth inhibition and cellular hypertrophy in cultured vascular smooth muscle cells. J Cell Biol 107: 771-780

14. Michel JB, Dussaule JC, Choudat L, Auzan C, Nochy D, Corvol P, Menard J (1985) Effects of antihypertensive treatment in one-clip, two kidney hypertension in rats. Kidney Int 29: 1011-20

15. Kincaid-Smith P (1980) Malignant hypertension: mechanisms and management. Pharmacol Ther 9: 245-69

16. Berry CL, Greenwald SE (1976) Effects of hypertension on the static mechanical properties and chemical composition of the rat aorta. Cardiovasc Res 10: 437-51

17. Wolinsky H (1970) Response of the rat aortic media to hypertension: morphological and chemical studies. Circ Res 26: 507-22

18. Wolinsky H (1971) Effects of hypertension and its reserval on the thoracic aorta of male and female rats. Morphological and chemical studies. Circ Res 28: 622-37

19. Lie JT (1980) The structure of the normal vascular system and its reactive changes In Juergens JL, Spittel Jr, Fairnbairn II J-F (eds) Allen-Barker-Hines, W.B. Saunders, Philadelphia 51-81

20. Churg J, Golstein MH (1995) Systemic hypertension and related vascular diseases. Section B: Pathological aspects of hypertension In Stehbens WE, Lie JT (eds) Vascular pathology. Chapman&Hall, London, pp. 571-84

21. Mark EJ (1984) Lung biopsy interpretation. Williams and Wilkins, Baltimore London, p 284

22. Bjornsson J, Edwards WD (1985) Primary pulmonary hypertension: a histopathologic study of 80 cases. Mayo Clin Proc 60: 16-25

23. Pietra GG, Edwards WD, Kay JM, Rich S, Kernis J, Schloo B, Ayres SM, Bergofsky EH, Brundage BH, Detre KM, et al (1989) Histopathology of primary pulmonary hypertension. A qualitative and quantitative study of pulmonary blood vessels from 58 patients in the National Heart, Lung, and Blood Institute, Primary Pulmonary Hypertension Registry. Circulation 80: 1198-206

24. Hosoda Y (1994) Pathology of pulmonary hypertension: a human and experimental study. Pathol Int 44: 241-67

25. Heath D, Wood EH, DuShane JW, Edwards JE (1959) The structure of the pulmonary trunk at different ages and in cases of pulmonary hypertension and pulmonary stenosis. J Path Bact 77: 443-54

26. Heath D (1972) Pulmonary hypertension in pulmonary parenchymal disease. Cardiovasc Clin 4: 79-96

27. Sato T, Akiba T, Suzuki H, Nakasato M, Sato S, Yoshikawa M, Yamaki S (1994) Histopathologic findings of lung vessels in five children with primary pulmonary hypertension. Tohoku J Exp Med 172: 9-15

28. Mesa RA, Edell ES, Dunn WF, Edwards WD (1998) Human immunodeficiency virus infection and pulmonary hypertension: two new cases and a review of 86 reported cases. Mayo Clin Proc 73: 37-45

29. Wagenvoort CA and Wagenvoort N (1977). Pathology of pulmonary hypertension. J Wiley & Sons New York

30. Haworth SG (1993) Pulmonary hypertension in childhood. Eur Respir J 6: 1037-43

31. Rabinovitch M, Haworth SG, Vance Z, Vawter G, Castaneda AR, Nadas AS, Reid LM (1980) Early pulmonary vascular changes in congenital heart disease studied in biopsy tissue. Hum Pathol 11: S499-S509

32. Aiello VD, Fukasawa S, da Silva MJ, Azeka E, Bosisio IB, Ebaid M, Higuchi ML (1997) Systematic quantification of the arteries in lung biopsies of patients with congenital heart defects and its contribution to the therapeutic management. Arq Bras Cardiol 68: 3-8

33. Yamaki S, Abe A, Endo M, Tanaka T, Tabayashi K, Takahashi T (1998) Surgical indication for congenital heart disease with extremely thickened media of small pulmonary arteries. Ann Thorac Surg 66: 1560-4

34. Liang MH, Stern S, Fortin PR, Louie DC, Marsh JD, Mudge GH Jr, Murphy G (1991) Fatal pulmonary venoocclusive disease secondary to a generalized venulopathy: a new syndrome presenting with facial swelling and pericardial tamponade. Arthritis Rheum 34: 228-33

35. Justo RN, Dare AJ, Whight CM, Radford DJ (1993) Pulmonary veno-occlusive disease: diagnosis during life in four patients. Arch Dis Child 68: 97-100

36. Ruchelli ED, Nojadera G, Rutstein RM, Rudy B (1994) Pulmonary veno-occlusive disease. Another vascular disorder associated with human immunodeficiency virus infection ? Arch Pathol Lab Med 118: 664-6

37. Escamilla R, Hermant C, Berjaud J, Mazerolles C, Daussy X (1995) Pulmonary veno-occlusive disease in a HIV-infected intravenous drug abuser. Eur Respir J 8: 1982-4

38. Palmer SM, Robinson LJ, Wang A, Gossage JR, Bashore T, Tapson VF (1998) Massive pulmonary oedema and death after prostacyclin infusion in a patient with pulmonary veno-occlusive disease. Chest 113: 237-40

39. Bourgeon R, Isman H, Bourgeon A (1986) Répercussions cave et sus hépatiques du kyste hydatique du foie. Explorations, thérapeutique. Chirurgie 112: 332-6

40. Naef M, Holzinger F, Glattli A, Gysi B, Baer HU (1998) Massive gastrointestinal bleeding from colonic varices in a patient with portal hypertension. Dig Surg 15: 709-12

41. Giovine S, Romano L, Aragiusto G, Scaglione M (1998) Budd-Chiari syndrome: retrospective study of 8 cases assessed with computerized tomography. Radiol Med (Torino) 96: 339-43

42. Cifuentes J, Viscarra M, Emilfork M (1991) Budd-Chiari syndrome. Rev Chil Pediatr 62: 260-3

43. Gentil-Kocher S, Bernard O, Brunelle F, Hadchouel M, Maillard JN, Valayer J, Hay JM, Alagille D (1988) Budd-Chiari syndrome in children: report of 22 cases. J Pediatr 113: 30-8

44. Okuda H, Yamagata H, Obata H, Iwata H, Sasaki R, Imai F, Okudaira M, Ohbu M, Okuda K (1995) Epidemiological and clinical features of Budd-Chiari syndrome in Japan. J Hepatol 22: 1-9

45. Okuda K, Kage M, Shrestha SM (1998) Proposal of a new nomenclature for Budd-Chiari syndrome: hepatic vein thrombosis versus thrombosis of the inferior vena cava at its hepatic portion. Hepatology 28: 1191-8

46. al-Dalaan A, al-Balaa S, Ali MA, Huraib S, Amin T, al-Maziad A, al-Fadda M (1991) Budd-Chiari syndrome in association with Behcet's disease. J Rheumatol 18: 622-6

47. Bayraktar Y, Balkanci F, Bayraktar M, Calguneri M (1997) Budd-Chiari syndrome: a common complication of Behcet's disease. Am J Gastroenterol 92: 858-62

48. Paliard P, Bretagnolle M, Collet P, Vannieuwenhyse A, Berger F (1983) Inferior vena cava thrombosis responsible for chronic Budd-Chiari syndrome during hepatic and digestive amyloidosis. Gastroenterol Clin Biol 7: 919-22

49. Altomonte L, Mingrone G, Gattini G, Pepe M, Magaro M (1979) Budd-Chiari syndrome in the course of polycythemia rubra vera. Presentation of a clinical case. Minerva Med 70: 3719-24

50. Foresti V, Ungaro A, Pediconi AM (1988) Budd-Chiari syndrome secondary to thrombosis of the inferior vena cava in myeloproliferative disease. Minerva Med 79: 477-80

51. Disney TF, Sullivan SN, Haddad RG, Lowe D, Goldbach MM (1984) Budd-Chiari syndrome with inferior vena cava obstruction associated with systemic lupus erythematosus. J Clin Gastroenterol 6: 253-6

52. Matsuura H, Matsumoto T, Hashimoto T (1983) Budd-Chiari syndrome in a patient with Sjogren's syndrome. Am J Gastroenterol 78: 822-5

53. Lalonde G, Theoret G, Daloze P, Bettez P, Katz SS (1982) Inferior vena cava stenosis and Budd-Chiari syndrome in a woman taking oral contraceptives. Gastroenterology 82: 1452-6

54. Ilan Y, Oren R, Shouval D (1990) Postpartum Budd-Chiari syndrome with prolonged hypercoagulability state. Am J Obstet Gynecol 162: 1164-5

55. Klein HH, de Vries H, de Vivie ER, Schuster R, Kreuzer H (1987) Budd-Chiari syndrome as a late complication following closure of an atrial septal defect. Z Kardiol 76: 371-4

56. Ishibe R, Maruko M, Tabata D, Toyohira H, Furuzono K, Nishimura A, Yoshida A (1990) Membranous obliteration of the inferior vena cava in the hepatic portion – postmortem study of a rapidly deteriorated aged case. Nippon Geka Gakkai Zasshi 91: 290-2

57. Ohtomo K, Furui S, Makita K, Yamauchi T, Kokubo T, Yashiro N, Itai Y, Iio M (1986) CT diagnosis of primary Budd-Chiari syndrome – membranous obstruction of the inferior vena cava. Radiat Med 4: 86-8

58. Kage M, Arakawa M, Kojiro M, Okuda K (1992) Histopathology of membranous obstruction of the inferior vena cava in the Budd-Chiari syndrome. Gastroenterology 102: 2081-90

59. Robotti GC, Meister F, Schroder R (1985) Budd-Chiari syndrome in liver echinococcosis. ROFO Fortschr Geb Rontgenstr Nuklearmed 142: 511-3

60. Khaldi F, Braham N, Ben Chehida F, Ben Jaballah N, Bennaceur B (1993) Hepatic hydatidosis and portal hypertension in children. Is it the Budd-Chiari syndrome? Ann Pediatr (Paris) 40: 631-4

61. Izard G, Houri R, Randrianasolo S, Gailleton R (1995) Acute Budd-Chiari syndrome of traumatic origin. Presse Med 24: 1209-10

62. Coue O, Fornes P, Paraf F, Couetil JP, Bruneval P (1996) Budd-Chiari syndrome secondary to post-traumatic stenosis of the inferior vena cava. Gastroenterol Clin Biol 20: 196-9

63. Markert DJ, Shanmuganathan K, Mirvis SE, Nakajima Y, Hayakawa M (1997) Budd-Chiari syndrome resulting from intrahepatic IVC compression secondary to blunt hepatic trauma. Clin Radiol 52: 384-7

64. Imakita M, Yutani C, Ishibashi-Ueda H, Hiraoka H, Naito H (1989) Primary leiomyosarcoma of the inferior vena cava with Budd-Chiari syndrome. Acta Pathol Jpn 39: 73-7

65. Nakajima Y, Baba S, Nagahama T, Tazaki H (1989) Renal cell carcinoma presenting as Budd-Chiari syndrome. Urol Int 44: 173-6

66. Fujita H, Kawata K, Sawada T, Mizutani T, Iwasaki Y, Shirono K, Kounosu H, Shirakata S (1993) Rhabdomyosarcoma in the inferior vena cava with secondary Budd-Chiari syndrome. Intern Med 32: 67-71

67. Miller WJ, Federle MP, Straub WH, Davis PL (1993) Budd-Chiari syndrome: imaging with pathologic correlation. Abdom Imaging 18: 329-35

XVII
Vascular tumours and tumour-like conditions

In this area the terminology is often confused, and even misleading. In many conditions, especially with regard to the benign lesions, the clinical and familial history are of great importance in diagnosis.

1 – Tumour-like conditions

Non-vascular tumours with a dominant vascular component

Some soft tissue tumours have a vascular component that appears predominant. Among these the following are the most common.

Angiolipoma

Although most frequent in the limbs, this tumour may occur at any site in the body. It is generally well defined and gives rise to single or multiple nodules located deep in the sub-cutaneous tissue. It may infiltrate nearby tissues and present an "invasive" pattern. Classical angiolipoma never recurs after complete excision.

Pathology and Differential diagnosis

Grossly, angiolipoma is a lobulated mass, yellowish on cut section. Histologically, it is made up of lobules of round or ovaladipocytes separated by angiomatous vessels. These are lined by flattened endothelial cells and may contain thrombi. In some instances, adipocytes may be spindle shaped and surround vascular channels, resembling angiosarcoma and Kaposi's sarcoma. Lack of endothelial cell atypia permits exclusion of angiosarcoma and in the skin Kaposi's sarcoma remains a superficial dermal tumour even in its nodular stage.

Angiomyolipoma

The renal cortex is the typical location. Involvement of the skin [1] and other viscera has been reported [2-4]. Multiple angiomyolipomas may be associated with pulmonary lymphangioleiomyomatosis [5, 6], arterial muscular fibrodysplasia, and tuberous sclerosis [7-9].

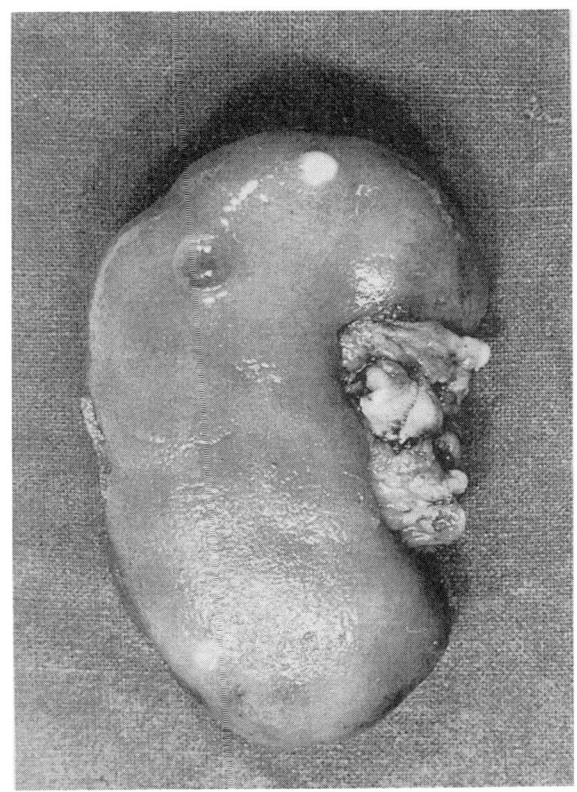

Fig. 1. Whitish single angiomyolipoma neighbouring an urinary cyst of the renal cortex

Pathology and Differential diagnosis

Round, sharply circumscribed, but non-capsulated, this tumour may be single (Fig. 1) or multiple (Fig. 2) giving rise to juxtaposed nodules of varying sizes, measuring from 0. 2 to 3 cm in diameter.

Histologically, it consists of a disorderly arrangement of thick-walled blood vessels, smooth muscle cells, and lipomatous lobules (Fig. 3-4-5). A few parenchymal elements may be incorporated at the margins of the nodules. Intratumour aneurysms may develop inside massive angiomyolipoma [10].

Angiofibroma and angiomyofibroblastoma

Juvenile angiofibroma or nasopharyngeal fibroma

Adolescent males are mostly affected, although some cases have been reported in females and in younger children [11]. The tumour appears as a lobulated mass

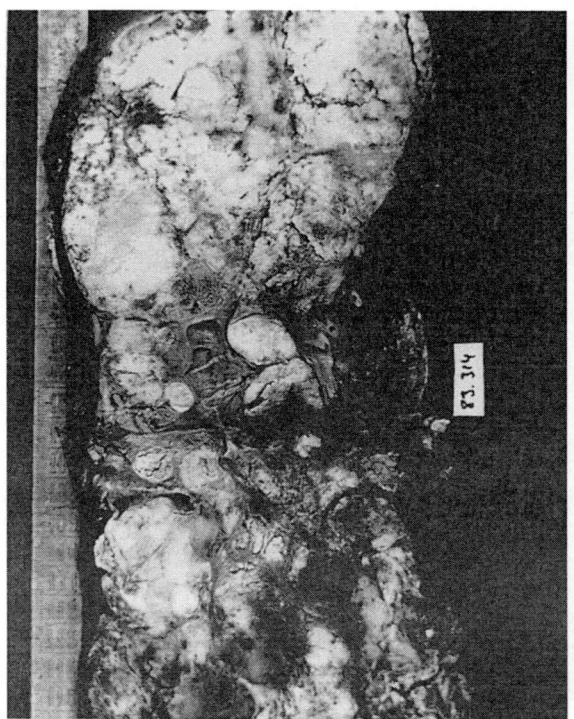

Fig. 2. Massive angiomyolipoma distorting the entirety of a kidney. Note diffuse haemorrhage

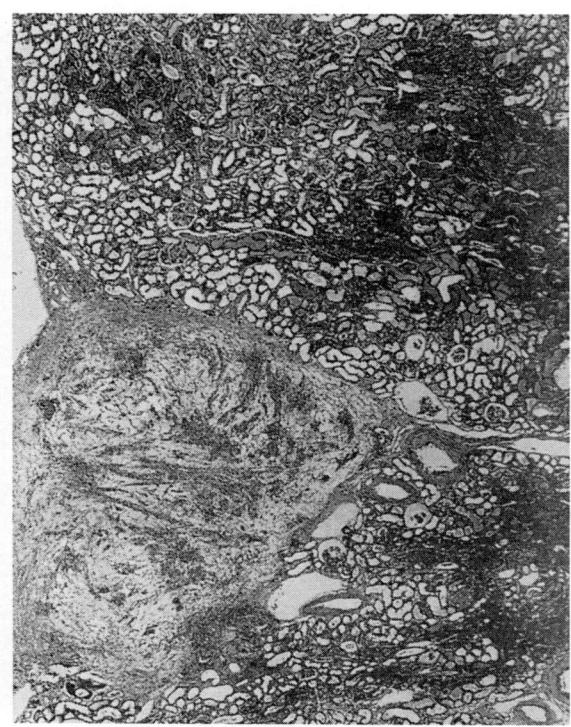

Fig. 3. Angiomyolipoma. Well-limited angiomyolipoma of the renal cortex. Masson's trichrome stain (Masson's trichrome)

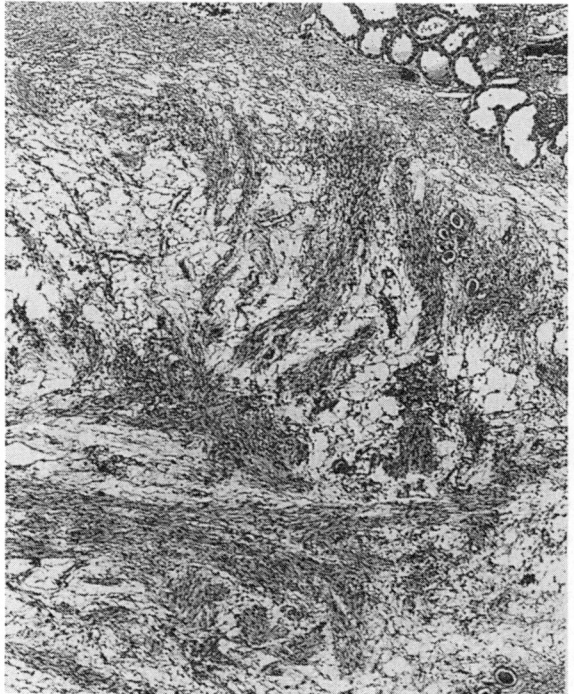

Fig. 4. Angiomyolipoma. Characteristic mixture of disorderly arranged thick-walled blood vessels interspersed with smooth muscle cells and lipomatous lobules. ...Masson's trichrome...

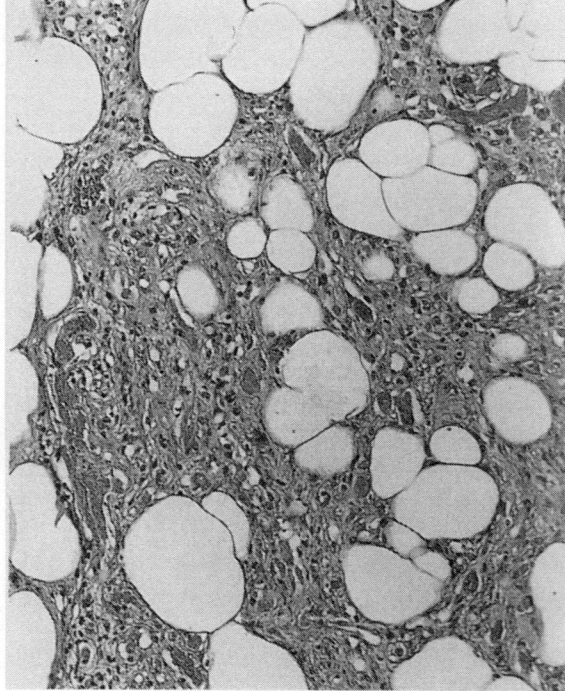

Fig. 5. Angiomyolipoma. In some areas, lipomatous and leimyomatous components predominate. ...Masson's trichrome...

obstructing the nasopharyngeal recesses or the choanae, compressing neighbouring structures and bleeding. These masses may occur in the nasal fossa or inside the naso-facial sinuses [12, 13]. Rapid growth may occur during puberty and the tumour is said to contain androgen receptors. Its growth rate may, at least in vitro, be reduced by antiandrogens such as cyproterone and flutamide. However, this has been disputed [14-16]. Surgical removal is indicated, but recurrence is frequent because of the anatomical site [17].

Pathology and differential diagnosis

The tumour is composed of cellular fibrous tissue criss-crossed by numerous vessels. These vessels, bordered by a flattened endothelium, may contain elastic fibers and smooth muscle cells in their wall. The overlying mucosa may display erosion and haemorrhage. The main differential diagnosis is angioleiomyoma, but pyogenic granuloma may cause confusion [18] and Castleman's disease may present in the nasopharynx [19].

Angiomyofibroblastoma

Only about 65 cases are documented in the literature [20]. This tumour occurs mostly in the female genital tract and usually presents as a painless mass in adult women (median age : 46 years).

Pathology and differential diagnosis

The tumour appears well delineated, measuring from 2 to 8 cm in its greatest dimension. Histologically, it is made up of spindled and epithelioid mesenchymal cells arranged in cords and nests around numerous small to medium-sized vessels. Mitotic activity ranges from 0 to 7 mitoses per 50 high-power fields (HPF) with no atypical figures. Intralesional fat may develop and become predominant. Tumour cells express vimentin, estrogen and progesterone receptor protein receptor, desmin (six of eight cases), CD31, CD34 and smooth muscle actin (one of seven cases). Image cytometry demonstrates a diploid DNA content [21-23]. Simple excision is the current treatment.

Vascular ectasias

This condition may affect arteries, veins, capillaries and lymphatic vessels. Acquired and congenital lymphangiectasias are discussed elsewhere (see chapters XIII-XIV).

Cutis marmorata telangiectatica congenita

This rare entity is characterized by a distinctive reticulated pattern that accentuates the superficial cutaneous vasculature. A case report in two sisters suggests a dominantly inherited trait with low penetrance [24]. There is no racial or sexual predilection. Lesions involve circumscribed areas of the skin (extremities, trunk, face, and scalp) but may be widespread. The lesions consist of livid, reticulated mottling of the skin. Telangiectasia, phlebectasia, and ulceration may occur. In 50% of patients, associated malformations have been reported [25-35] (Table 1). The lesions fade progressively during the early years of life but may persist into adulthood in about 15% of patients. Prognosis depends on the severity of associated anomalies.

Pathology and differential diagnosis

A skin biopsy specimen shows an increased number of widely dilated venules in the superficial dermis with a scanty infiltrate of lymphocytes around. Other vascular structures, such as capillaries and veins, may be involved. Some abnormal venules demonstrate a clearly increased number of pericytes. From the histological standpoint, the dilated venules in this condition are not readily distinguishable from telangiectases of other skin diseases and the differential diagnosis depends on ancillary clinical findings.

Generalized telangiectasia

This condition mainly involves the venous system of women in their thirties [36]. The lesions are bright red macula or plaques with venous lakes, stars or, rarely, varicosities around them. These lesions start in the lower limbs, progress steadily to involve the trunk arms and face, and persist over a period of years. Gastrointestinal bleeding has been reported [37].

Pathology and differential diagnosis.

Skin biopsy specimens show dilated venous vascular spaces. Elevated plaques or nodular lesions are often mistaken for haemangiomas.

Senile ectasia (Senile vascular naevus or cherry angioma)

This benign condition, of no clincial significance, affects middle-aged and elderly people. Small, raised, papillary, bright red or purplish lesions occur in the skin of the anterior surface of the trunk (Fig. 6) or

Table 1. Congenital malformations associated with cutis marmorata telangiectatica congenita

ASSOCIATED MALFORMATIONS	TYPES
Cardio-vascular	Atrial septal defect, Patent ductus arteriosus, Double aortic arch, Sturge-Weber syndrome, Haemangiomas, Phlebectasias, Varicosities, or Venous hypoplasia
Cerebral	Macrocephaly, Cerebrovascular anomalies
Ocular and oral	Glaucoma, Micrognathia, Cleft palate, Dental dystrophy
Anogenital	Imperforate anus, Absent clitoris, Rectovaginal and urethrovaginal fistulas
Visceral	Hepatomegaly
Endocrine	Congenital hypothyroidism
Muscular and skeletal	Widely spaced toes, Hemiatrophy or hemihypertrophy of a limb, Syndactyly, Transverse terminal limb defect (Adams-Oliver syndrome), Congenital generalized fibromatosis

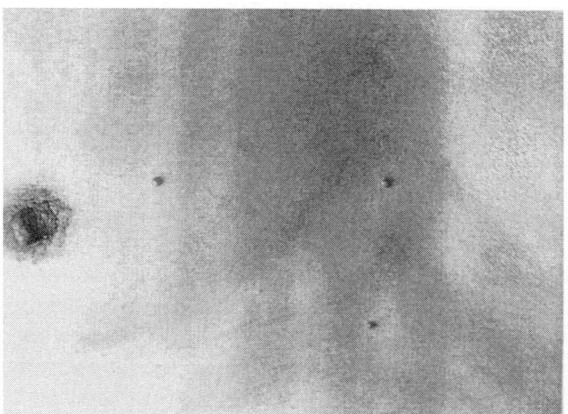

Fig. 6. Senile vascular ectasia. Three cherry angiomas on the anterior surface of the trunk of a 54 yo man

limbs. The lesions, usually multiple, vary from 0. 5 to 5 mm in diameter.

Pathology and differential diagnosis

The lesions look like small capillary angiomas but are made up of tufts of dilated capillaries (Fig. 7). The majority of the capillaries are fenestrated and histochemically react for carbonic anhydrase. They are surrounded by a hyalinized sheath containing an increased amount of collagen (type IV and type VI) [38, 39]. The surrounding dermis is elastotic.

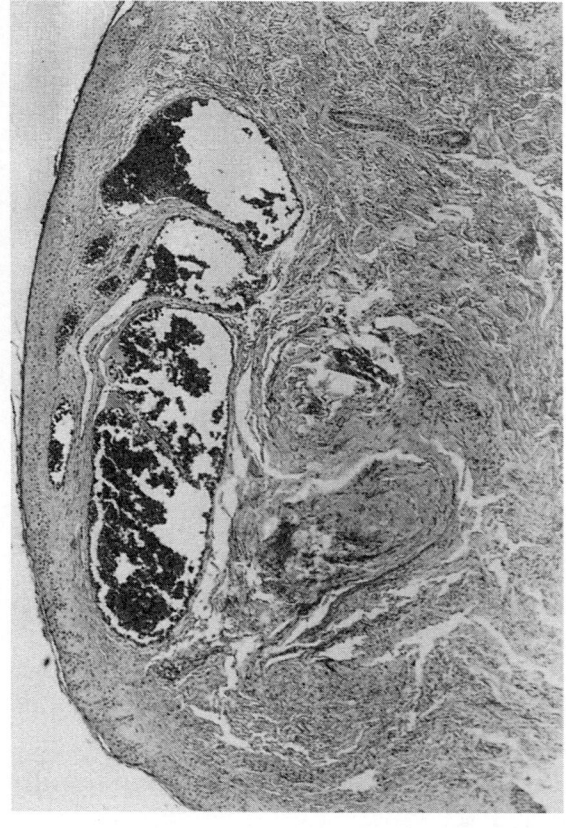

Fig. 7. Senile vascular ectasia. Tuft of dilated capillaries uplifing the epidermis. Haematoxylin, eosin and saffron stain. (HES)

Nevus araneus (Cutaneous arterial spider, pulsating telangiectasia, spider nevus)

This naevus consists of focal minute masses of subcutaneous small arteries or arterioles arranged in a radial fashion about a central core, so that the lesion looks like a spider [40]. It blanches with application of pressure, then reddens in a centrifugal direction when pressure is released. The lesions frequently pulsate. Nevus araneus often occurs onthe upper parts of the body (face, neck, upper chest and arms), but never where inherent vasoconstriction is strongest (hands, feet). Exceptionally, the distribution of lesions may affect one side of the body and in discrete fields (unilateral nevoid telangiectasia) [41]. Mucosal linings, including the digestive tract, may be involved. Single lesions are found in adults and children; they tend to appear suddenly, to fade rapidly, and to bleed if traumatised. Multiple lesions are associated with hepatic disease, hyperthyroidism, and pregnancy.

Pathology and differential diagnosis

A skin biopsy specimen displays dilated dermal thick-walled arterioles that communicate with a network of dilated superficial capillaries. This lesion should be distinguished from true capillary haemangioma.

Vascular reactive lesions

The vascular system is formed through a combination of vasculogenesis and angiogenesis. In vasculogenesis, blood vessels are formed *de novo* by the assembly of angioblasts. Angiogenesis strictly denotes new vessel formation from preexisting vasculature by the migration and proliferation of endothelial cells [42]. Under physiological conditions, angiogenesis is a highly regulated process and is under control of angiogenic stimulators and inhibitors. It plays a central role in organ development and reproduction, inflammation and vascular regeneration [43]. Unregulated angiogenesis occurs in pathological conditions. This process has been suggested as a key step in tumour growth, invasion, and metastases [44-46]. However, the nature of the newly-formed vessels is still debatable [47]. A major area of research is the development of factors that inhibit angiogenesis. Several modes of treatment, separately or combined, are under consideration and include agents that act directly on the tumor cells to prevent the release of angiogenic agents, drugs that inactivate already released angiogenic molecules, and agents that obliterate the endothelial cell response to angiogenic stimulators [48, 49]. The physiology of an-giogenesis is detailed elsewhere. Only reactive vascular lesions are discussed here.

Peliosis hepatis

The term "peliosis" designates the bluish colour of this liver lesion, which consists of blood-filled cavities scattered throughout the parenchyma. The condition also involves the spleen, lymph nodes, and other viscera [50]. A small lesion has no clinical effects, but large lesions may be associated with moderate jaundice, hepatosplenomegaly with portal hypertension, ascites, and oesophageal varices. Cases of angiosarcoma have been reported in patients with peliosis hepatis secondary to exposure to thorium dioxide [51].

In most cases, the cause is unknown. Table 2 summaries conditions or therapies in which peliosis hepatis has been observed [52, 53]. In patients with AIDS, *Rochalimaea henselae* (Bartonella), the cause of bacillary angiomatosis, may produce this lesion [54-58].

Pathology and differential diagnosis

When peliosis hepatis is extensive, the liver increases in volume and becomes soft to the touch. On cut section, there are numerous blood-filled cavities of variable size giving rise to an angiomatous pattern. The lesion consists of multiple irregularly distributed blood-filled cavities in the liver (Fig. 8). Some red blood cells may be present in Disse's space, in direct contact with the liver plates (Fig. 9), but sinusoidal endothelial cells do not show changes. No clear distinction can be made between peliosis and severe sinusoidal dilatation [59, 60]. Associated lesions include atrophy of the bordering liver cell plates and fibrotic thickening of the reticulin meshwork (Fig. 10). These give rise to a vascular-like channel limited by a fibrotic layer, mimicking a varicose vein. Thrombosis and segmentary endophlebitis may be seen in the sublobular veins, but complete obliteration never occurs. *Rochalimaea henselae* may be identified using the Warthin-Starry method (Fig. 11).

Peliosis hepatis should be distinguished from other conditions that interfere with the venous return at different levels, including the Budd-Chiari syndrome, veno-occlusive disease and post-irradiation liver. In these conditions, vascular changes are systematised or involve only the central areas of the hepatic lobule. These changes are diffuse in the Budd-Chiari syndrome but more focal in veno-occlusive disease and post-irradiation liver.

Table 2. Pathological entities associated with peliosis hepatis

POSSIBLE AETIOLOGIES	PATHOLOGICAL CONDITIONS
Infections	Bartonella *(Rochalimaea henselae)* infections, typhoid, tuberculosis, septicaemia
Immune-related conditions	Auto-immune diseases: Crohn's disease, Acquired immunodeficiency syndrome (AIDS)
Degradation of the general status	Severe cachexia
Hepatic and extrahepatic tumours	Adenoma, hepatocellular carcinoma, angiosarcoma, lymphangiomyomatosis, Hodgkin's disease, Castleman's disease
Drugs	Synthetic anabolic androgenic steroids, oral contraceptives, immunosuppresive therapy
Chemical agents	Chronic exposure to arsenic, thorium dioxide (thorotrast), vinyl chloride, copper sulfate

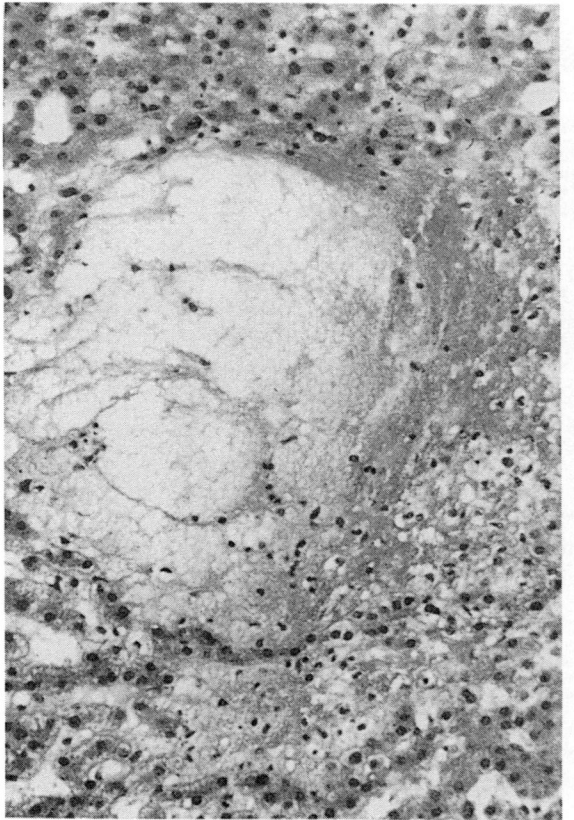
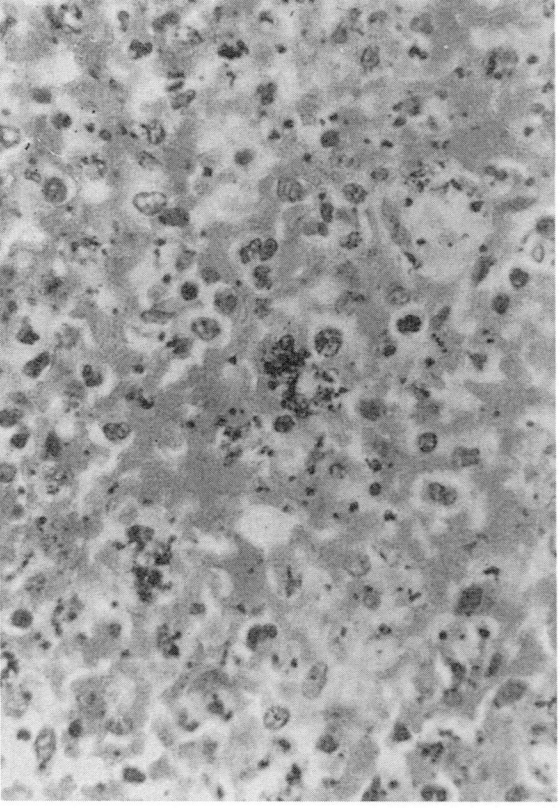

Fig. 8. Hepatic peliosis. Extensive peliosis with blood-filled cavities distorting the liver parenchyma. HES

Fig. 9. Hepatic peliosis. Red blood cells in Disse's space are in direct contact with the liver plate. HES

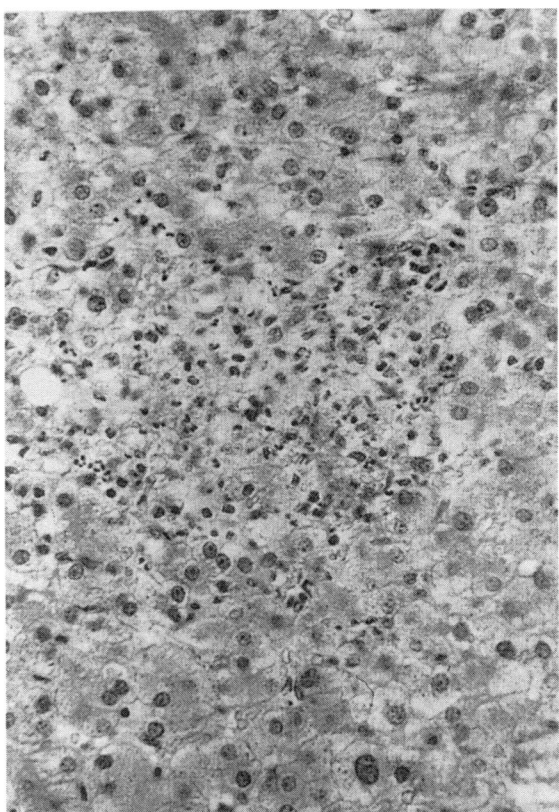

Fig. 10. Hepatic peliosis. Hepatocyte atrophy. HES

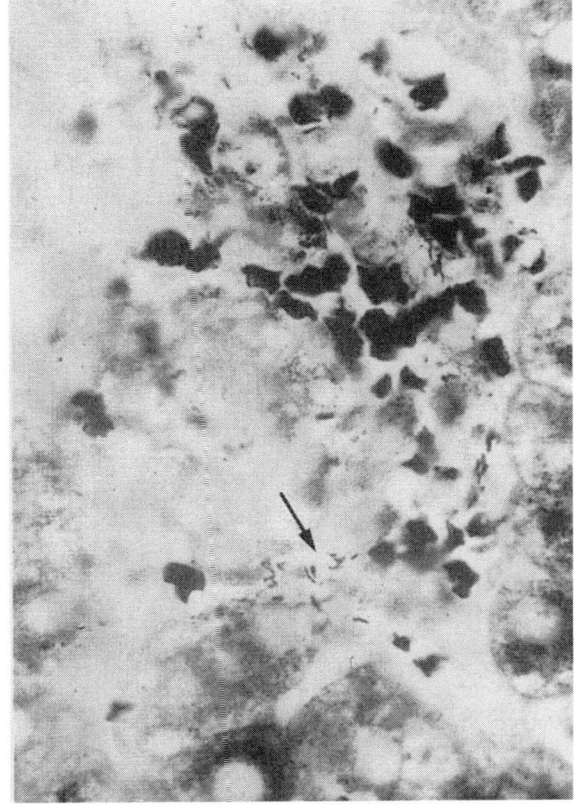

Fig. 11. Hepatic peliosis. Male AIDS patient. Presence of *Rochalimaea henselae* inside a peliosis hepatis lesion. Warthin-Starry stain (Courtesy Pr J. Amouroux)

Pyogenic granuloma (Granuloma pyogenicum)

This is a small rounded mass of highly vascular granulation tissue, frequently with an ulcerated surface, projecting from the skin or mucosa. The name reflects a mistaken view of a putative pathogenesis. About 30% of cases occur after trauma, growing rapidly in a few weeks. Association of pyogenic granuloma with pregnancy or oral contraceptive use suggests a hormone dependent process. The lesion occurs at any age in either sex and presents a predilection for the head and neck and the extremities. A pyogenic granuloma often appears as an exophytic sessile, red and strawberry-like nodule on the skin, gingival or oral mucosa and is often ulcerated but rarely pedunculated. Lesions may be multiple and disseminated. Around 1 to 5% of pregnant women develop these lesions in the gum, the so-called gingival pyogenic granuloma, epulis, gingival tumour of pregnancy, or granuloma gravidarum which often starts in the first trimester and regresses after delivery. An intravascular form of pyo-

genic granuloma has been reported in small to medium-sized veins [61]. No recurrence is seen after complete surgical excision. In rare cases, multiple satellite recurrent lesions may develop, especially in young patients with a primary lesion on the trunk. Multifocal pyogenic granulomas have been reported in patients receiving isotrentinoin (Accutane) for severe cystic acne. These regress after stopping isotrentinoin treatment [62].

Pathology and differential diagnosis

In the acute stage, cutaneous pyogenic granuloma consists of a lobulated polypoid dermal mass made up of numerous small proliferating blood capillaries (Fig. 12-13-14), often radiating from larger, more central vessels. The entirety is surrounded by extensive oedema with a dense acute and chronic inflammatory mantle. Some capillaries show leukocyte margination; others are clogged by fibrinous thrombi. The loose oedematous ground substance contains some monocytes and rare multinucleated giant cells.

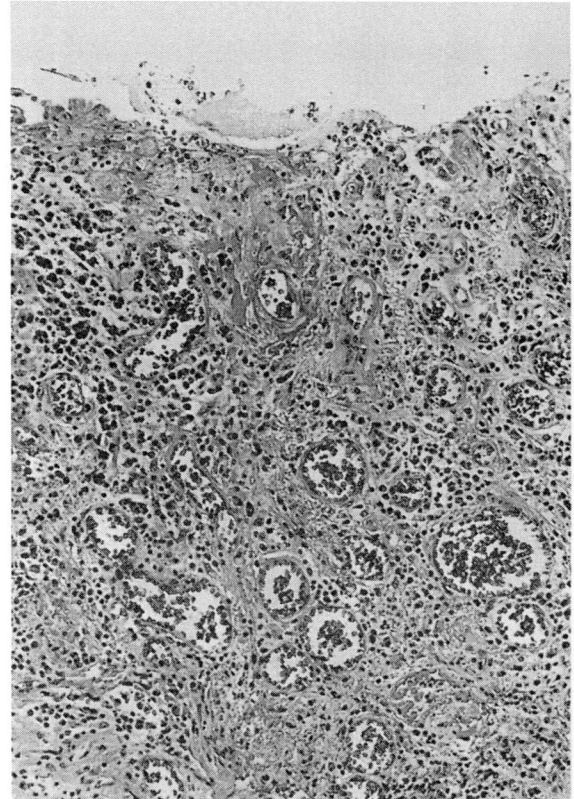

Fig. 12. Pyogenic granuloma. Acute stage. HES

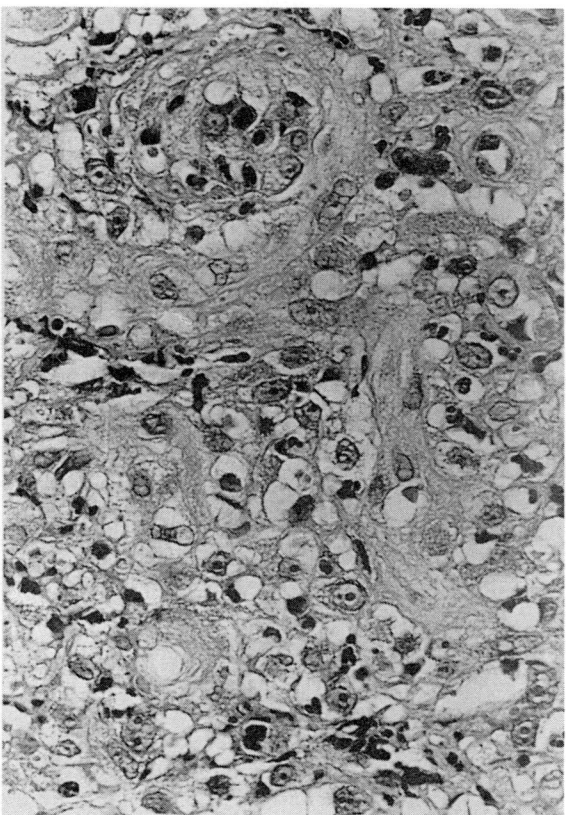

Fig. 13. Pyogenic granuloma. Acute stage. Proliferating blood capillaries are lined with plump endothelial cells. HES

These cells are interspersed with elongated or star-shaped fibroblasts. In the chronic stage, when the resorption of the inflammatory process is complete, this structure becomes a block of fibrous tissue containing well-differentiated capillaries (Fig. 15-16). Intravascular pyogenic granuloma appears as a polypoid nodule occluding the venous lumen. Histologically this lesion has the typical pattern of an usual pyogenic granuloma. In the acute stage, pyogenic granuloma may be misdiagnosed as acute angiitis. In the chronic stage, a re-epithelized pyogenic granuloma may simulate some infectious lesions (bacillary angiomatosis, Carrion's disease)or a vascular tumour (capillary haemangioma, well-differentiated angiosarcoma and the nodular stage of Kaposi's sarcoma). Bacillary angiomatosis displays foci of necrosis, especially when the lesion does not present surface ulceration. Carrion's disease only develops in endemic regions in South America. Capillary haemangioma is a true neoplasm made up of well-differentiated capillaries with swollen endothelial cells, pericytes and fibroblast-like cells.

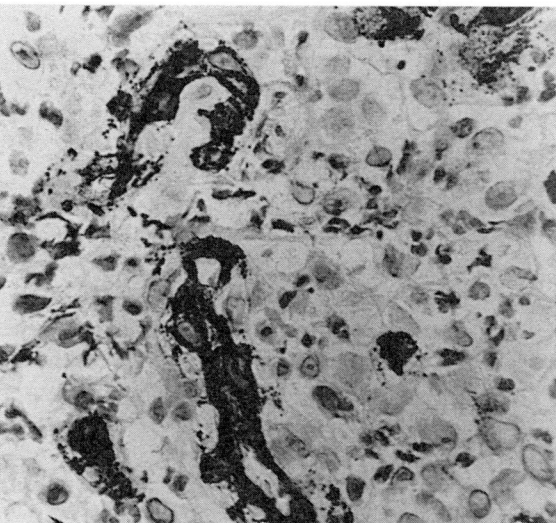

Fig. 14. Pyogenic granuloma. Acute stage. Hyperactive epithelioid endoenthelial cells reacting with factor VIII-Rag. Per-oxidase antiperoxidase immunohistochemical technique. (PAP)

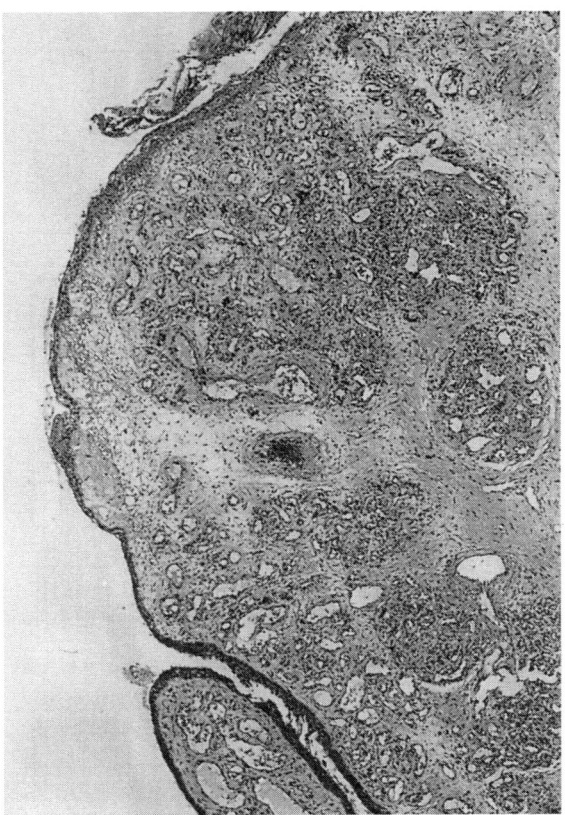

Fig. 15. Pyogenic granuloma. Chronic stage. Capillary angioma-like lesion. HES

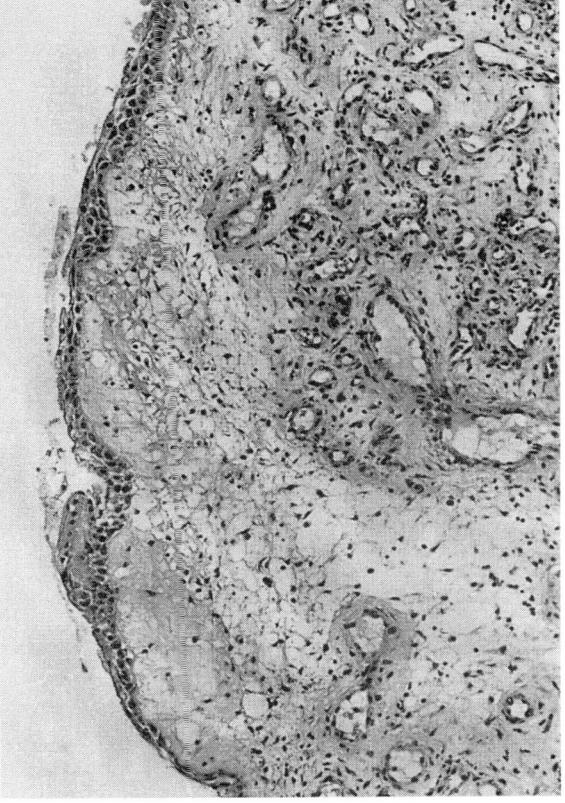

Fig. 16. Pyogenic granuloma. Chronic stage. Note well-differentiated capillaries. HES

Well-differentiated angiosarcoma has an infiltrative character with endothelial atypia and necrosis. Nodular Kaposi's sarcoma is criss-crossed by slit-like spaces, bordered by predominant spindle cells with extravasation of red blood cells. Periodic acid-Schiff-positive/diastase resistant eosinophilic hyaline globules are seen in the tumour cells.

Epithelioid haemangioma (Kimura's disease or angiolymphoid hyperplasia with esosinophilia)

The term "epithelioid haemangioma" unifies two possibly distinct clinical entities; Kimura's disease and angiolymphoid hyperplasia with esosinophilia (ALHE). Both conditions are characterised by proliferation of plump endothelial cells. There is marked inflammatory infiltration, vascular lesions suggesting small vessel trauma and presence of hyperplastic renin-secreting cells (angiotensin II is known to be angiogenic) [63]. Some clinical differences exist between Kimura's disease and angiolymphoid hyperplasia with esosinophilia (Table 3).

Kimura's disease is almost always seen in Asia, especially in Japan, and mostly affects male patients under 20 [64-66]. The disease appears as a nodule, measuring about 3 to 6 cm in diameter. The head and neck area are the most frequent sites, but the trunk and limbs may be involved. The lesion may be multifocal or bilateral and associated with frequent regional lymphadenopathy. Elevation of the serum IgE and peripheral blood eosinophilia are the common laboratory findings in about 80% of patients. Angiolymphoid "hyperplasia" with esosinophilia (ALHE) is sometimes called "hyperplasia"; the terms "inflammatory angiomatous nodules, atypical pyogenic granuloma, papular angioplasia, histiocytoid haemangioma" or "epithelioid haemangioma" have all been used. It has a world wide distribution, mostly affects adults in their third decade and has no sex predominance. Some patients report previous trauma at the site of the lesion. Systemic manifestations such as arterial hypertension, nephrotic syndrome and pseudo-Horton disease[67, 68] may be present.

Table 3. Clinical differences between Kimura's disease and angiolymphoid hyperplasia with esosinophilia (ALHE)

CLINICAL DIFFERENCES	KIMURA'S DISEASE	ANGIOLYMPHOID HYPERPLASIA WITH ESOSINOPHILIA (ALHE)
Distribution	Asia	Worldwide
Sex	Male	No sex predominance
Age	20	30-40
Location	Head, neck	Head, neck
Clinical aspect	Single, multiple, 3-6 cm	Single, multiple, 1 to 2 cm
Lymphadenopathy	+	+
Eosinophilia	Common	Less common
Serum IgE	Elevated	Normal
Course	Months to years	Months to years

The lesion appears as a painless, dull-red, usually single nodule in the head and neck area, measuring 1 to 2 cm in diameter. Multifocal lesions may occur. These nodules may merge to form bumpy plaques. Concomitant lymphadenopathy and an increased peripheral blood eosinophilia are noticed in a small proportion (less than 20%) of patients. The course of Kimura's disease and ALHE may last from months to years. Ulceration and bleeding are rare [69]. Some lesions regress spontaneously but complete surgical excision is the optimal management. Local recurrences arereported in up to one third of patients. In ALHE multifocal lesions are considered toresult from multicentricity rather than a metastatic process [70]

Pathology and differential diagnosis

Both Kimura's disease and ALHE have a predilection for the skin and subcutis. The major features of both Kimura's disease and ALHE consist of an inflammatory infiltrate dominated by eosinophils and lymphocytes and a reactive but inconspicuous vascular proliferation (Fig. 17-18-19-20). The lesions are surrounded by fibrosis. Early lesions present a more pronounced inflammatory reaction while later ones are more fibrotic. Lymphoid follicles are generally scattered through the lesion (Fig. 21). In Kimura's disease, the lesion may contain eosinophilic microabscesses (Fig. 22). The vessels are patent and epithelioid endothelial cells are not seen. In ALHE, the vascular proliferation is more prominent. Capillaries, although well formed, have immature features, most being bordered with epithelioid, plump endothelial cells (Fig.

23-24) that react with factor VIII-RAg. Renin-containing cells can be seen around abnormal vessels [63]. Necrosis and atypia are never seen. This vascular proliferation seems to develop radially from a medium-sized artery (Fig. 25) [71]. Ultrastructurally, there is a marked proliferation of both endothelial cells and pericytes. The solid cellular areas appear to be composed of solid vascular buds. A multi-layered basal lamina may enclose pericytes and external surfaces of endothelial cells [72]. In the subcutis, elastin stains identify both artery-like and vein-like vessels. In fact, morphological confusion exists. Other histological differential diagnoses encompass all vascular lesions displaying an epithelioid or histiocytoid endothelium, bacillary angiomatosis, verruga peruana or Carrion's disease. In these conditions, endothelial cells are more often plump than epithelioid. Occasionally, papillary endothelial hyperplasia, haemangioma, and lymphangioma may have a minor component which is epithelioid, but inflammatory infiltration is lacking. Neoplasms having epithelioid or histiocytoid endothelium include malignant endovascular papillary angioendothelioma or Dabska tumour, epithelioid haemangioendothelioma, spindle cell haemangioendothelioma, and angiosarcoma with epithelioid variant. In rare cases of angiolymphoid hyperplasia with eosinophilia, tufts of endothelial cells may simulate an adenocarcinomatous tumour embolus. However, negative reactivity with KL1 and EMA antibodies together with the presence of an inflammatory infiltrate help to confirm the diagnosis.

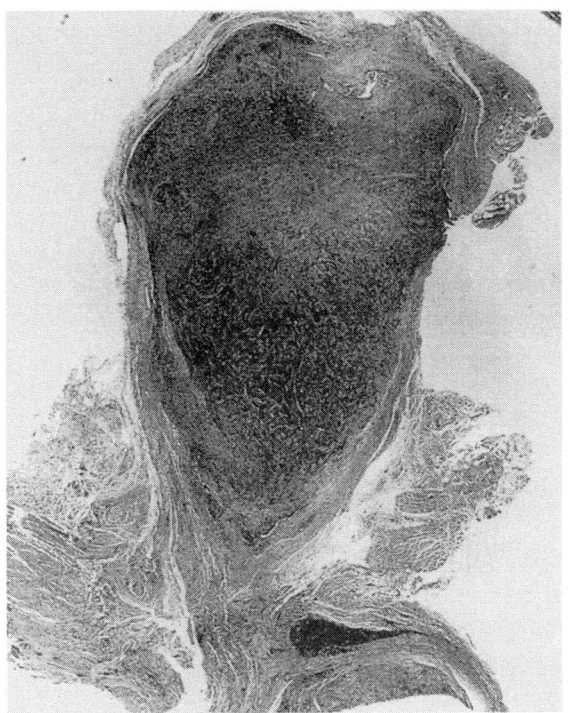

Fig. 17. Epithelioid haemangioma. Nodule resected from the forehead of a 40 yo man. HES

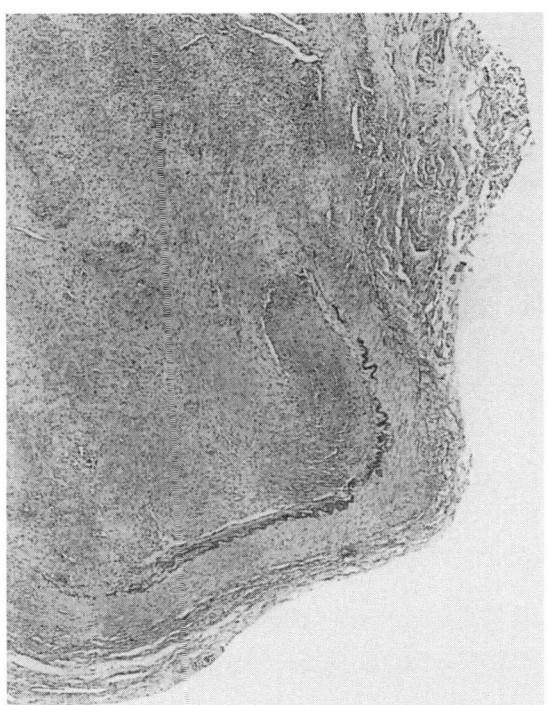

Fig. 18. Epithelioid haemangioma. Characteristic angiolymphoid hyperplasia with eosinophilia (ALHE) developed inside a ruptured frontal artery collateral. Note dilaceration of the internal elastic membrane. Orcein elastic stain (Orcein)

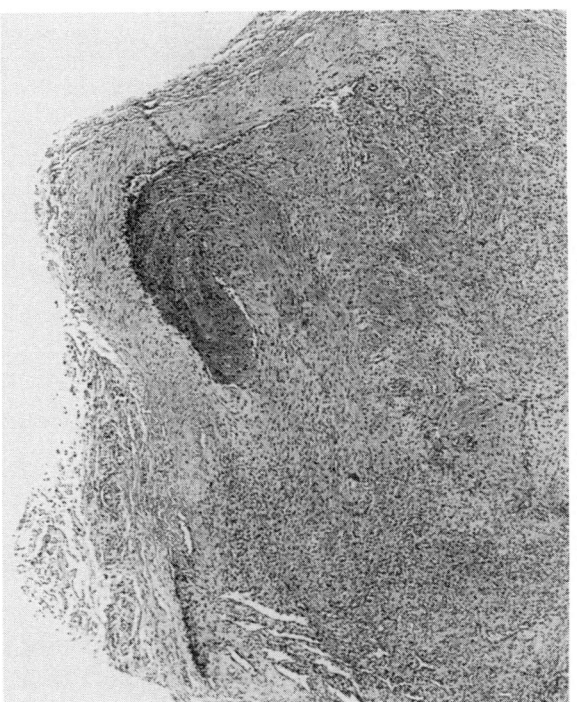

Fig. 19. Epithelioid haemangioma. ALHE. Vascular proliferation among a dense inflammatory infiltrate. HES

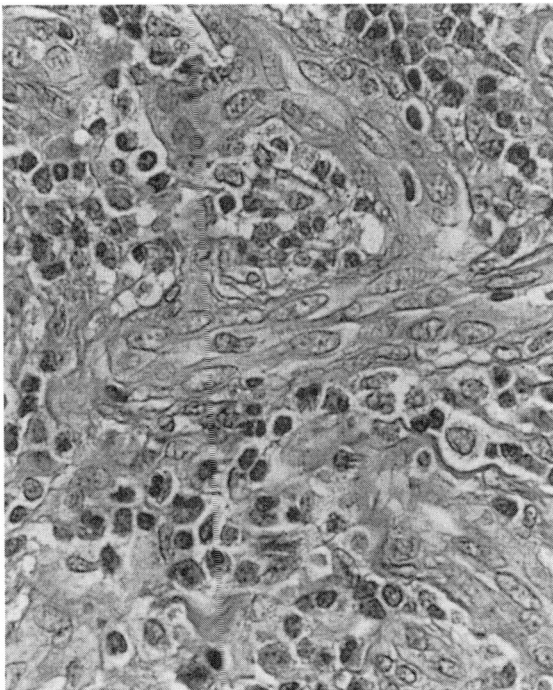

Fig. 20. Epithelioid haemangioma. ALHE. Newly-formed blood capillaries lined with plump endothelial cells. Note numerous eosinophils around. HES

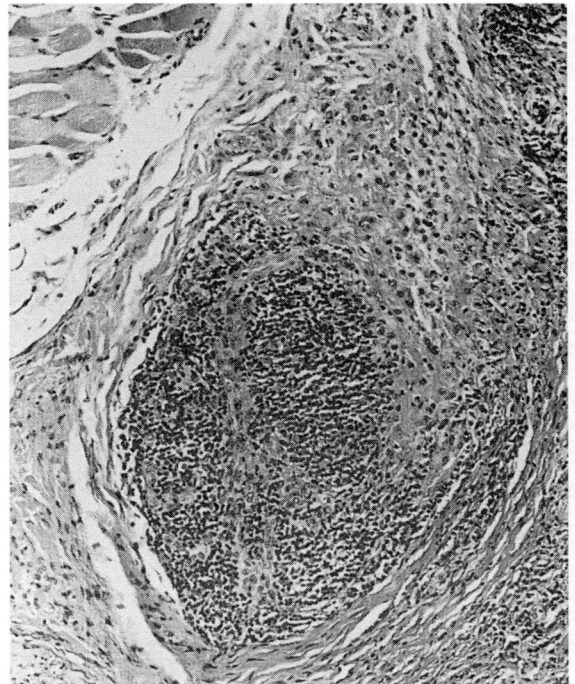

Fig. 21. Epithelioid haemangioma. AHLE. Lymphoid nodules in the adventitia. HES

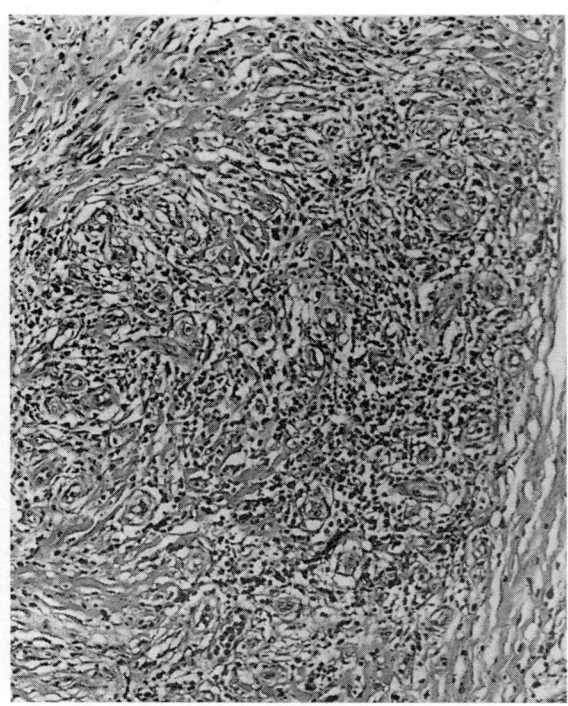

Fig. 22. Epithelioid haemangioma. Kimura's disease. Young 20-year-old asian man. Temporal nodule consisting of multiple abscess-like foci. HES

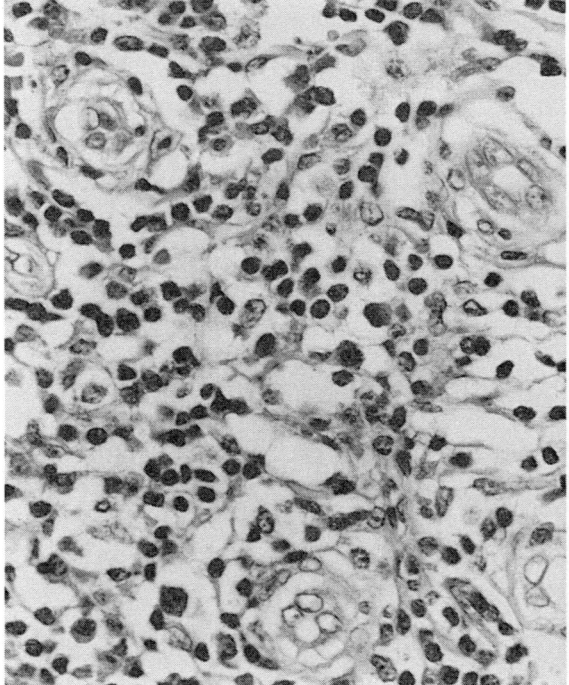

Fig. 23. Epithelioid haemangioma. Kimura's disease. Nodular proliferation of capillaries interspersed with eosinophils. HES

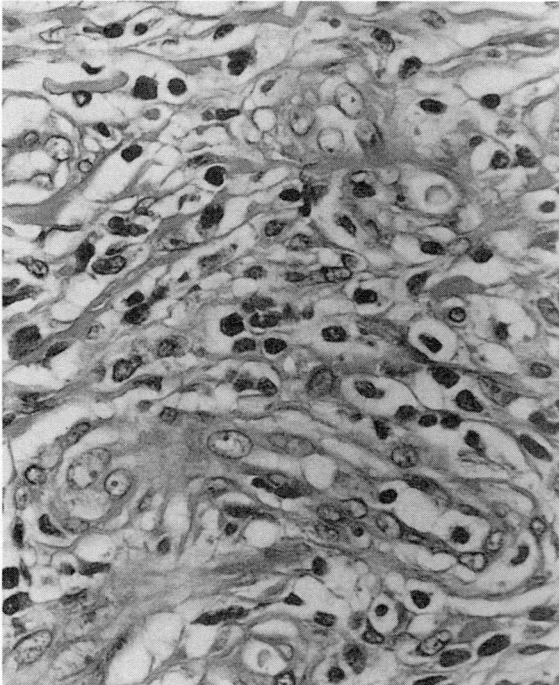

Fig. 24. Epithelioid haemangioma. Kimura's disease. Vascular proliferation is indistinguishable from that of AHLE. HES

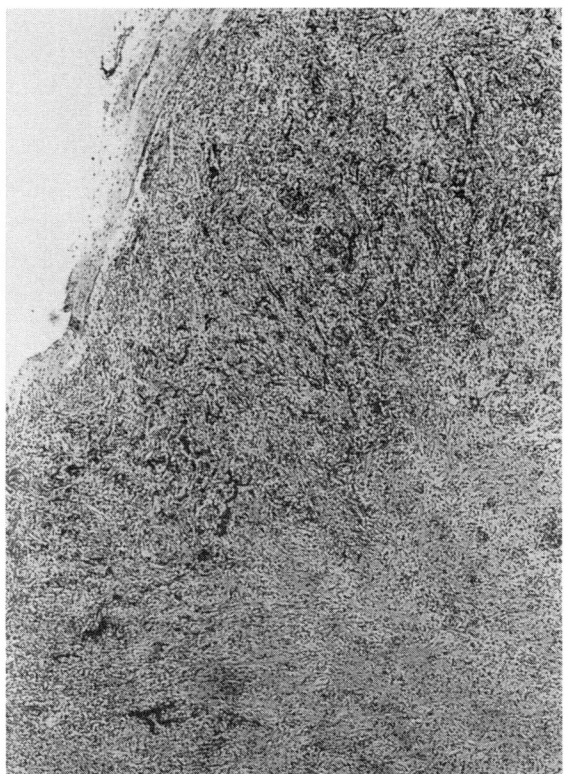

Fig. 25. Epithelioid haemangioma. Kimura's disease. Note radial disposition of proliferating vessels. HES

Miscellaneous tumour-like conditions of vessels

Intravascular papillary endothelial hyperplasia or Masson's tumour

This benign and relatively uncommon condition represents an exuberant but localised form of an organising vascular thrombus. It arises most often in the fourth and fifth decades with a slight female predilection. This lesion occurs frequently in the head and neck or extremities, presenting as a slow-growing solitary, firm, rather cystic bluish nodule. It has a good prognosis [73].

Pathology and differential diagnosis

Grossly, the lesion consists of a purple-red, multicystic mass containing clotted blood and surrounded by a fibrous capsule. Its diameter never exceeds 2 cm. Veins are most often involved by intravascular papillary endothelial hyperplasia (IPEH). The lesion, confined to the vascular lumen, is made up of vegetations, supported by a core of fibrin or hyalinized collagen and lined

with a single layer of flattened or plump factor VIII antigen-stained endothelial cells (Fig. 26-27-28). In some areas, vegetations appear to be free-floating within the vascular lumen (Fig. 29). Very rarely rupture of the vessel permits the process to spill over into extravascular surrounding tissues. IPEH may occur in a pre-existing vascular lesion such as an haemangioma, pyogenic granuloma, or vascular malformation. IPEH is distinguished from angiosarcoma by the following criteria: intraluminal-location, monolayer arrangement of the endothelial cells, absence of cellular necrosis and polymorphism and low mitotic rate [74].

Intravascular fasciitis

Nodular fasciitis may occur within blood vessels. In children and young adults, the upper limb, head and neck area are often involved [75], but cases have been reported in the foot and ankle [76].

Pathology and Differential diagnosis

Histologically, there is a spindle cell proliferation filling the lumen in masses or with a plexiform arran-

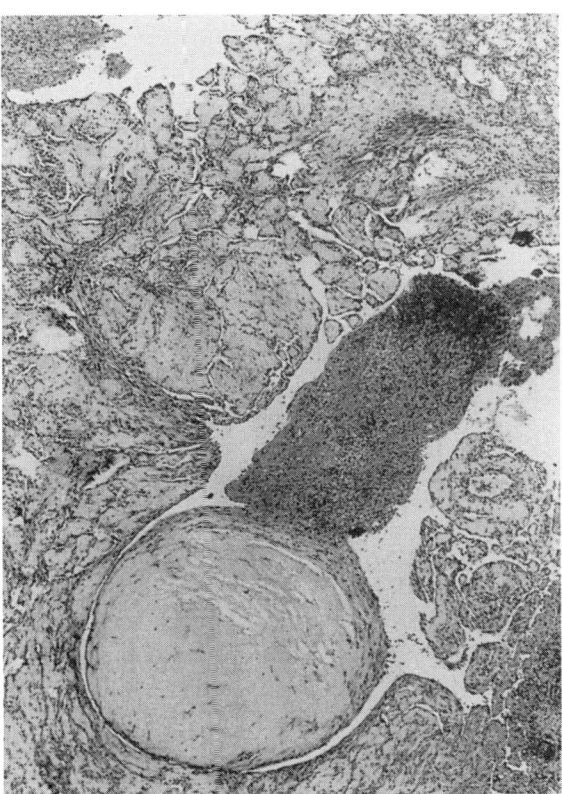

Fig. 26. Intravascular papillary endothelial hyperplasia developed in a venous lumen. Note a partially hyalinized thrombus. HES

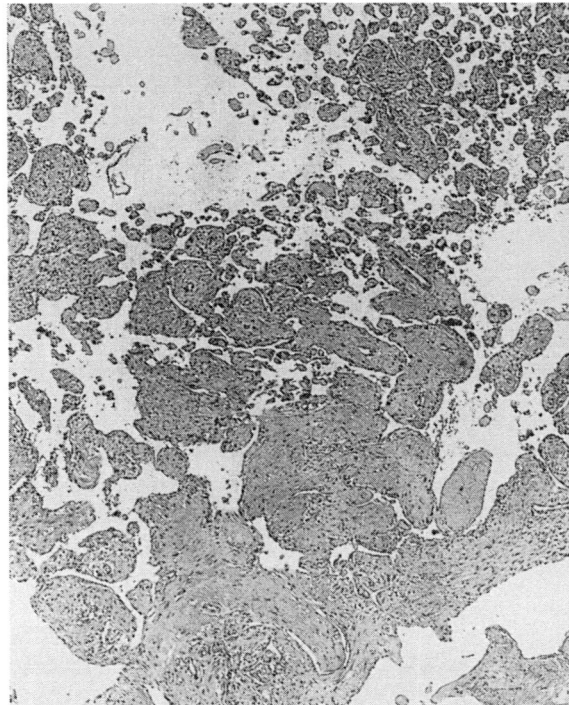

Fig. 27. Intravascular papillary endothelial hyperplasia. Organised thrombus with superficial vegetations. HES

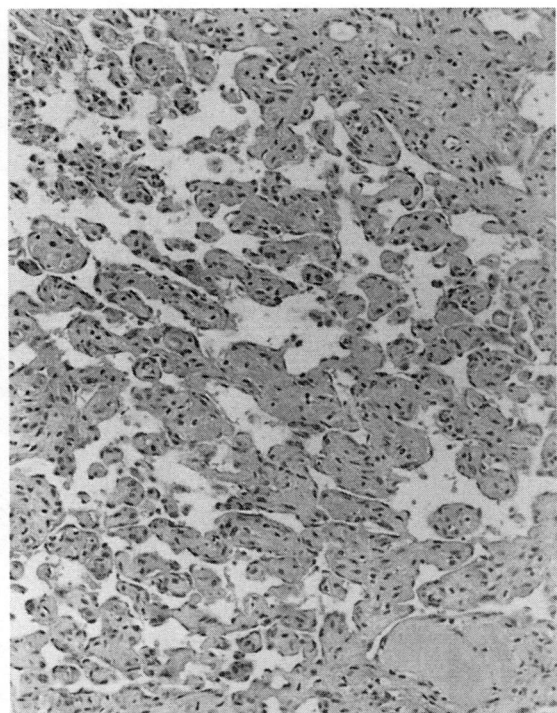

Fig. 28. Intravascular papillary endothelial hyperplasia. Histological incidence may give a free-floating pattern to the vegetations within the vascular lumen. HES

gement. Myofibroblasts, arranged in a loose storiform and fascicular pattern, occlude the vessel. The vessel wall and adjacent tissue may be invaded and mitoses may be present in a rapidly-growing lesion.

Malignant angioendotheliosis

This is a descriptive term for intravascular location of malignant lymphomas of B-cell or much more rarely, T-cell phenotype [77-81]. Clinically, most patients develop lesions in the skin and/or the central nervous system [82]. Skin involvement includes nodules and plaques scattered on the trunk and extremities associated with telangiectasia, ulceration and haemorrhage. Blindness, aphasia, headaches, and progressive paralysis reflect cerebral lesions.

Pathology and differential diagnosis

Histologically the lesion is made up of numerous dilated normal vessels. The lumen contains cells having the morphological features of activated mononuclear cells, some of which resemble endothelial cells. These cells may be few, or numerous and cohesive, mimicking a carcinomatous embolus (Fig. 30-31-32).Fibrin thrombi may be present. Immunohistochemistry is necessary for diagnosis.

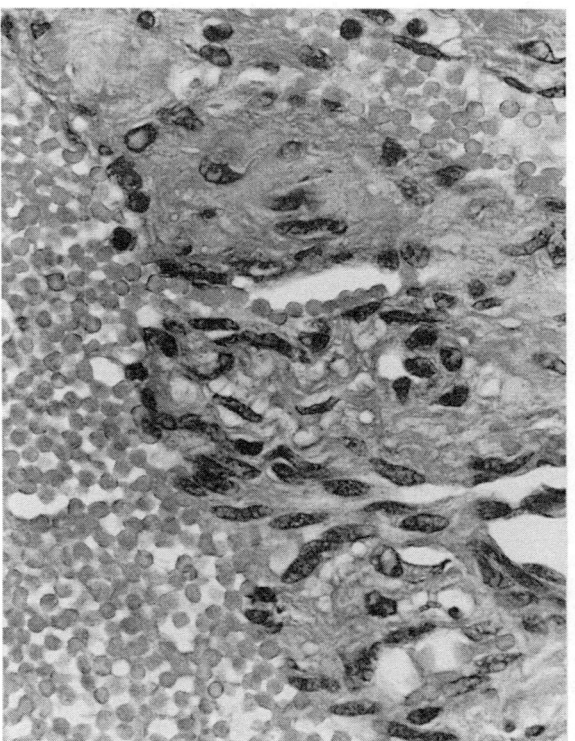

Fig. 29. Intravascular papillary endothelial hyperplasia. Vegetations lined with endothelial cells. HES

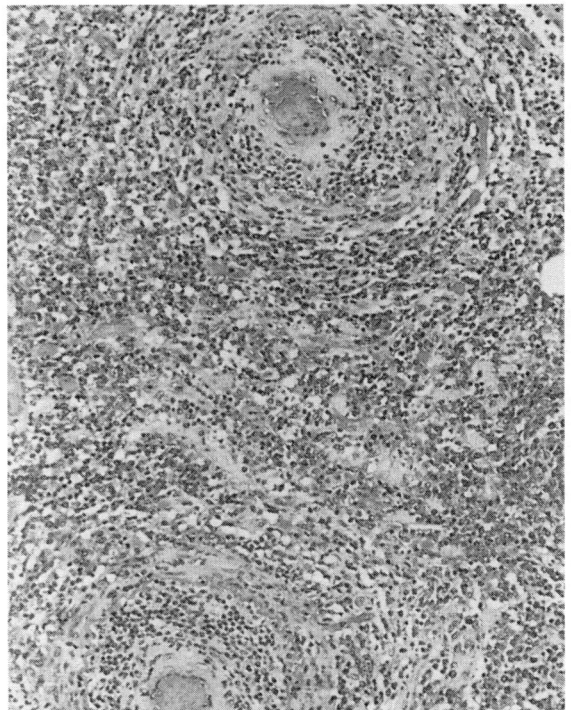

Fig. 30. Malignant angioendotheliosis. Male AIDS patient suffering from non-hodgkinian malignant lymphoma of the anus. Two muscular arteries invested by B lymphoma cells. HES (Courtesy Dr N. Lemarchand)

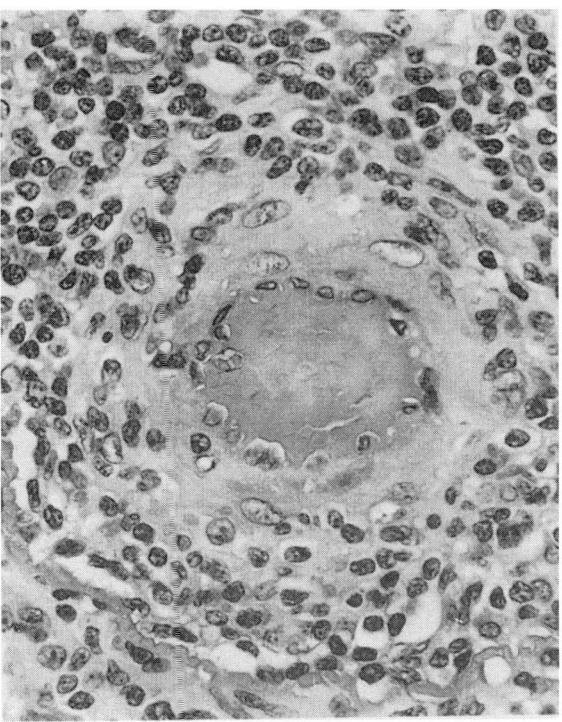

Fig. 31. Malignant angioendotheliosis. Medial infiltration of B-lymphoma cells. HES

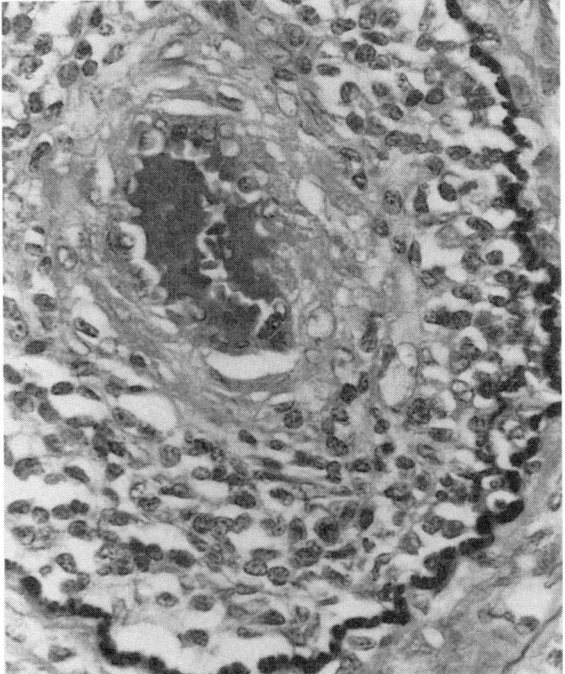

Fig. 32. Malignant angioendotheliosis. Elastin stain clearly evidences infiltration of the intima by lymphoma cells. Black line corresponds to the internal elatic membrane. Orcein

2 – Benign tumours of blood vessels

Haemangiomas

Haemangiomas make up 7.4% of all benign tumours in the general population [83].

Capillary haemangiomas

Capillary haemangiomas are most often recognised in the skin, subcutaneous tissues, and the mucous membranes (oral cavity and lips). The viscera (liver, spleen, and kidneys) may be involved. Skin haemangiomas are of two types; strawberry marks with the synonyms (tuberous or strawberry nevus, nevus vasculosus, juvenile haemangioma, hypertrophic angioma of infancy, or benign haemangioendothelioma of infancy) and cherry angiomas (senile ectasia, senile vascular nevus, Campbell-De Morgan spots). Most strawberry marks appear within a few weeks after birth, frequently in the head and neck, giving rise to irregularly-contoured bright red to purple lobules measuring a few millimeters to several centimeters in diameter. These lesions may either be level with the

skin surface or may bulge slightly but are rarely pedunculated. They enlarge rapidly over a period of several months, and begin to fade when the child is between one and three years old, then involute over a
period of years in 80% of cases, leaving a pigmented
scar. Cherry angiomas appear as small, slightly raised
red nodules scattered on the anterior surface of the
trunk or limbs. They mostly affect the middle-aged
and elderly.

Pathology and differential diagnosis

Capillary haemangiomas are usually well-defined but
nonencapsulated aggregates of capillaries, scattered or
grouped in lobules (Fig. 33-34). In the early stages,
vascular lumina are inconspicuous. With time, the capillaries become well-defined, delineated by a basal
membrane and separated by thin connective septa.
They are bordered by a thin endothelium. The endothelial cells appear immature and embryonic (Fig. 35-
36). Ultrastructurally, crystalloid inclusions (0.5 to
2.0 microns in diameter with parallel lamellar bands
with a regular periodicity of about 180 to 300) may be
seen while the typical rod-shaped tubulated Weibel-
Palade bodies are lacking [84]. Thrombosis and organisation and rupture of vessels causes fibrosis and accounts for the haemosiderin present.

Cavernous haemangioma (cavernoma)

Cavernous haemangiomas are less common than capillary haemangiomas and do not involute spontaneously. They may be part of a variety of dysmorphic
and hereditary syndromes, including the Maffuci,
Klippel-Trenaunay, and Parkes-Weber syndromes [85].

Usually present at birth, this tumour may not be
clinically evident until later in life. There is no sex
predilection. Almost any area of the body may be affected and clinical manifestations depend on the site
of the tumour. In the head and neck, large cavernous
haemangiomas may be associated with an arterio-venous fistula and erode the cranial vault. In the brain,
these haemangiomas are a potential source of increased intracranial pressure or haemorrhage and calcification [86-88]. A giant cavernous haemangioma may
cause the Kasabach-Merritt consumptive coagulopa-

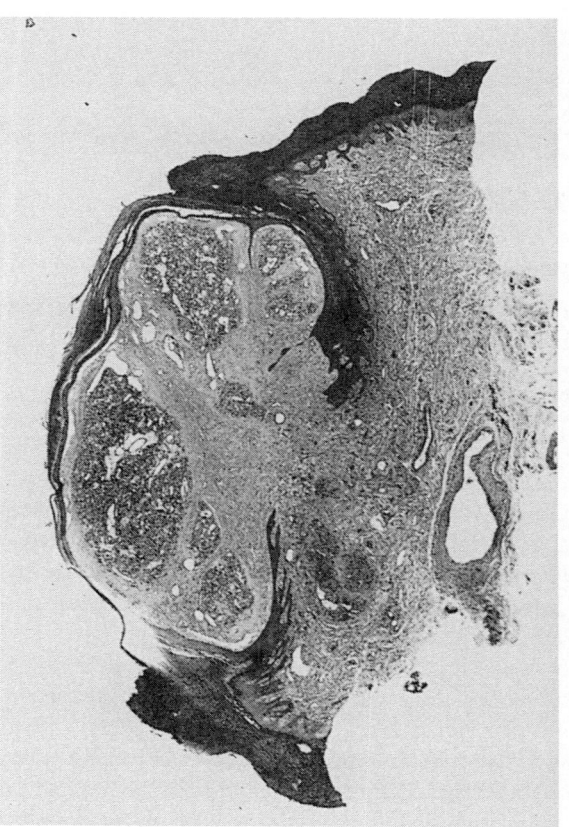

Fig. 33. Capillary haemangioma. Lobular pattern. HES

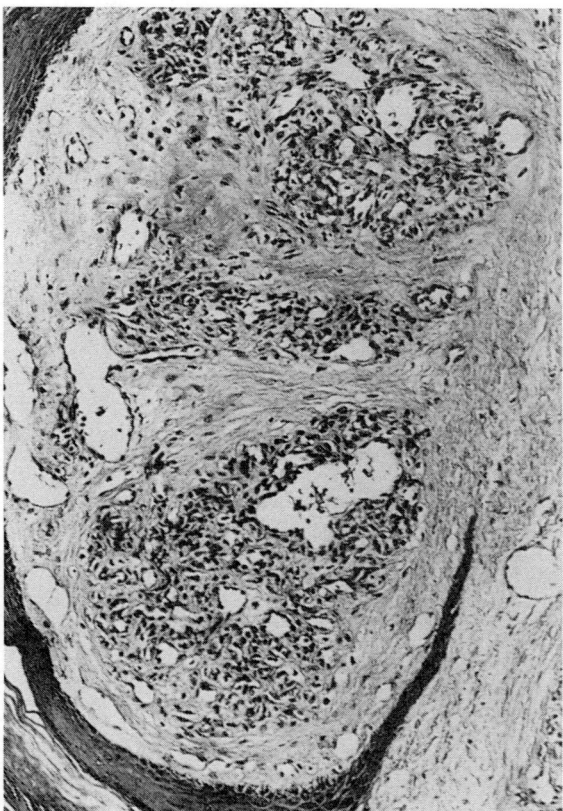

Fig. 34. Capillary haemangioma. Early stage with inconspicuous capillaries. HES

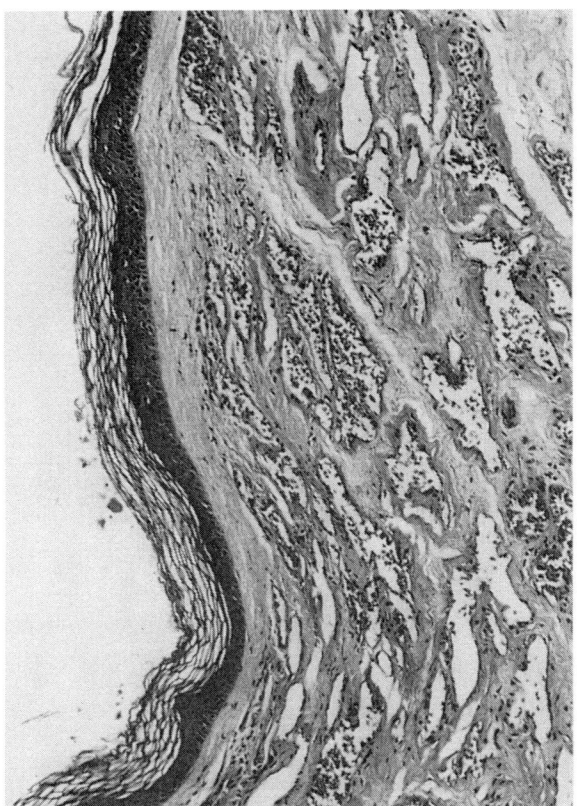

Fig. 35. Capillary haemangioma. Late stage with well-defined capillaries. HES

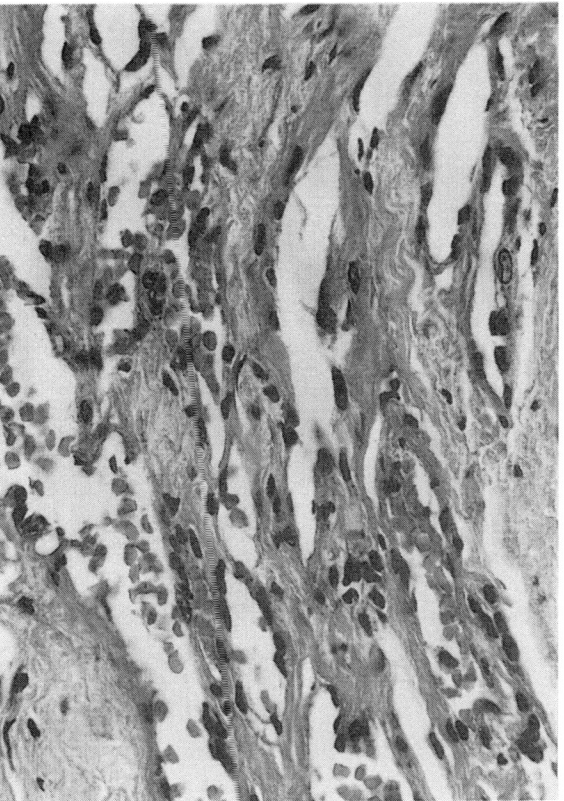

Fig. 36. Capillary haemangioma. Endothelial cells bordering the capillaries remain immature and embryonic. HES

thy syndrome [89, 90] to develop. Szlachetka [91] has suggested that this may occur in 1 in 300 of these lesions. However, as there are just over 200 cases in the literature and as the syndrome may occur with a number of vascular lesions, including haemangiopericytoma [92], it is clearly not a specific association. Indeed Enjolras et al [93] have suggested that although the syndrome will not occur with capillary haemangioma it may do so with tufted haemangioma or kaposiform haemangioendothelioma. It has been considered that cavernous haemangiomas may be precursor lesions for the development of an angiosarcoma [94], but little evidence supports this view.

Pathology and differential diagnosis

Grossly, a cavernous haemangioma appears as a reddish-black, soft, spongy haemorrhagic mass generally measuring less than 4 cm in diameter. Any part of the body may be affected: soft tissues, bones and viscera. Giant cavernous haemangiomas may affect large subcutaneous areas of the face, extremities (Fig. 37), or other regions of the body (Fig. 38), but are rare. Histologically, the mass is sharply defined, but not en-

capsulated, and is composed of large dilated thin-walled vessels and sinuses lined with a flattened endothelium. The wall of these spaces becomes thicker and hyalinized with time, with pericytes around (Fig. 39-40). In some areas, vascular channels are back-to-back, arranged in an intercommunicating sieve-like pattern producing a sinusoidal appearance [95]. Rare cases of cavernous haemangioma include a capillary component, but this combination is not rare in cavernous haemangiomas on the head and face of children. Organized thrombi can be seen with occasional central infarction (Fig. 41) The main differential diagnosis consists of ruling out an angiosarcoma, notably in the breast.

Haemangiomas with unusual clinical or histological patterns

Angiokeratoma

The term "angiokeratoma" is used to describe several distinct entities; these are the Mibelli type, the Fordyce type, the solitary and multiple nodular types,

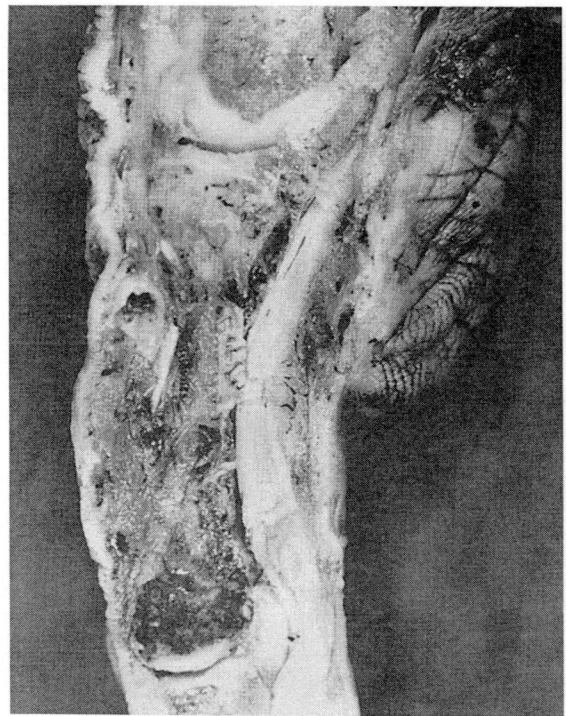

Fig. 37. Cavernous haemangioma of a finger

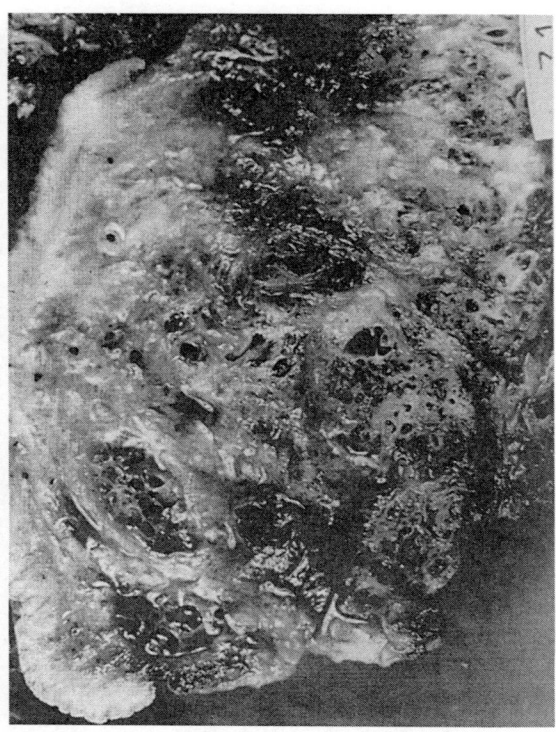

Fig. 38. Cavernous haemangioma. Large and deep involvement of the buttock. (Courtesy Dr Cl. Laurian)

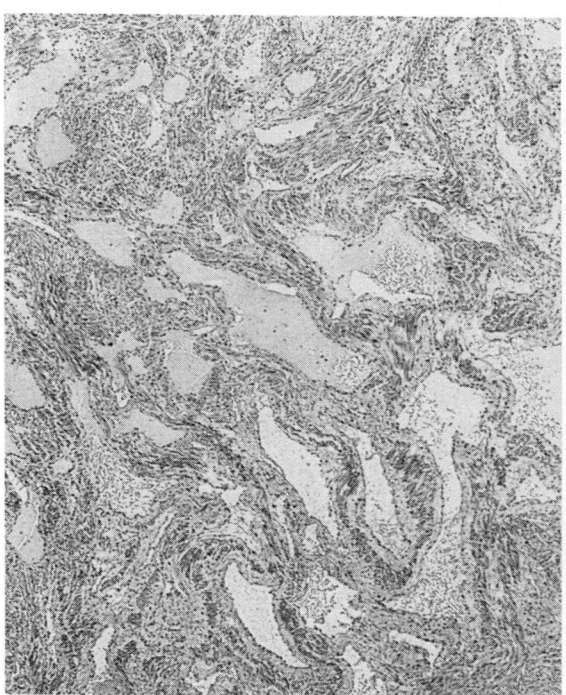

Fig. 39. Cavernous haemangioma of the index. Large vessels and sinuses engorged with red blood cells. HES

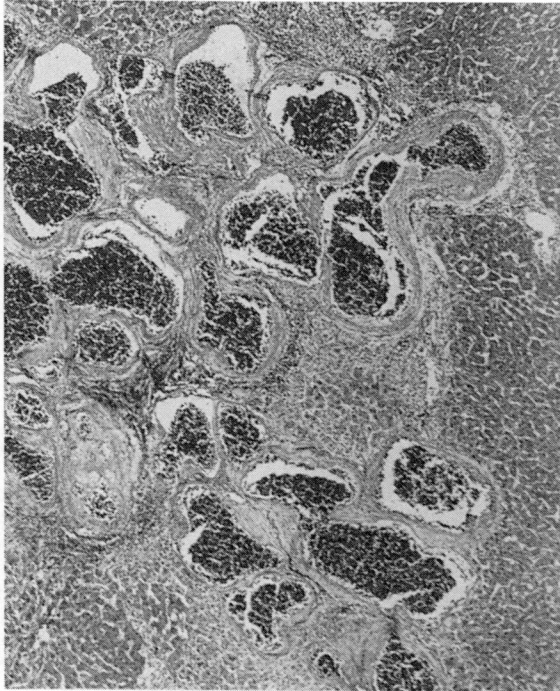

Fig. 40. Cavernous haemangioma of the liver. HES

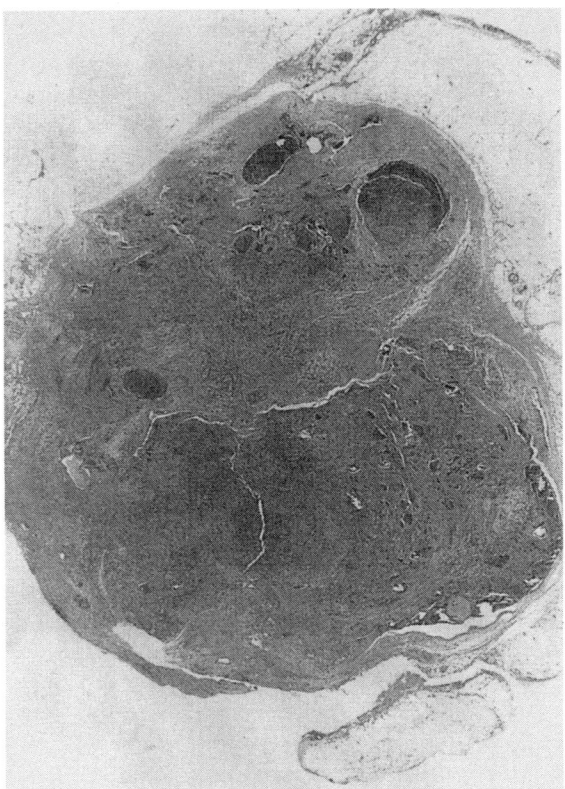

Fig. 41. Cavernous haemangioma. Central haemorrahge and thrombosis. HES

angiokeratoma cicumscriptum and angiokeratoma corporis diffusum [96].

- The Mibelli type occurs in the typical sites for chilblains (see chapter VII) and is a result of cold related vascular damage [97]. This type mostly affects girls and starts as reddish macules that evolve into red or purple keratotic papules, 2 to 5 mm in diameter. These lesions bleed readily and predominate in areas of bony prominences (fingers, toes, elbows and knees). An autosomal dominant mode of inheritance with variable penetrance is likely, as this condition may involve siblings or offspring.

- The "angiokeratoma of Fordyce" is a form of reactive vascular ectasia occurring in response to raised venous pressure, typically affecting the scrotum of men in the fourth decade, but also seen in young adults, children and rarely in the vulva. It consists of dome-shaped reddish papules, 2 to 4 mm in diameter, which may bleed profusely if injured.

- The solitary and multiple nodular types occur on the lower limbs of adolescents and young adults and are assumed to be a result of local elastic deficiencies.

- Angiokeratoma circumscriptum is a naevoid hamartoma associated with other congenital anomalies. It is the least common of all angiokeratomas and 50% of cases are present at birth or appear in infancy, with a predilection for girls. This lesion consists of verrucous dark red papules that merge into a large, solitary, linear, unilateral plaque, which may be large enough to involve a major part of a limb or a body region. The overlying skin tends to become keratotic. This change may be related to the presence of matrix metalloproteinase (MMP)-9 in the epidermal horny layer [98].

- Angiokeratoma corporis diffusum occurs in association with lysosomal enzyme disorders, usually α-glucosidase A deficiency [99] (See chapter XV). In the elderly, isolated angiokeratomas are frequently associated with conditions that cause local obstruction of venules. Patients may develop well-circumscribed reddish macules in the oral cavity [100] and the mucosa of the digestive tract.

- Solitary angiokeratoma is frequent and mostly affects adult in their third or fourth decades. This lesion may appear on any part of the body, especially in the lower extremities. It begins as a reddish spot that blanches under pressure and evolves to a reddish-brown keratotic papule. Sometimes a history of trauma is recorded at the site of the lesion. There is no tendency to involution and lesions may persist for life.

Pathology and differential diagnosis

The common features of the angiokeratomas consist of at least one widely dilated, thin-walled, endothelium-lined blood vessel in the upper dermis, enclosed by elongated rete ridges, focal acanthosis, papillomatosis and hyperkeratosis of the epidermis, and a thin band of collagen that separates the two structures. However, angiokeratomas have some differences that make them distinctive. Prominent compact orthokeratosis characterises angiokeratoma of Mibelli (Fig. 42). In the Fordyce type smooth muscle cells are prominent in the walls of the vascular spaces. The main differential diagnosis of angiokeratoma is lymphangioma circumscriptum, the characteristic valves of the lymphatics are useful in this regard.

Verrucous haemangioma

This appears at birth or soon thereafter as a solitary, brown to bluish-black lesion, usually on a lower extremity, but other areas may be involved (Fig. 43). A variant of verrucous haemangioma developed in the extremities is called "digital verucous fibroangioma" [101] and is thought to be a form of the Klippel-Trenaunay syndrome [102].

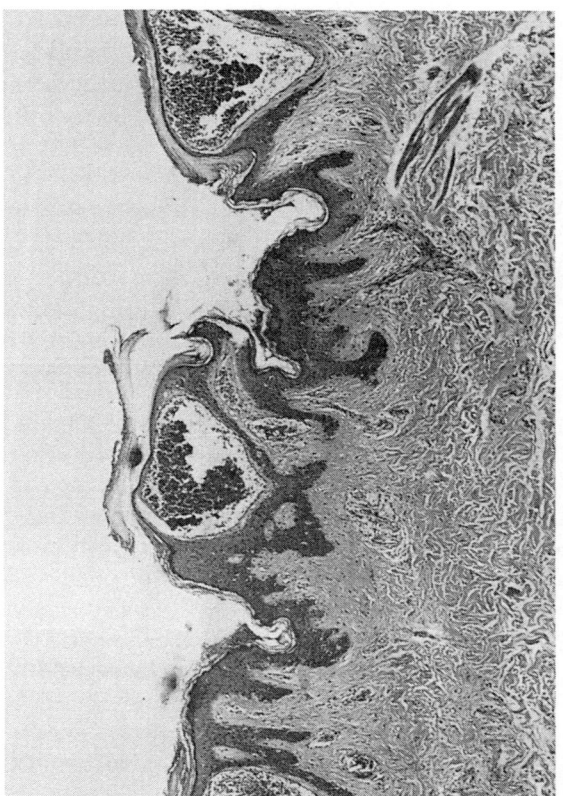

Fig. 42. Angiokeratoma of Mibelli. HES

Pathology and differential diagnosis

Histologically, verrucous haemangioma may present some similarities with angiokeratoma but angiomatous vessels appear deeper in the skin, distorting the dermis and subcutis (Fig. 44-45) [103, 104].

Angioma serpiginosum of Hutchinson

This is a rare vascular condition characterised by punctuate reddish macules, arranged in a serpiginous pattern. It is typically a lesion of childhood, with female predominance. It may involve any part of the body, especially the lower extremities and the buttocks. Multiple, punctuate, pinhead, red or purple lesions develop on a background of erythema or slight hyperpigmentation. These lesions coalesce to form patches that creep outward, hence the term "serpinosum". Association with retinal capillary aneurysms and neurological deficits has been reported [105]. In some patients, angioma serpiginosum may wax and wane for many years; in others it is progressive. Some cases are familial [106] with an autosomal dominant mode of inheritance.

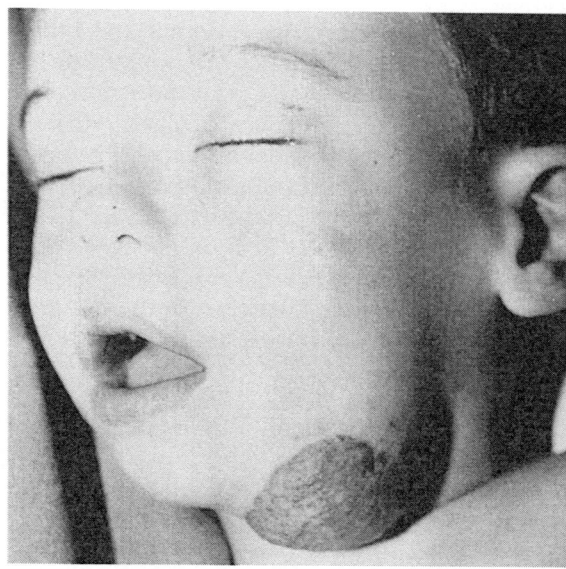

Fig. 43. Verrucous haemangioma of the chin of a 5 year-old boy. (Courtesy Dr P. Oger)

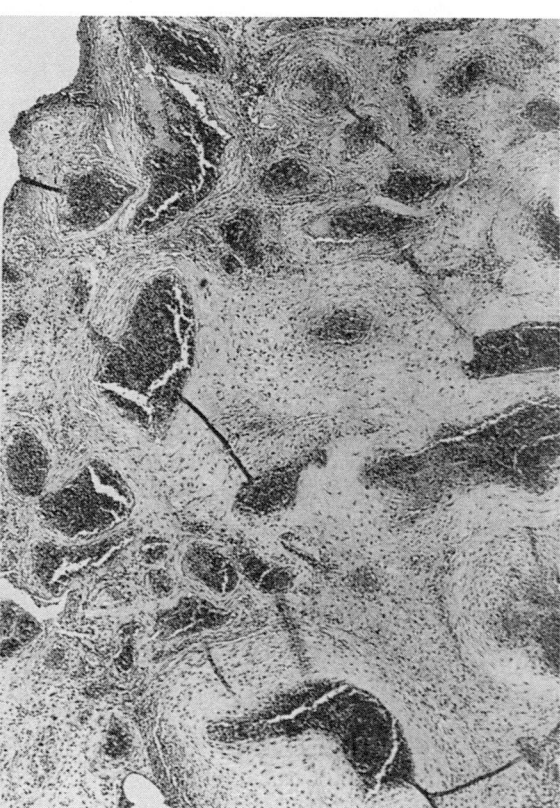

Fig. 44. Verrucous haemangioma. Angiomatous vessels extending to the subcutaneous tissues. HES

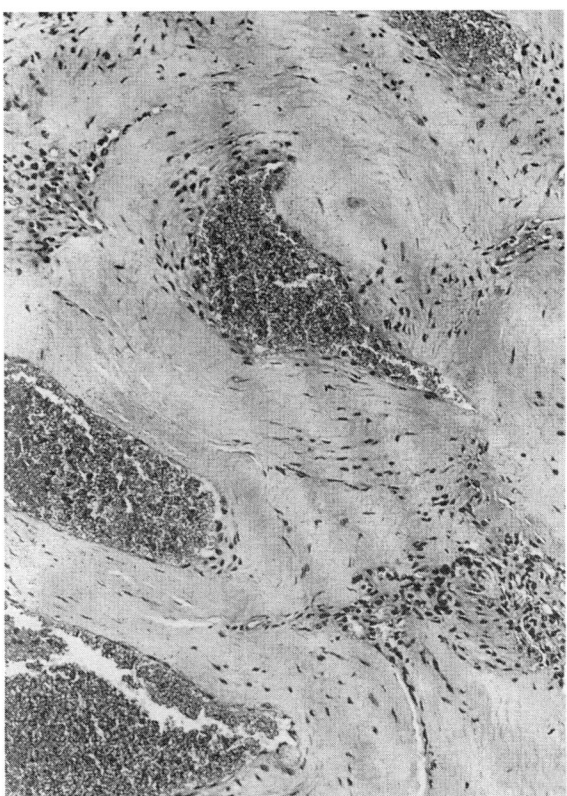

Fig. 45. Verrucous haemangioma. Angiomatous vessels are limited by a thick a hyalinized wall. HES

Pathology and differential diagnosis

Histologically, each lesion consists of a localized collection of dilated, well-formed capillaries in the dermal papillae, engorged with blood and lined with flattened endothelium. These vessels distort the superficial or mid-dermis. Ultrastructurally, the vessel walls have two distinct layers with fine fibrillar material internally and an outer layer of collagen. The endothelial cells have slit-like invaginations in the cytoplasm [107]. It may be impossible to distinguish these lesions from those in essential telangiectasia without the clinical context.

Targetoid haemosideric haemangioma

This rare haemangioma is characterized by a small, solitary, circular lesion with a raised purple centre and successive clear, ecchymotic haloes that expand centrifugally with time [108, 109]. Young and middle-aged patients are frequently affected, with a male predominance. This tumour usually develops on the trunk or extremities and often measures less than 1 cm in diameter.

Pathology and differential diagnosis

The haemangioma involves the dermis and subcutis. The histological pattern depends on the age of the lesion. In the early phase, the superficial portion is characterised by irregular, dilated vascular channels lined with plump, epithelioid, endothelial cells that focally form "hob-nail" papillary projections. There is no endothelial multilayering or tufting. Cytologic atypia is minimal or absent [110]. In the deep portion, there are anastomosing slit-like vascular channels that apparently dissect the collagen. The dermis often shows haemorrhage and infiltration of haemosiderin-loaded macrophages. In the intermediate phase the vascular channels are narrow with some spindle cells around them. In the late phase, the lesion is composed exclusively of narrow, empty, thin-walled anastomosing channels in the dermis and superficial subcutis. In some areas, collapse of the vascular lumen can create an impression of fibroblastic proliferation but immunohistochemistry shows variable reactivity of endothelial cells with CD31, CD34, Factor VIII-related antigen, and *Ulex europaeus* agglutinin-1. Smooth muscle actin-positive pericytes may be observed focally around some of the abnormal vascular spaces.

Targetoid haemangioma may simulate Kaposi's sarcoma, benign lymphangioendothelioma (acquired progressive lymphangioma) and epithelioid haemangioma. Kaposi's sarcoma can be ruled out on clinical grounds and the presence of epithelioid cells with papillary formations, extensive haemosiderin deposits, paucity of lymphocytes and plasma cells, and absence or paucity of hyaline globules [111]. Targetoid haemangioma can overlap epithelioid haemangioma but differs from the latter by its clinical annular appearance. Benign lymphangioendothelioma has a more extensive, slowly progressive lesion having the features of a large bruise-like macula [112]. This lesion does not contain red blood cells or haemosiderin deposits.

Glomeruloid haemangioma (Takatsuki syndrome, Crow-Fukase syndrome, plasma cell dyscrasia with polyneuropathy and endocrine disorders)

This is a variety of capillary haemangioma with a glomerulus-like arrangement of newly formed vessels. The tumour occurs as part of the POEMS syndrome, a complex syndrome characterised by polyneuropathy, organomegaly (hepatosplenomegaly, lymphadenopathy), endocrinopathy (amenorrhoea, gynaecomastia, glucose intolerance, hypothyroidism, adrenal insufficiency), M-protein (marrow plasmacytosis, paraproteinemia) and skin lesions (glomeruloid and cherry haemangiomas, acanthosis, hyperpigmentation, hypertrichosis) [113, 114]. It generally affects older patients but cases in their early twenties have been reported [115]. Enlarged lymph nodes in patients with POEMS frequently have the features of Castleman's disease [116, 117]. Glomeruloid haemangiomas are commonly multifocal, and develop as small papules scattered on the skin of the trunk or extremities. The viscera may be involved. More than 50% of endoneural blood vessels have a narrowed or closed lumen with thickened basement membranes [118]. Arterial occlusion is a recently documented feature of the syndrome [119, 120] and may be due to overproduction of vascular endothelial growth factor (VEGF).

Pathology and differential diagnosis

Glomeruloid haemangiomas are composed of dilated vascular spaces containing conglomerates of capillary loops resembling renal glomeruli (Fig. 46). These capillary loops are bordered by flat or plump endothelial cells and are surrounded by plump stromal cells with clear cytoplasm. Some of these contain eosinophilic Periodic acid-Schiff (PAS) – positive, diastase-resistant hyaline globules. In some areas, an intermediate pattern with cherry haemangiomas may be present. The differential diagnosis includes Kaposi's sarcoma, as hyaline globules are present in stromal cells. However, a glomeruloid haemangioma contains well-formed capillary loops and no spindle cellular component.

Microvenular haemangioma

This recently defined lesion [121-124] affects young adults and children of either sex (mean age: 29. 5 years). It appears as a small solitary nodule or plaque involving the extremities. A neoplastic nature for microvenular haemangioma is favoured by evidence of continued growth, but the natural history is not known.

Pathology and differential diagnosis

Histologically, this is an infiltrative proliferation of small irregularly anastomotic venules; some are dilated, others collapsed (Fig. 47-48-49). The endothelial lining appears regular without any atypia and is immunohistochemically positive for endothelial markers. Haemosiderin deposits may be present. Pathologists and clinicians should be aware of the infiltrative character of this type of haemangioma to avoid overdiagnosis and overtreatment [125].

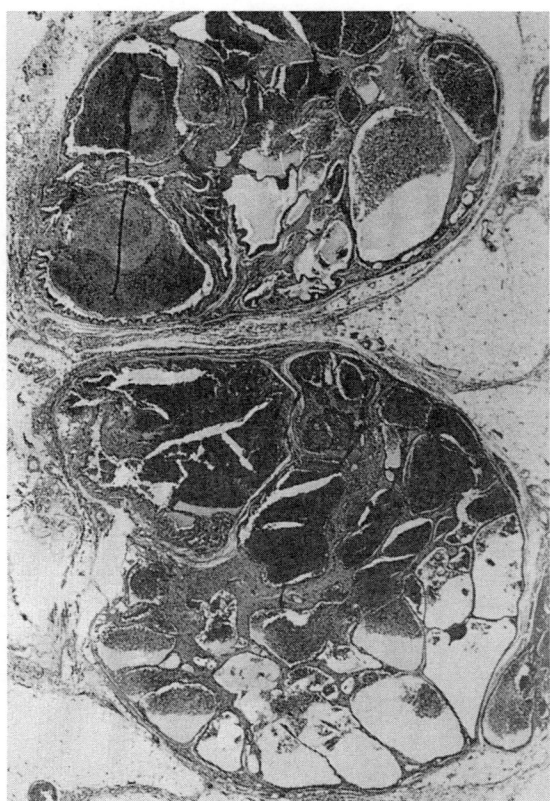

Fig. 46. Glomeruloid haemangioma. HES

Angioblastoma (Tufted angioma)

First reported by Nakagawa in 1949 as an angioblastoma [126], this slow-course tumour was rediscovered by MacMillan in 1971 [127] under the term "progressive capillary haemangioma". The lesion is characterised by packed lobules of immature endothelial cells scattered throughout the dermis giving an intradermal multinodular (cannon ball) pattern that compresses, indents and invaginates adjacent slit-like vessels.

Children are mainly affected, more rarely teenagers and young adults [128-133] without sex predilection. Any site may be affected. Angioblastomata appear as one or more red or purplish, slightly raised, indurated plaques, 2 to 10 cm in diameter, in a normal skin. They are sometimes painful on pressure. Occasionally, thrombocytopaenia may be found. In most cases, the lesions start insidiously and grow slowly for several years before stabilizing without involution. Some cases present a worryingly rapid phase with plaques increasing in size rapidly for weeks or

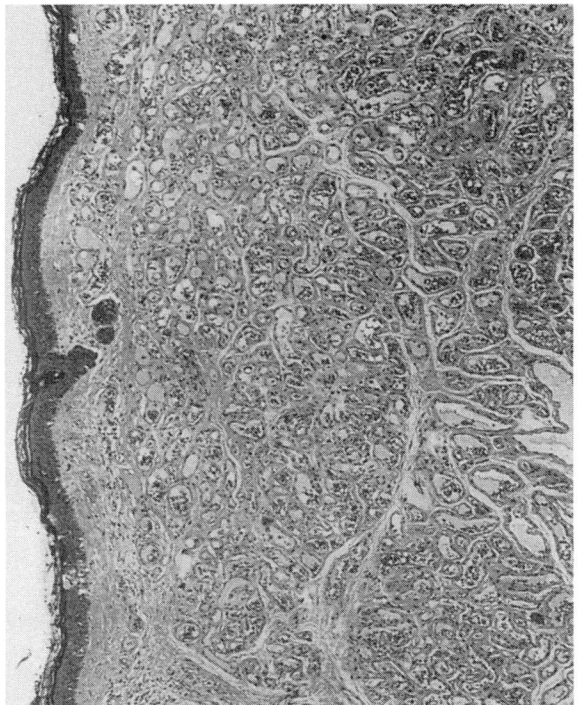

Fig. 47. Microvenular haemangioma. HES

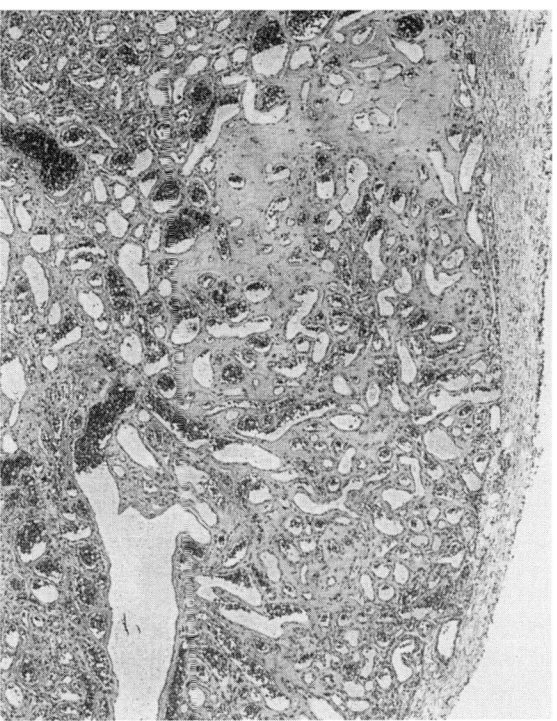

Fig. 48. Microvenular haemangioma. Infiltrating pattern should not be interpreted as malignant behavior. HES

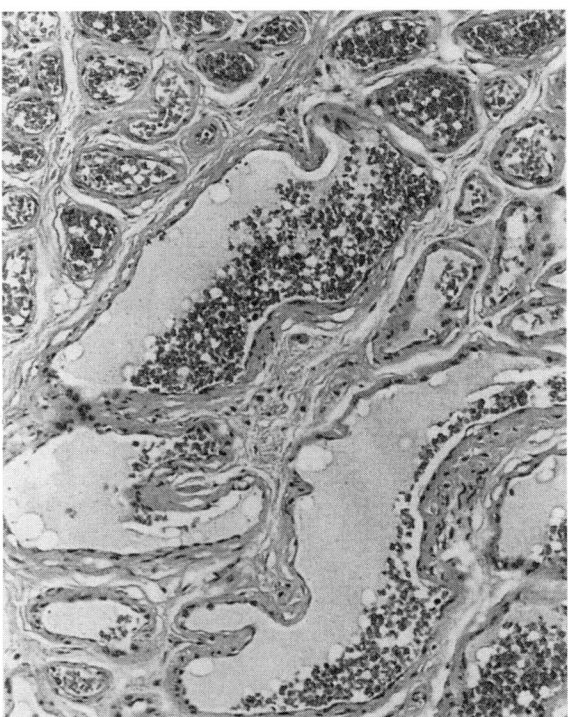

Fig. 49. Microvenular haemangioma. Venular-type angiomatous vessels. HES

months. Local recurrence may follow if excision is incomplete. There are isolated reports of familial incidence with an autosomal-dominant mode of inheritance [134], an association with lipodystrophy centrifugalis abdominalis [135], with pregnancy [136], and with liver transplantation [137]. Spontaneous regression has been reported [138, 139].

Pathology and differential diagnosis

The histological presentation is pathognomonic (Fig. 50-51-52). This tumour shares many of the histological features of a capillary haemangioma. It consists of multiple small tightly packed lobules of collapsed capillaries scattered throughout the dermis; some lobules abut on the epidermis, others overlap the subcutis and the underlying adipose tissue. The vascular slits are rimmed by cells indistinguishable cytologically from the cells that surround them and a giant-celled form exists [140]. Mitoses are rare. Mast cells may be present in and about the tumour. Haemosiderin pigment is seen. Immunohistochemistry demonstrates that most tumour cells are endothelial, reacting with CD 31 and for CD 34 and inconsistently with factor VIII Rag [126, 129]. Some intralobular cells are stained with alpha-smooth muscle actin indicating the participation of pericytes [128]. These data confirm the findings of Padilla et al [141] who suggested that the cellular proliferation is composed of both endothelial and perithelial cells. The negative staining of most endothelial cells for factor VIII underlines their immaturity [129]. No reactivity is seen with cytokeratin, common leukocyte antigen CD45 and desmin.

The differential diagnosis includes all vascular lesions with a lobular architecture, including bacillary angiomatosis, pyogenic granuloma, Kaposiform juvenile haemangioendothelioma (cellular capillary haemangioma), Kaposi's sarcoma and low-grade angiosarcoma. None of those entities displays the widespread, intradermal multinodular (cannon ball) pattern of tufted angioma. Bacillary angiomatosis contains scattered infiltrates of neutrophils, eosinophils and histiocytes. A search for rickettsiae is made by HES, Giemsa or Warthin-Starry staining techniques. Cellular capillary haemangioma or Kaposiform juvenile haemangioendothelioma [142] generally forms larger tumour lobules with an infiltrating pattern and harbours spindle cells. Kaposi's sarcoma and low-grade angiosarcoma do not commonly have a nodular pattern. Low-grade angiosarcoma is made up of anastomotic vessels lined with atypical endothelium [141].

Sclerosing haemangioma (Histiocytoma, fibroxanthoma, .alveolar angioblastoma, m.ast cell granuloma)

A sclerosing haemangioma consists of angiomatous vessels surrounded by various stages of fibrosis. In the lungs, sclerosing haemangioma presents as a solitary nodular or "coin" lesion developed most often in the lower lobe [143, 144]. However, lesions may be multiple and bilateral [145]. Sclerosing haemangioma has a significant female predilection and 80% of cases occur in middle-aged women (mean age 44 yrs). Expression of estrogen and progesterone receptors and 17-beta estradiol in this tumour has not been established consistently [146,147]. Although frequently asymptomatic [148], the tumour may cause haemorrhage.

The pathogenesis of sclerosing haemangioma is disputed and although it has been thought to result from a proliferation of undifferentiated epithelial mesenchymal tissue, with secondary vascular differentiation, most immunohistochemical and ultrastructural studies support the hypothesis that the tumour originates from type II pneumocytes and bronchiolar epithelial cells [149-151]. Leong et al [152] found the tumour cells to be clearly of epithelial origin in a study of 25 cases, using immunocytochemistry. Factor VIII-

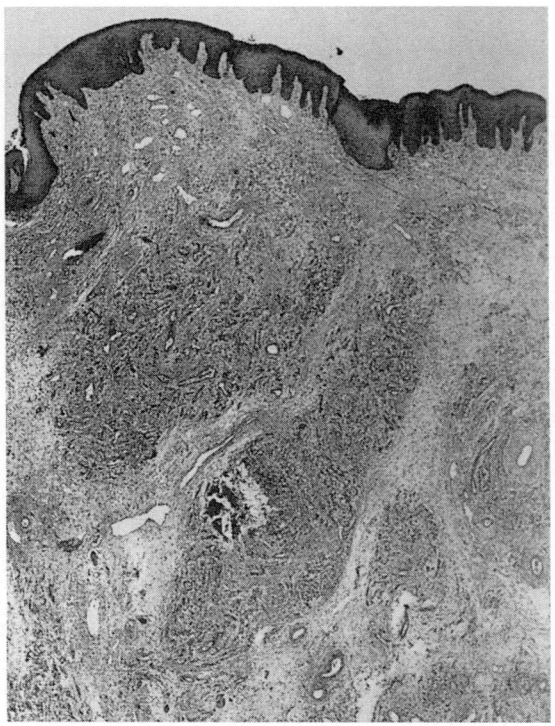

Fig. 50. Angioblastoma (tufted angioma) consisting of multiple packed capillary lobules. HES

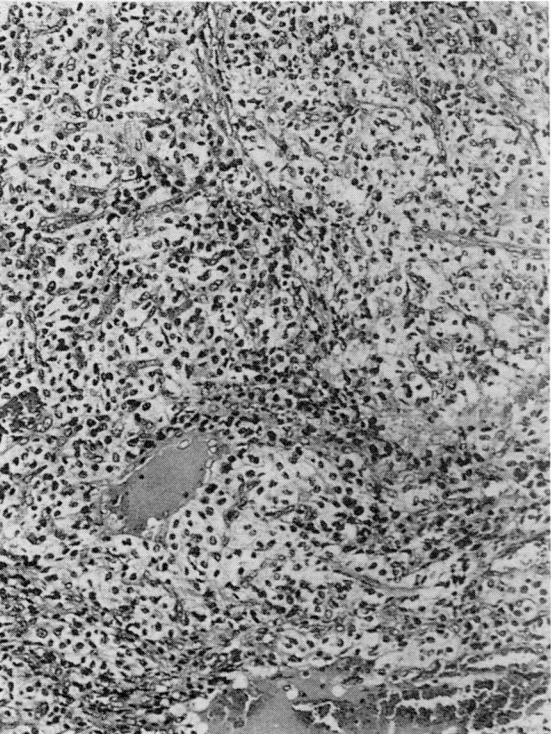

Fig. 51. Angioblastoma (tufted angioma). Vascular slits rimmed by pohyedral endothelial cells. HES

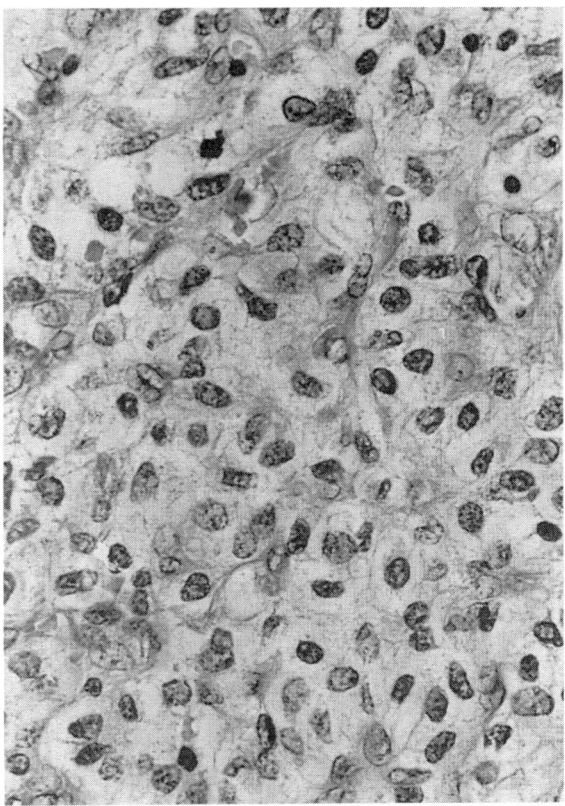

Fig. 52. Angioblastoma (tufted angioma). Pohyedral endothelial cells. HES

related antigen was negative. The natural history of this tumour is not established [153]. Chiba et al [154] suggested that this is a low-grade malignant tumuor as the cells displayed positive expression of the c-myc and p53 gene products.

Pathology and differential diagnosis

The lesion is a well-circumscribed, haemorrhagic, and occasionally calcified nodule. Histologically, there is a variegated appearance made up of papillae covered by prominent type II alveolar epithelioid cells, fibrotic areas containing haemangiomatous vessels, foam cells, cholesterol clefts, haemorrhage and haemosiderin deposits leading to aflorid granulomatous reaction in some instances [155].

The differential diagnosis includes inflammatory pseudotumour, benign clear cell "sugar" tumour, carcinoid and papillary carcinomas (metastatic thyroid or renal carcinoma). An inflammatory pseudotumour lacks papillary growth, vascular spaces and distinct epithelioid cells. In a benign clear cell tumour, the tumour cells have a clear, glycogen-rich cytoplasm. The

stroma contains delicate, thin-walled vessels or sinusoids in contrast with sclerosing haemangioma. Carcinoid tumours have an organoid, trabecular, rosette or spindle cell histological pattern. Papillary carcinomas have well defined cytological criteria.

3 – Benign tumours of lymphatic vessels or lymphangiomas

Tumours of lymphatic vessels are rare. Lymphangiomas encompass three main types: cavernous lymphangioma, lymphangioma circumscriptum (lymphangiectodes) andcystic lymphangioma (hygroma). A small percentage of cases may develop following radiation therapy or surgical block dissection of regional lymph nodes, but the vast majority are hamartomas. Association of lymphangiomas and haemangiomas, as well as the development of lymphangiomas in organs where lymph vessels are normally few or even absent, favors a failure of developmental control.

Cavernous lymphangioma

This lesion is evident at birth or soon after, with equal sex incidence. Cavernous lymphangioma may involve any part of the body; the most common sites include the head and neck, the axillae and scapulae, thighs, penoscrotal and vulvar regions [156]. In some areas, lesions are so superficial that the overlying skin or mucosa appears to be covered by vesicles or bullae. Other lesions may be deep-seated in soft tissues, bones, viscera and, rarely, the retroperitoneum. Clinical manifestations depend on the location. Occasionally, the tumour achieves considerable size and produces gross deformities in and about the involved parts, with lymphoedema and chylangiomas in the mesentery. Thrombosis, calcification, and periodic infection may occur, leading to enlargement and tenderness. Lymphangiomas frequently show a characteristic infiltrative spread, though this pattern does not indicate malignant transformation. Complications are ruptures, lymphorrhagia or chylous effusions, mechanical effects on the surrounding tissues and with lymphangiomas occurring in the intestinal canal, enteric loss of protein. Local recurrence after surgery may be expected due to poor marginal definition.

Pathology and differential diagnosis

Cavernous lymphangiomas are composed of a mass of massively dilated cystic cavities (Fig. 53). These cavities are delineated by a relatively scanty intervening connective tissue stroma and lined by flattened endothelial cells (Fig. 54). There may be budding and proliferation of fibrous tissue between the cavities. (Fig. 55). The smooth muscle contents of lymphangioma may very considerably and there may be muscle-free forms as well as true "muscular" lymphangiomata, sometimes arising from lymph trunks (Fig. 56). The stroma is either inconspicuous or infiltrated by large lymphoid follicles (Fig. 57). Combined haemolymphangiomas consist of vascular spaces engorged with red blood cells interspersed with lymphatic channels containing lymphocytes or mixtures of blood and lymph. The differentiation of retroperitoneal cystic lymphangiomata from lymph or chylous cysts is difficult and only of academic interest. However, lymphovascular cysts are easily differentiated from other vascular tumours.

Lymphangioma circumscriptum

This variety of cavernous lymphangioma often presents in infancy but may develop at any age. According to Mordehai et al [157], lymphangioma circumscriptum (LC) primarily affects the subcutaneous tissue in the form of cystic dilatation of lymphatic channels without systemic lymphatic communication. The skin lesions are probably secondary to the increased intraluminal pressure. LC may represent a rare complication of altered lymphatic drainage after surgery or cellulitis [158-161]. The proximal parts of the limbs and limb girdles are frequently involved. The lesions manifest as isolated or multiple verrucous vesicles or blebs in the skin, resembling warts. These nodules may form larger confluent masses. Puncture or injury of the lesions may release clear lymph or blood and drainage may continue for prolonged periods. Lymphangioma circumscriptum grows slowly over time. In vulval and perianal areas, long-term LC predisposes to development of squamous cell carcinoma [162, 163]. Occurrence of lymphangiosarcoma within a LC is an exceptional event [164]. The main treatment modality is surgical excision. Recurrences are not unusual and require re-excision.

Pathology and differential diagnosis

Histologically, lymphangioma circumscriptum is made up of a network of endothelium-lined lymphatic spaces, containing clear lymph with few lymphocytes. These spaces can be differentiated from capillaries only by the absence of red blood cells. Lymphangioma circumscriptum is usually located in

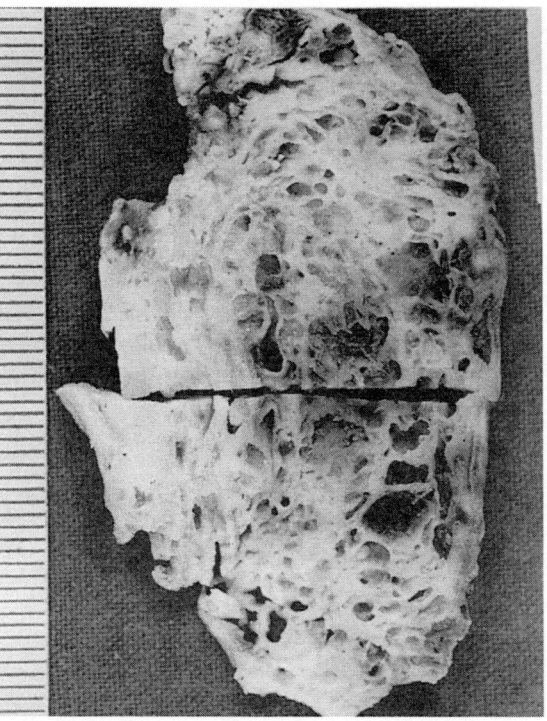

Fig. 53. Cavernous lymphangioma with spongy pattern. (Courtesy Dr E. Baviera)

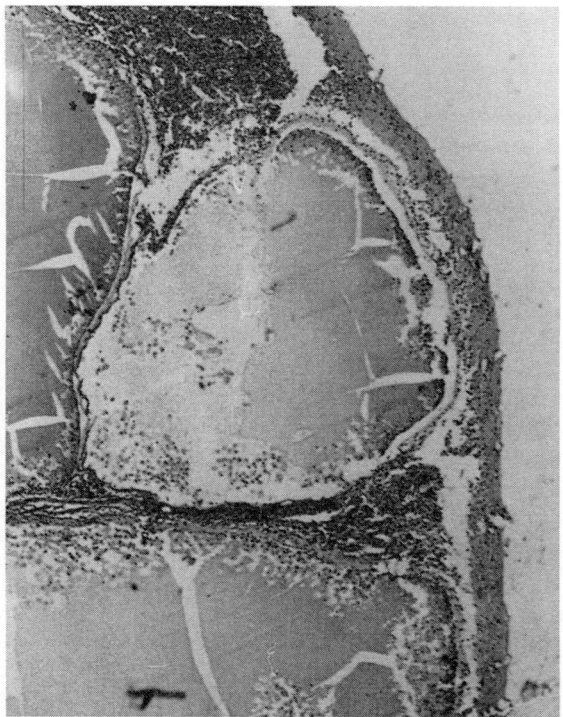

Fig. 54. Cavernous lymphangioma. Dilated lymphatic vessels delineated by scanty connective tissue. HES

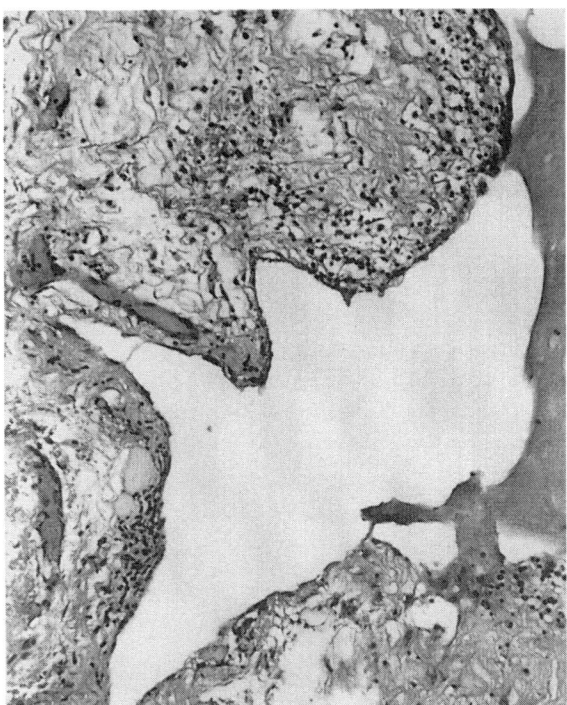

Fig. 55. Cavernous lymphangioma. Budding of connective tissue in the vascular lumen. HES

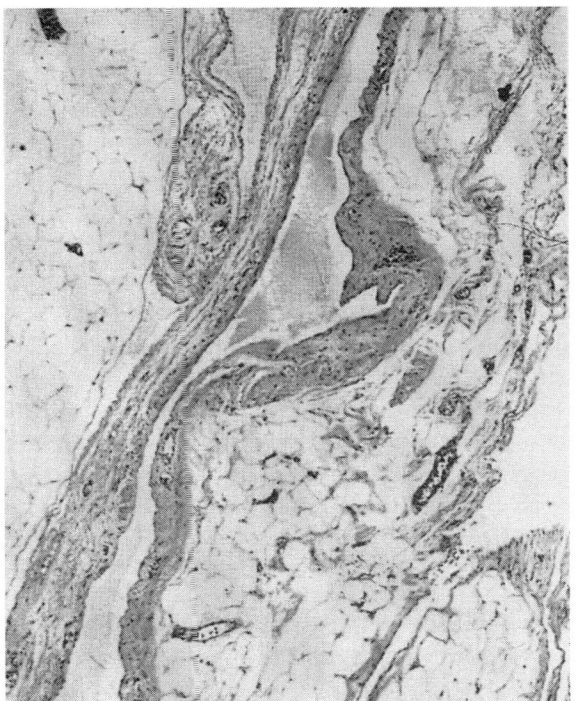

Fig. 56. Cavernous lymphangioma. Note hypertrophy of smooth muscle cells in the lymphatic vascular wall. HES

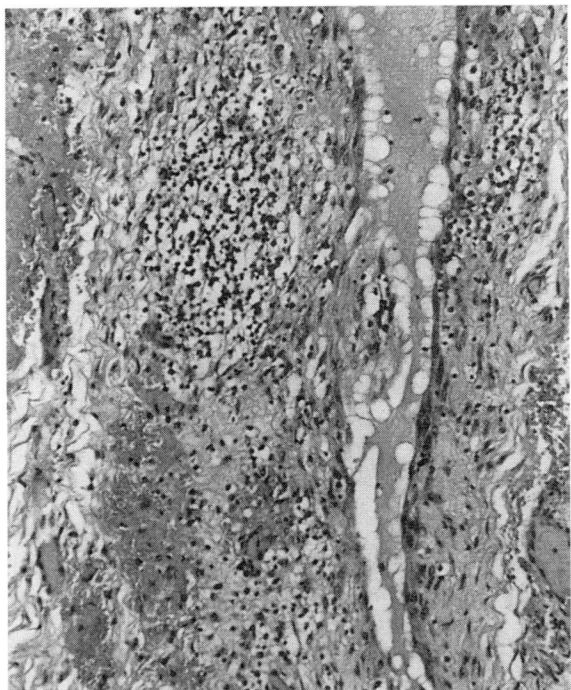

Fig. 57. Cavernous lymphangioma. Infiltrates of lymphocytes and lipophages in the lymphatic vascular wall. Note flattened endothelial cells. HES

the superficial dermis and often extends into the epidermis, which is frequently acanthotic.

Cystic lymphangioma or "cystic hygroma"

Hygromata arise from embryonic and jugular lymph sacs and are thus found mainly in the neck, in the region of the breast and axilla and in the mediastinum. This is a lesion of infancy, most commonly present shortly after birth with 40% presenting in the newborn period [165-167]. The most frequently involved sites are the neck area, axilla and groin but other sites have been reported [168-171]. Cystic lymphangioma usually presents as a large compressible cystic mass that transilluminates well. The clinical symptoms vary according to the location. Mediastinal lymphangioma may produce a compression syndrome [172]. Abdominal pain and transit disorders may unveil a mesenteric location and recurrent thrombo-embolic syndrome may result from retroperitoneal cystic lymphangioma (Fig. 58) [173, 174]. In neonates, cervical and axillary hygromas may be a cause of dystocia during delivery. Cervical and mediastinal hygromata may give rise to early respiratory insufficiency of the newborn or chylous effusion in the pericardium and pleura. Cystic lymphangioma may be associated with macroglossia, macrocheilia, macromelia of lymphangiomatous origin, Noonan's syndrome, the fetal-alcohol syndrome, the distichiasis-lymphoedema syndrome, familial pterygium colli and with Turner's syndrome (Fig. 59), trisomy 18 and trisomy 21 [165, 175].

Pathology and differential diagnosis

The gross aspect of lymphangioma varies according to its location, shape and the number of tumours; a solitary cyst, a grape-like polycystic mass, or a spongy tumour may be seen. Generally a solitary cyst measures from 5-10 cm in diameter but it can reach a considerable volume and contain a large quantity of lymph [169]. The cystic wall is thin, translucent, and poorly vascularized. The contents may be serous, chylous, especially when the cyst develops in the mesentery (Fig. 60), or even haemorrhagic when complications occur [176]. Histologically, cystic hygroma is almost indistinguishable from cavernous lymphangioma, but the thin-walled lymphatic vessels show marked cystic dilation (Fig. 61). Some smooth muscle cells are seen in the wall with lymphocyte infiltrates (Fig. 62-63). Sometimes, the endothelial cells hypertrophy, become cubical, and take on the appearance of glandular epithelium. They then react strongly with FVIII-RAg and CD 31 antibodies. The surrounding connective tissue shows oedema and lymphocytic infiltration.

Depending on location, differential diagnosis consists of ruling out an haemangioma, a mesothelial inclusion cyst, an hydatid cyst or other lymphatic lesions (lymphangiectasia, lymphangiomatosis, lymphangiomyomatosis). In general the contents of a cystic lymphangioma are free of red blood cells but they

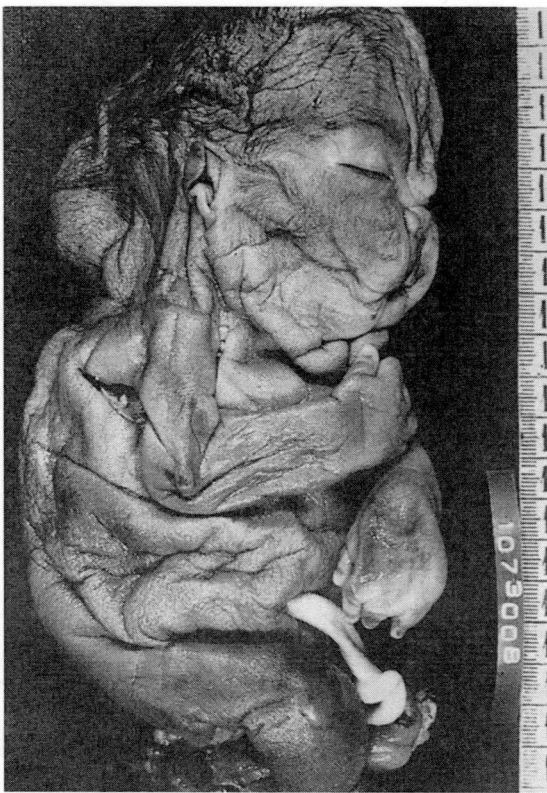

Fig. 59. Aborted fetus with Turner's syndrome. Note diffuse cystic hygroma involving the whole body. (Courtesy Dr A. Proust)

may be haemorrhagic when strangulation occurs. A mesothelial inclusion cyst has a lining non-reactive to FVIII-RAg. In countries where hydatid disease is prevalent, the preoperative diagnosis is more often hydatid cyst than cystic lymphangioma.

4 – Vascular tumours of intermediate malignancy

Spindle cell haemangioendothelioma

This tumour [177] is made up of masses of endothelial cells growing in and about vascular lumina and may develop in blood vessels and lymphatics (lymphangio-endothelioma). It mostly affects adults (mean age: 30-40 yrs). The most frequent locations are the hands, feet, and trunk. Clinically, it appears as a superficial, slow-growing, painless mass, measuring less than 2 cm in diameter, involving the skin and subcutis. The condition may be associated with pre-

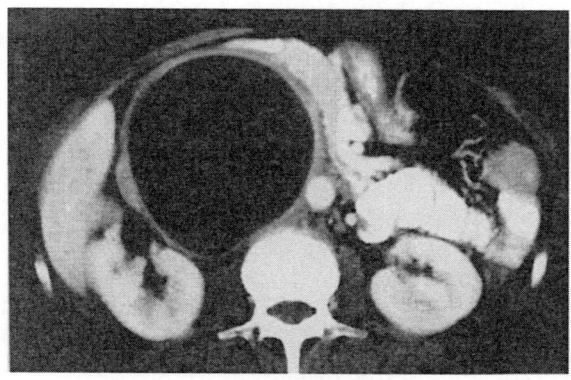

Fig. 58. Large retroperitoneal cystic lymphangioma. CT scan. (Courtesy Dr C. Gauthier)

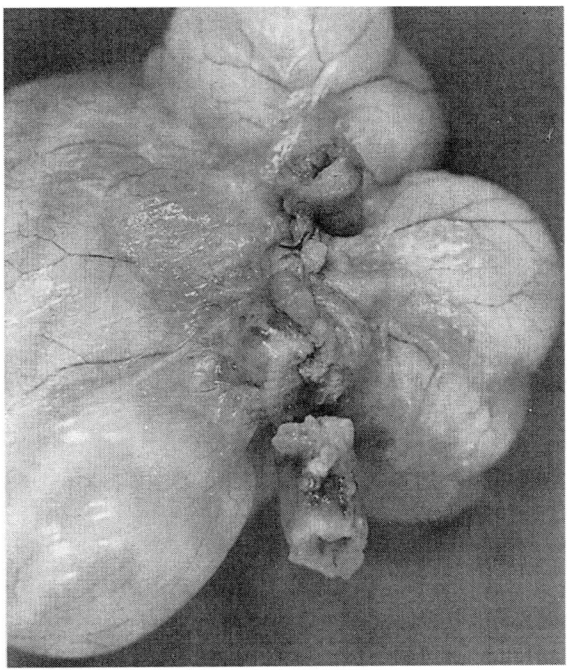

Fig. 60. Mesenteric cystic lymphangioma

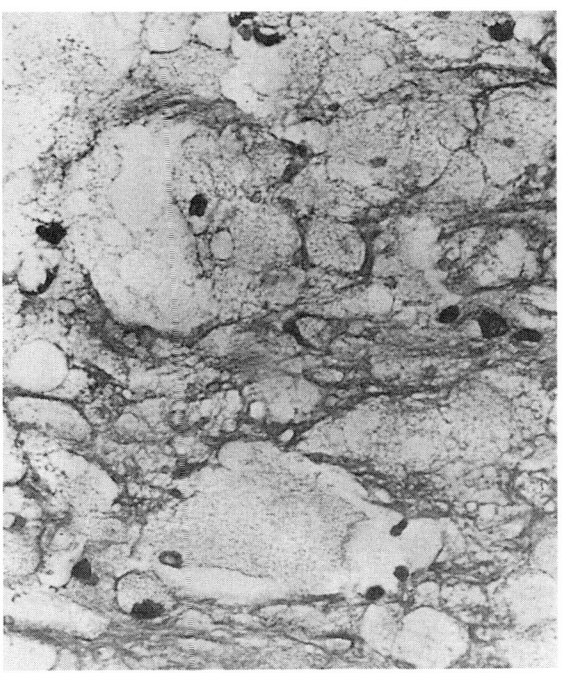

Fig. 61. Retroperitoneal cystic lymphangioma. Luminal aspect bordered by lipophages. HES

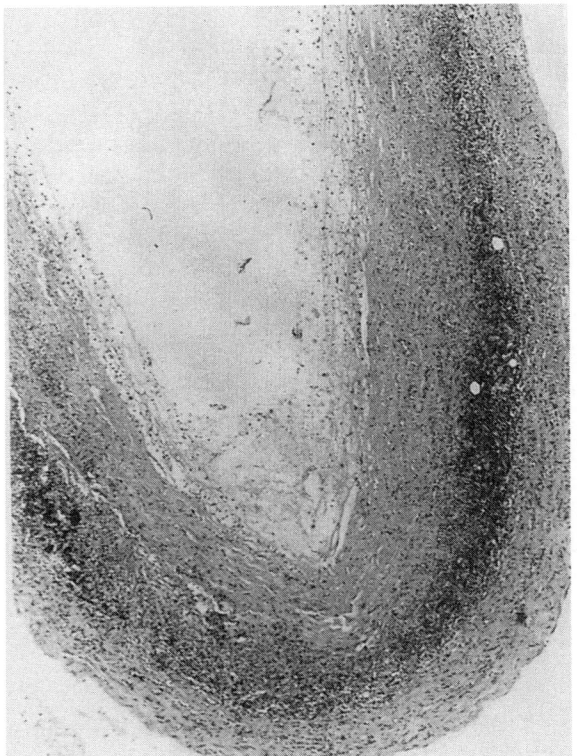

Fig. 62. Retroperitoneal cystic lymphangioma. Vascular wall displaying fibrosis with heavy lymphocyte infiltrates. HES

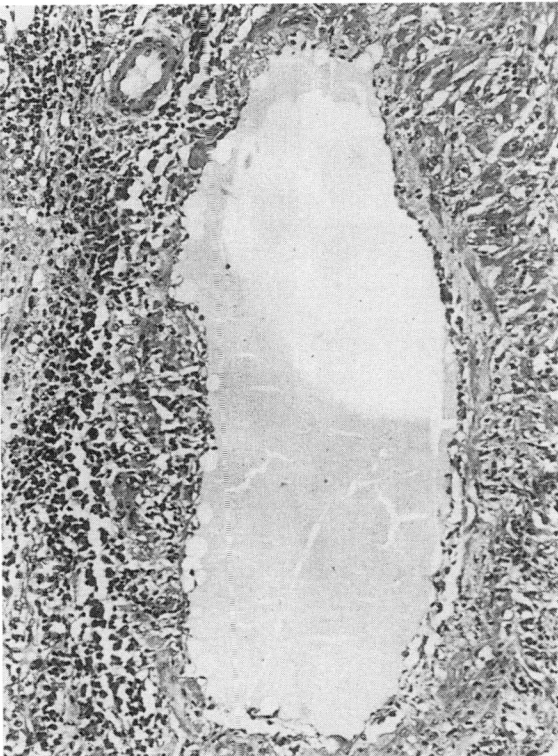

Fig. 63. Retroperitoneal cystic lymphangioma. Adventitial lymphatic collateral with lymphocyte infiltrates around. HES

existing vascular malformations or more complex syndromes including Maffuci's syndrome and the Klippel-Trenaunay syndrome [93, 178]. This condition is regarded as an intermediate grade between the well-differentiated haemangiomas and the frankly anaplastic angiosarcomas, as local recurrences involve about two-third of cases, but metastases rarely occur [177] although multifocality has been reported. Recent reports describe a benign course [179,180].

Pathology and differential diagnosis

Always well defined, this tumour has two components: cavernous vascular spaces and sheets or masses of spindle cells, which should not be confused with the cells of true angiosarcoma. Cavernous vascular spaces, similar to those seen in a cavernous haemangioma, may be lined with epithelioid endothelial cells that contain no intracytoplasmic PAS-positive diastase resistant hyaline globules. Spindle cell proliferation, with occasional atypical mitoses and some pleomorphism may mimic angiosarcoma and Kaposi's sarcoma. Transmission and scanning electron microscopic studies carried out by Imayama et al [181] demonstrated that the spindle cells appeared to be fibroblasts. These cells are characterized by phagocytic activity, the presence of many lysosomes, and factor XIIIa expression, but they develop the features of pericytes when they are close to the endothelial lining of well-developed vascular lumens.

Immunohistochemically, factor-VIII related antigen, CD34, vimentin, and lectin binding Ulex europaeus agglutinin 1 decorate the endothelial cells lining vascular spaces. Spindle cells in the solid areas are negative for these markers except for vimentin, but show divergent positive immunoreactions of HHF35, alpha-smooth muscle actin, desmin, and collagen type IV [182]. Flow cytometric study evidences a mostly diploid pattern suggesting SCH may be a benign lesion, probably a reactive process, rather than a low-grade angiosarcoma [182, 183].

Kaposiform infantile haemangioendothelioma

This haemangioma has Kaposi's sarcoma-like features with infiltrating nodules and locally aggressive behavior. Synonyms include epithelioid and spindle cell haemangioendothelioma, Kaposi-like infantile haemangioendothelioma, locally metastasizing vascular tumour, and angiosarcoma in infancy. Children in the first decade of life are mostly affected [184], but cases have been reported in adults [185]. This tumour develops in soft tissues (retroperitoneum, chest wall, scalp), and bone. Some cases are associated with the Kasabach-Merritt syndrome, lymphangiomatosis, or both [142, 184].

Locally aggressive behavior has helped to define this lesion as a borderline malignancy tumour [186]. Death frequently results from Kasabach-Merritt syndrome or complications of lymphangiomatosis, rather than the tumour burden *per se* [187]. Wide local excision, multiple excisions, even amputation are the appropriate treatments for most lesions. Radiation therapy, cyclophosphamide and interferon alpha-2a (presumably through the inhibition of angiogenesis) may be helpful [187, 188]. The histogenesis of the tumour is unknown.

Pathology and differential diagnosis

Crescentic well-formed capillaries are interspersed with sheets of plump, spindle endothelial cells, vaguely reminiscent of Kaposi's sarcoma lining slit-like spaces. Some vacuolated endothelial cells display epithelioid or histiocytoid features. Eosinophilic PAS-positive, diastase-resistant, hyaline globules and haemosiderin pigmentmay be present while mitoses are scattered. Nuclear atypia is minimal, mitotic figures are rare (1 to 6 mitoses in 10 high-power fields). Immunohistochemically, well-formed capillaries stain positively for all the vascular markers; however, endothelial cells lining the small slit-like and sieve-like vascular spaces do not stain for von Willebrand factor. Actin-positive pericytes may be seen. Neoplastic spindle cells stained only focally for CD34 and CD31 [185].

The differential diagnosis includes other paediatric vascular tumours, such as juvenile or infantile haemangioendothelioma and cellular haemangioma. The presence well-formed spindle cell fascicles delineating slit-like vascular spaces favors Kaposiform infantile haemangioendothelioma. Kaposiform haemangioendothelioma and Kaposi's sarcoma both display vascular slits with eosinophilic hyaline globules in some areas. They also present a similar immunohistochemical profile with common expression of CD34, XIIIA and FVIII-RAg to a lesser degree. Distinctive features of the Kaposiform lesion include the age of the patients, HIV-negativity, the usually deep-seated lesions, the lobulated architecture of the vascular proliferation, the lack of fusiform cells and inflammatory infiltrates. Spindle-cell haemangioendothelioma contains cavernous vascular spaces, but remains superficial. Tufted angioma or angioblastoma is distinctive from Kaposiform haemangioendothelioma because of the "cannonball" disposition of the well-organized capillaries in the dermis. This benign angioma lacks an infiltrative pattern. In the thyroid gland, pseudoinvasion in capsular veins by Hurthle cell carcinomas or follicular carcinomamay mimic Kaposiform haemangioendothelioma [189].

Endovascular papillary angioendothelioma (Dabska tumour)

This exceedingly rare tumour mainly affects infants and children, but cases have been reported in adults [190]. The tumour develops in the skin and subcutaneous tissues and infiltrates the underlying soft tissues. Dabska tumor may occur within a previous cavernous haemangioma [191]. Lymph node metastases have been reported in a small percentage of cases but no patient is reported to have died of the tumour [192], which some authors consider to be a very low-grade angiosarcoma. The histogenesis has been suggested to be from the "high" endothelial cells of the post-capillary venules [192].

Pathology and differential diagnosis.

The tumour is made up of intercommunicating vascular channels of varying calibre. Some are cavernous, others capillary-like. The vascular endothelium presents various patterns ranging from flattened lining to papillary or glomeruloid tufts supported by a hyaline core. The latter "match-head" or "hob-nail" appearance is a *sine qua non* of diagnosis. Endothelial cells may be regular, plump, epithelioid or columnar. Intravascular lymphocytes may be prominent. Several vascular tumors have EPA-like foci [193]. The differential diagnosis includes spindle cell haemangioendothelioma, epithelioid haemangioendothelioma and angiolymphoid hyperplasia with eosinophilia.

5 – Primary malignant tumours of vessels

Epithelioid haemangioendothelioma

Typically this tumour is characterized by a proliferation of epithelioid cells grouped in short trabeculae around vascular slits containing red blood cells. Epithelioid haemangioendothelioma (EHE) develops frequently in the lungs and soft tissues [194-196]. Other sites have also been reported, including bone, skin [197], the superior vena cava, the azygos vein [198, 199], liver [200-202], and duodenum [203]. Some of these lesions were probably metastatic. In the lungs, the age at the detection or onset of symptoms is 14-64 yrs (mean 44 yrs). Males are more likely to be detected by symptoms (50%) than are females (8%)[195]. Lesions may present as bilateral multiple nodular opacities. EHE is of low-grade malignancy [204]. Kitaichi et al [195] reported three cases of partial spontaneous regression in asymptomatic patients. In a series of 46 cases of epithelioid haemangioendothelioma of the soft tissues studied by Weiss et al [177], the short-term follow-up (average period: 48 months) has shown a recurrence rate in about 13%, a metastasis rate of 31% in regional lymph nodes, lung, liver and bone and a mortality rate in about 13% of cases.

Pathology and differential diagnosis

In the soft tissues, more than half of the cases involve a medium-sized or large vessel, most commonly a vein. In such tumours, well-defined vascular channels are inconspicuous, and the tumour cells are plump and often cubical, thus mimicking epithelioid cells. In the lungs, this tumour has a presentation similar to that of the so-called "pulmonary intravascular bronchiolo-alveolar tumour" described by Dail et al [205]. It consists of multiple hard, whitish, sometimes umbilicated nodules of variable size ranging from 0. 5 to 3 cm in diameter. Histologically, there is a proliferation of either epithelioid large cells or dendritic spindle or stellate cells. Epithelioid cells have vacuolated cytoplasm with a huge central nucleus. They are grouped in short trabeculae, jutting inside blood-filled vascular slits as polypoid formations. Cellular atypia is marked but mitoses are rare. The dendritic spindle or stellate cells may be isolated or arranged in clusters. Fibrosis predominates in the tumour, while its periphery is more cellular with marked vascular differentiation. Tumour cells react with FVIII-RAg, BNH9, UEA1 lectin and vimentin. Steroid receptor (17-beta estradiol) is inconsistently expressed [146]. Poor prognostic features include a predominance of spindle cells, cellular atypia, mitotic counts of greater than 1 mitosis per 10 high power fields (HPF) and necrosis. Differential diagnosis is from haemangioma and angiosarcoma. Marked cellular atypia helps to rule out haemangioma. Some epithelioid cells may be present inangiosarcoma but there is no tendency to nodularity. Fibrosarcoma, some carcinomas, especially intheliver (fibrolamellar hepatoma, cholangiocarcinoma) and metastatic carcinomas in the lungs have a different immunohistochemical profile with desmin, carcino-embryonic antigen, epithelial membrane antigen and cytokeratin [206].

Kaposi's sarcoma

First described by Kaposi in 1872 [207] and called "idiopathic pigment sarcoma of the skin", this is a multifocal malignant proliferation of vessels and mesenchymal cells containing haemorrhages with haemosiderin pigment deposits. There are four clinical forms with distinct ethnic and geographic distributions. The classic or European form of KS mostly affects Eastern European or Mediterranean peoples in their fifth and sixth decades. Clinically, this form consists of locally aggressive skin lesions with very rare visceral involvement [208, 209]. In sub-Saharan Central or equatorial Africa, Kaposi's sarcoma is endemic and accounts for up to 10% of all tumours. Clinically, African Kaposi's is similar to the European form but mostly affects young children and adults with a more aggressive course involving the viscera and lymph nodes, mimicking lymphoma. These lesions may precede cutaneous locations.

KS is common in the acquired immune deficiency syndrome. This form occurs in approximately one-third of AIDS patients. These are mostly young male adults (median age: 32 years), often practising homosexuals, and/or intravenous drug abusers [210]. There is no site of predilection for the lesions, which tend to disseminate widely. Most patients die of AIDS – related infectious complications rather than of KS *per se*. About one-third of these patients develop a second malignancy, usually malignant non-Hodgkin lymphoma or leukaemia [211, 212]. Cases of KS have been also reported in organ transplant recipients or in patients receiving immunosuppressive therapy [213-218]. Lesions are either cutaneous or widely metastatic, but often involute when immunosuppressive therapy is discontinued.

Clinically, early cutaneous lesions may resemble petechiae or consist of multiple red to purple flat nodules scattered on the lower limbs. Later, these nodules slowly increase in size and number and coalesce into plaques, measuring up to 10 cm or more in diameter. Over time, some regress while others appear, ulcerate, fungate, and tend to extend to more proximal sites. Usually the affected area may show lesions of different stages of development, interspersed with atrophic pigmented scars. Localized purpura and oedema occur with thrombosis in superficial veins. A variant of Kaposi's sarcoma is characterised by the appearance of "bulla-like" lesions (lymphangioma-like variant). This form occurs more often in men aged 59-80 years and is slowly progressive with localized or diffuse lesionsin the lower limbs [219]. In the lungs, KS has produced intrabronchial buds [220] and in the

digestive tract, the lesions may cause haemorrhage [221]. Cerebral involvement is common in patients with AIDS [222], and bone marrow involvement occurs in the disseminated form [223].

The course of Kaposi's sarcoma is variable. The patients may survive from 6 months from onset to 30 years or more [224]. Patients with cutaneous lesions alone may live for many years. Metastasis spread is by way of the lymphatics and deposits appear in almost any organ in the body.

There is controversy regarding the aetiolgy of KS and the origin of the tumour cells. Serological association of KS with cytomegalovirus was reported by Giraldo [225]. Herpesvirus-like inclusions have been found in tissue culture of KS [226], and in tumour cells [227]. Herpesvirus-like DNA sequences and human herpesvirus-8 (HHV-8) have been demonstrated in KS in patients with AIDS ; however, the role of the virus in KS development is still unknown [212, 228-230]. HPV16-like DNA transcripts are present in cases of AIDS and non-AIDS-related Kaposi's sarcoma [231] and induction of Kaposi's sarcoma-like lesions has been possible in transgenic mice with the HIV transactivating (Tat) gene. Furthermore, extracellular human immunodeficiency virus type 1 (HIV-1) Tat protein promotes growth of spindle cells derived from AIDS-associated Kaposi's sarcoma [232, 233]. The idea that the tumour is of viral origin has given rise to controversy [234]. The data suggest that growth factors released by T lymphocytes and the HIV Tat protein released (activated) by retrovirus-infected CD4+ T lymphocytes act together to induce the proliferation of Kaposi's sarcoma spindle cells. Experimentally, KS-derived spindle cells induce vascular lesions and display enhanced vascular permeability when inoculated subcutaneously in the nude mouse [235]. The origin of the tumour spindle cells has been attributed to many cell types: pericytes, fibroblasts, Schwann cell, multipotent mesenchymal cells [236] with potential differentiation into endothelial cells, pericytes and fibroblasts [227, 237], and endothelial cells.

Pathology and differential diagnosis

Histologically, all forms of Kaposi's sarcoma present a similar pattern. The early patch or nodular stage is characterized by jagged, thin-walled, dilated vascular spaces in the dermis, with interstitial inflammatory cells, extravasated red cells and haemosiderin pigment deposit. Between the vessels, there is an accumulation of spindle cells organized in short fascicles. The Gordon-Sweet staining technique reveals a vascular pattern of the reticulin network with tumour cells present on the luminal side of vessels. Tumour spindle cells have an indistinct, pale, eosinophilic cytoplasm with a centrally-placed nucleus. Some mitoses are present. A few cells contain eosinophilic hyaline globules, which are periodic acid-Schiff (PAS)-positive; these develop from either digested red blood cells [238] or an unknown proteinaceous glycoprotein. Extravasated red blood cells and haemosiderin pigment deposits are frequent in the lesion while lymphocytes and plasma cells, scattered in the nodule, predominate at its periphery. Haemosiderin pigment may be free in the stroma or present inside macrophages and tumour cells [239]. This finding validates interest in using Perls' reaction to identify early, noncharacteristic lesions [240]. This stage of Kaposi's sarcoma is the most difficult to recognize, as it mimics granulation tissue.

The plaque stage consists of multiple aggregates of spindle cells within the dermis. They are organized in fascicles or directional streams adjacent to primitive vascular slits lined with flattened endothelium. Extravasated red blood cells, lymphocytes and plasma cells are scattered throughout while haemosiderin pigment accumulates at the periphery of the ill-defined margins.

The mature patch or nodular stage is typified by a poorly circumscribed dermal mass made up of dispersed spindle cells, lymphocytes, plasma cells and numerous irregular slit-like spaces that lack an endothelial lining but contain extravasated red blood cells. At the periphery, haemorrhages and readily identifiable newly-formed capillaries may shadow the immature fibroblastic component. This appearance can be misinterpreted as a pyogenic granuloma.

Visceral involvement of KS parallels lymphatic distribution. Digestive involvement often affects the mucosa producing haemorrhagic polypoid lesions (Fig. 64-65-66-67-68). In the lungs, the tumour often develops externally along the bronchi and the parenchymal fibrous septa, and spreads over the pleura like the pulmonary lymphatics. This helps to explain the poor diagnostic performance of bronchial (20 to 60%) or transbronchial (13 to 17%) biopsies [220]. Cerebral involvement is common in patients with AIDS [222]. In the lymphangioma-like variant, the histological pattern is characterized by permeation of dermal collagen by labyrinthine vascular channels lined by a flattened endothelium [219]. In lymph nodes, lesions may involve either the paracortex or the capsule and septa.

Immunohistochemically, the vascular lining cells of KS displays reactivity with factor VIII related antigen [241], Ulex europeaus I lectin, BNH9, CD34,

HLA-DR and vimentin [242, 243] – the pattern seen in pyogenic granulomas, haemangiomas and angiosarcomas. Reactivity with CD34 is seen in all tumour spindle cells [244-246]. There is no reactivity with blood group antigens, alpha-actin smooth muscle cell, desmin, S100 protein and KL1 cytokeratin [236].

In general, the clinical context and immunohistochemical study help differentiate Kaposi's sarcoma from other entities. However, a solitary early patch or nodular lesion should be differentiated from pyogenic granuloma, which presents a shorter clinical history and lacks a spindle cell component. The differential diagnosis of plaque stage lesion should rule out a pyogenic granuloma and bacillary angiomatosis, acroangiodermatitis, lobular capillary haemangioma, targetoid haemangioma and angiosarcoma. In the late patch or nodular stage, the differential diagnosis includes hypervascularized spindle-celled tumours such as leiomyoma, haemorrhagic histiocytofibroma, dermatofibrosarcoma spindle cell haemangioendothelioma, malignant melanoma and even poorly-differentiated carcinoma. In lymph nodes, the differential diagnosis includes lymphadenitis, vascular transformation of lymph nodes, severe depletion of lymphoid tissue in lymph nodes in congenital immune deficiencies, chemotherapy for lymphoma and radiation the-

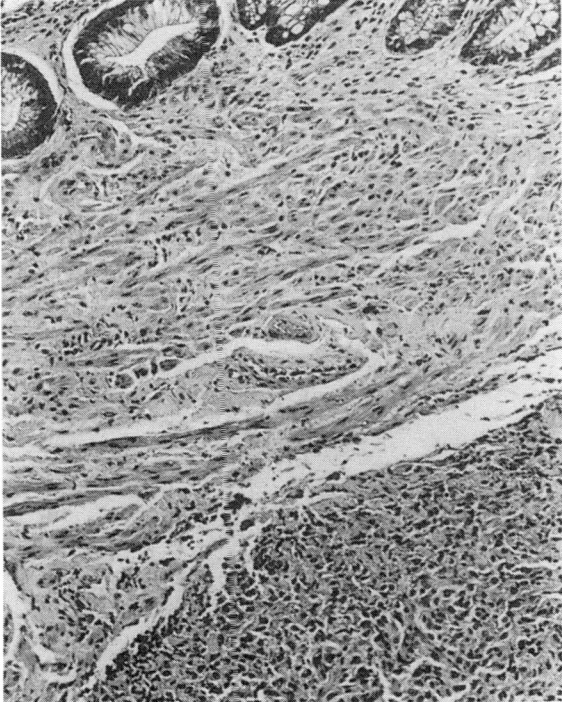

Fig. 64. Kaposi's sarcoma of the lower portion of the rectum in an AIDS patient. HES

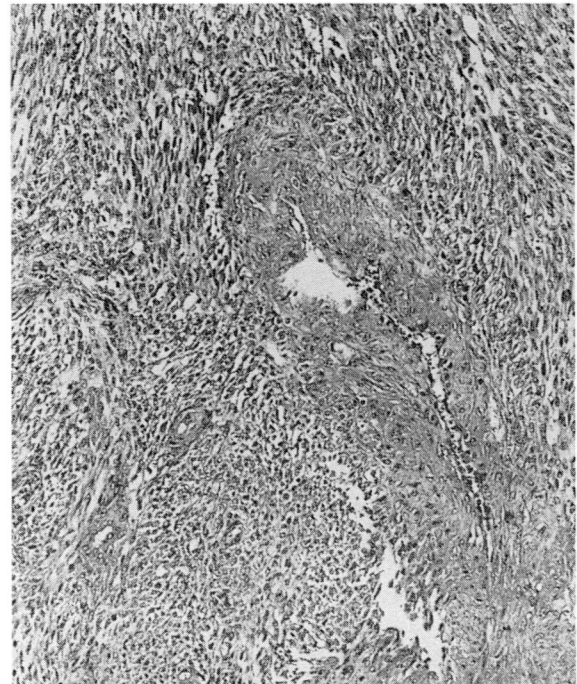

Fig. 65. Kaposi's sarcoma. Irregular slit-like spaces bordered by spindle cells. HES

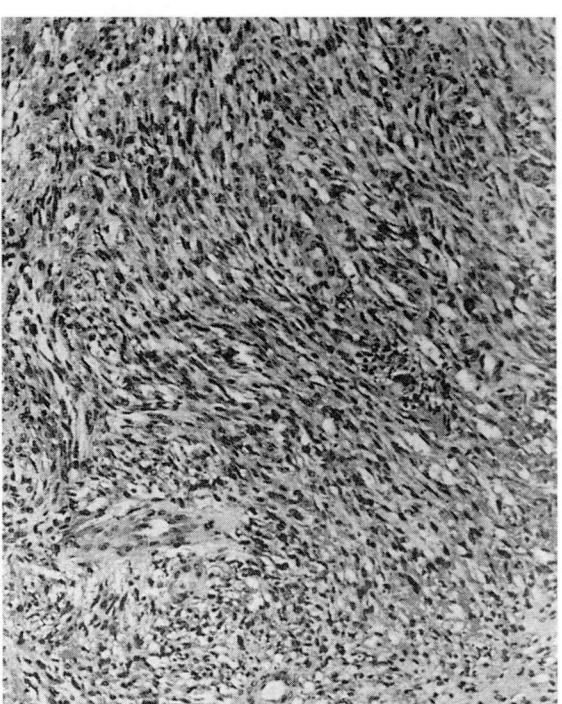

Fig. 66. Kaposi's sarcoma. Slit-like spaces limited by whorled spindle cells. HES

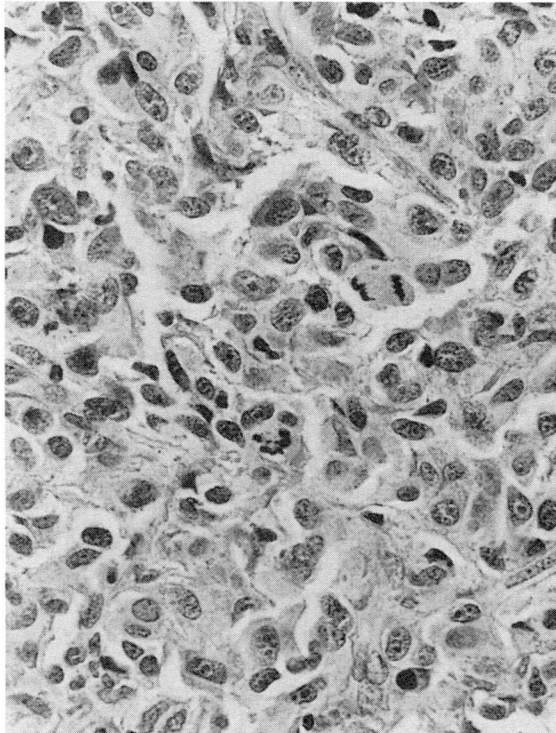

Fig. 67. Kaposi's sarcoma. Epithelioid tumour cells with nuclear atypias. Note multinucleation and atypical mitoses. HES

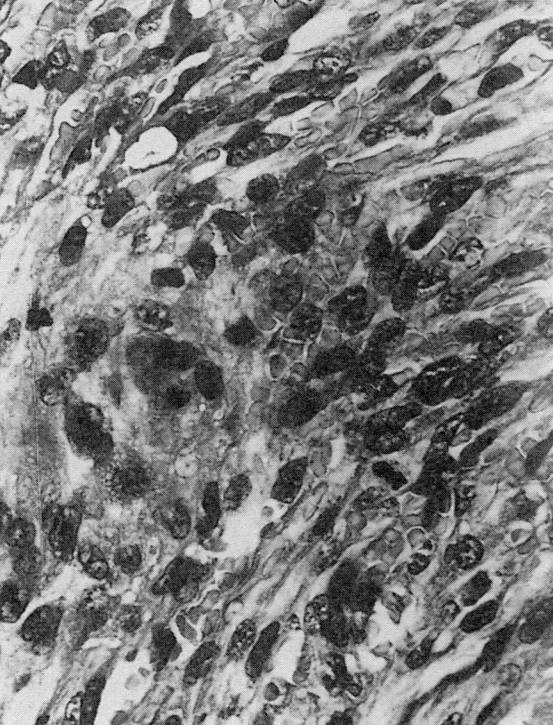

Fig. 68. Kaposi's sarcoma. Sarcomatous areas. HES

rapy. Radiation may affect the spleen and the collapsed vascular frame should not be mistaken for Kaposi's sarcoma. Thrombosed haemorrhoids in patients with AIDS should be differentiated from anal Kaposi's sarcoma.

Angiosarcoma

Angiosarcoma is a malignant vascular tumour, characterised by masses of endothelial cells displaying the cellular atypia and anaplasia. This general term "angiosarcoma" embraces all malignant endothelial tumours previously called haemangiosarcomas, lymphangiosarcomas, malignant haemangio- or lymphangio-endotheliomas [247, 248]. Primary angiosarcoma may affect both sexes and at all ages, and develops anywhere in the body but most often in the skin, soft tissue, breast, and liver. Other sites may be involved as well, including the spleen, bone marrow, lung, serous membranes and soft tissues. Gut involvement is exceptional [249, 250]. The tumour presents as a single or multiple, raised soft and bluish red plaque or nodule that tends to bleed and ulcerate. A thrill may be felt over the lesion. In the skin, angiosarcoma begins as small, sharply demarcated, asymptomatic multiple red nodules. These lesions progressively enlarge and become fleshy masses of pale gray-white, soft tissue. Central softening with necrosis and haemorrhage are frequent.

Angiosarcoma may develop on a pre-existing lymphoedematous background or other lesions including dysfunctional arteriovenous fistulae, cavernous haemangioma [94], cirrhosis, haemochromatosis or chronic hepatitis [251]. Association with radiation, foreign bodies of various natures (Dacron vascular prosthesis, metallic orthopedic appliances, a bullet, surgical sponges), chronic exposure to arsenic, polyvinyl chloride (PVC), thorium dioxide has been reported [252, 253]. There is a close association between angiosarcoma and human herpesvirus-8 (HHV8) infection, however the pathogenic role of HHV8 is doubtful [254]. Expression of steroid hormones receptors in mammary angiosarcoma is inconsistent in tumour cells, even though this tumour occurs mostly in women in their twenties or thirties or during pregnancy [255].

Lymphoedema associated angiosarcoma is a rare tumour that develops after prolonged lymphatic obstruction. Most cases occur in the oedematous arms of women who have had a mastectomy with axillary lymph node dissection and/or radiotherapy for carcinoma of the breast (Stewart-Treves syndrome) [256]

or in legs with chronic lymphoedema or elephantiasis [257-259] Approximately 400 cases of angiosarcoma associated with lymphoedema have been reported, of which 360 occurred after ipsilateral mastectomy. On the average, they appear from 10 to 20 years post-operatively with an average of 10 years 3 months [260]. Pathogenetically it seems that chronic lymphoedema, characterised histologically by lymphatic dilatation (lymphangectasia) leads first to proliferation of lymphatics (lymphangiomatosis) with possible slight endothelial atypia. Thereafter there is a gradual progression of increasing endothelial atypia, followed by multilayering, papillae formation and solid sheet-like tumour [261-263]. Clinically the affected arm undergoes acute swelling followed by the occurrence of dark red or purple macula or nodules with skin blisters. These lesions may coalesce, giving rise to a large mass. Ulceration and haemorrhage are frequent. Additional lesions occur in other parts of the limb and may spread to the trunk. Lesions may ulcerate, become necrotic and crusted. Involvement of an artery results in rupture with pseudoaneurysm and occlusion [264]. Both angiosarcoma developing in lymphoedema and isolated angiosarcoma have a very poor prognosis with local invasion, repeated local recurrence, rapid distal metastatic spread and a rapidly fatal course. Some patients survive only weeks or months. In some locations, especially the breast [265], most patients die within 2 years.

Pathology and differential diagnosis

Grossly, the tumour is an ill-defined lesion or mass, grayish in colour and soft in consistency. On cross section it contains haemorrhagic areas and translucent myxoid zones. Histologically, all degrees of differentiation may be found, ranging from a mass of vascular cavities (Fig. 69-70-71) to less differentiated sarcomatous areas containing no distinct vessels (Fig. 72-73). The pattern of angiosarcoma is highly variable, even within the same lesion. In some areas, proliferating vessels are arborizing and arranged in a retiform pattern, bordered by monomorphic hob-nail endothelial cells (Fig. 74) [266, 267]. In other areas, vascular cavities are lined with plump, monstrous but recognizable endothelial cells displaying marked anisocytosis, anisokaryosis and nuclear hyperchromatism (Fig. 75). Atypical mitoses are present and tumour cells may exhibit erythrophagocytosis (Fig. 76). In some areas, tumour cells pile up into papillary structures, jutting into the vascular lumen. A variant, epithelioid angiosarcoma, is composed of epithelioid cells with a large eosinophilic cytoplasm centred by vesicular nuclei containing prominent nucleoli. These

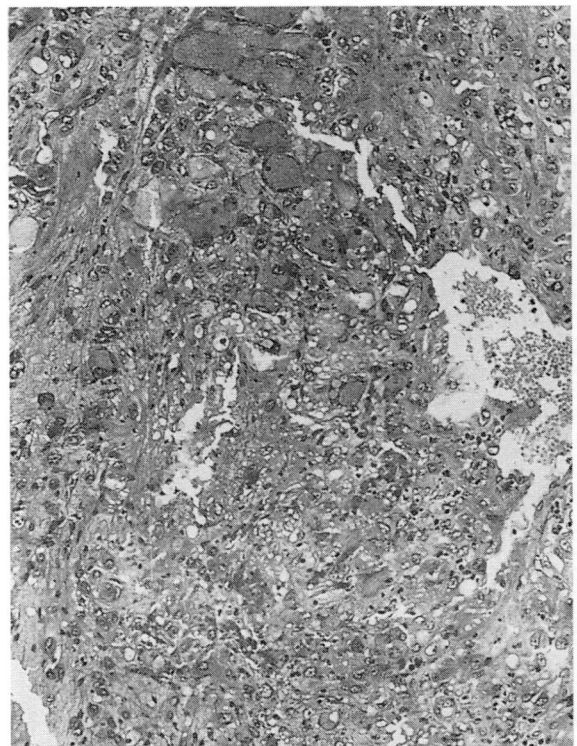

Fig. 69. Angiosarcoma. Low grade and well-differentiated tumour with area containing relatively well-defined vascular cavities. HES

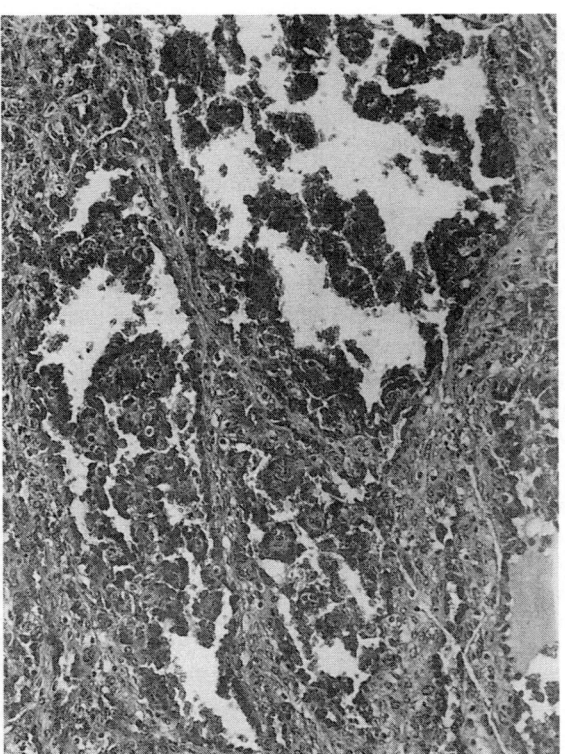

Fig. 70. Angiosarcoma. Low grade and well-differentiated tumour with cavernous pattern. HES

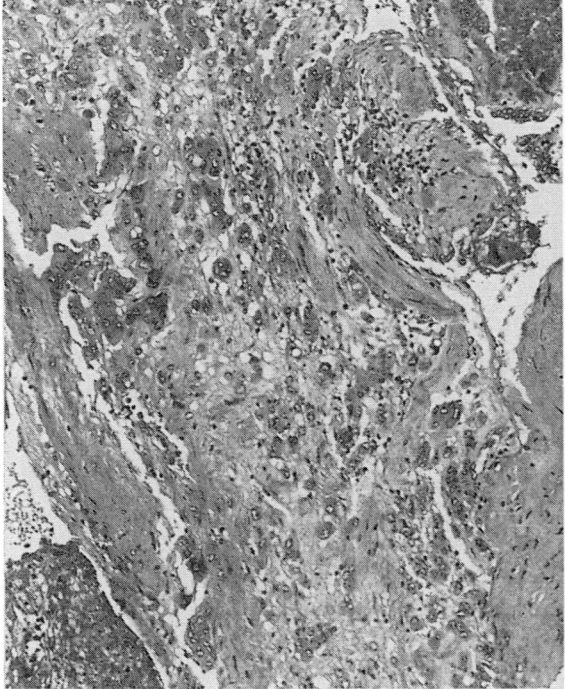

Fig. 71. Angiosarcoma. High grade, undifferentiated tumour with diffuse haemorrhage. HES

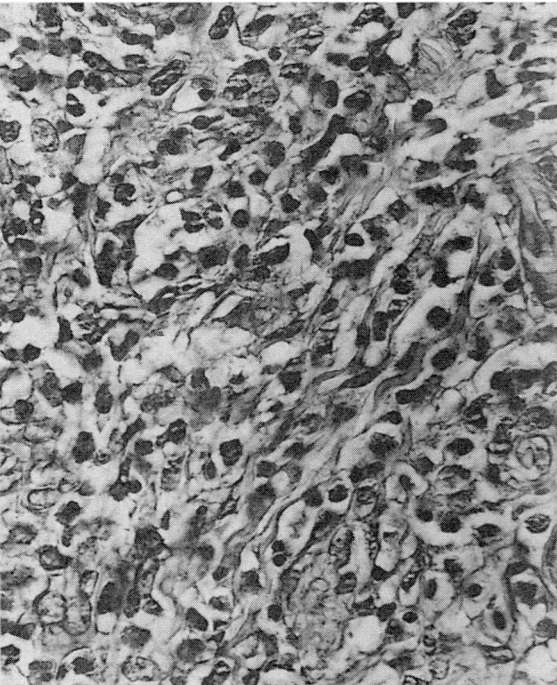

Fig. 72. Angiosarcoma. High grade tumour. Slit-like spaces lined with atypical endothelial cells. HES

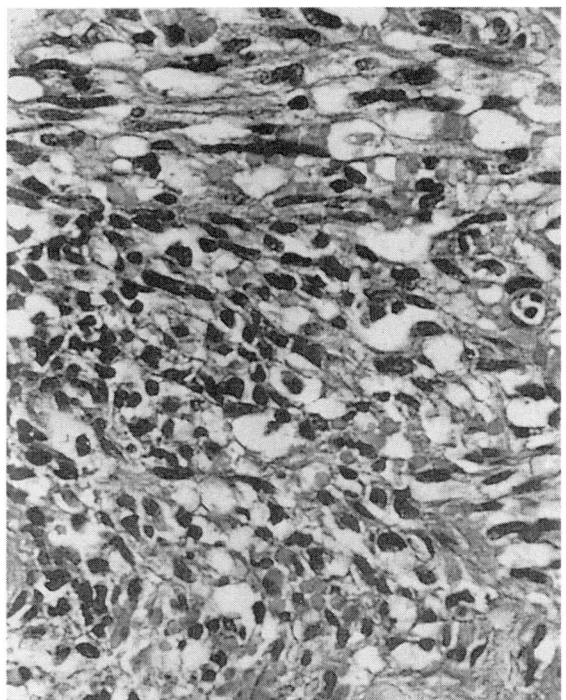

Fig. 73. Angiosarcoma. High grade tumour. Proliferating vessels bordered by hob-nailed endothelial cells. HES

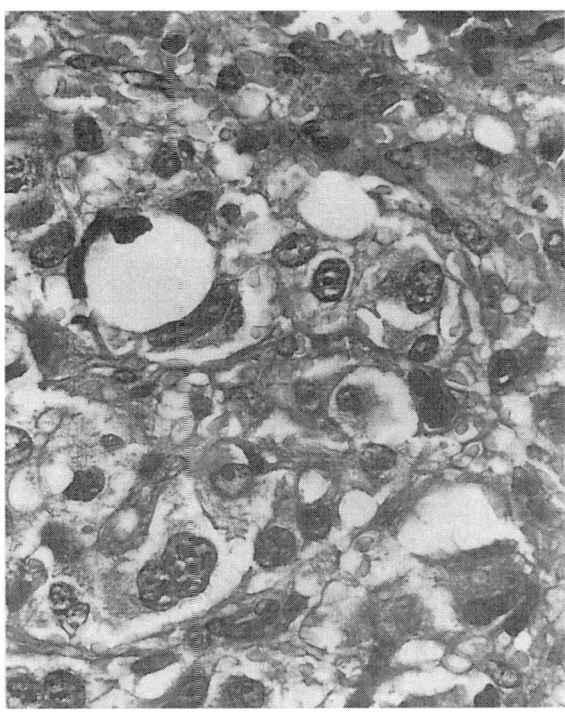

Fig. 74. Angiosarcoma. High grade tumour. Monstrous endothelial cells. HES

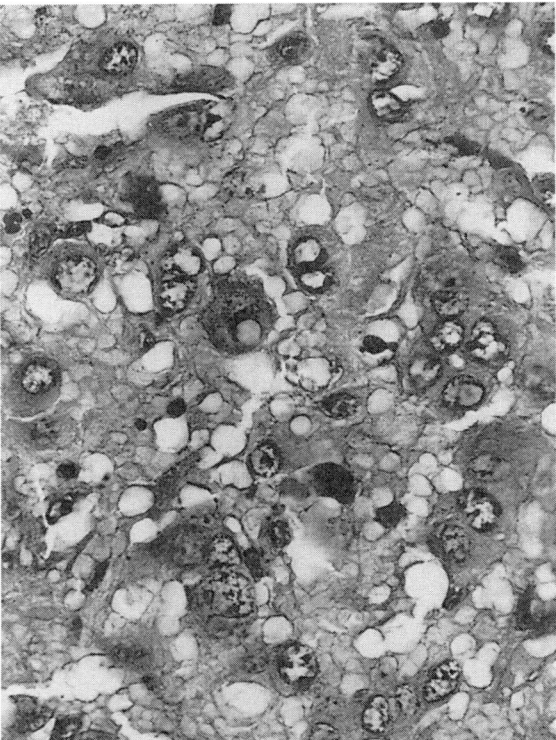

Fig. 75. Angiosarcoma. High grade tumour. Undifferentiated vascular cavities engorged with red blood cells. HES

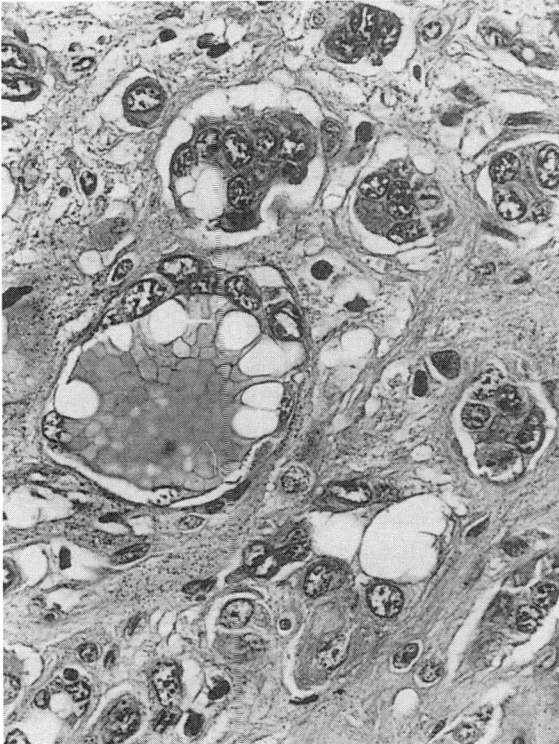

Fig. 76. Angiosarcoma. High grade tumour. Note erythrophagocytosis in tumour cells. HES

cells are arranged, for the most part, in solid sheets, and have small foci with a vascular architecture. The Gordon-Sweet silver impregnation technique unveils a reticulin network surrounding the vessels that are arranged in sinusoids or capillaries (Fig. 77). In solid areas, pleomorphism predominates with tumour giant cells, and atypical mitoses. Necrosis and haemorrhage with haemosiderin pigment are present in the stroma. Erythroblasts and megakaryocytes are often present in the tumour and its metastases. Distinction between isolated angiosarcomas and lymphangiosarcomas is impossible except in the presence of coexistent lymphoedema. Immunohistochemical study displayspositive reactivity oftumour cells with CD31, CD34, Ulex europaeus I lectin, BHN9 [268], laminine [269] and vimentin. This reactivity is variable with Factor VIII-related antigen and cytokeratin, especially for epithelioid angiosarcoma [270], and is negative with EMA. Electron microscopy reveals visible intercellular junctions, numerous micropycnotic vacuoles, and Weibel-Palade bodies. There is strong alkaline phosphatase and ATPase reactivity [247].

Superficial well-differentiated angiosarcoma may simulate a capillary haemangioma; areas of atypical proliferation, intraluminal pseudo-papillary masses, and anisocytosis and mitoses should be sought. Distinction from an angiomatosis may be difficult; the diffuse proliferation of variable sized blood vessels distributed uniformly throughout the tumour contrasts with a well-differentiated angiosarcoma, where vascular cavities present a heterogeneous distribution, being closely spaced in some areas, and widely separated in others. Early lesions of Kaposi's sarcoma containing many vessels should also be ruled out. A low-grade, well-differentiated angiosarcoma, such as spindle cell haemangioendothelioma, can be mistaken for Kaposi's sarcoma, which is often composed of multiple nodules, made up of spindle cells intermingled with newly-formed vessels, infiltrates of lymphocytes and plasma cells. Eosinophilic hyaline globules and haemosiderin pigment are seen in the tumour. The clinical context and immunohistochemical study help differentiate Kaposi's sarcoma. Serology frequently unveils an HIV-positivity [247].

Poorly-differentiated angiosarcomas must be differentiated from leiomyosarcomas, schwann cell sarcomas, and malignant melanomas. Immunolabelling most often results in negative reactivity with factor VIII related antigen but positive with UEA1 lectin. The differential diagnosis thus depends on the negativity of reactivity with alpha smooth muscle actin, desmin, S100 protein and HMB45. The lack of any immunolabelling by carcinoembryonic antigen, epi-

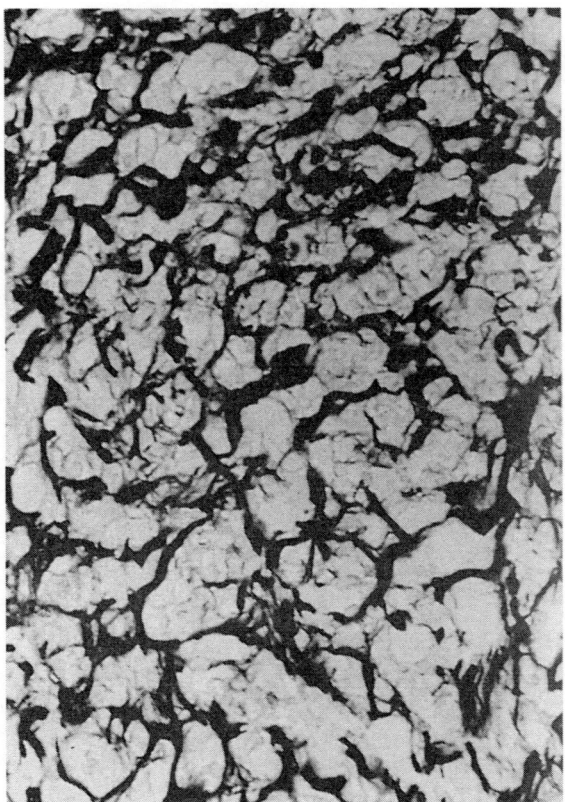

Fig. 77. Angiosarcoma. High grade tumour. Reticulin network surrounding the proliferating vessels. Gordon-Sweet stain

thelial membrane antigen and cytokeratin allows us to rule out an epithelial tumour. Some angiosarcomas may present epithelioid areas mimicking an epithelioid or histiocytoid haemangioendothelioma or a metastatic carcinoma [270]. Epithelioid or histiocytoid haemangioendothelioma is an intermediate malignancy tumour made up of cells with abundant, eosinophilic and often vacuolized cytoplasm, simulating a glandular differentiation. Mitoses are rare. Some tumour cells have the immunohistochemical and ultrastructural characteristics of histiocytes but the proliferation usually shows reactivity with factor VIII related antigen, UEA I lectin and cytokeratin as in epithelioid angiosarcoma.

6 – Secondary malignant tumours

Blood vessels are major routes for the dissemination of cancer. Exceptionally, great vessels may be involved with concomitant cardiac metastasis [271, 272].

Bibliography

1. Buyukbabani N, Tetikkurt S, Ozturk AS (1998) Cutaneous angiomyolipoma: report of two cases with emphasis on HMB-45 utility. J Eur Acad Dermatol Venereol 11: 151-4

2. Chaib E, Pugliese V, Garbugio-Filho V, Saad WA, Pinotti HW (1996) Angiomyolipoma of the liver. Int Surg 81: 320-2

3. Maesawa C, Tamura G, Sawada H, Kamioki S, Nakajima Y, Satodate R (1996) Angiomyolipoma arising in the colon. Am J Gastroenterol 91: 1852-4

4. Ito M, Sugamura Y, Ikari H, Sekine I (1998) Angiomyolipoma of the lung. Arch Pathol Lab Med 122: 1023-5

5. About I, Capdeville J, Voigt JJ, Bernard P, Michetti C, Faizon R (1994) Renal angiomyolipoma and pulmonary lymphangiomyomatosis: a non-fortuitous association. Rev Med Interne 15(4): 279-81

6. Tawfik O, Austenfeld M, Persons D (1996) Multicentric renal angiomyolipoma associated with pulmonary lymphangioleiomyomatosis: case report, with histologic, immunohistochemical, and DNA content analyses. Urology 48: 476-80

7. O'Hagan AR, Ellsworth R, Secic M, Rothner AD, Brouhard BH (1996) Renal manifestations of tuberous sclerosis complex. Clin Pediatr (Phila) 35: 483-9

8. Schuler GD, Boguski MS, Stewart EA, Stein LD, Gyapay G, Rice K, White RE, Rodriguez-Tome P, Aggarwal A, Bajorek E, Bentolila S, Birren BB, Butler A, Castle AB, Chiannilkulchai N, Chu A, Clee C, Cowles S, Day PJ, Dibling T, Drouot N, Dunham I, Duprat S, East C, Hudson TJ, et al (1996) A gene map of the human genome. Science 274(5287): 540-6

9. van Slegtenhorst M, de Hoogt R, Hermans C, Nellist M, Janssen B, Verhoef S, Lindhout D, van den Ouweland A, Halley D, Young J, Burley M, Jeremiah S, Woodward K, Nahmias J, Fox M, Ekong R, Osborne J, Wolfe J, Povey S, Snell RG, Cheadle JP, Jones AC, Tachataki M, Ravine D, Kwiatkowski DJ, et al (1997) Identification of the tuberous sclerosis gene TSC1 on chromosome 9q34. Science 277(5327): 805-8

10. De Wever W, Ghijselings L, Cassiman S, Baert AL (1996) Selective embolization of an aneurysm in a massive angiomyolipoma of the kidney. J Belge Radiol 79: 137-8

11. Schick B, Kahle G, Hassler R, Draf W (1996) Chemotherapy of juvenile angiofibroma—an alternative. HNO 44: 148-52

12. Mitskavich MT, Carrau RL, Snyderman CH, Weissman JL, Fagan JJ (1998) Intranasal endoscopic excision of a juvenile angiofibroma. Auris Nasus Larynx 25: 39-44

13. Tsunoda A, Kohda H, Ishikawa N, Komatsuzaki A (1998) Juvenile angiofibroma limited to the sphenoid sinus. J Otolaryngol 27: 37-9

14. Brentani MM, Butugan O, Oshima CT, Torloni H, Paiva LJ (1989) Multiple steroid receptors in nasopharyngeal angiofibromas. Laryngoscope 99: 398-401

15. Hagen R, Romalo G, Schwab B, Hoppe F, Schweikert HU (1994) Juvenile nasopharyngeal fibroma: androgen receptors and their significance for tumor growth. Laryngoscope 104: 1125-9

16. Gatalica Z (1998) Immunohistochemical analysis of steroid hormone receptors in nasopharyngeal angiofibromas. Cancer Lett 127: 89-93

17. Lantsov AA, Kovaleva LM, Ushakov VS, Mefodovskii AA (1998) Treatment results in patients with juvenile angiofibroma of the nasopharynx. Vestn Otorinolaringol 4: 12-4

18. el-Sayed Y, a -Serhani A (1997) Lobular capillary haemangioma (pyogenic granuloma) of the nose. J Laryngol Otol 111: 941-5

19. Tsai MH, Pai HH, Yen PT, Huang TS, Ho YS (1996) Nasopharyngeal Castleman's disease. J Formos Med Assoc 95: 877-80

20. Blake G, Char G, Williams E, Phillip H (1998) Angiomyofibroblastoma - a rare but distinct entity. West Indian Med J 47: 35-6

21. Laskin WB, Fetsch JF, Tavassoli FA (1997) Angiomyofibroblastoma of the female genital tract: analysis of 17 cases including a lipomatous variant. Hum Pathol 28: 1046-55

22. Sasano H, Date F, Yamamoto H, Nagura H (1997) Angiomyofibroblastoma of the vulva: case report with immunohistochemical, ultrastructural and DNA ploidy studies and a review of the literature. Pathol Int 47: 647-50

23. Takeshima Y, Shinkoh Y, Inai K (1998) Angiomyofibroblastoma of the vulva: a mitotically active variant ? Pathol Int 48: 292-6

24. Andreev VC, Pramatarov K (1979) Cutis marmorata telangiectatica congenita in two sisters. Br J Dermatol 101: 345-50

25. Del-Guidice SM, Nydorf ED (1986) Cutis marmorata telangiectatica congenita with multiple congenital anomalies. Arch Dermatol 122: 1060-1

26. Sato SE, Herschler J, Lynch PJ, Hodes BL, Fryczkowski AW, Schlosser HD (1988) Congenital glaucoma associated with cutis marmorata telangiectatica congenita: two case reports. J Pediatr Ophthalmol Strabismus 25: 13-7

27. Toriello HV, Graff RG, Florentine MF, Lacina S, Moore WD (1988) Scalp and limb defects with cutis marmorata telangiectatica congenita: Adams-Oliver syndrome ? Am J Med Genet 29: 269-76

28. Pehr K, Moroz B (1993) Cutis marmorata telangiectatica congenita: long-term follow-up, review of the literature, and report of a case in conjunction with congenital hypothyroidism. Pediatr Dermatol 10: 6-11

29. Simon MW, Moore AM 2d(1993) Cutis marmorata telangiectatica congenita. J Ky Med Assoc 91: 10-2

30. O' Toole EA, Deasy P, Watson R (1995) Cutis marmorata telangiectatica congenita associated with a double aortic arch. Pediatr Dermatol 12: 348-50

31. Chen CP, Chen HC, Liu FF, Jan SW, Chern SR, Wang TY, Hung HY (1997) Cutis marmorata telangiectatica congenita associated with an elevated maternal serum human chorionic gonadotrophin level and transitory isolated fetal ascites. Br J Dermatol 136: 267-71

32. Clayton-Smith J, Kerr B, Brunner H, Tranebjaerg L, Magee A, Hennekam RC, Mueller RF, Brueton L, Super M, Steen-Johnsen J, Donnai D (1997) Macrocephaly with cutis marmorata, haemangioma and syndactyly - a distinctive overgrowth syndrome. Clin Dysmorphol 6: 291-302

33. Morgan JM, Naisby GP, Carmichael AJ (1997) Cutis marmorata telangiectatica congenita with hypoplasia of the right iliac and femoral veins. Br J Dermatol 137: 119-22

34. Yeh YC, Wu KH, Chi CS (1997) Cutis marmorata telangiectatica congenita: report of one case. Chung Hua Min Kuo Hsiao Erh Ko I Hsueh Hui Tsa Chih 38: 223-5

35. Devillers AC, de Waard-van der Spek FB, Oranje AP (1999) Cutis marmorata telangiectatica congenita: clinical features in 35 cases. Arch Dermatol 135: 34-8

36. Swensson B, Swensson O, Haring G (1998) Progressive disseminated essential telangiectasia with conjunctival involvement. Klin Monatsbl Augenheilkd 212: 116-9

37. Checketts SR, Burton PS, Bjorkman DJ, Kadunce DP (1997) Generalized essential telangiectasia in the presence of gastrointestinal bleeding. J Am Acad Dermatol 37: 321-5

38. Tamm E, Jungkunz W, Marsch WC, Lutjen-Drecoll E (1992) Increase in types IV and VI collagen in cherry haemangiomas. Arch Dermatol Res 284: 275-82

39. Eichhorn M, Jungkunz W, Worl J, Marsch WC (1994) Carbonic anhydrase is abundant in fenestrated capillaries of cherry haemangioma. Acta Derm Venereol 74: 51-3

40. Enta T (1994) Dermacase. Nevus araneus (spider telangiectasia). Can Fam Physician 40: 1105, 1112

41. Selmanowitz VJ (1970) Unilateral nevoid telangiectasia. Ann Intern Med 73: 87-90

42. Beck L Jr, D'Amore PA (1997) Vascular development: cellular and molecular regulation. FASEB J 11(5): 365-73

43. Folkman J, Shing Y (1992) Angiogenesis. J Biol Chem 267: 10931-4

44. Gastl G, Hermann T, Steurer M, Zmija J, Gunsilius E, Unger C, Kraft A (1997) Angiogenesis as a target for tumor treatment. Oncology 54(3): 177-84

45. Uhr JW, Scheuermann RH, Street NE, Vitetta ES (1997) Cancer dormancy: opportunities for new therapeutic approaches. Nat Med 3: 505-9

46. Neitzel LT, Neitzel CD, Magee KL, Malafa MP (1999) Angiogenesis correlates with metastasis in melanoma. Ann Surg Oncol 6: 70-4

47. Maniotis AJ, Folberg R, Hess A, Seftor EA, Gardner LM, Pe'er J, Trent JM, Meltzer PS, Hendrix MJ (1999) Vascular channel formation by human melanoma cells in vivo and in vitro: vasculogenic mimicry. Am J Pathol 155: 739-52

48. Folkman J, Ingber D (1992) Inhibition of angiogenesis. Semin Cancer Biol 3: 89-96

49. Petruzzelli GJ (1996) Tumor angiogenesis. Head Neck 18: 283-91

50. Allimant P, Mangold J, Froelich N, Zachar D (1995) Splenic peliosis. Apropos of 2 cases. J Chir (Paris) 132: 451-3

51. Abe M, Wakasa H (1987) Thorostrast induced hepatic angiosarcoma with 39 years latency. Acta Pathol Jap 37: 1653-60

52. Molina T, Delmer A, Le Tourneau A, Texier P, Degott C, Audoin J, Zittoun R, Diebold J (1995) Hepatic lesions of vascular origin in multicentric Castleman's disease, plasma cell type: report of one case with peliosis hepatis and another with perisinusoidal fibrosis and nodular regenerative hyperplasia. Pathol Res Pract 191: 1159-64

53. Hamada K, Nakaya M, Shirayama R, Kobayashi H, Kasuga H, Narita N, Mishima K, Ichijima K (1997) Autopsy findings of retroperitoneal cystic tumor and peliosis hepatis in lymphangiomyomatosis. Nihon Kyobu Shikkan Gakkai Zasshi 35: 437-41

54. Slater LN, Welch DF, Min KW (1992) Rochalimaea hanselae causes bacillary angiomatosis and peliosis hepatis. Arch Intern Med 152: 602-6

55. Mainguene C, Moreau A, Hofman P, Milpied-Homsi B, Roulot D, Marullo S, Clauvel J-P, Lenne Y, Amouroux J (1993) Péliose bacillaire au cours du Sida. Etude anatomo-clinique de 2 observations. Ann Pathol 13: 341-5

56. Soe KL, Soe M, Gluud CN (1994) Liver pathology associated with anabolic androgenic steroids. Ugeskr Laeger 156: 2585-8

57. Staub PG, Leibowitz CB (1996) Peliosis hepatis associated with oral contraceptive use. Australas Radiol 40: 172-4

58. Ahsan N, Holman MJ, Riley TR, Abendroth CS, Langhoff EG, Yang HC (1998) Peloisis hepatis due to Bartonella henselae in transplantation: a hemato-hepato-renal syndrome. Transplantation 65: 1000-3

59. Zafrani ES, Cazier A, Baudelot AM, Feldmann G (1984) Ultrastructural lesions of the liver in human peliosis. A report of 12 cases. Am J Pathol 114: 349-59

60. Degott C, Potet F (1984) Péliose et dilatation sinusoïdale. Arch Anat Cytol Path 32: 296-300

61. Ulbright TM, Santa Cruz DJ (1980) Intravenous pyogenic granuloma. Cancer 45: 1646-52

62. Valentic JP, Barr RJ, WeinsteinGD (1983) Inflammatory neovascular nodules associated with oral isotrentinoin treatment of severe acne. Arch Dermatol 119: 871-2

63. Fernandez LA, Olsen TG, Barwick KW, Sanders M, Kaliszewski C, Inagami T (1986) Renin in angiolymphoid hyperplasia with eosinophilia. Its possible effect on vascular proliferation. Arch Pathol Lab Med 110: 1131-5

64. Chusid MJ, Rock AL, Sty JR, Oechler HW, Beste DJ (1997) Kimura's disease: an unusual cause of cervical tumour. Arch Dis Child 77: 153-4

65. Hareyama M, Oouchi A, Nagakura H, Asakura K, Saito A, Satoh M, Tamakawa M, Akiba H, Sakata K, Yoshida S, Koito K, Imai K, Kataura A, Morita K (1998) Radiotherapy for Kimura's disease: the optimum dosage. Int J Radiat Oncol Biol Phys 40: 647-51

66. Kini U, Shariff S (1998) Cytodiagnosis of Kimura's disease. Indian J Pathol Microbiol 41: 473-7

67. Ramos J, Girardot B (1994) Pseudo-Horton disease caused by angiolymphoid hyperplasia with eosinophilia. Arch Anat Cytol Pathol 42: 42-5

68. Altman DA, Griner JM, Lowe L (1995) Angiolymphoid hyperplasia with eosinophilia and nephrotic syndrome. Cutis 56: 334-6

69. Berney DM, Griffiths MP, Brown CL (1997) Angiolymphoid hyperplasia with eosinophilia in the colon: a novel cause of rectal bleeding. J Clin Pathol 50: 611-3

70. Ussmuller J, Donath K, Shimizu M, Bergmann I (1997) Differential diagnosis of tumorous space-occupying lesions of the parotid gland: angiolymphoid hyperplasia with eosinophilia and Kimura disease. Laryngorhinootologie 76: 110-5

71. Morton K, Robertson AJ, Hadden W (1987) Angiolymphoid hyperplasia with eosinophilia: Report of a case arising from the radial artery. Histopathology 11: 963-9

72. Kindblom LG, Fassina AS (1981) Angiolymphoid hyperplasia with eosinophilia of the skin. Light microscopic and ultrastructural study of 4 cases. Acta Pathol Microbiol Scand [A] 89: 271-83

73. Amerigo J, Berry CL (1980) Intravascular papillary endothelial hyperplasia in the skin and subcutaneous tissue. Virchows Arch [Pathol Anat] 387: 81-90

74. Garcia-Macias MC, Abad M, Alonso MJ, Flores T, Bullon A (1990) Masson's vegetant intravascular haemangioendothelioma. Fine needle aspiration cytology, histology and immunohistochemistry of a case. Acta Cytol 34: 175-8

75. Samaratunga H, Searle J, O'Loughlin B (1996) Intravascular fasciitis: a case report and review of the literature. Pathology 28: 8-11

76. Sticha RS, Deacon JS, Wertheimer SJ, Danforth RD Jr (1997) Intravascular fasciitis in the foot. J Foot Ankle Surg 36: 95-9

77. Bhawan J, Wolff SM, Ucci AA, Bhan AK (1985) Malignant lymphoma and malignant angioendotheliomatosis: one disease. Cancer 55: 570-6

78. Theaker JM, Gatter KC, Esiri MM, Easterbrook P (1986) Neoplastic angioendotheliosis – further evidence supporting a lymphoid origin. Histopathology 10: 1261-70

79. Wick MR, Rocamora A (1988) Reactive and malignant "angioendotheliomatosis": a discriminant pathologic study. J Cutan Pathol 15: 260-71

80. Croisile B, Tommasi M, Jouvet A, Truffert A, Trillet M, Aimard G (1990) Large-cell intravascular malignant lymphoma. Rev Neurol (Paris) 146: 184-90

81. Demolombe-Rague S, Pinede L, Ninet J, Bouchou K, Duhaut P, Berger F, Boucheron S, Rousset H, Pasquier J (1995) Intravascular malignant lymphoma (ex-malignant angioendotheliosis). 3 cases. Presse Med 24: 1689-93

82. Smadja D, Mas JL, Fallet-Bianco C, Meyniard O, Sicard D, de Recondo J, Rondot P (1991) Intravascular lymphomatosis (neoplastic angioendotheliosis) of the central nervous system: case report and literature review. J Neurooncol 11: 171-80

83. Burton BK, Schulz CJ, Angle B, Burd LI (1995) An increased incidence of haemangiomas in infants born following chorionic villus sampling (CVS). Prenat Diagn 15: 209-14

84. Pasyk KA, Grabb WC, Cherry GW (1983) Crystalloid inclusions in endothelial cells of cellular and capillary haemangiomas. A possible sign of cellular immaturity. Arch Dermatol 119: 134-7

85. de Felipe I, Quintanilla E (1997) Neurocutaneous syndromes with vascular alterations. Rev Neurol 25: S250-S258

86. Bizzozero L, Solaining Talamonti C, Villa F, Brusamolino R, Collice M (1997) Cavernous haemangioma of the skull. Case report and review of the literature. J Neurosurg Sci 41: 419-21

87. Demircan O, Sonmez H, Zeren S, Cosar E, Bicakci K, Ozkan S (1998) Diffuse cavernous haemangioma of the rectum and sigmoid colon. Dig Surg 15: 713-5

88. Lai PH, Hsu SS, Pan HB, Yang CF (1998) Intracranial cystic cavernous angioma: a case report. Kao Hsiung I Hsueh Ko Hsueh Tsa Chih 14: 593-8

89. Watzke HH, Linkesch W, Hay U (1989) Giant haemangioma of the liver (Kasabach-Merritt syndrome): successful suppression of intravascular coagulation permitting surgical removal.. J Clin Gastroenterol 11: 347-50

90. Mora A, Cortes C, Roige J, Noguer M, Camps MA, Margarit C (1995) Orthotopic liver transplant for giant cavernous haemangioma and Kasabach-Merritt syndrome. Rev Esp Anestesiol Reanim 42: 71-4

91. Szlachetka DM (1998) Kasabach-Merritt syndrome: a case review. Neonatal Netw 17: 7-15

92. Chung KC, Weiss SW, Kuzon WM Jr (1995) Multifocal congenital haemangiopericytomas associated with Kasabach-Merritt syndrome. Br J Plast Surg 48: 240-2

93. Enjolras O, Wassef M, Dosquet C, Drouet L, Fortier G, Josset P, Merland JJ, Escande JP (1998) Kasabach-Merritt syndrome on a congenital tufted angioma. Ann Dermatol Venereol 125: 257-60

94. Drouot F, Piard F, Thome C, Arnould L, Jacquot J. Ph, Bernard A, Michiels R (1990) Un cas d'angiosarcome hépatique développé sur un hémangiome caverneux préexistant. Ann Pathol 10: 336-40

95. Calonje E, Fletcher CDM (1991) Sinusoidal haemangioma. A distinctive benign vascular neoplasm within the group of cavernous haemangiomas. Am J Surg Pathol 15: 1130-5

96. Bisceglia M, Carosi I, Castelvetere M, Murgo R (1998) Multiple Forcyce-type angiokeratomas of the scrotum. An iatrogenic case. Pathologica 90: 46-50

97. Dave VK, Main RA (1972) Angiokeratoma of Mibelli with necrosis of the fingertips. Arch Dermatol 106: 726-8

98. Kobayashi T, Sakuraoka K (1998) A case of angiokeratoma circumscriptum: immunolocalization of matrix metalloproteinase (MMP)-9. J Dermatol 25: 391-4

99. Menkes DL, O'Neil TJ, Saenz KK (1997) Fabry's disease presenting as syncope, angiokeratomas, and spoke-like cataracts in a young man: discussion of the differential diagnosis. Mil Med 162: 773-6

100. Leung CS, Jordan RC (1997) Solitary angiokeratoma of the oral cavity. Oral Surg Oral Med Oral Pathol Oral Radiol Endod 84: 51-3

101. Kohda H, Narisawa Y (1992) Digital verrucous fibroangioma: a new variant of verrucous haemangioma. Acta Derm Venereol 72: 303-4

102. De Souza EM, Turini MA, Oliveira TC (1981) Verrucous hemangioma. Med Cutan Ibero Lat Am 9: 217-20

103. Rossi A, Bozzi M, Barra E (1989) Verrucous haemangioma and angiokeratoma circumscriptum: clinical and histologic differential characteristics. J Dermatol Surg Oncol 15: 88-91

104. Tan YY, Seah CS, Tan PH (1998) Verrucous haemangioma – a case report. Ann Acad Med Singapore 27: 255-7

105. Gautier-Smith PC, Sanders MD, Sanderson KV (1971) Ocular and nervous system involvement in angioma serpiginosum. Br J Ophthalmol 55: 433-43

106. Marriott PJ, Munro DD, Ryan T (1975) Angioma serpiginosum – familial incidence. Br J Dermatol 93: 701-6

107. Kumakiri M, Katoh N, Miura Y (1980) Angioma serpiginosum. J Cutan Pathol 7: 410-21

108. Tsang WYW, Chan JKC, Fletcher CDM (1991) Recently characterized vascular tumours of skin and soft tissues. Histopathology 19: 489-501

109. Perrin C, Rodot S, Ortonne JP, Michiels JF (1995) Targetoid hemosiderotic haemangioma. Ann Dermatol Venereol 122: 111-4

110. Guillou L, Calonje E, Speight P, Rosai J, Fletcher CD (1999) Hobnail haemangioma: a pseudomalignant vascular lesion with a reappraisal of targetoid hemosiderotic haemangioma. Am J Surg Pathol 23: 97-105

111. Krahl D, Petzoldt D (1994) Target-like hemosiderotic haemangioma. Further differential diagnosis of Kaposi sarcoma. Hautarzt 45: 34-7

112. Rapini RP, Golitz LE (1990) Targetoid hemosiderotic haemangioma. J Cutan Pathol 17: 233-5

113. Chan JK, Fletcher CD, Hicklin GA, Rosai J (1990) Glomeruloid haemangioma. A distinctive cutaneous lesion of multicentric Castleman's disease associated with POEMS syndrome. Am J Surg Pathol 14: 1036-46

114. Rongioletti F, Gambini C, Lerza R (1994) Glomeruloid haemangioma. A cutaneous marker of POEMS syndrome. Am J Dermatopathol 16: 175-8

115. Tuite PJ, Bril V (1997) POEMS syndrome in a 24-year-old man associated with vitamin B12 deficiency and a solitary lytic bone lesion. Muscle Nerve 20: 1454-6

116. Rose C, Mahieu M, Hachulla E, Facon T, Hatron PY, Bauters F, Devulder B (1997) POEMS syndrome. Rev Med Interne 18: 553-62

117. Yang SG, Cho KH, Bang YJ, Kim CW (1998) A case of glomeruloid haemangioma associated with multicentric Castleman's disease. Am J Dermatopathol 20: 266-70

118. Saida K, Kawakami H, Ohta M, Iwamura K (1997) Coagulation and vascular abnormalities in Crow-Fukase syndrome. Muscle Nerve 20: 486-92

119. Lesprit P, Authier FJ, Gherardi R, Belec L, Paris D, Melliere D, Schaeffer A, Godeau B (1996) Acute arterial obliteration: a new feature of the POEMS syndrome? Medicine (Baltimore) 75: 226-32

120. Soubrier M, Guillon R, Dubost JJ, Serre AF, Ristori JM, Boyer L, Sauvezie B (1998) Arterial obliteration in POEMS syndrome: possible role of vascular endothelial growth factor. J Rheumatol 25: 813-5

121. Hunt SJ, Santa Cruz DJ, Barr RJ (1991) Microvenular haemangioma. J Cutan Pathol 18: 235-40

122. Black RJ, McCusker GM, Eedy DJ (1995) Microvenular haemangioma. Clin Exp Dermatol 20: 260-2

123. Mentzel T, Calonje E, Fletcher CD (1994) Vascular tumors of the skin and soft tissue. Overview of newly characterized entities and variants. Pathologe 15: 259-70

124. Sanz-Trelles A, Ojeda-Martos A, Jimenez-Fernandez A, Vera-Casano A (1998) Microvenular haemangioma: a new case in a child. Histopathology 32: 89-90

125. Fukunaga M, Ushigome S (1998) Microvenular haemangioma. Pathol Int 48: 237-9

126. Jones EW, Orkin M (1989) Tufted angioma (angioblastoma). A benign progressive angioma, not to be confused with Kaposi's sarcoma or low-grade angiosarcoma. J Am Acad Dermatol 20: 214-25

127. MacMillan A, Champion RH (1971) Progressive capillary haemangioma. Br J Dermatol 85: 492-3

128. Croué A, Habersetzer M, Leclech C, Forest JL, Saint-André JP, Verret JL (1993) Tufted angioma. A benign vascular tumor not to be confused with Kaposi's sarcoma. Arch Anat Cytol Path 41: 159-63

129. Allen PW (1994) Three new vascular tumors-Tufted angioma, Kaposiform infantile haemangioendothelioma and Proliferative cutaneous angiomatosis. Int J Surg Pathol 2: 63-72

130. Mentzel T, Wollina U, Castelli E, Kutzner H (1996) Tufted haemangioma. Clinicopathologic and immunohistologic analysis of 5 cases of a distinct entity within the spectrum of capillary haemangioma. Hautarzt 47: 369-75

131. Catteau B, Enjolras O, Delaporte E, Friedel J, Brevière G, Wassef M, Lecomte-Houcke M, Piette F, Bergoend H (1998) Sclerosing tufted angioma. Apropos of 4 cases involving lower limbs. Ann Dermatol Venereol 125: 682-7

132. Descours H, Grezard P, Chouvet B, Labeille B (1998) Acquired tufted angioma in an adult. Ann Dermatol Venereol 125: 44-6

133. Wilmer A, Kaatz M, Bocker T, Wollina U (1999) Tufted angioma. Eur J Dermatol 9: 51-3

134. Heagerty AH, Rubin A, Robinson TW (1992) Familial tufted angioma. Clin Exp Dermatol 17: 344-5

135. Hiraiwa A, Takai K, Fukui Y, Adachi A, Fujii H (1990) Non regressing lipodystrophia centrifugalis abdominalis with angioblastoma (Nakagawa). Arch Dermatol 126: 206-9

136. Kim YK, Kim HJ, Lee KG (1992) Acquired tufted angioma associated with pregnancy. Clin Exp Dermatol 17: 458-9

137. Chu P, LeBoit PE (1992) An eruptive vascular proliferation resembling acquired tufted angioma in the recipient of a liver transplant. J Am Acad Dermatol 26: 322-5

138. Lam WY, Mac-Moune Lai F, Look CN, Choi PC, Allen PW (1994) Tufted angioma with complete regression. J Cutan Pathol 21: 461-6

139. Jang KA, Choi JH, Sung KJ, Moon KC, Koh JK (1998) Congenital linear tufted angioma with spontaneous regression. Br J Dermatol 138: 912-3

140. Gonzalez-Crussi F, Chou P, Crawford SE (1991) Congenital infiltrating giant cell angioblastoma, a new entity? Am J Surg Pathol 15: 175-83

141. Padilla RS, Orkin M, Rosai J (1987) Acquired "tufted" angioma (progressive capillary haemangioma). A distinctive clinicopathologic entity related to lobular capillary haemangioma. Am J Dermatopathol 9: 292-300

142. Zukerberg LR, Nickoloff BJ, Weiss SW (1993) Kaposiform haemangioendothelioma of infancy and childhood. An aggressive neoplasm associated with Kasabach-Merritt syndrome and lymphangiomatosis. Am J Surg Pathol 17: 321-8

143. Ballotta MR, Bianchini E, Borghi L, Rimondi AP (1996) Sclerosing haemangioma of the lung: a case report. Pathologica 88: 307-10

144. Fujiyoshi F, Ichinari N, Fukukura Y, Sasaki M, Hiraki Y, Nakajo M (1998) Sclerosing haemangioma of the lung: MR findings and correlation with pathological features. J Comput Assist Tomogr 22: 1006-8

145. Lee ST, Lee YC, Hsu CY, Lin CC (1992) Bilateral multiple sclerosing haemangiomas of the lung. Chest 101: 572-3

146. Katzenstein AL, Gmelich JT, Carrington CB (1980) Sclerosing haemangioma of the lung: a clinicopathologic study of 51 cases. Am J Surg Pathol 4: 343-56

147. Ohori NP, Yousem SA, Sonmez-Alpan E, Colby TV (1991) Estrogen and progesterone receptors in lymphangioleiomyomatosis, epithelioid haemangioendothelioma, and sclerosing haemangioma of the lung. Am J Clin Pathol 96: 529-35

148. Sugio K, Yokoyama H, Kaneko S, Ishida T, Sugimachi K (1992) Sclerosing haemangioma of the lung: radiographic and pathological study. Ann Thorac Surg 53: 295-300

149. Yousem SA, Wick MR, Singh G, Katyal SL, Manivel JC, Mills SE, Legier J (1988) So-called sclerosing haemangiomas of lung. An immunohistochemical study supporting a respiratory epithelial origin. Am J Surg Pathol 12: 582-90

150. Satoh Y, Tsuchiya E, Weng SY, Kitagawa T, Matsubara T, Nakagawa K, Kinoshita I, Sugano H (1989) Pulmonary sclerosing haemangioma of the lung. A type II pneumocytoma by immunohistochemical and immunoelectron microscopic studies. Cancer 64: 1310-7

151. Cheong PY, Lee CN, Wee A (1993) Sclerosing haemangioma of lung – case report with histologic, immunohistochemical and ultrastructural correlation. Ann Acad Med Singapore 22: 960-3

152. Leong AS, Chan KW, Seneviratne HS (1995) A morphological and immunohistochemical study of 25 cases of so-called sclerosing haemangioma of the lung. Histopathology 27: 121-8

153. Niho S, Suzuki K, Yokose T, Kodama T, Nishiwaki Y, Esumi H (1998) Monoclonality of both pale cells and cu-

boidal cells of sclerosing haemangioma of the lung. Am J Pathol 152: 1065-9

154. Chiba W, Sawai S, Yasuda Y, Wazawa H, Matsubara Y, Ikeda S (1995) Positive expression of c-myc and p53 products in two cases of pulmonary sclerosing haemangioma. Nihon Kyobu Shikkan Gakkai Zasshi 33: 1348-54

155. Moran CA, Zeren H, Koss MN (1994) Sclerosing haemangioma of the lung. Granulomatous variant. Arch Pathol Lab Med 118: 1028-30

156. Brown JV, Stenchever MA (1989) Cavernous lymphangioma of the vulva. Obstet Gynecol 73: 877-9

157. Mordehai J, Kurzbart E, Shinhar D, Sagi A, Finaly R, Mares AJ (1998) Lymphangioma circumscriptum. Pediatr Surg Int 13: 208-10

158. Leshin B, Whitaker DC, Foucar E (1986) Lymphangioma circumscriptum following mastectomy and radiation therapy. J Am Acad Dermatol 15: 1117-9

159. Ambrojo P, Cogolludo EF, Aguilar A, Sanchez Yus E, Sanchez de Paz F (1990) Cutaneous lymphangiectases after therapy for carcinoma of the cervix—a case with unusual clinical and histological features. Clin Exp Dermatol 15: 57-9

160. Weyers W, Nilles M, Konig M (1990) Lymphangioma circumscriptum cysticum following surgical and radiologic therapy. Hautarzt 41: 102-4

161. Buckley DA, Barnes L (1996) Vulvar lymphangiectasia due to recurrent cellulitis. Clin Exp Dermatol 21: 215-6

162. Wilson GR, Cox NH, McLean NR, Scott D (1993) Squamous cell carcinoma arising within congenital lymphangioma circumscriptum. Br J Dermatol 129: 337-9

163. Short S, Peacock C (1995) A newly described possible complication of lymphangioma circumscriptum. Clin Oncol (R Coll Radiol) 7: 136-7

164. King DT, Duffy DM, Hirose FM, Gurevitch AW (1979) Lymphangiosarcoma arising from lymphangioma circumscriptum. Arch Dermatol 115: 969-72

165. Anderson NG, Kennedy JC (1992) Prognosis in fetal cystic hygroma. Aust N Z J Obstet Gynaecol 32: 36-9

166. Thompson DM, Kasperbauer JL (1994) Congenital cystic hygroma involving the larynx presenting as an airway emergency. Natl Med Assoc 86: 629-32

167. Gimeno Aranguez M, Colomar Palmer P, Gonzalez Mediero I, Ollero Caprani JM (1996) The clinical and morphological aspects of childhood lymphangiomas: a review of 145 cases. An Esp Pediatr 45: 25-8

168. Silvestre de Sacy V, Keilani K, Duron J, Vayre P (1992) Lymphangiome du mésentère. Une cause rare de syndrome douloureux abdominal aigu chez l'adulte. J Chir (Paris) 129: 78-80

169. El Mansouri A (1996) Le lymphangiome kystique du mésentère. Sem Hôp Paris 72: 373-4

170. Di Carlo I, Gayet B (1996) Lymphangioma of the diaphragm (first case report). Surg Today 26: 199-202

171. Anadol AZ, Oguz M, Bayramoglu H, Edali MN (1998) Cystic lymphangioma of the spleen mimicking hydatid disease. J Clin Gastroenterol 26: 309-11

172. Icard P, Le Rochais JP, Galateau F, Jehan A, Martel B, Brun J, Evrard C (1998) Cystic lymphangioma of the mediastinum. Apropos of 3 cases, review of the literature. Ann Chir 52: 629-34

173. Desoutter P, Cohen Solal JL, Chabouis C, Loisel JC, Vuong Ngoc P, Choffel C, Kohlmann G (1983) A rare cause of recurring thromboembolism: retroperitoneal cystic lymphangioma. Ann Radiol (Paris) 26: 522-4

174. Hayashi J, Yamashita Y, Kakegawa T, Ogata M, Nakashima O (1994) A case of cystic lymphangioma of the pancreas. J Gastroenterol 29: 372-6

175. Reichler A, Bronshtein M (1995) Early prenatal diagnosis of axillary cystic hygroma. J Ultrasound Med 14: 581-4

176. Houissa H, Jouini M, Kacem M, Safta ZB, Belaid S (1994) Le lymphangiome kystique splénique: une location exceptionnelle. Ann Gastroenterol Hépatol 30: 215-7

177. Weiss SW, Enzinger FM (1986) Spindle cell haemangioendothelioma: a low-grade angiosarcoma resembling a cavernous haemangioma and Kaposi's sarcoma. Am J Surg Pathol 10: 521-30

178. Fanburg JC, Meis-Kindblom JM, Rosenberg AE (1995) Multiple enchondromas associated with spindle-cell haemangioendotheliomas. An overlooked variant of Maffucci's syndrome. Am J Surg Pathol 19: 1029-38

179. Fletcher CD, Beham A, Schmid C (1991) Spindle cell haemangioendothelioma: a clinicopathological and immunohistochemical study indicative of a non-neoplastic lesion. Histopathology 18: 291-301

180. Ding J, Hashimoto H, Imayama S, Tsuneyoshi M, Enjoji M (1992) Spindle cell haemangio-endothelioma: probably a benign vascular lesion not a low-grade angiosarcoma. A clinicopathological, ultrastructural and immunohistochemical study. Virchows Arch A Pathol Anat Histopathol 420: 77-85

181. Imayama S, Murakamai Y, Hashimoto H, Hori Y (1992) Spindle cell haemangio-endothelioma exhibits the ultrastructural features of reactive vascular proliferation rather than of angiosarcoma. Am J Clin Pathol 97: 279-87

182. Fukunaga M, Ushigome S, Nikaido T, Ishikawa E, Nakamori K (1995) Spindle cell haemangioendothelioma: an immunohistochemical and flow cytometric study of six cases. Pathol Int 45: 589-95

183. Hisaoka M, Kouho H, Aoki T, Hashimoto H (1995) DNA flow cytometric and immunohistochemical analysis of proliferative activity in spindle cell haemangio-endothelioma. Histopathology 27(5): 451-6

184. Tsang WY, Chan JK (1991) Kaposi-like infantile haemangioendothelioma. A distinctive vascular neoplasm of the retroperitoneum. Am J Surg Pathol 15: 982-9

185. Mentzel T, Mazzoleni G, Dei Tos AP, Fletcher CD (1997) Kaposiform haemangioendothelioma in adults. Clinicopathologic and immunohistochemical analysis of three cases. Am J Clin Pathol 108: 450-5

186. Beaubien ER, Ball NJ, Storwick GS (1998) Kaposiform haemangioendothelioma: a locally aggressive vascular tumor. J Am Acad Dermatol 38: 799-802

187. Deb G, Jenkner A, De Sio L, Boldrini R, Bosman C, Standoli N, Donfrancesco A (1997) Spindle cell (Kaposiform) haemangioendothelioma with Kasabach-Merritt syndrome in an infant: successful treatment with alpha-2A interferon. Med Pediatr Oncol 28: 358-61

188. Ezekowitz RA, Mulliken JB, Folkman J (1992) Interferon alfa-2a therapy for life-threatening hemangiomas of infancy. N Engl J Med 326: 1456-63

189. Baloch ZW, LiVolsi VA (1998) Intravascular Kaposi's-like spindle cell proliferation of the capsular vessels of follicular-derived thyroid carcinomas. Mod Pathol 11: 995-8

190. Dabska M (1969) Malignant endovascular papillary angioendothelioma of the skin in childhood. Clinicopathologic study of 6 cases. Cancer 24: 503-10

191. Argani P, Athanasian E (1997) Malignant endovascular papillary angioendothelioma (Dabska tumor) arising within a deep intramuscular haemangioma. Arch Pathol Lab Med 121: 992-5

192. Manivel JC, Wick MR, Swanson PE, Patterson K, Dehner LP (1986) Endovascular papillary angioendothelioma of childhood: a vascular lesion possibly characterized by "high" endothelial cell differentiation. Hum Pathol 17: 1240-4

193. Fukunaga M (1998) Endovascular papillary angioendothelioma. Pathol Int 48: 840-1

194. Kilpatrick SE, Koplyay PD, Ward WG, Richards F 2nd (1998) Epithelioid hemangioendothelioma of bone and soft tissue: a fine-needle aspiration biopsy study with histologic and immunohistochemical confirmation. Diagn Cytopathol 19: 38-43

195. Kitaichi M, Nagai S, Nishimura K, Itoh H, Asamoto H, Izumi T, Dail DH (1998) Pulmonary epithelioid haemangioendothelioma in 21 patients, including three with partial spontaneous regression. Eur Respir J 12: 89-96

196. Horio H, Nomori H, Fuyuno G, Kobayashi R, Morinaga S, Suemasu K (1998) A case of pulmonary epithelioid haemangioendothelioma diagnosed by video-assisted thoracoscopic biopsy. Kyobu Geka 51: 753-7

197. Kato N, Tamura A, Okushiba M (1998) Multiple cutaneous epithelioid haemangio-endothelioma: a case with spindle cells. J Dermatol 25: 453-9

198. Nataf P, Regnard JF, Solvignon F, Bruneval P, Faucher JN, Levasseur P (1989) Epithelioid haemangioendothelioma of the azygos vein. Arch Mal Cœur Vaiss 82: 1919-22

199. Ferretti GR, Chiles C, Woodruff RD, Choplin RH (1998) Epithelioid haemangio-endothelioma of the superior vena cava: computed tomography demonstration and review of the literature. J Thorac Imaging 13: 45-8

200. Bancel B, Patricot LM, Caillon P, Ducerf C, Pouyet M (1993) Hémangioendothéliome épithélioïde hépatique. Un cas avec transplantation hépatique. Revue de la littérature. Ann Pathol 13: 23-8

201. den Bakker MA, den Bakker AJ, Beenen R, Mulder AH, Eulderink F (1998) Subtotal liver calcification due to epithelioid haemangioendothelioma. Pathol Res Pract 194: 189-94

202. Horejsova M, Naprstkova J, Vyhnanek F, Wohl R (1998) Epithelioid haemangio-endothelioma of the liver. Accidental detection of a solitary focus resembling a hepatic cyst. Cas Lek Cesk 137: 476-8

203. Panzini L, Homer RJ (1998) Duodenal haemangioendothelioma: a case report. Am J Gastroenterol 93: 832-3

204. Dietze O, Davies SE, Williams R, Portmann B (1989) Malignant epithelioid haemangio-endothelioma of the liver: a clinicopathologic and histochemical study of 12 cases. Histopathology 15: 225-37

205. Dail DH, Liebow AA, Gmelich JT, Friedman PJ, Miyai K, Myer W, Patterson SD, Hammar SP (1983) Intravascular, bronchiolar, and alveolar tumor of the lung (IVBAT). An analysis of twenty cases of a peculiar sclerosing endothelial tumor. Cancer 51(3): 452-64

206. Weiss SW, Ishak KG, Dail DH, Sweet DE, Enzinger FM (1986) Epithelioid haemangioendothelioma and related lesions. Semin Diagn Pathol 3: 259-87

207. Kaposi M (1872) Idiopathisches multiples pigmentsarkom der haut. Archiv Dermatol Syphilis 4: 265-73

208. Santucci M, Pimpinelli N, Moretti S, Giannotti B (1988) Classic and immunodeficiency-associated Kaposi's sarcoma. Arch Pathol Lab Med 112: 1214-20

209. Iscovich J, Boffetta P, Brennan P (1999) Classic Kaposi's sarcoma as a first primary neoplasm. Int J Cancer 80: 173-7

210. Dawkins FW, Delapenha RA, Frezza EE, Green WR, Hardy C, Frederick WR, Manns A (1998) HIV-1-associated Kaposi's sarcoma in a predominantly black population at an inner city hospital. South Med J 91: 546-9

211. Goedert JJ, Cote TR, Virgo P, Scoppa SM, Kingma DW, Gail MH, Jaffe ES, Biggar RJ (1998) Spectrum of AIDS-associated malignant disorders. Lancet 351(9119): 1833-9

212. Hermans P (1998) Epidemiology, etiology and pathogenesis, clinical presentations and therapeutic approaches in Kaposi's sarcoma: 15-year lessons from AIDS. Biomed Pharmacother 52: 440-6

213. Erban SB, Sokas RK (1988) Kaposi's sarcoma in an elderly man with Wegener's granulomatosis treated with cyclophosphamide and corticosteroids. Arch Intern Med 148: 1201-3

214. Audoin AF, Lopes P, Lenne Y (1988) Sarcome de Kaposi du col utérin associé à un condylome atypique chez une femme transplantée cardiaque. Arch Anat Cytol Path 36: 226-8

215. Shmueli D, Shapira Z, Yussima A, Nakache R, Ral Z, Shaharabani E (1989) The incidence of Kaposi's sarcoma in renal transplant patients and its relation to immunosuppression. Transplant Proc 21: 3209-10

216. Puy-Montbrun T, Pigot F, Vuong PN, Ganansia R, Denis J (1991) Kaposi's sarcoma of the colon in a young HIV-negative woman with Crohn's disease. Dig Dis Sci 36: 528-31

217. Guo WX, Antakly T, Cadotte M, Kachra Z, Kunkel L, Masood R, Gill P (1996) Expression and cytokine regulation of glucocorticoid receptors in Kaposi's sarcoma. Am J Pathol 148: 1999-2008

218. Eberhard OK, Kliem V, Brunkhorst R (1999) Five cases of Kaposi's sarcoma in kidney graft recipients: possible influence of the immunosuppressive therapy. Transplantation 67: 180-4

219. Cossu S, Satta R, Cottoni F, Massarelli G (1997) Lymphangioma-like variant of Kaposi's sarcoma: clinicopathologic study of seven cases with review of the literature. Am J Dermatopathol 19: 16-22

220. Kambouchner M, Amouroux J (1994) Atteintes pulmonaires au cours de l'infection par le virus de l'immunodéficience humaine. Deuxième partie: Complications non infectieuses. Ann Pathol 14: 221-6

221. Friedman SL, Wright TL, Altman DF (1985) Gastrointestinal Kaposi's sarcoma in patients with acquired immunodeficiency syndrome: An autopsy series. Hum Pathol 16: 102-8

222. Ariza A, Kim JH (1988) Kaposi's sarcoma of the dura mater. Hum Pathol 19: 1461-3

223. Teh BS, Lu HH, Lynch GR, Banez E, Kroll MH (1999) AIDS-related Kaposi's sarcoma involving bone and bone marrow. South Med J 92: 61-4

224. Just Sarobe M, Ribera Pibernat M, Lopez Cabrerizo MP, Urrutia de Diego A, Ferrandiz Foraster C (1998) Classical Kaposi sarcoma of aggressive course. Rev Clin Esp 198: 95-8

225. Giraldo G, Beth E, Huang ES (1980) Kaposi's sarcoma and its relationship to cytomegalovirus (CMV) III – CMV DNA and CMV early antigens in Kaposi's sarcoma. Int J Cancer 26: 23-9

226. Giraldo G, Beth E (1972) Sarcome de Kaposi: présence de virus type herpès en culture de tissu dans 5 cas différents. CR Acad Sci (Paris) 275: 289-92

227. Walter P, Philippe E, Khalil Th, Nguemby-Mbina C, Chamlian A (1984) Le sarcome de Kaposi. Un néoplasme vasculaire présumé d'origine virale. Caractères histologiques et ultrastructuraux. Ann Pathol 4: 19-25

228. Chang Y, Cesarman E, Pessin MS, Lee F, Culpepper J, Knowles DM, Moore PS (1994) Identification of Herpesvirus-like DNA sequences in AIDS-associated Kaposi's sarcoma. Science 266: 1865-9

229. Ensoli B, Sirianni MC (1998) Kaposi's sarcoma pathogenesis: a link between immunology and tumor biology. Crit Rev Oncog 9: 107-24

230. Sturzl M, Ensoli B (1999) Big but weak: how many pathogenic genes does human herpesvirus-8 need to cause Kaposi's sarcoma ? Int J Oncol 14: 287-9

231. Huang YQ, Li JJ, Rush MG, Poiesz BJ, Nicolaides A, Jacobson M, Zhang WG, Coutavas E, Abbot MA, Friedman-Kien AE (1992) HPV-16-related DNA sequences in Kaposi's sarcoma. Lancet 339: 515-8

232. Albini A, Barillari G, Benelli R, Gallo RC, Ensoli B (1995) Angiogenic properties of human immunodeficiency virus type 1 Tat protein. Proc Natl Acad Sci USA 92: 4838-42

233. Fiorelli V, Barillari G, Toschi E, Sgadari C, Monini P, Sturzl M, Ensoli B (1999) IFN-gamma induces endothelial cells to proliferate and to invade the extracellular matrix in response to the HIV-1 Tat protein: implications for AIDS-Kaposi's sarcoma pathogenesis. J Immunol 162: 1165-70

234. Cohen J (1995)Controversy: Is KS really caused by new Herpesvirus ? Science 268: 1847-8

235. Masood R, Cai J, Zheng T, Smith DL, Naidu Y, Gill PS (1997) Vascular endothelial growth factor/vascular permeability factor is an autocrine growth factor for AIDS-Kaposi sarcoma. Proc Natl Acad Sci U S A 94: 979-84

236. Brooks JJ (1992) Kaposi's sarcoma and Kaposi's-like lesions in AIDS InWeinstein RS, Graham AR (eds) Advances in Pathology and Laboratory Medicine, vol. 5, Mosby-Year Book, Saint Louis, p 307

237. Niemi M, Mustakallio K (1965) The fine structure of the spindle cells in Kaposi's sarcoma. Acta Pathol Microb Scand 63: 567-75

238. Fukunaga M, Silverberg SG (1991) Hyaline globules in Kaposi's sarcoma: A light microscopic and immunohistochemical study. Mod Pathol 4: 187-90

239. Ravisse P (1984) Histopathologie du sarcome de Kaposi. Bull Soc Path Ex 77: 533-45

240. Yamashita JT, Valente NYS, Nagasse I, Michalany NS (1995) Intérêt de la coloration de Perls dans le diagnostic histologique du sarcome de Kaposi. Ann Pathol 15: 115-8

241. Nadji M, Morales AR, Ziegles-Weissman J, Penneys NS (1981) Kaposi's sarcoma: immunohistologic evidence for an endothelial origin. Arch Pathol Lab Med 105: 274-5

242. Beckstead JH, Wood GS, Fletcher V (1985) Evidence for the origin of Kaposi's sarcoma from lymphatic endothelium. Am J Pathol 119: 294-300

243. Bendelac A, Kanitakis J, Chouvet B, Viac J, Thivolet J (1985) Sarcome de Kaposi: Etude immunohistochimique comparative et intérêt histopronostique des marqueurs endothéliaux. Ann Pathol 5: 45-52

244. Nickoloff BJ (1991) The human progenitor cell antigen (CD34) is localized on endothelial cells, dermal dendritic cells and perifollicular cells in formalin-fixed normal skin, and on proliferating endothelial cells and stromal spindle-shaped cells in Kaposi's sarcoma. Arch Dermatol 127: 523-9

245. Kostianovsky M, Lamy MY, Greco MA (1992) Immunohistochemical and electron microscopic profiles of cutaneous Kaposi's sarcoma and bacillary angiomatosis. Ultrastruct Pathol 16: 629-40

246. Kanitakis J, Narvaez D, Claudy A (1996) Expression of the CD34 antigen distinguishes Kaposi's sarcoma from pseudo-Kaposi's sarcoma (acroangiodermatitis). Br J Dermatol 134: 44-6

247. Chomette G, Diebold J (1987) Tumeurs et pseudotumeurs vasculairesIn Camilleri JP, Berry CL, Fiessinger J-N, Bariety J (ed)Les maladies de la paroi artérielle, Flammarion, Paris, p 625

248. Enzinger FM, Weiss SW (1988) Soft tissue tumors, CV Mosby, Saint Louis

249. Hofman P, Bernard JL, Michiels JF, Saint-Paul MC, Rampal A, Benchimol D, Loubière R (1991) Angiosarcome primitif du côlon. Etude anatomo-clinique à propos d'un cas. Ann Pathol 11: 25-30

250. Deléaval JP, Peter MY, Laurencet F, Fontolliet C (1991) Angiosarcome multicentrique intestinal. A propos d'un cas. Ann Pathol 11: 342-4

251. Locker GY, Doroshow JH, Zwelling LA, Chabner B (1979) The clinical features of hepaticangiosarcoma: A report of 4 cases and a review of the English literature. Medicine 58: 48-64

252. Nanus DM, Kelsen D, Clark DG (1987) Radiation induced angiosarcoma. Cancer 60: 777-9

253. Meis-Kindblom JM, Kindblom LG (1998) Angiosarcoma of soft tissue: a study of 80 cases. Am J Surg Pathol 22: 683-97

254. Lasota J, Miettinen M (1999) Absence of Kaposi's sarcoma-associated virus (human herpes-8) sequences in angiosarcoma. Virchows Arch 434: 51-56

255. Brentani MM, Pacheco MM, Oshima CT, Nagai MA, Lemos LB, Goes JC (1983) Steroid receptors in breast angiosarcoma. Cancer 51: 2105-11

256. Stewart FW, Treves N (1948)Lymphangiosarcoma in post-mastectomy lymphedema: a report of six cases in elephantiasis chirurgica. Cancer 1: 64-81

257. Faggioli GL, Bertoni F, Bacchini P, Stella A, Gessaroli M, Gargiulo M (1989) Angiosarcoma in a limb with arteriovenous fistulas and elephantiasis. Int Angiol 8: 161-70

258. Lasa MV, Mateo P, Bascon N, Baquedano J, Fuertes F, Lopez P, Esco R (1995) Lymphangiosarcoma in a chronic lymphedematous limb: a case report. Tumori 81: 381-2

259. Sinclair SA, Sviland L, Natarajan S (1998) Angiosarcoma arising in a chronically lymphoedematous leg. Br J Dermatol 138: 692-4

260. Martin MB, Kon ND, Kawamoto EH, Myers RT, Sterchi JM (1984) Post mastectomy angiosarcoma. Am Surg 10: 541-5

261. Brostrom LA, Nilsonne U, Kronberg M, Soderberg G (1989) Lymphangiosarcoma in chronic hereditary oedema (Milroy's disease). Ann Chir Gynaecol 78: 320-3

262. Chen KT, Bauer V, Flam MS (1991) Angiosarcoma in postsurgical lymphedema. An unusual occurrence in a man. Am J Dermatopathol 13: 488-92

263. Bisceglia M, Attino V, D'Addetta C, Murgo R, Fletcher CD (1996) Early stage Stewart-Treves syndrome: report of 2 cases and review of the literature. Pathologica 88: 483-90

264. Kogon B, Kabeer M, Sawchuk AP, Dalsing M, Billings S (1998) Angiosarcoma presenting as an occluded popliteal artery pseudoaneurysm. J Vasc Surg 27: 970-3

265. Page DL, Anderson TJ (1987) Diagnosis histopathology of the breast. Churchill Livingstone, Edinburgh London Melbourne NewYork

266. Calonje E, Fletcher CD, Wilson-Jones E, Rosai J (1994) Retiform haemangioendothelioma. A distinctive form of

low-grade angiosarcoma delineated in a series of 15 cases. Am J Surg Pathol 18: 115-25

267. Duke D, Dvorak A, Harris TJ, Cohen LM (1996) Multiple retiform haemangio-endotheliomas. A low-grade angiosarcoma. Am J Dermatopathol 18: 606-10

268. Schammel DP, Tavassoli FA (1998) Uterine angiosarcomas: a morphologic and immunohistochemical study of four cases. Am J Surg Pathol 22: 246-50

269. Sastre-Garau X, Thiery JP, Ovtracht L, Gallet C, Quintana E, Laurent M (1992) Angiosarcome des tissus mous de l'enfant. Caractères immunohistochimiques et ultra-structuraux. Ann Pathol 12: 34-40

270. Eusebi V, Carcangiu ML, Dina R, Rosai J (1990) Keratin-positive epithelioid angiosarcoma of thyroid. A report of four cases. Am J Surg Pathol 14: 737-47

271. Borit A, Nezelof C (1976) Embolism of the heart and the aorta, from a rhabdomyosarcoma. Arch Anat Cytol Pathol 24: 295-6

272. Takamori S, Hayashi A, Tayama K, Mitsuoka M, Tamura K, Shirouzu K (1998) Resection of malignant fibrous histiocytoma invading the thoracic aorta. Nippon Kyobu Geka Gakkai Zasshi 46: 825-8

XVIII
Tumours of vessel wall components and vascular related structures

1 – Tumours of vessel wall components

Benign tumours

Angioleiomyoma (Vascular leiomyoma, Angiomyoma)

Most angioleiomyomas develop from the smooth muscle cells of the media or adventitia, most frequently in a subcutaneous vein, but larger veins (hepatic, femoral) may be involved. The tumour affects patients between the fourth and sixth decades with a predilection for females. The most frequent locations are in the legs and arms [1-3]. Other sites include the skin, nasal mucosa or the pharyngeal space [4-7]. An angioleiomyoma appears as a circumscribed mass, usually measuring about 2 cm in diameter, rarely larger than 4-5 cm. Pain, present in half of the cases, may be exacerbated by menses, pregnancy, pressure and changes in temperature. Simple excision is adequate treatment.

Pathology and differential diagnosis

Angioleiomyoma is a round encapsulated nodule, whitish on cut section (Fig. 1). Histologically, it is comprised of interlacing bundles of smooth muscle cells (Fig. 2), criss-crossed by thick-walled vessels (Fig. 3). In areas of myxoid change, hyalinization may be present. Serial sections permit identification of the transitional zone between the tumour and the vascular wall (Fig. 4) that often surrounds the tumour. Angioleiomyoma should be distinguished from leiomyoma developed from the arrectores pilora of the dermis, neuroma and neurofibroma. Some so-called angioleiomyomas involving the inferior vena cava are extensions of uterine leiomyomas and are best referred to as intravenous leiomyomatosis. Karyotypic abnormalities, such as chromosomal rearrangements (6p, 13q, and 21q) and t(X; 10)(q22; q23.2) translocation, have been reported in primary short-term cultured cells from an angiomyoma [8].

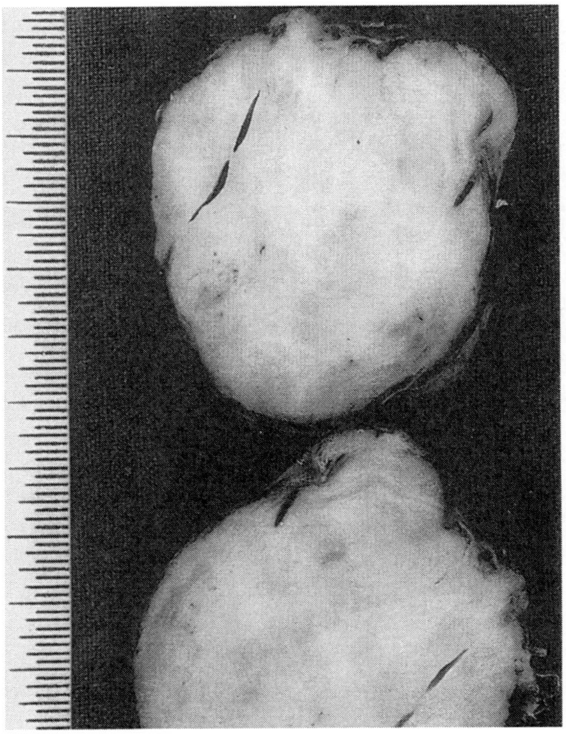

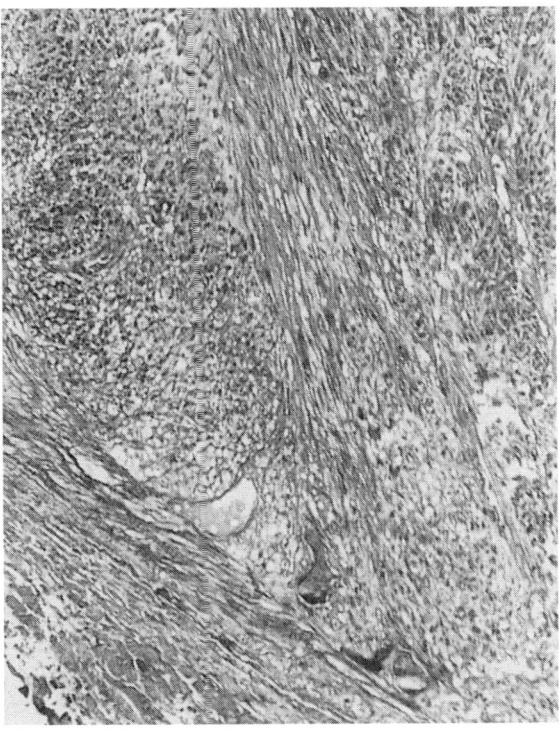

Fig. 1. Angioleiomyoma. Cut section. (Courtesy Dr J. Khalifé)

Fig. 2. Angioleiomyoma. Hyperplastic smooth muscle cells arranged in interlacing bundles. Haematoxylin, eosin and saffron stain. (HES)

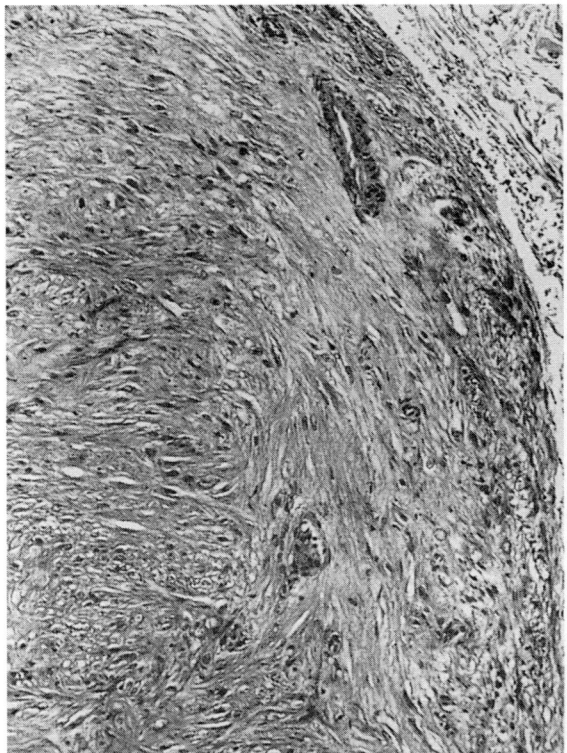

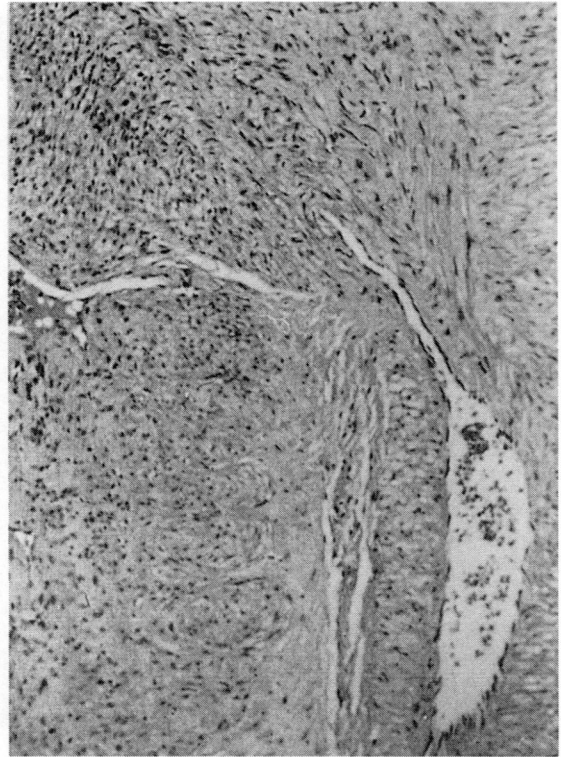

Fig. 3. Angioleiomyoma. Thick-walled vessels criss-crossing the tumour. HES

Fig. 4. Angioleiomyoma. Transitional zone between the tumour and the media of the surrounding artery. HES

Other miscellaneous benign tumours

These are extremely rare. Gough and Moreano [9] and Ramphal et al [10] reported two cases of primary myxoma involving the ascending aorta and the right femoral vein respectively. Its histological features resemble those of a cardiac myxoma. Mai et al [11] described a case of mobile, tender, encapsulated myxolipoma ("angiomyxolipoma") of a vessel of the spermatic cord. A few examples of fibrous histiocytomas of the aortic adventitia have been reported and cured by surgical resection.

Glomus tumour

The origin of glomus tumours is a matter of controversy; Masson [12, 13] suggested an origin from the "neuro vascular glomi", with non-cutaneous lesions arising from ectopic glomi. Stout [14] contended that this tumour derives from pericytes – thus a glomus tumour is thought to be closely related to haemangiopericytoma. However, ultrastructural studies support a smooth muscle cell origin [15, 16]. Both myocytes

and neural elements are seen in histological sections and this is confirmed by immunohistochemistry. A close relationship between glomus cells and myocytes has been suggested with transformation from one type to the other [13, 17]. A further hypothesis suggests that glomus tumours result from permanent hyperplasia of glomus cells with enlargement of the normal glomus, secondary to ischaemic vascular disorders [18, 19].

Glomus tumours are relatively common. They occur at all ages with a peak from 30 to 40 years and there is often a long history (7-10 years) before intervention [20, 21]. There is no sex predilection and familial cases are well documented [22]. A glomus tumour may occur at any almost cutaneous site, but most often develops in the distal phalanx of the finger in the nail bed, or in the palm. An exquisite pain, radiating throughout the whole limb, exacerbated by exposure to cold or tactile stimulation, may occur for some time before the tumour becomes visible. It appears as a firm, small nodule, rarely exceeding 1 cm in diameter. Usually reddish-blue or purple, it may change colour when irritated during the course of clinical examination. An underlying scalloped bone defect is often found on X-ray in digital cases [21]. In a small proportion of cases, glomus tumours may be multiple and associated with other vascular malformations. Benign familial glomus tumours are transmitted as an autosomal dominant trait, but are only manifest in those who inherit the gene from their father [23]. The gene has recently been mapped to 11q22.3-q23. Extracutaneous locations include the muscles and aponeuroses, and various viscera including the mediastinum, lungs, stomach, rectum, mesentery, renal capsule, uterine cervix and vulva. The spinal cord may be affected [24]. In bones (Fig. 5), glomus tumours have been reported to be preceded by trauma (phalanx, pubis, femur, fibula) [13, 25-27]. Complete surgical excision eliminates the symptoms and local recurrence (about 10%) only follows inadequate excision. True malignant transformation is exceedingly rare [28].

Pathology and differential diagnosis

The tumour appears as a round and well-circumscribed nodule (Fig. 6). Histologically, it consists of a proliferation of small, globoid, cubic or oval cells centered by punched-out round nuclei with faintly eosinophilic stained cytoplasm (Fig. 7-8). Rarely are tumour cells elongated, spindle-shape (Fig. 9). The cells are devoid of glycogen. They form packed areas around variably structured arterioles or veins with a normally flat endothelium and anastomotic ribbon-like sheets surrounded by myxoid or hyalinized stroma. No demonstrable elastic lamellae are seen in the vessels, and in some areas the glomus cells may extend to and abut on the endothelial lining. Gordon-Sweet's stain shows a delicate reticulin meshwork enclosing each tumour cell individually. An ill-defined collagen capsule containing small vessels and nerves is seen at the periphery and the appearance mimics an hypertrophied peripheral neuromyovascular glomus.

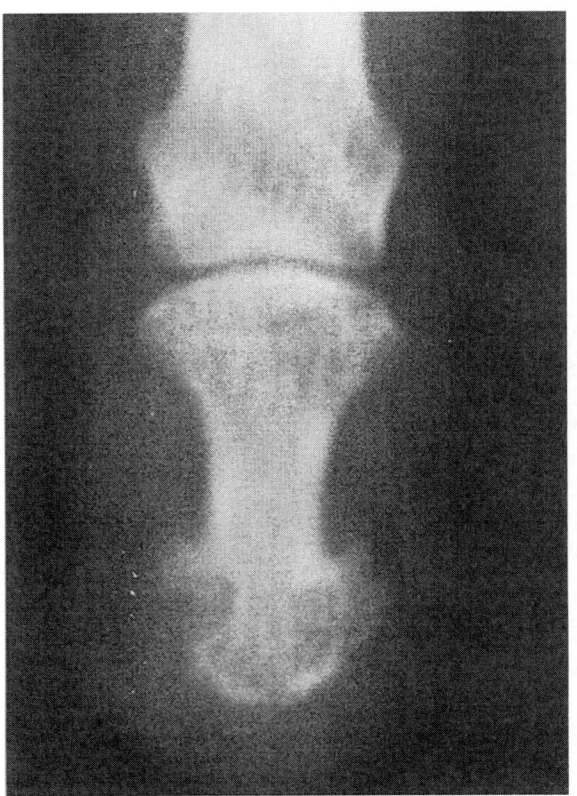

Fig. 5. Radiograph of the ungual phalanx eroded by a glomus tumour. (Courtesy Dr A. Mazabraud)

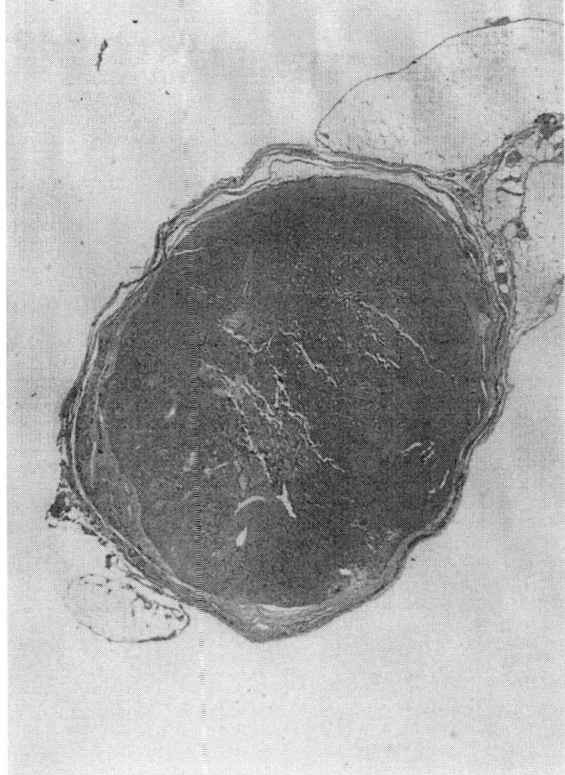

Fig. 6. Well-circumscribed glomus tumour of the ungual phalanx. HES

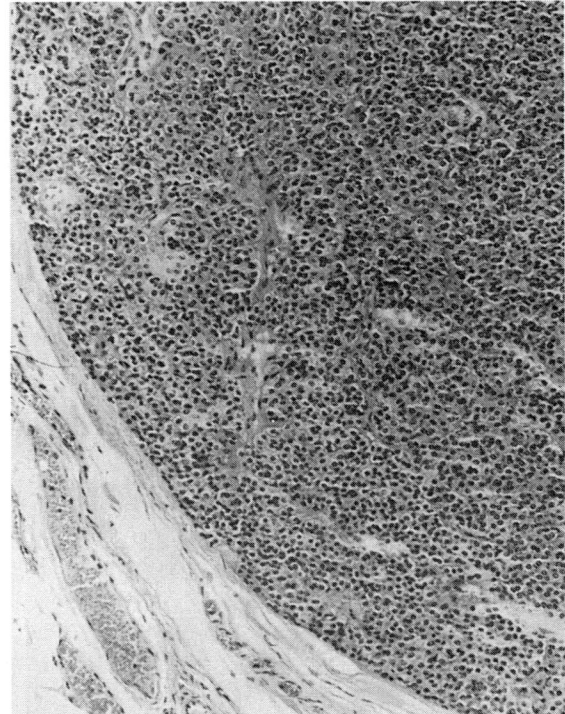

Fig. 7. Glomus tumour. Proliferation of packed small glomic cells. HES

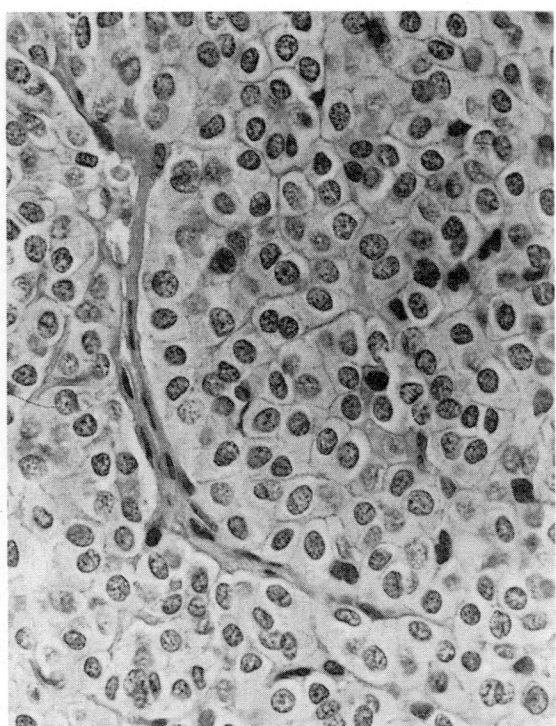

Fig. 8. Glomus tumour. Glomic tumour cells centered by punched-out round nuclei. HES

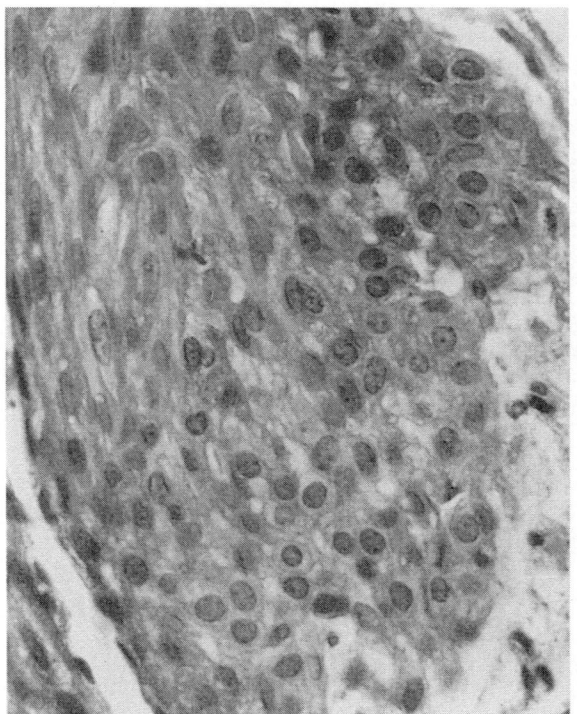

Fig. 9. Glomus tumour. Elongated, spindle-shape glomic cells with two regular mitotic figures. HES

Some variants exist. A compact glomus tumour is almost devoid of stroma; there are glomus tumours with a myxoid stroma, glomus tumours with prominent vascular ectasia (glomangioma) (Fig. 10) and glomus tumours rich in smooth muscle cells (glomangiomyoma). In the epithelioid variant, the tumour cells present both epithelioid and myoid features. Some cells are small with dark round nuclei and scanty cytoplasm; others are large, polygonal or spindle-shaped, with abundant eosinophilic cytoplasm and irregular nuclei (Fig. 11-12) [29]. In glomangioma, hyalinization of vessel walls (Fig. 13) and calcified thrombi may be present. In the rarest subtype, the large hyperplastic smooth muscle cells merge with the surrounding normal glomus cells. Immunohistochemistry displays reactivity with vimentin and alpha2– smooth muscle actin in all cases and desmin in 73% of cases. Reactivity with cytokeratin and S100 protein is negative in all instances [30]. The location and symptomatology of a glomus tumour are clearly important in differential diagnosis. This includes cutaneous adnexal tumour with ductal differentiation, an epithelioid leiomyoma (leiomyoblastoma), an haemangiopericytoma, a non-chromaffin paraganglioma (chemodectoma) when the tu-

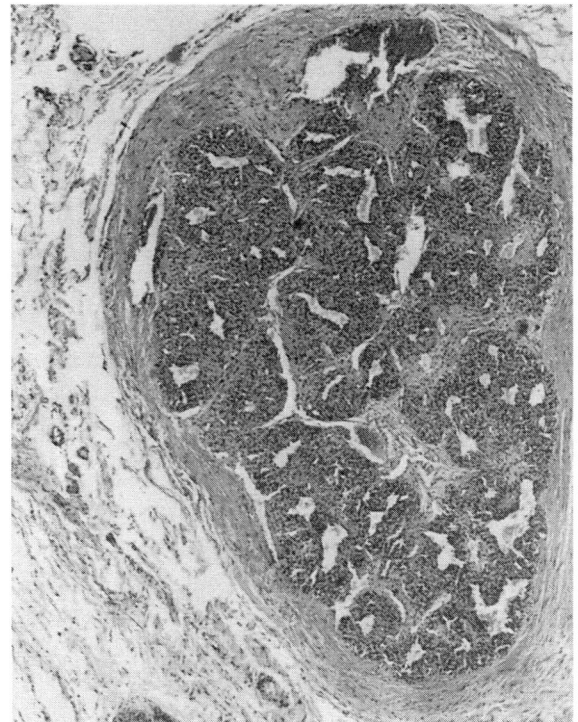

Fig. 10. Glomangioma with ectatic vessels. HES

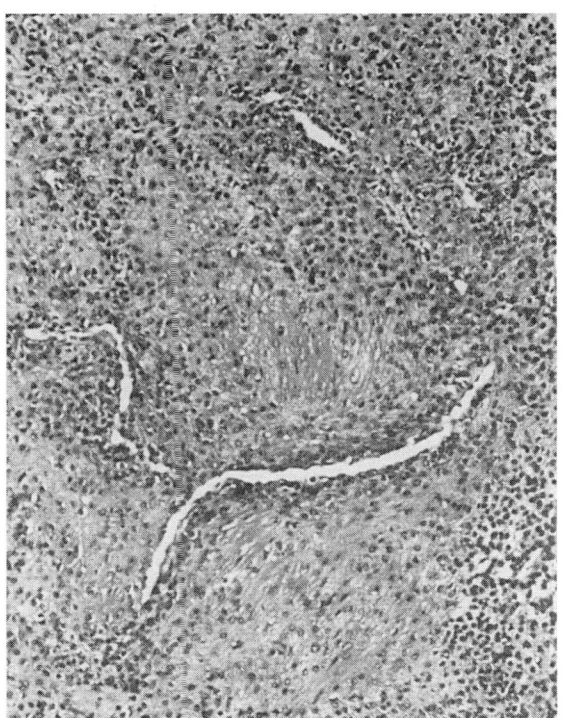

Fig. 11. Glomangioma. Epithelioid variant. HES

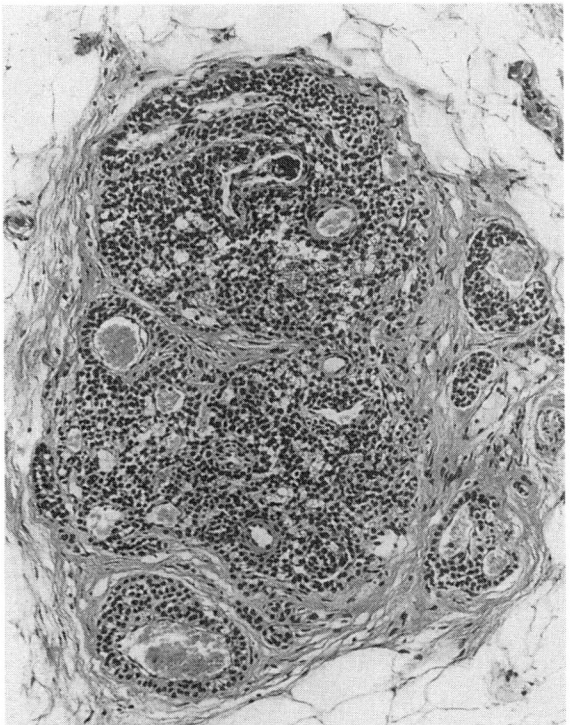

Fig. 12. Glomangioma. Epithelioid variant. HES

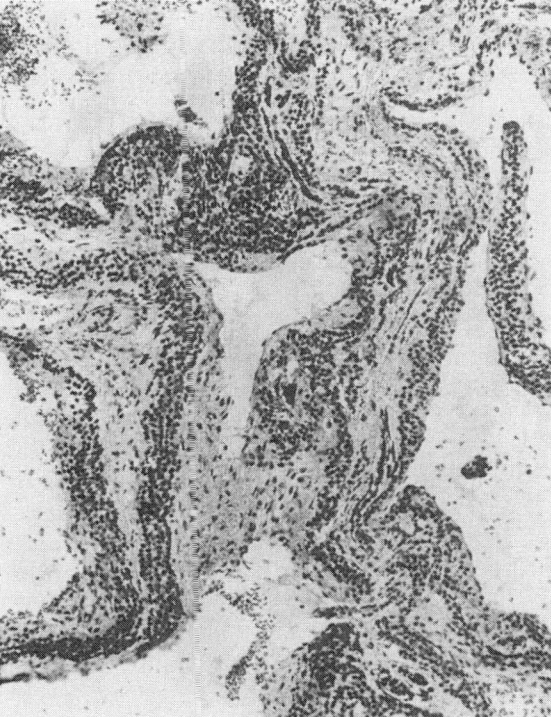

Fig. 13. Glomangioma. Note hyalinization of vascular wall. HES

mour is highly vascular, and a hypervascularized naevocellular naevus. In an epithelioid leiomyoma, tumour cells are larger and more eosinophilic. The tumour cells of an epithelioid leiomyoma or an haemangiopericytoma usually show organoid arrangement around vessels. A glomus tumour in the bones of the digits should not be misinterpreted as an haemangio-endothelioma, which has a poor prognosis and should be treated by amputation [27]. In a non-chromaffin paraganglioma (chemodectoma), tumour cells are larger but have an ill-defined cytoplasm. The cells are enclosed by vessels, unlike those in a glomus tumour and haemangiopericytoma. A naevocellular nevus may mimic a glomus tumour when melanocytes surround vascular slits, but melanocytes are larger and frequently pleomorphic. An epithelial tumour can be ruled out by immunohistochemistry.

Haemangiopericytoma

This lesion is produced by proliferation of the pericapillary cells or pericytes of Zimmerman [31]; contractile, modified smooth muscle cells are arranged in an interlacing network around the outer aspect of the basement membrane of capillary vessels. This rare tumour affects all ages, with a peak between 40 to 50 years. There is a predilection for men, generally in the ratio of 2: 1. Congenital hemangiopericytoma has been described [32, 33]. Haemangiopericytoma may develop almost anywhere in the body – skin, breasts, nose and paranasal sinuses, orbits, meninges, soft tissues, lungs, kidneys, gut, mesentery and peritoneum (Fig. 14), uterus, and spinal cord have all been reported [34-38], but the most common locations are the lower extremities and the retroperitoneum. Bone involvement is rare but the pelvis, femur, ankle and foot, skull and vertebrae have been involved [27, 39-41]. Haemangiopericytoma presents as a slow-growing, painless, highly vascular mass. Occasionally, a bruit can be heard. Associated hypoglycaemia [42, 43], a masculinization syndrome, and abnormal secretion of renin with hypertension and hypokalaemia [44] and a Kasabach-Merritt syndrome [32] have been reported in some cases. The tumours may recur after local excision and as many as 50% of malignant haemangiopericytomas metastasize within a period of 5 years to the lungs, and liver, and, less commonly, to the bone and regional lymph nodes [45]. Location is an important prognostic factor [46]. Malignant haemangiopericytoma frequently occurs in the lower extremities, especially in the thigh. Hemangiopericytomas of the nose and paranasal sinuses are

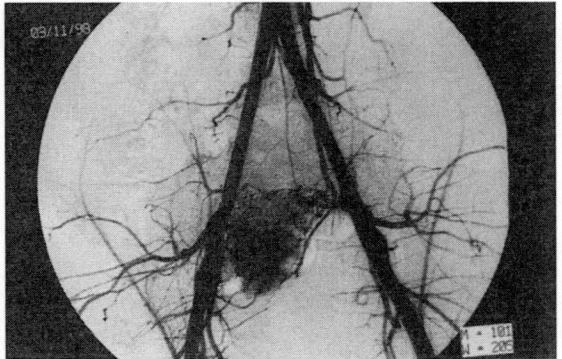

Fig. 14. Haemangiopericytoma. 25 yo woman patient. Pelvic haemangiopericytoma with rich vascularization evidenced by selective angiogram. (Courtesy Dr R. Baumer)

thought to behave less aggressively than those occurring in other parts of the body. Lymph node metastasis is rare and elective neck dissection is not indicated [47]. Hatva et al [48] recently demonstrated an upregulation of the endothelial cell mitogen vascular growth factors (VEGF) and its two receptor tyrosine kinases VEGFR-1(FLT1) and VEGFR-2(KDR) in hemangiopericytomas. These substances are known to stimulate angiogenesis and are up-regulated during the malignant progression of gliomas.

Pathology and differential diagnosis

The tumour is usually a well circumscribed nodule surrounded by a thin capsule (Fig. 15). Usually from 2 to 5 cm in diameter, it rarely reaches 10 cm. On cut section, it is grayish-white to reddish-brown and hypervascular. Haemorrhage and cyst formation may be present. Histologically, the tumour consists of a monomorphous proliferation of ovoid, round, or spindle-shaped cells having little eosinophilic cytoplasm and a centrally-placed, ovoid, and clear nucleus. These cells are packed around numerous anastomosing thin-walled sinusoidal vessels with a staghorn or antlerlike configuration, and are lined by a single endothelial layer (Fig. 16). Some myocytes are present at the outer aspect of the basement membrane. Reticulin stains helps demonstrate that the tumour cells are outside the basement membrane of the endothelium and hence are pericytes rather than endothelial cells. A reticulin meshwork, radiating from vessels, encloses each tumour cell (Fig. 17). In solid areas, vascular cavities are compressed by elongated tumour cells, which display a palisading arrangement of their nuclei. The stroma may contain mucoid material intermingled with some lymphocyte infiltrates. A lipomatous component may be present [49]. Calcification is exceptional. Ultrastructural study

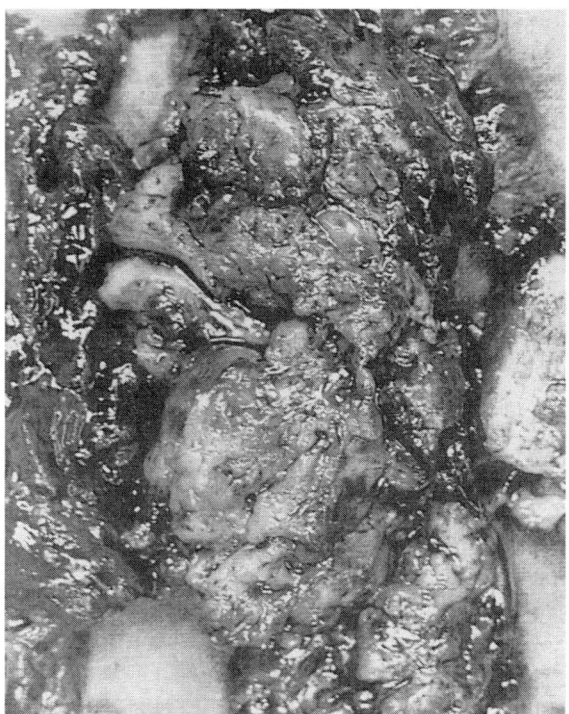

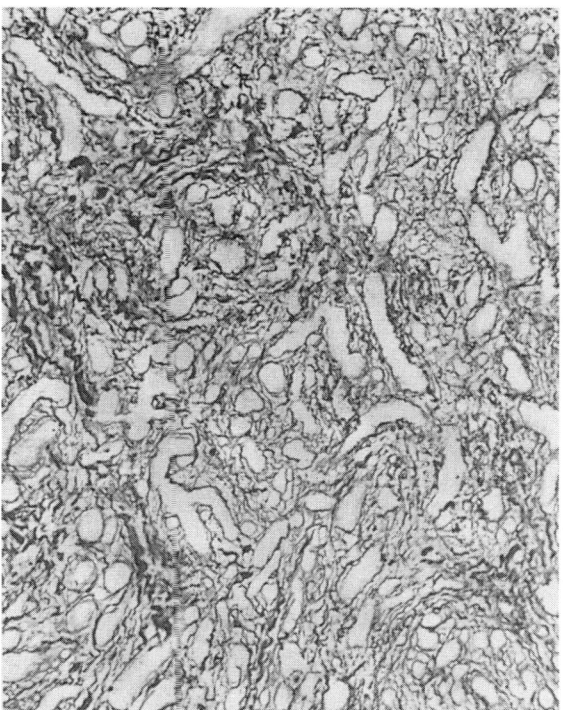

Fig. 15. Haemangiopericytoma. Peritoneal haemangiopericytoma made up of circumscribed masses bulging from the surrounding tissue

Fig. 17. Haemangiopericytoma. Reticulin meshwork radiating from vessels enclosing each tumour cell. Gordon-Sweet stain

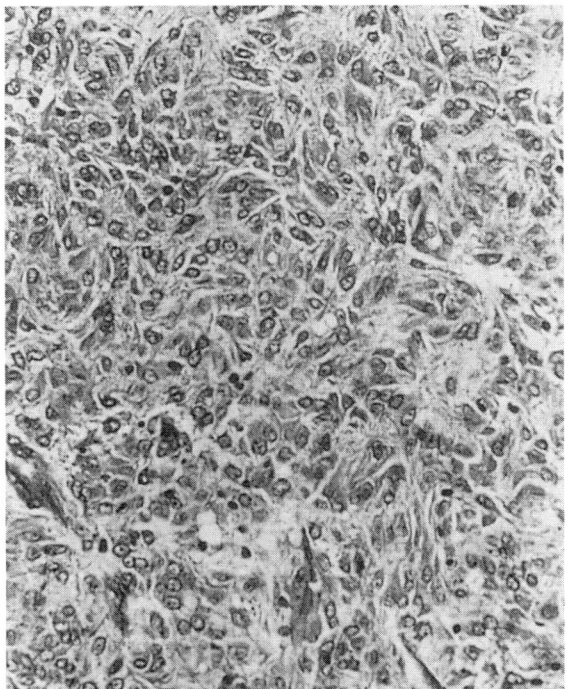

Fig. 16. Haemangiopericytoma. Ovoid or spindle-shaped tumour cells surrounding small thin-walled sinusoidal vessels. HES

clearly traces the pericytic nature of the tumour cells [50, 51], which are separated from the endothelial lining by a basement membrane. Their cytoplasm contains small bundles of filaments. Immunohistochemistry shows reactivity of tumour cells for vimentin with or without associated positivity for CD34 and CD57. Hemangiopericytoma lacks other immunodeterminants of epithelial, neural differentiation. Alpha-smooth muscle actin isotype may be focally positive [52-54]. A subpopulation of tumour cells also expresses F-XIII and HLA-DR antigens [55]. These tumour cells are clearly different from endothelial cells (Fig. 18)

The diagnosis of benign versus malignant haemangiopericytoma may be very difficult and some tumours that recur and metastasize have an innocent appearance. Distinction can be made by an extensive study of the cellular pattern (cellularity, cellular differentiation and pleomorphism, number of mitotic figures), the nature of the stromal changes (haemorrhage, necrosis) and the vascular invasion [56]. Malignant tumours are usually larger (measuring more than 10 cm diameter).

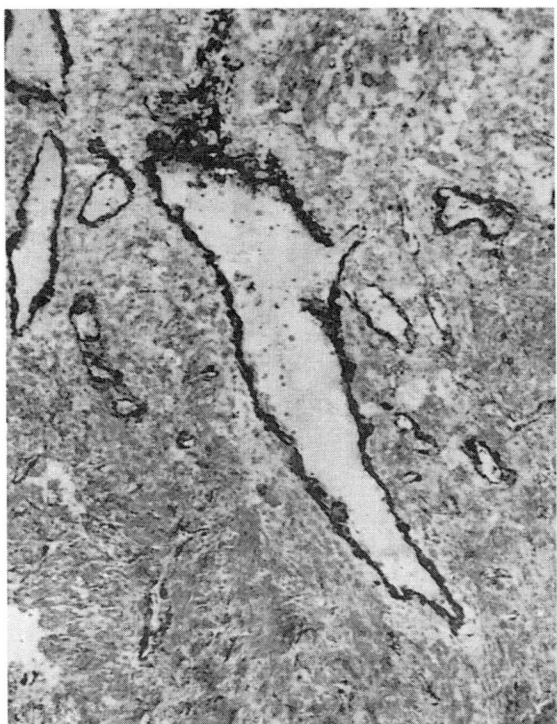

Fig. 18. Haemangiopericytoma. Endothelial cells lining the sinusoidal vessels are labelled by factor VIII related antigen (FVIIIR-Ag). Peroxidase-antiperoxidase immunohistochemical technique (PAP)

Hypercellularity and greater cellular polymorphism are frequent, as is vascular invasion, stromal haemorrhage and necrosis. Recurrences and metastasis are likely when the tumour has 4 or more mitotic figures per 10 high power fields. In differential diagnosis, the vascular component of haemangiopericytoma may suggest a glomus tumour, a vascularized leiomyoma, an haemangioma or a renal renin glomerular tumour. In the last instance the clinical history will be different (arterial hypertension, high renin). Palisading nuclei in compact areas may mimic a schwanoma. Dural-based or "central" hemangiopericytomas (cHPCs) should be differentiated from meningiomas. Neurofibromatosis 2 (NF2) gene analysis and cytogenetic study may be helpful in distinguishing the two entities. No NF2 mutations are found in either central HPCs or peripheral HPCs, whereas 35% of meningiomas present NF2 gene alterations [57]. Cytogenetic studies on meningioma demonstrate monosomy or partial deletion of chromosome 22 in 60% ; conversely, hemangiopericytomas never present monosomy 22, but are hyperdiploid [58]. A case of hemangiopericytoma with translocation t(13; 22) (q22; q11) has been reported by Limon et al [59].

Distinction from a poorly differentiated solid angiosarcoma is afforded by the reticulin staining pattern, which shows the tumour cells in a perivascular reticulin sheath. Some soft tissue tumours can present a focal haemangiomatous pattern: these include malignant fibrous histiocytoma, which is more pleomorphic and contains foamy histiocytes interspersed with giant cells; extra-skeletal mesenchymal chondrosarcoma, which is made up of well differentiated cartilage and areas of spindle cell proliferation; and synovial sarcoma, which is usually multinodular, and painful, and which harbors a focal biphasic pattern characterized by the presence of muco-secreting glands. Myxoid liposarcoma should be excluded when the interstitial mucoid material is abundant.

Lymphangiopericytoma

Some authors regard this tumour as having a semi-malignant potential but too few reports exist to define the clinical course, prognosis, and treatment of the lesion [60, 61]. Histologically, it consisted of cords of cells resembling pericytes arranged around endothelial-bordered vascular slits and circumscribed by a lymphatic plexus.

Malignant tumours

Angioleiomyosarcoma

This is a rare tumour which develops from smooth muscle cells of the intima or media. All patients are adults. Clinically, the symptoms depend on the location: chest pain, cough, haemoptysis and acute pulmonary oedema, dyspnoea, and tachycardia may all occur. A venous origin is five times more common than an arterial one. The inferior vena cava, especially in its superior part, is by far the most common site, and is involved in half of the cases seen [62-66]. In a series of 89 cases of leiomyosarcomas of the inferior vena cava reviewed by Kieffer et al [67], the mean age at presentation was 54,3 yr with a female predominance (F/M: 3.9). Occlusion gives rise to a Budd-Chiari syndrome. Leiomyosarcoma is rare in the superior vena cava and in the low-pressured pulmonary vessels [68-70]. Involvement of the peripheral veins often presents no remarkable symptomatoly [71]. Some reports on arterial leiomyosarcomas dealt with the aorta, the carotid, and the subclavian artery [72, 73]. For great vessels, the tumour can be diagnosed by intraluminal catheter suction biopsy [74, 75]. In bones, leiomyosarcoma arise from the intraosseous vascular smooth muscle cells. Radiographically, the tumour appears osteolytic with a geographic or moth-eaten appearance and is devoid of sclerotic margin [76]. Local growth and metastases leading to obstruction of the cardiac outflow are fatal. Recurrences and regional extensions to the viscera and the retroperitoneum are rapid and constant after resection. Metastasis to the lumbar vertebrae causes lumbago, pain and paraplagia. Primary renal vein leiomyosarcoma can obstruct the infrahepatic inferior vena cava (IVC) by endoluminal propagation [77]. In the vena cava, intraluminal extension involves the right sided cardiac cavities, resulting in thrombosis and obstruction. Embolism occurs in the pulmonary arteries; metastases are multiple and frequent. The prognosis of leiomyosarcoma of the inferior vena cava is poor; the location is dangerous and the state of differentiation usually poor. The frequency of metastases reported is more than 35% [78]. Arterial leiomyosarcoma may leak leading to an inflammatory aneurysm [79].

Pathology and differential diagnosis

The tumour often presents as a stenotic mass infiltrating the vessel wall and extending into neighboring viscera. Rarely, a bud protrudes into the lumen and the atrial cavities. The morphological pattern is that of any leiomyosarcoma of smooth muscle; it is made up of interlacing bundles of smooth muscle cells having an eosinophilic cytoplasm and a blunt-ended nucleus (Fig. 19-20). Nuclear palisading may be present. Periodic acid-Schiff staining may show perinuclear glycogen vacuoles. It is difficult to confirm malignancy when tumour cells appear regular and mitoses are rare (Fig. 21-22-23) but haemorrhage, necrosis, a pleomorphic pattern, and the presence of mitotic activity (more than 5 mitoses per ten high power fields) are suggestive of aggressive behavior. The differential diagnosis consists of ruling out other vascular sarcomas. Immunohistochemical study helps to identify the cellular types.

Other miscellaneous sarcomas

Vascular sarcomas may arise from any component of the wall. Occasionally, a tumour of vascular cell origin may be associated with a vascular prothesis [80]. The diagnosis of intimal sarcoma can be made on material obtained from vascular unblocking procedures.

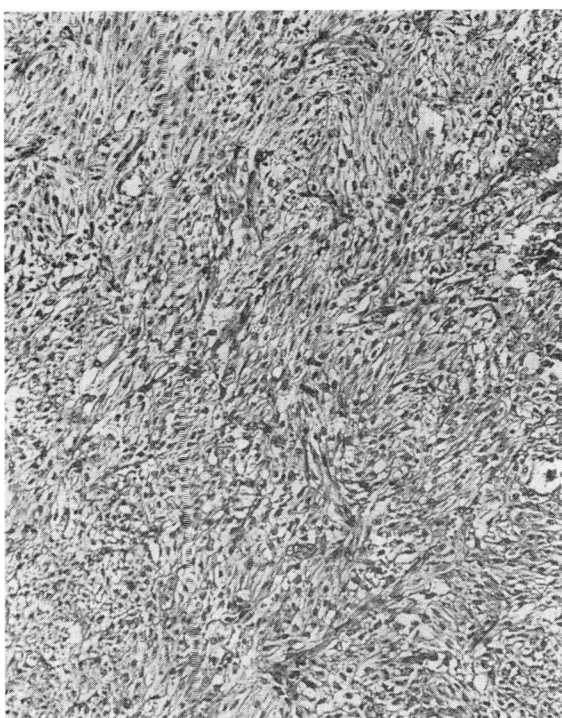

Fig. 19. Angioleiomyosarcoma. Leiomyosarcoma of the renal vein. Note tumour hypercellularity. HES

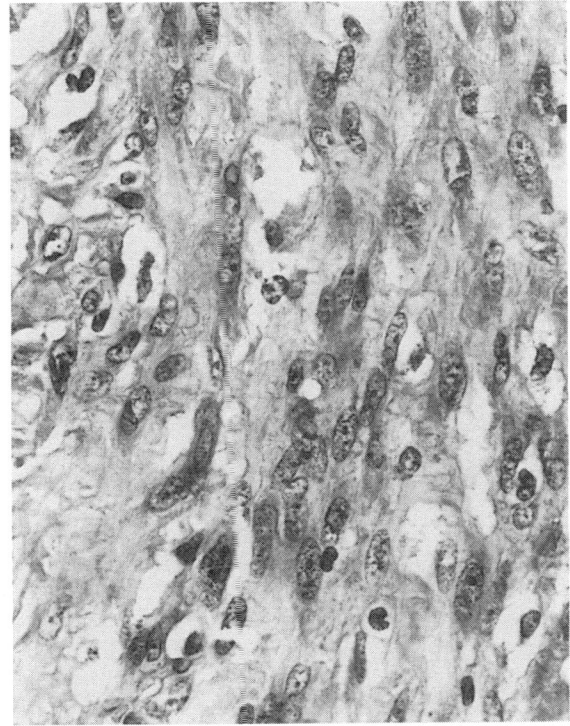

Fig. 20. Angioleiomyosarcoma. Leiomyosarcoma of the renal vein made up of interlacing bundles of atypical smooth muscle cells. HES

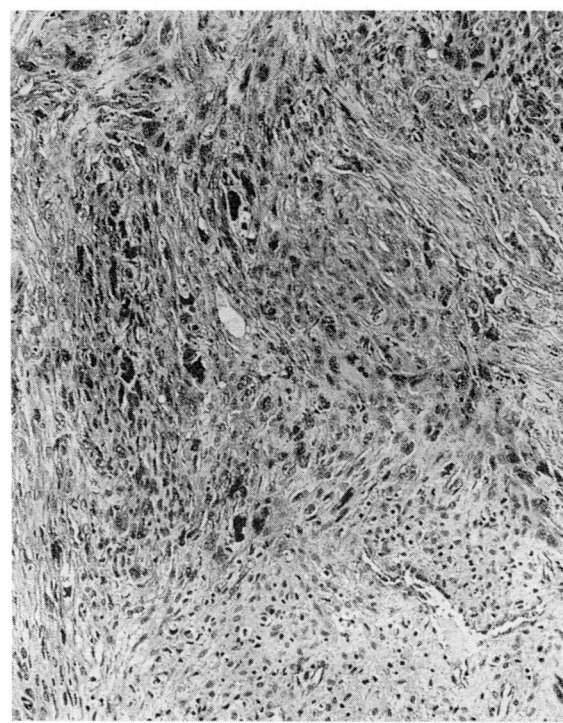
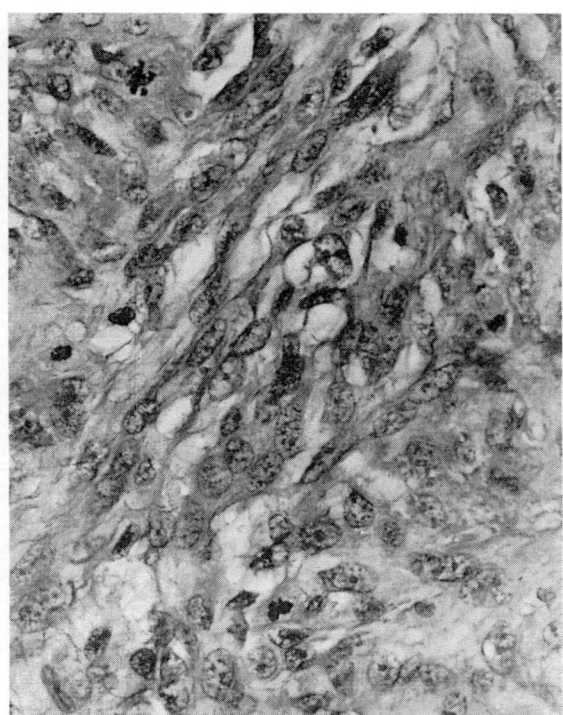

Fig. 21-22. Angioleiomyosarcoma. Leiomyosarcoma of the renal vein. Sarcomatous smooth muscle cells centered by blunt-ended nuclei. HES

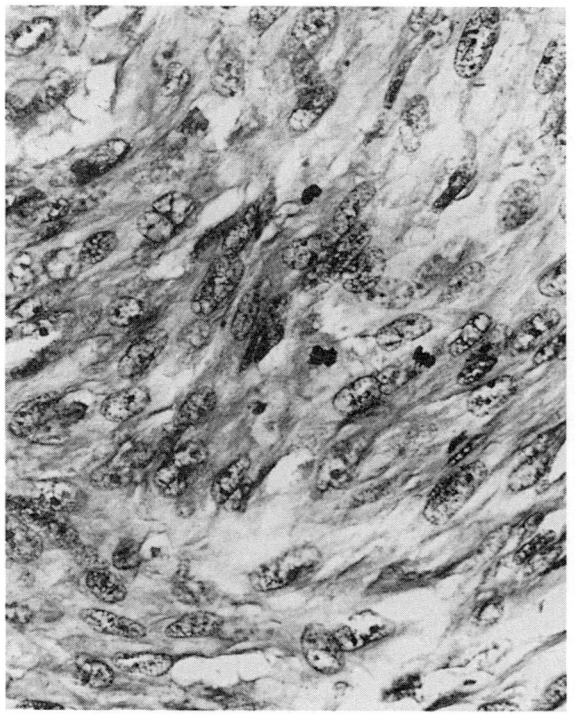

Fig. 23. Angioleiomyosarcoma. Leiomyosarcoma of the renal vein. Aggressive tumour behavior evidenced by the presence of mitotic activity. HES

Pathology and differential diagnosis

Vascular sarcomas usually resemble parietal thrombi protruding into the arterial lumen. Very often they creep along the arterial wall, separating the intima from the underlying layers. This kind of spreading brings about the appearance often described as "intimal sarcoma", (Fig. 24-25) which mostly occurs in the aorta. One third of the cases involve the descending aorta. Histologically, the nature of the proliferation may vary; a poorly differentiated fibroblastic sarcoma made up of spindle cells with varying degrees of atypia, pleomorphism and necrosis is perhaps commonest (Fig. 26-28). Fibroxanthosarcoma and malignant fibrous histiocytomas may harbour epithelioid tumour cells. Angiosarcomas, comprised of haphazardly arranged spindle cells and giant cells displaying aberrant differentiation, are seen in this pattern, and malignant mesenchymoma, rhabdomyosarcoma, chondrosarcoma, and osteosarcoma may all present in this way [81, 82].

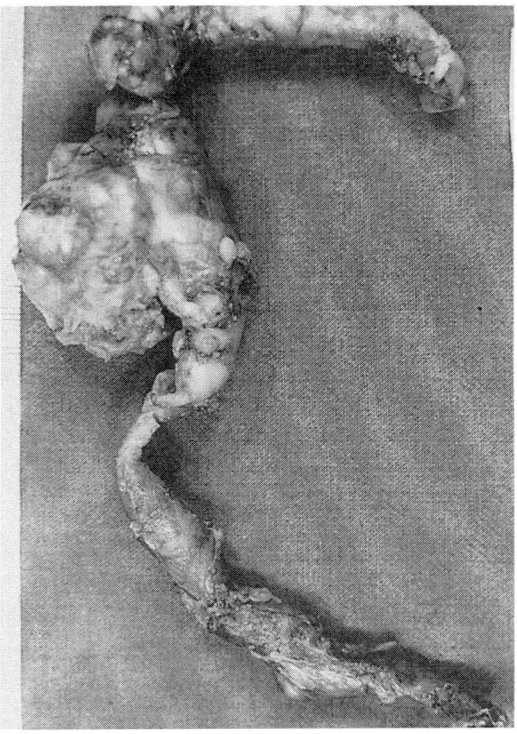

Fig. 24. Vascular sarcoma. Sarcoma of the external saphenous vein in a woman. (Courtesy Dr Ch. Lebard)

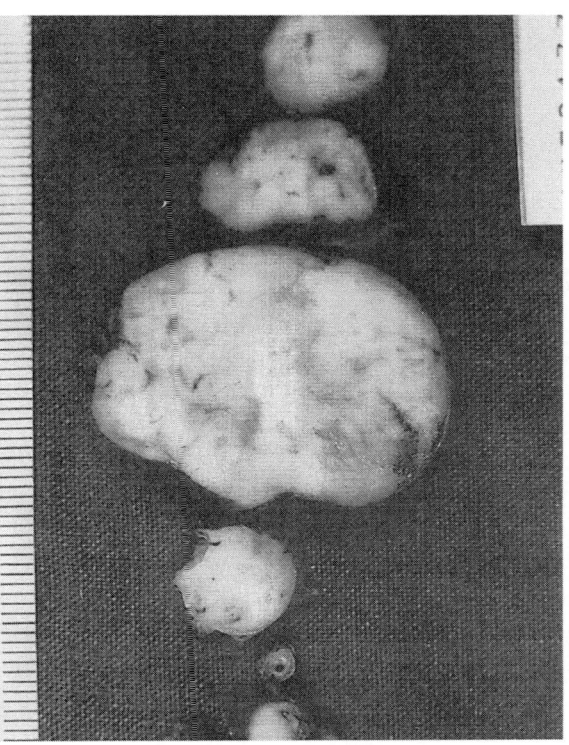

Fig. 25. Vascular sarcoma. Sarcoma of the external saphenous vein. Cut section

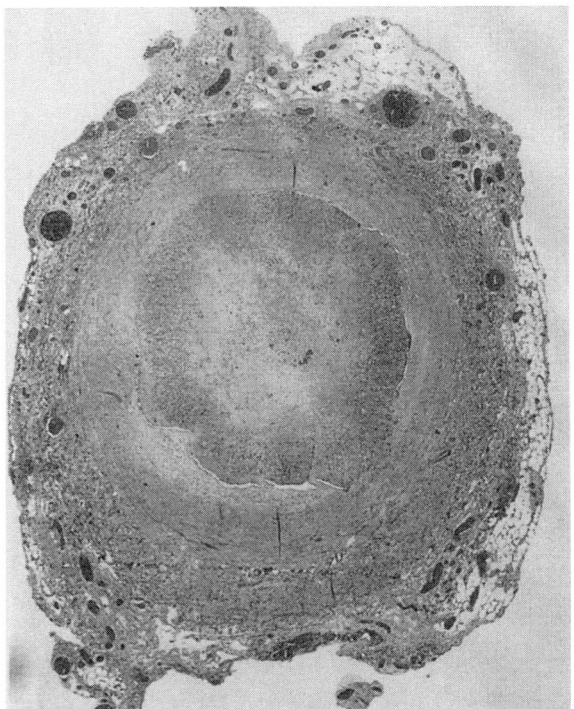

Fig. 26. Vascular sarcoma. Occlusive pleomorphic sarcoma thickening the intima. HES

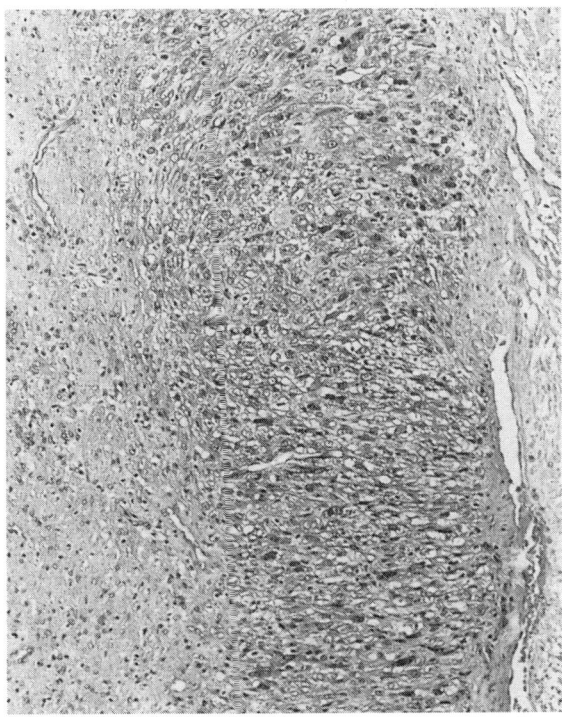

Fig. 27. Vascular sarcoma. Intimal pleomorphic sarcoma. HES

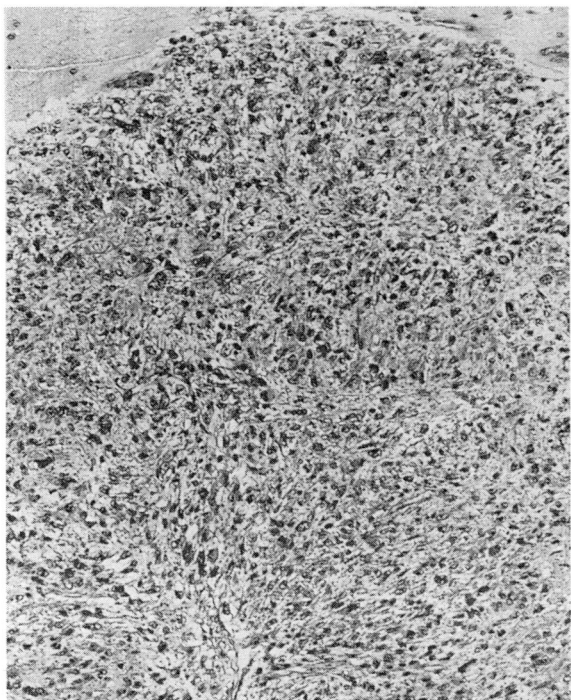

Fig. 28. Vascular sarcoma. Intimal pleomorphic sarcoma showing marked cellular atypia. HES

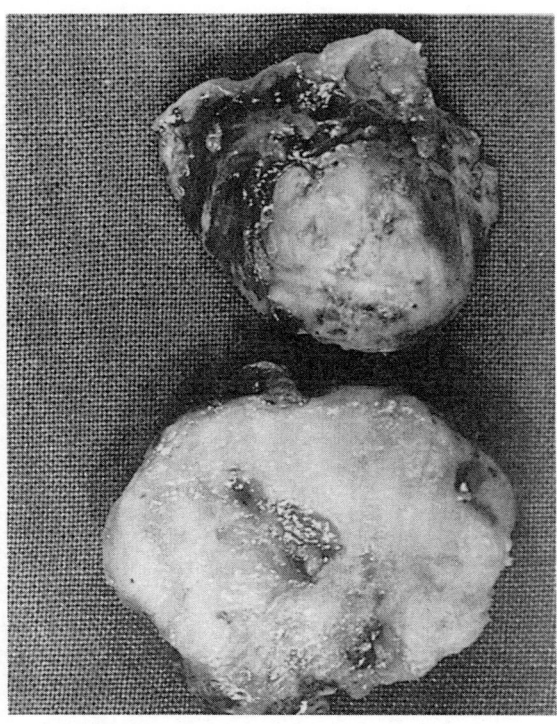

Fig. 29. Renin-secreting cell tumour of the kidney. (Courtesy Dr E. Baviera)

2 – Tumours of vascular-related structures

Juxtaglomerular renin-secreting tumour

This benign renal tumour is rare. Controversy exists regarding its origin, which derives from the renin-secreting cells of the juxtaglomerular apparatus. It is considered to be an hamartoma [83]. Clinical presentation is characterized by arterial hypertension together with a high plasma renin, hyperaldosteronism and hypokalaemia. Teenagers represent the largest single population with JCT (39%) and approximately two-thirds of the entire population are female. Renal angiography is initially negative in more than half the cases. Computerized tomography often demonstrates a renal mass even when other imaging studies remain negative. Postoperatively, the blood pressure is promptly normalized and the plasma renin activity level decreased. Recurrences or metastasis have never been reported, even after a mean follow-up of 98 months (range 24 to 204) [84-90].

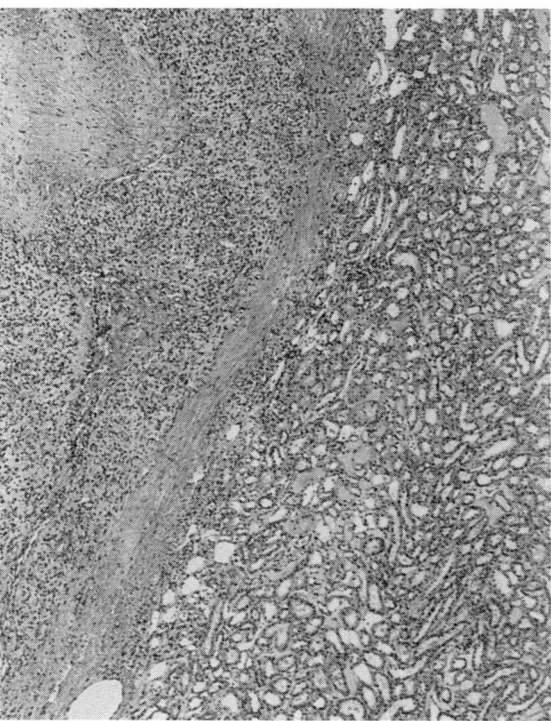

Fig. 30. Renin-secreting cell tumour of the kidney. Well-limited tumour with well-preserved renal parenchyma beyond. HES

Pathology and differential diagnosis

In the kidney, the tumour is small, measuring from 2mm to 4 cm in diameter. It is yellowish in colour with some haemorrhagic areas, polylobular, and well-delineated from the surrounding parenchyma (Fig. 29). Histologically, there is a well-limited and vascularised proliferation of cells having an endocrine pattern, made up of secreting cells resembling the epithelioid cells of a normal juxtaglomerular apparatus (Fig. 30-31). The cells have a polyhedral clear, eosinophilic and finely granular cytoplasm with a central round, regular nucleus. No atypia or mitoses are seen. There is a reticulin network, which continues the basal lamina of stromal capillaries and encloses nests of tumour cells or individual cells, mimicking an haemangiopericytoma (Fig. 32) with similar reticulin meshwork enclosing each tumour cell (Fig. 33). In some areas, the tumour cells are elongated, spindle-shaped (Fig. 34-35) and interspersed with numerous mastocytes easily recognizable in Giemsa staining (Fig. 36) [91]. Some tumours present a tubular

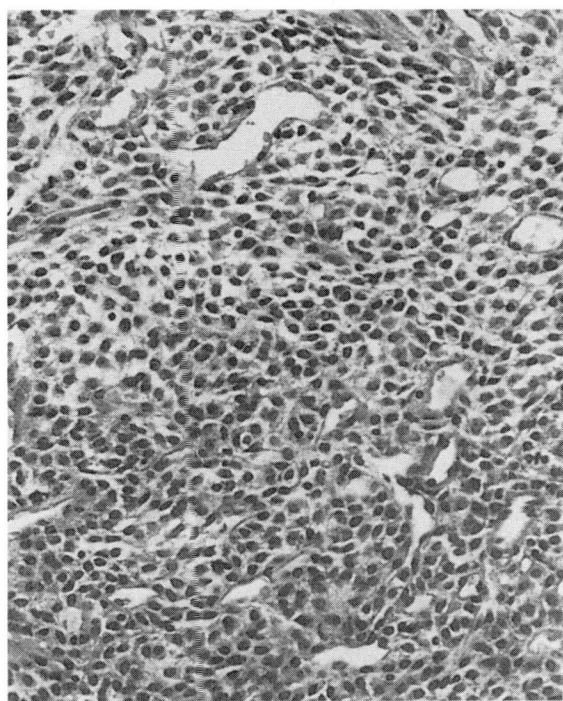

Fig. 32. Renin-secreting cell tumour of the kidney. Area displaying a pattern mimicking an haemangiopericytoma. HES

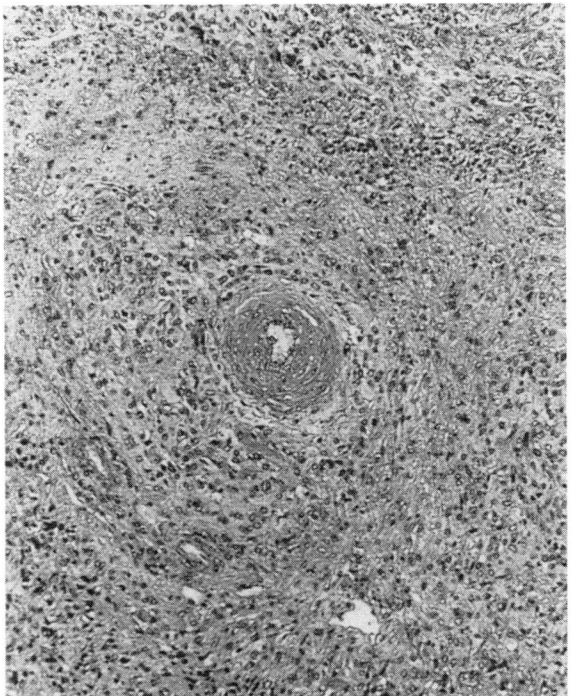

Fig. 31. Renin-secreting cell tumour of the kidney. Regular tumour cells arranged in trabeculae separated by numerous anastomotic capillaries. HES

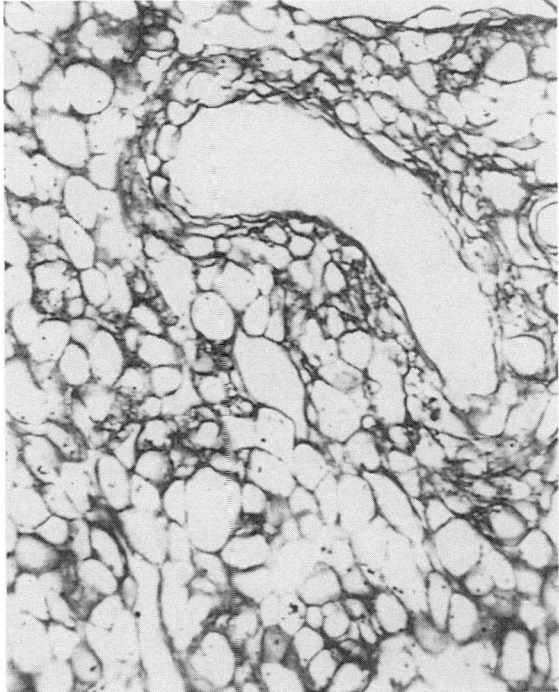

Fig. 33. Renin-secreting cell tumour of the kidney. Reticulin meshwork surrounding tumour cells presenting a pattern similar to that of an haemangiopericytoma

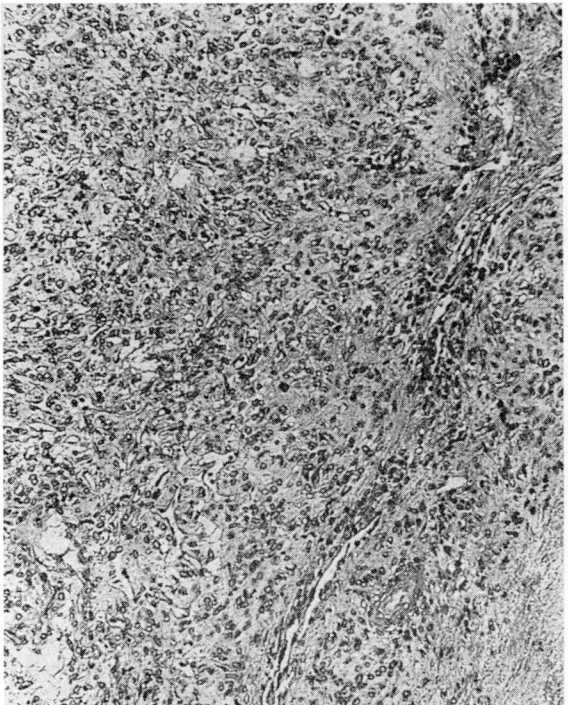

Fig. 34. Renin-secreting cell tumour of the kidney. Elongated tumour cells. HES

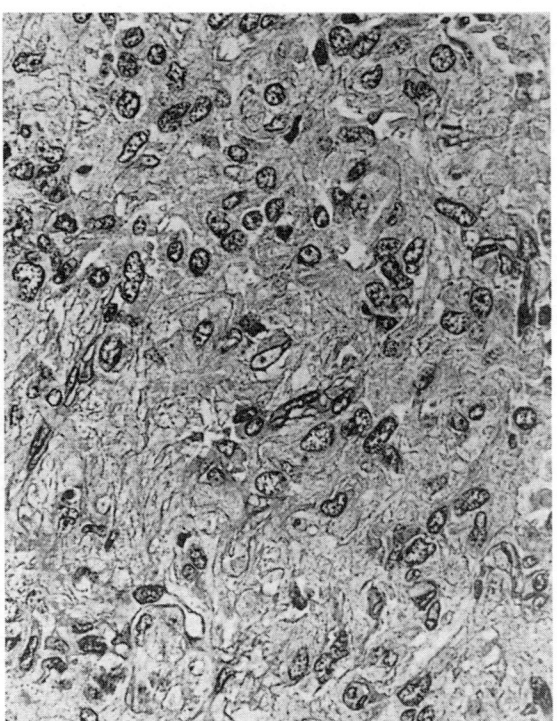

Fig. 35. Renin-secreting cell tumour of the kidney. Spindle-shaped tumour cells. HES

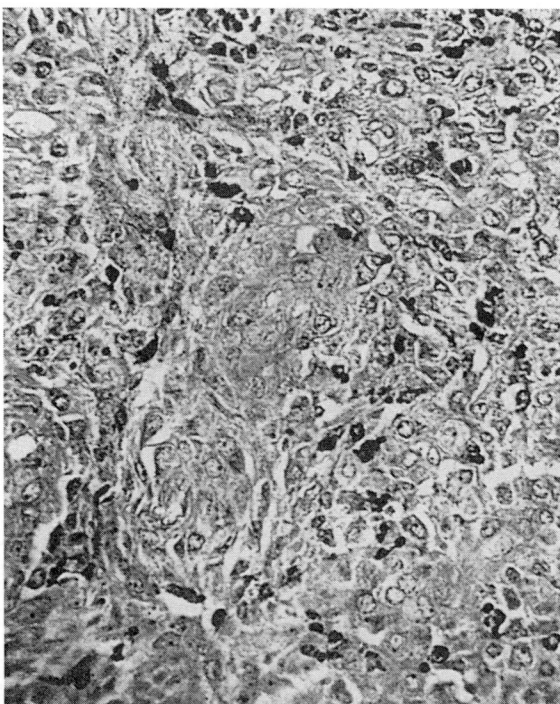

Fig. 36. Renin-secreting cell tumour of the kidney. Numerous mastocytes are present within the tumour. Giemsa

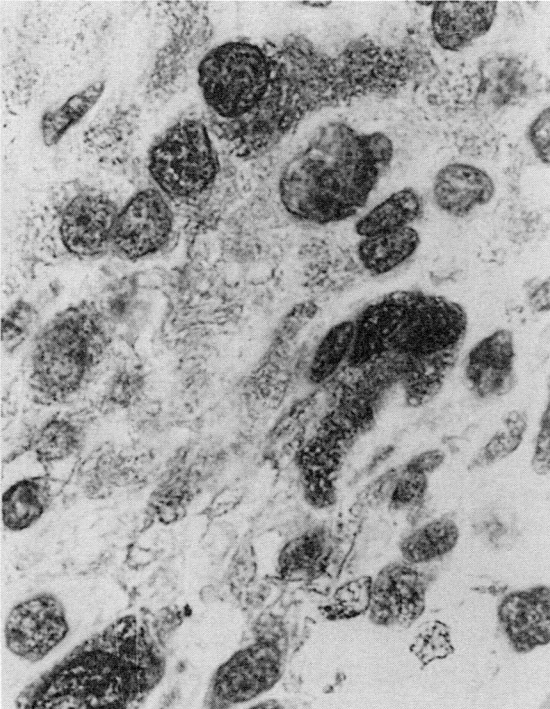

Fig. 37. Renin-secreting cell tumour of the kidney. Strong reactivity of tumour cells with renin antibody. PAP

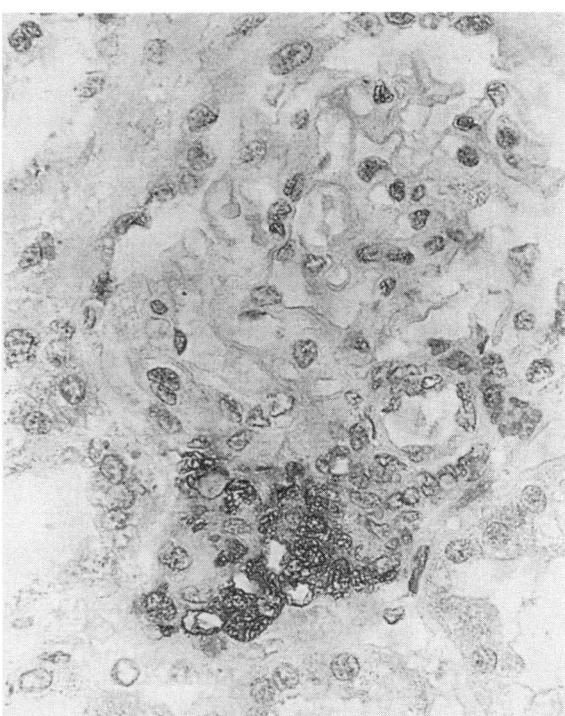

Fig. 38. Renin-secreting cell tumour of the kidney. Hyperplasia of the glomerular renin-secreting-apparatus cells in the neighbouring renal parenchyma. PAP

differentiation with nerve fibers inside [92-94], others a papillary pattern. Electron microscopy helps identify typical rhomboid granules corresponding with the specific granules of juxtaglomerular cells [95]. Immunohistochemical study displays a strong reactivity of tumour cells with renin antiserum (Fig. 37-38) [96-98].

Differential diagnosis consists of ruling out an haemangiopericytoma. Juxtaglomerular renin-secreting tumours present a different clinical and biological pattern, although some rare haemangiopericytomata may secrete renin as exceptionally do other renal tumours (nephroblastomas, adenocarcinomas) and extrarenal tumours (broncho-pulmonary cancers, ovarian, fallopian and pituitary tumours, alveolar sarcomas, epithelioid sarcoma, leiomyosarcoma) [44, 99, 100]. Immunohistochemical findings are totally different. Moreover, mastocytes are present in great abundance in renin-secreting tumours. Hayami et al [101] described a case of juxta-glomerular cell tumour without hypertension, unlike all previously reported cases.

Tumours of the paraganglia

The paraganglia are clusters of neuroendocrine cells dispersed throughout the body; innervation is both sympathetic and parasympathetic. Some terms are uniformly used, neuroendocrine tumours of the adrenal medulla are phaeochromocytomas and tumours arising in extra-adrenal paraganglia are paragangliomas but some authors designate all of these tumours as "paragangliomas"; others differentiate functioning tumours (extra-adrenal phaeochromocytomas) from non-functioning ones (paragangliomas) [102].

Pheochromocytoma

Although only about 0.1 to 0.3% of hypertensive patients have an underlying phaeochromocyoma, its curability and the fact that the hypertension can be fatal when the tumour remains unrecognized make diagnosis important. Ninety percent of phaeochromocyomas occur sporadically in adults (40 to 60 years) with a slight predilection for women. About one-third of patients experience paroxysmal hypertension, precipitated by nervousness, anxiety, exercise, and changes in posture. In another third, the hypertension is intermittent; in the remaining third, it is sustained without paroxysms. Ten percent of patients have puffy, red, or cyanotic hands. A sudden release of catecholamines may precipitate congestive heart failure, provoke ventricular fibrillation by direct toxicity, or may induce vasomotor constriction of the myocardial circulation, leading to myocardial infarction and even death. Pheochromocytoma is rarely observed during pregnancy and not easily diagnosed, especially since the clinical manifestations may mimic common gravid hypertension [103]. Occasionally, a phaeochromocyoma produces other biogenic steroids or peptides, ACTH, erythropoietin, prostaglandins, a parathormone-like substance and renin [99]. Association with Cushing's syndrome or some other endocrinopathy is possible. Around 10% of cases occur as part of familial syndromes including von Hippel-Lindau disease (14%) and the familial multiple endocrine neoplasm (MEN) syndrome with an autosomal dominant trait inheritance [104, 105]. In these instances, the tumour develops in childhood, with a strong male preponderance. Phaeochromocyomas and medullary thyroid carcinomas are also part of the multiple endocrine neoplasm or MEN II (Sipple's) syndrome, sometimes referred to as MEN 2A and MEN 2B or the "medullary thyroid carcinoma-phaeochromocyoma" syndrome

[106] characterized by mutations of the receptor tyrosine kinase (RET) proto-oncogene on chromosome 10; the mutant gene can be found in these concomitant tumours [107].

Most tumours are larger than 2 cm and 90% occur in the medulla of the adrenals with a preponderance on the right. Bilaterality is present in 10-15% of cases. This frequency is higher for phaeochromocyomas in the other familial syndromes (70%) [104]. Extraadrenal phaeochromocyomas mostly occur in young adults (20-30) with no sex predisposition. These tumours develop wherever chromaffin tissue exists, or in any paraganglia along the sympathetic chain, most often below the diaphragm [102]. Most of them are densely adherent to adjacent vessels and difficult to remove. Multifocality is evident in 15 to 25% of patients. Two to ten percent of adrenal phaeochromocyoma are malignant. This frequency is higher in extra-adrenal tumours (20-40%). Some malignancy markers have been suggested: MIB-1 labelling index, male gender, extra-adrenal location, tumour weight, and young age [108]. Metastases in lymph nodes, liver, lungs, and bones may be functional. They should be differentiated from multiple, independently-born tumours, especially when they are in a site normally devoid of chromaffin tissue [109]. Survival after metastatic spread rarely exceeds 3 years.

Pathology and differential diagnosis

Grossly, these tumours are firm, and tan-red on cross section. Their diameter varies from 1 to 6 cm. The histological pattern varies. They are made up of large, mature-appearing medullary cells with basophilic cytoplasm containing secretory granules (Fig. 39-40-41). In some areas, tumour cells are syncytia-like with indistinct contours or spindle-shaped. They are arranged in cords or clusters (zellballen) surrounded by a hypervascularized stroma containing a delicate reticulin meshwork (Fig. 42) Catecholamine-containing neurosecretory granules are found in most tumour cells. Mitoses may be present in an overtly pleomorphic and anaplastic form. Occasionally, tumour cells can be found lying in the capillaries or sinusoids. However, not all these aspects are reliable criteria for diagnosing malignant phaeochromocyoma. Histological diagnosis of a rare malignant tumour is not possible; local invasion is unreliable and the only good evidence of malignancy is metastasis (Fig. 43).

Other tumours of the extra-adrenal paraganglia

Tumours arising in paravertebral paraganglia and, rarely, the bladder, are innervated by the sympathetic nervous system and are chromaffin positive. About 50% of these "chromaffin paragangliomas" secrete catecholamines.

Chemodectomas are tumours of ganglion cells that sense oxygen and carbon dioxide levels in the blood. These are found in relation to the great vessels (aortico-pulmonary or aortic bodies located predominantly near the ligamentum arteriosum, carotid bodies, jugulotympanic ganglia, ganglion nodosum of the vagus nerve) and in clusters located in the head and neck (mouth, nose, nasopharynx, larynx, and orbits). These paraganglia are innervated by the parasympathetic nervous system, and their tumours are referred to as nonchromaffin paragangliomas. They infrequently release catecholamines. Inhabitants of altitudes higher than 2000 meters above sea level are predisposed to chemodectomas with an evident female predominance (8.3: 1), low rate of bilaterality (5%), and a family history. Three percent of these tumours are malignant [110]. Development of metastases is the only formal proof of malignancy as histology cannot distinguish between benign and malignant chemodectomas [111].

Paragangliomas are also rare. They occur in the sixth decade of life with a slight predilection for women. They usually develop sporadically and singly. Familial cases, transmitted by autosomal dominant trait, are part of the multiple endocrine neoplasm (MEN) II syndrome; the tumours may be multiple and sometimes bilaterally symmetric [112, 113]. The most frequent location is the carotid body. Tumours of other ganglia are rare. A tumour of the jugular glomus may penetrate the middle ear. For tumours located at the skull base, surgical treatment is disappointing. Recurrence often follows incomplete resection [114]. Despite their benign pattern, many metastasize to local and distant sites. About 50% ultimately prove fatal, largely because of infiltrative growth, 30% are malignant and overall about 16 % metastasize widely, causing death [115-117]

Pathology and differential diagnosis

Grossly, these tumours measure 2 to 3 cm and rarely exceed 6 cm in diameter. Surrounded by a thin capsule, they are red-pink to brown on cross section (Fig. 44). Haemorrhage may be present. The histological, immunopathological and ultrastructural pattern of paragangliomas is identical whatever their location. They are composed of lobules or nests (zellballen) of predominant ovoid cells enclosed by trabeculae of fibrous and sustentacular elongated cells (Fig. 45-46-47). The tumour cells have abundant, clear or granular, eosinophilic cytoplasm centered by rather

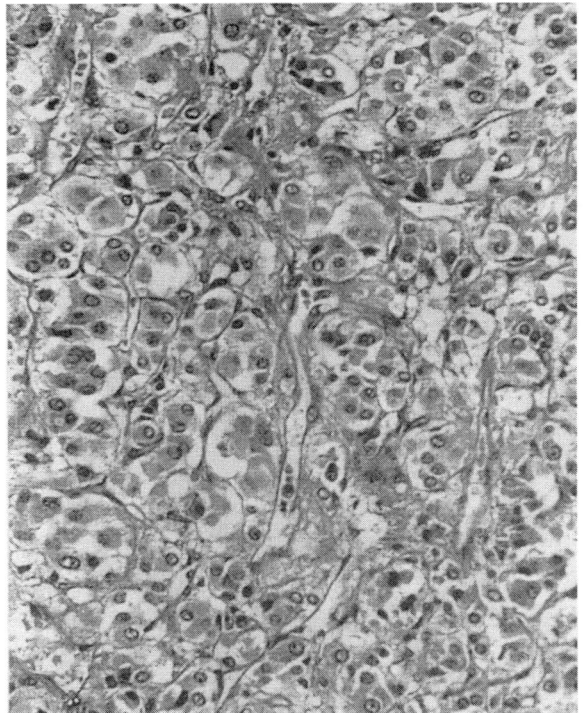

Fig. 39. Phaemochromocytoma made up of large, mature-appearing medullary cells. HES

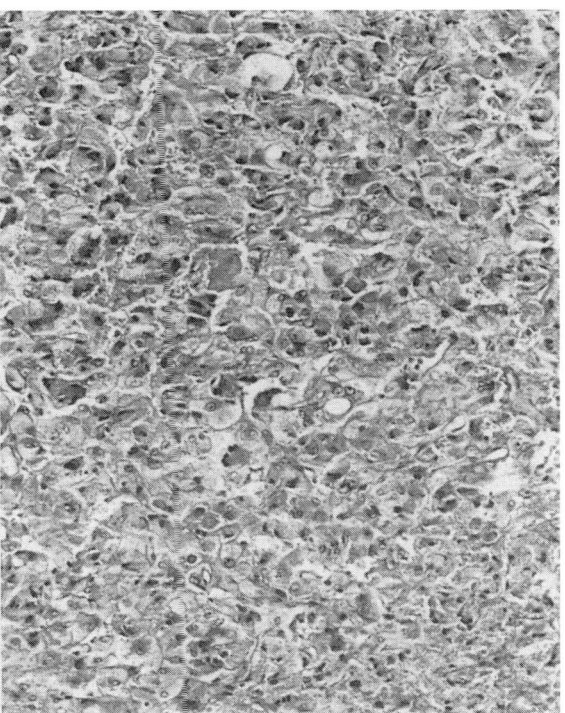

Fig. 40. Phaemochromocytoma. Tumour cells have a basophilic cytoplasm containing secretory granules. HES

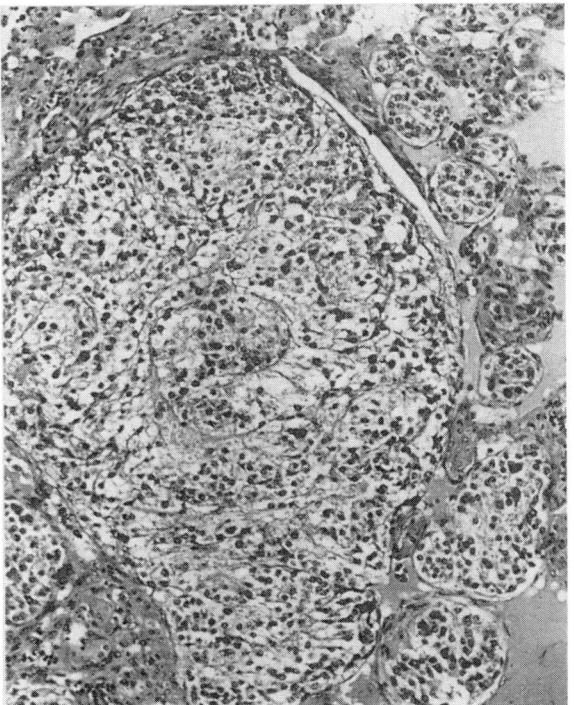

Fig. 41. Phaemochromocytoma. Tumour cells tumour trabeculae protruding in surrounding vascular lumen. HES

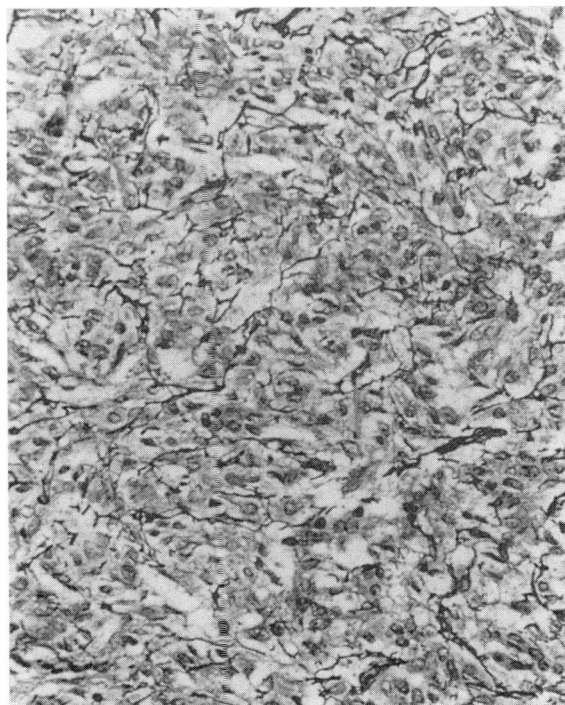

Fig. 42. Phaemochromocytoma. Fine reticulin meshwork enclosing tumour cell trabeculae. Gordon-Sweet

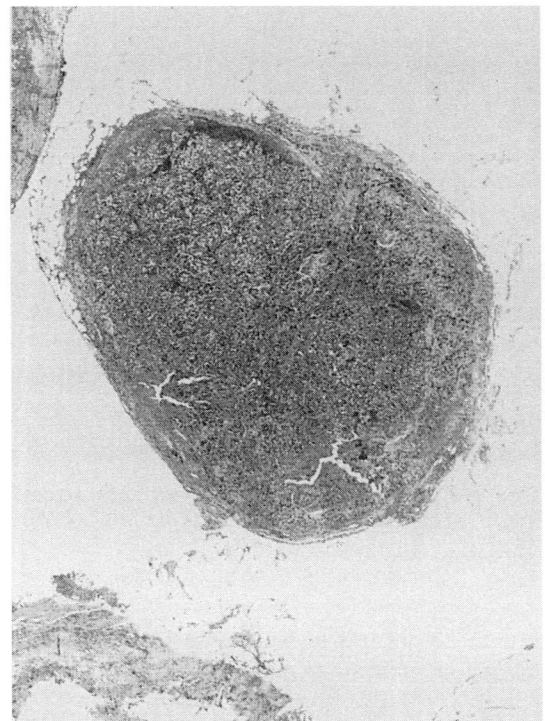

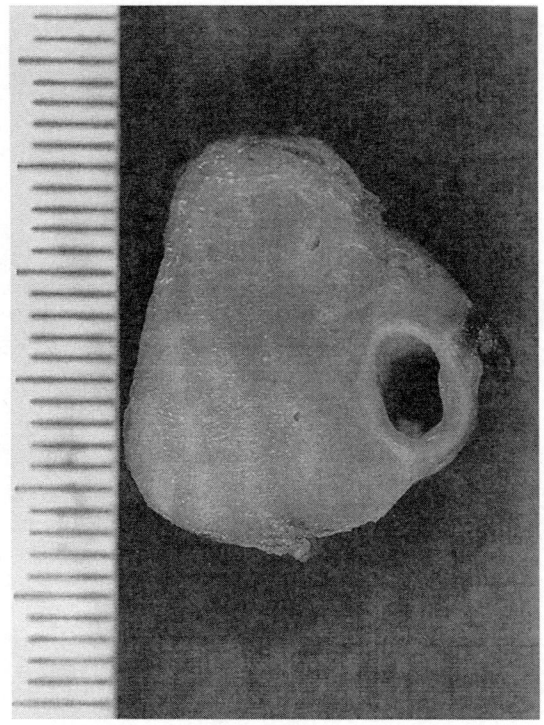

Fig. 43. Phaemochromocytoma. Peritoneal metastatic malignant phaemochromocytoma. HES

Fig. 44. Paraganglioma of the carotid tripod. (Courtesy Pr J-M Cormier)

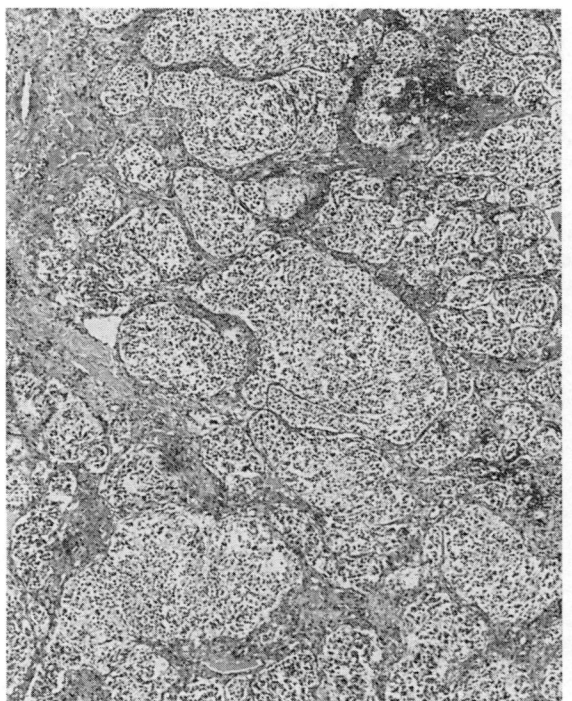

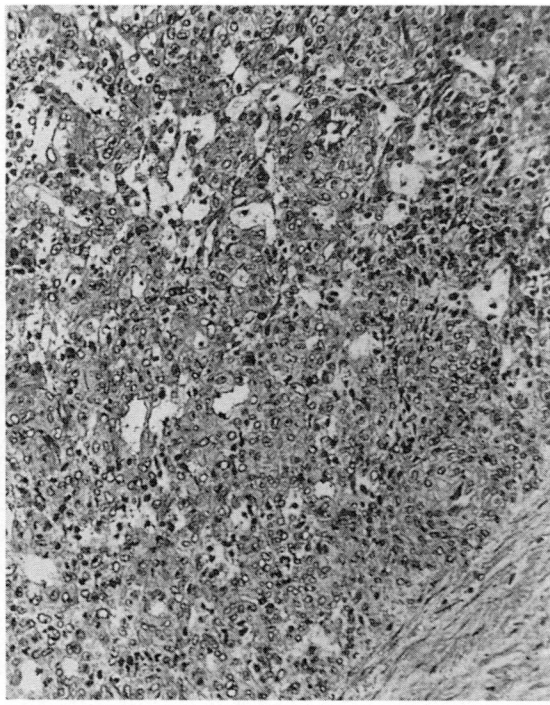

Fig. 45. Paraganglioma of the carotid tripod made up of a nest of ovoid cells enclosed by large fibrotic strands. HES

Fig. 46. Paraganglioma of the carotid tripod. Note interspersed clear sustentacular cells throughout the tumour. HES

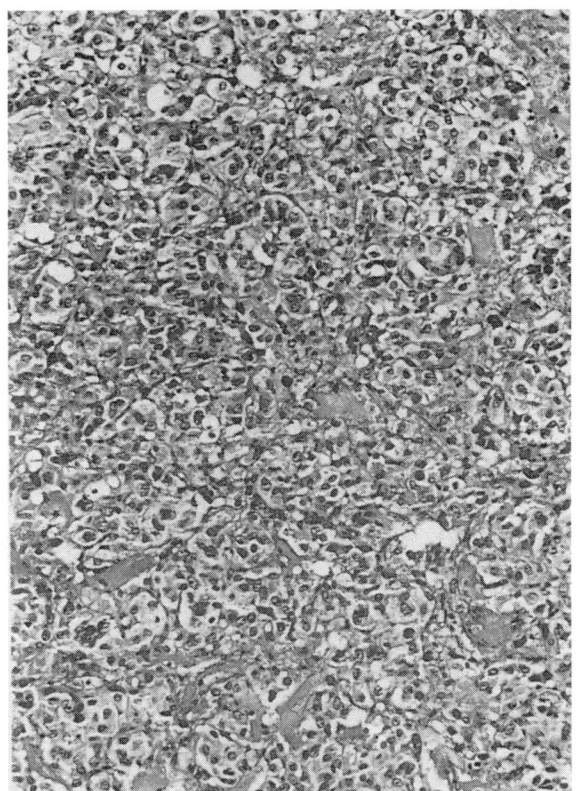

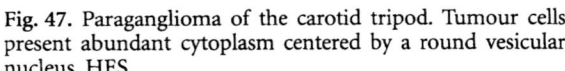

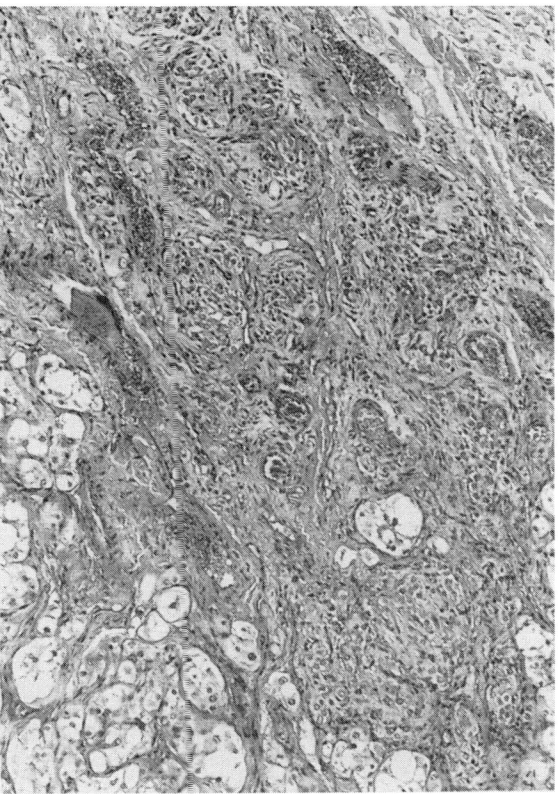

Fig. 47. Paraganglioma of the carotid tripod. Tumour cells present abundant cytoplasm centered by a round vesicular nucleus. HES

Fig. 48. Paraganglioma of the carotid tripod. Spindle-shaped tumour cells. HES

uniform, round to ovoid, sometimes vesicular, nuclei. Sometimes the cells are spindle-shaped (Fig. 48). Unfortunately, it is almost impossible to judge the clinical course of a paraganglioma on histological grounds; pleomorphism, even vascular invasion are unreliable criteria [118]. Electron microscopy often discloses well-demarcated neuroendocrine granules in paravertebral tumours, but they tend to be scant in nonfunctioning tumours. However, the cells in most tumours are argyrophilic and reactive to antibodies directed against neuron-specific enolase, as well as serotonin, gastrin, somatostatin, and bombesin.

Bibliography

1. Martinez JA, Quecedo E, Fortea JM, Oliver V, Aliaga A (1996) Pleomorphic angioleiomyoma. Am J Dermato-pathol 18: 409-12
2. Kataoka M, Yano H, Fukunaga T, Masumi S (1997) Giant vascular leiomyoma in the hand. Scand J Plast Reconstr Surg Hand Surg 31: 91-3
3. Hanft JR, Carbonell JA, Do HQ (1997) Angioleiomyoma of the lower extremity. J Am Podiatr Med Assoc 87: 388-91
4. Nall AV, Stringer SP, Baughman RA (1997) Vascular leiomyoma of the superior turbinate: first reported case. Head Neck 19: 63-7
5. Melgarejo Moreno P, Hellin Meseguer D, Sarroca Capell E (1997) Angioleiomyoma of the inferior nasal turbinate. A case report and review of the literature. Acta Otorrinolaringol Esp 48: 571-3
6. Fuse T, Yoshida S, Sakakibara A, Motoyama T (1998) Angiomyoma of the retropharyngeal space. J Laryngol Otol 112: 290-3
7. Heffernan MP, Smoller BR, Kohler S (1998) Cutaneous epithelioid angioleiomyoma. Am J Dermatopathol 20: 213-7
8. Sonobe H, Ohtsuki Y, Mizobuchi H, Toda M, Shimizu K (1996) An angiomyoma with t(X; 10) (q22; q23.2). Cancer Genet Cytogenet 90: 54-6
9. Gough J, Moreano W (1974) Primary myxoma of the aorta. J Clin Pathol 27: 806-7
10. Ramphal PS, Spencer HW, Mitchell DI, Denbow C (1998) Myxoma of right femoral vein origin presenting as a right atrial mass with syncope. J Thorac Cardiovasc Surg 116: 655-6

11. Mai KT, Yazdi HM, Collins JP (1996) Vascular myxolipoma ("angiomyxolipoma") of the spermatic cord. Am J Surg Pathol 20: 1145-8

12. Masson P, Géry L (1927) Les tumeurs glomiques sous-cutanées en dehors des doigts (angio-neuromyomes artériels). Anat Path 4: 153-165

13. Enzinger FM, Weiss SW (1988) Soft tissue tumors, CV Mosby, Saint Louis

14. Stout AP (1956) Tumours featuring pericytes: glomus tumour and haemangiopericytoma. Lab Invest 5: 217-23

15. Venkatachalam MA, Greally JC (1969) Fine structure of glomus tumour: similarity of glomus cells to smooth muscle. Cancer 23: 1176-84

16. Miettinen M, Lehto VP, Virtanen I (1983) Glomus tumor cells: evaluation of smooth muscle and endothelial cell properties. Virchows Arch B Cell Pathol Incl Mol Pathol 43: 139-49

17. Granter SR, Badizadegan K, Fletcher CD (1998) Myofibromatosis in adults, glomangiopericytoma, and myopericytoma: a spectrum of tumors showing perivascular myoid differentiation. Am J Surg Pathol 22: 513-25

18. Ichinose H, Hewitt RL, Drapanas T (1971) Minute pulmonary chemodectomas. Cancer 28: 692-700

19. Roujeau J, Derba C (1975) Hyperplasie des organes chémo-recepteurs ou micro-chémodectomes intra-pulmonaires. A propos de 3 observations. Arch Anat Path 23: 233-6

20. Shih TT, Sun JS, Hou SM, Huang KM, Su TT (1996) Magnetic resonance imaging of glomus tumour in the hand. Int Orthop 20: 342-5

21. Van Geertruyden J, Lorea P, Goldschmidt D, de Fontaine S, Schuind F, Kinnen L, Ledoux P, Moermans JP (1996) Glomus tumours of the hand. A retrospective study of 51 cases. J Hand Surg [Br] 2: 257-60

22. Oosterwijk JC, Jansen JC, van Schothorst EM, Oosterhof AW, Devilee P, Bakker E, Zoeteweij MW, van der Mey AG (1996) First experiences with genetic counselling based on predictive DNA diagnosis in hereditary glomus tumours (paragangliomas). J Med Genet 33: 379-83

23. van der Mey AG, Frijns JH, Cornelisse CJ, Brons EN, van Dulken H, Terpstra HL, Schmidt PH (1992) Does intervention improve the natural course of glomus tumors? A series of 108 patients seen in a 32-year period. Ann Otol Rhinol Laryngol 101: 635-42

24. Bao YH, Ling F (1997) Classification and therapeutic modalities of spinal vascular malformations in 80 patients. Neurosurgery 40: 75-81

25. Billard F, Dumollard JM, Cucherousset J, Boucheron S, Baril (1991) Deux tumeurs vasculaires bénignes de la capsule du rein. Ann Pathol 11: 266-70

26. Simmons TJ, Bassler TJ, Schwinn CP, Forrester DM (1992) Case report 749: Primary glomus tumor of bone. Skeletal Radiol 21: 407-9

27. Mazabraud A (1994) Anatomie pathologique osseuse tumorale. Springer-Verlag, Paris Berlin Heidelberg New York Londres Tokyo Hong Kong Barcelone Budapest

28. Wetherington RW, Lyle WG, Sangueza OP (1997) Malignant glomus tumor of the thumb: a case report. J Hand Surg [Am] 22: 1098-102

29. Pulitzer DR, Martin PC, Reed RJ (1995) Epithelioid glomus tumor. Hum Pathol 26: 1022-7

30. Nuovo MA, Grimes MM, Knowles DM (1990) Glomus tumours: a clinicopathologic and immunohistochemical analysis of forty cases. Surg Pathol 3: 31-45

31. Stout AP, Murray MR (1942) Haemangiopericytoma: a vascular tumour featuring Zimmermann's pericytes. Ann Surg 116: 26-33

32. Chung KC, Weiss SW, Kuzon WM Jr (1995) Multifocal congenital hemangiopericytomas associated with Kasabach-Merritt syndrome. Br J Plast Surg 48: 240-2

33. Bosch AM, Hack WW, Ekkelkamp S (1998) Congenital hemangiopericytoma: two case reports. Pediatr Surg Int 13: 211-2

34. Mariotti E, Ruelle A, Boccardo M (1984) Spinal hemangiopericytoma. Description of a clinical case. Rev Neurol 54: 411-8

35. Bastin KT, Mehta MP (1992) Meningeal hemangiopericytoma: defining the role for radiation therapy. J Neurooncol 14: 277-87

36. Kauffmann E, Buffin RP, Dabrowski A, Delobelle-Deroide A, Lmrabet H (1995) Uterine hemangiopericytomas. Two case reports. J Gynecol Obstet Biol Reprod (Paris) 24: 149-54

37. Grimsley BR, Loggie BW, Goco IR (1997) Hemangiopericytoma: an unusual cause of upper gastrointestinal hemorrhage. Am Surg 63: 248-51

38. Schick B, Brors D, Draf W (1998) Experiences with hemangiopericytoma in cranial base surgery. Laryngorhinootologie 77: 256-63

39. Rao CR, Naresh KN, Pattabhiraman V, Prabhakaran PS, Hazarika D (1994) Hemangiopericytoma of bone – a case report. Indian J Cancer 31: 264-7

40. Chiodi E, Centanni F, Gattazzo D (1998) Multiple hemangiopericytoma of the left ankle and foot. Magnetic resonance study and surgical findings in a case. Radiol Med (Torino) 95: 237-9

41. Lafond-Kim GM, Disler DG, Hou J, Riben MW, Jennings TA (1998) Osseous hemangiopericytomas of unsuspected intracranial origin. Skeletal Radiol 27: 98-102

42. Hoog A, Sandberg Nordqvist AC, Hulting AL, Falkmer UG (1997) High-molecular weight IGF-2 expression in a haemangiopericytoma associated with hypoglycaemia. APMIS 105: 469-82

43. Pavelic K, Cabrijan T, Hrascan R, Vrkljan M, Lipovac M, Kapitanovic S, Gall-Troselj K, Bosnar MH, Tomac A, Grskovic B, Karapandza N, Pavelic LJ, Kurslin B, Spaventi S, Pavelic J (1998) Molecular pathology of hemangiopericytomas accompanied by severe hypoglycemia: oncogenes, tumor-suppressor genes and the insulin-like growth factor family. J Cancer Res Clin Oncol 124: 307-14

44. Yokoyama H, Yamane Y, Takahara J, Yoshinouchi T, Ofuji TA (1979) A case of ectopic renin-secreting orbital haemangiopericytoma associated with juvenile hypertension and hypokalemia. Acta Med Okayama 33: 315-22

45. Velasco A, Mora X, Baeza R, Guzman S (1993) Hemangiopericytoma: report of 4 cases. Rev Med Chil 121: 1305-8

46. Kiefer T, Wertzel H, Freudenberg N, Hasse J (1997) Long-term survival after repetitive surgery for malignant hemangiopericytoma of the lung with subsequent systemic metastases: case report and review of the literature. Thorac Cardiovasc Surg 45: 307-9

47. Reiner SA, Siegel GJ, Clark KF, Min KW (1990) Hemangiopericytoma of the nasal cavity. Rhinology 28: 129-36

48. Hatva E, Bohling T, Jaaskelainen J, Persico MG, Haltia M, Alitalo K (1996) Vascular growth factors and receptors in capillary hemangioblastomas and hemangiopericytomas. Am J Pathol 148: 763-75

49. Nielsen GP, Dickersin GR, Provenzal JM, Rosenberg AE (1995) Lipomatous hemangiopericytoma. A histologic, ultrastructural and immunohistochemical study of a

unique variant of hemangiopericytoma. Am J Surg Pathol 19: 748-56

50. Chomette G, Auriol M, Terreau Y (1978) Héman-giopéricytome malin: à propos de l'analyse ultrastructurale et histoenzymologique d'une observation. Ann Anat Pathol 23: 41-51

51. Nunnery EW, Kahn LB, Reddick RL, Lipper S (1981) Haemangiopericytoma: a light microscopic and ultrastructural study. Cancer 47: 906-14

52. Eichhorn JH, Dickersin GR, Bhan AK, Goodman ML (1990) Sinonasal haemangiopericytoma. A reassessment with electron microscopy, immunohistochemistry and long-term follow-up. Am J Surg Pathol 14: 856-66

53. Nappi O, Ritter JH, Pettinato G, Wick MR (1995) Hemangiopericytoma: histopathological pattern or clinicopathologic entity? Semin Diagn Pathol 12: 221-32

54. Middleton LP, Duray PH, Merino MJ (1998) The histological spectrum of hemangiopericytoma: application of immunohistochemical analysis including proliferative markers to facilitate diagnosis and predict prognosis. Hum Pathol 29: 636-40

55. Nemes Z (1992) Differentiation markers in hemangiopericytoma. Cancer 69: 133-40

56. Nguyen GK, Neifer R (1985) The cells of benign and malignant haemangiopericytomas in aspiration biopsy. Diagnostic cytopathology 1: 327-31

57. Joseph JT, Lisle DK, Jacoby LB, Paulus W, Barone R, Cohen ML, Roggendorf WH, Bruner JM, Gusella JF, Louis DN (1995) NF2 gene analysis distinguishes hemangiopericytoma from meningioma. Am J Pathol 147: 1450-5

58. Zattara-Cannoni H, North MO, Gambarelli D, Figarella-Branger D, Graziani N, Grisoli F, Vagner-Capodano AM (1996) The contribution of cytogenetics to the histogenesis of meningeal hemangiopericytoma. J Neurooncol 29: 137-42

59. Limon J, Rao U, Dal Cin P, Gibas Z, Sandberg AA (1986) Translocation (13; 22) in hemangiopericytoma. Cancer Genet Cytogenet 21: 309-18

60. Cornog JL Jr, Enterline HT (1966) Lymphangiomyoma, a benign lesion of chyliferous lymphatics synonymous with lymphangiopericytoma. Cancer 19: 1909-30

61. Cabanne F, Renault P, Michiels R, Dusserre P, Justrabo E, Bastien H (1971) Lymphangiomyoma or lymphangiopericytoma. Laval Med 42: 431-7

62. Chomette G (1985) Compressions et obstructions de la veine cave inférieure: aspects anatomo-pathologiques In Kieffer E (ed.) Chirurgie de la veine cave inférieure et de ses branches. Expansion Scientifique Française Paris, 132-40

63. Courtin P, Stankowiak C, Dumont A, Servais B, Sault MC, Gosselin B (1991) Leiomyosarcome de la veine cave supérieure. Ann Pathol 11: 261-5

64. Fedorov VD, Tsvirkun VV, Skuba ND (1998) Diagnosis and treatment of leiomyosarcomas of inferior vena cava. Khirurgiia (Mosk) 9: 21-5

65. Rasaretnam R, Gunatunga CK, Seneviratne RH (1998) Leiomyosarcoma of the inferior vena cava. Ceylon Med J 43: 41-2

66. Hines OJ, Nelson S, Quinones-Baldrich WJ, Eilber FR (1999) Leiomyosarcoma of the inferior vena cava: prognosis and comparison with leiomyosarcoma of other anatomic sites. Cancer 85: 1077-83

67. Kieffer E, Berrod JL, Chomette G (1985) Primary tumors of the inferior vena cava In Berhan JJ, Yao JST (eds) Surgery of the veins. Grune and Straton Grune, Orlando, 423-43

68. Eng J, Murday AJ (1992) Leiomyosarcoma of the pulmonary artery. Ann Thorac Surg 53: 905-6

69. Schlittenbauer M, Muller KM (1996) Angioleiomyosarcoma of the lung – primary tumor or metastasis. Pneumologie 50: 215-8

70. Babatasi G, Massetti M, Galateau F, Khayat A (1998) Leiomyosarcoma of the pulmonary veins extending into the left atrium or left atrial leiomyosarcoma: multimodality therapy. J Thorac Cardiovasc Surg 116: 665-7

71. Stambuk J, Oddo D, Perez R, Bravo M (1993) Leiomyosarcoma of the saphenous vein. Rev Med Chil 121: 673-6

72. Glock Y, Laghzaoui A, Wang J, Delisle MB, Bachaud JM, Massabuau P, Roux D, Fournial G (1997) Fissured leiomyosarcoma of the descending thoracic aorta. Apropos of a case and review of the literature. Arch Mal Cœur Vaiss 90: 1317-20

73. Novak K, Hajek M, Hassan A (1998) Brachial plexus paralysis due to leiomyosarcoma of the subclavian artery successfully treated by surgery. Rozhl Chir 77: 95-7

74. Shimoda H, Oka K, Otani S, Hakozaki H, Yoshimura T, Okazaki H, Nishida S, Tomita S, Oka T, Kawasaki T, Mori N (1998) Vascular leiomyosarcoma arising from the inferior vena cava diagnosed by intraluminal biopsy. Virchows Arch 433: 97-100

75. Yamada K, Kamei S, Yasuda F, Isaka N, Yada I, Nakano T (1998) Primary leiomyosarcoma of the pulmonary artery confirmed by catheter suction biopsy. Chest 113: 555-6

76. Wirbel RJ, Verelst S, Hanselmann R, Remberger K, Kubale R, Mutschler WE (1998) Primary leiomyosarcoma of bone: clinicopathologic, immunohistochemical, and molecular biologic aspects. Ann Surg Oncol 5: 635-41

77. Lipton M, Sprayregen S, Kutcher R, Frost A (1995) Venous invasion in renal vein leiomyosarcoma: case report and review of the literature. Abdom Imaging 20: 64-7

78. Panebianco V, Grasso A, Ferreri ME, Puzzo L, Pistritto A, Blandino R, Poli A, Calanducci F, Messina D, Minutolo V, et al (1994) Leiomyosarcoma of the inferior vena cava: description of a new case and review of the literature. G Chir 15: 492-4

79. Mikami Y, Manabe T, Lie JT, Sakurai T, Endo K (1997) Intramural sarcoma of the carotid artery with adventitial inflammation and fibrosis resembling 'inflammatory aneurysm'. Pathol Int 47: 569-74

80. Weinberg DS, Maini BS (1980) Primary sarcoma of the aorta associated with a vascular prosthesis: a case report. Cancer 15: 398-40

81. Crum CP, Feldman PS, Nolan SP (1978) Primary fibroxanthosarcoma of the thoracic aorta. Virchows Arch A Pathol Pathol Anat 379: 351-8

82. Uruma T, Yagi T, Tanabe N, Chou K, Hiroshima K, Kakusaka I, Nagao K, Kuriyama T (1993) A case of primary pulmonary artery sarcoma. Nippon Kyobu Shikkan Gakkai Zasshi 31(6): 785-789

83. Gherardi GJ, Arya S, Hichler RB (1974) Juxtaglomerular body tumour: A rare occult but curable cause of lethal hypertension. Hum Pathol 5: 236-40

84. Tetu B, Totovic V, Bechtelsheimer H, Smend J (1984) Tumeur rénale à sécrétion de rénine. A propos d'un cas avec étude ultrastructurale et immunohistochimie. Ann Pathol 4: 55-59

85. Ducret F, Pointet P, Lambert C, Pin J, Baret M, Botta JM, Mutin M, Colon S, Vincent M (1991) Renin secreting tumor and severe hypertension. Apropos of a new case. Nephrologie 12: 17-24

86. McVicar M, Carman C, Chandra M, Abbi RJ, Teichberg S, Kahn E (1993) Hypertension secondary to renin-secreting juxtaglomerular cell tumor: case report and review of 38 cases. Pediatr Nephrol 7: 404-12

87. Corvol P, Pinet F, Plouin PF, Bruneval P, Menard J (1994) Renin-secreting tumors. Endocrinol Metab Clin North Am 23: 255-70

88. Caregaro L, Menon F, Gatta A, Amodio P, Armanini D, Fallo F, Corona MC, Pescarini L, Ruol A (1994) Juxtaglomerular cell tumor of the kidney. Clin Exp Hypertens 16: 41-53

89. Chung CT, Chen JW, Wu TR, Chen KK, Wang JH, Yang AH, Chang MS (1994) Secondary hypertension due to renin secreting tumor: a case report. Chung Hua I Hsueh Tsa Chih (Taipei) 54: 188-92

90. Ouchi H, Fujimoto K, Matsuura K (1996) Juxtaglomerular cell tumor: a case report. Hinyokika Kiyo 42: 303-6

91. Baldet P, Mimran A (1977) So-called juxtaglomerular benign tumor of the kidney with renin secretion. Optical and ultrastructural study. Ann Anat Pathol (Paris) 22: 21-40

92. Philips G, Mukherjee TM (1972) A juxtaglomerular cell tumour: light and electron microscopic studies of a renin-secreting kidney tumour containing both juxtaglomerular cells and mast cells. Pathology 4: 193-204

93. Barajas L, Bennett CM, Connor G, Lindstrom RR (1977) Structure of a juxtaglomerular cell tumour: the presence of a neural component. A light and electron microscopic study. Lab Invest 37: 357-68

94. Baldet P, Mimran A, Granier M, Dupont M (1983) Histologic and ultrastructural forms of benign tumors of the kidney with renin secretion. Functional implications. Ann Pathol 3: 225-34

95. Camilleri JP, Hinglais N, Bruneval P, Bariety J, Tricottet V, Rouchon M, Mancilla-Jimenez R, Corvol P, Menard J (1984) Renin storage and cell differentiation in juxtaglomerular cell tumors: an immunohistochemical and ultrastructural study of three cases. Hum Pathol 15: 1069-79

96. Camilleri JP, Phat VN, Bariety J, Corvol P, Menard J (1980) Use of a specific antiserum for renin detection in human kidney. J Histochem Cytochem 28: 1343-6

97. Phat VN, Camilleri JP, Bariéty J, Galtier N, Baviera E, Corvol P, Ménard J (1981) Immunohistochemical characterization of renin-containing cells in the human juxta-glomerular apparatus during embryonal and fetal development. Lab Invest 45: 387-90

98. Lindop GBM, Stewart JA, Downie TT (1983) The immunocytochemical demonstration of renin in a juxtaglomerular cell tumour in light and electron microscopy. Histopathol 7: 421-31

99. Gaudemar M, Bruneval P, Camilleri JP (1988) Tumor syndromes with inappropriate renin secretion. Diagnostic criteria and review of published cases. Ann Pathol 8: 83-90

100. Steffens J, Girardot P, Bock R, Braedel HU, Alloussi S, Ziegler M (1992) Carcinoma of the kidney with production of renin. A special form of hypertension. Ann Urol (Paris) 26: 5-9

101. Hayami S, Sasagawa I, Suzuki H, Kubota Y, Nakada T, Endo Y (1998) Juxta-glomerular cell tumor without hypertension. Scand J Urol Nephrol 32: 231-3

102. Whalen RK, Althausen AF, Daniels GH (1992) Extra-adrenal pheochromocytoma. J Urol 147: 1-10

103. Castaigne V, Afriat R, Cambouris-Perrine S, Radu S, Desdouit J, Freund M (1998) Pheochromocytoma associated with pregnancy. Report of 2 cases and review of the literature. J Gynecol Obstet Biol Reprod (Paris) 27: 622-4

104. Chew SL, Dacie JE, Reznek RH, Newbould EC, Sheaves R, Trainer PJ, Lowe DG, Shand WS, Hungerford J, Besser GM, et al (1994) Bilateral phaeochromocytomas in von Hippel-Lindau disease: diagnosis by adrenal vein sampling and catecholamine assay. Q J Med 87: 49-54

105. Carney JA (1998) Familial multiple endocrine neoplasia syndromes: components, classification, and nomenclature. J Intern Med 243: 425-32

106. Eng C, Clayton D, Schuffenecker I, Lenoir G, Cote G, Gagel RF, van Amstel HK, Lips CJ, Nishisho I, Takai SI, Marsh DJ, Robinson BG, Frank-Raue K, Raue F, Xue F, Noll WW, Romei C, Pacini F, Fink M, Niederle B, Zedenius J, Nordenskjold M, Komminoth P, Hendy GN, Mulligan LM, et al (1996) The relationship between specific RET proto-oncogene mutations and disease phenotype in multiple endocrine neoplasia type 2. International RET mutation consortium analysis. JAMA 276: 1575-9

107. Morrison PJ, Nevin NC (1996) Multiple endocrine neoplasia type 2B (mucosal neuroma syndrome, Wagenmann-Froboese syndrome). J Med Genet 33: 779-82

108. Clarke MR, Weyant RJ, Watson CG, Carty SE (1998) Prognostic markers in pheochromocytoma. Hum Pathol 29: 522-6

109. Brown CL (1981) Endocrine pathology in Paediatrics In Berry C (ed.) Paediatric pathology. Springer-Verlag, Berlin, Heidelberg, NewYork, p571

110. Rodriguez-Cuevas S, Lopez-Garza J, Labastida-Almendaro S (1998) Carotid body tumors in inhabitants of altitudes higher than 2000 meters above sea level. Head Neck 20: 374-8

111. Defraigne JO, Limet R (1997) Lymphatic, hepatic and osseous metastasis of a carotid chemodectoma. Apropos of a case. J Chir (Paris) 134: 336-9

112. Ophir D (1991) Familial multicentric paragangliomas in a child. J Laryngol Otol 105: 376-80

113. Chow SN, Seear M, Anderson R, Magee F (1998) Multiple pulmonary chemodectomas in a child: results of four different therapeutic regimens. J Pediatr Hematol Oncol 20: 583-6

114. Anand VK, Leonetti JP, al-Mefty O (1993) Neurovascular considerations in surgery of glomus tumors with intracranial extensions. Laryngoscope 103: 722-8

115. Gaylis H, Mieny CJ (1977) The incidence of malignancy in carotid body tumours. Br J Surg 64: 885-9

116. Bernard RP (1992) Carotid body tumors. Am J Surg 163: 494-6

117. Fruhwirth J, Koch G, Hauser H, Gutschi S, Beham A, Kainz J (1996) Paragangliomas of the carotid bifurcation: oncological aspects of vascular surgery. Eur J Surg Oncol 22: 88-92

118. Capella C, Riva C, Cornaggia M, Chiaravalli AM, Frigerio B, Solcia E (1988) Histopathology, cytology and cytochemistry of pheochromocytomas and paragangliomas including chemodectomas. Pathol Res Pract 183: 176-87

Annex I
Laboratory handling of vascular specimens

The examination protocol to be used for vascular specimens will depend on the surgical techniques used in obtaining them [1] and the clinical context in which they are taken. They will thus be considered in a number of clinical or surgical contexts.

1 – Products obtained during the re-establishment of a vascular lumen

The end products of vascular obstruction are usually localised thrombus or an embolus.

1.1. Determine the anatomical configuration of the specimen. A thrombus or embolus may be either cylindrical or oval-shaped. Search for non-haemorrhagic material that may be of neoplastic or exogenous origin (foreign bodies).

1.2. Count the number of tissue fragments. Record their dimensions.

1.3. When the clinical context suggests that an infectious process is involved, remove a fragment of the blood clot for microbiological study.

1.4. Fix the remains of the specimen.

1.5. For cylindrical-shaped specimens, make cross sections perpendicular to the main axis of the specimen. Small specimens should be blocked whole.

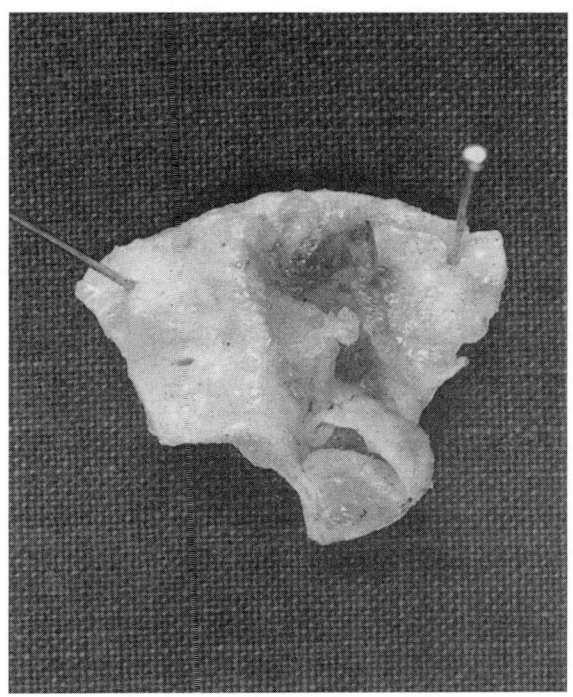

Fig. 1. Endarterectomy core

2.4. Make sections of the specimen perpendicular to its main axis (Fig. 2). Locate areas of dissection beneath plaques of atheroma.

2.5. Block specimens in transverse sections.

2 – Endarterectomy

The specimen consists of the diseased intima (Fig. 1) and a part of the media of an artery, or the thickened internal capsule of a prosthesis.

2.1. Establish the anatomical orientation of the surgical specimen using anatomical markers.

2.2. Measure the specimen and describe the type of lesion present (atherosclerotic plaques, calcifications, ulceration or parietal thrombi etc.).

2.3. Fix the specimen. X-ray to see whether decalcification is necessary (a simple "Faxitron®" radiograph will suffice).

3 – Biopsies

The surgical specimen should include the three coats of the blood vessel wall.

3.1. Check the anatomical configuration of the specimen. The surgeon should indicate one end of the specimen (proximal or distal) with a suture thread.

3.2. Depending on the clinical context, prepare specimens for special examination (ultrastructural study, immunohistochemistry).

3.3. Two protocols may be followed:

3.3.1. **Protocol 1.** This protocol is recommended when the blood vessel has a small calibre (Fig. 3) or when it is already opened longitudinally.

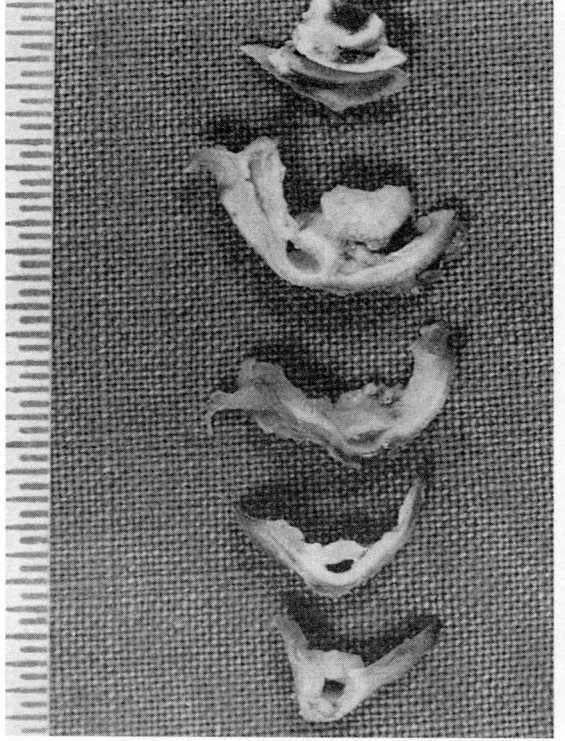

Fig. 2. Endarterectomy core.Perpendicular sections to the axis help identify intraplaque dissection

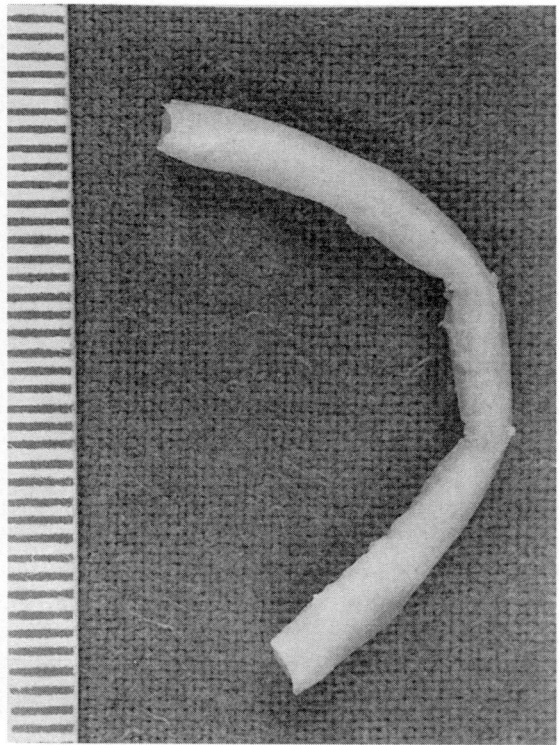

Fig. 3. Vascular biopsy

a) Cut 0.3 cm thick sections from the specimen. Number them (Fig. 4). Make a description of these sections (calibre, lumen, intimal lesions, parietal dissection). For short segment of small-calibre blood vessels (like the temporal artery) it is preferable to leave the vascular segment as it is. This makes it easier for the technician to grasp the specimen with forceps and to orient it appropriately for embedding in paraffin. Serial sections should be made.

b) Check to see whether decalcification is necessary. Include these cuts in their cross-section.

3.3.2. **Protocol 2.** This protocol is indicated especially for the examination of specimens with an abnormal configuration (loop, kink, coarctation, and varicosities).

a) Catheterise the vessel with the stylet.

b) Incise the specimen in a sagittal section.

c) Make a description of this section: calibre, lumen, valvular structures, the vascular wall.

d) Include each half of the surgical specimen. Block each section sagitally.

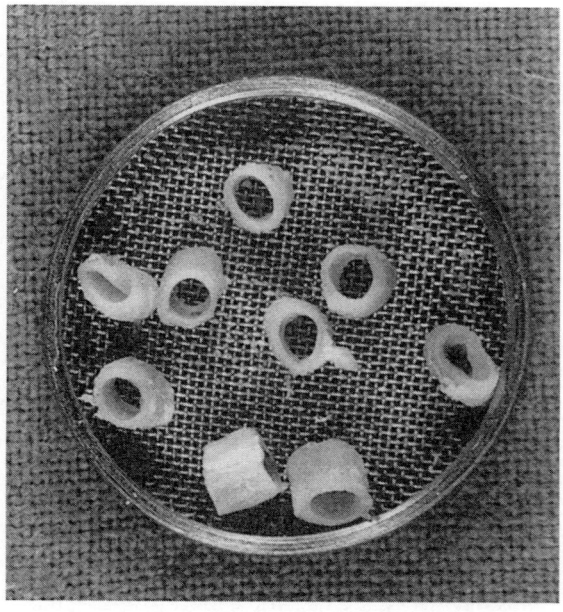

Fig. 4. Vascular biopsy. Study protocol 1. Cut sections perpendicular to the main axis, 0.3 cm thick, transferred to a metallic cassette before paraffin blocking processing

4 – Resection of vascular prostheses

4.1. Establish the anatomical configuration and orientation of the surgical specimen.

4.2. Measure the specimen (length, diameter). Describe the outer aspect or external capsule.

4.3. If the clinical context suggests an infected graft, use sterile techniques to obtain a fragment of the prosthesis for microbiological examination. Prepare specimens for special studies (ultrastructure, immunohistochemistry).

4.4. Use one of the two study protocols intended for biopsy and biopsy-resections of vascular specimens.

4.4.1. **Protocol 1.** When the lumen of the vascular graft or prosthesis is obliterated, cut 0.3 cm thick small sections perpendicular to the main axis of the specimen. Describe these sections carefully: the nature of the lumen, internal capsule or neo-intima, wall of the prosthesis, external capsule, etc. Block a few cuts in their cross-section for histology.

4.4.2. **Protocol 2.** This protocol is particularly recommended for studying anastomoses between the prosthesis and the recipient blood vessel. When the lumen of the natural graft or prosthesis remains patent, incise the specimen along its main axis after catheterising it (Fig. 5). Identify the intimal flap then the vascular and the prosthetic sides (Fig. 6). Make longitudinal sections through the anastomotic line (Fig. 7). Block the areas of anastomosis sagittally in paraffin after removing the surgical thread with pointed scissors; thread will damage the microtome blade, and tear and distort the sections. At the intermediate portion of the vascular graft or of the prosthesis, make cross-sections perpendicular to its main axis. Include them in their cross-section.

4.4.3. After having sampled the specimen for light microscopy, corrosion of the soft tissues surrounding the prosthesis is best achieved by immersing the remaining portion of the operative specimen into a solution of 50% hydrochloric acid for 1 to 2 days. Describe the gross aspect of the now denuded prosthesis noting perforations, dilatation etc.

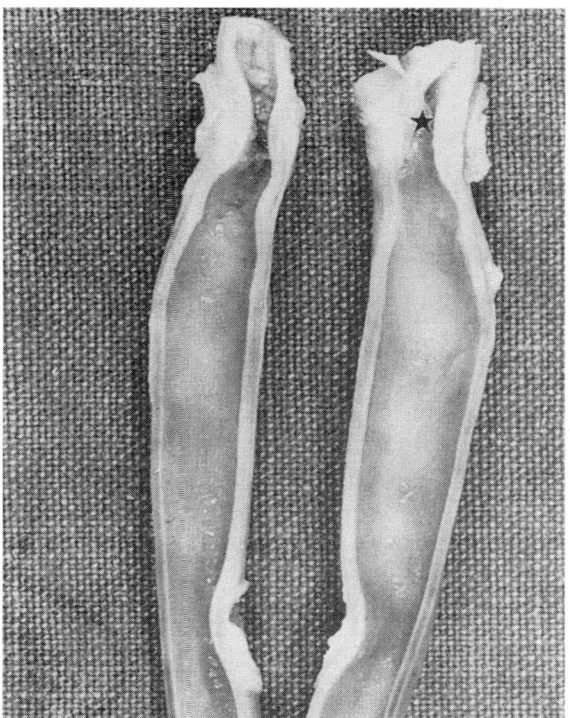

Fig. 5. PTFE vascular graft specimen opened longitudinally. (star): intimal flap

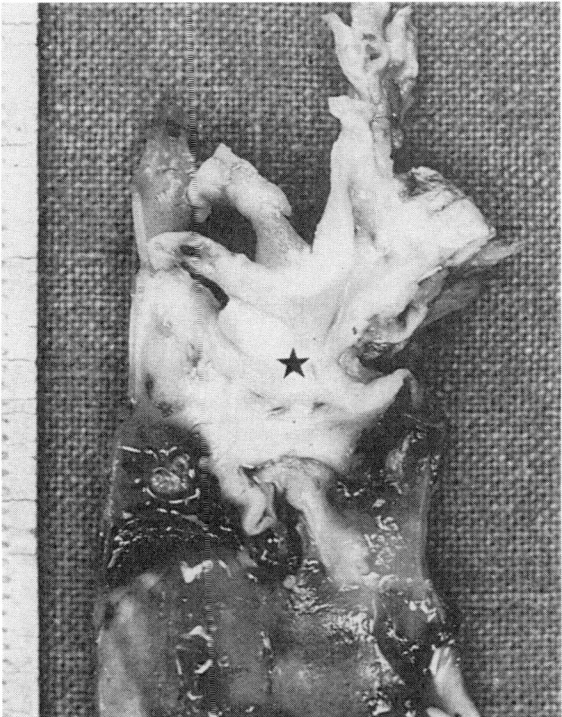

Fig. 6. Anastomotic point of a PTFE prosthesis with non occluding thrombus developed next to a large whitish intimal flap (star)

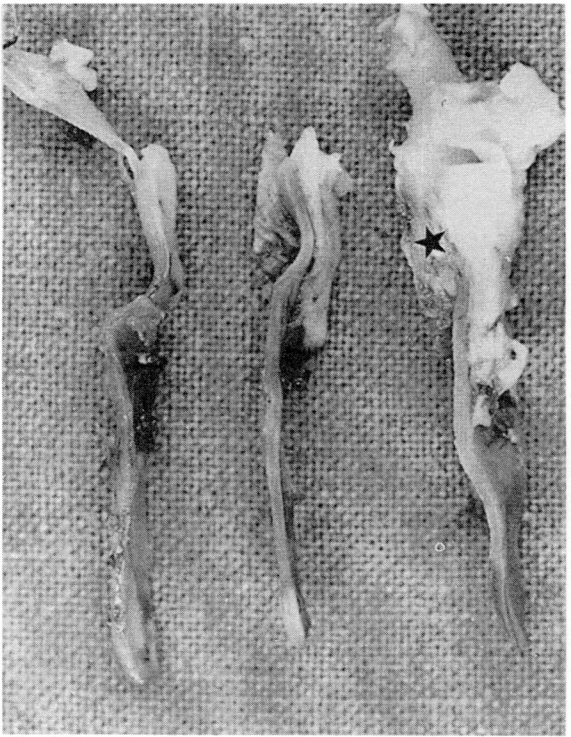

Fig. 7. Longitudinal sections of the anastomotic point buried by an intimal flap (star) sliding from the recipient arterial side

5.2.1. X-ray the specimen. Identify the stent wire, its type (simple or covered) and configuration (Palmaz, Wallstent, Gianturco, Strecker endoprostheses etc.) (Fig. 9).

5.2.2. Make a longitudinal incision on the external aspect or adventitia of the stented vascular segment, parallel to the blood flow.

5.2.3. With the use of a needle-nosed wire cutter, complete the opening by cutting the wire rings. Care should be taken to preserve the intima and media.

5.2.4. Describe the gross aspect of the lumen, the different vascular layers around and between the stent wire. Photograph the luminal aspect (Fig. 10).

5.2.5. Carry on in the same way to perform cross sections of the stented segment.

5.2.6. Samples of the upper and lower ends of the stented segment should include non-adjacent stented areas, as for the anastomotic zones of a vascular prosthesis.

5.2.7. Remove the cut stent wire from the vascular wall before the specimen is processed for light and electron microscopy.

5 – Vascular stents

Study of the vascular response to stent insertion is hampered by difficulties in sectioning metal and vascular tissue without distortion of the tissue stent interface. A special technique using resin embedding and thin sectioning of the specimen with the stent wires in place has been suggested [2]. In daily practice, the removal of metal wires from the tissue sampling before histological processing appears adequate. Vascular specimens related to stent insertion are of two types; the isolated stent and the stent in situ.5.1. Isolated thrombosed stent

5.1.1. Detach the thrombus from the stent wire (Fig. 8).

5.1.2. Identify the stent wire, its type and configuration

5.1.3. Examine the clot by standard histological methods.

5.2. Stented vascular specimen

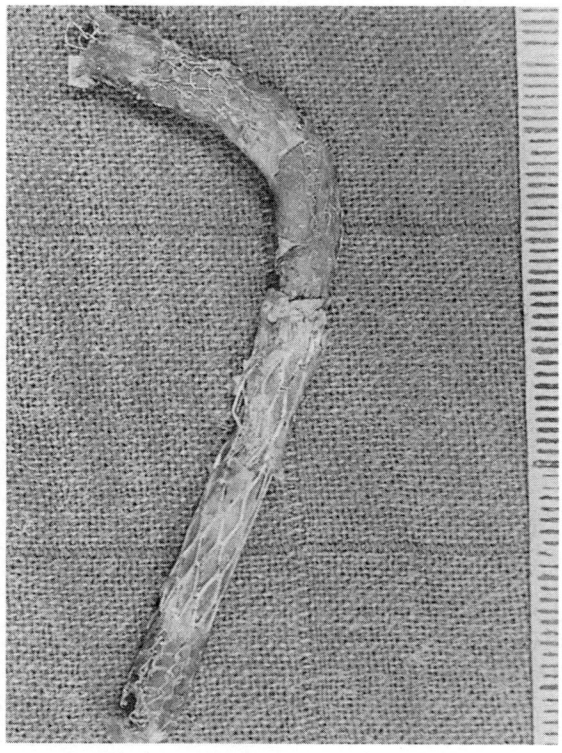

Fig. 8. Detached thrombosed stent

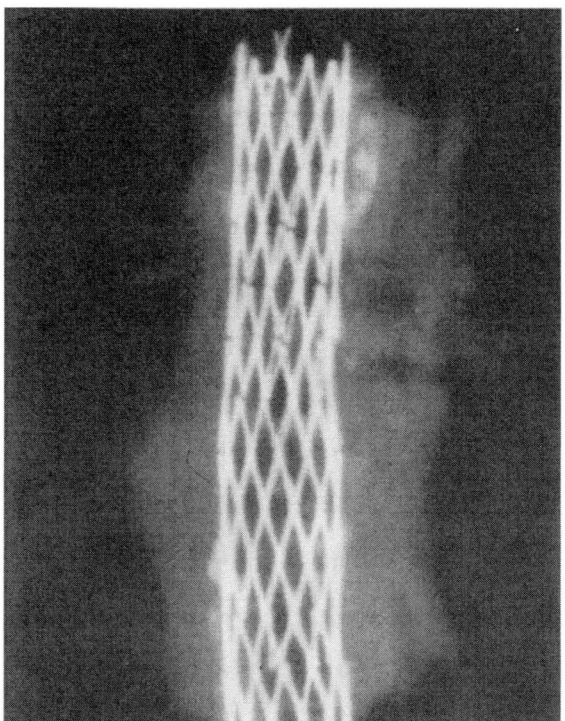

Fig. 9. Stented vascular resection specimen. A specimen radiograph permits identification of the in place stent wire

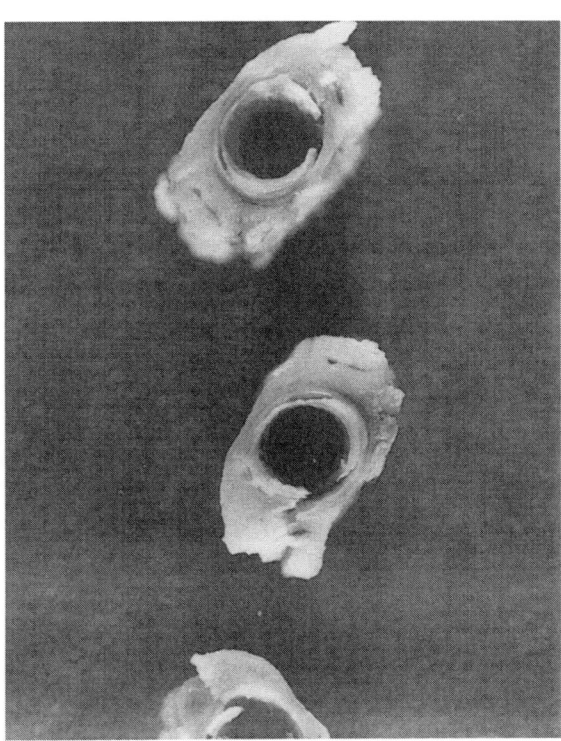

Fig. 10. Cut sections of the stented vessel devoid of wire rings

6 – Limb amputation specimens for gangrene and extensive thrombosis

6.1. Amputation of the upper arm and forearm

6.1.1. It is preferable to dissect the operative specimen before fixation (Fig. 11). Identify the type of amputation (inferior half of upper arm, forearm) descriptively and with measurements of distance from remaining joints.

6.1.2. Measure the length of the operative specimen. Orient it (anterior and posterior faces, medial and external borders).

6.1.3. Dissection of the brachial artery

a) Place the specimen on a corkboard, the medial face upwards. Identify the internal border of the superior surgical section; the brachial artery is visible at this level. Using a felt-tip pen with permanent ink, mark the middle A of the internal border of this section. At the elbow fold, draw an horizontal line connecting the external condyle D to the internal condyle E to of the humerus. Divide this segment into three equal parts EB, BC and CD by marking two points B and C respectively.

b) Draw the segments AB and BC.

c) Incise the skin and the aponeurosis of the biceps along the segment AB.

d) Reflect the anterior border of the muscle. The neuro-vascular bundle appears under a thin aponeurosis. Two veins that communicate with each other like a ladder flank the brachial artery (1-1'); one of these receives the basilic vein; the ulnar nerve is posterior to the artery.

6.1.4. Dissection of the inferior part of the brachial artery.

a) Rotate the operative specimen, the elbow fold upwards. Extend the incision AB to BC.

b) Section the communicating vein at the elbow fold and the aponeurotic expansion of the biceps. The brachial tripod, flanked by two veins, is located between the median nerve, which is medial, and the tendon of the biceps muscle, which is lateral.

6.1.5. Dissection of the arteries of the forearm.

a) Identify the radial (F) and the ulnar (G) styloid processes. Draw the segments CF and BG.

b) Isolate the radial artery (2,2'). From the brachial tripod, incise the skin along the segment CF. The radial artery appears under an aponeurosis, deep to the supinator longus.

c) Isolate the ulnar artery (3,3'). From the brachial tripod, incise the skin along the segment BG. The ulnar artery is deep to the flexor carpi ulnaris. The ulnar nerve lies deeper than the artery.

6.2. Amputation of the hand

6.2.1. Orient the operative specimen by identifying the fingers (I, II, III, IV, V).

6.2.2. Describe the lesions: nails, free extremities, dorsal and palmar faces, the surgical section.

6.2.3. Dissection of the superficial palmar arch (Fig. 11-12-13).

a) On the palmar face of the hand, draw a horizontal segment HI parallel to the segment FG. H corresponds to the internal border of the base of the thumb. Delineate the parallelogram FGHI. After the skin incision, remove the soft tissues of the superior half of the metacarpus by shaving the palmar face of the metacarpal bones.

b) Pin the cutaneo-muscular flap on a corkboard. Frontal sections allow us to identify the ulnar artery on the internal border, and the radial artery on the external border.

6.2.4. Dissection of the perforating branches of palmar interosseous arteries and the deep palmar arteries.

a) Remove the soft tissues of each intermetacarpal space [1-4] in the sagittal plane by shaving the lateral sides of the metacarpal bones. The soft tissues of each intermetacarpal space contain the perforating branches of the interosseous palmar arteries and the deep branches of the palmar arteries.

b) Frontal sections allow identification of the vessels.

6.2.5. Dissection of digital vessels.Proceed in the same way as for finger amputation specimens.

6.3. Digits (finger or toe) amputation

6.3.1. Verify the anatomical configuration of the operative specimen: side, site (I, II, III, IV, V)

6.3.2. Make a description of the digit (finger or toe), the nail, its free end and its dorsal aspect. Describe the plantar or palmar aspects and the proximal surgical section (Fig. 14).

6.3.3. Fix the specimen.

6.3.4. Make either transverse sections perpendicular to the great axis of the digit or a longitudinal section involving the great axis of the digit by using an electric saw (Fig. 15). Separate the soft tissues from the underlying bone. Block these small cuts in their cross section to examine the digital arteries and the distal blood vessels; two veins flank each digital artery. Soften the nail by immersing it in a potash solution

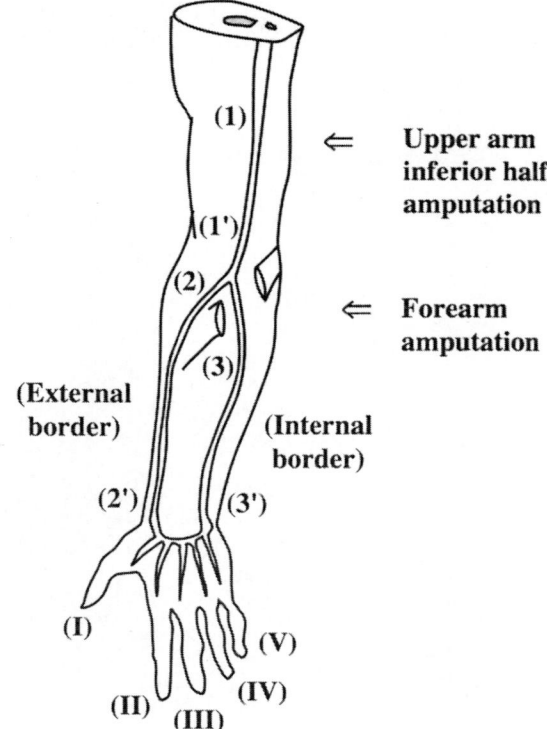

Fig. 11. Diagram of the arterial paths in an amputation specimen of the right upper limb with anterior face upward. Brachial (1,1'), radial (2,2') and ulnar (3,3') arteries

for 30 minutes before paraffin blocking. Bone samples must be decalcified.

6.4. Trans-metatarsal guillotine or forefoot amputation

6.4.1. Orient the surgical specimen appropriately by identifying the different toes (I, II, III, IV, V). Describe the gross aspect of lesions present: anatomical configuration and lesions (Fig. 16).

6.4.2. Using a surgical knife, divide the specimen in the sagittal plane, shaving the lateral edges of the 1st, 2nd, 3rd, 4th and 5th metatarsal bones. These sagittal sections make it possible to separate the soft tissue from the 1st, 2nd, 3rd and 4th metatarsal spaces (Fig. 17). This tissue contains the plantar interosseous arteries, the deep communicating branches and the common plantar digital arteries.

6.4.3. Examination of blood vessels of the 1st, 2nd, 3rd and 4th metatarsal interspaces (Fig. 18) may be made with sections perpendicular to their main axis. Include these sections in their cross-section.

6.4.4. Amputate toes. Proceed as described in the protocol for digit amputation.

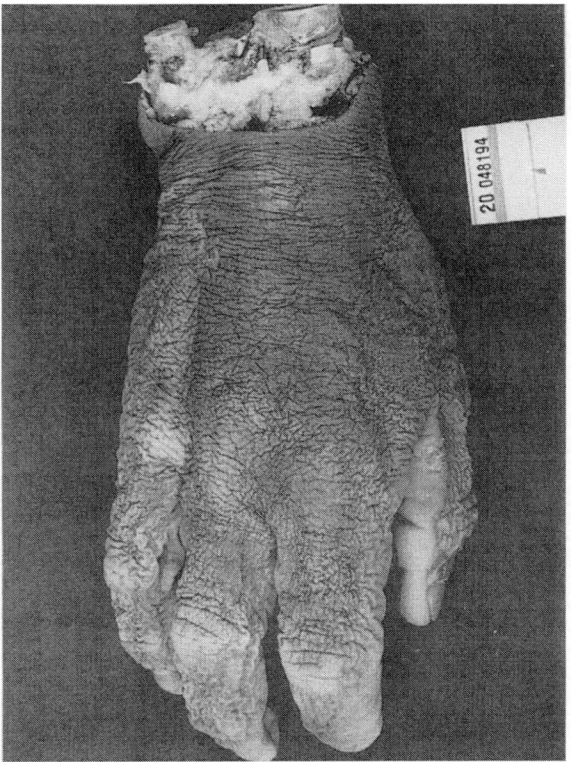

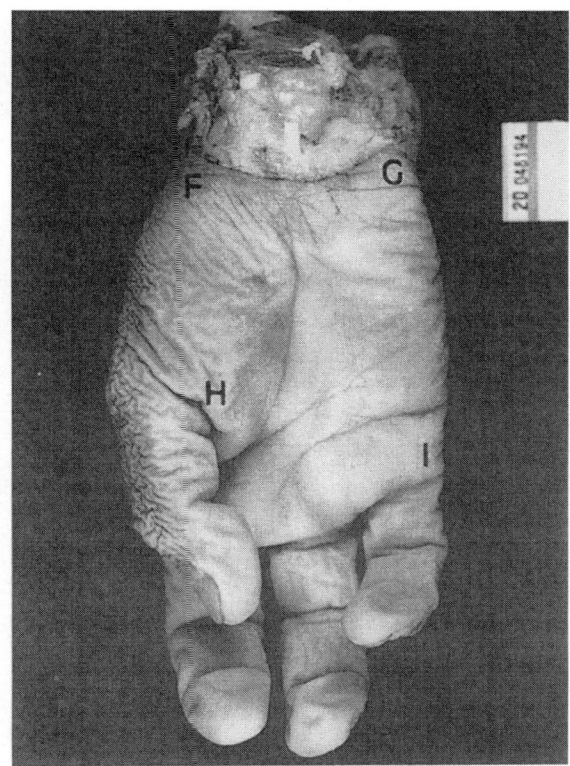

Fig. 12. Hand amputation for recurrent angiosarcoma of finger IV already resected one year ago. Note former surgical incision along the 4th metacarpal space

Fig. 13. Dissection of the superficial palmar arch

6.5. Amputation of the lower limb

6.5.1. Determine the surgical procedure performed in descriptive terms (Fig. 19); amputation at the lower third of the thigh (A) (Fig. 20), superior two thirds (A') of the leg, middle one-third (A") of the leg (Fig. 21) etc. Measurements from remaining joints are valuable.

6.5.2. Dissection of the neurovascular bundles of an amputation at the lower third of the thigh or at the junction of the upper third with the lower two-thirds of the leg. It is preferable to dissect these structures in an unfixed surgical specimen.

a) Note the length of the specimen. Identify anatomical structures.

b) Identify and surgically place markers.

1) Place the specimen on a corkboard, posterior surface facing upwards. Identify the midpoint of the posterior section of the specimen. This point corresponds to the location of the deep femoral artery (profunda femoris) (A) or the popliteal artery (A') at the popliteal pit (Fig. 22).

2) Identify the heel. Mark its midpoint (B).

3) Turn over the surgical specimen, the internal side facing upwards. Identify the internal malleolus. Locate point D 2 cm below the posterior edge of the internal or medial malleolus.

4) Turn over the specimen, the tibial border facing upwards. Identify the external or lateral malleolus. Locate point E 2 cm below the posterior border of the external malleolus.

5) Identify the head of the fibula. Mark the midpoint (F) of the segment connecting the styloid process of the fibula to the anterior tibial tubercle.

6) Place specimen anterior face facing upwards. Mark point G at the midpoint of the segment connecting the anterior borders of the internal or medial (D) and external or lateral (E) malleolus.

c) Dissection of the posterior arteries of the leg (popliteal, posterior tibial and peroneal) (Fig. 23-24-25).

1) Using a felt-tip pen with permanent ink, draw a line from the midpoint of the popliteal pit (point A')

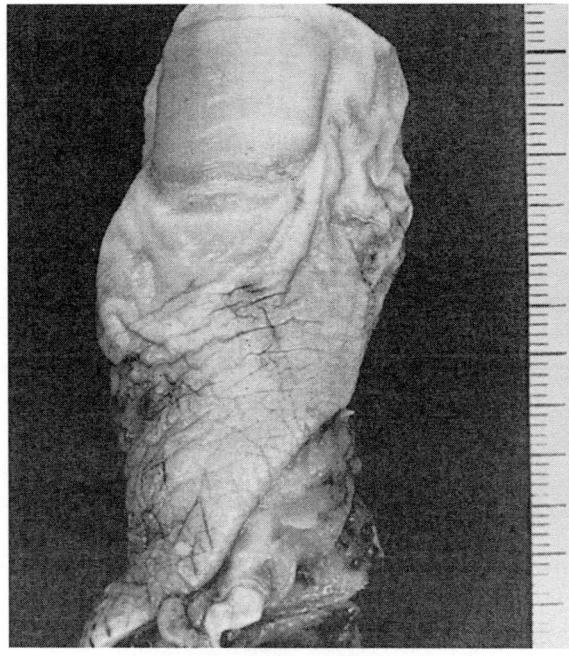

Fig. 14. Accidental amputation of the thumb

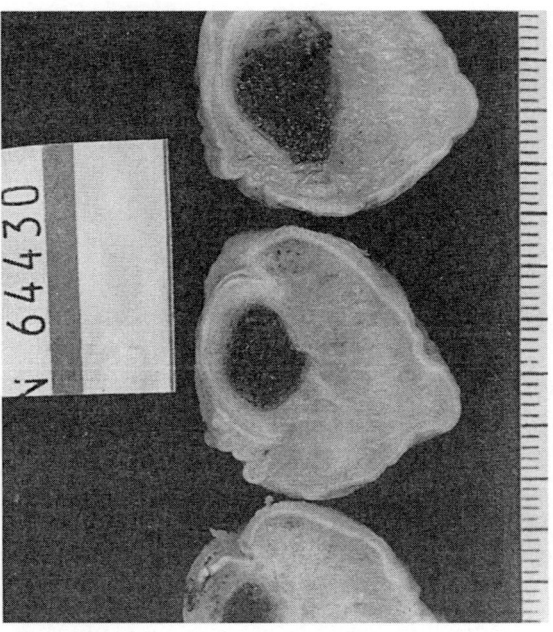

Fig. 15. Accidental amputation of the thumb. Transversal sections perpendicular to the main axis of the digit

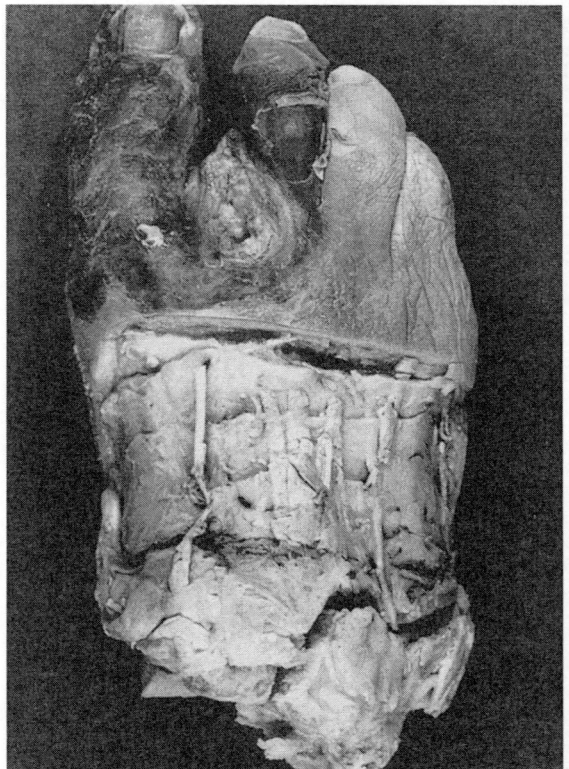

Fig. 16. Transmetatarsal guillotine amputation of the anterior two-thirds of the right foot for recurrent cholesterol embolism with gangrene in a diabetic patient having previously had an amputation of the toe for the same cause

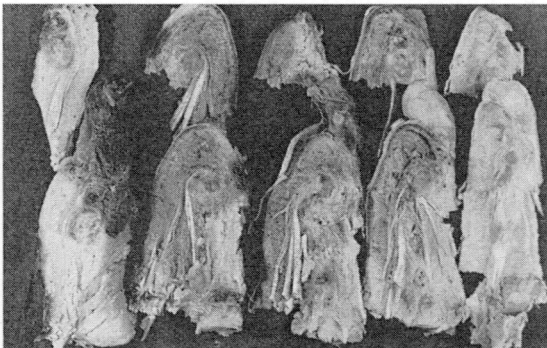

Fig. 17. Transmetatarsal guillotine amputation of the anterior two-thirds of the right foot. 1st, 2nd, 3rd, 4th and 5th metatarses with corresponding toes and soft tissues

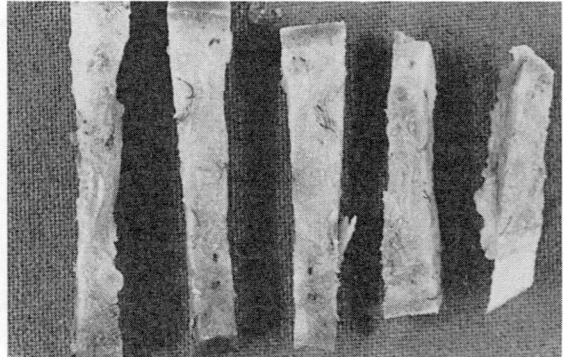

Fig. 18. Transmetatarsal guillotine amputation of the anterior two-thirds of the right foot. Soft tissues of 1st, 2nd, 3rd and 4th metatarsal interspaces

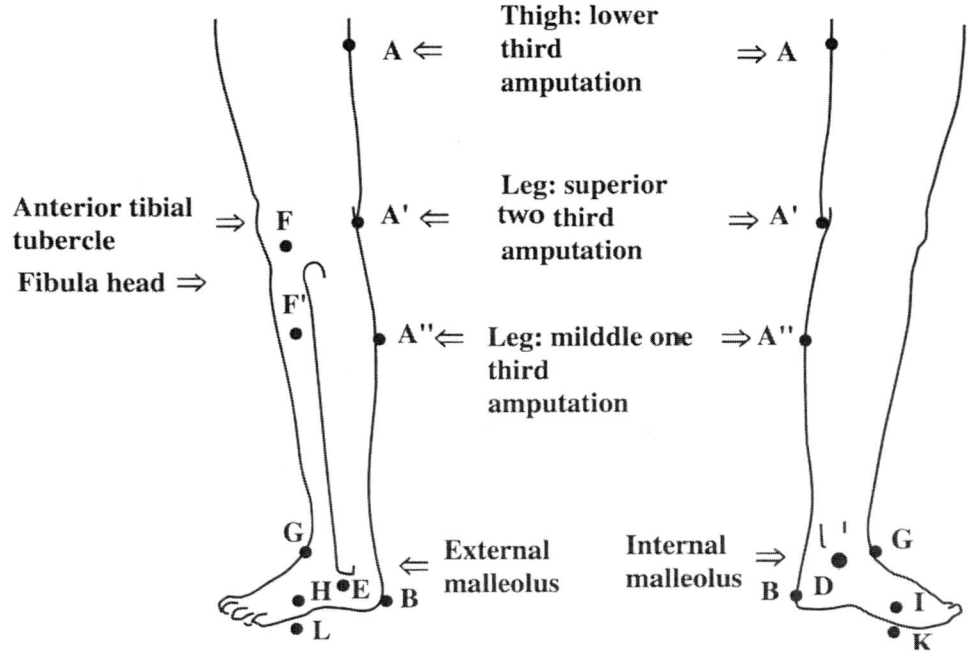

Fig. 19. Amputation of the lower limb: types of amputation

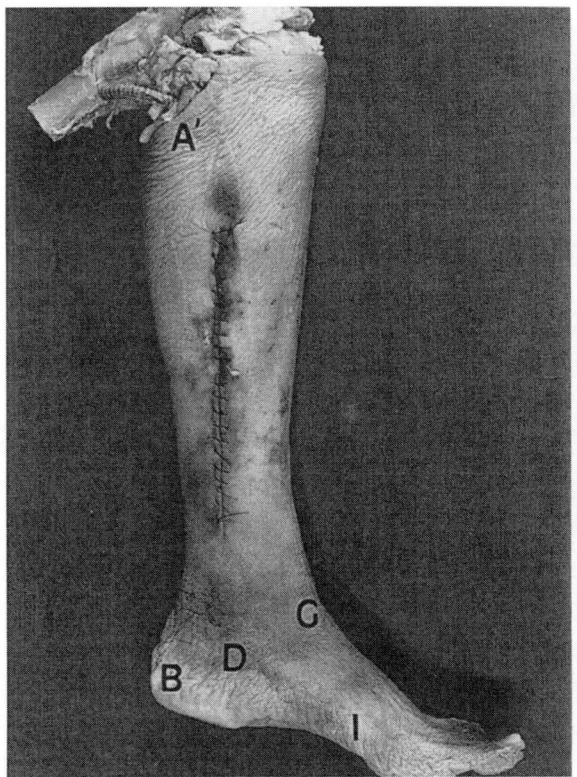

Fig. 20. Lower third amputation of the left thigh for gangrene of the left leg secondary to thrombosis of a long femoro-tibial prosthetic bypass. Soft tissues already removed from the bone. Internal side

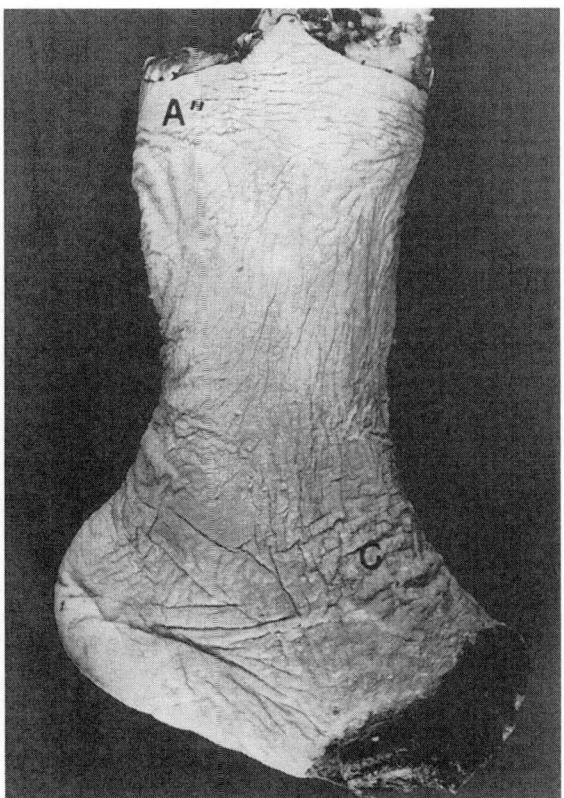

Fig. 21. Lower third amputation of the right leg. Soft tissues already removed from the bone. External side

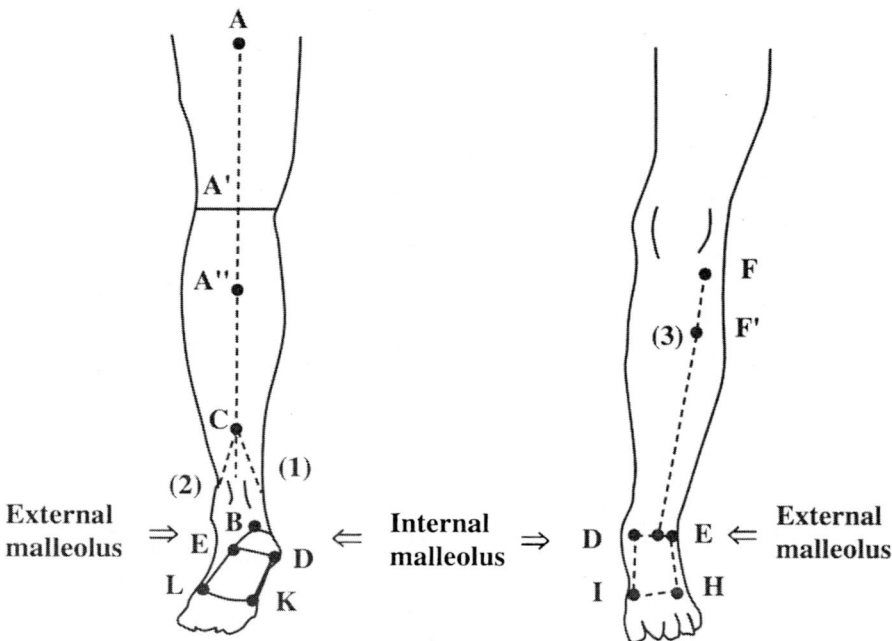

Fig. 22. Diagram of the arterial paths in an amputation specimen of the left lower limb

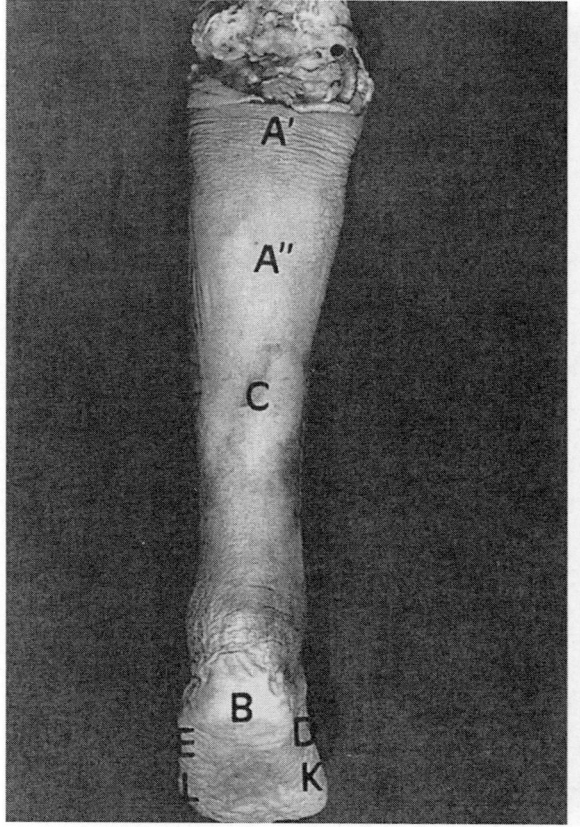

Fig. 23. Lower third amputation of the left thigh. Posterior aspect

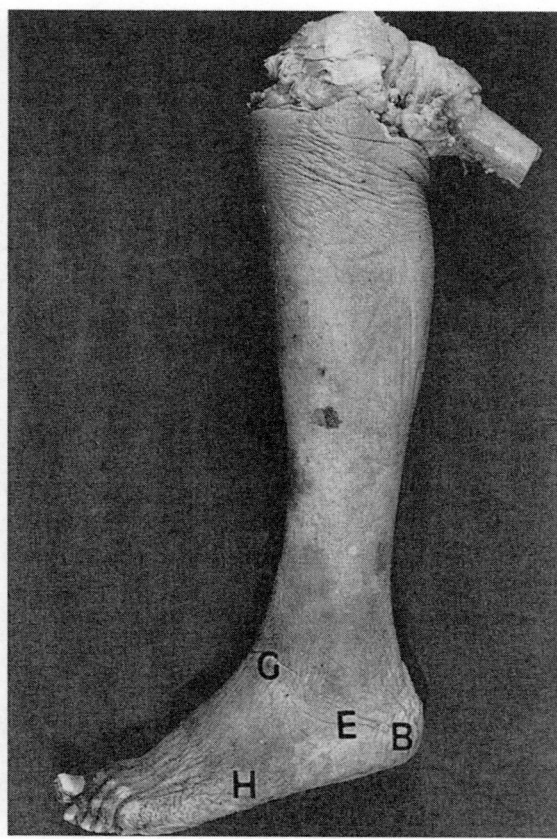

Fig. 24. Lower third amputation of the left thigh. External aspect.

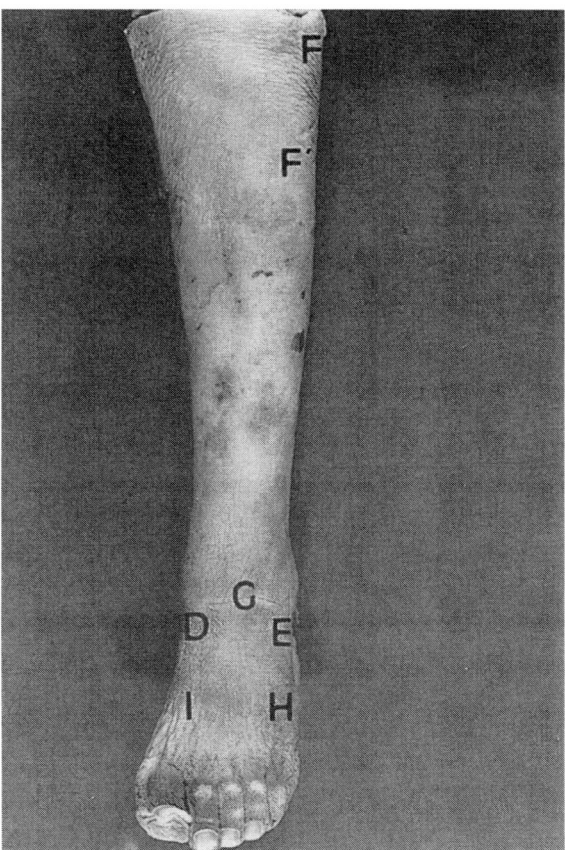

Fig. 25. Lower third amputation of the left thigh. Anterior aspect

d) Dissection of the anterior tibial artery of the leg.

1) Make an incision from points F to G. Section the extensor digitorum communis, tibialis anterior and extensor digitorum longus muscles respectively. This incision exposes the anterior tibial artery. Dissect the vessel down to point G.

2) Remove these vessels and fix them separately after orientating them.

e) Removal of dorsalis pedis artery.

1) Draw a line (HI) parallel to the line connecting the anterior borders of the external and internal malleoli (ED), crossing through the upper end of the first metatarsal bone.

2) Using a scalpel, remove the cutaneous trapezoid EDHI outlined by these two parallel lines and the internal and external borders of the foot. The dorsalis pedis blood vessels are located in the deeper portion of this specimen.

3) Spread out this specimen after appropriate orientation on a corkboard. Immerse this preparation in fixative. Make sections perpendicular to the pathway of the pedal blood vessels. Block these in their cross-section.

e) Removal of internal and external plantar vessels.

1) Turn plantar aspect of foot upwards. Draw two lines parallel to the anterior border of the foot, one crossing through the medial and lateral malleolus (DE), the other through the upper end of the first matatarsal bone (KL).

2) Remove the cutaneous trapezoid DELK outlined by these two parallel lines and the two internal and external borders of the plantar surface of the foot while shaving the bone. The inner half of this rectangle contains the internal plantar blood vessels, the outer half the external plantar vessels (Fig. 26).

to the midpoint of the heel (point B). Identify the dividing line between the upper two-thirds and lower one-third of segment AB. Mark point C at this division.

2) Make an incision of the skin surface from A to C, then make 2 oblique incisions from C to D and from C to E.

3) Beginning with the upper surgical section, incise the skin along the segment AC. Dissect the deep femoral (A) and popliteal (A') arteries down to where they cross the sciatic nerve. Continue to dissect the posterior tibial vessels from point C to point D and the peroneal vessels up to point C to point E.

4) At the incision CD, section the soleus, gastrocnemius and flexor digitorum longus muscles respectively. This incision exposes the posterior tibial artery.

5) At the incision CE, section the soleus and the flexor hallucis longus muscles respectively. This incision exposes the peroneal artery.

6) Remove the different vessels and, after orientating, fixate them separately.

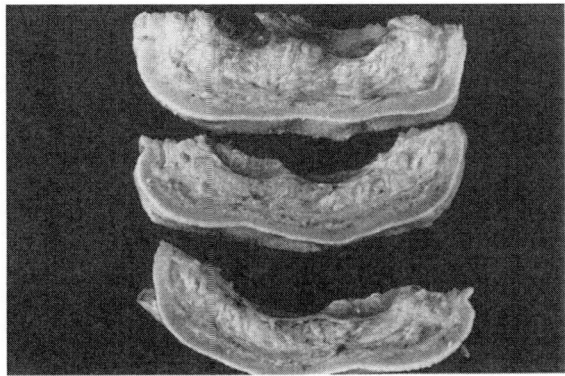

Fig. 26. Removal of the plantar vessels

3) Fix and remove the plantar blood vessels in the same way as for the anterior tibial vessels.

6.5.3. Dissection of the neurovascular bundles of a leg amputated through the middle third of the leg.

a) The skin incisions are similar to those for the amputated specimen of the lower one-third of the thigh. In this case, point A" corresponds to the midpoint of the posterior border of the surgical specimen, point F' to the midpoint of the segment connecting the anterior borders of the tibia and the fibula.

b) Removal of the anterior and posterior blood vessels of the leg is performed by the same method used for a biopsy or biospy-resection of vascular specimens.

c) Examination of the forefoot and of the toes is done by the protocol described above.

7 – Vascular injection

Vascular injection is essential in identifying angiodysplasia and the origin of obscure haemorrhages. Macroscopic and microscopic techniques can be used. We use the following technique for digestive resections (colon) and hysterectomy specimens [3].

7.1. Injection of the vascular network

7.1.1. Surgical help is necessary for good results and the vascular pedicles should be identified by means of a thread on the unfixed specimen.

7.1.2. Introduce a small catheter in each main vessel (artery, vein). Hold each catheter in place with a surgical clamp. Attach a syringe containing a permanent ink to each catheter (red ink in an artery, Indian ink in a vein) (Fig. 27-28).

7.1.3. Inject the ink. The pressure used is approximately 150 and 100 mmHg respectively in an artery and a vein.

7.1.4. Clamp the vascular pedicles to prevent leakage.

7.2. Fix the specimen by standard techniques

7.2.1. Once the specimen is fixed, opening, gross description and histological sampling can be carried out according to standard protocols.

7.3. Clearing

7.3.1. Dehydrate the specimen in 3 baths of 70%, 90% and absolute ethylic alcohol; each lasts 24 hours.

7.3.2. Clear the specimen in 2 successive baths of toluene; the first bath lasts at least 24 hours.

7.4. Examination

7.4.1. Place the cleared specimen in a flat glass tank containing toluene. Examine the vascular net-

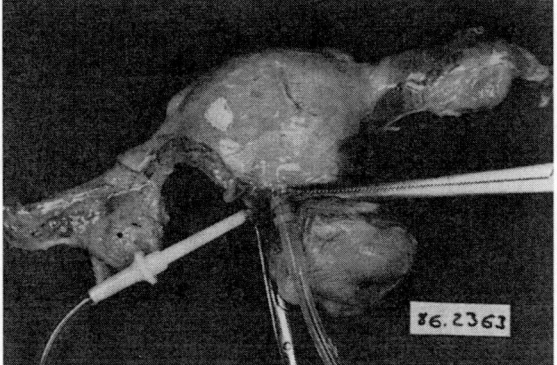
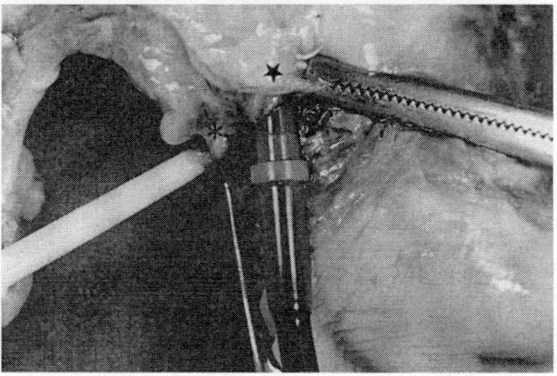

Fig. 27-28. Vascular injection of uterine vessels.(asterisk) : uterine artery; (Star): uterine vein

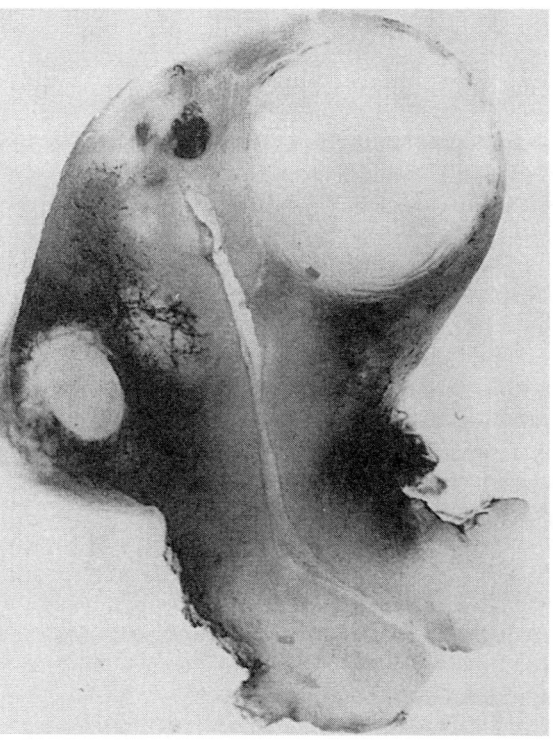

Fig. 29. Vascular injection of uterine vessels. "Cleared" specimen

work above an illuminated X-ray viewing screen (Fig. 29). Photograph the specimen by installing the scree Mn horizontally under the camera. Sample specimens for histological study. Block into paraffin directly (clearing is the last step of classical tissue processing).

7.4.2. The remains of the specimen can be kept in toluene. For practical purposes, the injected specimen can be extracted from the toluene and left exposed to the air. Once this has evaporated, the specimen loses its transparency and recovers the appearance of a dried fixed specimen.

Bibliography

1. Vuong PN, Baviéra E, Houissa-Vuong S (1986) Protocole d'étude en Anatomie et Cytologie Pathologiques. Vigot, Paris. p.364
2. Malik N, Gunn J, Holt CM, Shepherd L, Francis SE, Newman CMH, Crossman DC, Cumberland DC (1998) Intravascular stents: a new technique for tissue processing for histology, immunohistochemistry, and transmission electron microscopy. Heart 80: 509-16
3. Vuong PN, Proust A, Guillet JL, Benamour JM, Lucas M, Vaury Ph, Baviera E (1994) Angiodystrophie utérine responsable de métrorragies récidivantes, une nouvelle entité anatomo-pathologique. Gynécologie 2: 230-6.

Annex II
Pathological interpretation of vascular specimens and immunohistochemistry of vessels

1 – Interpretation of vascular specimens

Clinical information

As in any field of Pathology, interpretation of vascular specimens should be done in a clear clinical context. Adequate patient identification and a concise clinical history, radiological results, and accounts of previous therapy should accompany the vascular specimen. References to previous pathological examinations and suggested diagnosis should be made. An operative surgical report is of great help when specimens are multiple.

Diagnostic evaluation

It is prudent to follow a number of steps in evaluating a vascular specimen ; some of the steps are self-evident but should be in the protocol.

Thrombus

Organisation

Evaluating the degree of organisation helps to date the mass.

Embolus versus thrombus

An embolus is generally a simple thrombus but may contain cholesterol crystals, calcified material, tissue fragments or foreign bodies. A local thrombus usually adheres to the intima, which may be thickened by fibrosis or atherosclerotic plaques.

Vascular wall

Type of vessel

Identify the type of vessel. Stenosis cannot be evaluated in open vessels.

Vascular architecture

Identify the lumen. Measure the thickness of the intima, media and adventitia.

Measurements

The normal diameter and length of vessels are seldom investigated fully. Standards used by anatomists, radiologists, surgeons and pathologists vary. Moreover, these values depend on multiple variables including age, gender, race, height, and weight. Commonly, an ectatic artery has a calibre two or three times greater and is 1.5 to 1.7 times longer than a normal one. In the aorta, an aneurysm should not be diagnosed unless the distended segment is 1.5 times that of the normal diameter.

Patch-grafts, vascular grafts and prostheses

Patch-grafts

Identification of the suture stitches and the surrounding foreign body granulomas can define the contours of a patch-graft.

Vascular grafts and prostheses

Evaluate the degree of stenosis at anastomotic lines (foreign body granulomas, intimal flap). Identify internal and external junctional zones and the lumen. Serial sections help locate the area of deterioration of prosthetic fibers visible under polarised light.

Vascular tumours

Hypervascular tissue versus true vascular tumour

1) Rule out normally hypervascular tissue, such as erectile tissue. Check the location of the specimen (nasal mucosa, corpora cavernosum or spongiosum, clitoris).

2) Rule out tumour-like conditions: vascular ectasia, some vascular changes in viscera (peliosis hepatis, parenchymal collapse with accentuation of the vascular framework, vascular transformation of lymph node sinuses), inflammatory or pyogenic granulomas, bacillary angiomatosis.

3) Identify primary non-vascular tumours having a hypervascular pattern. Search for predominant tissue component (adipose, fibrous tissue).

True vascular tumour

1) Identify the types of vessel involved. A combination of various kinds of vessels often suggests a congenital lesion.

2) Locate the site of proliferation (lumen, vascular wall, and perivascular tissues). An intraluminal tumour should be distinguished from an organised thrombus or embolus, or a tumour embolus. An extraluminal tumour may develop from various components of the vascular wall or from special vascular structures, such as vasoactive tissues.

2 – Immunohistochemistry of vessels

Many useful antibodies are now commercially available in forms suitable for use in formalin-fixed tissue and frozen sections. Histochemistry may thus help to identify different cellular components of vessels [1-3].

Endothelium

Vascular endothelial cells play important roles in coagulation, fibrinolysis, inflammation, immunity, the regulation of vascular tone and in a wide variety of synthetic and metabolic functions. These activities result in the expression of specific proteins and receptors. Endothelial cells express Factor VIII-related antigen (FVIIIRAg), Ulex europaeus I agglutinin (AEAI) and blood group antigens together with platelet endothelial adhesion molecule-1 and EN-4 antigen (see, for example, Slomp et al 1996) [4]. HLA-DR antigen, BMA120, ICAM-1 and cytokeratins 8 and 18 may also be expressed.

2.1.1. Factor FVIII-RAg is composed of three functionally distinct components: factor VIIIC or coagulation factor, factor VIIIR (von Willebrand factor), and antihemophilic factor A or antihemophilic globulin A (ALF VIII). In normal human tissues, ALF VIII is evidenced in vascular endothelial cells, megakaryocytes, platelets and mastocytes. ALF VIII synthesis can be demonstrated in cultured endothelial cells. The staining of endothelial cells with antibodies to FVIII-related antigen (FVIII-Rag) has been disappointing, with reports of poor staining and of cross reaction with carcinomas [5] (Fig. 1).

2.1.2. Ulex europaeus I agglutinin (AEAI) is a lectin extracted from a plant of the genus Ulex (gorse) binding to some alpha-L-fucose-containing glycocompounds. The agglutinin binds to blood group O expressing blood group H substance in endothelial cells. The staining pattern is more intense than with FVIII-RAg, especially in small vessels. Ulex europaeus agglutinin shows variable staining of angiosarcoma cells [6-15].

2.1.3. Monoclonal antibodies to ABH blood group isogentigens are available in forms applicable to routinely processed formalin-fixed, paraffin-embedded tissue and consistently stain endothelial cells without prior trypsin digestion. Antibodies to A, B and H antigens stain the endothelial lining of blood and lymphatic vessels. However, they are not endothelial

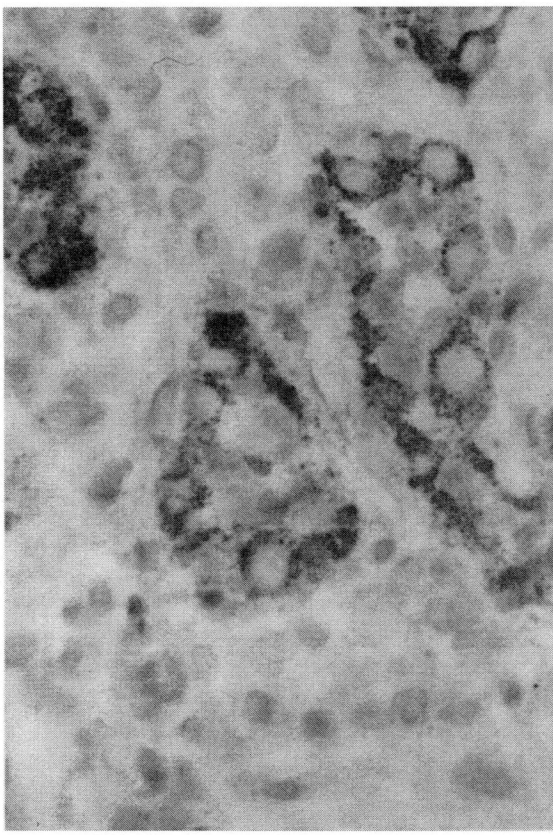

Fig. 1. Granular labelling of endothelial cells by factor VIII related antigen (FVIIIR-Ag). Peroxidase-antiperoxidase immunohistochemical technique (PAP)

cell-specific, binding to squamous cell carcinomas and synovial sarcomas and to neoplasms arising from colonic epithelium [16-19].

2.1.4. In normal human tissues HLA-DR antigens (Class II) have a limited distribution. HLA-DR antigen is expressed by endothelial cells and cells having an immune function (activated B and T-lymphocytes, monohistiocytes) as well as melanocytes [20], and smooth muscle cells [21]. HLA-DR is clearly not a specific endothelial marker.

2.1.5. Monoclonal BMA120 antibody (Behring Diagnostics) recognises a 200 KD endothelial antigen distinct from FVIIIRAg. Good results are obtained in paraffin-embedded tissue. It is reported to produce stronger staining in angiosarcoma than either Ulex or FVIIIRAg.

2.1.6. Monoclonal antibodies to ICAM-1 (intercellular adhesion molecule)-1 CD54 are also excellent markers of endothelium. They are now available in forms suitable for formalin-fixed material (Dakopatts, Immunotech, Novacastra) [22-,24].

2.1.7. Recently, a monoclonal antibody raised to CD31 (JC70) has been found to be more reliable than current endothelial markers (Fig. 2-3) [25]. Some normal endothelial cells express cytokeratins 8 and 18 [26]. In some vascular tumours, this reactivity may lead to misinterpretation as carcinoma.

Smooth muscle cells

Vascular smooth muscle cells contain more α-smooth muscle actin (Fig. 4) and vimentin (Fig. 5), and less desmin than ordinary smooth muscle [27]. A monoclonal smooth muscle actin antibody is now commercially available and can be used in formalin-fixed tissue [28]. It stains glomic cells and pericytes positively [29, 30].

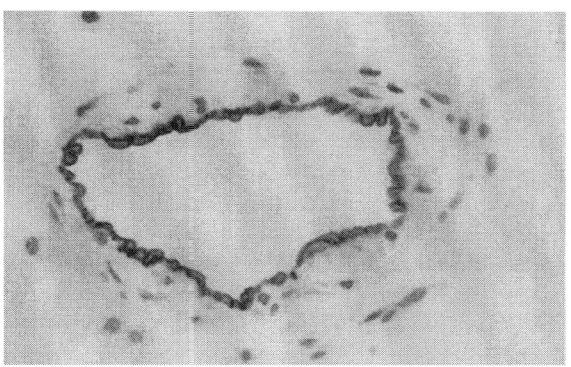

Fig. 3. CD31 labelling helps identify endothelial cells decorating newly-formed blood capillaries inside a breast adenocarcinoma. PAP

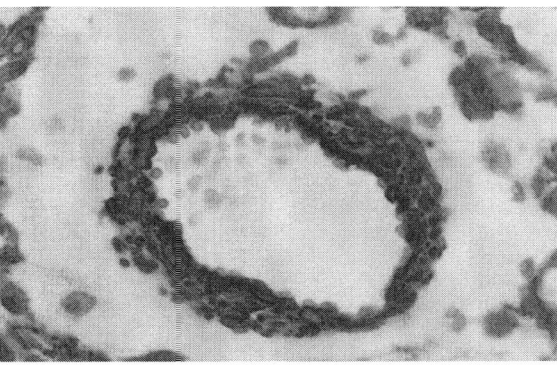

Fig. 4. Strong reactivity of smooth muscle cells and pericytes to alpha smooth muscle actin antibody. PAP

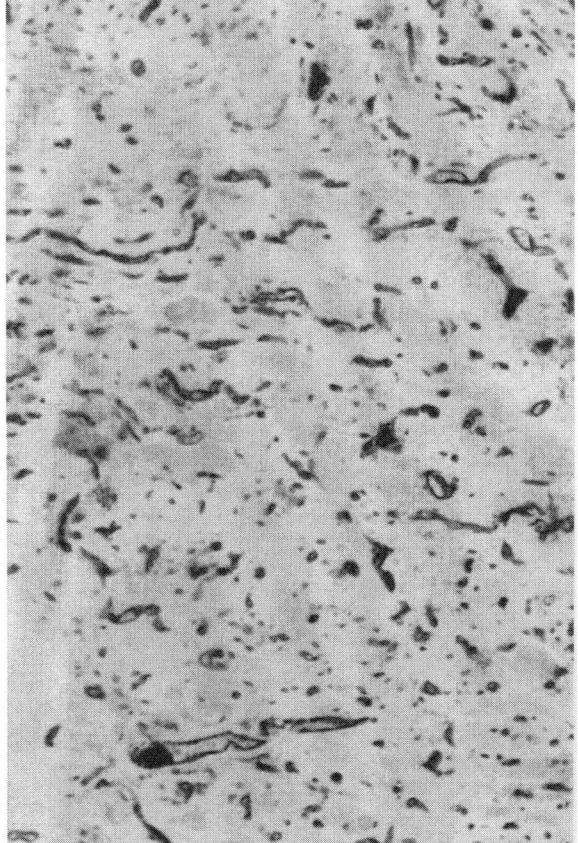

Fig. 2. CD31 labelling of endothelial cells of an arteriole. PAP

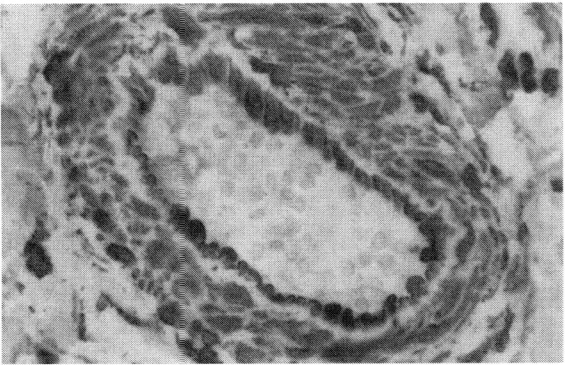

Fig. 5. Labelling of smooth muscle cells, pericytes and endothelial cells by vimentin antibody. PAP

Basement membrane

The basement membrane can be demonstrated by antibodies directed against laminin or type IV collagen. Identification of tumour emboli in blood or lymphatic channels can be facilitated in this way [31-33]. In theory, laminin immunoreactivity should help to differentiate lymphatics from blood capillaries, since the former lack a true basement membrane, but larger lymphatics, including those within lymph nodes, and some lymphangiomas stain with laminin. It is doubtful whether laminin immunoreactivity can be used routinely for the identification of small vascular channels [34].

Bibliography

1. Andrews BS, Shadforth M, Cunningham P, Davis JS 4th (1981) Demonstration of a C1q receptor on the surface of human endothelial cells. J Immunol 127: 1075-80

2. Groger M, Sarmay G, Fiebiger E, Wolff K, Petzelbauer P (1996) Dermal microvascular endothelial cells express CD32 receptors in vivo and in vitro. J Immunol 156: 1549-56

3. Kim-Schulze S, McGowan KA, Hubchak SC, Cid MC, Martin MB, Kleinman HK, Greene GL, Schnaper HW (1996) Expression of an estrogen receptor by human coronary artery and umbilical vein endothelial cells. Circulation 94: 1402-7

4. Slomp J, Gittenberger-deGroot AC, van Munsteren JC, Huysmans HA, van Bockel JH, van Hinsbergh VW, Poelmann RE (1996) Nature and origin of the neointima in whole vessel wall organ culture of the human saphenous vein. Virchows Arch 428: 59-67

5. Parums DV, Cordell JL, Micklem K, Heryet AR, Gatter KC, Mason DY (1990) JC70: a new monoclonal antibody that detects vascular endothelium associated antigen on routinely processed tissue sections. J Clin Pathol 43: 752-7

6. Holthöfer H, Virtanen I, Kariniemi AL, Hormia M, Linder E, Miettinen A (1982) Ulex europaeus I lectin as a marker for vascular endothelium in human tissues. Lab Invest 47: 60-6

7. Yonezawa S, Nakamura T, Irisa S, Otsuji Y, Sato E (1983) Ulex europaeus agglutinin I staining of human glomerular lesions using a highly sensitive immunoperoxidase method in paraffin sections. Nephron 35: 187-9

8. Roussel F (1985) Immunoperoxidase labelling of blood vessels by 3 lectins: Ulex europaeus I, Lotus tetragonolobus, Dolichos biflorus. C R Seances Soc Biol Fil 179: 59-69

9. Roussel F, Tayot J (1987) Evonymus europaeus agglutinin as a marker of endothelial cells in the human. Acta Anat (Basel) 129: 92-5

10. Gnepp DR (1987) Vascular endothelial markers of the human thoracic duct and lacteal. Lymphology 20: 36-43

11. Hultberg BM, Svanholm H (1989) Immunohistochemical differentiation between lymphangiographically verified lymphatic vessels and blood vessels. Virchows Arch A Pathol Anat Histopathol 414: 209-15

12. Walker RA (1989) The use of lectins in histopathology. Pathol Res Pract 185: 826-35

13. Ito N, Nishi K, Kawahara S, Okamura Y, Hirota T, Rand S, Fechner G, Brinkmann B (1990) Difference in the abi-

14. Laitinen L, Hormia M, Virtanen I (1990) Psophocarpus tetragonolobus agglutinin reveals N-acetyl galactosaminyl residues confined to endothelial cells and some epithelial cells in human tissues. J Histochem Cytochem 38: 875-84

15. Miettinen M, Lindenmayer AE, Chaubal A (1994) Endothelial cell markers CD31, CD34, and BNH9 antibody to H- and Y-antigens – evaluation of their specificity and sensitivity in the diagnosis of vascular tumors and comparison with von Willebrand factor. Mod Pathol 7: 82-90

16. Oriol R, Cooper JE, Davies DR, Keeling PWN (1984) ABH antigens in vascular endothelium and some epithelial tissues of baboons. Lab Invest 50: 514-8

17. Lee B/AKC, DeLellis RA, Wolfe HJ (1986) Intramammary lymphatic invasion in breast carcinomas. Evaluation using ABH isoantigens as endothelial markers. Am J Surg Pathol 10: 589-94

18. Perlman EJ, Epstein JI (1990) Blood group antigens expression in dysplasia and adenocarcinoma of the prostate. Am J Surg Pathol 14: 810-8

19. Kirkeby S, Mandel U, Vedtofte P (1993) Identification of capillaries in sections from skeletal muscle by use of lectins and monoclonal antibodies reacting with histo-blood group ABH antigens. Glycoconj J 10: 181-8

20. Brocker EB, Suter L, Sorg C (1984) HLA-DR antigen expression in primary melanomas of the skin. J Invest Dermatol 82: 244-7

21. Bendelac A, Kanitakis J, Chouvet B, Viac J, Thivolet J (1985) Sarcome de Kaposi: Etude immunohistochimique comparative et intérêt histoprognostique des marqueurs endothéliaux. Ann Pathol 5: 45-52

22. Dougherty GJ, Murdoch S, Hogg N (1988) The function of human intercellular adhesion molecule-1 (ICAM-1) in the generation of an immune response. Eur J Immunol 18: 35-9

23. Caughman SW, Li LJ, Degitz K (1992) Human intercellular adhesion molecule-1 gene and its expression in the skin. J Invest Dermatol 98: S61-S65

24. Almenar-Queralt A, Duperray A, Miles LA, Felez J, Altieri DC (1995) Apical topography and modulation of ICAM-1 expression on activated endothelium. Am J Pathol 147: 1278-88

25. Page C, Rose M, Yacoub M, Pigott R (1992) Antigenic heterogeneity of vascular endothelium. Am J Pathol 141: 673-83

26. Jahn L, Fouquet B, Roche K, Franke WW (1987) Cytokeratins in certain endothelial and smooth muscle cells in two taxonomically distant vertebrate species, Xenopus laevis and man. Differentiation 36: 234-54

27. Gabbiani G, Schmid E, Winter S (1981) Vascular smooth muscle cells differ from other smooth muscle cells: predominance of vimentin filaments and a specific type actin. Proc Natl Acad Sci 78: 298-302

28. Skalli O, Ropraz P, Trzeciak A, Benzonana G, Gillessen D, Gabbiani G (1986) A monoclonal antibody against alpha smooth muscle actin. A new probe for smooth muscle differentiation. J Cell Biol 103: 2787-96

29. Vici M, Pasquinelli G, Preda P, Martinelli GN, Gibellini D, Freyrie A, Curti T, D'Addato M (1993) Electron microscopic and immunocytochemical profiles of human subcutaneous fat tissue microvascular endothelial cells. Ann Vasc Surg 7: 541-8

30. Lantuejoul S, Isaac S, Pinel N, Negoescu A, Guibert B,

Brambilla E (1997) Clear cell tumor of the lung: an immunohistochemical and ultrastructural study supporting a pericytic differentiation. Mod Pathol 10: 1001-8

31. Lee AK, Delellis RA, Silverman ML, Wolfe HJ (1986) Lymphatic and blood vessel invasion in breast carcinoma. A useful prognostic indicator. Hum Pathol 17: 984-7

32. Ordonnez NG, Brooks T, Sharon T, Batsakis JG (1987) Use of Ulex Europeaus Agglutinin I in the identification of lymphatic and blood vessel invasion in previously stained microscopic slides. Am J Surg Pathol 11: 543-50

33. Schmidt D, von Hochstetter AR (1995) The use of CD31 and collagen IV as vascular markers. A study of 56 vascular lesions. Pathol Res Pract 191: 410-4

34. Listrom MB, Fenoglio-Preiser CM (1988) Does laminin immunoreactivity really distinguish between lymphatics and blood vessels. Surg Pathol 1: 71-4

Index

A

A-beta-lipoproteinaemia 400
Abnormal cellular infiltrations 60
— Eosinophilic vasculitis 60
— Foam-cell vasculitis 62
— Granulomatous vasculitis 61
— Leukocytoclastic vasculitis 60
— Lymphocytic vasculitis 60
— Rejection-type vasculitis 61
— Giant cell vasculitis 61
Abnormal deposits 48
— fibrinoid 48
— calcification 48
Acetylcholine 18
Acid lipase 397
Acquired
— coarctation 59
— lymphangiectasia 342
Acromegaly 410
Acute vascular purpura 244
Advanced glycosylation end (AGE) products 73
Adventitia 7
Adventitial
— cystic degeneration of vessels 99
— thickening 47
Ageing of vessels 25
— arteries 27
— erectile tissue 31
— lymph vessels 32
— microvasculature 30
— veins 30
Agonal clot 37
Ainhum 110
Alipoprotein CII deficiency (Type I) 398
Alkaptonuria 378
Allergic granulomatosis 255
Allergic granulomatous angiitis 255
Allografts 303
Alterations in caliber 50
— Aneurysm 51
— Dissecting aneurysm or haematoma 52
— Ectasia 50
— Poststenotic dilatation 52
— Posttraumatic or false aneurysm 52
Alveolar angioblastoma 456
Amantadine hydrochloride (1-Adamantanamine) 154
American trypanosomiasis 175
Amino-acid and protein metabolism 400
Amoebic infections 177
Amyloidosis 401
Anaphylactoid purpura 244
Anastomosis
— arterial 292
— End-to-end 292
— End-to-side 292
— Rupture 302
— Side-to-side 292
Anderson-Fabry's disease 371
Aneurysms 215,217
— acquired 218
— arterial 217
— atherosclerotic 218
— berry 217
— caused by fibromuscular dysplasia 220
— congenital cerebral 217
— dissecting 223
— false 293
— formation in vascular access 314
— inflammatory 219
— microaneurysms of Charcot Bouchard 217
— poststenotic aneurysms 221
— posttraumatic or false 220
— syphilitic 219
— venous 222
Angiitis
— Allergic granulomatous 255
— Leukocytoclastic 241
Angioblastoma 454
— Alveolar 456
Angiodysplasia 103
— acquired 103
— digestive tract 104
— uterine 106
— Veno-lymphatic 108
Angiodystrophy 103
— uterine 106
Angioendotheliosis
— malignant 446
Angiokeratoma 449
— circonscriptum 451
— corporis diffusum 371,451
— Fordyce type 451
— Mibelli type 451
— solitary 451
— solitary and multiple nodular types 451
Angioleiomyoma 481
Angioleiomyosarcoma 488
Angiolipoma 433
Angiolymphoid hyperplasia with esosinophilia 441
Angioma
— tufted 454
— Cherry 435
— serpiginosum of Hutchinson 452
Angiomatosis 360
— Bacillary (epithelioid) 171
— Encephalo-facial 356
— Encephalotrigeminal 356
— Cutaneomeningospinal 357
— Retinocerebral 374
Angiomyofibroblastoma 433, 435
Angiomyolipoma 433
Angiomyoma 481
Angiomyxolipoma 482
Angio-osteohypertrophy syndrome 354
Angioplasty 297
— Endoluminal vascular stenting 298
— Laser 299
— Patch-graft 300
— Percutaneous transluminal 297
— Rotating shaver 300
Angiosarcoma 467
Angiostrongyliasis 181
— A.cantonensis 181
— A.costaricensis 181
Ankylosing spondylitis 248
Anomalies

— great systemic veins 368
— great vessels 361
— innominate artery 365
— pulmonary artery 366
— truncus brachiocephalicus 365
Anomalous innominate artery or truncus brachiocephalicus 365
Ante-mortem thrombus 37
Antineutrophil cytoplasmic autoantibody (ANCA) associated vasculitis 239,253
Aorta
— dissection 223
— thoracic 362
Aortic coarctation 362,363
Arterial
— anastomosis 292
— pulmonary hypertension 422,426
— steal syndrome 313
Arteries 3
— ageing 27
— architectural variations 7
— Dilatation and tortuosity 59
— Elastic 7
— innervation 8
— Innominate 365
— Internal mammary 7
— Muscular 6
— Recipient 302
— vascularity 8
Arteriogenic impotence
Arterioles 12
Arteriopathy
— Cerebral autosomal dominant with subcortical infarcts and leukoencephalopathy (CADASIL) 371
— Competition cyclist 131
— Plexiform 423
— Segmental mediolytic 102
Arteriovenous anastomoses or fistulae 14,18, 56,225
— acquired 57,225
— congenital 56,229
— Pathology 327,342
Arteritis
— Cranial 257
— Giant cell 257
— Granulomatous 257
— Takayasu's 262
Ascariasis 182
Aspergillosis 185
Ataxia-telangiectasia 378
Atherosclerosis 69
— Aneurysms 218
— Complicated lesions 76
— development in bypasses 303
— Fibroatheromas 75
— Fibrolipidic plaques 75
— Gelatinous plaques 75
— Haemorrhage 78
— in veins 84
— Lipid and fatty streaks 74
— Lipid deposits 74
— Outcome 79
— Pathogenesis 73
— Peripheral cholesterol embolization 80

— Plaque disruption or ulceration 78
— Regression 79
— Thrombosis 79
Atresia of aortic arch 365
Autografts 303
Autosomal disorders 369
Azygos drainage of the inferior vena cava 368

B

Bacillary (epithelioid) angiomatosis
Bancroftian and Malayan filariasis 178
Bartonella bacilliformis 170
Bartonellosis 170
Bassen-Kornweig syndrome 400
Behçet's disease or syndrome 269
Bejel 168
Benign lymphangioendothelioma 358
Berry aneurysms 217
Bilharziasis 182
Biological grafts 303
Blastomycosis 188
Blue rubber-bleb nevi syndrome 381
Bluefarb-Stewart syndrome 315
Blunt injury to vessels 121
Bourneville's disease 377
Bovine brucellosis 172
Bradikinin 18
Budd-Chiari syndrome 427
Buerger's disease 271
Burns 146
Bury's disease 275
Bypass 300
— healing of sutures and lines of anastomosis 300
— adaptation to the neighbouring tissue and the recipient artery 302
— general complications 302

C

Calabar swelling 180
Calcification 405
— Idiopathic arterial calcification of infancy 405
Candidiasis or Candidosis 185
Capillaries 12
— Continuous 13
— Fenestrated 13
— Sinusoids or sinusoid 13
— structure 13
Capillary haemangiomas 447
Carbohydrate metabolism 395
Carotid sinus 18
Catheterisation
Cat-scratch disease or fever 172
Cavernoma 448
Cavernosal artery insufficiency 346
Cavernous haemangiomas 448
Cavernous lymphangioma 457
Cell-mediated vasculitis 239
Cenuriasis or Cenurosis 183
Cerebral autosomal dominant arteriopathy with subcortical infarcts and leukoencephalopathy (CADASIL) 371
Cerebrotendinous xanthomatosis 400

Cervical rib syndrome 125
Cestodes 183
Chagas disease 175
Changes in vascular dimensions 215
— Aneurysms 215
— Dilatation or dilation and tortuosity 59
Charles operation 319
Chemodectomas 496
Cherry angioma 435
Chilblain 147
Chlamydia pneumoniae infection 173
Cholesterol storage disease 400
Christian's disease 276
Chronic injury of vessels 124
Chronic venous insufficiency 333
Churg-Strauss syndrome 255
Classic polyarteritis nodosa 265
Coagulation thrombus 37
Coarctation 57
— congenital 57
— acquired 59
— Aortic 362,363
Cobb's syndrome 357
Cocaine 156
Cockett's syndrome 133
Coeliac compression syndrome 133
Coenurosis 183
Cogan's syndrome 272
Coiling 230
Collecting lymph vessels 21
Combined hyperlipidaemia (TypeV) 399
Competition cyclist arteriopathy 131
Complex or polygenic inheritance 381
Compression injury 121
Compression syndrome of the innominate veins 133
Congenital
— dysplastic angiectasia 354
— coarctation 57
— angiodysplasia 360
Congenital heart diseases 425
Congestive heart failure 314
Conglutination thrombus 37
Continuous capillaries 13
Contrast media 156
Copper metabolism 406
Corpus cavernosum recti 15
Corrosive and freezing agents 154
Costo-clavicular syndrome 125
Coxsackie virus infection 165
Cranial arteritis 257
Craniofacial dysostosis 373
Crepe-type prostheses (Wesolowki's prostheses) 308
Cri-du-chat syndrome 369
Cross-over anatomosis 15
Crouzon's syndrome 373
Crow-Fukase syndrome 453
Cushing's syndrome 410
Cutaneomeningospinal angiomatosis 357
Cutaneous arterial spider 437
Cutis hyperelastica 374
Cutis laxa 383
Cutis marmorata telangiectatica congenita 435
Cystic hygroma 459

Cystic medial necrosis 102
Cytogenetic disorders 369
Cytomegalovirus infection 166

D

D Trisomy (D1,13,13-15) 369
Dabska tumour 463
Dacron (polyethylene teraphthalate) 306,309
Deceleration 121
Deficiencies
— Acid lipase 397
— Familial alipoprotein CII (Type I) 398
— Familial lecithin-cholesterol acyltransferase (LCAT) 400
— Familial lipoprotein lipase (Type II) 397
— Lipoprotein 399
— Lysosomal enzymes of lipid metabolism 396
— Vitamin C 407
— Vitamin D 407
— Vitamin E 407
Dermatochalasis 383
Developmental anomalies of vessels 351,353
Diabetes mellitus 73,407
Diabetic macroangiopathy 407
Diabetic microangiopathy 408
Diffuse haemangioma 360
Dilatation and tortuosity of vessels 59
— arteries 59
— lymphatics 60
— veins 59
Dipetalonemiasis 178
Direct antibody attack-mediated vasculitis 239,251
Direct blow 121
Dirofilariasis 179
Diseases
— Amino-acid and protein metabolism 401
— Anderson-Fabry's 371
— Behçet's 269
— Bourneville's 377
— Buerger's 271
— Bury's 275
— Carbohydrate metabolism 395
— Cat-scratch 172
— caused by bacteria 170
— caused by fungi 184
— caused by parasites 175
— caused by Treponema 168
— Chagas 175
— cholesterol storage 400
— Christian's 276
— Endocrine 407
— Fabry's 371
— Farber's 396
— Fish-eye disease 399
— Gaucher's 396
— Gilchrist's disease 188
— Hereditary diseases of vessels 351
— Horton's 257
— Hutchinson-Gilford 377
— Kawasaki's 252
— Kimura's 441
— Kussmaul's 265

— Light chain deposition 404
— Lipid metabolism 396
— Luzt-Splendore-Almeida's 187
— Mineral metabolism 405
— Osler's 376
— Osler-Rendu-Weber 376
— Phytanic acid storage 400
— Primary pulmonary veno-occlusive 333
— Pulseless 262
— Raynaud's 342
— Refsum's 401
— Sickle cell 381
— Sturge-Weber 356
— Takayasu's 262
— Tangier disease 399
— Vibration-induced 148
— Vitamin metabolism 405
— von Hippel-Lindau 374
— Weber-Christian 276
Disorders
— Autosomal 369
— Cytogenetic 369
— Sex chromosome 370
— Metabolic 393,395
— Endocrine 393
— Copper metabolism 406
— Vitamin 407
Dissecting aneurysm or haematoma 52,223
Dissection
— aorta 223
— medium, small arteries and veins 225
Disseminated intravascular coagulation (DIC) 206
Disseminated lipogranulomatosis 396
Dolichomega-arteries 29
Double inferior vena cava 369
Down's syndrome 369
Drug reactions 243
Dys-beta-lipoproteinaemia (Type III) 399
Dyschondroplasia with
— vascular hamartomas 357
— haemangiomas 357

E

E Trisomy (17,18,16-18) 369
Ectasia 50
— lymphangiectasia 50
— telangiectasia 50
Edwards' syndrome 369
Effects of physical and chemical agents on vessels 139
— X-Ray 141
— Lasers 144
— Other radiation 144
— Chemical agents and drugs 154
Ehlers-Danlos syndrome 371,374
Elastic arteries 7
Elastic lamellae 4
Elastoma 401
Electric shock and Lightning injury 149
Embolism 38,41
Embolism 38,41,199,208,360
— peripheral arterial 208
— pulmonary thrombo-embolic syndrome 208

Embolus 208
— Air and gas 209
— Amniotic fluid and placental material 211
— Bone marrow 211
— cholesterol crystals 81,208
— composition 208
— Detached thrombus 208
— Fat 209
— Foreign bodies 209
— Microbial and parasitic pathogens 212
— Tumour cells 209
— versus thrombus 521
Encephalo-facial angiomatosis 356
Encephalotrigeminal angiomatosis 356
Endarterectomy 505
— Semi-closed 294
— Open 294
Endocrine diseases and disorders 393,407
— Hyperparathyroidism 410
— Acromegaly 410
— Cushing's syndrome 410
— Myxoedema 409
— Diabetes mellitus 407
Endofibrosis of the external iliac artery 131
Endoluminal vascular stenting 298
Endophlebosclerosis 30,332
Endothelial cell 3
— Junctional complexes 3
— Weibel-Palade bodies 3
— Injury 201
— changes 42
Endothelial injury 201
Endothelium-derived nitic oxide 18
Endothelium-derived relaxing factor (EDRF) 18
Endovascular papillary angioendothelioma 463
End-to-end anastomosis 292
Eosinophilic meningitis 181
Eosinophilic vasculitis 60
Epiloia 377
Epithelioid haemangioendothelioma 463
Epithelioid haemangioma 441
Epstein-Barr virus (EBV) DNA 98
Erectile vascular tissue 16
— ageing 31
— clitoris 16
— corpora cavernosum or spongiosum 16
— Pathology 327,346
— vasculogenic impotence 32
Ergotamine 154
Erythema elevatum diutinum 274
Erythema nodosum 274
Erythema pernio 147
Erythromelalgia 146
Essential mixed cryoglobulinaemic vasculitis 250
Expanded reinforced porous prostheses 308
Expanded tetrafluoroethylene prostheses (ePTFE) 310
External iliac artery 131
Extracellular matrix 5

F

Fabry's disease 371
Factor VIII-related antigen (FVIIIRAg) 522

False aneurysm 52,220,293
Familial disorders associated with low levels of low density liporoteins 400
— hypo-beta-proteinaemia 400
— a-beta-lipoproteinaemia 400
Farber's disease
Fenestrated capillaries 13
Fever
— Cat-scratch 172
— Malta 172
— Mediterranean 172
— Undulant 172
— Trench 171
Fibrillar proteins 401
Fibrinoid necrosis 419,424
Fibromuscular dysplasia 91,220
Fibrous endophlebitis 30,332
Fibroxanthoma 456
Fiessinger-Leroy-Reiter syndrome 248
Filament proteins 5
— actin 5
— desmin 5
— intermediate 5
— myosin 5
— vimentin 5
Fish-eye disease 399
Fistula 303
Flame naevus 353
Foam-cell vasculitis 62
Fragile X syndrome 370
Frostbite 148
Fucosidosis 396
Fugitive swelling 180
Fundamental lesions in vascular pathology 35
Fungi 184

G

Gangrene 204
Gaucher's disease 396
Generalized telangiectasia 435
Giant cell arteritis 257
Giant cell vasculitis 61
Gilchrist's disease 188
Glomeruloid haemangioma 453
Glomus tumour 484
Glucosyl ceramide lipidosis 396
Glues 64
Glycogen storage diseases 395
Glycolipid lipidosis 371
Goodpasture's syndrome 251
Grafts and prostheses 63,521
— Adaptation of synthetic bypass grafts 64
— Changes at anastomotic lines 63
Granuloma faciale 276
Granuloma pyogenicum 439
Granulomatous vasculitis 61
— arteritis 257
— Phlebitis 182
Great systemic veins 368

H

Haemangiectatic hypertrophy 354
Haemangioendothelioma 460
— Spindle cell 460
— Kaposiform infantile 460
— epithelioid (EHE) 463
Haemangiomas 447
— Capillary 447
— Cavernous 448
— Glomeruloid 453
— Microvenular 454
— Targetoid haemosideric 453
— verrucous 451
Haemangiomatosis
— Pulmonary capillary 384
Haemangiomatous syndromes 354
Haemangiopericytoma 486
Haemorrhagic fever 165
Haemorrhoids 344
Heat stroke 146
Henoch-Schönlein purpura 244
Hepatitis B and C microscopic polyarteritis
Hereditary diseases of vessels 351
Hereditary haemorrhagic telangiectasia 376
Herpes virus infections 166
High flow arterial priapism 347
High pressure impact damage and compression 152
Histiocytoma 456
Histology of vessels 1
Histoplasmosis 188
HIV infection 168
HLA-DR antigens (Class II) 522
Homocystinuria 378,407
Homogentisuria 378
Horton's disease 257
H-shaped arteriovenous anastomosis 16
Human herpesvirus-8 (HHV8) 166
Hunter's syndrome 371
Hurler and Scheie's syndrome 379
Hutchinson-Gilford disease 377
Hyalinosis 29
Hyperabduction syndrome 125
Hypercalcaemia
— Idiopathic infantile 405
Hypercholesterolaemia (Type II) 399
Hypercholesterolemic xanthomatosis 374
Hypercoagubility 201
Hyperlipidaemiae 72
Hyperlipoproteinaemias 397
— Familial alipoprotein CII deficiency (Type I) 398
— Familial combined hyperlipidaemia (TypeV) 399
— Familial dys-beta-lipoproteinaemia (Type III) 399
— Familial hypercholesterolaemia (Type II) 399
— Familial hypertriglyceridaemia (Type IV) 399
— Familial lipoprotein lipase deficiency (Type I) 397
— Multiple lipoprotein-type hyperlipidaemia 399
Hyperoxaluria
— Secondary 405
Hyperparathyroidism 410
Hyperplastic phlebitis 332
Hypersensitivity vasculitis 241,244
Hypertension 72,417
— arterial pulmonary 422

— Systemic arterial 419
— venous pulmonary 426
Hypertensive cardiomegaly 420
Hypertensive encephalopathy 421
Hyperthermic injuries 146
Hypertonic solutions 154
Hypertriglyceridaemia (Type IV) 399
Hypertrophic cardiomyopathy 404
Hypo-alpha-lipoproteinaemia 400
Hypo-beta-proteinaemia 400
Hypocomplementemic vasculitis 242
Hypothermic injuries 147

I

I-cell disease 395
Idiopathic arterial calcification of infancy 405
Idiopathic infantile hypercalcaemia 405
Immersion foot 147
Immune complex-mediated vasculitis 239,241
Immunohistochemistry
— Basement membrane 524
— endothelium 522
— smooth muscle cells 523
— vessels 519
Immunologic vasculitis 241
Incorporation of foreign material within the vascular wall 62
— Glues 64
— Patch-grafts 63
— Suture threads 62
— Vascular grafts and prostheses 63,521
Infectious diseases caused by 163
— Bacteria 170
— Fungi 184
— Parasites 175
— Rickettsiae 168
— Treponema 168
— Viruses 165
Infectious vasculitis 241
Influenza 165
Infracardiac veins 9
Injuries of vessels caused by
— Ultrasound 146
— Hyperthermic 146
— Hypothermic 147
— Electric shock and Lightning 149
Innominate artery 365
Innominate veins 133
Insufficiency
-Cavernosal artery 346
-Chronic venous 333
Internal mammary artery 7
Interrupted aortic arch 365
Intima 3
Intimal
— hyperplasia 44,64,293,422
— thickening 44,419
— sarcoma 489
— flap 64
— fibroelatosis 423
Intravascular fasciitis 445
Intravascular papillary endothelial hyperplasia 39,445

Ischaemic heart syndromes 83
Isolated visceral vasculitis 268

J

Junctional complexes 3
— gap 3
— intermediate 3
— nexus 3
— tight 3
Juvenile angiofibroma 433
Juxtaglomerular apparatus 420
Juxtaglomerular rennin-secreting tumour 492

K

Kaposiform angiodermatitis 315
Kaposiform infantile haemangioendothelioma 460
Kaposi's sarcoma 464
Kasabach-Merritt syndrome 406
Kawasaki's disease 252
Kimura's disease 441
Kinking 230
Klippel-Trenaunay-Weber syndrome 354
Knitted prostheses (DeBakey's ultra-light prostheses) 308
Kussmaul's disease 265

L

Laboratory handling of vascular specimens 503
Larsen's syndrome 401
Laser angioplasty 299
Lecithin-cholesterol acyltransferase (LCAT) deficiency 400
Left superior vena cava (Left SVC) 368
Leishmaniasis or Leishmaniosis 176
Lejeune syndrome 369
Leprosy 173
Leptospirosis 174
Leukocytoclastic angiitis or vasculitis 60,241
Light chain deposition disease 404
Limb amputation 509
— digits (finger or toe) 510
— hand 510
— lower limb 511
— trans-metatarsal guillotine or forefoot 510
— upper arm and forearm 510
Lipid metabolism 396
Lipoprotein deficiencies 399
— Hypo-alpha-lipoproteinaemia 399
— Familial hypo-alpha-lipoproteinaemia 400
— Familial lecithin-cholesterol acyltransferase (LCAT) deficiency 400
— Fish-eye disease 399
— Tangier disease 399
Lipoprotein lipase deficiency (Type II) 397
Lipoproteins and alipoproteins 397
Listeriosis 174
Livedo reticularis 81
Loiasis 180
Louis-Bar syndrome 378
Low flow veno-occlusive priapism 347
Luzt-Splendore-Almeida's disease 187

Lymph cysts 342
Lymphangiectasia 32,353
Lymphangiectasis 353
Lymphangioleiomyomatosis 359
Lymphangiomas 457
— cavernous 457
— circumscriptum 458
— Cystic lymphangioma 459
Lymphangiomatosis 358
Lymphangiomatous syndromes
Lymphangiomyoma 359
Lymphangiopericytoma 359,488
Lymphangiosclerosis 32
Lymphangiosis 336
Lymphangitis 336
Lymphatic vessels 20
— ageing 32
— benign tumours 457
— capillaries 20
— collecting 21
— Dilatation and tortuosity 60
— effects of cold and heat 148
— Pathology 327,336
— Trauma 124
— trunks 22
Lymphectasia 353
Lymphocele 342
Lymphocytic vasculitis 60
Lymphoedema 336
— acquired 337
— primary 336
Lysosomal enzymes of lipid metabolism 396

M

Maffucci's syndrome 357
Malaria 176
Malignant angioendotheliosis 446
Malta fever 172
Mansonelliasis or Mansonelliasis ozzardi 178
Marfan's syndrome 375
Maroteaux-Lamy syndrome 379
Martin-Bell syndrome 370
Mason's tumour 39,445
Mast cell granuloma 456
Measles 165
Media 4
Medial changes 47
— calcification 29
— degeneration 102
— hypertrophy 422
— thickening 47,419
— thinning 47
Medionecrosis aortae idiopathica cystica 102
Mediterranean fever 172
Menke's syndrome 406
Metabolic disorders 393,395
Methyl-malonic acidaemia 407
Microaneurysms of Charcot Bouchard 217
Microcirculation 12
— ageing 30
Microscopic polyarteritis 255
Microvenular haemangioma 454

Mineral metabolism 405
Mixed thrombus 37
Monckeberg's medial calcific sclerosis 29
Moniliasis 185
Monoclonal antibodies raised to
— ABH blood group isogentigens 522
— BMA120 522
— CD31 (JC70) 522
— ICAM-1 (intercellular adhesion molecule)-1 CD54 522
Morquio A and Morquio B syndromes 379
Moyamoya disease 98
Mucocutaneous lymph node syndrome 252
Mucoid degeneration of the media 102
Mucolipidoses 395
— Mucolipidosis II 395
— Mucolipidosis III 395
— Mucolipidosis IV 395
— Fucosidosis 396
Mucopolysaccharidoses 378
— MPSI 379
— MPS IV 379
— MPS VI 379
Mucormycosis 186
Multiple lipoprotein-type hyperlipidaemia 399
Muscular arteries 6
Muscular venules 14
Myxoedema 409
Myxoma 482

N

Naevus or Nevus
— araneus 437
— Flame 353
— flammeus 353
— Spider 437
— telangiectaticus 353
Nasopharyngeal fibroma 433
Necrotizing vasculitis 419
Nematodes 178
— filarial nematodes 178
— non-filarial nematodes 181
Nerve fibers 8
— myelinated 8
— non-myelinated 8
Neurofibromatosis 375
Neuronal ceroid lipofuscinosis 397
Neurovascular glomus 18
Nevus araneus 437
Nodal angiomatosis 339
Nodular nonsuppurative panniculitis 276
Nodular vasculitis 276
Non-atherosclerotic and non-vasculitic diseases 89
— Adventitial cystic degeneration of vessels 99
— Agiodystrophy 103
— Ainhum 110
— Angiodysplasia 103
— Cystic medial necrosis 102
— Fibromuscular dysplasia 91
— Medial degeneration 102
— Medionecrosis aortae idiopathica cystica 102
— Moyamoya disease 98

— Mucoid degeneration of the media 102
— Segmental arterial mediolysis 102
— Segmental mediolytic arteriopathy 102
Noonan's syndrome 376
North American blastomycosis 188
Nutcracker syndrome 134

O

Obstructive endarteritis 44
Obstructive membranes in the inferior vena cava 333
Ochronosis 378
Oculovestibulo-auditory syndrome 272
Onchocerciasis 179
Open endarterectomy 294
Operative pathology 289
Operative procedures for
— lymphoedema 318
— veins 316
Osler's disease 376
Osler-Rendu-Weber disease 376
Osseous metaplasia 29
Osteogenesis imperfecta 384
Oxalosis 380
— Secondary 405
Ozzardi's filariasis 178

P

Paget – von Schrötter syndrome 125
Papova virus infection 165
Paracoccidioidomycosis 187
Paraganglia 18
Paragangliomas 496
— Chromaffin 496
Patau's syndrome 369
Patch-grafts 63
— angioplasty 300
Patent ductus arteriosus 361
Pathological interpretation of vascular specimens 519
Peliosis hepatis 437
Pelvic congestion syndrome 335
Penta X syndrome 370
Percutaneous angioscopy 297
Percutaneous transluminal angioplasty 297
Peri-adventitia 7
Pericytic venules 14
Peripheral cholesterol embolization 80
Perniosis 147
Pheochromocytoma 495
Phlebitis 329
— granulomatous 182
— hyperplastic 30,332
Phlebosclerosis 30,332
Phlegmasia cerulea dolens 204
Phycomycosis 186
Phytanic acid storage disease 400
Pinta 168
Pipestem arteries 29
Plasma cell dyscrasia with polyneuropathy and endocrine disorders 453
Plexiform arteriopathy 424
POEMS syndrome 453

Polyaneurysmal dystrophy 29
Polyarteritis nodosa 265
Polyethylene terepthalate (PET) prostheses 308
Popliteal artery entrapment syndrome 127
Portal hypertension 427
Postcapillary venules 14
Post-coarctation surgery 421
Post-mortem clot 37
Postphlebitic syndrome 333
Poststenotic aneurysms 221
Poststenotic dilatation 52
Posttraumatic aneurysms 52,220
Pregnancy 410
Priapism
— low flow veno-occlusive 347
— high flow arterial 347
Primary hyperoxaluria 380
Primary angiitis of the central nervous system 268
Primary pulmonary veno-occlusive disease 333
Products obtained during the re-establisment of a vascular lumen 505
Progeria 377
Progressive lymphangioma 358
Progressive systemic sclerosis 108
Prostheses 306
— behaviour 309
— changes in shape or size 302
— pathology 306
— synthetic 307
— types 306
Protozoa 175
Pseudo-Hurler dystrophy 395
Pseudo-Kaposi's sarcoma 315
Pseudoxanthoma elasticum 401
Psoriatic arthritis 249
Pulmonary
— aortic window 362
— capillary haemangiomatosis 384
Pulmonary aortic window 362
Pulmonary artery 366
— anomalies 366
Pulmonary capillary haemangiomatosis 384
Pulmonary thrombo-embolic syndrome 208
Pulmonary vein 10
Pulsating haematoma 220
Pulsating telangiectasia 437
Pulseless disease 262
Pyoderma gangrenosum 276
Pyogenic granuloma 439

R

Raynaud's phenomenon and Raynaud's disease 342
Recipient artery 64,302
Red (coagulation) thrombus 37
Re-establishment of vascular patency 296
Refsum's disease 401
Regional granulomatous lymphadenitis 172
Reiter's syndrome 248
Rejection-type vasculitis 61,256
— hyperacute 256
— acute 257
— subacute 257

— chronic 257
Relapsing polychondritis 249
Resection of vascular prostheses 507
Retinocerebral angiomatosis 374
Rheumatoid arthritis (RA) 248
Rochalimaea henselae (Bartonella) 437
Rotating shaver angioplasty 300
Rubella 165
Rupture 42
— adventitia 42
— anastomosis 302
— complete rupture 42
— intima 42
— intima and media 42
Rupture of anastomosis 302

S

Sarcoidosis 274
Scalenus anticus syndrome 125
Scedosporium apiospermum infection 188
Schistosomiasis 182
Scleroprotein 27
Sclerosing haemangioma 456
Sclerotherapy 316
Secondary hyperoxaluria or oxalosis 405
Segmental
— arterial mediolysis 102
— mediolytic arteriopathy 102
— vascular ectasias 424
Selenium deficiency 407
Semi-closed endarterectomy 294
Senile ectasia 435
Senile vascular naevus 435
Seronegative spondyloarthropathies 248
Serum sickness 243
Sex chromosome disorders 370
Sickle cell disease 381
Side-to-side anastomosis 292
Silicosis 154
Single-gene mutations 371
— Autosomal dominant diseases 371
— Autosomal recessive anomalies 378
— X-linked anomalies 371
Sinusoids or sinusoid capillaries 13
Small lymphatics 20
Smoking 72
Smooth muscle cell 5
Sneddon's syndrome 81
Soleus syndrome 134
Sparganosis 183
Specialized vascular structures 14
Spider nevus 437
Spindle cell haemangioendothelioma 460
Sporotrichosis 188
Stents 508
Stretch and tear injuries 122
Stripping of varicose veins 317
Structure of vessels 3
Sturge-Kalischer-Weber syndrome 365
Sturge-Weber syndrome or disease 356
Subendothelial layer 4
Supracardiac veins 9

Supravalvular aortic stenosis 384
Surgical procedures and techniques 291,293
Suture threads 62
Syndromes
— Angio-osteohypertrophy 354
— Arterial steal 313
— Bassen-Kornweig 400
— Behçet's 269
— Blue rubber-bleb nevi 381
— Bluefarb-Stewart 315
— Budd-Chiari 427
— Cervical rib 125
— Churg-Strauss 255
— Cobb's 357
— Cockett's 133
— Coeliac compression 133
— Cogan's 272
— Costo-clavicular 125
— cri-du-chat 369
— Crouzon's 373
— Crow-Fukase 453
— Cushing's 410
— Down's 369
— Edwards' 369
— Ehlers-Danlos 371,374
— Fiessinger-Leroy-Reiter 248
— Fragile X 370
— Goodpasture's 251
— Haemangiomatous 354
— Hunter's 371
— Hurler and Scheie's 379
— Hyperabduction 125
— Ischaemic heart 83
— Kasabach-Merritt 406
— Klippel-Trenaunay-Weber 354
— Larsen's 401
— Louis-Bar 378
— Lymphangiomatous 358
— Maffucci's 357
— Marfan's 375
— Maroteaux-Lamy 379
— Martin-Bell 370
— Menke's 406
— Morquio A and Morquio B 379
— Mucocutaneous lymph node 252
— Noonan's 376
— Nutcracker 134
— Oculovestibulo-auditory 272
— Paget – von Schrötter 125
— Patau's 369
— Pelvic congestion 335
— Penta X 370
— POEMS 453
— Popliteal artery entrapment 127
— Postphlebitic 333
— Pulmonary thrombo-embolic 208
— Reiter 248
— Scalenus anticus 125
— Sneddon's 81
— Soleus 134
— Sturge-Kalischer-Weber 365
— Sturge-Weber 356
— Takatsuki 453

— Thoracic outlet 124
— Turner's 370
— Venous compression 133
— Vuong-Proust 106
— Werner's 381
— XO 370
— XXXXY 370
Syphilitic vasculitis 169
Systemic arterial hypertension 419
Systemic hyperthermia 146
Systemic lupus erythematosus 245

Tumours of vascular-related structures 479,492
— Paraganglia 495
— Juxtaglomerular rennin-secreting tumour 492
Turner's syndrome 370

T

Takatsuki syndrome 453
Takayasu's arteritis or disease 262
Tangier disease 399
Targetoid haemosideric haemangioma 453
Teflon (polytetrafluoroethylene) prostheses 306,310
Telangiectases 353
Telangiectasia lymphatica 353
Temporal arteritis 257
Temporary cavitation 123
Thompson's technique 319
Thoracic outlet syndrome and related conditions 124
Thromboangiitis obliterans (TAO) 271
Thrombo-endarterectomy (TEA) 293
Thrombolysis 37
Thrombosis 199,201,302
— arterial 201
— venous 201,202,204
— lymphatic 206
— concomitant arterial,venous and lymphatic 206
Thrombus 37,79,521
— Embolus versus thrombus 521
— evolution 37
— homogenisation 38
— mixed 37
— organization 39,41,521
— red (coagulation) 37
— types 37
— white (conglutination) 37
Thrush 185
Tortuosity 230
Toxocariasis 181
Trauma 119
— Closed trauma or blunt injury 121
— Complications 124
— Direct trauma 121
— Open trauma or wounding 121
— Veins and lymphatic vessels 124
Trematodes 182
Trench fever 171
Trench foot 147
Treponema 168
Trisomy 369
— D (D1,13,13-15, Patau's syndrome) 369
— E (17,18,16-18, Edward's syndrome) 369
— 21 (Down's) 369
Truncus brachiocephalicus 365
Tuberculosis 174
Tuberous sclerosis 377
Tufted angioma

U

Ulex europaeus I agglutinin (AEAI) 522
Ultrasound injuries 146
Undulant fever 172
Urticarial vasculitis 242

V

Varicella-zoster virus 166
Varicocele 335
Varicose veins 330
Vasa vasora 8
Vascular
— access 310,313
— ageing 25
— anomalies associated with complex or polygenic inheritance 381
— anomalies associated with cytogenetic disorders 369
— anomalies associated with single-gene mutations 371
— anomalies related to environmental influences 385
— biopsies 505
— bypass 300
— catheter procedures 291
— clamping 291
— Developmental anomalies 351
— ectasias 435
— exposure and mobilisation 291
— grafts and prostheses 63,521
— in metabolic and endocrine disorders 393
— incision 291
— injection technique 516
— leiomyoma 481
— ligation 291
— occlusion 291
— proliferation in lymph nodes 339
— prostheses 306,507
— pulmonary sling 367
— puncture 291
— reactive lesions 437
— rings 365
— suture 292
— transformation of lymphatic node sinuses 339
— trauma 119
— tumour-like conditions 431,433
— tumours 431,521
— wounding 121
Vascular changes caused by lasers 144
Vasculitis 237
— Antineutrophil cytoplasmic autoantibody (ANCA) associated 239
— associated with connective tissue diseases 245
— associated with miscellaneous disorders 279
— associated with neoplasms 249
— caused by Pinta, Yaws and Bejel 168
— Cell-mediated 239,253
— Direct antibody attack-mediated 239,251
— Eosinophilic 60

— Essential mixed cryoglobulinaemic 250
— Foam-cell 62
— Giant cell 61
— Granulomatous 61
— Hypersensitivity 241,244
— Hypocomplementemic 242
— Immune complex-mediated 239,241
— Immunologic 241
— Infectious 241
— Isolated visceral 268
— Leukocytoclastic 60,241
— Lymphocytic 60
— Necrotizing 419
— Nodular 276
— of unknown origin 257
— Rejection-type 61,256
— Syphilitic 169
— Urticarial 242
Vasculogenic impotence 32,346
— Inflow disorder 346
— Outflow disorder 347
— Failure to fill 346
Vasculomegaly 230
Vasculopathy
— X-Ray induced or post-radiation 141
Vasoactive intestinal polypeptide (VIP) 18
Veins 8,30
— ageing 30
— architectural variations 10
— Dilatation and tortuosity 59
— hypertrophy 30
— Infracardiac 9
— pathology 327,329
— Phlebitis 329
— pulmonary 10
— structure 8
— Supracardiac 9
— trauma 124
— Varicose 330
— Vena cava 10
Velvet prostheses 308
Vena cava
— Azygos drainage in the inferior vena cava 368
— Double inferior vena cava 369
— intraluminal interruption 317
— juxta-cardiac segment 10
— Left superior (Left SVC) 368
— Obstructive membranes in the inferior vena cava 333
— surgery 317
Venofibrosis 30,332
Venous
— aneurysms 222
— atherosclerosis 314
— chronic insufficiency 333
— compression syndromes 133
— gangrene 204
— hypertension 314

— hypertrophy 332
— plexuses 10
— pulmonary hypertension 426
— valve reconstruction 318
Venules 14
— Pericytic 14
— Muscular 14
— Postcapillary 14
Verrucous haemangioma 451
Vessels
— Developmental anomalies 351
— tumours of intermediate malignancy 460
— benign tumours 447
— primary malignant tumours 463
— secondary malignant tumours 470
— tumours of vessel wall components 479,481
— Hypertension 72,417
Vibration-induced vascular diseases 148
Vinyl chloride (chloroethylene) 154
Viral hepatitis 166
Visceral larva migrans 181
Vitamin metabolism 405
Vitamine disorders 407
— Vitamin B12 related metabolic defects with methyl-malonic acidaemia and homocystinuria (Cbl-C typs) 407
— Vitamin C deficiency 407
— Vitamin D overdosage or deficiency 407
— Vitamin E deficiency 407
von Hippel-Lindau disease 374
Vuong-Proust syndrome 106

W

Weber-Christian disease 276
Wegener's granulomatosis 253
Weibel-Palade bodies 3
Werners' syndrome 381
White thrombus 37
Williams syndrome 384
Woven prostheses 308

X

Xenografts 303
XO syndrome 370
X-Ray induced or post-radiation vasculopathy 141
XXXXY syndrome 370

Y

Yaws 168

Z

Zahn bands 37
Zygomycosis 186

Composition, photogravure et impression
JOUVE, 18, rue Saint-Denis, 75001 PARIS
N° 283780J — Dépot légal : Mars 2002